Early Breast Cancer

Early Breast Cancer
From Screening to Multidisciplinary Management

Third Edition

Edited by

John R. Benson MA DM (Oxon), MD (Cantab), FRCS (Eng), FRCS (Ed)
Cambridge Breast Unit, Addenbrooke's Hospital, Cambridge, UK
University of Cambridge and Anglia Ruskin University, Cambridge, UK

Gerald Gui MS, FRCS, FRCS (Ed)
Breast Unit, The Royal Marsden NHS Trust, London, UK

Todd M. Tuttle MD, MPH
Masonic Cancer Center, University of Minnesota, Minneapolis, MN, USA

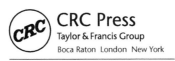

CRC Press
Taylor & Francis Group
Boca Raton London New York

CRC Press is an imprint of the
Taylor & Francis Group, an **informa** business

CRC Press
Taylor & Francis Group
6000 Broken Sound Parkway NW, Suite 300
Boca Raton, FL 33487-2742

First issued in paperback 2019

© 2013 by Taylor & Francis Group, LLC
CRC Press is an imprint of Taylor & Francis Group, an Informa business

No claim to original U.S. Government works

Typeset by Exeter Premedia Services Pvt Ltd., Chennai, India

ISBN-13: 978-1-84184-885-3 (hbk)
ISBN-13: 978-0-367-38046-5 (pbk)

Visit the Taylor & Francis Web site at
http://www.taylorandfrancis.com

and the CRC Press Web site at
http://www.crcpress.com

Contents

Contributors

Sausan Abouharb
Division of Cancer Medicine, The University of Texas MD Anderson Cancer Center, Houston, TX, USA

Steven D. Allen
Royal Marsden Hospital, London, UK

Alice O. Andrews
The Dartmouth Institute for Health Policy & Clinical Practice, Dartmouth College, Lebanon, NH, USA

Evdokia Arkoumani
The Michael Letcher Dept of Cellular Pathology, The Princess Alexandra Hospital NHS Trust, Essex, UK

Jane Barker
North Bristol Breast Cancer Unit, North Bristol NHS Trust, Southmead, Bristol, UK

Susan J. Barter
Cambridge University Hospitals NHS Foundation Trust and the University of Cambridge, Cambridge, UK

John R. Benson
Cambridge Breast Unit,
Addenbrooke's Hospital, Cambridge, UK
University of Cambridge and
Anglia Ruskin University, Cambridge, UK

Richard J. Bleicher
Department of Surgical Oncology, Fox Chase Cancer Center, Philadelphia, PA, USA

Patrick Borgen
Brooklyn Breast Cancer Program
Maimonides Medical Center
Brooklyn, NY, USA

Peter D. Britton
Cambridge University Hospitals NHS Foundation Trust, Cambridge, UK

Pauline J. Carder
Bradford Teaching Hospitals NHS Foundation Trust, Bradford, UK

Massimiliano Cariati
Division of Cancer Studies, King's College London, London, UK

Jenny C. Chang
The Methodist Cancer Center, Houston, TX, USA

K.L. Cheung
Division of Breast Surgery, University of Nottingham, UK

Rosanna C. Ching
Department of Plastic Surgery, Addenbrooke's Hospital, Cambridge University Hospitals NHS Foundation Trust, Cambridge, UK

Catharine F. Clay
The Dartmouth Institute for Health Policy & Clinical Practice, Lebanon, NH, USA

Charlotte Coles
Addenbrooke's Hospital, Cambridge
University Hospitals NHS Foundation Trust, Cambridge, UK

Thomas Conner
Department of Radiology, Northwick Park Hospital, Harrow, UK

Erika Denton
Norfolk and Norwich University Hospitals NHS Foundation Trust, Norwich, UK

Laura S. Dominici
Department of Surgery, Brigham and Women's Hospital, Boston, MA, USA

Sue K. Down
Addenbrooke's Hospital, Cambridge University Hospitals Foundation Trust, Cambridge, UK

Ian O. Ellis
Histopathology Department,
The University of Nottingham
and Nottingham University Hospitals NHS Trust, Nottingham, UK

Tim Emory
Department of Radiology, University of Minnesota Medical School, Minneapolis, MN, USA

Claudia Engeler
Department of Radiology, University of Minnesota Medical School, Minneapolis, MN, USA

Francisco J. Esteva
Department of Breast Medical Oncology, The University of Texas
MD Anderson Cancer Center, Houston, TX, USA

D. Gareth Evans
St. Mary's Hospital, Manchester, UK

Maisam Z. Fazel
Heatherwood & Wexham Park Hospital NHS Foundation Trust,
Windsor, UK

Chris I. Flowers
H Lee Moffitt Cancer Center and Research Institute,
Tampa, FL, USA

Pranjali V. Gadgil
University of Texas Health Science Center,
San Antonio, TX, USA

Hannah Gay
Royal Marsden Hospital, London, UK

Mehra Golshan
Department of Surgery, Brigham and Women's Hospital,
Boston, MA, USA

Gerald Gui
Breast Unit, The Royal Marsden NHS Trust, London, UK

Mattia Intra
European Insititue of Oncology, Milan, Italy

Angela Ives
School of Surgery, The University of Western Australia,
Crawley, WA, Australia

Ismail Jatoi
University of Texas Health Science Center
San Antonio, Texas, USA

Stephen R.D. Johnston
The Royal Marsden NHS Foundation Trust,
The Institute of Cancer Research, London, UK

V. Craig Jordan, OBE
Georgetown Lombardi Comprehensive Cancer Center,
Washington DC, USA

Martin Keisch
Cancer Healthcare Associates, Miami, FL, USA

Starr Koslow
Weill Medical College of Cornell University, The New York
Presbyterian Hospital, New York, NY, USA

Ian Kunkler
University of Edinburgh, Western General Hospital,
Edinburgh, UK

Jessica Kuehn-Hajder
Department of Radiology, University of Minnesota Medical
School, Minneapolis, MN, USA

Michael D. Lagios
Stanford University School of Medicine, Stanford, CA, USA

Gill Lawrence
West Midlands Cancer Intelligence Unit,
University of Birmingham, Birmingham, UK

R.C.F Leonard
Department of Surgery and Cancer, Imperial College London,
London, UK

Rebecca Llewellyn-Bennett
School of Clinical Sciences, University of Bristol,
Research and Teaching, Bristol Royal Infirmary, Bristol, UK

Andreas Makris
Mount Vernon Hospital, Northwood, Middlesex, UK

Charles M. Malata
Cambridge Breast Unit & Department of Plastic Surgery
Addenbrooke's Hospital
Cambridge University Hospitals NHS Foundation Trust
Cambridge, UK

J. Mathew
Division of Breast Surgery, University of Nottingham, UK

Anthony J. Maxwell
Department of Radiology, Royal Bolton Hospital, Bolton, UK

Russell E. McDaniel
Georgetown Lombardi Comprehensive Cancer Center,
Washington DC, USA

Michael J. Michell
King's College Hospital NHS Foundation Trust,
London, UK

Mukesh Mukesh
Cambridge University Hospitals NHS Foundation Trust,
Cambridge, UK

Animesh J. K. Patel
Department of Plastic Surgery, Addenbrooke's Hospital,
Cambridge University Hospitals NHS Foundation Trust,
Cambridge, UK

Julietta Patnick
NHS Cancer Screening Programmes, Sheffield, UK

Sarah Pinder
Division of Cancer Studies, King's College London, Guy's
Hospital, London, UK

Vassilis Pitsinis
Cambridge Breast Clinic at Mediterraneo Hospital,
Athens, Greece

Linda J. Pointon
The Royal Marsden NHS Foundation Trust, London, UK

Elena Provenzano
Addenbrooke's Hospital, Cambridge University Hospitals NHS Foundation Trust, Cambridge, UK

Anand Purushotham
Division of Cancer Studies, King's College London, Guy's & St Thomas' NHS Foundation Trust, London, UK

Sabrina Rajan
Cambridge University Hospitals NHS Foundation Trust, Cambridge, UK

Emad A. Rakha
Department of Histopathology, City Hospital, The University of Nottingham and Nottingham University Hospitals NHS Trust, Nottingham, UK

J.S. Ries-Filho
Department of Pathology, Memorial Sloan-Kettering Cancer Center, New York, NY, USA

Mark Robson
Clinical Genetics Service, Memorial Sloan-Kettering Cancer Center, Weill Cornell Medical College, New York, NY, USA

Christobel Saunders
School of Surgery, The University of Western Australia, Crawley, WA, Australia

Amanda Shewbridge
Guy's & St Thomas' NHS Foundation Trust, London, UK

Melvin J. Silverstein
Hoag Memorial Hospital Presbyterian, CA, USA
Keck School of Medicine, CA, USA

Rache M. Simmons
Weill Medical College of Cornell University, The New York Presbyterian Hospital, New York, NY, USA

Baljit Singh
Department of Pathology, New York University Langone Medical Center, New York, NY, USA

Cath Taylor
Florence Nightingale School of Nursing and Midwifery, Kings College London, London, UK

Kathryn Taylor
Cambridge University Hospitals NHS Foundation Trust, Cambridge, UK

William Teh
Department of Radiology, Northwick Park Hospital, Harrow, UK

G.A. Thomas
Department of Surgery and Cancer, Imperial College London, London, UK

Hazel Thornton
Department of Health Sciences, University of Leicester, Leicester, UK

Todd M. Tuttle
Masonic Cancer Center, University of Minnesota, Minneapolis, MN, USA

Lisardo Ugidos
The Methodist Cancer Center, Houston, TX, USA

Jayant S. Vaidya
University College London, London, UK

Jajini Susan Varghese
University of Cambridge, Cambridge, UK
Department of Plastic Surgery, Royal Free Hospital, London, UK

Dale Collins Vidal
The Dartmouth Institute for Health Policy & Clinical Practice, Lebanon, NH, USA

Clive A. Wells
Department of Pathology, University College Hospital, London, UK

Rebecca Wight
Department of Surgery, Maimonides Medical Center, Brooklyn, NY, USA

Paul M. Wilkerson
Breakthrough Breast Cancer Research Centre, Institute of Cancer Research, London, UK

A. Robin M. Wilson
Department of Clinical Radiology, The Royal Marsden, Surrey, UK

Zoë Ellen Winters
School of Clinical Sciences, University of Bristol, Director of the Breast Reconstruction Patient Reported and Clinical Outcomes Research group, Research and Teaching, Bristol Royal Infirmary, Bristol, UK

Gordon C. Wishart
Anglia Ruskin University, Cambridge, UK

Preface

Worldwide breast cancer remains the most common malignancy in women, with over 1.3 million cases diagnosed annually and about 400,000 deaths from the disease. Globally, one-quarter of new female cancers have breast as the primary site, although this figure is up to one-third in the United Kingdom where the lifetime risk is 1 in 8. The annual number of cases has almost doubled over the past 3 decades within the United Kingdom (UK) where half of breast cancers are diagnosed within the screening age bracket. Introduction of the National Health Service Breast Screening Programme led to a surge in incidence of the disease which was confined to women of initial screening age. Rates have now fallen slightly for this age group but increased for women aged 65–69 years with age extension of screening. Breast cancer is a disease predominantly found in postmenopausal women, and the rising incidence of breast cancer during the 1990s has been attributed to increased usage of hormone replacement therapy amongst affluent women. One-quarter of women aged 45–69 years took exogenous hormones at the start of the millennium, but this dramatically halved after 2002 and continues to fall. This reduction in hormone replacement therapy usage resulted in a transient decrease in breast cancer incidence after 2002 amongst white American women, but this decline has not persisted.

Though more than three-quarters of breast cancers occur in women over 50 years of age, the disease occurs frequently in women under 35 years where genetic factors predominate etiologically. Breast cancers are now recognized to display epigenetic phenomena, which permit changes in gene expression without DNA sequence alterations, and to act translators between environment and genome.

Despite a higher prevalence of breast cancer in wealthy countries, incidence rates are rising steadily in less affluent societies, with contraction of historical differences in breast cancer rates based on income levels. Those countries which had moderate or low rates are now experiencing rapid rate increases which have more than doubled in Japan over the past 40 years and are rising inexorably in conurbations of mainland China. The high incidence rates within major industrialized nations have been attributed to lifestyle factors which now have relevance to increasing rates amongst the emerging economies. These include changes in reproductive behaviour, altered dietary habits (increased consumption of polyunsaturated fats and alcohol), physical inactivity, and hormone replacement therapy usage. These are all potentially modifiable risk factors with the opportunity to impact favourably not only on incidence but also treatment outcomes and mortality. Indeed, there are claims that up to one-third of breast cancer cases in developed countries could be prevented by adoption of a healthier lifestyle with maintenance of optimum body weight and regular exercise. Obese patients may benefit from extended endocrine treatments due to higher risk of recurrence in those with estrogen receptor-positive disease, though ironically obesity may partially offset the therapeutic benefit of adjuvant hormonal therapies.

Mortality rates for breast cancer have fallen over the past two decades despite the continued rise in incidence. This is testimony to the success of interventional strategies such as screening and adjuvant systemic therapies which permit diagnosis of breast cancer prior to de novo formation of micrometastases or obliteration of established foci of disease at distant sites. It is this burden of micrometastatic disease outside the breast and regional tissues that represents the most fundamental and challenging aspect of treatment for breast cancer—a disease which is heterogeneous with a variable and unpredictable natural history. We have entered a new era in breast cancer management where disease is "small" and more likely to be confined to the breast and regional nodes. Some of these tumours will have minimal proclivity for hematogenous dissemination and formation of micrometastases at an early stage in the neoplastic process. By contrast, some patients have micrometastatic diseases which can remain dormant and be activated many years after the diagnosis. A spectrum or intermediate paradigm is emerging which encompasses this variable capacity to form distant micrometastatic foci. Modern methods of molecular profiling may permit tumors to be assigned to one or other group based on biological behavior with appropriate intensities of locoregional and systemic treatments.

The latest overview by the Early Breast Cancer Trialists' Collaborative Group has confirmed an overall survival benefit at 15 years from local radiation treatment to either the breast following breast conservation therapy or the chest wall after mastectomy. Though these survival benefits are relatively modest, they emphasize the importance of surgery and radiotherapy, and there is a risk that "minimal effective treatments" may compromise locoregional control in some patients. It is essential that all forms of breast conservation surgery achieve histologically negative margins and that radiobiological equivalence to conventional external beam therapy is demonstrable for newer techniques of breast irradiation. Skin-sparing mastectomy represents the latest phase in the development of progressively less mutilating forms of mastectomy for breast cancer treatment. The oncological equivalence of skin-sparing mastectomy to standard forms of modified radical mastectomy has never been validated in prospective controlled trials, but this procedure appears safe in terms of local recurrence. Sentinel lymph node biopsy has revolutionized surgical management of breast cancer and has generated more questions than answers with ongoing intense debate following publication of the seminal American College of Surgeons Oncology Group Trial Z0011.

Systemic therapies target microscopic foci of tumor, and their modes of action are increasingly based on an understanding of the biological events underlying disordered growth patterns. The primary action of chemotherapeutic agents is to indiscriminately kill cancer cells by dislocating biochemical pathways, interfering with DNA repair processes and inducing apoptosis. A more selective approach is possible with the newer biological response modifiers which exploit natural growth regulatory mechanisms and target pathways at the level of ligand, growth factor receptor, or intracellular signal transduction. These translational approaches are exemplified by agents such as trastuzumab which may be administered either concomitantly or sequentially with conventional chemotherapy to maximize efficiency and minimize compound toxicity. A small number of well-designed trials with adequate power may provide more definitive answers to key clinical questions with less reliance on meta-analysis of many imperfect and potentially flawed trials.

Management of breast cancer is centred around the multidisciplinary team; this multidisciplinary approach facilitates optimum clinical decision-making with input from various specialities, including surgery, radiology, pathology, radiation/medical oncology, genetics, and plastic surgery. This pan-integration of diagnostic and therapeutic modalities is epitomized by breast cancer, and routine practice within a framework of local, national, and international guidelines has improved treatment outcomes and quality of life for this group of patients.

Early Breast Cancer: From Screening to Multidisciplinary Management was conceived by the late Guidubaldo Querci della Rovere (Uccio), a dear friend and colleague who died of cancer in 2009. The book discusses the principles and practice of breast cancer management within the context of the multidisciplinary team working with respect to both screen-detected and symptomatic disease. The text does not provide exhaustive coverage within the field but discusses key areas of contemporary interest and potential controversy. *Early Breast Cancer* aims to provide the reader with sound understanding and critical insight into many aspects of the disease from epidemiology, genetics, and screening to pathology, diagnosis, treatment, and prevention. This latest edition continues the general ethos of the second edition with an emphasis on breast cancer screening and continued development of the multidisciplinary team. There are dedicated chapters on shared decision-making and

informed consent together with the role of the "modern" breast care nurse. This latter group of healthcare workers have become increasingly important in delivery of high quality breast care service and ensuring that experience along the potentially complex patient pathway is facilitated.

Clinical practice takes place within an increasingly litigious and regulated working environment. Furthermore, there are shifting social and ethical mores coupled with increased patient rights and expectations. The advent of the Internet has allowed ease of access to unprecedented volumes of "literature" on breast cancer with emergence of "webwise" patients who come to the clinic forearmed with information. It is particularly important that less highly specialized clinicians who work in the field of breast disease maintain a critical and up-to-date knowledge base and can make sensible judgements and appropriate clinical decisions. Breast cancer is a global disease, and *Early Breast Cancer* draws on the expertise of leading specialists from three continents, many of whom have personal experience of working in developing countries with limited healthcare resources and organization. The recent economic downturn has led to contraction of private insurance plans and rationing of state-funded healthcare in the West. This has implications for several aspects of care for breast cancer patients including screening strategies, inclusion of sophisticated investigations into routine diagnostic workup (e.g., magnetic resonance imaging), access to immediate breast reconstruction, and availability of some anticancer agents.

This is an intermediate-sized text which complements more comprehensive tomes covering breast diseases in general. It should be of value to not only established practitioners but also trainees and clinical nurse practitioners. It may also be of assistance to basic research scientists at the laboratory-clinical interface and other professionals involved in the management and care of patients with breast cancer or survivors of this common but enigmatic disease.

John R. Benson
Gerald Gui
Todd M. Tuttle

Foreword

Writing a foreword to a medical textbook as a layperson turns out to be a more difficult undertaking than I thought. I was pleased to be asked by my Cambridge colleague, John R. Benson, to do what sounded like a simple and interesting task. Sitting down to read the proof chapters of this third edition, I realized that the task was, indeed, extremely interesting but not at all simple. One cannot write a peer review if one is not a peer, so I have torn up my first draft, written in the dispassionate style of the scientist I once was, and instead I will talk straight onto the page.

I have not read every word of every chapter of this comprehensive treatise on early breast cancer, nor would I understand it all if I did, but I have dipped in enough to recognize the high quality of the contributions, the enormous range of digestible and authoritative information the book contains, and the painstaking work the editors must have done to hone authors' drafts into such polished accounts.

It is not for me to hold forth on the great advances in diagnosis and treatment that have led to the dramatic improvement in breast cancer outcomes we have seen in recent years, although with my background as a chemist I can appreciate and applaud the brilliance of the research that underpins the rapidly increasing understanding of the molecular changes that characterize breast tumors. Science has paid off—increasingly tailoring the right drug to the right patient at the right time—and Herceptin will always stand a pioneer success for stratified medicine.

However, what I can say is something from the perspective of being a woman who has had a major brush with cancer, albeit not of the breast but of the bladder, and the daughter of a man who died of lung cancer in the 1970s, and also from my experience of the excellent breast services at Addenbrooke's Hospital.

A diagnosis of cancer is always a shock, and whoever invented the phrase "cancer journey" was spot on. Step by step, you go along the road from the first realization that something is wrong, through the flurry of early tests, the anxious waits, the breaking of the bad news, the preoperative assessments and treatments, the surgery, the postoperative therapy, and then the gradual recovery, until months or even years later you achieve—if you are fortunate, as increasing numbers of women who have had breast cancer are—a new normality infused with a pleasant flush of gratitude for being alive and well.

Step by step along this cancer journey, you walk metaphorically—or literally in the case of the nurses who get you out of bed and tottering down the ward the day after your operation—hand in hand with a large and expert multidisciplinary team. Reading this book made me realize just how large and expert the teams who look after women with breast cancer are. Some of them become friends, some of them you never see as a patient, but around you are medical and clinical oncologists, radiologists and radiographers, histopathologists, breast and plastic surgeons, specialist nurses, physiotherapists, dieticians and nutritionists, and those who provide expert psychological support where it is needed. There is a chapter in this book on the role of a breast care nurse, who can do so much for the psychological and emotional needs of women following a diagnosis of breast cancer. Breast cancer services have led the way in a holistic and multidisciplinary approach to the treatment of disease.

They have also led the field in patient-centered services. My father went bravely down his lung cancer journey to death before the "maximum tolerable" paradigm for cancer surgery of the 1960s had changed to the "minimum effective treatment" of today. Now women are offered the choice between mastectomy and breast-conserving surgery, and breast reconstructive surgery can restore their confidence in their body image after what is often a difficult time with no hair and no energy.

In the previous edition of this book, "informed consent" was a new chapter. Six years on, much has changed in terms of the doctor–patient relationship, and this edition has a chapter on shared decision-making from the renowned group at the Dartmouth Institute in New Hampshire. I have worked on shared decision-making between clinicians and men with a diagnosis of early prostate cancer, and I know how much more confident patients who are active participants in decisions about their treatment are.

I salute the range of professionals who have written this book, whose work has constantly and consistently increased survival rates for breast cancer and improved life after breast cancer by giving women more confidence as they travel along their personal cancer journeys.

Mary Archer, DBE

1   An introduction to screening for breast cancer

Linda J. Pointon and Sue K. Down

INTRODUCTION

The mortality rate of breast cancer has fallen in the last 20 years, but it is still the leading cause of death from cancer among women in the United Kingdom (UK). In 2009, over 48,000 cases were diagnosed and there were nearly 13,000 deaths (1–4). The etiology of the disease is not fully understood although the risk is known to be associated with increasing age, reproductive practices and family history. Screening for breast cancer has been shown to advance the diagnosis of the disease which can lead to more successful treatment and therefore reduced mortality. This chapter details the evidence upon which breast screening has been introduced on a national scale, with particular reference to the UK.

All screening programs should satisfy the Wilson–Jungner criteria set out by the World Health Organization (5):

- The condition being screened for should be an important health problem.
- The natural history of the condition should be well understood.
- There should be a detectable early stage.
- Treatment at an early stage should be of more benefit than at a later stage.
- A suitable test should be devised for the early stage.
- The test should be acceptable.
- Intervals for repeating the test should be determined.
- Adequate health service provision should be made for the extra clinical workload resulting from screening.
- The risks, both physical and psychological, should be less than the benefits.
- The costs should be balanced against the benefits.

Although breast cancer is a significant health problem, its natural history is not well understood. The disease may be initiated by atypical changes within breast cells which then progress to a preinvasive stage where the carcinoma cells are confined to the duct system. This may then become invasive and begin to invade the surrounding tissue, and thereafter possibly spread to the lymph nodes or other secondary sites within the body. However, invasive disease can also arise *de novo* and there is evidence to suggest that certain invasive breast cancers may regress spontaneously (6).

Breast tumors may disseminate at different stages in their natural history. In some women, and for some types of tumor, this could take years while in others the metastatic spread may take only weeks depending on the aggressiveness of the cancer. Some studies have suggested that tumor grade increases exponentially with size (7,8). Ideally, screening should detect tumors while they are still small and before any metastases

have developed (9). In order for screening to be effective, the disease must have a recognizable early stage. In the case of breast cancer this is the preclinical detectable phase where a tumor can be seen on a mammogram but before it becomes palpable (about 1 cm in diameter). Tumors in this phase are more likely to be non-invasive or, if already invasive, less likely to have regional or distant spread.

For screening to be beneficial, treating breast cancer at this earlier stage must improve prognosis compared with treatment of more advanced cancers. However, it is not appropriate to compare the survival of women having screen-detected cancers with that of those who present symptomatically with the effect of various biases not being removed. Figure 1.1 illustrates the stages the disease passes through as it progresses (10). Lead-time bias occurs because survival time is measured from the time of diagnosis. As screening will advance the date of diagnosis, the survival time will automatically be longer even if there is no effect on the actual date of death. Also, less aggressive, slower-growing cancers will spend more time in the preclinical detectable phase than fast-growing cancers which are more likely to present symptomatically. Screening will therefore detect proportionally more of the slow-growing or non-invasive cancers which in turn have a better prognosis. This is known as length bias. There is also the problem of selection bias in which those who attend for screening are more likely to be health-conscious than those who refuse and will probably have a better prognosis anyway. These biases can be removed by comparing the mortality incidence in a population which was offered screening with that in a population which was not offered screening, in the context of a randomized controlled trial.

The suitability of any screening test depends on its accuracy. It must be able to detect the majority of women who have breast cancer (high sensitivity) and therefore give few false-negative results, as well as to eliminate most of those women who do not have the disease (high specificity) thereby minimizing the number of false-positive results. Sensitivity is defined as the proportion of all those women with breast cancer who test positive; specificity is defined as the proportion of all those without the disease who test negative. Ideally, both sensitivity and specificity should be 100% but there is an inevitable compromise, as no test is perfect and these two parameters are inversely related to one another. Different screening modalities will be discussed in more detail later.

For public health, the acceptability of a screening test by the general population is of paramount importance and will be reflected by the rate of compliance with invitation to screening. Compliance levels in the range of 80–90% have been

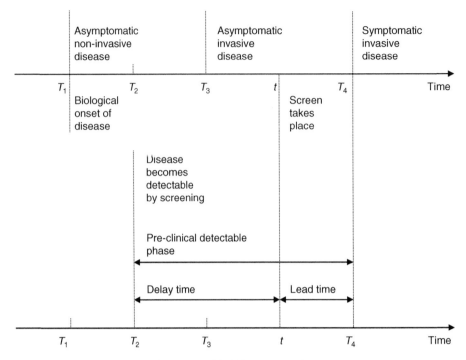

Figure 1.1 Model of disease progression.

documented in Sweden (11). A minimum level of 70% compliance has been shown to be effective in reducing breast cancer mortality in the target population (12). Latest figures show that an acceptance rate of 73.3% has been achieved in the UK as a whole, although there are regional differences and specific groups where attention is needed (13,14). A new project addressing this issue is discussed later in this chapter.

Screening must be repeated at regular intervals to ensure its effectiveness, as the risk of developing breast cancer increases with age. Moreover, the growth rate of the disease is variable and there has to be a compromise taking into account the cost and practicality of screening too frequently while aiming to minimize the number of cancers which escape detection by screening. In the UK, the interval was initially set to three years which reflected the 33-month interval in the Swedish Two-County Trial, with a recommendation for more research into the screening interval. In the UKCCCR (UK Coordinating Committee on Cancer Research) Breast Screening Frequency Trial, 76,000 women were randomized to either three-yearly or annual screening (15). The Nottingham Prognostic Index (NPI) was used to compare predicted mortality in the two groups. Although tumors diagnosed in the annual mammography group were of significantly smaller size, no overall improvement in predicted mortality was seen. The screening interval in the National Health Service Breast Screening Programme (NHSBSP) therefore remains unchanged at three years.

Another important consideration for a screening test is that it should do no harm, either physical or psychological. The potential physical hazards from screening by mammography are the risk from ionizing radiation (X-rays) and unnecessary surgical procedures resulting from an overdiagnosis of tumors which may never have become invasive in a patient's lifetime. The radiation risk from mammography has been much reduced especially with the introduction of digital mammography. Due to technical advances the maximum dose for standard two-view studies is now 4.5–4.7 mGy for screen-film mammograms and 3.7 mGy for digital mammograms (compared with 2–3 cGy in the past) (16,17). Screening women aged 47–73 at three-yearly intervals using screen-film mammography is estimated to induce 0.3–0.6 breast cancers per 1000 women (18). Annual/biennial digital screening from 40 to 74 years would induce 0.86 cancers per 1000 women (19). It is estimated that for every 14,000 women screened in England, 35 lives are saved and one fatal breast cancer is induced (20). Psychological hazards associated with screening include anxiety and distress associated with false-positive mammograms, though studies to date have shown mixed results regarding persistent anxiety and depression in those patients who are recalled but eventually have negative results (21,22).

High-quality screening techniques and highly trained technical and radiological staff should minimize the risk of overdiagnosis. Ideally, the recall rate should be as low as possible. A study which analyzed data from a UK breast screening program (NHSBSP) and Swedish Two-County Trial estimated that between 2 and 2.5 lives are saved for each case overdiagnosed in the above-50 age group (23). It is also important that adequate assessment and treatment facilities exist to ensure that women are seen as quickly as possible. In addition, there is a range of non-invasive and minimally invasive investigative techniques which should be employed to reduce the risk of unnecessary open surgical biopsies. These include ultrasound, spot views, micromagnification, fine needle aspiration, needle core biopsy, and vacuum-assisted biopsy. These techniques have collectively reduced the benign biopsy rate in many units.

Screening for breast cancer was introduced in the UK in 1988 following the recommendations of the Forrest Report (24). The NHSBSP initially offered single mediolateral oblique view mammography to women aged 50–64 years with an interval of three years. Following ongoing research and evaluation, the program is currently being expanded to invite women in the age of 47–73 years. Furthermore, two-view digital mammography will be offered at all screens.

SCREENING MODALITIES

There are three potential mass screening tools: mammography, clinical examination by trained staff, and breast self-examination. Mammography has been shown to be effective in reducing breast cancer mortality. The Swedish Two-County Trial (25) used single mediolateral oblique view film mammography alone and achieved a mortality reduction of 32% in women aged 40–74 years. The sensitivity was 91–100% for women aged above 50 years and 83% for women in the 40–49 age group. This may be due to denser breast tissue in younger women and sensitivity could possibly be improved by using the two-view film mammography. The main reason for using a single view only was the perceived need in the 1970s to minimize the radiation dose. However, as already discussed, with modern mammography techniques, this risk is now considered insignificant. A study of one- versus two-view mammography (26) has shown that adding a second (craniocaudal) view increases the sensitivity of screening during the prevalence round of a population screening program from 83% to 89%. Moreover, the recall rate was reduced from 8.8% to 6.6%. Therefore, mammography, particularly with two views, is an effective, acceptable, and sensitive method for primary screening.

In addition, the Digital Mammographic Imaging Screening Trial (DMIST) reported increased diagnostic accuracy for digital mammography over film mammography in certain groups of women (27). Digital mammography is also known to reduce the radiation dose required for screening (17), and is now being introduced into screening units throughout the UK.

The effectiveness of clinical breast examination (CBE) alone has not been tested, although some trials have used it in conjunction with mammography. In Edinburgh, between 1979 and 1981, a randomized controlled trial compared CBE alternating with and without mammography, to no screening (28). Compliance was poor within this study (61%) and there is no conclusive evidence to show that clinical examination is effective in reducing mortality. Interestingly, a Canadian trial conducted between 1980 and 1985 compared mammography and CBE with CBE alone, and reported no difference in mortality (29). A large randomized trial in the Philippines comparing CBE to no screening was discontinued due to poor compliance (30). Further trials are ongoing in Egypt and India (31). One analysis has shown the sensitivity of mammography to be 63% and of clinical examination, 40% (32).

Breast self-examination (BSE) has been evaluated in two large population-based studies in China and Russia (33,34). In the Russian trial, the cohort practicing BSE detected a significantly higher number of breast cancers, but this was not the case in the Chinese study from Shanghai. Neither study found a difference in overall mortality incidence from breast cancer when BSE was used as a screening tool and more women in the BSE groups of both trials underwent benign biopsies than in control groups. BSE is therefore not recommended as a single screening modality for breast cancer (35).

Magnetic resonance imaging (MRI) has been shown to have high sensitivity for detecting abnormalities in the breast.

However, specificity is lower than for mammography, resulting in a higher number of false-positive results and benign biopsies (36). In addition, the cost of MRI is significantly higher than that of mammography due to equipment requirements and analysis time (37). In general, the population at the greatest risk of breast cancer is that which comprises women over the age of 50 years. No studies have been conducted to assess the efficacy of MRI for women in this age group with an average breast cancer risk. As mammography has been shown to be a much cheaper, quicker, and more effective modality for breast screening, it is not appropriate to consider MRI as an alternative mass screening tool.

However, MRI has a particular application in screening younger women (age less than 50 years) who are at high genetic risk of developing breast cancer. In these younger premenopausal women, breast tissue can be radiologically dense and mammograms more difficult to interpret. There is a recognized need to screen women at high risk of breast cancer as the disease may develop at an earlier age than in the general population, but there are concerns about repeated radiation exposures. With the advent of genetic testing, groups of women at high risk have been identified, for whom conventional mammography alone is not a satisfactory method of screening for breast cancer. MRI avoids radiation exposure while providing high sensitivity in detecting breast cancer, even in the mammographically dense breast. Several studies have confirmed that the sensitivity of MRI is higher than that of mammography (77–94% vs. 33–59%), although the specificity of MRI is lower than mammography (63–89.8% vs. 77–95%) (the UK MARIBS study (38), the Dutch MRISC study (39), the Italian HIBCRIT study (40)). Annual screening, with a combination of mammography and MRI, of high risk women therefore increases sensitivity for cancer detection, while achieving acceptable specificity. Current guidelines from the UK National Institute for Health and Clinical Excellence recommend annual MRI surveillance from the age of 30 years for women at high risk of developing familial breast cancer (41), and the NHSBSP has now commenced MRI screening of higher-risk women (42).

Another group that is considered at a high risk of breast cancer has women who have been previously exposed to supradiaphragmatic radiotherapy for Hodgkin's disease. Breast screening is currently recommended from the age of 25 years, or 8 years following first irradiation, whichever is the later. Imaging should be by annual MRI from 25 to 39 years, with the addition of annual mammography in the 40–50 years age group to improve sensitivity (42). Women over the age of 50 have routine three-yearly screening.

EVIDENCE FOR MORTALITY REDUCTION FROM RANDOMIZED CONTROLLED TRIALS

The Health Insurance Plan (HIP) of Greater New York was the first trial of breast cancer screening (12). The population consisted of approximately 62,000 women aged 40–64 years who were selected from 23 of the 31 HIP medical centers. From each group, two systematic random samples of women with membership in HIP for at least a year were selected and entered into the program from December 1963 to June 1966. These two groups then formed the study and control populations. The study group was offered screening by clinical examination and two-view mammography first at entry to the trial and then yearly for the next three years. The control group was not invited to screening. The compliance at the first screen was 67%, and 80% of these women attended the first annual repeat examination, 75% the second, and 69% the third. Overall, 40% attended all four screens. Ten years after the start of the trial, the breast cancer mortality reduction in the study group was 30%, whereas after a more prolonged follow-up to 18 years, the reduction was around 25%.

The Swedish two county study took place in Östergotland and Kopparberg counties, Sweden (25). Women aged 40–74 were entered into the program from 1977 to 1981. The trial group was randomized by population cluster rather than by individual, and subsequent analyses have shown the loss of power to be minimal. In Östergotland, one cluster in each block of two was randomized to screening and in Kopparberg it was two clusters in each block of three. This resulted in a study group of 77,080 and a control group of 55,985. Women aged 40–49 were invited to screening by one-view mammography alone every 24 months, and those in the age range 50–74 were invited every 33 months on average. The control group was not invited to screening in the initial study. In 1985, after four rounds of screening in the younger age range, three in the 50–69 range, and two in the 70–74 range, the control group was invited to screening. All breast cancers in both arms of the trial diagnosed between randomization and the end of the first screen of the controls were included in the final analysis of the trial results. Compliance levels were high and for women under 70 years, participation was consistently about 90% at all screens. For women aged between 70 and 74 years, the participation rate was 79% for the first screening round and 67% for the second. Consequently no further invitations were issued to this age group. The first set of results of the study obtained before the controls were invited to screening, were published in 1985 and showed a mortality rate reduction of 31% in the study group. After 30 years, the main findings of the trial remain unchanged with a mortality reduction in the study group of 31% [Relative risk (RR) = 0.69, 95% confidence interval (CI) 0.56–0.84] (43).

The Malmo screening trial started in October 1976 and aimed to determine whether breast cancer mortality level in women over 45 could be reduced by mammographic screening (44). All women born during 1908–1932 were identified from the population registry of Malmo, Sweden. Half the women in each birth year cohort were randomly selected as the study group and invited to mammographic screening at intervals of 18–24 months. The remaining women were allocated to the control group and were not offered screening. In the first two rounds, two views were taken. In subsequent rounds either both views or just the oblique was taken depending on the density of the breasts. The attendance rate was higher in the first round (74%) than in subsequent rounds (70%) and higher among younger than among older women. The predetermined termination date for the trial was 31 December 1986, at which time no significant reduction in mortality was seen in the study group. In fact, during the first seven calendar years of the screening program, the cumulative number of deaths from breast cancer was higher in the study group than in the controls, although by the end of the trial this situation had been reversed. The Malmo study suffered from loss of power due not only to the attendance rate but also to dilution of the control group. A random sample of 500 of the control group showed that 24% had undergone mammography during the study period.

The randomized controlled trial in Edinburgh, Scotland (28) has been described previously. Like the two-county study, population clusters (general practices) rather than individuals, were randomized. There were initial concerns that cluster randomization did not achieve comparability between the two groups in terms of factors such as cardiovascular mortality, although with adjustments for socioeconomic status using logistic regression, these differences disappeared. After 14 years, there was a significant reduction of 29% in the mortality rate of those invited for screening (RR = 0.71, 95% CI 0.53–0.95) (45).

In Stockholm, Sweden, a randomized controlled trial was begun in March 1981 to compare single view mammography with no intervention in women aged 40–64 years (46). Selection was done individually by birth date with 40,000 women randomized to the study population and 20,000 controls. The study group was invited twice to attend for mammography with a screening interval of about 30 months. The compliance was over 80% in the first and second screening rounds with little difference between the age groups. After the second round was completed in 1985, the control group was invited for one screen by mammography where the compliance was approximately 77%. After an 11-year follow-up, there was a nonsignificant reduction of 26% (RR = 0.74, CI 0.5–1.1) in the mortality rate. However, in the age group of 50–64 years, a significant 38% reduction in mortality was observed (CI 0.38–1.0). In the 40–49 age group, no effect on mortality was seen (RR = 1.08, CI 0.54–2.17).

The Canadian National Breast Screening Study (CNBSS) was planned in the late 1970s and started screening women in January 1980. The study was in two parts and had different screening regimens for women aged 40–49 years (47) and those aged 50–59 years (48). In the younger age group, 50,430 women with no history of breast cancer and who had not undergone mammography in the previous 12 months were invited to an initial physical examination. At this initial visit, half were then randomly assigned to the study group who would be offered annual mammography and physical examination (MP group) and the other half to the control group who would be returned to usual community care (UC group) with annual follow-up by mailed questionnaire. The first 62% of the study women were eligible for a four-year program; the rest were offered a three-year program. All women were taught BSE and the mean follow-up time was 8.5 years. Over 90% of women in each group attended the screening sessions or returned the annual questionnaires, or both over two to five years. The ratio of the proportions of death from breast cancer in the MP group compared with the UC group was 1.36 (95% CI 0.84–2.21) which was not a significant difference. The study concluded that screening with mammography and physical examination had no impact on the rate of death from breast cancer after seven years.

The entry criteria and randomization techniques were the same in the older age group (48). In this part of the study, 39,405 women attended the initial physical examination and were randomly assigned to undergo either annual mammography and physical examination (MP group) or annual physical examination only group). The first two-thirds of women who entered the study were offered five annual screens and the rest were offered four. Again, these older women were taught BSE at the initial examination and were followed up for an average of 8.3 years. Over 85% of women in each group attended the screening sessions after the initial screen. The survival rates were similar in the two groups and women whose cancer had been detected by mammography alone had the highest survival rates. The ratio of the proportions of death from breast cancer in the MP group compared with the annual physical examination only group was 0.97 (95% CI 0.62–1.52) but these differences were not significant. The conclusions for this older cohort were similar to those for the younger age group but critics have pointed out that the quality of the mammography, as assessed by independent review, was unacceptably poor and therefore any conclusions must be tentative (49). There were also some concerns about the randomization process although these have been discounted after formal investigation (50). Further interrogation has also shown that a significant number of women in the control groups underwent private screening mammograms outside of the trial during the study period (51).

Recruitment of women aged 39–59 years to the screening trial in Gothenburg, Sweden, started in December 1982. Approximately 21,000 women were randomly allocated to the study group and 30,000 to the controls. The randomization was done largely by individual in the age range 40–49 years and by cluster from 50 to 59 years, according to day of birth. The study group was invited to two-view mammography at intervals of 18 months, while the control group was not screened. The compliance rate for the first round was 84% with a mortality reduction of 14% although this result was not significant. The control group was invited to screening from November 1987 onward and the screening phase continued until 1991. Follow-up to assess effects on breast cancer mortality continued until the end of December 1996; overall there was a nonsignificant reduction in the mortality rate of 21–24% after 13 years of follow-up, with a reduction in mortality for the 39–49 years age group of 31% (RR = 0.69, CI 0.45–1.05) (52).

The randomized, controlled UK Age trial investigated the effect of mammographic screening from 40 years of age on breast cancer mortality (53). Women aged 39–41 years were randomized to either invitation for annual mammography (54,000) or no intervention (107,000). Compliance was 68% for the first round and 69% for subsequent rounds, which reflects national rates (54). The trial ran from 1991 to 2004, and included women up to 48 years of age. After 10 years' follow-up, there was a nonsignificant mortality reduction of 17% (RR = 0.83, 95% CI 0.66–1.04). A subsequent analysis emphasized that very few women in the control arm underwent screening mammography out of the trial (55) and this was therefore not a confounding factor.

The results of all these randomized controlled trials are summarized in Table 1.1.

EFFECTS OF AGE

The most important risk factor for breast cancer is age. Therefore, screening should not only target those most likely to develop breast cancer but also consider those groups of women whose prognosis will be improved by early detection.

The Swedish Two-County study is the only randomized trial to have analyzed the mortality benefit in the older age group (aged 65–74 years) and shows a mortality reduction of 32% (RR = 0.68, 95% CI 0.51–0.89) (56). However, for women aged 70 years and older, there is generally little data available. An overview of the Swedish randomized screening trials (57) suggested that screening has no impact on mortality in this age group (RR = 1.12, 95% CI 0.73–1.72) but further research is needed.

The issue of screening women in the younger age range from 40 to 49 years was investigated by the Canadian NBSS study (47) and the UK Age Trial (53); both offered annual mammography and have been described previously. The Canadian trial showed no benefit from screening in this age group, while the UK study found a nonsignificant 17% reduction in mortality with annual screening. Concerns over widespread population screening of women in this age range relate to lower efficacy, increased radiation exposure, and the likelihood of false positives leading to psychological distress (58). As discussed in an earlier section (Introduction), the advent of digital mammography has increased the sensitivity for younger women and reduced the radiation dosage. Studies of radiation risk have concluded that the chance of inducing breast cancer from doses used in annual mammography is extremely small and is outweighed by the reported mortality benefit (19,20). Further analysis of the Age Trial data has demonstrated that the false-positive rate in this age group was comparable with that of the national screening program (59); 4.9% for the prevalence screen and 3.2% for incidence screens.

Table 1.1 Randomized Controlled Trials of Breast Cancer Screening with Mammography

Study	Year Started	Age Group (yrs)	Approx. No. of Subjects (Total)	% Mortality Reduction	95% CI
HIP, New York (12)	1963	40–64	62,000	25	Not stated
Two-county, Sweden (25)	1977	40–74	133,000	30	(15 to 42)
Malmo, Sweden (44)	1976	45–69	42,000	4	(−35 to 32)
Edinburgh, Scotland (45)	1979	45–64	45,000	17	(−18 to 42)
Stockholm, Sweden (46)	1981	40–64	60,000	29	(−20 to 60)
NBSS (1), Canada (47)	1980	40–49	50,000	−36	(−121 to 16)
NBSS (2), Canada (47)	1980	50–59	39,000	3	(−52 to 38)
Gothenburg (52)	1982	40–59	50,000	14	(−37 to 46)
UK Age trial (53)	1991	39–48	161,000	17	(−34 to 4)

Abbreviations: HIP, Health Insurance Plan; NBSS, National Breast Screening Study.

Some of the trials already described have included women in the younger age range, and sub-group analyses have generally shown that with high-quality mammography and a 12–18 month screening interval, there may be some benefit to screening younger women. The HIP study shows an overall mortality reduction across all ages, but questions the utility of screening the under 50s at randomization as most of the benefit in this group was seen in cancers actually diagnosed after the age of 50 years (12). An overview of the Swedish trials demonstrated a 23% mortality reduction in women aged 40–49 at randomization with a median follow-up time of 12.8 years and a screening interval of 18–24 months (60). The Gothenburg trial found a 31% mortality benefit in this age group for the screened population compared with the controls where two-view mammography was used and an 18-month screening interval was strictly adhered to (52). It is evident from the Swedish two-county study that the mortality benefit is smaller and occurs later than it does in the above-50 age group (25).

Combining all of the available data, a meta-analysis of the major trials has shown that for women aged 39–49 years, screening mammography every 1–2 years results in a 15% decrease (RR = 0.85, CI 0.75–0.96) in breast cancer mortality after a maximum of 20 years' follow-up (61). A retrospective review of screening women aged 40–49 years in Sweden from 1986–2005 has suggested a reduction in the mortality rate of 26% (RR = 0.74, CI 0.66–0.83) with 16 years' follow-up (62).

The NHSBSP is currently conducting a randomization project examining the benefits and harms associated with extending the age range for breast screening to 47–73 years.

HOW DOES SCREENING WORK?

As neither the causal pathways for breast cancer nor the means of preventing it are known, the only intervention possible at the moment in healthy women to improve mortality from breast cancer is screening. Trials of chemoprevention agents involving tamoxifen, raloxifene, and exemestane have shown reduction in the incidence of invasive breast cancers for moderate- to high-risk women (63–67). However, all these agents have side effects which make it difficult to justify their use in an otherwise healthy population.

Although treatments continue to improve, prognosis rapidly worsens with increasing tumor burden. Screening can advance the diagnosis so that a cancer is treated at an early stage with a greater chance of success. This is reflected in the earlier stage of tumors detected in the study group in the Swedish two-county trial (9). The progression of the disease is shown in Figure 1.1 (10). The lead time is the interval between the time when a prevalent case is detected by screening and the time when that case would otherwise have become clinically incident. The longer the lead time for a given case, the better one would expect the prognosis to be. If the cancer is not detected until it becomes clinically detectable, the lead time is zero. The lead time for an individual case is unobservable but the distribution of lead times is dependent on the distribution of the time spent in the preclinical detectable phase (sojourn time). The sojourn time is also unobservable but may be estimated using the method of Walter and Day (10). The method will also provide an estimate of the sensitivity of the screen and these may be used to estimate the optimum screening regimen and the potential gains in terms of mortality. For example, if the sojourn time is long, the maximum possible lead time is correspondingly long. If the sojourn time is short, however, the potential benefit from screening is smaller and screening must take place more frequently to increase the probability that the preclinical disease is detected before it becomes clinically apparent.

DETECTION STATUS

In a screening trial, breast cancers can be detected in seven different ways: symptomatically in the control group; after randomization but before screening; at the first (prevalence) screen; at later (incidence) screens; in the intervals between screens; in women who refused screening; or after the trial has finished in the study or the control group. In a routine screening program, not a randomized trial, there are four possible modes of detection: at screening (prevalence or incidence), in the interval between screens, and in refusers. In the Swedish two-county trial, a cancer was classified as being in a refuser if it was diagnosed after the woman did not attend a screen to which she was invited but before the invitation to the next. Interval cancers are those that appear symptomatically between screens, after a negative screen. Table 1.2 shows the number of deaths from breast cancer by age and detection mode and also the relative risk of mortality by detection mode in the Swedish two-county trial. The cancer detection rate at the first two screens is shown in

---

Table 1.2 Breast Cancer Deaths/Cases by Age Group and Detection Mode and Relative Risk by Detection Mode

| Detection Mode | Breast Cancer Deaths/Cases in Age Group | | | | | Relative Risk |
	40–49	50–59	60–69	70–74	Total	
PSP	32/160	73/315	90/419	40/146	234/1040	1.00
Before screening[a]	1/6	3/5	3/12	1/4	8/27	NK
First screen	5/39	13/102	20/184	10/101	48/436	0.57
Later screens	9/110	12/156	15/183	6/52	42/501	0.69
Interval 0–11 months	7/32	3/19	2/23	0/2	12/76	0.80
Interval 12–23 months	10/43	7/35	7/36	2/11	26/125	
Interval 24+ months	6/12	10/32	8/34	2/9	26/87	
Interval (time not known)	0/4	0/4	0/2	0/0	0/10	
Refuser	4/10	15/28	20/49	23/50	62/137	1.46
After screening[b]	0/0	0/0	0/0	8/30	8/30	NK
Total ASP	42/256	3/381	75/523	52/259	232/1419	0.70

[a]Between randomization and commencement of screening.
[b]In women aged 70–74 after routine screening ceased in this group.
Abbreviations: ASP, active study population (i.e., invited to screening); NK, not known; PSP, passive study population (i.e., not invited to screening).

Table 1.3. Detection rates increase steadily with age. Although the detection rate at the prevalence screen was higher, Table 1.2 shows that the relative risk of mortality is lower than for subsequent screens. This is likely to be due to length bias. Many slow-growing cancers, which may have been present for years, will be detected at the first screen and these will have a far better prognosis than the more aggressive fast-growing tumors. Thus, length bias can be largely eliminated by defining the so-called "unbiased set" of all tumors diagnosed up to and including the last screen but excluding those diagnosed at the first. The improvement in the cancer to biopsy ratio is partly due to increasing expertise as the trial progresses and partly because, at the first screen, more minimally invasive and non-invasive lesions will be picked up.

In younger women there is a predominance of deaths from interval cancers, whereas in older women there are more deaths in the refuser category. This is due to the fact that interval cancers are more common in younger women and that older women are more likely to be refusers, rather than age variation in case fatalities. A good means for expressing interval cancer rates is to express them as a proportion of the underlying incidence that will be expected in the absence of screening (in a trial this is given by the control group incidence). Proportionate incidence rates for interval cancers in the Swedish two-county study are shown in Table 1.4. For women over age 50, these results have been used to set targets in the UK national program. The incidence rates for younger women (under 50) are notably higher than for women over 50.

Both the lower cancer detection rates and the higher interval cancer rates underline the difficulty of effective screening for women below 50 years of age. They provide an explanation for the smaller mortality reduction that is generally seen.

TUMOR CHARACTERISTICS

There has been a debate in the past as to whether breast cancer is systemic from the outset and size is merely a marker of the age of the tumor or whether breast cancer is a progressive disease. It is clear that most breast tumors grow and lymph nodes become positive with time, although there is also evidence to suggest that certain invasive tumors may regress spontaneously (6). It is unclear whether other features of the tumor such as grade, DNA ploidy, and pathological type also change with time. Although it is not expected that individual tumor cells change their nature, many tumors are heterogeneous and contain several cell types with different intrinsic behavior. It is therefore reasonable to surmise that as time goes on, the more aggressive component multiplies faster.

There is some evidence that breast cancer is a systemic disease from the outset (68–70). The National Surgical Adjuvant

Table 1.3 Cancer Detection Rate in the Swedish Two-County Study

Screen	Cancer Detection Rate/ 1000 Women Screened	Cancers/ Open Biopsy
Prevalence	6.1	0.50
First incidence	3.4	0.75

Table 1.4 Control Incidence of Breast Cancer by Age at Randomization, with Screening Prevalence and Interval Incidence as a Percentage of Control Incidence, by Age, and by Screening Round in the Swedish Two-County Study

Age Group	Control Incidence[a]	Interval Incidence in Year[b]			Screening Prevalence[c]
		1	2	3 or more	
First interval					*First round*
40–49	1.05	46	53		2.09
50–59	1.87	10	28	52	4.67
60–69	2.50	17	27	57	8.80
70–74	2.99	8	44	48	12.15
Second interval					*Second round*
40–49	As above	66	41		2.65
50–59		19	35	62	3.03
60–69		9	31	43	4.89
70–74					7.50
Third interval					*Third round*
40–49	As above	22	109		2.16
50–59		23	40	85	3.74
60–69		24	22	26	5.07
70–74					
Overall					*Overall*
40–49	As above	45	62		2.30
50–59		17	34	63	3.84
60–69		17	27	46	6.41
70–74		8	44	48	10.13

[a]Incidence per 1000 woman years.
[b]As a percentage of control incidence; for the age group 40–49 only given years 1 and 2+.
[c]Prevalence per 1000 women.

Breast & Bowel Project (NSABP) B-06 study of ipsilateral breast tumor recurrence (IBTR) found that although the frequency of IBTR was reduced when patients treated by lumpectomy also received breast irradiation, the distant disease-free survival was no different from those who received lumpectomy alone (71). The size of the original tumor was an important predictor of distant disease-free survival, but when adjusted for IBTR, this relationship disappeared. Fisher concluded that IBTR and axillary lymph node invasion are merely markers for the risk of developing distant metastases rather than a clinically significant cause of distant disease.

Evidence of progressive disease comes from the Swedish two-county trial (11) and the New York HIP screening trial (12) which show a deficit of both deaths and advanced cancers (by size and lymph node status) in the group invited to screening. This phenomenon would not be observed if breast cancer was not a progressive disease in which the process can be halted by early detection. If the other, more controversial progression hypothesis is considered, that of changing grade and defining two populations of tumors, one "young" (screened) and one "old" (unscreened), there is always an excess of grade 3 tumors in the latter group. It may be argued, however, that this is due to length bias. Removal of the prevalence screen eliminates (for the most part) the length bias. After doing so in the Swedish two-county study, there was still an excess of grade 3 tumors in the unscreened group, suggesting that this "drift" indeed occurs (8).

The three prognostic factors which are most commonly considered for a breast tumor are its size, nodal status, and an underlying measure of malignant potential such as histological grade. The nodal status is an indication of how far a tumor has spread. If the lymph nodes are negative, then the tumor is more likely to remain localized to the breast. If it spreads to the lymph nodes, the prognosis will be worse; if distant metastases are present, the prognosis is very poor. Grade is a measure of the aggressiveness of a tumor. Grade 1 tumors have the best prognosis as they tend to be slow growing (well differentiated), whereas grade 3 tumors are notably more aggressive (poorly differentiated). However, grade is assigned by an individual pathologist and it can be subjective. In the Swedish two-county study, grade was assessed independently by one pathologist in each county and the grade distributions were different. This is more likely to be a reflection of the differences between the two pathologists rather than differences in the tumor populations. However, the effect of grade on prognosis was much the same, suggesting that the pathologists were measuring the same phenomenon but scoring it differently. The prognostic importance of these three factors, when considered together, is given in Table 1.5 (8).

In the same study, detection status was found to be significantly correlated with each of the tumor attributes: size, nodal status, and grade. Screen-detected cancers are more likely to be small and have a favorable nodal status and grade, all of which indicate a good prognosis. Tumors in the groups of refusers are larger, of worse grades, and are more likely to have positive nodes or distant metastases. There is no apparent reason to expect the cancers in the refusers to have a poorer grade than those detected at screening unless the grade is not static for each tumor but deteriorates as the tumor grows. This could

be explained if tumors have a mixture of poorly- and well-differentiated cells; the poorly-differentiated cells are expected to multiply more quickly. In order to test this, an unbiased set was required so that two groups of tumors could be compared

Table 1.5 Estimates of Relative Hazard Based on Proportional Hazards Regression, with Each Factor Adjusted for the Others, and for Age and County, in the Swedish Two-County Study

Factors/Category	Hazard Ratio	(95% CI)
Size (mm)		
1–9	1.00	
10–14	1.57	(0.94–2.63)
15–19	1.84	(1.11–3.07)
20–29	3.23	(1.99–5.23)
30–49	5.35	(3.28–8.74)
50+	9.97	(6.04–16.4)
Lymph node status		
Negative	1.00	
Positive or distant metastases	3.20	(2.6–3.9)
Histological type		
Others[a]	1.00	
Ductal grade 1	0.75	(0.45–1.27)
Ductal grade 2	1.24	(0.85–1.80)
Ductal grade 3	2.06	(1.44–2.93)
Ductal grade unspecified	1.56	(0.83–2.92)
Lobular	1.19	(0.76–1.86)
Medullary	0.94	(0.50–1.78)
Missing size, lymph node status, or type	3.84	(3.21–4.58)

[a]Others include ductal carcinoma *in-situ*, mucinous carcinoma, tubular carcinoma, and other carcinomas.

Table 1.6 Percentage Distributions of Grade, Nodal Status, and Size of Invasive Tumors Diagnosed in Women Aged 40–69 in the ASP and the PSP After the Prevalence Screen in the Swedish Two-County Study

| Factors/Category | Group | | |
	ASP	PSP	Overall
Grade			
1	21.3	16.8	19.3
2	38.7	34.7	36.9
3	40.0	48.5	43.8
Number of cases	600	493	1093
Nodal status			
Negative	68.2	54.5	62.0
Positive	27.6	39.8	33.2
Distant metastases	4.2	5.7	4.8
Number of cases	670	558	1228
Tumor size (mm)			
1–9	18.0	7.1	13.0
10–14	22.4	15.4	19.3
15–19	20.5	19.7	20.0
20–29	23.2	29.0	25.9
30–49	10.5	20.0	14.9
50+	5.4	8.8	7.0
Number of cases	704	590	1294

Abbreviations: ASP, active study population (i.e., invited to screening); PSP, passive study population (i.e., not invited to screening).

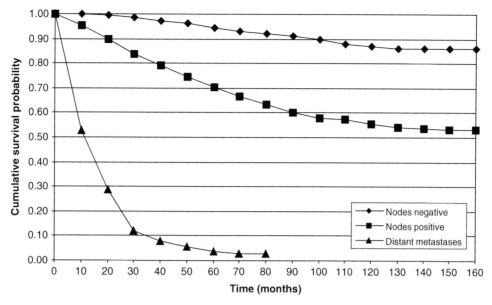

Figure 1.2 Cumulative probability of survival by nodal status.

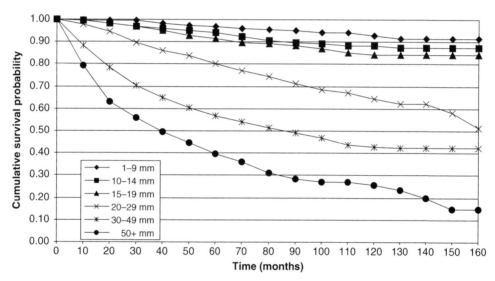

Figure 1.3 Cumulative probability of survival by size.

whose only major difference was that one was detected at an earlier stage. In the study and control groups, non-invasive (*in situ*) cancers were excluded, and also those occurring in women aged 70–74 years at entry to the trial as they were invited to only two screening rounds. Cancers that occurred before or at the prevalence round were omitted to avoid length bias in the study group. The tumor characteristics of the two groups were then compared: these are shown in Table 1.6. The distributions of grade were indeed different in the two groups indicating that grade does deteriorate as tumors grow. When grade was controlled for size however, there was no significant difference between the two groups. One could thus consider the effect of early detection on size to secondarily be influenced by grade.

Overall, it was found that size, grade, and nodal status are significantly and independently related to each other and to detection mode. All three prognostic factors are more favorable in tumors which are detected earlier, but although screen detected tumors tend to have a lower grade there are still considerable numbers of high-grade lesions (grade 3). Figures 1.2–1.5 show the survival probabilities plotted against time by nodal status, tumor size, grade, and detection status (9). It is clear that all of these factors have a considerable effect on survival.

TARGETS AND MONITORING

The NHSBSP was introduced in 1988, based on the recommendations of the Forrest report published in 1987 (24). A study conducted later showed that breast cancer–specific mortality decreased by 35% in England and Wales between 1989 and 2006 over this period, with a decrease of 40% in the 50–69 year age group (72). It has been estimated that about 6–30% of the observed reduction in breast cancer mortality is due to screening, with the remainder attributable to other factors, including improved adjuvant therapies (20,73,74).

However, despite advances in treatment, the UK breast cancer mortality rate still remains among the highest in Europe (75).

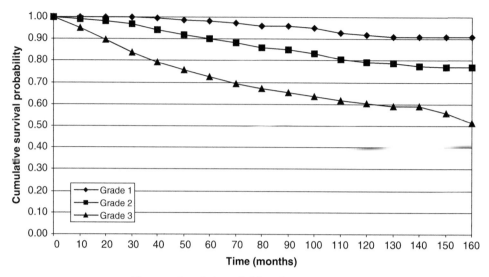

Figure 1.4 Cumulative probability of survival by grade.

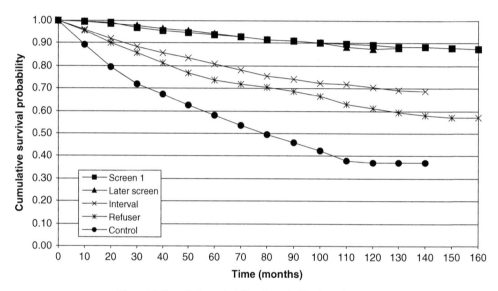

Figure 1.5 Cumulative probability of survival by detection status.

There is evidence to suggest that this is due to poor one-year survival, and that increasing awareness and early detection of breast cancers will improve mortality rates (76).

The Department of Health produced an outline of strategies aimed at improving cancer outcomes in the UK, with the aim of achieving mortality rates comparable with the best in Europe (77). The document highlights the importance of raising public awareness, and the value of screening programs in promoting earlier diagnosis of cancer. At present, approximately one-third of breast cancers are diagnosed through the NHSBSP and these cancers have a better prognosis than symptomatic tumors due principally to earlier stage at presentation (78).

The overall effectiveness of any screening program will depend directly on the proportion of the target population attending for screening and therefore compliance is another important interim measurement. Every effort must be made to ensure that the population lists used are accurate and that every woman who is invited is both alive and resident in the catchment area. Recently, efforts have been made to increase

the acceptance rate for breast screening in certain geographical areas of the UK, and for specific ethnic groups which have historically had low uptake rates for screening interventions (13).

Table 1.7 summarizes the target of attainment levels for the UK program in 2010–2011 (13) from which it can be seen that the program has met or exceeded all predefined set targets. The latter are continually updated by quality assurance committees to maintain standards of care and improve the performance of the screening program.

CONCLUSION

The NHS breast screening program has played an important role in decreasing breast cancer mortality in the UK since its inception in 1988. It is currently introducing extension which will broaden the range invited for screening. In addition, the program has incorporated screening of women at high risk for breast cancer and the annual cost of the program is estimated to be £96 million per year.

Despite its proven benefits, screening also has a downside and carries risks related to radiation exposure, overdiagnosis,

Table 1.7 Screening Quality Targets and Achievements in 2010–2011

Measure	First Screen (50–70)		Subsequent Screen (50–70)	
	Target	Achievement	Target	Achievement
Acceptance rate at first invitation (%)	≥70.0	69.7	–	82.1
Recall rate (%)	<10.0	8.3	<7.0	3.2
Benign biopsies per 1000 women screened	<3.6	1.9	<2.0	0.5
Invasive cancer detection rate per 1000 women screened	>2.7	6.0	>1.65	6.2
In situ rate per 1000 women screened	>0.4	2.0	>0.5	1.4
Invasive cancers <15 mm per 1000 women screened	>1.5	3.0	>1.7	3.3
Standardized detection ratio	≥1.0	1.47	≥1.0	1.44
Total number of women screened	–	331,222	–	1,623,593

and psychological effects. It is essential that women invited for screening are fully informed about its potential advantages and disadvantages.

There are known to be discrepancies in the uptake of screening by region and ethnic background. This is being addressed with the introduction of a public health project employing patient advocates to advise women from ethnic minorities about breast screening, and to provide community breast screening awareness sessions.

It is possible that as treatments improve in the future and mortality rates continue to fall, breast screening will have less of an impact and may ultimately not be required (20,79). Ongoing audit and research will be required to continue to demonstrate the efficacy of breast screening (see chapter 6).

REFERENCES

1. Office for National Statistics. Statistical Bulletin. Cancer registrations in England 2009. Published 20 July 2011.
2. Information and Statistics Division, NHS Scotland. Cancer Incidence in Scotland (2009). Published 30 August 2011.
3. Welsh Cancer Intelligence and Surveillance Unit. Cancer Incidence in Wales 2006–2010. 2002. Published 24 January 2012.
4. Northern Ireland Cancer Registry. Cancer Incidence and Mortality 1993–2009. [Available from: www.qub.ac.uk/research-centres/nicr/CancerData/OnlineStatistics/Breast]
5. Wilson JMG, Jungner G. Principles and Practice of Screening for Disease. Geneva: World Health Organisation, 1968; WHO Public Health Paper 34.
6. Zahl PH, Gøtzsche PC, Mæhlen J. Natural history of breast cancers detected in the Swedish mammography screening programme: a cohort study. Lancet Oncol 2011; 12: 1118–24.
7. Tubiana M, Koscielny S. Natural history of human breast cancer: recent data and clinical implications. Breast Cancer Res Treat 1991; 18: 125–40.
8. Tabar L, Fagerberg G, Chen HH, Duffy SW, Gad A. Tumour development, histology and grade of breast cancers: prognosis and progression. Int J Cancer 1996; 66: 413–19.
9. Tabar L, Fagerberg G, Day NE, Duffy SW, Kitchin RM. Breast cancer treatment and natural history: new insights from results of screening. Lancet 1992; 339: 412–14.
10. Walter SD, Day NE. Estimation of the duration of a pre-clinical disease state using screening data. Am J Epidemiol 1983; 118: 865–86.
11. Tabar L, Fagerberg G, Duffy SW, et al. Update of the Swedish two-county program of mammographic screening for breast cancer. Radiol Clin North Am 1992; 30: 187–210.
12. Shapiro S. Periodic screening for breast cancer: the HIP Randomized Controlled Trial. Health Insurance Plan. J Natl Cancer Inst Monogr 1997: 27–30.
13. NHS Breast Screening Programme Annual Review 2011: 2010–2011 breast screening statistics.
14. National Cancer Intelligence Network. Second All Breast Cancer Report 2007. Published June 2011.
15. Breast Screening Frequency Trial Group. The frequency of breast cancer screening: results from the UKCCCR Randomised Trial. Eur J Cancer 2002; 38: 1458–64.
16. Young KC, Burch A, Oduko JM. Radiation doses received in the UK Breast Screening Programme in 2001 and 2002. Br J Radiol 2005; 78: 207–18.
17. Hendrick RE, Pisano ED, Averbukh A, et al. Comparison of acquisition parameters and breast dose in digital mammography and screen-film mammography in the American College of Radiology Imaging Network digital mammographic imaging screening trial. Am J Roentgenol 2010; 194: 362–9.
18. Berrington de González A. Estimates of the potential risk of radiation-related cancer from screening in the UK. J Med Screen 2011; 18: 163–4.
19. Yaffe MJ, Mainprize JG. Risk of radiation-induced breast cancer from mammographic screening. Radiology 2011; 258: 98–105.
20. Screening for Breast Cancer in England: Past and Future. Advisory Committee on Breast Cancer Screening. NHSBSP Publication No 61, 2006.
21. Brett J, Bankhead C, Henderson B, Watson E, Austoker J. The psychological impact of mammographic screening. A systematic review. Psychooncology 2005; 14: 917–38.
22. Brewer NT, Salz T, Lillie SE. Systematic review: the long-term effects of false-positive mammograms. Ann Intern Med 2007; 146: 502–10.
23. Duffy SW, Tabar L, Olsen AH, et al. Absolute numbers of lives saved and overdiagnosis in breast cancer screening, from a randomized trial and from the Breast Screening Programme in England. J Med Screen 2010; 17: 25–30.
24. Forrest APM. Breast Cancer Screening. Report to the Health Ministers of England, Wales, Scotland and Northern Ireland by a working group chaired by Sir Patrick Forrest London: HMSO, 1987.
25. Tabar L, Vitak B, Chen HH, et al. The Swedish Two-County Trial twenty years later. Updated mortality results and new insights from long-term follow-up. Radiol Clin North Am 2000; 38: 625–51.
26. Warren RML, Duffy SW, Bashir S. The value of the second view in screening mammography. Br J Radiol 1996; 69: 105–8.
27. Pisano ED, Gatsonis C, Hendrick E, et al. Digital Mammographic Imaging Screening Trial (DMIST) Investigators Group. Diagnostic performance of digital versus film mammography for breast-cancer screening. N Engl J Med 2005; 353: 1773–83.
28. Alexander F, Anderson TJ, Brown HK, et al. The Edinburgh randomised trial of breast cancer screening: results after 10 years of follow-up. Br J Cancer 1994; 70: 542–8.
29. Miller AB, To T, Baines CJ, Wall C. Canadian National Breast Screening Study-2: 13-year results of a randomized trial in women aged 50–59 years. J Natl Cancer Inst 2000; 92: 1490–9.
30. Pisani P, Parkin DM, Ngelangel C, et al. Outcome of screening by clinical examination of the breast in a trial in the Philippines. Int J Cancer 2006; 118: 149–54.
31. US Preventive Services Task Force. Screening for breast cancer: U.S. Preventive Services Task Force recommendation statement. Ann Intern Med 2009; 151: 716–26.
32. Shen Y, Zelen M. Screening sensitivity and sojourn time from breast cancer early detection clinical trials: mammograms and physical examinations. J Clin Oncol 2001; 19: 3490–9.
33. Semiglazov VF, Manikhas AG, Moiseenko VM, et al. Results of a prospective randomized investigation [Russia (St.Petersburg)/WHO) to evaluate the significance of self-examination for the early detection of breast cancer. Vopr Onkol 2003; 49: 434–41.

34. Thomas DB, Gao DL, Ray RM, et al. Randomized trial of breast self-examination: final results. J Natl Cancer Inst 2002; 94: 1445–57.

35. Kösters JP, Gøtzsche PC. Regular self-examination or clinical examination for early detection of breast cancer. Cochrane Database Syst Rev 2003: CD003373.

36. Orel SG. MR imaging of the breast. Radiol Clin North Am 2000; 38: 899–913.

37. Griebsch I, Brown J, Boggis C, et al. Cost effectiveness of screening with contrast enhanced magnetic resonance imaging vs X-ray mammography of women at a high familial risk of breast cancer. Br J Cancer 2006; 95: 801–10.

38. Leach MO, Boggis CR, Dixon AK, et al. MARIBS Study Group. Screening with magnetic resonance imaging and mammography of a UK population at high familial risk of breast cancer: a prospective multicentre cohort study (MARIBS). Lancet 2005; 365: 1769–78.

39. Kriege M, Brekelmans CT, Obdeijn IM, et al. Factors affecting sensitivity and specificity of screening mammography and MRI in women with an inherited risk for breast cancer. Breast Cancer Res Treat 2006; 100: 109–19.

40. Sardanelli F, Podo F, Santoro F, et al. High Breast Cancer Risk Italian 1 (HIBCRIT-1) Study. Multicenter surveillance of women at high genetic breast cancer risk using mammography, ultrasonography, and contrast-enhanced magnetic resonance imaging (the high breast cancer risk italian 1 study): final results. Invest Radiol 2011; 46: 94–105.

41. NHS National Institute for Health and Clinical Excellence (NICE) Clinical Guideline 41: Familial Breast Cancer. October 2006.

42. Technical Guidelines for Magnetic Resonance Imaging for the Surveillance of Women at Increased Risk of Developing Breast Cancer. NHS Cancer Screening Programmes, March 2012 (NHSBSP Publication No 68).

43. Tabár L, Vitak B, Chen TH, et al. Swedish two-county trial: impact of mammographic screening on breast cancer mortality during 3 decades. Radiology 2011; 260: 658–63.

44. Andersson I, Aspegren K, Janzon L, et al. Mammographic screening and mortality from breast cancer: the Malmö mammographic screening trial. BMJ 1988; 297: 943–8.

45. Alexander FE, Anderson TJ, Brown HK, et al. 14 years of follow-up from the Edinburgh randomised trial of breast-cancer screening. Lancet 1999; 353: 1903–8.

46. Frisell J, Lidbrink E, Hellström L, Rutqvist LE. Followup after 11 years–update of mortality results in the Stockholm mammographic screening trial. Breast Cancer Res Treat 1997; 45: 263–70.

47. Miller AB, Baines CJ, To T, Wall C. Canadian National Breast Screening Study: 1. Breast cancer detection and death rates among women aged 40 to 49 years. CMAJ 1992; 147: 1459–76.

48. Miller AB, Baines CJ, To T, Wall C. Canadian National Breast Screening Study: 2. Breast cancer detection and death rates among women aged 50 to 59 years. CMAJ 1992; 147: 1477–88.

49. Baines CJ, Miller AB, Kopans DB, et al. Canadian National Breast Screening Study: assessment of technical quality by external review. AJR Am J Roentgenol 1990; 155: 743–7.

50. Bailar JC 3rd, MacMahon B. Randomization in the Canadian National Breast Screening Study: a review for evidence of subversion. CMAJ 1997; 156: 193–9.

51. Goel V, Cohen MM, Kaufert P, MacWilliam L. Assessing the extent of contamination in the Canadian National Breast Screening Study. Am J Prev Med 1998; 15: 206–11.

52. Bjurstam N, Björneld L, Warwick J, et al. The gothenburg breast screening trial. Cancer 2003; 97: 2387–96.

53. Moss SM, Cuckle H, Evans A, et al. for the Trial Management Group. Effect of mammographic screening from age 40 years on breast cancer mortality at 10 years' follow-up: a randomised controlled trial. Lancet 2006; 368: 2053–60.

54. Johns LE, Moss SM; Trial Management Group. Randomized controlled trial of mammographic screening from age 40 ('Age' trial): patterns of screening attendance. J Med Screen 2010; 17: 37–43.

55. Kingston N, Thomas I, Johns L, Moss S; Trial Management Group. Assessing the amount of unscheduled screening ("contamination") in the control arm of the UK "Age" Trial. Cancer Epidemiol Biomarkers Prev 2010; 19: 1132–6.

56. Tabar L, Fagerberg G, Chen HH, et al. Efficacy of breast cancer screening by age. New results from the Swedish Two-County Trial. Cancer 1995; 75: 2507–17.

57. Nyström L, Andersson I, Bjurstam N, et al. Long-term effects of mammography screening: updated overview of the Swedish randomised trials. Lancet 2002; 359: 909–19.

58. Harris KM, Vogel VG. Breast cancer screening. Cancer Metastasis Rev 1997; 16: 231–62.

59. Johns LE, Moss SM; Age Trial Management Group. False-positive results in the randomized controlled trial of mammographic screening from age 40 ("Age" trial). Cancer Epidemiol Biomarkers Prev 2010; 19: 2758–64.

60. Larsson LG, Andersson I, Bjurstam N, et al. Updated overview of the Swedish Randomized Trials on Breast Cancer Screening with Mammography: age group 40–49 at randomization. J Natl Cancer Inst Monogr 1997: 57–61.

61. Nelson HD, Tyne K, Naik A, et al. U.S. Preventive Services Task Force. Screening for breast cancer: an update for the U.S. Preventive Services Task Force. Ann Intern Med 2009; 151: 727–37, W237–42.

62. Hellquist BN, Duffy SW, Abdsaleh S, et al. Effectiveness of population-based service screening with mammography for women ages 40 to 49 years: evaluation of the Swedish Mammography Screening in Young Women (SCRY) cohort. Cancer 2011; 117: 714–22.

63. Fisher B, Costantino JP, Wickerham DL, et al. Tamoxifen for the prevention of breast cancer: current status of the National Surgical Adjuvant Breast and Bowel Project P-1 study. J Natl Cancer Inst 2005; 97: 1652–62.

64. Veronesi U, Maisonneuve P, Rotmensz N, et al. Italian Tamoxifen Study Group. Tamoxifen for the prevention of breast cancer: late results of the Italian Randomized Tamoxifen Prevention Trial among women with hysterectomy. J Natl Cancer Inst 2007; 99: 727–37.

65. Powles TJ, Ashley S, Tidy A, Smith IE, Dowsett M. Twenty-year follow-up of the Royal Marsden randomized, double-blinded tamoxifen breast cancer prevention trial. J Natl Cancer Inst 2007; 99: 283–90.

66. Vogel VG, Costantino JP, Wickerham DL, et al. Effects of tamoxifen vs raloxifene on the risk of developing invasive breast cancer and other disease outcomes: the NSABP Study of Tamoxifen and Raloxifene (STAR) P-2 trial. JAMA 2006; 295: 2727–41.

67. Goss PE, Ingle JN, Ales-Martinez JE, et al. Exemestane for breast-cancer prevention in postmenopausal women. N Engl J Med 2011; 364: 2381–91.

68. Fisher B, Redmond C, Fisher ER. The contribution of recent NSABP clinical trials of primary breast cancer therapy to an understanding of tumor biology–an overview of findings. Cancer 1980; 46: 1009–25.

69. Connor RJ, Chu KC, Smart CR. Stage-shift cancer screening model. J Clin Epidemiol 1989; 42: 1083–95.

70. Ahmed MI, Lennard TW. Breast cancer: role of neoadjuvant therapy. Int J Surg 2009; 7: 416–20.

71. Fisher B, Anderson S, Fisher ER, et al. Significance of ipsilateral breast tumour recurrence after lumpectomy. Lancet 1991; 338: 327–31.

72. Autier P, Boniol M, La Vecchia C, et al. Disparities in breast cancer mortality trends between 30 European countries: retrospective trend analysis of WHO mortality database. BMJ 2010; 341: c3620.

73. Patnick J. Breast and cervical screening for women in the United Kingdom. Hong Kong Med J 2000; 6: 409–11.

74. Blanks RG, Moss SM, McGahan CE, Quinn MJ, Babb PJ. Effect of NHS breast screening programme on mortality from breast cancer in England and Wales, 1990–8: comparison of observed with predicted mortality. BMJ 2000; 321: 665–9.

75. Sant M, Allemani C, Santaquilani M, et al. EUROCARE Working Group. EUROCARE-4. Survival of cancer patients diagnosed in 1995–1999. Results and commentary. Eur J Cancer 2009; 45: 931–91.

76. Thomson CS, Forman D. Cancer survival in England and the influence of early diagnosis: what can we learn from recent EUROCARE results? Br J Cancer 2009; 101: S102–9.

77. Improving outcomes: a strategy for cancer. Department of Health publication, January 2011.

78. Nagtegaal ID, Allgood PC, Duffy SW, et al. Prognosis and pathology of screen-detected carcinomas: how different are they? Cancer 2011; 117: 1360–8.

79. Jatoi I. The impact of advances in treatment on the efficacy of mammography screening. Prev Med 2011; 53: 103–4.

2 Mammographic density as an early indicator of breast cancer

Jajini Susan Varghese

INTRODUCTION

The mammogram depicts the constituent tissues of the normal breast and is taken to show various features of pathology. This technique is now widely used in the early diagnosis of breast cancer through population screening. The appearance of normal breast parenchyma on a mammogram varies among women as it depends on the relative proportions of fibroglandular dense tissue that appears light on a mammogram ("dense area") and fat tissue that appears dark ("non-dense area"). Mammographic density is most popularly expressed as "percent density" which is the area of dense tissue divided by the total breast area and multiplied by one hundred.

Since the 1970s and the early observations made by Wolfe, there has been considerable interest in why some women have greater proportions of dense tissue than others. He described four categories for separating women with differing amounts of dense tissue and proposed a relationship between the densest mammographic pattern and breast cancer risk (1). Figure 2.1 shows a group of four right breast mammograms that illustrate the Wolfe grades. Even though this was extensively debated in the literature for two decades, greater credence has been given to this hypothesis in the past few years. It is now widely recognized that the densest mammographic patterns express a four- to six-fold increased risk of breast cancer when compared with the least dense ones.

RELATIONSHIP BETWEEN MAMMOGRAPHIC DENSITY AND BREAST CANCER RISK

Mammographic density has been shown to be one of the most powerful independent predictors of breast cancer with over 50 studies published in the past three decades which report a strong dose–response relationship between mammographic density and breast cancer. This is regardless of the classification methods used and the type of study, be it an incidence or prevalence study (2). Women in whom more than 75% of the breast appears dense have a 4.64 fold (95% CI 3.64–5.91) increased risk of breast cancer compared with women in the least dense category (<5%) (3). This increase in risk is seen both before and after menopause. Moreover, the densest pattern is also found to be associated with high-grade tumors and ductal carcinoma *in situ* (4). Large tumors are independently associated with the densest pattern and this is found to be due to a combination of impaired sensitivity and the association with higher grades of tumor (5).

BIOLOGICAL BASIS FOR THE ASSOCIATION BETWEEN BREAST DENSITY AND BREAST CANCER

The mechanisms through which mammographic density affects breast cancer risk are not well understood. Li et al. studied randomly selected breast tissue blocks obtained through forensic autopsy and found that increased mammographic density is associated with a higher proportional area occupied by nuclei, both epithelial and non-epithelial; collagen; and glandular tissue (6).

Breast cancers originate in epithelial cells, so increased amounts of fibroglandular tissue may reflect a greater number of cells that are at risk of carcinogenesis and/or an increased rate of epithelial proliferation (7). In line with this reasoning, some have suggested that the total area of dense breast tissue is a measure of cumulative exposure to mitogens such as estrogens and other hormones, or growth factors that are known to have a proliferative effect on breast tissue (8). This supports the hypothesis that many of the established breast cancer risk factors may influence risk through their effect on density (9).

Although the number of epithelial and duct lobular units has been observed to increase with percent density, increase in the fibrous component is proportionately greater (11-fold increase) and may therefore contribute more to variations in percent density (6,10). The exact role of fibrous elements in carcinogenesis remains unclear but it has been suggested that the stromal tissue may provide a supportive microenvironment for the development of cancer (11,12).

MEASURES OF MAMMOGRAPHIC DENSITY

These lines of evidence collectively suggest that the relationship between percent density and breast cancer may be more closely related to the absolute volume of dense tissue in the breasts. Although percent density is the most commonly used measure to quantify mammographic density, to make relevant etiological inferences, the association it has with absolute dense area and the non-dense area is also important (13,14). As percent density is a ratio of the absolute dense area and total breast area (which includes the non-dense area) an increase in percent density could reflect an increase in the absolute dense area or a decrease in the non-dense area of the breasts, or both. Moreover, a given area of dense tissue in a small breast would represent a higher percent density value compared with the same area of dense tissue within a larger breast.

Measuring the area occupied by dense tissue in a three-dimensional organ is far from ideal. A report from the United Kingdom (UK) MARIBS study showed that MRI percent density volume was reasonably correlated with percent density when measured as a proportion (r = 0.76) (15). MRI dense tissue volume was also correlated with the absolute dense area (r = 0.61). It is anticipated that with the development of new automated measurements based on estimation of the volume of dense tissue, the accuracy of breast cancer risk prediction

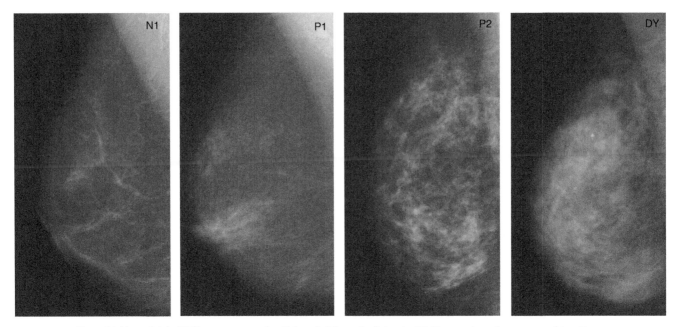

Figure 2.1 Normal right MLO mammograms (mediolateral oblique view) showing Wolfe parenchymal mammographic patterns.

could be increased. At present, due to dual considerations of cost and ease of measurement, area measurement based on mammography remains the most prevalent technique used for the characterization of mammographic density.

ASSOCIATION BETWEEN MAMMOGRAPHIC DENSITY AND KNOWN RISK FACTORS FOR BREAST CANCER
Mammographic Density and Age
Percent density decreases with increasing age, and after adjusting for rising body mass index (BMI) and menopause (both decrease percent density) an annual within-woman rate of decline of 1.4% (95% CI 1.2–1.6) at age 50 has been reported (16). This decrease in percent density is partly as a result of a decrease in dense tissue [annual decrease of 1.6 cm^2 (95% CI 1.2–1.9)] but, more importantly is a consequence of an increase in the non-dense area which has been observed to increase at twice the rate [after controlling for BMI (annual increase of 3.4 cm^2; 95% CI 2.7–4.1)]. The age at which percent density ceased to decline was around 65 years of age (16).

This pattern contrasts with an increasing breast cancer risk with age. This opposing trend may be explained by the observation that changes in percent density with age parallel changes in the rate of "breast tissue aging" proposed by Pike (17–19). The process of "breast tissue aging" is thought to be related to effects of hormones on the kinetics of breast epithelial cells and the accumulation of genetic damage. Rate of aging and percent density, both have been noted to be highest between menarche and first birth, fall slightly after pregnancy, and are lowest after the menopause perhaps suggesting that influences in the early stages of breast development may be more relevant in the development of breast cancer.

Mammographic Density and BMI
Percent density shows an inverse relationship with BMI with a unit increase in BMI estimated to be associated with approximately 2% decrease in percent density. Although any association between BMI and the absolute dense area has been inconclusive, a link between BMI and the non-dense area of the breast has been consistently affirmative in all studies examining this association. This is perhaps not surprising, since with increasing levels of obesity, the breast becomes infiltrated with fat, in common with other organs. BMI is thus a negative confounder which must be adjusted for when assessing effects on percent density (20).

The inverse association between BMI and percent density parallels the protective effect on breast cancer among premenopausal women. However, among postmenopausal women, higher BMI is associated with an increase in breast cancer risk (thought to be related to changes in estrogen levels) whereas it decreases percent density. Although BMI is correlated with both mammographic density and breast cancer risk, evidence suggests that this risk is not mediated through changes in percent density. Boyd et al. have conducted a nested case–control study, which suggests that percent density does not mediate any association between BMI and breast cancer risk as adjustment for percent density strengthens the association between these two factors (20).

Mammographic Density and Reproductive Factors
Evidence that breast tissue is hormonally responsive is supported by consistent associations linking age, menopause, BMI (through increased local estrogen conversion in fatty tissue), and hormone replacement therapy (HRT) induced changes. Among women of a similar age, those who are postmenopausal have lower percent density and a lower risk of breast cancer compared with premenopausal women. In a study, the onset of menopause was associated with a 2.4% (95% CI −1.4 to −3.4) fall in percent density, which can be attributed both to a decline in absolute dense area of 3.3 cm^2 (95% CI −4.8 to −1.8) together with an increase in the non-dense area of 4.2 cm^2 (95% CI 0.9–7.4) (16). There is also

some evidence to suggest that changes in mammographic density associated with menopause may be more pronounced in women with a clearly defined predisposition to breast cancer (21).

Nulliparous women have long been recognized to be at a higher risk for breast cancer than parous women and generally have denser breasts. A study by Boyd et al. revealed that an average 2% decrease in percent density was observed with each pregnancy (7). Among parous women, later age at first full-term pregnancy is also associated with higher density and a greater risk of breast cancer (22,23).

INTERVENTIONS THAT CHANGE MAMMOGRAPHIC DENSITY

Hormone Replacement Therapy

Mammographic density is modulated by interventions that affect breast cancer risk. Thus anti-estrogen therapies reduce both breast cancer risk (22,24–27) and mammographic density (26), whereas estrogen–progestin replacement therapy increases breast cancer risk (28) and density (29,30). Observational studies suggest that use of combination (estrogen and progestin) HRT may have a greater impact on percent density than estrogen alone. Greendale et al. reported that administration of estrogen alone for a two-year period only resulted in a nonsignificant increase in percent density, whereas a larger statistically significant increase in percent density (approximately 3–5%) was seen with combination therapy (29). Similar results were reported from the Women's Health Initiative study. Interestingly, compared with never-users of HRT, those women who used HRT before the menopause were twice as likely to have a higher percent density (OR = 2.53, 95% CI 1.31–4.87) (31).

Although combination HRT increases both percent density and breast cancer risk, there is no clear evidence indicating that any increased risk is mediated through changes in density. In a nested case–control study conducted by Boyd and colleagues (9), current users of HRT were found to have an increased risk of breast cancer (OR 1.26, 95% CI 1.0–1.6) which showed little change on adjustment for percent density (OR 1.19, 95% CI 0.9–1.5). These findings suggest that the pathway through which exogenous hormones influence breast cancer risk may be independent of percent density (17).

Tamoxifen

Interventional studies have shown that administration of tamoxifen (selective estrogen receptor modulator) substantially reduces percent density (24,26,32). The International Breast Intervention Study reported a decrease of 13.7% in percent density compared with a 7.3% decrease observed in the placebo arm over a period of 4.5 years (24). This decrease in percent density was significantly associated with reduced breast cancer risk (26).

GENETIC BASIS OF MAMMOGRAPHIC DENSITY

A small twin study first showed how the degree of similarity in mammographic parenchymal patterns was greater for monozygotic than dizygotic twins (33). Further compelling evidence for a genetic susceptibility to mammographic density came from a study of 571 pairs of monozygotic and 380 pairs of dizygotic twins recruited from the Australian Twin Registry and North American Twin Registry (34). Based on the assumptions of a classical twin model and after adjustments for age, BMI, and other measured covariates, the patterns of familial correlation were consistent with additive genetic effects and accounted for 60–70% of the variance in mammographic density measures. The high heritability estimates for mammographic density and its strong association with breast cancer risk (which cannot be explained by common lifestyle risk factors) led to the hypothesis that a component of the association between mammographic density and breast cancer risk might be explained by a shared genetic basis. This was supported by the observation from a combined genome-wide association study of mammographic density, that the single nucleotide polymorphism (SNP) rs10995190 in intron 4 of *ZNF365*, a known breast cancer SNP, is also associated with mammographic density, in the same direction as the corresponding breast cancer risk (35). Moreover, after adjustment for mammographic density, this breast cancer association was attenuated, suggesting that the change in level of risk was indeed mediated through change in density.

To further test the hypothesis that genetic factors might contribute to the association between mammographic density and breast cancer, a recent case–control study involved calculation of genetic risk scores for individuals based on the number of percent density SNPs each individual was carrying and its effect size (36). These scores were found to be predictive of an individual's breast cancer status indicating that partial overlap exists between the set of genetic variants involved in breast density and those involved in breast cancer risk. Hence, the well-established correlation between these two traits appears genuine and not a consequence of confounding factors.

MAMMOGRAPHIC DENSITY AS AN EPIDEMIOLOGICAL TOOL

It is being increasingly recognized that mammographic density is a biomarker of risk and can provide useful surrogate information prior to development of cancer in an individual woman. More exhaustive studies should be able to identify further loci which might be involved in the regulation of breast density. Identification of genetic factors, even those which contribute minimal effects, can suggest new underlying causal mechanisms, which in turn may inform the development of cancer prevention strategies for the general population. In the future it is possible that a set of SNPs strongly associated with breast density could also be used in conjunction with other breast cancer risk factors to stratify younger women who may benefit from early screening.

As higher degrees of mammographic density are relatively common in the general population, this factor could account for a substantial proportion of breast cancer cases (2). Moreover, mammographic density is potentially modifiable. The possibility of bringing about a downward shift in global breast density distribution remains an exciting possibility and could theoretically lead to a reduction of overall breast cancer rates. Improved methods for automated measurement need to be developed in the future for estimation of this particular biomarker of risk.

ACKNOWLEDGMENTS
I thank Dr Ruth Warren for her contribution toward the preparation of this manuscript.

REFERENCES
1. Wolfe JN. Breast patterns as an index of risk for developing breast cancer. AJR Am J Roentgenol 1976; 126: 1130–7.
2. McCormack VA, dos Santos Silva I. Breast density and parenchymal patterns as markers of breast cancer risk: a meta-analysis. Cancer Epidemiol Biomarkers Prev 2006; 15: 1159–69.
3. Vachon CM, van Gils CH, Sellers TA, et al. Mammographic density, breast cancer risk and risk prediction. Breast Cancer Res 2007; 9: 217.
4. Sala E, Solomon L, Warren R, et al. Size, node status and grade of breast tumours: association with mammographic parenchymal patterns. Eur Radiol 2000; 10: 157–61.
5. Sala E, Warren R, McCann J, et al. Mammographic parenchymal patterns and breast cancer natural history–a case-control study. Acta Oncol 2001; 40: 461–5.
6. Li T, Sun L, Miller N, et al. The association of measured breast tissue characteristics with mammographic density and other risk factors for breast cancer. Cancer Epidemiol Biomarkers Prev 2005; 14: 343–9.
7. Martin LJ, Boyd NF. Mammographic density. Potential mechanisms of breast cancer risk associated with mammographic density: hypotheses based on epidemiological evidence. Breast Cancer Res 2008; 10: 201.
8. Kerlikowske K, Shepherd J, Creasman J, et al. Are breast density and bone mineral density independent risk factors for breast cancer? J Natl Cancer Inst 2005; 97: 368–74.
9. Boyd NF, Martin LJ, Li Q, et al. Mammographic density as a surrogate marker for the effects of hormone therapy on risk of breast cancer. Cancer Epidemiol Biomarkers Prev 2006; 15: 961–6.
10. Gertig DM, Stillman IE, Byrne C, et al. Association of age and reproductive factors with benign breast tissue composition. Cancer Epidemiol Biomarkers Prev 1999; 8: 873–9.
11. Bhowmick NA, Neilson EG, Moses HL. Stromal fibroblasts in cancer initiation and progression. Nature 2004; 432: 332–7.
12. Bissell MJ, Weaver VM, Lelievre SA, et al. Tissue structure, nuclear organization, and gene expression in normal and malignant breast. Cancer Res 1999; 59: 1757–1763s.
13. Haars G, van Noord PA, van Gils CH, Grobbee DE, Peeters PH. Measurements of breast density: no ratio for a ratio. Cancer Epidemiol Biomarkers Prev 2005; 14: 2634–40.
14. Stone J, Ding J, Warren RM, Duffy SW, Hopper JL. Using mammographic density to predict breast cancer risk: dense area or percentage dense area. Breast Cancer Res 2010; 12: R97.
15. Thompson DJ, Leach MO, Kwan-Lim G, et al. Assessing the usefulness of a novel MRI-based breast density estimation algorithm in a cohort of women at high genetic risk of breast cancer: the UK MARIBS study. Breast Cancer Res 2009; 11: R80.
16. McCormack VA, Perry NM, Vinnicombe SJ, dos SS, I. Changes and tracking of mammographic density in relation to Pike's model of breast tissue aging: a UK longitudinal study. Int J Cancer 2010; 127: 452–61.
17. Martin LJ, Minkin S, Boyd NF. Hormone therapy, mammographic density, and breast cancer risk. Maturitas 2009; 64: 20–6.
18. Pike MC, Krailo MD, Henderson BE, Casagrande JT, Hoel DG. 'Hormonal' risk factors, 'breast tissue age' and the age-incidence of breast cancer. Nature 1983; 303: 767–70.
19. Pike MC, Pearce CL, Wu AH. Prevention of cancers of the breast, endometrium and ovary. Oncogene 2004; 23: 6379–91.
20. Boyd NF, Martin LJ, Sun L, et al. Body size, mammographic density, and breast cancer risk. Cancer Epidemiol Biomarkers Prev 2006; 15: 2086–92.
21. Boyd NF, Melnichouk O, Martin LJ, et al. Mammographic density, response to hormones, and breast cancer risk. J Clin Oncol 2011; 29: 2985–92.
22. Maskarinec G, Pagano I, Lurie G, Kolonel LN. A longitudinal investigation of mammographic density: the multiethnic cohort. Cancer Epidemiol Biomarkers Prev 2006; 15: 732–9.
23. Vachon CM, Kuni CC, Anderson K, Anderson VE, Sellers TA. Association of mammographically defined percent breast density with epidemiologic risk factors for breast cancer (United States). Cancer Causes Control 2000; 11: 653–62.
24. Cuzick J, Warwick J, Pinney E, Warren RM, Duffy SW. Tamoxifen and breast density in women at increased risk of breast cancer. J Natl Cancer Inst 2004; 96: 621–8.
25. Cuzick J, Sestak I, Baum M, et al. Effect of anastrozole and tamoxifen as adjuvant treatment for early-stage breast cancer: 10-year analysis of the ATAC trial. Lancet Oncol 2010; 11: 1135–41.
26. Cuzick J, Warwick J, Pinney E, et al. Tamoxifen-induced reduction in mammographic density and breast cancer risk reduction: a nested case-control study. J Natl Cancer Inst 2011; 103: 744–52.
27. Fisher B, Powles TJ, Pritchard KJ. Tamoxifen for the prevention of breast cancer. Eur J Cancer 2000; 36: 142–50.
28. Beral V. Breast cancer and hormone-replacement therapy in the Million Women Study. Lancet 2003; 362: 419–27.
29. Greendale GA, Reboussin BA, Slone S, et al. Postmenopausal hormone therapy and change in mammographic density. J Natl Cancer Inst 2003; 95: 30–7.
30. Vachon CM, Sellers TA, Vierkant RA, Wu FF, Brandt KR. Case-control study of increased mammographic breast density response to hormone replacement therapy. Cancer Epidemiol Biomarkers Prev 2002; 11: 1382–8.
31. Sala E, Warren R, McCann J, et al. High-risk mammographic parenchymal patterns, hormone replacement therapy and other risk factors: a case-control study. Int J Epidemiol 2000; 29: 629–36.
32. Brisson J, Brisson B, Cote G, et al. Tamoxifen and mammographic breast densities. Cancer Epidemiol Biomarkers Prev 2000; 9: 911–15.
33. Kaprio J, Alanko A, Kivisaari L, Standertskjold-Nordenstam CG. Mammographic patterns in twin pairs discordant for breast cancer. Br J Radiol 1987; 60: 459–62.
34. Boyd NF, Dite GS, Stone J, et al. Heritability of mammographic density, a risk factor for breast cancer. N Engl J Med 2002; 347: 886–94.
35. Lindstrom S, Vachon CM, Li J, et al. Common variants in ZNF365 are associated with both mammographic density and breast cancer risk. Nat Genet 2011; 43: 185–7.
36. Varghese JS, Thompson DJ, Michailidou K, et al. Mammographic breast density and breast cancer: evidence of a shared genetic basis. Cancer Res 2012; 72: 1478–84.

3 Genetic predisposition and breast screening

D. Gareth Evans

INTRODUCTION

Breast cancer is the commonest malignancy affecting women of whom one in eight will develop the disease in their lifetime. The annual incidence of breast cancer in England and Wales is 48,000 and 12,000 die each year of this disease (1). According to official statistics the United Kingdom (UK) has a relatively poor record on survival from breast cancer compared with Continental Europe and the United States (US). Nonetheless there has been a 40% reduction in mortality within the UK since the mid-1980s though smaller improvements in survival have been documented in other parts of the world over the past 30 years. The fall in mortality from breast cancer within the UK can be attributed to the combined impact of breast cancer screening (and earlier detection of the disease) and the introduction of adjuvant systemic therapies including both chemotherapy and hormonal treatments. In particular the pioneering work with tamoxifen and the early clinical enthusiasm for this drug may account for the improved mortality figures in the UK (which may become evident in other countries at a future stage).

Prognosis of breast cancer is determined by a combination of tumor size, grade, and axillary lymph node status; small tumors (<1 cm) and a favorable histology (grade I, special types) with no lymph node involvement are associated with a five-year survival in excess of 90%.

Racial and cultural factors appear to influence breast cancer predisposition. Incidence of the disease is relatively low in Chinese and other Asian groups for whom family history may be more significant.

RISK FACTORS
Family History

Family history can be a highly significant factor in predisposition to breast cancer with about 4–5% of cases being attributed to inheritance of high-risk autosomal dominant genes (2,3). Hereditary factors are likely to have a role in the remaining sporadic cases, but their contribution is still difficult to determine on an individual basis. Cowden's disease in which individuals have substantial macrocephaly and cutaneous features is almost unique in having a phenotypic expression of an underlying genetic abnormality which gives rise to an external marker of risk (4). In order to assess the likelihood of there being a predisposing gene in a family it is necessary to analyze the cancer pedigree with construction of a family tree. Inheritance of a germ-line mutation or deletion of a predisposing gene leads to the development of the disease at a relatively young age and often subsequent occurrence of cancer in the contralateral breast. Some gene mutations may confer susceptibility to other cancers such as ovary, prostate, pancreas, or sarcomas (5–8). Multiple primary cancers in a single individual or related early-onset cancers in a pedigree are suggestive of a predisposing gene. To illustrate the importance of age, it is estimated that over 25% of breast cancers occurring below 30 years of age are due to a mutation in a dominant gene compared with 1% for cases above 70 years of age (3). The important features in a family tree are therefore as follows:

1. Age at onset
2. Bilateral disease
3. Multiple cases in a family (particularly on one side predominantly)
4. Other related early-onset tumors
5. Number of unaffected individuals (large families are more informative)

There are few families for whom a dominant pattern of inheritance can be confidently predicted. In such families it can be assumed that unaffected relatives have a 50% chance of inheriting the faulty gene as all genes come in pairs. For example when four first-degree relatives (FDRs) with early-onset or bilateral breast cancer exist within a single blood line of a family, the daughter or sister of an affected case will have a 50% risk of inheriting the high risk predisposition. Epidemiological studies have shown that about 50–85% of individuals with mutations in predisposing genes develop breast cancer in their lifetime. Therefore, unless there is a strong family history involving both maternal and paternal relatives the maximum risk counseled is 40–45%. Breast cancer genes can be inherited through the paternal line and a dominant history on the father's side of the family will give at least a 20–25% lifetime risk to the daughters.

Other Risk Factors (Table 3.1)

Nongenetic or environmental risk factors relate principally to the hormonal environment of breast tissue. A woman will derive maximal benefit from never ovulating—breast cancer is very uncommon in Turner's (XO) syndrome. A relatively high degree of protection is afforded by minimizing the period of ovulation prior to a woman's first pregnancy and therefore late menarche combined with an early first full-term pregnancy reduces the subsequent risk of breast cancer. Exposure of relatively immature breast tissue to estrogen (especially unopposed) increases risk, whereas progesterone associated with pregnancy is protective and may induce terminal differentiation in pluripotential stem cells. Pregnancy transforms breast parenchymal cells into a more stable state where proliferation

Table 3.1 Factors Associated with an Increased Risk
of Breast Cancer

Family history
Early menarche (<12 years)
Late first pregnancy (after 28 years)
Current use of an OCP and for 10 years after
Nulliparity
Late menopause
Prolonged use of HRT
Significant weight gain in adult life
Indolent lifestyle
Proliferative breast disease on biopsy (not benign disease such as a
　fibroadenoma)
Increased mammographic density

Abbreviations: HRT, hormone replacement therapy; OCP, oral contraceptive
pill.

in the second half of the cycle is less. There is now convincing evidence that current use of the oral contraceptive pill is associated with a 20% increase in risk and this persists for 10 years post use (9). Though the estrogen component of the oral contraceptive pill suppresses ovulation, proliferation of breast cancer cells is stimulated. The continued rise in the incidence of breast cancer may be a consequence of greater numbers of women delaying their first full-term pregnancy combined with a more prolonged use of the oral contraceptive pill. This trend is most apparent in the well-educated professional classes who may already possess an elevated background risk for breast cancer. Early menopause is protective and reduces cumulative estrogen exposure. Other factors such as the number of pregnancies and breastfeeding may have a small protective effect. There is some controversy over the use of hormone replacement therapy (HRT), particularly in breast cancer patients. Prolonged use of HRT for more than 10 years after the menopause is associated with a significant increase in risk. However, shorter treatment duration may still confer an increased risk on individuals with a family history of breast cancer (10).

Dietary factors have some role in determining breast cancer risk with epidemiological studies confirming that diets low in animal fats from dairy produce and red meat are associated with marginal risk reductions. Previous breast biopsies revealing proliferative changes such as atypical hyperplasia (lobular or ductal) increase breast cancer risk significantly and these histopathological changes may be a manifestation of alterations at the genetic level in gene mutation carriers (11,12).

RISK ESTIMATION

In the absence of a dominant family history risk estimation is based on large epidemiological studies which have revealed a 1.5 to 3.0-fold elevated risk for individuals with a single affected relative (2,3). It is important to distinguish between lifetime and age-specific risks. For example some studies quote an increased risk of nine fold or greater for an FDR with bilateral disease or a personal history of proliferative breast disease. However in the latter case, risk decreases with increasing time since diagnosis and with a prolonged follow-up eventually returns to near-normal levels (11). If cumulative lifetime risk is calculated from these risk estimates multiplied by the overall

lifetime incidence of 1 in 9–10, some women will apparently have a lifetime risk of breast cancer in excess of 100%. Risk estimates for individual factors are not multiplicative and may not be additive in a simple arithmetic manner. Perhaps the most accurate way to assess risk is to define the strongest single factor which for breast cancer is usually family history. When the level of risk is based on this factor alone, minor adjustments can be made to incorporate other factors. However, it seems unlikely that these additional factors will influence risks to any great extent in the presence of predisposing genes with a high degree of penetrance. Rather than determining the absolute risk of development of breast cancer they may advance or delay the onset of disease. The effects of nonhereditary elements of risk can only be assumptive rather than calculated in objective terms. Although some studies suggest an increased risk attributable to these nonhereditary factors in family history cases, these may merely represent the earlier expression of the gene. Therefore risk assessments will generally range between 40% and 1 in 12 (8%) though lower risks are sometimes sited. Higher risks may be applicable when a woman has a 40% genetic risk and is found to have a germline mutation, to have an inherited high-risk allele or to have proliferative breast disease.

BREAST CANCER RISK OVER TIME
Risk Estimation Models
Initially, the two most frequently used models were the Gail model and the Claus model.

The Gail Model
The Gail model was originally designed to determine the eligibility criteria for the Breast Cancer Prevention Trial, and has since been modified (in part to adjust for race) (13,14) and made available on the National Cancer Institute web site (http://bcra.nci.nih.gov/brc/q1.htm). The model has been validated in a number of settings and probably works best in general assessment clinics (15), where family history is not the main reason for referral. The major limitation of the Gail model is the inclusion of only FDRs, which results in underestimating risk in the 50% of families with cancer in the paternal lineage and also takes no account of age of onset of breast cancer (15,16). As such it performed less well in our own validation set from a family history clinic (Table 3.2), substantially underestimating risk overall in most subgroups and groups assessed.

Claus Model
Three years after publication of the model, lifetime risk tables for most combinations of affected first- and second-degree relatives were published (3). Although these do not give figures for some combinations of relatives, for example mother and maternal grandmother, an estimation of this risk can be garnered by using the mother–maternal aunt combination. An expansion of the original Claus model estimates breast cancer risk in women with a family history of ovarian cancer (17). The major drawback of the Claus model is that it does not include any of the nonhereditary risk factors. Concordance of the Gail and Claus models has been shown to be relatively poor (16,18–21). While the tables make no adjustments for unaffected relatives the computerized version is able to reduce

the likelihood of the "dominant gene" with an increasing number of affected women. However, the tables give consistently higher risk figures than the computer model suggesting that either a population risk element is not added back into the calculation or that the adjustment for unaffected relatives is made from the original averaged figure rather than assuming that each family will have already had an "average" number of unaffected relatives (16). The latter appears to be the likely explanation as inputting families with zero unaffected female relatives gives risk figures close to the Claus table figure. Another potential drawback of the Claus tables is that these reflect risks for women in the 1980s in the US. These are lower than the current incidence in both North America and most of Europe. As such an upward adjustment of 3–4% for lifetime risk is necessary for lifetime risks below 20%. Our own validation of the Claus computer model showed that it substantially underestimated risks in the family history clinic. However, manual use of the Claus tables provided accurate risk estimation (Table 3.2). A modified version of the Claus model has now been validated as "Claus extended," by adding the risk for bilateral disease, ovarian cancer, and three or more affected relatives (21).

BRCAPRO Model

Parmigiani et al. developed a Bayesian model that incorporated details like published *BRCA1* and *BRCA2* mutation frequencies, cancer penetrance in mutation carriers, cancer status (affected, unaffected, or unknown), and age of the consultee's first- and second-degree relatives (22). An advantage of this model is that it includes information on both affected and unaffected relatives. In addition, it provides estimates for the likelihood of finding either a *BRCA1* or *BRCA2* mutation in a family. An output that calculates breast cancer risk using the likelihood of *BRCA1/2* can be utilized. None of the nonhereditary risk factors can yet be incorporated into the model (Table 3.2). The major drawback from the breast cancer risk assessment aspect is that no other "genetic" element is allowed for (16). As such in breast-cancer-only families it will underestimate the risk. As such BRCAPRO model produced the least accurate breast cancer risk estimation from our family history clinic validation. It predicted only 49% of the breast cancers that actually occurred in the screened group of 1900 women (16).

Cuzick–Tyrer Model

No single model integrated family history, surrogate measures of endogenous estrogen exposure, and benign breast disease in a comprehensive fashion. The Cuzick–Tyrer model (23) based partly on a dataset acquired from the International Breast Cancer Intervention Study (IBIS) and other epidemiological data has now done this (17). The major advantage over the Claus model and BRCAPRO is that the model allows for the presence of multiple genes of differing penetrance. It does give a readout of BRCA1/2, but also allows for a lower penetrance BRCAX.

Table 3.2 Family History and Other Known Risk Factors and their Incorporation into Existing Risk Models

	RR at Extreme	Gail	Claus	BRCAPRO Ford	Cuzick–Tyrer	BOADICEA
Prediction						
Follow-up study (E/O)		0.48	0.56	0.49	0.81	Not assessed
95% confidence interval		(0.54–0.90)	(0.59–0.99)	(0.52–0.80)	(0.85–1.41)	Not assessed
Personal information						
Age (20–70 yrs)	30	Yes	Yes	Yes	Yes	Yes
Body mass index	2	No	No	No	Yes	No
Alcohol intake (0–4 units) daily	1.24	No	No	No	No	No
Hormonal/reproductive factors						
Menarche	2	Yes	No	No	Yes	No
First live birth	3	Yes	No	No	Yes	No
Menopause	4	No	No	No	Yes	No
HRT	2	No	No	No	Yes	No
OCP	1.24	No	No	No	No	No
Breast feeding	0.8	No	No	No	No	No
Plasma estrogen	5	No	No	No	No	No
Personal breast disease						
Breast biopsies	2	Yes	No	No	Yes	No
Atypical ductal hyperplasia	3	Yes	No	No	Yes	No
Lobular carcinoma *in situ*	4	No	No	No	Yes	No
Breast density	6	Yes/No	No	No	Yes/No	No
Family history						
First-drgree relatives	3	Yes	Yes	Yes	Yes	Yes
Second -drgree relatives	1.5	No	Yes	Yes	Yes	Yes
Third -drgree relatives		No	No	No	No	Yes
Age of onset of breast cancer	3	No	Yes	Yes	Yes	Yes
Bilateral breast cancer	3	No	No	Yes	Yes	Yes
Ovarian cancer	1.5	No	No	Yes	Yes	Yes
Male breast cancer	3	No	No	Yes	No	Yes

Abbreviations: E/O, expected over observed cancer ratio (all models assessed underestimated cancer occurrence); OCP, oral contraceptive pill.

As can be seen in Table 3.2, the Cuzick–Tyrer model addresses many of the pitfalls of the previous models, significantly, the combination of extensive family history, endogenous estrogen exposure, and benign breast disease (atypical hyperplasia). In our original validation the Cuzick–Tyrer model performed by far the best in estimating the breast cancer risk (16).

Model Validation

The goodness of fit and discriminatory accuracy of the above four models was assessed using data from 1317 women. The main analysis was on 1933 women attending our family history evaluation and screening program in Manchester, UK, who underwent ongoing screening; of these 52 developed cancer (16). All models were applied to these women over a mean follow-up of 5.27 years to estimate the risk of breast cancer. The ratios of expected numbers of breast cancers to observed numbers of breast cancers [95% confidence interval (CI)] were 0.48 (0.37–0.64) for Gail, 0.56 (0.43–0.75) for Claus, 0.49 (0.37–0.65) for Ford, and 0.81 (0.62–1.08) for Cuzick–Tyrer (Table 3.2). The accuracy of the models for individual cases was evaluated using Receiver Operating Characteristics (ROC) curves. These showed that the area under the curve was 0.735 for Gail, 0.716 for Claus, 0.737 for Ford, and 0.762 for Cuzick–Tyrer. The Cuzick–Tyrer model was the most consistently accurate model for prediction of breast cancer. Gail, Claus, and Ford all significantly underestimated risk although with a manual approach the accuracy of Claus tables may be improved by making adjustments for other risk factors ("Manual Method") by subtracting from the lifetime risk for a positive endocrine risk factor (e.g., a lifetime risk may change from 1 in 5 to 1 in 4 with late age of first pregnancy). The Gail, Claus, and BRCAPRO models all underestimated risk particularly in women with a single FDR affected with breast cancer. Cuzick–Tyrer and the Manual model were both accurate in this subgroup. Conversely, all the models accurately predicted risk in women with multiple relatives affected with breast cancer (i.e., two FDRs and one first-degree plus two other relatives). This implies that the effect of a single affected FDR is higher than may have been previously thought. The Gail model is likely to have underestimated in this group as it does not take into account age of breast cancer and most women in our single FDR category had a relative diagnosed at less than 40 years of age. The Ford, Cuzick–Tyrer, and Manual models were the only models to accurately predict risk in women with a family history of ovarian cancer. As these were the only models to take account of ovarian cancer in their risk assessment algorithm, this confirmed that ovarian cancer has a significant effect on breast cancer risk.

The Gail, Claus, and BRCAPRO models all significantly underestimated risk in women who were nulliparous or whose first live birth occurred after the age of 30 years. Moreover, the Gail model appeared to increase risk with pregnancy at age below 30 years in the familial setting. It is not clear why such a modification to the effects of age at first birth should be made unless it is as a result of modifications to the model made after early results suggested an increase with BRCA1/2 mutation carriers. However, the Gail model has determined an apparent increase in risk with early first pregnancy and it would appear to be misplaced from our results, and from subsequent studies published on BRCA1/2. Furthermore, Gail, Claus, and BRCAPRO models also underestimated risk in women whose menarche occurred after the age of 12. The Cuzick–Tyrer and Manual models accurately predicted risk in these subgroups. These results suggest that age at first live birth has also an important effect on breast cancer risk, while age at menarche perhaps has a lesser effect. The effect of pregnancy at age below 30 years appeared to reduce risk by 40–50% compared with an older first pregnancy or late age/nulliparity whereas at the extremes of menarche there was only a 12–14% effect. Our study remains the only one to validate these risk models prospectively and clearly further such studies are necessary to gauge the accuracy of these and newer models. Indeed the tendency to modify models to adapt for new risk factors without prospective validation in an independent dataset is a problem and can lead to erroneous risk prediction.

BOADICEA Model

Using segregation analysis a group in Cambridge, UK, has derived a susceptibility model (BOADICEA, Breast and Ovarian Analysis of Disease Incidence and Carrier Estimation Algorithm) in which susceptibility is explained by mutations in BRCA1 and BRCA2 together with a polygenic component reflecting the joint multiplicative effect of multiple genes of small effect on breast cancer risk (24). The group has shown that the overall familial risks of breast cancer predicted by the model are close to those observed in epidemiological studies. The predicted prevalence of BRCA1 and BRCA2 mutations among unselected cases of breast and ovarian cancer was also consistent with observations from population-based studies. They also showed that their predictions were closer to the observed values than those obtained using the Claus model and BRCAPRO. The predicted mutation probabilities and cancer risks in individuals with a family history can now be derived from this model. Early validation studies have been carried out on mutation probability but not yet cancer risk prediction (25).

BREAST CANCER GENES

The hereditary component of breast cancer is likely to result from multiple different predisposing genes conferring risks which may be as little as a 1.05 relative risk up to genes which confer a lifetime risk of up to 85%. Attention has tended to focus on two high-risk predisposing genes; the first on the long arm of chromosome 17 (BRCA1) (26) and the other on the long arm of chromosome 13 (BRCA2) (27). These genes have an estimated population frequency of 0.2% and are thought to account for over 80% of highly penetrant inherited breast cancer. The majority of families with a combination of breast and ovarian cancer are linked to BRCA1 with mutations thereof causing the disease. However, 20% of families with breast and ovarian cancer may have mutations in BRCA2 (28,29) and mutations in one or other of these two genes account for most, if not all, breast/ovarian cancer predisposition (28). Furthermore, the occurrence of two or more cases of epithelial ovarian cancer within a family is highly suggestive of BRCA1 involvement. There is increasing evidence that families with BRCA1 and BRCA2 involvement have differential susceptibilities to ovarian cancers. The associated cumulative lifetime risks across all the linked families for mutations of BRCA1 and BRCA2 are

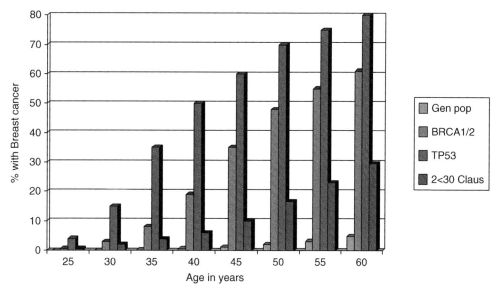

Figure 3.1 Age-specific penetrance for breast cancer in carriers of *BRCA1/BRCA2* and *TP53* mutations. 2<30 = 2 first-degree relatives (e.g., mother and daughter or two sisters, with breast cancer aged below 30 years % risk. *Source*: Adapted from Ref. (6).

85% (breast) and 60% (ovarian) (28,30) and 85% (breast) and 10–20% (ovary) (15) respectively (Fig. 3.1). Two subsets of mutation probably exist, one of which results predominantly in ovarian cancer risk, whereas the other confers a relatively low risk of ovarian predisposition (31). It may transpire that nearly all of these so-called site-specific ovarian cancer families are caused by *BRCA1* mutations. This is supported by evidence from several areas including (*i*) long–term follow-up of site-specific families (32), (*ii*) new cancers in families from the UKCCCR (UK Coordinating Committee on Cancer Research) familial ovarian cancer study (B Ponder/P Pharoah – personal communication), and (*iii*) linkage and mutation analysis within families (28,29,33,34). Controversy persists over the true cumulative lifetime risk associated with mutations of *BRCA1* and *BRCA2*. Though initial studies in selected groups revealed high levels of risk, subsequent population studies have shown risks as low as 40% (35). However, large scale studies are consistent with higher risk estimates for both genes (36). In reality the risk will depend on the method of ascertainment and whether other genetic modifiers exist in the family (36,37).

The *TP53* gene on chromosome 17p is known to predispose to early breast cancer (5) and germline mutations of this gene account for over 70% of cases of the Li–Fraumeni syndrome (38). However, the overall contribution of Li-Fraumeni to breast cancer incidence is probably minimal except in patients diagnosed below 31 years of age (39). Carriage of the ataxia telangiectasia muted (ATM) gene is associated with a two to five fold risk of breast cancer (40,41). Though the carrier frequency for this gene was estimated to be as high as 2%, (it is now known to be about 0.5%) this was based on five complementation groupings and the disease is now known to be caused by a single gene on chromosome 11q (42). The PTEN gene on chromosome 10 is linked to Cowden's disease (43), but neither this gene nor the ATM gene account for high-risk families. Other genes which might be implicated in breast cancer are being actively sought and it is likely that several other predisposing genes remain to be identified. Table 3.3 lists known hereditary conditions and location of genes

predisposing to breast cancer. This includes genes in the moderate (BRIP, PALB2) (44,45) and high-risk categories, but not the gene locations (>20) (common Single Nucleotide Polymorphisms) associated with lower (1.05–1.5) relative risks (37,46,47).

For the majority of women it will only be possible to derive an estimate of lifetime risk which will ultimately depend upon whether a gene mutation exists within the family and whether an individual has inherited this. Genetic testing has the potential to significantly modify risk estimates by confirming the presence of or excluding a particular germline mutation. In the latter case, risk is only reduced significantly and confidently by demonstrating the absence of a known family mutation.

COMMUNICATION OF RISK

Risk can be expressed either as a cumulative lifetime risk or as a risk over a specific period of time. Thus a woman from a breast cancer family with young-onset disease may have a lifetime risk of 40%. However, if she has already reached 60 years of age and remains disease free her chance of carrying a gene mutation is only 20% as more than 60% would have developed breast cancer by the age of 60 years in the presence of a genetic predisposition. Moreover there is only a 10% chance of having a hereditary form of breast cancer in her remaining life consistent with the gradual equalization of risk toward normal in patients over 60 years of age with a strong family history of breast cancer. Thus communication of risk to women must incorporate these concepts of time dependence and residual lifetime risk. Some women may prefer to have information on annual risk which is approximately 1% per year from the late 20s for an individual from a dominant family with a 50% chance of inheriting the gene.

OPTIONS

The options available for a woman with a significantly increased risk of breast cancer remain limited. Some women ignore this risk and prefer to "bury their head in the sand" and avoid seeking any professional advice. Others are rendered disillusioned,

Table 3.3 Hereditary Conditions Predisposing to Breast Cancer

Gene	Other Tumor % of Susceptibility	Population Frequency (%)	Proportion of Breast Cancer (%)	Proportion of HPHBC (%)	Proportion of Familial Breast Cancer Risk (%)	Lifetime Risk in Women (RR, %)
BRCA1 AD	Ovary/prostate Colorectal	0.1	1.5	40	5–10	60–85
BRCA2 AD	Ovary/prostate Pancreas HoZ-Fanconi (AR)	0.1	1.5	40	5–10	50–85
TP53 LFS AD	Sarcoma, glioma Adrenal	0.0025	0.02	2	0.1	80–90
PTEN Cowden's AD	Thyroid Colorectal	0.0005	0.004	0.3	0.02	25–50
CHEK2	Colorectal, prostate	0.5	0.5	0	2	18–20 (2.0)
ATM AD & AR	HoZ (AR) Lymphoma, leukemia	0.5	0.5	0	2	20
STK11 AD	Colorectal	0.001	0.001	0.6	0.04	50
BRIP1	HoZ-Fanconi (AR)	0.1	0.1	0	0.4	20 (2.0)
PALB2	HoZ-Fanconi (AR)	0.1	0.1	0	0.4	20 (2.0)
RAD51C	HoZ-Fanconi (AR)	0.1	0.1	0	0.2	?20 (2.0)
20 SNPs Refs (37,41–43)		25–46	0.5	0	12	11–13 (1.1–1.3)
Totals		80 for any	5	83	37	

Abbreviations: AD, autosomal dominant; AR, autosomal recessive; HeZ, heterozygous; HPHBC, highly penetrant hereditary breast cancer (e.g., >3 affected relatives); HoZ, homozygous; LFS, Li–Fraumeni syndrome; SNP, single nucleotide polymorphism.

confused, or even skeptical by enthusiastic doctors. While the efficacy of screening young women remains controversial with mammography and is expensive with MRI, a degree of circumspection is appropriate when advocating screening for this subgroup of women at a higher risk. Nonetheless, many women are prepared to accept any intervention which may be associated with potential benefits in terms of reduction in mortality.

The options are as listed below:

1. No action
2. Try to reduce risks
3. Early detection of tumors (screening)
4. Removal of risk

Try to Reduce Risks

The following methods may help reduce breast cancer risks:

1. Plan family early
2. Avoid OCP and HRT
3. Follow a good diet

Some doctors may advocate these:

1. Delaying menarche
2. Artificial early menopause (oophorectomy)
3. Antiestrogen therapy (tamoxifen)

The identification of a group of women at high risk increases the probability of a sufficient number of events occurring (i.e., development of breast cancer) to justify prevention trials as a worthwhile intervention. Four major trials of prevention with tamoxifen have now been published (48–52). Tamoxifen had already been shown to reduce the risk of contralateral breast cancer in affected women and the large American National Surgical Adjuvant Breast and Bowel Project (NSABP) P1 trial was the first to show a reduction in risk of breast cancer in asymptomatic women (at increased lifetime risk) by 40–50% (50). Tamoxifen is generally well tolerated, although hot flushes and other menopausal symptoms are common and there are increased risks of thromboembolic events and endometrial cancer. The IBIS-1 study showed a 30–40% reduction in breast cancer risk, but a rise in all-cause mortality (50–53). As a result, tamoxifen was not licensed for prevention in the UK and Europe but does have a license in North America. Longer–term follow-up of the International IBIS-1 trial now suggests that the risk–benefit ratio may well be in favor of chemoprevention in women at increased risk who are still premenopausal (54,55). A study comparing tamoxifen with raloxifene in America, the STAR trial showed no overall difference in prevention between the two drugs (56). Raloxifene may well be the drug of choice in postmenopausal women (55). Other studies that are underway involve reduction in fat intake in Canada and administration of retinoids in Italy. A high-risk trial RAZOR has been piloted in the UK involving switching off the ovaries with zoladex (Goserelin®, AstraZeneca, Alderley Park, Cheshire, UK) and protecting the bones (and breasts) with raloxifene. Variations of this are being undertaken in the US and mainland Europe. Recruitment to these trials in women at high risk for breast cancer has been disappointing and this may be due to a reluctance to be randomized to placebo (57).

An alternative strategy particularly in *BRCA1* carriers is to opt for early risk-reducing salpingo-oophorectomy at about 40 years of age. This can reduce breast cancer risk by around 50% (58) and indeed earlier oophorectomy may well reduce the risk further. Nonetheless, the effects of an early menopause and doubts over long–term HRT have to be considered if the primary purpose is breast cancer prevention.

Early Detection of Tumors (Screening)

Methods that help detect the presence of tumors early include the following.

1. Regular self-examination.
2. Annual mammography screening from 35 to 40 years or five years before the earliest cancer in family. This may be partly replaced by the following:
   a) Annual ultrasound.
   b) MRI scanning

It is likely that annual screening will identify over 60% of cancers in young women (59,60), but interval cancers do occur. The young breast is denser and more difficult to interpret. However, as relative risk to the general population at age 35 may be 40 fold, this group needs to be treated as a special case. Although the first evidence for a significant survival advantage emerged some years ago for the general population under 50 years (61,62), the frequency of disease is probably too low to justify screening on economic grounds. However, our own work has shown that impalpable small lesions are detected in the 35–49 year age group and that similar detection rates to the NHS Breast Screening Programme are attainable by targeted screening (63). There are also the first signs of a mortality benefit, although this may not be the case for *BRCA1* carriers who appear to have a worse prognosis (60,63–65). Mammography may eventually be replaced by other more sensitive techniques such as MRI in *BRCA1/2* mutation carriers (66–69), but the costs and scarcity of scanners may make MRI unviable outside a very high-risk group. MRI screening is recommended in the UK for *BRCA1/2* and *TP53* mutation carriers aged 30–49 as well as for individuals without mutations who are at a very high risk (www.nice.org.uk) (70). In the US, a lifetime risk in excess of 25% is sufficient for MRI. Currently most countries are combining mammography with MRI even in mutation carriers, particularly from the age of 40 years (70). The very small dose of radiation involved with mammography has only a small theoretical risk of inducing a breast cancer (71). Even cumulatively this is unlikely to cause more than an extra breast cancer in one in every 10,000 women. This is not really comparable to a 40% lifetime risk. However, known carriers of *TP53* and *ATM* gene mutations should probably not be screened with mammography and there is now some doubt about carriers of *BRCA2*. *BRCA2* interacts with a protein involved in DNA repair and as such carriers may be more susceptible to radiation-induced damages (72). Women screened for breast cancer may undergo fine needle aspiration or open biopsy for screen-detected lumps which are entirely benign. This will be associated with at least a small degree of psychological and physical morbidity, but in experienced hands the risks of unnecessary biopsy are small (73).

Removal of Risk
Risk Reducing Mastectomy

This is often perceived as a rather drastic measure and was more commonly practiced in the US than Europe until the 1990s (74). For those women with a particularly high risk, this option of risk reduction should be considered and sensitively discussed with the patient (70). The usual procedure undertaken for prophylaxis has been a subcutaneous mastectomy which preserves the nipple–areola complex and therefore leaves behind a small amount of sub-areola breast tissue (75). The placement of implants within a subpectoral muscular pocket has greatly improved cosmetic results and ensures that any residual breast tissue lies anterior to the prosthesis, which may otherwise mask any tumor. For those women who opt for a mastectomy, the surgical procedure should be a complete mastectomy preserving most of the breast envelope but sacrificing the nipple–areola complex (skin-sparing mastectomy). This may be a more appropriate operation from an oncological point of view. Nonetheless, there is evidence from a study involving almost 1000 women carried out at the Mayo Clinic that breast cancer risks can be reduced by 90% when subcutaneous mastectomy is undertaken as a prophylactic procedure (74). Further studies have now confirmed the benefits of surgical prophylaxis in *BRCA1* and *BRCA2* mutation carriers (76,77). It remains unclear whether there are any long–term sequelae of preventative surgery; it is essential that women are prepared psychologically for bilateral prophylactic mastectomy and have realistic expectations of cosmetic results which may not always be satisfactory to any individual woman. The attendant risks of general anesthesia (especially if concomitant medical problems) and surgery must be taken into account when making a final decision about prophylactic mastectomy. Studies have shown significant reduction in levels of anxiety in cancer-related worry in women opting for prophylactic mastectomy compared with those who do not (78). Women at high risk are increasingly opting for prophylactic mastectomy within the UK and it is important that comprehensive protocols which include psychological assessment are available to prepare women prior to surgery (70,79). As genetic testing becomes more widely available with identification of women whose lifetime risk approaches 80–90%, demand for risk-reducing mastectomy is likely to increase. A report from our own group and another from a Dutch group indicate uptake rates of around 50% in unaffected mutation carriers (80,81). Women at a high risk for breast cancer are more likely to choose risk-reducing surgery than prevention trials (57).

The subpopulation of women who might benefit from presymptomatic genetic testing is difficult to define. Any individual could, in principle, undergo mutation testing for either *BRCA1* or *BRCA2* (or both), but detection of mutations would be very low unless those individuals were identified as being at an increased risk for a genetic fault and hence breast cancer in the first place. Those individuals without any family history of breast or ovarian cancer will have no alteration to their lifetime risk from a negative screen. Furthermore, these women will not be in screening programs outside the NHS Breast Screening Programme where screening commences at 47–50 years of age. It is doubtful whether those individuals with one or two relatives with breast cancer will benefit much in terms of reassurance from a negative genetic screen. Currently, the target population is at-risk relatives and families with four or more cases of breast cancer under 60 years or ovarian cancer at any age. There must be an affected family member alive who is willing to provide a blood sample for mutation screening. These criteria will eventually be extended to allow for testing of much smaller aggregations of breast cancer cases, especially with the advent of next-generation sequencing technology. It is estimated that only one in every 1000 individuals come from families suitable for genetic testing at the present time and 3% at most of breast cancer cases could be prevented by testing for BRCA1 and BRCA2 mutations. There may be potential cost savings from withdrawal of women who test negative from existing surveillance programs.

THE GENETIC TESTING PROGRAM

Genetic testing for BRCA1 and BRCA2 mutations was mainly carried out to develop a test for at-risk relatives. With the advent of poly ADP-ribose polymerase (PARP) inhibitor treatments which may have a synthetic lethal effect on tumors in mutation carriers as well as greater uptake of risk-reducing surgery among affected women the need to drive personal decision making has come more to the fore. Therefore, who should be offered genetic testing and how should this be carried out? Clearly, testing cannot be offered on demand to all individuals requesting screening for BRCA1 or BRCA2 mutations. This will entail a significant expansion of current laboratory services together with the peritest counseling which is a crucial aspect of genetic screening. A more realistic approach is to offer testing to those individuals with a family history of breast or ovarian cancer. Approximately, one in 9–10 women develop breast cancer in their lifetime and thus many women will have some family history of the disease. Even if access is restricted to those with a more significant history there will be a potentially huge demand. What will a positive or negative screen mean for a woman? Those individuals in the general population without a family history have less than 0.1% chance of carrying a mutation in the BRCA1 gene. Therefore a negative screen will not reduce their breast cancer risk even if the sensitivity of the test were 100%. An individual with an FDR with breast cancer at age 45 years whose lifetime risk is one in six will derive no meaningful reduction in their chance of developing breast cancer. Even where there is a strong family history of breast and ovarian cancer, mutation testing at 90% sensitivity will not lead to a risk reduction which justifies cessation of screening or prophylactic intervention. It will appear logical therefore to offer a predictive test only when a mutation has been identified in a family and shown to have relevance to disease causation. This will allow those family members without a mutation to be completely reassured and permit informed risk estimates of breast and ovarian cancer to those with a mutation. A large number of population studies have attempted to determine the proportion of early-onset breast cancer (39,82,83) and ovarian (34,84) cancer caused by BRCA1 mutations (assuming a sensitivity of mutation detection as low as 70%). However several populations exhibit a significant "founder" effect whereby a limited number of mutations account for a large proportion of hereditary disease (85,86). This is particularly true for the Ashkenazi Jews among whom three distinct mutations are

Table 3.4 Summary of Potential Problems in Identifying an Appropriate Target Population

- Too much demand for too little yield
- Residual risk (population risk or still above) for women who test negative
- Unknown psychological sequelae
- Economic cost benefit only if management is changed

found in 2.5% of the entire population (86). Were the population frequency of other BRCA1/2 mutations to be the same as in the non-Jewish population (0.2%) testing for three mutations would account for over 90% of highly penetrant families. Work done by our own group has shown that a significant proportion of the smaller aggregations are due to these founder mutations (87). Population testing is therefore likely to have a higher predictive value in the Jewish community and because of the relatively high frequency of mutations within this group, testing of unaffected individuals without a known family history of breast cancer is feasible (Table 3.4).

UPTAKE OF GENETIC TESTING AND OUTCOME

Once a mutation has been found this can be offered to the extended family. Early surveys indicated that approximately 60% of women would accept the offer of BRCA1 gene testing (88,89). This figure came from our own preliminary data, based on 75 individuals distributed amongst five families (90), in addition to population studies and a clinical survey (91,92). A longer–term follow-up of nonresearch families suggests an uptake of around 60% in women and 15–20% in men at 50% risk (90,93).

Evidence to date suggests that techniques such as gene sequencing combined with an analysis for large rearrangements such as Multiplex Ligation Dependent Probe Amplification (MLPA, MRC-Holland Willem Schoutenstraat 6, 1057 DN Amsterdam the Netherlands) will detect 90–95% of BRCA1 and BRCA2 mutations (29,94). Should these techniques become widely available expansion of the number of genetic counselors and appropriately trained clinicians will be essential if at-risk individuals are to be adequately prepared for predictive testing. Funding will have to be made available not only to carry out testing but also to make provision for the consequences of genetic testing.

Genetic testing is difficult to cost; commercial laboratories in the US such as MYRIAD and their UK subsidiary Lab 21 charge a total of around $3000 (£1800) for initial complete screening of BRCA1 and BRCA2 genes. Once a specific mutation is identified for that family, subsequent tests are charged at a much lower rate of about $400. In the UK the comparable NHS service lab costs are £600 for a complete screen of BRCA1/2 and £120 for subsequent testing. These costs are likely to reduce drastically with next-generation sequencing technology. Screening for founder mutations is relatively cheaper. Thus it costs approximately £120 to screen for the three common mutations (185 del AG, 5382 ins C, and 6174 del T) within the Ashkenazi Jewish population which is potentially very cost-effective. Cost analysis undertaken by our own group for the non-Jewish population has also shown a significant cost benefit (using a 10% testing threshold) if over 40% of women choose risk-reducing surgery and those individuals deemed to be at low risk are discharged from screening (60% uptake of testing). The current threshold for initiating testing in the UK is 20% (70), although this is currently under review.

Cost savings will only be forthcoming if management is changed as a consequence of genetic testing. This is unlikely to be the case for women outside families with proven *BRCA1/2* mutations; testing unaffected women who have no knowledge of the family mutation (if one exists) may not alter their breast cancer risk in a practically meaningful way. An exception to this in the non-Jewish population will be a woman contemplating risk-reducing mastectomy who may be sufficiently reassured by a negative *BRCA1/2* test to abandon surgery. Even within the Jewish population exclusion of the three common mutations does not equate with minimal risk. Though a large proportion of hereditary risk is excluded family history of breast cancer still confers increased risk and new mutations can occur within the Jewish population.

Whilst there is still a need to assess the likelihood of a *BRCA1/2* mutation prior to mutation testing, the use of genetic testing prediction models is necessary. The simple-to-use Manchester manual model has compared well with computer models in this respect (Tables 3.5 and 3.6) (22,24,25,94–96).

CONCLUSION

Cancer genetics has emerged as a new specialty over the last decade with familial risk clinics being established across Europe and North America. Categorization of individuals into high,

Table 3.5 Manchester Scoring System for Identification of a Pathogenic BRCA1/2 Mutation

	BRCA1	BRCA2
FBC <30	6	5
FBC 30–39	4	4
FBC 40–49	3	3
FBC 50–59	2	2
FBC >59	1	1
MBC <60	5 (if *BRCA2* tested)	8
MBC >59	5 (if *BRCA2* tested)	5
Ovarian cancer <60	8	5 (if *BRCA1* tested)
Ovarian cancer >59	5	5 (if *BRCA1* tested)
Pancreatic cancer	0	1
Prostate cancer <60	0	2
Prostate cancer >59	0	1

Scores for each cancer in a direct lineage are summated. A score of 10 is equivalent to a 10% chance of identifying a mutation in each gene. A combined score of 20 points will qualify for NHS testing at the 20% threshold. *Abbreviations*: FBC, female breast cancer; MBC, male breast cancer.

Table 3.6 Calculated Adjustments to the Manchester Score for Predicting *BRCA*1 and *BRCA*2 Mutations According to Pathology and Receptor Status of Breast Cancer in the Index Case and the Presence of Ovarian Cancer in Family

Pathology	BRCA1 Adjustment	BRCA2 Adjustment	Notes
Breast			
Her2+	−4[a]	0	No other alteration to score on the basis of pathology needed
Lobular	−2	0	Add or subtract ER status
DCIS only (no invasive cancer)	−1	0	Add or subtract ER status
LCIS only (no invasive cancer)	−4[a]	0	No other adjustment
Grade 1 IDC	−2	0	Add or subtract ER status
Grade 2 IDC	0	0	Add or subtract ER status
Grade 3 IDC	+2	0	Add or subtract ER status
ER positive	−1	0	Add or subtract grade
ER negative	+1	0	Add or subtract grade
Grade 3 triple negative	+4[a]	0	No other alteration to score on the basis of pathology needed
Ovary			
Epithelial (endometrioid, serous, clear cell, NOS) Granulosa cell	0 no change to MS	0	No adjustment to ovarian score, i.e., 5 points for cancers >59 years for each gene.
Mucinous	No score given for index case or other relative	No score given for index case or other relative	Do not include in scoring at all
Borderline	No score given for index case or other relative	No score given for index case or other relative	Do not include in scoring at all
Germ cell tumors except granulosa cell	No score given for index case or other relative	No score given for index case or other relative	Do not include in scoring at all

[a]These adjustments are final and no further adjustment based on other pathological features is necessary.

Abbreviations: DCIS, ductal cell carcinoma *in situ*; ER, estrogen receptor; IDC, invasive ductal carcinoma; LCIS, lobular carcinoma *in situ*; NOS, not otherwise specified.

Examples

1. Grade 3 ER positive would score +1 (+2 for grade 3, and −1 for ER pos).
2. Grade 3 ER negative would score +3 (+2, +1) unless triple negative (+4) 4 points added to total score.
3. Grade 1 ER positive scores −3 (−2, −1) 3 points deducted from total score.
4. Grade 2 but no receptor status known (0), no adjustment.
5. Lobular carcinoma ER positive would score −3 (−2, −1).

moderate, and average (low) risk groups has permitted genetic testing to be targeted to those most likely to benefit (70).

Genetic testing is likely to become more widely available with improvements in molecular biological techniques and the discovery of the remaining genes which predispose to breast cancer.

REFERENCES

1. CR-UK, Cancer Stats Incidence - UK. Cancer Research UK 2008. [Available from: www.cancerresearchuk.org] 2009. http://info.cancerresearchuk.org/cancerstats/types/breast/index.htm?script=true] [Accessed 01/07/2011].
2. Newman B, Austin MA, Lee M, King M. Inheritance of human breast cancer: Evidence for autosomal dominant transmission in high-risk families. Proc Natl Acad Sci USA 1988; 85: 3044–8.
3. Claus EB, Risch N, Thompson WD. Autosomal dominant inheritance of early onset breast cancer. Cancer 1994; 73: 643–51.
4. Nelen MR, Padberg GW, Peeters EAJ, et al. Localisation of the gene for cowden disease to chromosome lOq22–23. Nat Genet 1996; 13: 114–16.
5. Malkin D, Li FP, Strong LC, et al. Germline p53 mutations in cancer families. Science 1990; 250: 1233–8.
6. The Breast Cancer Linkage Consortium. Cancer risks in BRCA2 mutation carriers. The Breast Cancer Linkage Consortium. J Natl Cancer Inst 1999; 91: 1310–16.
7. Thompson D, Easton DF; Breast Cancer Linkage Consortium. Cancer incidence in BRCA1 mutation carriers. J Natl Cancer Inst 2002; 94: 1358–65.
8. van Asperen CJ, Brohet RM, Meijers-Heijboer EJ, et al. Netherlands Collaborative Group on Hereditary Breast Cancer (HEBON). Cancer risks in BRCA2 families: estimates for sites other than breast and ovary. J Med Genet 2005; 42: 711–19.
9. Collaborative Group on Hormonal Factors in Breast Cancer. Breast cancer and hormonal contraceptives: collaborative reanalysis of individual data on 53,297 women with breast cancer and 100,239 women without breast cancer from 54 epidemiological studies. Lancet 1996; 347: 1713–27.
10. Steinberg KK, Thacker SB, Smith J, et al. A meta-analysis of the effect of oestrogen replacement therapy on the risk of breast cancer. JAMA 1991; 1985–90.
11. Dupont WD, Page DL. Relative risk of breast cancer varies with time since diagnosis of atypical hyperplasia. Hum Pathol 1989; 20: 723–5.
12. Scolnick MH, Cannon-Albright LA, Goldgar DE, et al. Inheritance of proliferative breast disease in breast cancer kindreds. Science 1990; 250: 1715–21.
13. Gail MH, Brinton LA, Byar DP, et al. Projecting individulized probabilities of developing breast cancer for white females who are being examined annually. J Natl Cancer Inst 1989; 81: 1879–86.
14. Costantino JP, Gail MH, Pee D, et al. Validation studies for models projecting the risk of invasive and total breast cancer incidence. J Natl Cancer Inst 1999; 91: 1541–8.
15. Euhus DM, Leitch AM, Huth JF, Peters GN. Limitations of the Gail model in the specialized breast cancer risk assessment clinic. Breast 2002; 8: 23–7.
16. Amir E, Evans DG, Shenton A, et al. Evaluation of breast cancer risk assessment packages in the family history evaluation and screening programme. J Med Genet 2003; 40: 807–14.
17. Claus EB, Risch N, Thompson WD. The calculation of breast cancer risk for women with a first degree family history of ovarian cancer. Breast Cancer Res Treat 1993; 28: 115–20.
18. McTiernan A, Kuniyuki A, Yasui Y, et al. Comparisons of two breast cancer risk estimates in women with a family history of breast cancer. Cancer Epidemiol Biomarkers Prev 2001; 10: 333–8.
19. McGuigan KA, Ganz PA, Breant C. Agreement between breast cancer risk estimation methods. J Natl Cancer Inst 1996; 88: 1315–17.
20. Tischkowitz M, Wheeler D, France E, et al. A comparison of methods currently used in clinical practice to estimate familial breast cancer risks. Ann Oncol 2000; 11: 451–4.
21. van Asperen CJ, Jonker MA, Jacobi CE, et al. Risk estimation for healthy women from breast cancer families: new insights and new strategies. Cancer Epidemiol Biomarkers Prev 2004; 13: 87–93.
22. Parmigiani G, Berry DA, Aquilar O. Determining carrier probabilities for breast cancer susceptibility genes BRCA1 and BRCA2. Am J Hum Genet 1998; 62: 145–8.
23. Tyrer J, Duffy SW, Cuzick J. A breast cancer prediction model incorporating familial and personal risk factors. Stat Med 2004; 23:1111–30.
24. Antoniou AC, Pharoah PP, Smith P, Easton DF. The BOADICEA model of genetic susceptibility to breast and ovarian cancer. Br J Cancer 2004; 91: 1580–90.
25. Simard J, Dumont M, Moisan AM, et al. Evaluation of BRCA1 and BRCA2 mutation prevalence, risk prediction models and a multistep testing approach in French-Canadian families with high risk of breast and ovarian cancer. J Med Genet 2007; 44: 107–21.
26. Miki Y, Swensen J, Shattuck-Eidens D, et al. A strong candidate for the breast and ovarian cancer gene BRCA1. Science 1994; 266: 66–71.
27. Wooster R, Bignell G, Lancaster J, et al. Identification of the breast cancer susceptibility gene BRCA2. Nature 1995; 378: 789–92.
28. Ford D, Easton M, Stratton S, et al. Genetic heterogeneity and penetrance analysis of the BRCA1 and BRCA2 genes in breast cancer families. Am J Hum Genet 1998; 62: 676–89.
29. Evans DGR, Young K, Bulman M, Shenton A, Lalloo F. Mutation testing for BRCA1/2 in ovarian cancer families: use of histology to predict status. Clin Genet 2008; 73: 338–45.
30. Easton DF, Ford D, Bishop DT. Breast and ovarian cancer incidence in BRCA1 mutation carriers. Am J Hum Genet 1994; 56: 265–71.
31. Gayther SA, Mangion J, Russell P. Variations of risks of breast and ovarian cancer associated with different germline mutations of the BRCA2 gene. Nat Genet 1997; 15: 103–5.
32. Evans DGR, Donnai D, Ribeiro G, Warrell D. Ovarian cancer family and prophylactic choices. J Med Genet 1992; 29: 416–18.
33. Steichen-Gersdorf E, Gallion HH, Ford D, et al. Familial site specific ovarian cancer is linked to BRCA1 on 17q12–21. Am J Hum Genet 1994; 55: 870–5.
34. Risch HA, McLaughlin JR, Cole DEC, et al. Prevalence and penetrance of germline BRCA1 and BRCA2 mutations in a population series of 649 women with ovarian cancer. Am J Hum Genet 2001; 68: 700–10.
35. Ramus SJ, Harrington PA, Pye C, et al. Contribution of BRCA1 and BRCA2 mutations to inherited ovarian cancer. Hum Mutat 2007; 28: 1207–15.
36. Evans DG, Shenton A, Woodward E, et al. Penetrance estimates for BRCA1 and BRCA2 based on genetic testing in a clinical cancer genetics service setting. BMC Cancer 2008; 8: 155.
37. Turnbull C, Ahmed S, Morrison J, et al. Genome-wide association study identifies five new breast cancer susceptibility loci. Nat Genet 2010; 42: 504–7.
38. Varley JM, Evans DGR, Birch JM. Li-Fraumeni syndrome -A molecular and clinical review. Br J Cancer 1997; 76: 1–14.
39. Evans DG, Moran A, Hartley R, et al. L long term outcomes of breast cancer in women aged 30 years or younger, based on family history, pathology and BRCA1/BRCA2/TP53 status. Br J Cancer 2010; 102: 1091–8.
40. Swift ML, Reitnauer PJ, Morrell D, Chase CL. Breast and other cancers in families with ataxia telangiectasia. N Engl J Med 1987; 316: 1289–94.
41. Renwick A, Thompson D, Seal S, et al. Breast Cancer Susceptibility Collaboration (UK). ATM mutations that cause ataxia-telangiectasia are breast cancer susceptibility alleles. Nat Genet 2006; 38: 873–5.
42. Savitsky K, Bar-Shira A, Gilad S, et al. A single ataxia telangectasia gene with a product similar to PI-3 kinase. Science 1995; 268: 1749–53.
43. Liaw D, Marsh DJ, Li J, et al. Germline mutations of the PTEN gene in Cowden disease, an inherited breast and thyroid cancer syndrome. Nat Genet 1997; 16: 64–7.
44. Seal S, Thompson D, Renwick A, et al. Truncating mutations in the Fanconi anemia J gene, BRIP1, are low penetrance breast cancer susceptibility alleles. Nat Genet 2006; 38: 1239–41.
45. Rahman N, Seal S, Thompson D, et al. PALB2 which encodes a BRCA2-interacting protein is a breast cancer susceptibility gene. Nat Genet 2007; 39: 165–7.
46. Meindl A, Hellebrand H, Wiek C, et al. Germline mutations in breast and ovarian cancer pedigrees establish RAD51C as a human cancer susceptibility gene. Nat Genet 2010; 42: 410–14.
47. Easton DF, Pooley KA, Dunning AM, et al. A genome-wide association study identifies multiple novel breast cancer susceptibility loci. Nature 2007; 447: 1087–93.
48. Powles TJ, Tillyer CR, Jones AL, et al. Prevention of breast cancer with tamoxifen an update on the royal marsden hospital pilot programme. Eur J Cancer 1990; 26: 680–4.
49. Fisher B, Constantino JP, Wickerham DL, et al. Tamoxifen for prevention of breast cancer: Report of the national surgical adjuvant breast and bowel project P-1 study. J Natl Cancer Inst 1998; 90: 1371–87.

50. Powles TJ, Eeles R, Ashley S, et al. Interim analysis of the incidence of breast cancer in the royal marsden hospital tamoxifen randomised chemoprevention trial. Lancet 1998; 352: 98–101.

51. Veronesi U, Maisonneuve P, Costa A, et al. Prevention of breast cancer with tamoxifen: preliminary findings from the Italian randomised trial among hysterectomised women. Lancet 1998; 352: 93–7.

52. IBIS Investigators. First results from the International Breast Cancer Intervention Study (IBIS-1): a randomised prevention trial. Lancet 2002; 360: 817–24.

53. Cuzick J, Powles T, Veronesi U, et al. Overview of the main outcomes in breast cancer prevention. Lancet 2003; 361: 296–300.

54. Cuzick J, Forbes JF, Sestak I, et al. International Breast Cancer Intervention Study I Investigators. Long-term results of tamoxifen prophylaxis for breast cancer–96-month follow-up of the randomized IBIS-I trial. J Natl Cancer Inst 2007; 99: 272–82.

55. Cuzick J, DeCensi A, Arun B, et al. Preventive therapy for breast cancer: a consensus statement. Lancet Oncol 2011; 12: 496–503.

56. Vogel VG, Constantinoi JP, Wicherham DL, et al. Effects of tamoxifen vs raloxifene on the risk of developing invasive breast cancer and other disease outcomes: the NSABP Study of Tamoxifen and Raloxifene (STAR) P-2 trial. JAMA 2006; 295: 2727–41.

57. Evans DG, Harvie M, Bundred N, Howell A. Uptake of breast cancer prevention and screening trials. J Med Genet 2010; 47: 853–5.

58. Rebbeck TR, Lynch HT, Neuhausen SL, et al. Reduction in cancer risk after bilateral prophylactic oophorectomy in BRCA1 and BRCA2 mutation carriers. N Engl J Med 2002; 346: 1616–22.

59. Tabar L, Faberberg G, Day NE, Holmberg L. What is the optimum interval between mammographic screening examinations? An analysis based on the Swedish two county breast cancer screening trial. Br J Cancer 1987; 56: 547–51.

60. Tabar L, Fagerberg G, Chen HH, et al. Efficacy of breast cancer screening by age. Cancer 1995; 75: 2507–17.

61. FH01 Collaborative Teams. Mammographic surveillance in women younger than 50 years who have a family history of breast cancer: tumour characteristics and projected effect on mortality in the prospective, single-arm, FH01 study. Lancet Oncol 2010; 11: 1127–34.

62. Report of the Coordinating Group for breast cancer screening, Falun meeting, Falun, Sweden. Breast screening with mammography in women 40–49 years. Int J Cancer 1996; 68: 693–9.

63. Lalloo F, Boggis CRM, Evans DGR, et al. Screening by mammography women with a family history of breast cancer. Eur J Cancer 1998; 34: 937–40.

64. Moller P, Borg A, Evans DG, et al. Survival in prospectively ascertained familial breast cancer: Analysis of a series stratified by tumour characteristics, BRCA mutations and oophorectomy. Int J Cancer 2002; 101: 555–9.

65. Maurice A, Evans DGR, Shenton A, et al. The Screening of women aged less than 50 years at increased risk of breast cancer by virtue of their family history. Eur J Cancer 2006; 42: 1385–90.

66. Leach MO, Boggis CR, Dixon AK, et al. MARIBS Study Group. Screening with magnetic resonance imaging and mammography of a UK population at high familial risk of breast cancer: a prospective multicentre cohort study (MARIBS). Lancet 2005; 365: 1769–78.

67. Kuhl CK, Schrading S, Leutner CC, et al. Mammography, breast ultrasound, and magnetic resonance imaging for surveillance of women at high familial risk for breast cancer. J Clin Oncol 2005; 23: 8469–76.

68. Warner E, Plewes DB, Hill KA, et al. Surveillance of BRCA1 and BRCA2 mutation carriers with magnetic resonance imaging, ultrasound, mammography, and clinical breast examination. JAMA 2004; 292: 1317–25.

69. Kriege M, Brekelmans CT, Boetes C, et al. Efficacy of MRI and mammography for breast-cancer screening in women with a familial or genetic predisposition. N Engl J Med 2004; 351: 427–37.

70. McIntosh A, Shaw C, Evans G, et al. (2006) Clinical Guidelines and Evidence Review for The Classification and Care of Women at Risk of Familial Breast Cancer, London: National Collaborating Centre for Primary Care/University of Sheffield. NICE guideline CG041. www.nice.org.uk update of CG014 2004.

71. Law J. Cancers detected and induced in mammographic screening: new sceeening schedules and younger women with family history. Br J Radiol 1997; 70: 60–62.

72. Andrieu N, Easton DF, Chang-Claude J, et al. Effect of chest X-rays on the risk of breast cancer among BRCA1/2 mutation carriers in the IBCCS Study. J Clin Oncol 2006; 24: 3361–6.

73. Moller P, Evans G, Maehle L, Lalloo F, Heimdal KR. Use of cytology to diagnose hereditary breast cancer. Dis Markers 1999; 15: 212–16.

74. Hartmann LC, Schaid DJ, Woods JE, et al. Efficacy of bilateral prophylactic mastectomy in women with a family history of breast cancer. N Engl J Med 1999; 340: 77–8.

75. Goodnight JE, Quagliani JM, Morton DL. Failure of subcutaneous mastectomy to prevent the development of breast cancer. J Surg Oncol 1984; 26: 198–201.

76. Meijers-Heijboer EJ, van Geel B, van Putten WLJ, et al. Breast cancer after prophylactic bilateral mastectomy in women with a BRCA1 or BRCA2 mutation. N Engl J Med 2001; 345: 159–64.

77. Evans DGR, Baildam AD, Anderson E, et al. Risk reducing mastectomy: outcomes in 10 European centres. J Med Genet 2009; 46: 54–8.

78. Hatcher MB, Falowfield L, A'Hern B. The psychosocial impact of bilateral prophylactic mastectomy: prospective study using questionnaires and semistructured interviews. Br Med J 2001; 322: 1–7.

79. Lalloo F, Baildam A, Brain A, et al. Preventative mastectomy for women at high risk of breast cancer. Eur J Surg Oncol 2000; 26: 711–13.

80. Meijers-Heijboer EJ, Verhoog LC, Brekelmans CTM, et al. Presymptomatic DNA testing and prophylactic surgery in families with a BRCA1 or BRCA2 mutation. Lancet 2000; 355: 2015–20.

81. Evans DG, Lalloo F, Ashcroft L, et al. Uptake of risk reducing surgery in unaffected women at high risk of breast and ovarian cancer is risk, age and time dependent. Cancer Epidemiol Biomarkers Prev 2009; 18: 2318–24.

82. Fitzgerald MG, MacDonald DJ, Krainer M, et al. Germ-line BRCA1 mutations in Jewish and non-Jewish women with early onset breast cancer. N Engl J Med 1996; 334: 143–9.

83. Langston AA, Malone KE, Thompson JD, et al. BRCA1 mutations in a popu lation based sample of young women with breast cancer. N Engl J Med 1996; 334: 137–42.

84. Stratton J, Gayther SA, Russell P, et al. Contribution of BRCA1 mutations to ovarian cancer. N Engl J Med 1997; 336: 1125–30.

85. Thorlacius S, Olafsdottir G, Tryggvadottir L, et al. A single BRCA2 mutation in male and female breast cancer families from Iceland with varied cancer phenotypes. Nat Genet 1996; 13: 117–19.

86. Tonin P, Weber B, Proffit K, et al. Frequency of recurrent BRCA1 and BRCA2 mutations in the Ashkenazi Jewish breast cancer families. Nat Med 1996; ll: 1179–83.

87. Lalloo F, Cochrane S, Bulman B, et al. An evaluation of common breast cancer mutations within a population of Ashkenazi Jews. J Med Genet 1998; 35: 10–12.

88. Watson M, Murday V, Lloyd S, et al. Genetic testing in breast/ovarian cancer (BRCA1)families. Lancet 1995; 346: 583.

89. Lerman C, Narod S, Schulman K, et al. BRCA1 testing in families with hereditary breast ovarian cancer. A prospective study of patient decision making and outcomes. JAMA 1996; 275: 1928–9.

90. Evans DGR, Binchy A, Shenton A, Hopwood P, Craufurd D. Ten year follow up study of predictive testing for BRCA1 in five large BRCA1 linked families. Clin Genet 2009; 75: 124–32.

91. Lerman C, Daly M, Masny A, Bashem A. Attitudes about genetic testing for breast ovarian cancer susceptibility. J Clin Oncol 1994; 12: 843–50.

92. Mohammed S, Barnes C, Watts S, Michie S, Hodgson S. Attitudes to predictive testing for BRCAI. J Med Genet 1995; 32: 140A.

93. Brooks L, Lennard F, Shenton A, et al. BRCA1/2 predictive testing: a study of uptake in two centres. Eur J Hum Genet 2004; 12: 654–62.

94. Evans DG, Lalloo F, Cramer A, et al. Addition of pathology and biomarker information significantly improves the performance of the Manchester scoring system for BRCA1 and BRCA2 testing. J Med Genet 2009; 46: 811–17.

95. Antoniou AC, Hardy R, Walker L, et al. Predicting the likelihood of carrying a BRCA1 or BRCA2 mutation: validation of BOADICEA, BRCAPRO, IBIS, Myriad and the Manchester scoring system using data from UK genetics clinics. J Med Genet 2008; 45: 425–31.

96. Amir E, Freedman OC, Seruga B, Evans DG. Assessing women at high risk of breast cancer: a review of risk assessment models. J Natl Cancer Inst 2010; 102: 680–91.

4 Application of new genomic technologies to breast cancer risk assessment

Mark Robson

INTRODUCTION

Genetic factors significantly influence the risk of breast cancer. A family history of breast cancer is well known to be one of the most important risk factors for the disease. Numerous studies have shown that women with an affected first-degree relative are at approximately twofold increased risk, and that risk increases with increasing numbers of affected relatives, as well as with decreasing age at diagnosis among those relatives (1). Linkage studies and candidate gene studies have defined several genes that confer an increased risk for cancer when mutated in the germline. These are well-described in a previous chapter (chap. 3 Genetic Predisposition and Breast Screening). Broadly speaking, these genes can be classified as high- or moderate-penetrance genes. High-penetrance genes, such as *BRCA1* and *BRCA2*, are rare (population heterozygote prevalence <0.1%) and confer up to 10-fold increased risk for breast cancer. These genes are responsible for autosomally dominant breast cancer predisposition syndromes. Moderate-penetrance genes, such as *BRIP1* and *PALB2*, are also rare. Mutations in these genes are generally associated with relative risks of 2–3, similar to that resulting from a family history of breast cancer. However, because of incomplete penetrance, families transmitting mutations in these genes may not manifest a pattern of breast cancer diagnoses that suggests an inherited predisposition. Mutations in some genes, such as *CHEK2*, appear to confer higher relative risks in familial than in unselected ascertainments, suggesting that other loci exist which modify the risk that results from the mutation.

Although mutations in high- and moderate-penetrance genes are clearly associated with breast cancer risk, they are too rare to explain the *heritability* of breast cancer. Heritability can be defined as the proportion of variance in risk that can be explained by genetic factors. One way of calculating heritability is by comparing the risk of a disease in monozygotic and dizygotic twins of an affected individual. Lichtenstein et al. performed a classic study of over 44,000 pairs of twins in Scandinavia, of which 9512 pairs included at least one individual diagnosed with cancer. For breast cancer, they calculated a relative risk of 5.2 for sisters in monozygotic twin pairs, versus 2.8 in dizygotic twins (2). In this analysis, the heritability of breast cancer was 27% (95% CI 4–41%). This degree of variance is clearly not explained by known mutations.

GENOME-WIDE ASSOCIATION STUDIES

After publication of the first human genome sequence, investigators began to catalog the extent of normal human genetic variation through collaborations such as the International HapMap project and, subsequently, the 1000 Genomes project (3,4). One of the most remarkable findings of these efforts has been the sheer degree of inter-individual variation among humans. The HapMap project, for example, has delineated over 3.1 million loci where there are single nucleotide variants with minor allele frequencies of greater than 5% (4). The investigators estimate that these single nucleotide polymorphisms (SNPs) constitute only 25–30% of the common variants in the human genome. However, because of linkage disequilibrium, most of the remainder of the common variants are strongly correlated with the HapMap SNPs and can be *imputed* from them.

Since the genetic contribution to variance in the risk of breast cancer cannot be explained by mutations in known susceptibility genes, a number of investigators reasoned that common variants could be responsible (the *common disease–common variant hypothesis*). The development of technologies that rapidly genotype large numbers of individuals at large numbers of loci gave rise to the era of genome-wide association studies (GWAS) that were intended to test this hypothesis and define the responsible variants. GWAS are essentially case–control studies that compare the frequencies of hundred of thousands to millions of different genetic variants in affected and unaffected individuals (5). The approach has proven to be enormously successful, and as of the second quarter of 2011 there were 1449 published associations for 237 traits, including breast cancer (http://www.genome.gov/gwastudies/; accessed April 14, 2012). Nonetheless, there are significant limitations to GWAS. First, the number of comparisons requires a high level of stringency in reporting statistical significance, to avoid false discovery. For discovery studies, a P value for comparison of 10^{-7} or greater is usually required (6), and even at this level a number of loci that are significant in the first stage of a study do not replicate in subsequent validation phases. There are two implications of this. The first is that a number of loci that do influence risk may fail to rise to the level of significance required, and thus be missed. The second is that the loci that are identified may have associated odds ratios that are at the higher end of their actual effect sizes. This phenomenon is known as "the winner's curse," and has implications for the use of published odds ratios in risk prediction models. Another limitation of GWAS is that they are not able to identify associations with rare variants (minor allele frequencies less than 5%), even with large numbers of cases and controls. This has implications for the problem of "missing heritability," to be discussed later. Third, it appears that the variants discovered through GWAS are not, in most cases, the causal variants that are actually responsible for the increase in risk. In fact, the exploration of mechanisms by which common variants influence risk remains an active, and challenging, field of study (7).

GENOME-WIDE ASSOCIATION STUDIES IN BREAST CANCER

A number of consortia have reported GWAS that seek to define the genetic architecture of common breast cancer susceptibility. The main results of these studies are presented in Table 4.1 and described in the following text. Broadly speaking, the studies can be categorized as discovery or validation studies, with a subset of more recent studies directed toward defining differential associations with different breast cancer subtypes. The discovery sets are described in more detail later.

Easton et al. reported the first breast cancer GWAS in 2007 (8). In the first stage, they genotyped 408 United Kingdom (UK) familial breast cancer cases and 400 controls at 266,722 loci. After excluding genotyping failures, the final analysis included 390 cases and 364 controls typed at 205,586 loci. The 12,711 SNPs that were most significantly different between cases and control were then analyzed in a second stage of 3990 different UK breast cancer cases and 3916 controls, with 10,405 SNPs being considered in the final analysis. Combining stage I and stage II, a single SNP (rs2981582) reached genome-wide significance. In a third stage, the top 30 SNPs from stage I and II were evaluated in a combined ascertainment of 22 case–control studies, consisting of 21,860 cases of invasive breast cancer, 988 cases of carcinoma in situ, and 22,578 controls. Six SNPs reached a significance level of 10^{-5} in this third stage, all of which reached 10^{-7} in a combined analysis of all three stages. Five of the six most significant SNPs are within genes or within blocks of genes that contain linkage disequilibrium. One SNP, however, lies in a "gene desert" in 8q24 where there are no known genes. Presumably, the causative variant in this area has an influence on the regulation of a gene or genes important in breast cancer development. Indeed, the region may be of more general relevance to carcinogenesis, since SNPs in the same region have been associated with increased risks at other cancer sites (9). The most significant SNP, rs2981582, is within the *FGFR2* gene, which had not been associated with breast cancer before this study.

Hunter et al. reported in 2007 the results of a GWAS that used 1183 women from the Nurses' Health Study cohort with postmenopausal breast cancer and 1185 matched controls, all of whom were of self-described European ancestry (10). These women were genotyped at 528,173 SNPs. Six SNPs were significantly different between cases and controls at P values of less than 10^{-5}. Two of these (rs1219648 and rs2420946) are also within the *FGFR2* gene, and are tightly correlated with the rs2981582 SNP described by Easton (r2 = 1.0). The most significant stage I SNPs were evaluated in a second stage analysis comprised of 1176 cases and 2072 controls taken from within three different cohort studies. Although rs1219648 was highly significantly correlated with case status (P values of the order 10^{-10}), the value was lower than required to declare significance using a conservative Bonferroni correction.

Also in 2007, Stacey et al. described the results of a GWAS that studied 1600 Icelandic individuals with breast cancer and 11,563 controls in the discovery phase, genotyping 311,524 SNPs in stage I (11). SNPs from the 10 most significant loci were then analyzed in replication sets from Iceland, Europe,

and European-Americans from the United States. Two SNPs (rs13387042, 2q35 and rs3803662, 16q12) showed significant associations in all analyses. This study was particularly significant as it was the first to note that these variants were associated with estrogen receptor (ER) positive breast cancer, but not ER negative cancer, suggesting that the influence of common variants on breast cancer risk could be subtype specific. A follow-up analysis from the Breast Cancer Association Consortium, however, found that rs13387042 was associated with increased risks of both ER-positive and ER-negative breast cancer (12). Stacey et al. also noted a signal from an SNP in the 5q12 which did not reach genome-wide significance in their replication phases, but that was also somewhat correlated in GWAS from other groups. In a follow-up analysis of 5028 cases and 32,090 controls of European ancestry, the relevance of 5p12 SNPs rs4415084 and rs10941679 was demonstrated more definitively (13). Again, the association was confined to ER-positive breast cancer. In fact, a follow-up study by the Breast Cancer Association Consortium suggested that the association was largely with progesterone receptor positive cancers, with a stronger association with lower grade tumors (14). In this analysis, the group also evaluated the subtype specificity of rs1219648 in *FGFR2* and found that the risk of this SNP was also confined to ER-positive cancer.

Gold et al. performed a GWAS in 249 non-*BRCA* mutation carrying familial breast cancer cases and 299 controls (all of Ashkenazi Jewish ancestry), in an attempt to reduce bias that could be introduced into GWAS by unrecognized population substratification (15). The investigators analyzed the top 343 SNPs in two separate replication sets of Ashkenazi cases and controls. As with the previous GWAS, the *FGFR2* locus was significantly associated (rs1078806), although other loci from previous studies were not. This group also identified a second locus on 6q22 (*ECHDC1; RNF146*). This SNP did not replicate in a later study (16).

In 2009, Zheng et al. reported the first GWAS in a non-European population, analyzing 1505 Chinese women with breast cancer and 1522 controls in stage I, followed by replication of the top 29 SNPs in an independent set of 1554 cases and 1576 controls and then third stage of 3472 cases and 900 controls (17). One SNP was consistently associated across all three stages, rs2046210 at 6q25, close to *ESR1/C6orf97*. The SNP was associated with increased risks of both ER-positive and ER-negative breast cancer, and was also associated with risk (*albeit* less strongly) in a small replication cohort of United States (US) women of European ancestry.

Also in 2009, Thomas et al. described a follow-up study exploring a larger number of SNPs from the original NCI Cancer Genetic Markers of Susceptibility initiative reported by Hunter et al. in 2007 (18). In this follow-on study, 30,278 SNPs from stage I were evaluated in an additional 4434 cases and 4547 controls from a number of prospective US studies, and the top 24 SNPs from stage II were studied in another 5223 cases and 4078 controls. This study confirmed the significance of loci identified in preceding studies, including 5p12, and also identified two new regions of interest at 1p11 (rs11249433) and 14q24 (rs999737, *RAD51L*). These new regions were subsequently replicated in a large study from the Breast Cancer Association Consortium (19), which also indicated that the 1p11 association was stronger for ER-positive cancers,

Table 4.1 Results of Genome-Wide Association Studies in Breast Cancer

Paper	Type	Discovery Population	SNP	Gene	Position	OR per-allele	HetOR	HomOR
Easton 2007 (8)	Discovery	UK	rs2981582	FGFR2	10q26	1.26 (1.23–1.30)	1.23 (1.18–1.28)	1.63 (1.53–1.72)
Easton 2007 (8)	Discovery	UK	rs12443621	TNRC9/TOX3	16q12	1.11 (1.08–1.140)	1.14 (1.09–1.20)	1.23 (1.17–1.30)
Easton 2007 (8)	Discovery	UK	rs8051542	TNRC9/TOX3	16q12	1.09 (1.06–1.13)	1.10 (1.05–1.16)	1.19 (1.12–1.27)
Easton 2007 (8)	Discovery	UK	rs889312	MAP3K1/MEKK	5q	1.13 (1.10–1.16)	1.13 (1.09–1.18)	1.27 (1.19–1.36)
Easton 2007 (8)	Discovery	UK	rs3817198	LSP1	11p	1.07 (1.04–1.11)	1.06 (1.02–1.11)	1.17 (1.08–1.25)
Easton 2007 (8)	Discovery	UK	rs13281615	None	8q	1.08 (1.05–1.11)	1.06 (1.01–1.11)	1.18 (1.10–1.25)
Hunter 2007 (10)	Discovery	US (European)	rs2420946	FGFR2	10q26	1.32 (1.17–1.49)	1.24 (1.03–1.50)	1.79 (1.40–2.28)
Hunter 2007 (10)	Discovery	US (European)	rs10510126	None	10q	0.62 (0.51–0.75)	0.59 (0.48–0.72)	0.59 (0.26–1.34)
Hunter 2007 (10)	Discovery	US (European)	rs12505080	None	4p	0.93 (0.81–1.06)	1.22 (1.02–1.45)	0.51 (0.35–0.73)
Hunter 2007 (10)	Discovery	US (European)	rs17157903	RELN	7q	1.35 (1.14–1.600)	1.60 (1.31–195)	0.77 (0.42–1.41)
Hunter 2007 (10)	Discovery	US (European)	rs1219648	FGFR2	10q26	1.32 (1.17–1.49)	1.23 (1.04–1.48)	1.79 (1.41–2.28)
Hunter 2007 (10)	Discovery	US (European)	rs7696175	TLR1/TLR6	4p	0.98 (0.87–1.10)	1.39 (1.15–1.58)	0.86 (0.67–1.09)
Stacey 2007 (11)	Discovery	Iceland	rs13387042	None	2q35	1.20 (1.14–1.26)		
Stacey 2007 (11)	Discovery	Iceland	rs3803662	TNRC9/TOX3	16q12	1.28 (1.21–1.35)		
Gold 2008 (15)	Discovery	US (Ashkenazi)	rs2180341	ECHDC1; RNF146	6q22	1.41 (1.25–1.59)	1.53 (1.32–1.77)	1.51 (1.10–2.08)
Gold 2008 (15)	Discovery	US (Ashkenazi)	rs1078806	FGFR2	10q	1.26 (1.13–1.40)	1.32 (1.13–1.54)	1.40 (1.16–1.69)
Stacey 2008 (13)	Discovery	European ancestry	rs4415084	MRPS30	5p12	1.16 (1.10–1.21)		
Stacey 2008 (13)	Discovery	European ancestry	rs10941679	MRPS30	5p12	1.19 (1.13–1.26)		
Zheng 2009 (17)	Discovery	Chinese	rs2046210	ESR1/C6orf97	6q	1.29 (1.21–1.37)		
Milne 2009 (12)	Replication	European and Asian	rs13387042	None	2q35	1.13 (1.11–1.16)	1.09 (1.05–1.3)	1.28 (1.22–1.34)
Thomas 2009 (18)	Replication	US (European)	rs2981579	FGFR2	10q26		1.17 (1.07–1.27)	1.46 (1.30–1.62)
Thomas 2009 (18)	Replication	US (European)	rs3803662	TNRC9/TOX3	16q12		1.16 (1.07–1.27)	1.55 (1.34–1.78)
Thomas 2009 (18)	Replication	US (European)	rs16886165	MAP3K1/MEKK	5q		1.23 (1.12–1.35)	1.65 (1.30–2.10)
Thomas 2009 (18)	Replication	US (European)	rs1562430	None	8q		0.84 (0.77–0.92)	0.79 (0.71–0.89)
Thomas 2009 (18)	Replication	US (European)	rs13387042	None	2q35		0.80 (0.73–0.87)	0.74 (0.67–0.83)
Thomas 2009 (18)	Replication	US (European)	rs3817198	LSP1	11p		1.02 (0.96–1.08)	1.12 (1.02–1.23)
Thomas 2009 (18)	Replication	US (European)	rs4415084	MRPS30	5p12		1.09 (1.03–1.17)	1.20 (1.11–1.31)
Thomas 2009 (18)	Replication	US (European)	rs10941679	MRPS30	5p12		1.12 (1.03–1.22)	1.20 (1.03–1.41)
Thomas 2009 (18)	Discovery	US (European)	rs11249433	None	1p11		1.16 (1.09–1.24)	1.30 (1.19–1.41)
Thomas 2009 (18)	Discovery	US (European)	rs999737	RAD51L	14q24		0.94 (0.88–0.59)	0.70 (0.62–0.80)
Thomas 2009 (18)	Discovery	US (European)	rs7716600	MRPS30	5p12		1.10 (1.04–1.17)	1.28 (1.13–1.45)
Thomas 2009 (18)	Discovery	US (European)	rs2067980	MRPS30	5p12		1.08 (1.02–1.15)	1.29 (1.09–1.52)
Ahmed 2009 (20)	Discovery	European and Asian	rs4973768	SLC4A7/NEK10	3p24	1.11 (1.08–1.13)	1.12 (1.08–1.17)	1.23 (1.17–1.29)
Ahmed 2009 (20)	Discovery	European and Asian	rs6504950	COX11/STXBP4	17q23	0.95 (0.92–0.97)	0.96 (0.92–0.99)	0.89 (0.83–0.95)
Turnbull 2010 (21)	Replication	UK	rs2981579	FGFR2	10q26	1.43 (1.35–1.53)		
Turnbull 2010 (21)	Replication	UK	rs3803662	TNRC9/TOX3	16q12	1.30 (1.22–1.39)		
Turnbull 2010 (21)	Replication	UK	rs889312	MAP3K1/MEKK	5q	1.22 (1.14–1.30)		
Turnbull 2010 (21)	Replication	UK	rs1562430 (r2 0.42 with rs13281615)	none	8q24	1.17 (1.10–1.25)		
Turnbull 2010 (21)	Replication	UK	rs13387042	none	2q35	1.21 (1.14–1.29)		
Turnbull 2010 (21)	Replication	UK	rs909116 (r2 0.23 with rs3817198)	LSP1	11p	1.17 (1.10–1.24)		

(Continued)

Table 4.1 Results of Genome-Wide Association Studies in Breast Cancer (*Continued*)

Paper	Type	Discovery Population	SNP	Gene	Position	OR per-allele	HetOR	HomOR
Turnbull 2010 (21)	Replication	UK	rs3757318 (r2 0.088 with rs2046210)	ESR1/C6orf97	6q25	1.30 (1.17–1.46)		
Turnbull 2010 (21)	Replication	UK	rs4973768	SLC4A7/NEK10	3p24	1.16 (1.10–1.24)		
Turnbull 2010 (21)	Replication	UK	rs1156287 (r2 0.91 with rs6504950)	COX11/STXBP4	17q23	0.91 (0.85–0.97)		
Turnbull 2010 (21)	Replication	UK	rs8009944 (r2 0.13 with rs999737)	RAD51L	14q24	0.88 (0.82–0.95)		
Turnbull 2010 (21)	Replication	UK	rs11249433	NOTCH2	1p11.2	1.08 (1.02–1.15)		
Turnbull 2010 (21)	Replication	UK	rs10931936 (r2 0.08 with rs1045485)	CASP8	2	0.88 (0.82–0.94)		
Turnbull 2010 (21)	Discovery	UK	rs1011970	CDKN2A/B	9p21	1.20 (1.11–1.30)	1.19 (1.08–1.31)	1.45 (1.13–1.86)
Turnbull 2010 (21)	Discovery	UK	rs614367	none	11q13	1.15 (1.10–1.20)	1.16 (1.10–1.23)	1.27 (1.10–1.47)
Turnbull 2010 (21)	Discovery	UK	rs10995190	ZNF365	10q21	0.76 (0.70–0.84)	0.77 (0.69–0.86)	0.55 (0.40–0.77)
Turnbull 2010 (21)	Discovery	UK	rs2380205	ANKRD16/FBXO18	10	0.94 (0.91–0.98)	0.95 (0.90–1.01)	0.89 (0.82–0.95)
Turnbull 2010 (21)	Discovery	UK	rs704010	ZMIZ1	10q22	1.07 (1.03–1.11)	1.11 (1.05–1.17)	1.13 (1.04–1.21)
Antoniou 2010 (23)	Discovery	UK (ER negative)	rs8170	MERIT 40	19p13	1.21 (1.07–1.37)		
Antoniou 2010 (23)	Discovery	UK (ER negative)	rs2363956	MERIT 40	19p13	0.83 (0.75–0.920)		
Cai 2011 (29)	Discovery	Asian	rs10822013	ZNF365	10q21		1.12 (1.06–1.18)	1.21 (1.13–1.29)
Fletcher 2011 (26)	Replication	UK	rs13387042	None	2q35	0.86 (0.82–0.90)	0.83 (0.77–0.90)	0.75 (0.68–0.82)
Fletcher 2011 (26)	Replication	UK	rs4973768	SLC4A7/NEK10	3p24	1.14 (1.09–1.19)	1.17 (1.08–1.26)	1.29 (1.18–1.42)
Fletcher 2011 (26)	Replication	UK	rs4415084	MRPS30	5p12	1.17 (1.11–1.22)	1.23 (1.14–1.32)	1.33 (1.21–1.47)
Fletcher 2011 (26)	Replication	UK	rs6900157 (r2 0.92 with rs2046210)	ESR1/C6orf97	6q25	1.13 (1.05–1.22)	1.14 (1.03–1.27)	1.28 (1.09–1.50)
Fletcher 2011 (26)	Replication	UK	rs1562430 (r2 0.42 with rs13281615)	None	8q24	0.86 (0.82–0.90)	0.84 (0.78–0.90)	0.74 (0.67–0.81)
Fletcher 2011 (26)	Replication	UK	rs1219648	FGFR2	10q26	1.31 (1.25–1.37)	1.31 (1.24–1.39)	1.72 (1.60–1.86)
Fletcher 2011 (26)	Replication	UK	rs999737	RAD51L	14q24	0.89 (0.82–0.97)	0.94 (0.85–1.05)	0.69 (0.55–0.87)
Fletcher 2011 (26)	Replication	UK	rs4783780 (r2 0.97 with rs12443621)	TNRC9/TOX3	16q12	1.16 (1.10–1.21)	1.14 (1.06–1.23)	1.34 (1.22–1.46)
Fletcher 2011 (26)	Discovery	UK	rs865686	None	9q31	0.89 (0.85–0.92)	0.90 (0.86–0.96)	0.77 (0.71–0.84)
Fletcher 2011 (26)	Discovery	UK	rs9393938	ESR1	6q25	1.18 (1.11–1.26)	1.18 (1.10–1.27)	1.40 (1.07–1.83)
Fletcher 2011 (26)	Discovery	UK	rs3734805	ESR1	6q25	1.19 (1.11–1.27)	1.20 (1.12–1.29)	1.31 (0.99–1.73)
Figueroa 2011 (19)	Replication	European and Asian	rs999737	RAD51L	14q24	0.92 (0.90–0.94)		
Figueroa 2011 (19)	Replication	European and Asian	rs11249433	NOTCH2	1p11.2	1.10 (1.07–1.12)		
Milne 2011 (14)	Replication	European and Asian	rs10941679	MRPS30	5p12	1.11 (1.08–1.14)		
Campa 2011 (16)	Replication	US (European)	rs11249433	NOTCH2	1p11.2	1.09 (1.05–1.14)	1.10 (1.03–1.18)	1.19 (1.09–1.30)
Campa 2011 (16)	Replication	US (European)	rs1045485	CASP8	2	0.91 (0.85–0.97)	0.91 (0.85–0.98)	0.79 (0.62–1.00)

(*Continued*)

Table 4.1 Results of Genome-Wide Association Studies in Breast Cancer (*Continued*)

Paper	Type	Discovery Population	SNP	Gene	Position	OR per-allele	HetOR	HomOR
Campa 2011 (16)	Replication	US (European)	rs13387042	none	2q35	0.85 (0.81–0.88)	0.78 (0.67–0.79)	0.73 (0.67–0.79)
Campa 2011 (16)	Replication	US (European)	rs4973768	SLC4A7/NEK10	3p24	1.08 (1.04–1.13)	1.07 (1.00–1.14)	1.17 (1.08–1.27)
Campa 2011 (16)	Replication	US (European)	rs4415084	MRPS30	5p12	1.08 (1.03–1.12)	1.14 (1.07–1.22)	1.14 (1.05–1.24)
Campa 2011 (16)	Replication	US (European)	rs10941679	MRPS30	5p12	1.12 (1.07–1.17)	1.13 (1.06–1.20)	1.25 (1.12–1.39)
Campa 2011 (16)	Replication	US (European)	rs889312	MAP3K1/MEKK	5q	1.10 (1.05–1.15)	1.09 (1.03–1.16)	1.23 (1.11–1.36)
Campa 2011 (16)	Replication	US (European)	rs2046210	ESR1/C6orf97	6q25	1.10 (1.05–1.15)	1.11 (1.04–1.18)	1.20 (1.10–1.31)
Campa 2011 (16)	Replication	US (European)	rs13281615	none	8q24	1.09 (1.05–1.13)	1.09 (1.02–1.16)	1.19 (1.09–1.29)
Campa 2011 (16)	Replication	US (European)	rs3750817	FGFR2	10q26	0.86 (0.82–0.90)	0.85 (0.79–0.91)	0.74 (0.67–0.81)
Campa 2011 (16)	Replication	US (European)	rs2981582	FGFR2	10q26	1.21 (1.16–1.26)	1.16 (1.09–1.24)	1.48 (1.36–1.61)
Campa 2011 (16)	Replication	US (European)	rs999737	RAD51L	14q24	0.91 (0.86–0.95)	0.93 (0.87–0.99)	0.77 (0.67–0.89)
Campa 2011 (16)	Replication	US (European)	rs3803662	TNRC9/TOX3	16q12	1.16 (1.11–1.21)	1.14 (1.07–1.21)	1.38 (1.25–1.52)
Campa 2011 (16)	Replication	US (European)	rs6504950	COX11/STXBP4	17q23	0.92 (0.88–0.97)	0.92 (0.87–0.98)	0.85 (0.76–0.96)
Haiman 2011 (25)	Discovery	African, European (ER negative)	rs10069690	TERT-CLPTM1L	5p15	1.18 (1.13–1.25)	1.15 (1.06–1.23)	1.46 (1.29–1.64)
Ghoussaini 2012 (28)	Discovery	European, Asian	rs10771399	PTHLH/PTHrP	12p11	0.85 (0.83–0.88)		
Ghoussaini 2012 (28)	Discovery	European, Asian	rs1292011	None	12q24	0.92 (0.91–0.94)		
Ghoussaini 2012 (28)	Discovery	European, Asian	rs2823093	None	21q21	0.94 (0.92–0.96)		
Long 2012 (30)	Discovery	Asian	rs9485372	TAB2	6q25	0.90 (0.87–0.92)	0.89 (0.85–0.94)	0.80 (0.75–0.86)
Long 2012 (30)	Discovery	Asian	rs9383591	ESR1	6q25	0.88 (0.84–0.93)		
Long 2012 (30)	Discovery	Asian	rs7107217	None	11q24	1.08 (1.05–1.11)		
Stevens 2012 (24)	Replication	European and Asian	rs8170	MERIT 40	19p13.1	1.22 (1.13–1.31) "Triple negative"		
Lambrechts 2012 (22)	Replication	European and Asian	rs1011970	CDKN2A/B	9p21	1.08 (1.05–1.11)		
Lambrechts 2012 (22)	Replication	European and Asian	rs10995190	ZNF365	10q21	0.88 (0.85–0.90)		
Lambrechts 2012 (22)	Replication	European and Asian	rs704010	ZMIZ1	10q22	1.07 (1.05–1.10)		
Lambrechts 2012 (22)	Replication	European and Asian	rs614367	None	11q13	1.21 (1.17–1.24)		

particularly of lobular histology and lower grade. The 14q24 SNP was associated with all tumor types, including "triple negative" breast cancer.

By this time, it was clear that the effect sizes associated with most common variants were very small, and that it would require large validation sets to confirm or refute the significance of weaker signals identified in the first stage of GWAS. To this end, Ahmed et al. reported in 2009 a deeper exploration of the first breast cancer GWAS reported in 2007 by Easton et al. and the Breast Cancer Association Consortium (20). A group of 814 SNPs from the first two stages of the original GWAS were studied in a third stage of 3878 cases and 3928 controls. The three SNPs that were significant at $P < 10^{-5}$ were then evaluated in a fourth replication stage of 36,141 controls and 33,134 cases. Two of these SNPs (rs4973768 and rs6504950) replicated in stage 4, but a third SNP did not, despite "surviving" three stages of analysis (underscoring the risk of false discovery even with stringent statistical correction for multiple comparisons). Stage 4 of this large study included a significant number of Asian cases and controls, allowing cross-ethnicity comparisons of effect. For both of the new SNPs, the effects in Europeans and Asians appeared similar.

In a further effort to increase sample size and thus power to detect associations, Turnball and colleagues conducted a new GWAS, genotyping 582,886 SNPs in 3659 cases of familial breast cancer and 4897 controls (21). The most significant associations from stage I were evaluated in an additional 12,576 cases and 12,223 controls. There was confirmatory evidence of association for previously reported loci, although only 7 of 12 reached a significance level of $P < 10^{-4}$. The calculated odds ratios were generally higher than in the previous population-based studies, consistent with the hypothesis that the effects of risk alleles will be greater in women with a family history of disease. Another 15 SNPs outside of previously reported regions were taken to stage 2, and six of these replicated at appropriate levels of significance. Two of these SNPs were highly correlated, so this effort led to the identification of five new regions, one on chromosome 9 (linked to *CDKN2A* and *CDKN2B*), three on chromosome 10, and one on chromosome 11. Four of these SNPs were replicated by the Breast Cancer Association Consortium (rs1011970, 9p21; rs10995190, 10q21; rs704010, 10q22; rs614367, 11q13) (22). The 11q13 locus appeared to be exclusively associated with hormone receptor–positive cancer. None of these variants replicated in the Asian studies of the Breast Cancer Association Consortium, but both sample size and minor allele frequencies were too low to confidently exclude an effect.

The search for common variants modifying risk in *BRCA1* and *BRCA2* mutation carriers could be expected to reveal loci that would confer susceptibility in the general population. A publication by Antoniou et al. and the Consortium for Investigation of Modifiers of BRCA (CIMBA) confirmed this hypothesis when a group of SNPs delineating a locus on 19p13 was found to modify risk in *BRCA1* mutation carriers (whose breast cancer is most commonly ER negative) and to be associated with risk of ER-negative disease in the general population (23). In fact, two SNPs (rs8170 and rs2363956) seemed to be independently associated, with the strength of association being strongest for "triple negative" breast cancer. In fact, a follow-up analysis by the Breast Cancer Association

Consortium found that rs8170 was only associated with an increased risk for triple negative disease, and that the association with ER-negative disease was lost once "triple negative" cases were excluded (24). These SNPs were not significant in unselected sporadic breast cancer cases, further demonstrating the relevance of tumor subtyping and supporting the hypothesis of differing susceptibility loci for different subtypes.

The 19p13 locus was the first found to be specifically associated with ER-negative breast cancer. Previously identified loci increased the risk of either ER-positive and ER-negative disease or ER-positive disease alone. In part, this may have been because previous discovery studies of unselected breast cancer cases were comprised of subjects who mostly had ER positive disease, consistent with the distribution of ER expression in sporadic breast cancer. To further explore the genetic architecture of susceptibility to ER negative disease, Haiman et al. performed a GWAS of women with ER negative disease of either African (1004 cases and 2745 controls) or European (1718 cases and 2745 controls) ancestry (25). Stage 2 replication was conducted in 2292 cases and 16,901 controls of European ancestry. The methodology for this study was slightly different from the previous one in that results from GWAS performed previously (on different platforms) were combined and, for one component of the analysis, publicly available control data were used. Only 1 SNP (rs10069690, *TERT-CLPTM1L*) reached genome-wide significance in the combined results. This locus appeared to be particularly associated with "triple negative" disease, similar to the observation with the 19p13 locus.

In 2011, Fletcher et al. reported the results of a GWAS in which the discovery stage was conducted on an ascertainment of UK women, most of whom had experienced two primary breast cancers or had a family history of the disease (26). Stage 1 data were combined with publicly available data from NCI Cancer Genetic Markers of Susceptibility. Stage I genotyping analyzed 300,298 SNPs, after quality control exclusions. Stage 2 and 3 replications were performed on two different ascertainments of sporadic UK breast cancer patients. In addition to replicating previously reported loci, this study identified a new locus on 9q31.2 (rs865686). In addition, there was a strong suggestion of association at 6q25.1, although the most associated SNP (rs9383938) is only weakly correlated with the SNP reported by Zheng et al.

Also in 2011, Campa et al. reported a large replication study of 17 SNPs in the Breast and Prostate Cancer Cohort Consortium, with the primary intent of the study being to evaluate interactions between known risk SNPs and classical epidemiological breast cancer risk factors (16). Three previously reported SNPs (rs3817198, *LSP1*; rs2075555, *COL1A1*; rs2180341, *RNF146*) did not replicate. No significant interactions were identified between the known risk factors and published SNPs. However, a meta-analysis of GWAS seeking loci associated with mammographic breast density (a strong breast cancer risk factor) found correlation between mammographic density and rs10995190 (*ZNF365*) (27), an SNP found by Turnball to be associated with sporadic breast cancer risk (21).

Ghoussanini et al. continued the approach of exploring SNPs identified in earlier GWAS through replication in the expanding set of studies participating in the Breast Cancer

Association Consortium (28). They selected 72 SNPs from two earlier UK GWAS and studied their effects in a further 54,588 invasive cases, 2401 in situ cases, and 58,098 controls from 41 case–control studies, combined with publicly available data from seven additional breast cancer GWAS (which required imputation in a number of studies). Three new loci were identified, one of which (rs10771399, 12p11) was associated with ER positive and ER negative breast cancer and two of which (rs1292011, 12q24; rs2823093, 21q21) were associated only with ER positive disease. There were several studies of women of Asian ancestry and in these studies only rs10771399 replicated.

In 2011, Cai et al. reported a four-stage GWAS from the Asia Breast Cancer Consortium (29), extending the work reported in 2009 by Zheng et al. (17). In this extension, the top 49 SNPs from stage 1 (conducted in 2062 cases and 2066 controls from Shanghai) were evaluated in an additional 15,339 cases and 15,036 controls from different East Asian countries. This analysis demonstrated a highly significant association with rs10822013 (10q21.2, *ZNF365*), seen in both ER negative and ER positive cases. In 2012, Long reported an even larger GWAS from the same consortium (30). Stage 1 was performed in 2918 Chinese women with breast cancer and 2324 community controls. Subsequent replications were conducted in nearly 20,000 cases and nearly 20,000 controls from Chinese, Korean, and Japanese ascertainments. This study identified two more SNPs on 6q25 (rs9485372, *TAB2*; rs9383951, *ESR1*) that are not correlated with the rs2046210 SNP previously reported by this group. This larger study also suggested association with rs7107217 on 11q24.3. None of these SNPs have yet been evaluated in European or other non-Asian populations.

Summary of GWAS Studies

Since publication of the first breast cancer GWAS in 2007, increasingly large association studies have been conducted and have defined a number of loci that are associated with breast cancer with a high degree of statistical confidence (Table 4.2). Many of these loci have been replicated in different ascertainments. The true causal variants are unknown for most of these loci, although there are putative gene associations with many. A number of studies have indicated that some of these loci are associated with both ER positive and ER negative disease, while others are only associated with ER positive cancers (31–34). One locus, on 19p13, seems to be specifically associated with "triple negative" breast cancer, although other common loci are also associated with this subtype (35). Large studies have been conducted in European and East Asian populations, but no large discovery studies and few replication studies have been performed in individuals of African ancestry or other ethnicities (35). A number of replication studies (and two discovery GWAS) have been conducted in carriers of *BRCA1* or *BRCA2* mutations, and have shown that common susceptibility alleles identified in GWAS of sporadic or familial breast cancer have generally similar effects in women with these rare high-penetrance alleles (36–43), both in terms of effect size and subtype associations. As noted, the 19p13 locus was first identified in a *BRCA1* GWAS, likely because of the predominance of ER negative tumors in women with *BRCA1* mutations.

The associations between common variants and breast cancer risk are incontrovertible. However, the degree of risk associated with each locus/SNP is relatively small and the known associations only account, in aggregate, for a limited amount of the known heritability of breast cancer. There are a number of hypotheses that attempt to explain the discrepancy. The most common explanation holds that there are more common variants to be found, but that their effect sizes are such that the published studies have been underpowered to discover them. A competing hypothesis is that there are multiple rare variants that contribute to the genetic architecture of common disease, and that GWAS are limited in their ability to detect such variants (44). Some prominent researchers have pointed out that genetic interactions are not taken into account in current estimates of heritability, and that the number of variants contributing to risk may be less than believed (and, therefore, the proportion of heritability that has been explained may be greater than believed) (45). Whatever be the reason, it is clear that GWASs, although very successful, have not resolved the genetic architecture of common diseases, including breast cancer.

APPLICATION OF GWAS FINDINGS TO BREAST CANCER RISK PREDICTION

Although the known breast cancer risk loci do not explain all of the heritability of breast cancer, it remains possible that what is known could be sufficient to improve the prediction of individual breast cancer risk. Before the genomics era, a number of risk prediction models were derived from conventional epidemiological risk factors. The performance of these models has been thoroughly reviewed (46,47). Two main metrics are used to evaluate risk prediction models, although both have significant limitations in a clinical context (48). *Discriminatory accuracy* is the ability of a model to discriminate between individuals with or without the condition in question. It is usually measured by means of the concordance statistic (*c* statistic), which is nearly identical to the area under the curve (AUC) of the receiver operating characteristic (ROC) curve for the "test." Simplistically, the discriminatory accuracy is the likelihood that an individual with the condition in question will be predicted to have a higher "score" on the model than a randomly selected unaffected individual from the test population. Discriminatory accuracy is one of the more commonly reported metrics, perhaps in part because it can be calculated from case–control studies. The other metric is the *calibration* of the model, measured by the ratio of observed cases in a cohort to the number that are predicted by the model. Although this is arguably a more important metric from a clinical perspective, it is much more difficult to calculate from case–control data. Ideally, prospectively followed cohorts of initially unaffected individuals would be used to identify improvements in model calibration.

A number of studies have evaluated whether genomic information, either alone or as a supplement to existing models, could improve breast cancer risk prediction. Gail performed theoretical assessments of the addition of the seven earliest risk SNPs to the Breast Cancer Risk Assessment Tool (BCRAT, also known as "Gail model") (49,50). He calculated that a seven-SNP model alone would have a discriminatory accuracy less than that of the BCRAT (0.574 vs. 0.607), and that the

Table 4.2 Loci Identified Through Genome-Wide Association Studies as Relevant to Breast Cancer Risk

Chromosome	Gene	SNP	Paper	Comment
1p11.2	NOTCH2	rs11249433	Thomas 2009 (18)	
1p11.2	NOTCH2	rs11249433	Turnbull 2010 (21)	
1p11.2	NOTCH2	rs11249433	Figueroa 2011 (19)	
1p11.2	NOTCH2	rs11249433	Campa 2011 (16)	
2q33	CASP8	rs1045485	Cox 2007	
2q33	CASP8	rs10931936	Turnbull 2010 (21)	r2 0.08 with 1045485
2q33	CASP8	rs1045485	Campa 2011 (16)	
2q35	None	rs13387042	Stacey 2007 (11)	
2q35	None	rs13387042	Milne 2009 (12)	
2q35	None	rs13387042	Thomas 2009 (18)	
2q35	None	rs13387042	Turnbull 2010 (21)	
2q35	None	rs13387042	Fletcher 2011 (26)	
2q35	None	rs13387042	Campa 2011 (16)	
3p24	SLC4A7/NEK10	rs4973768	Ahmed 2009 (20)	
3p24	SLC4A7/NEK10	rs4973768	Turnbull 2010 (21)	
3p24	SLC4A7/NEK10	rs4973768	Fletcher 2011 (26)	
3p24	SLC4A7/NEK10	rs4973768	Campa 2011 (16)	
4p	TLR1/TLR6	rs12505080	Hunter 2007 (10)	
4p	TLR1/TLR6	rs7696175	Hunter 2007 (10)	
5p12	MRPS30	rs10941679	Stacey 2008 (13)	
5p12	MRPS30	rs10941679	Thomas 2009 (18)	
5p12	MRPS30	rs10941679	Milne 2011 (14)	
5p12	MRPS30	rs10941679	Campa 2011 (16)	
5p12	MRPS30	rs2067980	Thomas 2009 (18)	
5p12	MRPS30	rs4415084	Stacey 2008 (13)	
5p12	MRPS30	rs4415084	Thomas 2009 (18)	
5p12	MRPS30	rs4415084	Fletcher 2011 (26)	
5p12	MRPS30	rs4415084	Campa 2011 (16)	
5p12	MRPS30	rs7716600	Thomas 2009 (18)	
5p12	MRPS30	rs9790879	Turnbull 2010 (21)	r2 0.48 with 10941679
5p15	TERT-CLPTM1L	rs10069690	Haiman 2011 (25)	
5q	MAP3K1/MEKK	rs889312	Easton 2007 (8)	
5q	MAP3K1/MEKK	rs889312	Turnbull 2010 (21)	
5q	MAP3K1/MEKK	rs889312	Campa 2011 (16)	
5q	MAP3K1/MEKK	rs16886165	Thomas 2009 (18)	
6q22	RNF146	rs2180341	Gold 2008 (15)	
6q25	ESR1/C6orf97	rs2046210	Zheng 2009 (17)	
6q25	ESR1/C6orf97	rs2046210	Campa 2011 (16)	
6q25	ESR1/C6orf97	rs3757318	Turnbull 2010 (21)	r2 0.088 with 2046210
6q25	ESR1/C6orf97	rs6900157	Fletcher 2011 (26)	r2 0.92 with 2046210
6q25	ESR1	rs3734805	Fletcher 2011 (26)	
6q25	ESR1	rs9393938	Fletcher 2011 (26)	
6q25	ESR1	rs9393591	Long 2012 (30)	
6q25	TAB2	rs9485372	Long 2012 (30)	
7q	RELN	rs17157903	Hunter 2007 (10)	
7q	RELN	rs6964587	Milne 2011 (14)	
8q24	None	rs13281615	Easton 2007 (8)	
8q24	None	rs13281615	Campa 2011 (16)	
8q24	None	rs1562430	Thomas 2009 (18)	r2 0.42 with 13281615
8q24	None	rs1562430	Turnbull 2010 (21)	r2 0.42 with 13281615
8q24	None	rs1562430	Fletcher 2011 (26)	r2 0.42 with 13281615
9p21	CDKN2A/B	rs1011970	Turnbull 2010 (21)	
9p21	CDKN2A/B	rs1011970	Lambrechts 2012 (22)	
9p31	None	rs865686	Fletcher 2011 (26)	
10p15	ANKRD16/FBX018	rs2380205	Turnbull 2010 (21)	
10q	None	rs10510126	Hunter 2007 (10)	
10q21	ZNF365	rs10822013	Cai 2011 (29)	
10q21	ZNF365	rs10995190	Turnbull 2010 (21)	
10q21	ZNF365	rs10995190	Lambrechts 2012 (22)	
10q22	ZMIZ1	rs704010	Turnbull 2010 (21)	
10q22	ZMIZ1	rs704010	Lambrechts 2012 (22)	
10q26	FGFR2	rs2981582	Easton 2007 (8)	

(*Continued*)

Table 4.2 Loci Identified Through Genome-Wide Association Studies as Relevant to Breast Cancer Risk (*Continued*)

Chromosome	Gene	SNP	Paper	Comment
10q26	FGFR2	rs2981582	Turnbull 2010 (21)	
10q26	FGFR2	rs2981579	Thomas 2009 (18)	
10q26	FGFR2	rs2981579	Turnbull 2010 (21)	
10q26	FGFR2	rs1219648	Hunter 2007 (10)	
10q26	FGFR2	rs1219648	Fletcher 2011 (26)	
10q26	FGFR2	rs1078806	Gold 2008 (15)	
10q26	FGFR2	rs3750817	Campa 2011 (16)	
11p	LSP1	rs3017198	Easton 2007 (8)	
11p	LSP1	rs3817198	Thomas 2009 (18)	
11p	LSP1	rs909116	Turnbull 2010 (21)	r2 0.23 with 3817198
11q13	None	rs614367	Turnbull 2010 (21)	
11q13	None	rs614367	Lambrechts 2012 (22)	
11q24	None	rs710727	Long 2012 (30)	
12p11	PTHLH/PTHrP	rs10771399	Ghoussaini 2012 (28)	
12q24	None	rs1292011	Ghoussaini 2012 (28)	
14q24	RAD51L	rs999737	Thomas 2009 (18)	
14q24	RAD51L	rs999737	Fletcher 2011 (26)	
14q24	RAD51L	rs999737	Figueroa 2011 (19)	
14q24	RAD51L	rs999737	Campa 2011 (16)	
14q24	RAD51L	rs8009944	Turnbull 2010 (21)	r2 0.13 with 999737
16q12	TNRC9/TOX3	rs12443621	Easton 2007 (8)	
16q12	TNRC9/TOX3	rs4783780	Fletcher 2011 (26)	r2 0.97 with 12443621
16q12	TNRC9/TOX3	rs3803662	Stacey 2007 (11)	
16q12	TNRC9/TOX3	rs3803662	Thomas 2009 (18)	
16q12	TNRC9/TOX3	rs3803662	Turnbull 2010 (21)	
16q12	TNRC9/TOX3	rs3803662	Campa 2011 (16)	
17q23	COX11/STXBP4	rs6504950	Ahmed 2009 (20)	
17q23	COX11/STXBP4	rs6504950	Campa 2011 (16)	
17q23	COX11/STXBP4	rs1156287	Turnbull 2010 (21)	r2 0.91 with 6504950
19p13	MERIT40	rs8170	Antoniou 2010 (23)	
19p13	MERIT40	rs8170	Stevens 2012 (24)	
19p13	MERIT40	rs2363956	Antoniou 2010 (23)	

addition of seven SNPs to the BCRAT would have limited impact on discriminatory accuracy (0.632 vs. 0.607). When he assessed the impact of adding SNPs to BCRAT on clinical endpoints (threshold for tamoxifen chemoprevention and decision to undergo mammogram screening), he found limited impact on the number of projected life-threatening events. He did note that a number of individuals would be considered to belong to different risk categories if absolute risk were calculated with a combined model. He calculated that 9.27% of those with a BRCAT risk of less than 1.5% would be above that threshold with the SNP-enhanced model, and 21.2% of the women with a risk above 1.5% would be reclassified lower. This would be clinically relevant because it could alter recommendations (e.g., for pharmacological risk reduction) in the reclassified women. Our group essentially confirmed Gail's predictions in a group of 519 unaffected BRCA mutation–negative women who were genotyped at 15-risk SNPs (51). The discriminatory accuracy of a calculated cumulative genomic risk (CGR) score was only 0.55, but using the CGR to adjust risk from empiric models such as BCRAT and Tyrer–Cuzick would lead to changes in recommendations for chemoprevention in 11–19% of subjects and for MRI screening in 8–32%. The CGR was not correlated with the risks estimated by empiric models, consistent with the findings of Campa et al. that risk genotypes are not correlated with traditional risk factors (16).

Three other large studies have evaluated the performance of risk prediction models that incorporate risk SNPs. Wacholder et al. combined risk factor information with genotypes at 10 SNPs in 5590 cases and 5998 controls from four US cohort studies and a European case–control study (52). The inclusion of genotype information improved the AUC of a more traditional risk model from 0.58 to 0.618, and reclassified slightly more than half of subjects into a different quintile of risk. The AUC for the SNP model alone was 0.597. As with earlier studies, a significant proportion of individuals were reassigned higher or lower categories of risk with the model that included both genetic and nongenetic factors. Mealiffe et al. evaluated the addition of seven risk SNPs to Gail model risk in a group of 1664 cases and 1636 controls from the Women's Health Initiative (53). They found that adding SNPs to the Gail model improved its discriminatory accuracy (0.594 vs. 0.557 for Gail alone) and led to significant improvement in classification as measured by the Net Reclassification Improvement (NRI), a newer metric proposed by Pencina et al. (54). Finally, Darabi et al. have recently described the performance of a comprehensive model including mammographic density, body mass index, and a "Swedish Gail model" combined with 18 breast cancer risk SNPs in a group of 1569 postmenopausal women with breast cancer and 1730 controls (55). Discriminatory accuracy improved from 0.55 to 0.62, with significant values for NRI in all categories of risk.

Consistent conclusions flow from the aggregate results of the studies described earlier, as well as those of smaller studies and theoretical calculations (56–61). Risk models based on genotyping for known risk SNPs have very modest discriminatory accuracy and do not discriminate better than existing models based on clinical risk factors. However, the addition of genotype information to existing models does improve the discriminatory accuracy of those models, and seems to improve absolute risk estimation (as measured by NRI), at least when considering whether women are assigned appropriate risk categories. The degree to which genotyping improves the calibration of existing models, in terms of individual absolute risk prediction, is unclear. However, including a genomic risk term into a risk prediction model would clearly alter recommendations for pharmacological risk reduction, and potentially for screening interventions such as MRI (or potentially even mammography) in a non-trivial fraction of women. The degree to which this would improve individual outcomes and more global public health is not clear, and the role of genotype-informed risk prediction remains an area of active discussion, even controversy (62,63).

CONCLUSION

A large number of studies have established without a doubt that common genomic variation is associated with variation in breast cancer risk. The mechanism by which the identified variants (or the loci they tag) contribute to risk is the subject of active research, but for most SNPs the explanation for association remains unknown. Despite considerable effort, the SNPs identified so far do not explain most of the variation calculated as being due to inherited factors. There are a number of possible explanations for this, one of these being that the "common disease, common variant" model is too simplistic to explain the heritability of common diseases such as breast cancer. Now that the "post-GWAS" era has arrived, investigators have turned toward using fine mapping to identify the causal variants associated with the risk SNPs and next-generation sequencing to search for rare variants that may be associated with risk.

While the basic work of explaining the genetic architecture of breast cancer continues, clinicians are evaluating whether the discoveries that have been made so far can be applied to patient care. It appears that genomic risk resulting from common variation is independent of risk conferred by traditional risk factors, which raises the possibility of combined models that could be more accurate than the existing prediction models. The gains appear to be quite modest on an overall basis, but the observation that a significant proportion of women are assigned to different risk categories by combined models is important, since such reclassification could have a significant impact on management recommendations. Determining whether such genomically informed decisions would improve overall outcomes would require large randomized studies that are unlikely to be performed in today's funding environment. Without such studies, genomic risk prediction for breast cancer is likely to remain an unrealized goal in the near future.

REFERENCES

1. Pharoah PD, Day NE, Duffy S, Easton DF, Ponder BA. Family history and the risk of breast cancer: a systematic review and meta-analysis. Int J Cancer 1997; 71: 800–9.

2. Lichtenstein P, Holm NV, Verkasalo PK, et al. Environmental and heritable factors in the causation of cancer–analyses of cohorts of twins from Sweden, Denmark, and Finland. N Engl J Med 2000; 343: 78–85.

3. Consortium GP, Durbin RM, Abecasis GR, et al. A map of human genome variation from population-scale sequencing. Nature 2010; 467: 1061–73.

4. Consortium IH, Frazer KA, Ballinger DG, et al. A second generation human haplotype map of over 3.1 million SNPs. Nature 2007; 449: 851–61.

5. Manolio TA. Genomewide association studies and assessment of the risk of disease. N Engl J Med 2010; 363: 166–76.

6. Thomas DC, Haile RW, Duggan D. Recent developments in genomewide association scans: a workshop summary and review. Am J Hum Genet 2005; 77: 337–45.

7. Freedman ML, Monteiro ANA, Gayther SA, et al. Principles for the post-GWAS functional characterization of cancer risk loci. Nat Genet 2011; 43: 513–18.

8. Easton DF, Pooley KA, Dunning AM, et al. Genome-wide association study identifies novel breast cancer susceptibility loci. Nature 2007; 447: 1087–93.

9. Ghoussaini M, Song H, Koessler T, et al. Multiple loci with different cancer specificities within the 8q24 gene desert. J Natl Cancer Inst 2008; 100: 962–6.

10. Hunter DJ, Kraft P, Jacobs KB, et al. A genome-wide association study identifies alleles in FGFR2 associated with risk of sporadic postmenopausal breast cancer. Nat Genet 2007; 39: 870–4.

11. Stacey SN, Manolescu A, Sulem P, et al. Common variants on chromosomes 2q35 and 16q12 confer susceptibility to estrogen receptor-positive breast cancer. Nat Genet 2007; 39: 865–9.

12. Milne RL, Benítez J, Nevanlinna H, et al. Risk of estrogen receptor–positive and –negative breast cancer and single–nucleotide polymorphism 2q35-rs13387042. J Natl Cancer Inst 2009; 101: 1012–18.

13. Stacey SN, Manolescu A, Sulem P, et al. Common variants on chromosome 5p12 confer susceptibility to estrogen receptor-positive breast cancer. Nat Genet 2008; 40: 703–6.

14. Milne RL, Goode EL, Garcia-Closas M, et al. Confirmation of 5p12 as a susceptibility locus for progesterone-receptor-positive, lower grade breast cancer. Cancer Epidemiol Biomarkers Prev 2011; 20: 2222–31.

15. Gold B, Kirchhoff T, Stefanov S, et al. Genome-wide association study provides evidence for a breast cancer risk locus at 6q22.33. Proc Natl Acad Sci USA 2008; 105: 4340–5.

16. Campa D, Kaaks R, Le Marchand L, et al. Interactions between genetic variants and breast cancer risk factors in the breast and prostate cancer cohort consortium. J Natl Cancer Inst 2011; 103: 1252–63.

17. Zheng W, Long J, Gao YT, et al. Genome-wide association study identifies a new breast cancer susceptibility locus at 6q25.1. Nat Genet 2009; 41: 324–8.

18. Thomas G, Jacobs KB, Kraft P, et al. A multistage genome-wide association study in breast cancer identifies two new risk alleles at 1p11.2 and 14q24.1 (RAD51L1). Nat Genet 2009; 41: 579–84.

19. Figueroa JD, Garcia-Closas M, Humphreys M, et al. Associations of common variants at 1p11.2 and 14q24.1 (RAD51L1) with breast cancer risk and heterogeneity by tumor subtype: findings from the Breast Cancer Association Consortium. Hum Mol Genet 2011; 20: 4693–706.

20. Ahmed S, Thomas G, Ghoussaini M, et al. Newly discovered breast cancer susceptibility loci on 3p24 and 17q23.2. Nat Genet 2009; 41: 585–90.

21. Turnbull C, Ahmed S, Morrison J, et al. Genome-wide association study identifies five new breast cancer susceptibility loci. Nat Genet 2010; 42: 504–7.

22. Lambrechts D, Truong T, Justenhoven C, et al. 11q13 is a susceptibility locus for hormone receptor positive breast cancer. Hum Mutat 2012; 33: 1123–32.

23. Antoniou AC, Wang X, Fredericksen ZS, et al. A locus on 19p13 modifies risk of breast cancer in BRCA1 mutation carriers and is associated with hormone receptor-negative breast cancer in the general population. Nat Genet 2010; 42: 885–92.

24. Stevens KN, Fredericksen Z, Vachon CM, et al. 19p13.1 Is a triple-negative-specific breast cancer susceptibility locus. Cancer Res 2012; 72: 1795–803.

25. Haiman CA, Chen GK, Vachon CM, et al. A common variant at the TERT-CLPTM1L locus is associated with estrogen receptor-negative breast cancer. Nat Genet 2011; 43: 1210–14.

26. Fletcher O, Johnson N, Orr N, et al. Novel breast cancer susceptibility locus on 9q31.2: results of a genome-wide association study. J Natl Cancer Inst 2011; 103: 425–35.

27. Lindstrom S, Vachon CM, Li J, et al. Common variants in ZNF365 are associated with both mammographic density and breast cancer risk. Nat Genet 2011; 43: 185–7.

28. Ghoussaini M, Fletcher O, Michailidou K, et al. Genome-wide association analysis identifies three new breast cancer susceptibility loci. Nat Genet 2012; 44: 312–18.

29. Cai Q, Long J, Lu W, et al. Genome-wide association study identifies breast cancer risk variant at 10q21.2: results from the Asia Breast Cancer Consortium. Hum Mol Genet 2011; 20: 4991–9.

30. Long J, Cai Q, Sung H, et al. Genome-wide association study in east Asians identifies novel susceptibility loci for breast cancer. PLoS Genet 2012; 8: e1002532.

31. Broeks A, Schmidt MK, Sherman ME, et al. Low penetrance breast cancer susceptibility loci are associated with specific breast tumor subtypes: findings from the Breast Cancer Association Consortium. Hum Mol Genet 2011; 20: 3289–303.

32. Garcia-Closas M, Chanock S. Genetic susceptibility loci for breast cancer by estrogen receptor status. Clin Cancer Res 2008; 14: 8000–9.

33. Garcia-Closas M, Hall P, Nevanlinna H, et al. Heterogeneity of breast cancer associations with five susceptibility loci by clinical and pathological characteristics. PLoS Genet 2008; 4: e1000054.

34. Reeves GK, Travis RC, Green J, et al. Incidence of breast cancer and its subtypes in relation to individual and multiple low-penetrance genetic susceptibility loci. JAMA 2010; 304: 426–34.

35. Stevens KN, Vachon CM, Lee AM, et al. Common breast cancer susceptibility loci are associated with triple-negative breast cancer. Cancer Res 2011; 71: 6240–9.

36. Antoniou AC, Beesley J, McGuffog L, et al. Common breast cancer susceptibility alleles and the risk of breast cancer for BRCA1 and BRCA2 mutation carriers: implications for risk prediction. Cancer Res 2010; 70: 9742–54.

37. Antoniou AC, Kartsonaki C, Sinilnikova OM, et al. Common alleles at 6q25.1 and 1p11.2 are associated with breast cancer risk for BRCA1 and BRCA2 mutation carriers. Hum Mol Genet 2011; 20: 3304–21.

38. Antoniou AC, Sinilnikova OM, McGuffog L, et al. Common variants in LSP1, 2q35 and 8q24 and breast cancer risk for BRCA1 and BRCA2 mutation carriers. Hum Mol Genet 2009; 18: 4442–56.

39. Antoniou AC, Spurdle AB, Sinilnikova OM, et al. Common breast cancer-predisposition alleles are associated with breast cancer risk in BRCA1 and BRCA2 mutation carriers. Am J Hum Genet 2008; 82: 937–48.

40. Couch FJ, Gaudet MM, Antoniou AC, et al. Common variants at the 19p13.1 and ZNF365 loci are associated with ER subtypes of breast cancer and ovarian cancer risk in BRCA1 and BRCA2 mutation carriers. Cancer Epidemiol Biomarkers Prev 2012; 21: 645–57.

41. Engel C, Versmold B, Wappenschmidt B, et al. Association of the variants CASP8 D302H and CASP10 V410I with breast and ovarian cancer risk in BRCA1 and BRCA2 mutation carriers. Cancer Epidemiol Biomarkers Prev 2010; 19: 2859–68.

42. Gaudet MM, Kirchhoff T, Green T, et al. Common genetic variants and modification of penetrance of BRCA2-associated breast cancer. PLoS Genet 2010; 6: e1001183.

43. Wang X, Pankratz VS, Fredericksen Z, et al. Common variants associated with breast cancer in genome-wide association studies are modifiers of breast cancer risk in BRCA1 and BRCA2 mutation carriers. Hum Mol Genet 2010; 19: 2886–97.

44. Manolio TA, Collins FS, Cox NJ, et al. Finding the missing heritability of complex diseases. Nature 2009; 461: 747–53.

45. Zuk O, Hechter E, Sunyaev SR, Lander ES. The mystery of missing heritability: genetic interactions create phantom heritability. Proc Natl Acad Sci USA 2012; 109: 1193–8.

46. Anothaisintawee T, Teerawattananon Y, Wiratkapun C, Kasamesup V, Thakkinstian A. Risk prediction models of breast cancer: a systematic review of model performances. Breast Cancer Res Treat 2011; 133: 1–10.

47. Meads C, Ahmed I, Riley RD. A systematic review of breast cancer incidence risk prediction models with meta-analysis of their performance. Breast Cancer Res Treat 2012; 132: 365–77.

48. Janes H, Pepe MS, Bossuyt PM, Barlow WE. Measuring the performance of markers for guiding treatment decisions. Ann Intern Med 2011; 154: 253–9.

49. Gail MH. Discriminatory accuracy from single-nucleotide polymorphisms in models to predict breast cancer risk. J Natl Cancer Inst 2008; 100: 1037–41.

50. Gail MH. Value of adding single-nucleotide polymorphism genotypes to a breast cancer risk model. J Natl Cancer Inst 2009; 101: 959–63.

51. Comen E, Balistreri L, Gönen M, et al. Discriminatory accuracy and potential clinical utility of genomic profiling for breast cancer risk in BRCA-negative women. Breast Cancer Res Treat 2011; 127: 479–87.

52. Wacholder S, Hartge P, Prentice R, et al. Performance of common genetic variants in breast-cancer risk models. N Engl J Med 2010; 362: 986–93.

53. Mealiffe ME, Stokowski RP, Rhees BK, et al. Assessment of clinical validity of a breast cancer risk model combining genetic and clinical information. J Natl Cancer Inst 2010; 102: 1618–27.

54. Pencina MJ, D'Agostino RB, D'Agostino RB, Vasan RS. Evaluating the added predictive ability of a new marker: from area under the ROC curve to reclassification and beyond. Stat Med 2008; 27: 157–72; discussion 207-12.

55. Darabi H, Czene K, Zhao W, et al. Breast cancer risk prediction and individualised screening based on common genetic variation and breast density measurement. Breast Cancer Res 2012; 14: R25.

56. Hartman M, Suo C, Lim WY, et al. Ability to predict breast cancer in Asian women using a polygenic susceptibility model. Breast Cancer Res Treat 2011; 127: 805–12.

57. Mihaescu R, Moonesinghe R, Khoury MJ, Janssens AC. Predictive genetic testing for the identification of high-risk groups: a simulation study on the impact of predictive ability. Genome Med 2011; 3: 51.

58. Pashayan N, Duffy SW, Chowdhury S, et al. Polygenic susceptibility to prostate and breast cancer: implications for personalised screening. Br J Cancer 2011; 104: 1656–63.

59. So HC, Kwan JS, Cherny SS, Sham PC. Risk prediction of complex diseases from family history and known susceptibility loci, with applications for cancer screening. Am J Hum Genet 2011; 88: 548–65.

60. Sueta A, Ito H, Kawase T, et al. A genetic risk predictor for breast cancer using a combination of low-penetrance polymorphisms in a Japanese population. Breast Cancer Res Treat 2012; 132: 711–21.

61. Zheng W, Wen W, Gao YT, et al. Genetic and clinical predictors for breast cancer risk assessment and stratification among Chinese women. J Natl Cancer Inst 2010; 102: 972–81.

62. Chatterjee N, Park JH, Caporaso N, Gail MH. Predicting the future of genetic risk prediction. Cancer Epidemiol Biomarkers Prev 2011; 20: 3–8.

63. van Zitteren M, van der Net JB, Kundu S, et al. Genome-based prediction of breast cancer risk in the general population: a modeling study based on meta-analyses of genetic associations. Cancer Epidemiol Biomarkers Prev 2011; 20: 9–22.

5 Endocrine prevention of breast cancer

Russell E. McDaniel and V. Craig Jordan, OBE

INTRODUCTION

The idea of prevention of breast cancer is not new, but significant practical progress has been made, through translational research, to make the idea feasible in some women. It is now possible to reduce the incidence of breast cancer through the inhibition of estrogen action.

Professor Antoine Lacassagne (1) stated a vision for the prevention of breast cancer at the annual meeting of the American Association of Cancer Research in Boston in 1936.

> "*If one accepts the consideration of adenocarcinoma of the breast as the consequence of a special hereditary sensibility to the proliferative actions of oestrone, one is led to imagine a therapeutic preventative for subjects predisposed by their heredity to this cancer. It would consist – perhaps in the very near future when the knowledge and use of hormones will be better understood – in the suitable use of a hormone antagonistic or excretory, to prevent the stagnation of oestrone in the ducts of the breast.*"

But no agent that was "antagonistic to prevent the stagnation of oestrone in the breast" was available for clinical trial until tamoxifen (2,3). Tamoxifen (Fig. 5.1) became the "antiestrogen" of choice because (*i*) there was a large body of basic biological evidence that this was a valid hypothesis to test; (*ii*) tamoxifen was noted to reduce the incidence of contralateral breast cancer when used as an adjuvant therapy to treat micrometastases from the ipsilateral primary tumor and most importantly (*iii*) there was a huge and expanding clinical experience with tamoxifen as a long-term treatment for node-positive and node-negative breast cancer. The latter point was important as the majority of patients with estrogen receptor (ER)-positive node-negative breast cancers are cured by surgery (plus radiation) alone. So five years of adjuvant tamoxifen was essentially being used in the majority of "well women" (4,5).

In this chapter, the changing fashions in endocrine chemoprevention are described. These have occurred because of significant advances in our understanding of the pharmacology of the drug group the "nonsteroidal antiestrogens" (6) that underwent a metamorphosis in the mid 1980s (7) to become the new drug group, the selective estrogen receptor modulators (SERMs) (8,9). This laboratory work on SERM action and the finding that antihormone resistance in breast cancer is not static but evolves (10,11) ultimately led to discovery (rediscovery?) of a new biology of estrogen action—estrogen-induced apoptosis (12). Remarkably, this conversation between the laboratory and the clinical research community now provides a fascinating insight into a paradoxical clinical finding in the Women's Health Initiative (WHI) trial of conjugated equine estrogen (CEE) alone in hysterectomized postmenopausal women in their late 60s. Since dogma dictates that estradiol is the survival signal that fuels breast cancer cell replication, the WHI trial unexpectedly noted a significant decrease in the incidence of breast cancer during CEE treatment and for the six years after treatment stops (cumulative annualized incidence of 151 invasive breast cancers with CEE treatment as opposed to 199 invasive breast cancers with placebo) (13). These data might provide a starting point for consideration of estrogen-induced apoptosis as a chemoprevention strategy in the future.

THE LINK BETWEEN ESTROGEN AND BREAST CANCER

The topic has been reviewed (14) in the referred research literature so only essential facts will be considered here. The link between estrogen action for breast cancer growth, the tumor prior to treatment, ER, and five years of adjuvant tamoxifen therapy to block tumor growth is compelling and proven in randomized clinical trials (15). The findings can be simply summarized: breast tumors that are ER negative do not respond to tamoxifen treatment, tamoxifen dramatically reduces recurrence and mortality during 5 years of treatment for patients with ER-positive breast cancer, and this is maintained for at least 15 years following completion of therapy. Tamoxifen reduces the incidence of contralateral breast cancer by 50% and this is sustained but tamoxifen also increases the incidence of endometrial cancer in postmenopausal women (and mortality). The negative actions of adjuvant tamoxifen, such as deaths from endometrial cancer or thromboembolic disease, do not affect the overall benefit of treatment (15) but do impact on the use of tamoxifen for chemoprevention. Profound target-site-specific actions of tamoxifen on the uterus in the recent overview (15) recapitulate and confirm findings from translational research with tamoxifen completed in the 1980s (16,17). There is thus recognition of a small but significant increase in the incidence of endometrial cancer in postmenopausal women treated with tamoxifen. This finding eventually resulted in the paradigm shift away from tamoxifen to new opportunities but this advances our story too quickly. In the 1980s, tamoxifen was the only medicine available for testing therapeutic and chemopreventive strategies with SERMs in the 1990s. The clinical community advanced with a responsibility to weigh risks and benefits in clinical trials to ensure the safety and long-term health of women at risk for breast cancer.

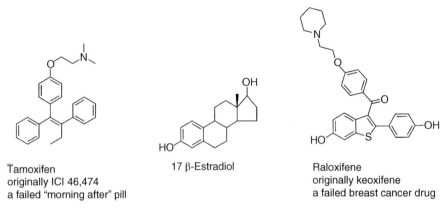

Tamoxifen
originally ICI 46,474
a failed "morning after" pill

17 β-Estradiol

Raloxifene
originally keoxifene
a failed breast cancer drug

Figure 5.1 A comparison of the structures of the potent steroidal estrogen 17β-estradiol and the nonsteroidal antiestrogens (now called SERMs) tamoxifen and raloxifene. Tamoxifen and raloxifene are both approved in the United States (US) for the reduction of risk for breast cancer in high risk pre- and postmenopausal women or postmenopausal women alone respectively.

The treatment trials' database and translational research were essential to address the hypothesis that tamoxifen, a nonsteroidal antiestrogen, could effectively block the genesis and growth of ER-positive breast cancer but would be ineffective against the growth of ER-negative disease. Nevertheless in the 1980s, estrogen was also considered to be an essential component of women's health, maintaining bone density and preventing coronary heart disease. Thus, if tamoxifen, an antiestrogen, prevented the development and growth of ER-positive breast cancer in half a dozen high-risk women per year per 1000 (18), hundreds of other women in the selected population might subsequently develop osteoporosis and coronary heart disease. The intervention with tamoxifen would be detrimental to public health. The good news was that tamoxifen was not an antiestrogen everywhere; it was the lead compound of a class of drug that selectively modulated ER target tissues around the body. This discovery ultimately facilitated the development of a new strategy for the utilization of SERMs as chemopreventives in breast cancer.

SERM ACTION IN THE LABORATORY

The original work to investigate the target site pharmacology of tamoxifen in the laboratory was to provide a database with which to predict clinical outcomes and safety for future chemoprevention trials. Historically in the 1960s, there was general interest in the chance finding that nonsteroidal antiestrogens lowered circulating cholesterol. Unfortunately, severe toxicological findings were an issue for some compounds because of their ability to increase the level of circulatory desmosterol, which was associated with cataract formation. This toxicity made a search for safer antiestrogens imperative (2). The discovery of ICI 46474 (Fig. 5.1), the pure trans isomer of the substituted triphenylethylene that was to become tamoxifen, was notable because there was a low conversion to desmosterol though circulating cholesterol was lowered profoundly in rats (19). Indeed the first patent application for tamoxifen in the United Kingdom (UK) in 1965 stated the following (2):

> "*The alkene derivatives of the invention are useful for the modification of the endocrine status in man and animals and they may be useful for the control of hormone-dependent tumours or for the management of the sexual cycle and aberrations thereof. They also have useful hypocholesterolaemic activity.*"

However, the patent was denied in the United States (US)and the statements concerning breast cancer had to be removed initially as the claim was considered to be "fantastic" and without experimental evidence. The patent for tamoxifen in the US was finally awarded in 1986 just at the time that the National Cancer Institute recommended adjuvant tamoxifen as the standard of care for patients with ER-positive breast cancer (20).

Parenthetically, all studies conducted in the senior author's laboratory during the 1970s and 1980s on the application of tamoxifen for the treatment and prevention of breast cancer in the US and UK were at a time of no patent protection in the US. No other company exploited the findings as no one cared because it was unlikely to be a successful therapeutic strategy!

During the 1980s, the Wisconsin Tamoxifen study followed up the question of tamoxifen treatment lowering circulating cholesterol in postmenopausal patients (21,22) and noted a decrease in low density lipoprotein cholesterol but no effect on high density lipoprotein cholesterol. There was certainly some initial enthusiasm that there would be a significant decrease in coronary heart disease but despite some encouraging reports (23–25) no consistent decrease in coronary events has been noted in the Oxford Overview Analysis for tamoxifen treatment.

Tamoxifen maintains bone density in ovariectomized rats (26–28) and this counterintuitive laboratory result for an "antiestrogen" formed the scientific basis for the Wisconsin Tamoxifen Study. The clinical study was a placebo controlled double blind trial to establish the actions of two years of tamoxifen on bone density in postmenopausal patients with node-negative breast cancer (at the time of recruitment, these patients were several years post diagnosis and surgery and no adjuvant treatment was the standard of care). Tamoxifen significantly improved bone density compared with placebo treatment (29).

Thus tamoxifen was estrogen-like, lowering circulating cholesterol and estrogen-like, maintaining bone density; so tamoxifen might provide benefit for women enrolled in a chemoprevention trial. The anticancer actions of tamoxifen were well established and supported by the inhibition of mammary carcinogenesis in rat (30,31) and mouse (32) models. But an

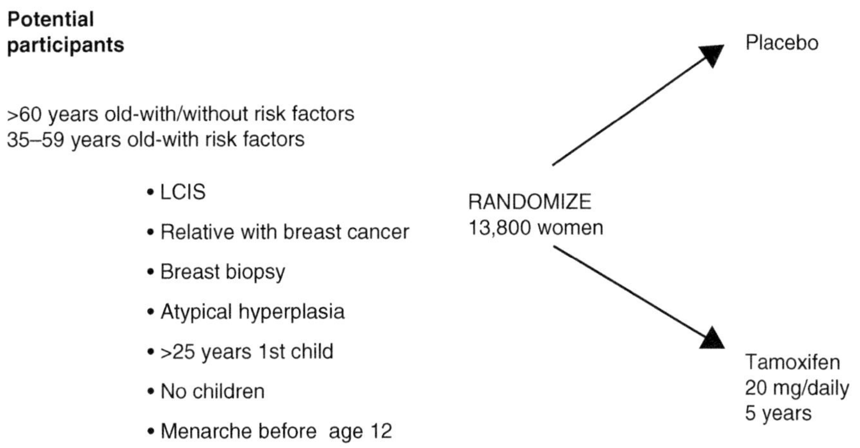

Potential participants

>60 years old-with/without risk factors
35–59 years old-with risk factors

- LCIS
- Relative with breast cancer
- Breast biopsy
- Atypical hyperplasia
- >25 years 1st child
- No children
- Menarche before age 12

RANDOMIZE
13,800 women

Placebo

Tamoxifen
20 mg/daily
5 years

Figure 5.2 The risk requirements for recruitment to the National Surgical Breast and Bowel Project (NSABP)/National Cancer Institute (NCI) study P-1 to determine the worth of tamoxifen for preventing breast cancer in high-risk pre- and postmenopausal women (38).

increase in the incidence of endometrial cancer was a predictable concern, based on earlier work (16,17) before major clinical trials of chemoprevention in breast cancer started. Also the finding that tamoxifen was a hepatocarcinogen in specific rat strains (33) was of significance from a toxicology point of view and for safety reasons in any chemopreventive trial. However, no evidence either at that time (34,35) or subsequently has emerged which demonstrates hepatocarcinogenesis in humans with the use of tamoxifen.

The first pilot chemoprevention study was initiated by Trevor Powles at the Royal Marsden Hospital in the early 1980s (36). This study grew over the years of accrual and interestingly showed benefit at 20 years for those women taking tamoxifen for eight years following recruitment (37). However, the pivotal chemoprevention study was the Fisher P-1 study (Fig. 5.2) conducted by the National Surgical Advent Breast and Bowel Project (NSABP) (38). This landmark study was an adequately powered prospective, placebo controlled trial primarily used by the Food and Drug Administration (FDA) as evidence to approve tamoxifen for the reduction of risk of breast cancer in pre- and postmenopausal women at high risk for the disease.

There are significant benefits for women at risk for breast cancer nested within the results of the P-1 prevention trial during treatment with tamoxifen. There were fewer fractures but this was not significant overall. Tamoxifen reduces ER-positive invasive breast cancer incidence by 50% and the same is true for ductal carcinoma *in situ* (DCIS) (38). Benefits from breast chemoprevention last for years following cessation of treatment (39) and this has been confirmed by others (40). This is clearly a consistent long-term "antitumor action" of tamoxifen which is imprinted following therapy and is analogous to the sustained antitumor effect of tamoxifen following adjuvant treatment (15,41). We will comment further on the new concept of "imprinting" in the section "SERM Summary".

Despite extensive testing, tamoxifen is seen as presenting the well woman with significant risks such as endometrial cancer and blood clots (although only in postmenopausal women) (Fig. 5.3) (38). There is also the nagging concern about rat hepatocarcinoma. Tamoxifen has a human carcinogen black box designation in the US. With all these uncertainties, clearly

another strategy for chemoprevention was necessary for an appropriate science-based advance in public health. This was obvious (7) even before the NSABP trial had been launched in the early 1990s (38) but tamoxifen was the only medicine available with sufficient clinical trial experience to move forward into chemoprevention. Nevertheless, the recognition of SERMs in the laboratory (7) also catalyzed a change in the development of another nonsteroidal antiestrogen, keoxifene (Fig. 5.1). Keoxifene was initially investigated in the 1980s as a competitor for tamoxifen as a breast cancer drug, but failed to advance in development and was abandoned in clinical trials (42). Surprisingly, keoxifene also maintained bone density in rats similar to tamoxifen but was significantly less uterotrophic than the latter (26,43) which would translate to a reduced risk of endometrial cancer in all subsequent clinical trials. The name was changed from keoxifene to raloxifene (Fig. 5.1).

Keoxifene prevented mammary cancer in rats but because of poor pharmacokinetics and rapid excretion keoxifene does not have the sustained actions of tamoxifen (31) and continuous therapy was necessary. Thus the scene was set for a move away from a broad therapeutic strategy with tamoxifen administered to high-risk populations where a few ER-positive invasive breast cancers can be prevented but most women are exposed to side effects with no benefit to balance the risks. In response, a "roadmap" was created based on laboratory science and the emerging clinical trial data that would significantly advance women's health.

USE OF SERMs TO PREVENT MULTIPLE DISEASES IN WOMEN

A plan to prevent breast cancer as a public health initiative was initially described at the First International Chemoprevention meeting in New York in 1987 (44). It was reasonable simply to state the proposal, published from the 1987 meeting (44) and subsequently to refine and present again at the annual meeting of the American Association for Cancer Research in San Francisco in 1989 (7). "*The majority of breast cancer occurs unexpectedly and from unknown origin. Great efforts are being focused on the identification of a population of high-risk women to test "chemopreventive" agents. But, are resources being used less than optimally? An alternative would be to seize on the*

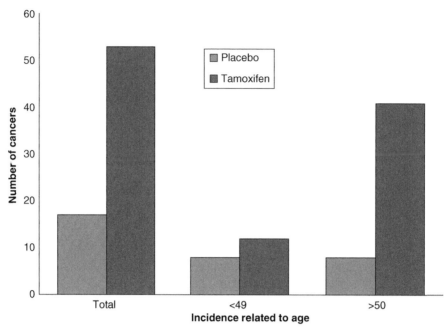

Figure 5.3 The total and age-related incidence of endometrial cancer in the NSABP/NCI P-1 chemoprevention trial (39). Premenopausal women have no increased risk of developing endometrial cancer during or following five years of tamoxifen treatment.

developing clues provided by an extensive clinical investigation of available antioestrogens. Could analogues be developed to treat osteoporosis or even retard the development of atherosclerosis? If this proved to be true, then a majority of women in general would be treated for these conditions as soon as menopause occurred. Should the agent also retain anti-breast tumour actions, then it might be expected to act as a chemosuppressive on all developing breast cancers if these have an evolution from hormone-dependent disease to hormone-independent disease. A bold commitment to drug discovery and clinical pharmacology will potentially place us in a key position to prevent the development of breast cancer by the end of this century (44)." The vision of the concept was refined and focused by 1990 (7). "We have obtained valuable clinical information about this group of drugs that can be applied in other disease states. Research does not travel in straight lines and observations in one field of science often become major discoveries in another. Important clues have been garnered about the effects of tamoxifen on bone and lipids, so apparently, derivatives could find targeted applications to retard osteoporosis or atherosclerosis. The ubiquitous application of novel compounds to prevent diseases associated with the progressive changes after menopause may, as a side effect, significantly retard the development of breast cancer. The target population would be postmenopausal women in general, thereby avoiding the requirement to select a high-risk group to prevent breast cancer." This concept is exactly what has been translated to clinical practice (45,46): use a SERM (raloxifene) to treat osteoporosis and reduce the incidence of breast cancer as a beneficial side effect (45–47).

THE SERMS SURFACE IN CLINICAL PRACTICE

Raloxifene is the pioneering SERM approved for the prevention of osteoporosis around the world. The pivotal registration trial was the Multiple Outcomes of Raloxifene Evaluation (MORE) trial. Raloxifene reduced spine fractures by 50% compared with placebo (47). A separate analysis of breast cancer incidence demonstrated a 76% decrease in the incidence of invasive breast cancer (Fig. 5.4) over the three-year evaluation. There was no increase in endometrial cancer but DCIS remained unaffected (45). A long running trial, Raloxifene Use for the Heart (RUTH), to examine whether coronary heart events could be reduced in high-risk populations, did not show any benefit for raloxifene (48). Looked at another way, it showed little harm, but coronary heart disease (CHD) in a high-risk population was unaffected.

The use of estrogen-like medicines to treat and prevent osteoporosis in the postmenopausal woman demands a long-term therapy—perhaps an indefinite therapy. The extension trial to MORE was Continuing Outcomes Relevant to Evista (CORE) (46). An evaluation of both breast cancer and endometrial cancer in the CORE trial confirmed a sustained efficacy to prevent the development of breast cancer over the nine years of raloxifene treatment (Fig. 5.5) and this effect was entirely expressed in the prevention of ER-positive disease with no effect on the development of ER-negative disease.

Not unexpectedly, the promising data from the MORE trial (45) would propel raloxifene into a head to head study comparing tamoxifen with raloxifene for chemoprevention in high-risk postmenopausal women (Fig. 5.6). The Study of Tamoxifen and Raloxifene (STAR) trial illustrates several important lessons; however the dramatic decrease in invasive breast cancer noted in the MORE trial (raloxifene reducing the risk of ER-positive breast cancer by 90% and a 76% reduction of any newly diagnosed invasive breast cancer) (45) was not noted in the STAR trial with raloxifene. There was no difference between the incidence of breast cancer during treatment with tamoxifen or raloxifene (49) notwithstanding the

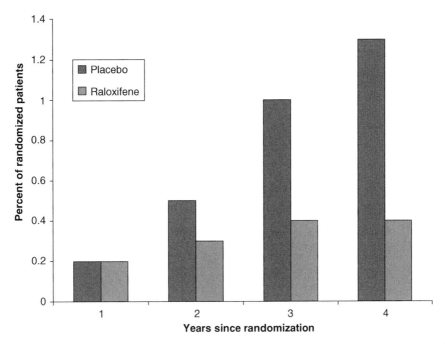

Figure 5.4 The annual accumulative incidence breast cancers represented as a percent of affected randomized patients in the Multiple Outcomes of Raloxifene Evaluation (MORE) trial that randomized women with an increased risk for osteoporotic fractures to placebo (2576 women) or raloxifene (5129 women) (45).

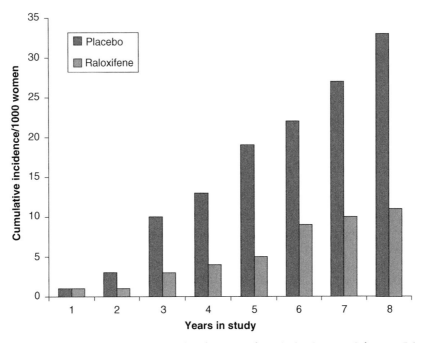

Figure 5.5 The cumulative incidence of invasive breast cancer for the combined MORE and Continuing Outcomes Relevant to Evista (CORE) studies. Shown are patients at high risk for osteoporotic fractures receiving either placebo or raloxifene (60 mg daily) (46).

presumed 50% decrease based on the results from the P-1 trial (38,39). Raloxifene had a very low proliferative effect on the uterine epithelium when compared with tamoxifen and this translated to fewer hysterectomies in the raloxifene-treated women (49). Additionally, there were fewer thrombotic events with raloxifene and fewer operations for cataracts (see earlier concerns with the triphenyl ethylene based nonsteroidal anti-estrogens (2)). Overall raloxifene seems to be equivalent to tamoxifen as a chemopreventive for invasive breast cancer but

is less effective than tamoxifen at controlling the development of DCIS. Nevertheless, raloxifene confers greater safety.

However, the importance of long-term follow-up for clinical trials is illustrated by the STAR trial. A re-evaluation of the STAR trial three years after stopping five years of treatment showed that although tamoxifen retained its "imprinting" as an antitumor agent raloxifene did not. Raloxifene was only 78% as effective at reducing primary breast cancer incidence as tamoxifen. These clinical data reflect the superiority

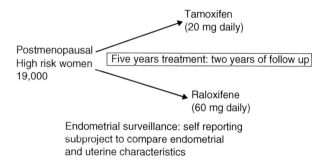

Figure 5.6 The design of the Study of Tamoxifen and Raloxifene (STAR). The STAR trial for postmenopausal women at an elevated risk for breast cancer had fewer serious side effects when taking raloxifene but a similar reduction in the incidence of breast cancer (49). However, after stopping the SERM treatment, the antitumor action of raloxifene was not maintained (50); so a continuous treatment with raloxifene was recommended (as this is the approval for the treatment and prevention of osteoporosis).

of tamoxifen in preclinical studies (31,50) and based on the raloxifene extension study, this agent (46) may need to be given indefinitely to prevent both osteoporosis and breast cancer.

INNOVATIONS IN SERM DEVELOPMENT

The story of the initial discovery and clinical application of the SERMs, tamoxifen and raloxifene, can be partially attributed to the play of chance; the right people were in the right place at the right time and willing to seize an opportunity that ultimately resulted in progress in medicine and pharmaceutical profits. The profits are necessary to permit progress in medicine. This is not a new idea and was stated as being essential by Professor Paul Ehrlich in the late 19th century for the successful development of what was the first chemical therapy for any disease (51). The anti-syphilitic Salvarsan™ (606; Hoechst) was discovered through systematic organic synthesis and testing of hundreds of compounds in appropriate animal models of human disease. But syphilis would not have been conquered if the pharmaceutical company Hoechst had not developed the drug. Without successful drug development, there would be no medicines. This fact is critical to the next part of the SERM story.

There has been considerable innovation by pharmaceutical chemists to refine the selectivity of SERMs and advance in the creation of the ideal SERM. The goal is illustrated in Figure 5.7. Numerous compounds have been synthesized and tested in preclinical studies but it is not our intention to survey progress in the laboratory here. This progress has been documented elsewhere (52,53). Rather, four SERMs are selected for consideration: ospemifene, arzoxifene, bazedoxifene, and lasofoxifene (Fig. 5.8). The reason for the selection of these four is that significant progress has been made in completed clinical trials of these drugs.

Ospemifene

Ospemifene (FC-1271a) is a new SERM that has shown estrogen-like effects in bone marrow (54), enhancing osteoblast formation *in vitro* by a mechanism unlike that of raloxifene. Ospemifene, Z-2-(4-(4-chloro-1,2-diphenyl-but-1-enyl)phenoxy) ethanol) is a metabolite of toremifene (55). Ospemifene

also has estrogenic activity in the vaginal epithelium, though not in the endometrium, suggesting its application as a treatment for vaginal dryness associated with menopause (56,57). Ospemifene has been shown to inhibit the growth of the ER-positive MCF-7 cells in culture (56).

Preclinical studies *in vivo* have shown ospemifene to prevent bone loss and increase bone strength in ovariectomized rats and to have a benefit in lowering serum cholesterol levels (58).

Phase I, II, and III clinical trials have been carried out with ospemifene (55) with no significant toxicity evident. Phase II trials (56,59) and a phase III trial (60) indicate that ospemifene is effective for treating vulvar and vaginal atrophy in postmenopausal women. Ospemifene's estrogen-like activity on the vagina improved symptoms of vaginal dryness, unlike raloxifene (61).

Arzoxifene

Arzoxifene (LY353381) is a potent SERM that was evaluated by Eli Lilly and Company (62). This SERM binds to the estrogen receptor alpha with higher affinity than raloxifene (62–64). It was found to have antagonistic effects on the uterus while being 30–100 times more potent than raloxifene in the prevention of body weight, bone, and serum cholesterol changes secondary to ovariectomization of rats (65). Furthermore, arzoxifene and its metabolite, demethylated arzoxifene, have been shown to not have a proliferative effect on endometrial tissue while protecting the bone.

In clinical trials, arzoxifene has shown promise for treatment of osteoporosis. In a phase III trial (66), arzoxifene treatment of postmenopausal osteoporotic women increased spine and hip bone density. Other trials have suggested that arzoxifene was effective against vertebral fractures but not nonvertebral fractures.

In spite of arzoxifene's encouraging preclinical and early clinical findings, arzoxifene is not on the market and is not being developed. Arzoxifene has some adverse effects in common with all SERMs such as hot flashes, increased risk of venous thromboembolic events, and cramps. In addition, a phase III breast cancer clinical trial was stopped because "*Arzoxifene was statistically significantly inferior to tamoxifen with regard to progression-free survival and other time-to-event parameters, although tumor response was comparable between the treatments*" (67). Arzoxifene has not been developed further.

Bazedoxifene

Bazedoxifene, a SERM for the treatment and prevention of osteoporosis in postmenopausal women (as well as, in combination with conjugated equine estrogens, for treatment of menopausal symptoms (68)), is currently approved for use in the European Union (EU) and it is under review by the US' Food and Drug Administration. This SERM, developed from a collaborative effort between Wyeth Pharmaceuticals and Ligand Pharmaceuticals, has a binding affinity for ERα about 10-fold lower than 17β-estradiol (69,70). Preclinical studies on bazedoxifene have been two-tiered: those studying bazedoxifene alone as treatment and as a preventative agent for osteoporosis and those of bazedoxifene in combination with conjugated estrogens. Bazedoxifene alone shows its efficacy in maintaining

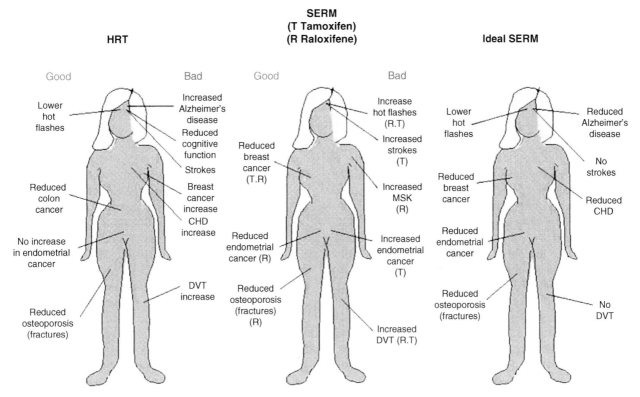

Figure 5.7 A comparison of the good and bad aspects of hormone replacement therapy (HRT) and current selective estrogen receptor modulators (SERMs) tested in postmenopausal women. On the right is the ideal SERM of the future. *Source*: From Ref. (95).

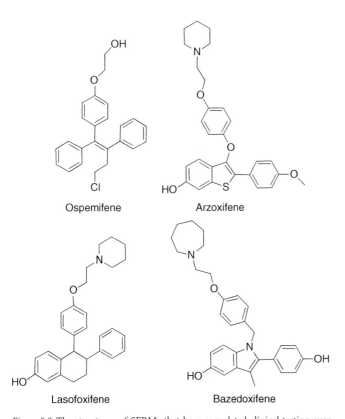

Figure 5.8 The structures of SERMs that have completed clinical testing over the last decade. Arzoxifene has not been pursued for clinical use and ospemifene is targeted for an application for vaginal atrophy. Lasofoxifene is the newest SERM thus far to attain the pharmacological profile of an ideal SERM (Fig. 5.7). Bazedoxifene is targeted for treatment and prevention for osteoporosis, or with conjugated equine oestrogen as an estrogen replacement therapy for hot flashes.

bone mass in doses as low as 0.1 mg/kg/day in ovariectomized rats (69,70). This bone preservation is comparable to that of raloxifene and lasofoxifene (71,72).

Combination studies have been carried out on bazedoxifene given with a mixture of the 10 principal conjugated estrogens (CEs) in Premarin® (Pfizer Pharmaceuticals; New York, NY). Bazedoxifene (3.0 mg/kg) was given in tandem with the CE. Bazedoxifene antagonized CE-induced dose-dependent increase in uterine weight to control levels (73).

Bazedoxifene has gone through several phase III clinical trials. It has been shown to reduce bone turnover and to prevent bone loss without undue endometrial, ovarian, and breast risks (74,75). Another phase III study showed that bazedoxifene reduced the incidence of vertebral fractures as compared with placebo (76). Among high-risk women for breast cancer, bazedoxifene significantly lowered the risk of nonvertebral fracture relative to both placebo and raloxifene (77). Bazedoxifene is considered to be well tolerated; serious adverse events and discontinuations are similar to those of a placebo group (77). Any increased risks of venous thromboembolism are similar to raloxifene and lasofoxifene (78,79). Bazedoxifene is considered safe regarding osteoporosis treatment and prevention (77) but cannot be considered a chemopreventive agent for breast cancer (76,77).

Lasofoxifene

Lasofoxifene is a SERM which binds with high affinity to the ER that is approved for the treatment of osteoporosis in the UK and EU but not currently in the US (80). Animal model studies of lasofoxifene have shown it to inhibit osteoclastogenesis, prevent bone loss, and reduce bone turnover (72,81).

Phase II and phase III clinical studies have confirmed improvements in bone mineral density (BMD). In one phase II study (82) one year's treatment with lasofoxifene showed significant improvement regarding lumbar spine BMD as compared with calcium and vitamin D. In another study, lasofoxifene acted positively by increasing BMD comparably to CEE (83).

Three phase III clinical studies have been carried out on lasofoxifene: The Postmenopausal Evaluation and Risk-Reduction with Lasofoxifene (PEARL) study, The Osteoporosis Prevention and Lipid Lowering (OPAL) study, and the Comparison of Raloxifene and Lasofoxifene (CORAL) study. The PEARL study found that both lumbar spine and femoral neck BMDs were increased after three years' treatment. Lasofoxifene also significantly reduced the risk of ER-positive breast cancer as compared with placebo (84–86). The OPAL trial tested three doses of lasofoxifene against placebo. All doses showed improved lumbar spine and hip BMD as compared with placebo (87). All doses also showed reduced serum levels of C-terminal telopeptide of type 1 collagen, serum osteocalcin, and no increase in breast density or pain (88). The CORAL study found that lasofoxifene maintained BMD in the lumbar spine better than raloxifene, with no difference in hip BMD; lasofoxifene also lowered total cholesterol more than raloxifene (89).

Lasofoxifene is a major advance toward improved potency and side effect profile. Lasofoxifene is 100 times more potent than raloxifene, but unlike the latter, lasofoxifene reduces the risk of coronary heart disease and strokes. Like raloxifene, lasofoxifene reduces the incidence of fractures and ER-positive breast cancers with no increase in the risk of endometrial cancer (79,86).

SERM SUMMARY

The practical application of SERMs for the chemoprevention of breast cancer has only resulted from the research philosophy first espoused by Professor Paul Ehrlich to achieve successful outcomes in experimental therapeutics, that is, the four Gs (in German): *Gluck* (luck), *Geduld* (patience), *Geshick* (skill), and *Geld* (money) (51). The discoveries with both tamoxifen and raloxifene, in the same laboratory, were not predictable. Some would say lucky. But with patience and skill over decades and the investment of money from philanthropy and the pharmaceutical industry to develop the new concepts further and "sell" the idea to physicians, millions of women are alive and millions more continue to benefit. The approved drugs, tamoxifen and raloxifene, are safe and effective if used in the correct manner for the right patients: tamoxifen for five years in high-risk premenopausal women (or the postmenopausal woman without a uterus) or raloxifene indefinitely in high-risk postmenopausal women. This therapeutic intervention will reduce the incidence of breast cancer in select populations. By contrast, 40 years ago there was nothing.

Unfortunately to advance further, it is unclear whether the new SERMs have the "uniqueness" to supersede raloxifene as the SERM of choice to prevent both osteoporosis and significantly reduce the risk of breast cancer. Arzoxifene can be viewed as a "long-acting raloxifene" but following completion

of clinical trials the decision was made not to seek FDA approval. In contrast, bazedoxifene for osteoporosis or bazedoxifene plus CEE to treat menopausal symptoms appears to hold merit for the postmenopausal women with a uterus. Bazedoxifene is approved in several countries. Ospemifene could have a "niche" application to ameliorate vaginal dryness, but an application to prevent breast cancer, like toremifene before, is unlikely without major clinical trials for chemoprevention, osteoporosis, or other indications. Lasofoxifene is approved in the EU but the drug has not been launched. The FDA has not approved lasofoxifene. It is all about *Geld* and the fear of financial failure by the pharmaceutical industry. The same was true for tamoxifen and raloxifene. Now the market may be overcrowded but there have been advances. The ideal SERM is illustrated in Figure 5.7 with the goal to achieve an improvement on raloxifene, the failed breast cancer drug. Raloxifene is seen to be a safe advance over tamoxifen as there is no endometrial cancer incidence and no rat hepatocarcinogenicity with the former. If we only focus on SERMs that have successfully moved to approval for osteoporosis (or hot flashes in the case of bazedoxifene) it is clear that lasofoxifene has solved additional issues by reducing strokes and reducing CHD. Significant progress has been made. The innovation of using CEE with bazedoxifene to protect the uterus (and breasts in early menopausal women) may yet prove to be useful as estrogen replacement therapy in younger postmenopausal women.

So if SERMs are currently optimal for the foreseeable future what about "no estrogen" at all. The aromatase inhibitors (AIs) have been rigorously tested in clinical trials of treatment and there is a recent trial of letrozole versus placebo in high-risk women that has shown promise for future consideration (91). However, despite claims about low incidence of side effects such as bone loss, joint pain, and vaginal dryness (with the attendant sexual issues), it would be hard to believe that the side effects of the many could ever outweigh the benefits of the few. If large populations are to benefit from AIs, issues of increased risk of CHD will again demand rigorous monitoring (91). Good quality of life is essential for any chemopreventive strategy. This was the basis some 60 years ago, for the introduction of estrogen replacement therapy/hormone replacement therapy (HRT) to improve quality of life for the many. Unfortunately, estrogen and HRT have a bad reputation relating to growth of breast cancer for the few (92). Nevertheless, there has been a recent surprise and once again science is poised to propel innovation forward and make progress.

The surprise was counterintuitive in the estrogen alone trial of the WHI (93). The finding that administration of CEE to postmenopausal hysterectomized women in their late 60s reduced the incidence of breast cancer for up to five years after stopping CEE (13) demands explanation. Clues as to the mechanisms for these paradoxical antitumor effects of low dose estrogen administration to women in their late 60s come from work of the mechanisms of antihormone resistance during long-term therapy (12). Two decades of laboratory study of the consequences of long-term SERM therapy demonstrated an evolution of types of resistance culminating in the discovery of a new biology of estrogen-induced apoptosis (94). It appears that five years of adjuvant antihormone therapy for breast cancer accelerates a process of breast cancer cell survival that is similar to what occurs over the 20 years with long-term estrogen deprivation following the menopause. Physiologically estrogen deprivation after the menopause needs decades to change the cell sensitivity from estrogen being a survival signal in breast cancer to an apoptotic trigger. In contrast it takes less than a decade to achieve the same effect on breast cancer with antihormone therapy. The WHI results and the associated laboratory evidence now pose a provocative dilemma in the era of "individualized" medicine. The application of low dose (physiological) estrogen-induced apoptosis has already moved successfully from the laboratory to clinical trial (95), and is being tested as a "purge strategy" for long-term AI adjuvant therapy with three-month drug holidays annually in the Study of Letrozole Extension (SOLE) trial (96). Maybe the era of individualized chemoprevention is soon to dawn as we piece together all the advances being made in cancer research and treatment. This era will deploy new knowledge of genetics, lifestyle, detection, and molecular medicine for the right preventive for the right women. If we can understand the mechanism of estrogen-induced apoptosis (97) as currently applied to second-line treatment after SERMs or AIs and use the knowledge to alternate or "purge" nascent breast cancer cells resistant to SERMs used as long-term preventatives with CEE for a few months, this new approach may be added to the armamentarium available to physicians as inexpensive but effective.

ACKNOWLEDGEMENTS

This work (VCJ) was supported by the Department of Defense Breast Program under Award number W81XWH-06-1-0590 Center of Excellence; subcontract under the SU2C (AACR) Grant number SU2C-AACR-DT0409; the Susan G Komen for the Cure Foundation under Award number SAC100009 and the Lombardi Comprehensive Cancer 1095 Center Support Grant (CCSG) Core Grant NIH P30 CA051008. The views and opinions of the author(s) do not reflect those of the US Army or the Department of Defense.

REFERENCES

1. Lacassagne A. Hormonal pathogenesis of adenocarcinoma of the breast. Am J Cancer 1936; 27: 217–25.
2. Jordan VC. Tamoxifen: a most unlikely pioneering medicine. Nat Rev Drug Discov 2003; 2: 205–13.
3. Jordan VC. Tamoxifen (ICI46,474) as a targeted therapy to treat and prevent breast cancer. Br J Pharmacol 2006; 147: S269–76.
4. Report from the Breast Cancer Trials Committee, Scottish Cancer Trials Office (MRC), Edinburgh. Adjuvant tamoxifen in the management of operable breast cancer: the Scottish Trial. Lancet 1987; 2: 171–5.
5. Fisher B, Costantino J, Redmond C, et al. A randomized clinical trial evaluating tamoxifen in the treatment of patients with node-negative breast cancer who have estrogen-receptor-positive tumors. N Engl J Med 1989; 320: 479–84.
6. Jordan VC. Biochemical pharmacology of antiestrogen action. Pharmacol Rev 1984; 36: 245–76.
7. Lerner LJ, Jordan VC. Development of antiestrogens and their use in breast cancer: eighth Cain memorial award lecture. Cancer Res 1990; 50: 4177–89.
8. Jordan VC. The science of selective estrogen receptor modulators: concept to clinical practice. Clin Cancer Res 2006; 12: 5010–13.
9. Jordan VC. Chemoprevention of breast cancer with selective oestrogen-receptor modulators. Nat Rev Cancer 2007; 7: 46–53.
10. Wolf DM, Jordan VC. A laboratory model to explain the survival advantage observed in patients taking adjuvant tamoxifen therapy. Recent Results Cancer Res 1993; 127: 23–33.
11. Yao K, Lee ES, Bentrem DJ, et al. Antitumor action of physiological estradiol on tamoxifen-stimulated breast tumors grown in athymic mice. Clin Cancer Res 2000; 6: 2028–36.
12. Jordan VC, Ford LG. Paradoxical clinical effect of estrogen on breast cancer risk: a "new" biology of estrogen-induced apoptosis. Cancer Prev Res (Phila) 2011; 4: 633–7.
13. LaCroix AZ, Chlebowski RT, Manson JE, et al. Health outcomes after stopping conjugated equine estrogens among postmenopausal women with prior hysterectomy: a randomized controlled trial. JAMA 2011; 305: 1305–14.
14. Jordan VC. A century of deciphering the control mechanisms of sex steroid action in breast and prostate cancer: the origins of targeted therapy and chemoprevention. Cancer Res 2009; 69: 1243–54.
15. EBCTG. Relevance of breast cancer hormone receptors and other factors to the efficacy of adjuvant tamoxifen: patient-level meta-analysis of randomised trials. Lancet 2011; 378: 771–84.
16. Gottardis MM, Robinson SP, Satyaswaroop PG, et al. Contrasting actions of tamoxifen on endometrial and breast tumor growth in the athymic mouse. Cancer Res 1988; 48: 812–15.
17. Fornander T, Rutqvist LE, Cedermark B, et al. Adjuvant tamoxifen in early breast cancer: occurrence of new primary cancers. Lancet 1989; 1: 117–20.
18. Gail MH, Brinton LA, Byar DP, et al. Projecting individualized probabilities of developing breast cancer for white females who are being examined annually. J Natl Cancer Inst 1989; 81: 1879–86.
19. Harper MJ, Walpole AL. A new derivative of triphenylethylene: effect on implantation and mode of action in rats. J Reprod Fertil 1967; 13: 101–19.
20. Consensus Conference. Adjuvant chemotherapy for breast cancer. JAMA 1985; 254: 3461–3.
21. Love RR, Newcomb PA, Wiebe DA, et al. Effects of tamoxifen therapy on lipid and lipoprotein levels in postmenopausal patients with node-negative breast cancer. J Natl Cancer Inst 1990; 82: 1327–32.
22. Love RR, Wiebe DA, Newcomb PA, et al. Effects of tamoxifen on cardiovascular risk factors in postmenopausal women. Ann Intern Med 1991; 115: 860–4.
23. Nordenskjöld B, Rosell J, Rutqvist LE, et al. Coronary heart disease mortality after 5 years of adjuvant tamoxifen therapy: results from a randomzed trial. J Natl Cancer Inst 2005; 97: 1609–10.
24. Hackshaw A, Roughton M, Forsyth S, et al. Long-term benefits of 5 years of tamoxifen: 10-year follow-up of a large randomized trial in women at least 50 years of age with early breast cancer. J Clin Oncol 2011; 29: 1657–63.
25. McDonald CC, Stewart HJ. Fatal myocardial infarction in the Scottish adjuvant tamoxifen trial. The Scottish Breast Cancer Committee. BMJ 1991; 303: 435–7.
26. Jordan VC, Phelps E, Lindgren JU. Effects of anti-estrogens on bone in castrated and intact female rats. Breast Cancer Res Treat 1987; 10: 31–5.
27. Turner RT, Wakley GK, Hannon KS, et al. Tamoxifen prevents the skeletal effects of ovarian hormone deficiency in rats. J Bone Miner Res 1987; 2: 449–56.
28. Turner RT, Wakley GK, Hannon KS, et al. Tamoxifen inhibits osteoclast-mediated resorption of trabecular bone in ovarian hormone-deficient rats. Endocrinology 1988; 122: 1146–50.
29. Love RR, Mazess RB, Barden HS, et al. Effects of tamoxifen on bone mineral density in postmenopausal women with breast cancer. N Engl J Med 1992; 326: 852–6.
30. Jordan VC. Effect of tamoxifen (ICI 46,474) on initiation and growth of DMBA-induced rat mammary carcinomata. Eur J Cancer 1976; 12: 419–24.
31. Gottardis MM, Jordan VC. Antitumor actions of keoxifene and tamoxifen in the N-nitrosomethylurea-induced rat mammary carcinoma model. Cancer Res 1987; 47: 4020–4.
32. Jordan VC, Lababidi MK, Langan-Fahey S. Suppression of mouse mammary tumorigenesis by long-term tamoxifen therapy. J Natl Cancer Inst 1991; 83: 492–6.
33. Greaves P, Goonetilleke R, Nunn G, et al. Two-year carcinogenicity study of tamoxifen in Alderley Park Wistar-derived rats. Cancer Res 1993; 53: 3919–24.
34. Jordan VC. What if tamoxifen (ICI 46,474) had been found to produce rat liver tumors in. 1973? A personal perspective. Ann Oncol 1995; 6: 29–34.
35. Jordan VC, Morrow M. Should clinicians be concerned about the carcinogenic potential of tamoxifen? Eur J Cancer 1994; 30A: 1714–21.

36. Powles TJ, Hardy JR, Ashley SE, et al. A pilot trial to evaluate the acute toxicity and feasibility of tamoxifen for prevention of breast cancer. Br J Cancer 1989; 60: 126–31.

37. Powles TJ, Ashley S, Tidy A, et al. Twenty-year follow-up of the Royal Marsden randomized, double-blinded tamoxifen breast cancer prevention trial. J Natl Cancer Inst 2007; 99: 283–90.

38. Fisher B, Costantino JP, Wickerham DL, et al. Tamoxifen for prevention of breast cancer: report of the national surgical adjuvant breast and bowel project P-1 Study. J Natl Cancer Inst 1998; 90: 1371–88.

39. Fisher B, Costantino JP, Wickerham DL, et al. Tamoxifen for the prevention of breast cancer: current status of the national surgical adjuvant breast and bowel project P-1 study J Natl Cancer Inst 2005; 97: 1652–62.

40. Cuzick J, Forbes JF, Sestak I, et al. Long-term results of tamoxifen prophylaxis for breast cancer–96-month follow-up of the randomized IBIS-I trial. J Natl Cancer Inst 2007; 99: 272–82.

41. (EBCTCG) EBCTCG. Effects of chemotherapy and hormonal therapy for early breast cancer on recurrence and 15-year survival: an overview of the randomised trials. Lancet 2005; 365: 1687–717.

42. Lewis JS, Jordan VC. Case histories: raloxifene. In: Taylor J, Triggle D, eds. Comprehensive Medicinal Chemistry II. Volume 8 Oxford, UK: Elsevier Limited, 2006: 103–21.

43. Black LJ, Jones CD, Falcone JF. Antagonism of estrogen action with a new benzothiophene derived antiestrogen. Life Sci 1983; 32: 1031–6.

44. Jordan VC. Chemosuppression of breast cancer with tamoxifen: laboratory evidence and future clinical investigations. Cancer Invest 1988; 6: 589–95.

45. Cummings SR, Eckert S, Krueger KA, et al. The effect of raloxifene on risk of breast cancer in postmenopausal women: results from the MORE randomized trial. Multiple Outcomes of Raloxifene Evaluation. JAMA 1999; 281: 2189–97.

46. Martino S, Cauley JA, Barrett-Connor E, et al. Continuing outcomes relevant to Evista: breast cancer incidence in postmenopausal osteoporotic women in a randomized trial of raloxifene. J Natl Cancer Inst 2004; 96: 1751–61.

47. Ettinger B, Black DM, Mitlak BH, et al. Reduction of vertebral fracture risk in postmenopausal women with osteoporosis treated with raloxifene: results from a 3-year randomized clinical trial. Multiple Outcomes of Raloxifene Evaluation (MORE) Investigators. JAMA 1999; 282: 637–45.

48. Barrett-Connor E, Mosca L, Collins P, et al. Effects of raloxifene on cardiovascular events and breast cancer in postmenopausal women. N Engl J Med 2006; 355: 125–37.

49. Vogel VG, Costantino JP, Wickerham DL, et al. Effects of tamoxifen vs raloxifene on the risk of developing invasive breast cancer and other disease outcomes: the NSABP Study of Tamoxifen and Raloxifene (STAR) P-2 trial. JAMA 2006; 295: 2727–41.

50. Vogel VG, Costantino JP, Wickerham DL, et al. Update of the national surgical adjuvant breast and bowel project Study of Tamoxifen and Raloxifene (STAR) P-2 trial: preventing breast cancer. Cancer Prev Res (Phila) 2010; 3: 696–706.

51. Baumler E. Paul Ehrlich: Scientist for Life. New York: Holmes & Meier, 1984: 288.

52. Jordan VC. Antiestrogens and selective estrogen receptor modulators as multifunctional medicines. 2. Clinical considerations and new agents. J Med Chem 2003; 46: 1081–111.

53. Jordan VC. Antiestrogens and selective estrogen receptor modulators as multifunctional medicines. 1. Receptor interactions. J Med Chem 2003; 46: 883–908.

54. Qu Q, Harkonen PL, Vaananen HK. Comparative effects of estrogen and antiestrogens on differentiation of osteoblasts in mouse bone marrow culture. J Cell Biochem 1999; 73: 500–7.

55. Gennari L, Merlotti D, Valleggi F, et al. Ospemifene use in postmenopausal women. Expert Opin Investig Drugs 2009; 18: 839–49.

56. Taras TL, Wurz GT, DeGregorio MW. In vitro and in vivo biologic effects of ospemifene (FC-1271a) in breast cancer. J Steroid Biochem Mol Biol 2001; 77: 271–9.

57. Voipio SK, Komi J, Halonen K, et al. Effects of ospemifene (FC-1271a) on uterine endometrium, vaginal maturation index, and hormonal status in healthy postmenopausal women. Maturitas 2002; 43: 207–14.

58. Qu Q, Zheng H, Dahllund J, et al. Selective estrogenic effects of a novel triphenylethylene compound, FC1271a, on bone, cholesterol level, and reproductive tissues in intact and ovariectomized rats. Endocrinology 2000; 141: 809–20.

59. Rutanen EM, Heikkinen J, Halonen K, et al. Effects of ospemifene, a novel SERM, on hormones, genital tract, climacteric symptoms, and quality of life in postmenopausal women: a double-blind,randomized trial. Menopause 2003; 10: 433–9.

60. Bachmann GA, Komi JO, Group OS. Ospemifene effectively treats vulvovaginal atrophy in postmenopausal women: results from a pivotal phase 3 study. Menopause 2010; 17: 480–6.

61. Komi J, Lankinen KS, Harkonen P, et al. Effects of ospemifene and raloxifene on hormonal status, lipids, genital tract, and tolerability in postmenopausal women. Menopause 2005; 12: 202–9.

62. Palkowitz AD, Glasebrook AL, Thrasher KJ, et al. Discovery and synthesis of [6-hydroxy-3-[4-[2-(1-piperidinyl)ethoxy]phenoxy]-2-(4-hydroxyphenyl)] b enzo[b]thiophene: a novel, highly potent, selective estrogen receptor modulator. J Med Chem 1997; 40: 1407–16.

63. Bryant HU, Glasebrook AL, Yang NN, et al. An estrogen receptor basis for raloxifene action in bone. J Steroid Biochem Mol Biol 1999; 69: 37–44.

64. Grese TA, Cho S, Finley DR, et al. Structure-activity relationships of selective estrogen receptor modulators: modifications to the 2-arylbenzothiophene core of raloxifene. J Med Chem 1997; 40:146–67.

65. Sato M, Turner CH, Wang T, et al. LY353381.HCl: a novel raloxifene analog with improved SERM potency and efficacy in vivo. J Pharmacol Exp Ther 1998; 287: 1–7.

66. Kendler DL, Palacios S, Cox DA, et al. Arzoxifene versus raloxifene: effect on bone and safety parameters in postmenopausal women with osteoporosis. Osteoporos Int 2011; 23: 1091–101.

67. Deshmane V, Krishnamurthy S, Melemed AS, et al. Phase III double-blind trial of arzoxifene compared with tamoxifen for locally advanced or metastatic breast cancer. J Clin Oncol 2007; 25: 4967–73.

68. Gruber C, Gruber D. Bazedoxifene (Wyeth). Curr Opin Investig Drugs 2004; 5: 1086–93.

69. Miller CP, Collini MD, Tran BD, et al. Design, synthesis, and preclinical characterization of novel, highly selective indole estrogens. J Med Chem 2001; 44: 1654–7.

70. Komm BS, Kharode YP, Bodine PV, et al. Bazedoxifene acetate: a selective estrogen receptor modulator with improved selectivity. Endocrinology 2005; 146: 3999–4008.

71. Black LJ, Sato M, Rowley ER, et al. Raloxifene (LY139481 HCl) prevents bone loss and reduces serum cholesterol without causing uterine hypertrophy in ovariectomized rats. J Clin Invest 1994; 93: 63–9.

72. Ke HZ, Paralkar VM, Grasser WA, et al. Effects of CP-336,156, a new, nonsteroidal estrogen agonist/antagonist, on bone, serum cholesterol, uterus and body composition in rat models. Endocrinology 1998; 139: 2068–76.

73. Kharode Y, Bodine PV, Miller CP, et al. The pairing of a selective estrogen receptor modulator, bazedoxifene, with conjugated estrogens as a new paradigm for the treatment of menopausal symptoms and osteoporosis prevention. Endocrinology 2008; 149: 6084–91.

74. Miller PD, Chines AA, Christiansen C, et al. Effects of bazedoxifene on BMD and bone turnover in postmenopausal women: 2-yr results of a randomized, double-blind, placebo-, and active-controlled study. J Bone Miner Res 2008; 23: 525–35.

75. Pinkerton JV, Archer DF, Utian WH, et al. Bazedoxifene effects on the reproductive tract in postmenopausal women at risk for osteoporosis. Menopause 2009; 16: 1102–8.

76. Silverman SL, Christiansen C, Genant HK, et al. Efficacy of bazedoxifene in reducing new vertebral fracture risk in postmenopausal women with osteoporosis: results from a 3-year, randomized, placebo-, and active-controlled clinical trial. J Bone Miner Res 2008; 23: 1923–34.

77. de Villiers TJ, Chines AA, Palacios S, et al. Safety and tolerability of bazedoxifene in postmenopausal women with osteoporosis: results of a 5-year, randomized, placebo-controlled phase 3 trial. Osteoporos Int 2011; 22: 567–76.

78. Grady D, Ettinger B, Moscarelli E, et al. Safety and adverse effects associated with raloxifene: multiple outcomes of raloxifene evaluation. Obstet Gynecol 2004; 104: 837–44.

79. Cummings SR, Ensrud K, Delmas PD, et al. Lasofoxifene in postmenopausal women with osteoporosis. N Engl J Med 2010; 362: 686–96.

80. UK Medicines Information New Drugs Online. New Drugs Online Report for lasofoxifene. Availabile from http://www.ukmi.nhs.uk/applications/ndo/record_view_open.asp?newDrugID=3184 Af] [Cited 2011, 29 September].

81. Maeda T, Ke HZ, Simmons H, et al. Lasofoxifene, a next generation estrogen receptor modulator: preclinical studies. Clin Calcium 2004; 14: 85–93.

82. Moffett A, Ettinger M, Bolognese M, et al. Lasofoxifene, a next generation SERM, is effective in preventing loss of BMD and reducing LDL-C in postmenopausal women. J Bone Min Res 2004; 19: S96.

83. Lee A, Radecki D, Wolter K. Lasofoxifene Phase II and Phase III clinical trial design and strategy. J Bone Min Res 2005; 20: M384.

84. Eastell R, Reid DM, Vukicevic S, et al. The effects of lasofoxifene on bone turnover markers: the PEARL trial. J Bone Min Res 2008; 23: 1287.

85. Cummings SR, Ensrud K, Delmas PD, et al. Lasofoxifene in postmenopausal women with osteoporosis. N Engl J Med 2010; 362: 686–96.

86. LaCroix AZ, Powles T, Osborne CK, et al. Breast cancer incidence in the randomized PEARL trial of lasofoxifene in postmenopausal osteoporotic women. J Natl Cancer Inst 2010; 102: 1706–15.

87. McClung M SE, Cummings S, et al. Lasofoxifene increased BMD of the spine and hip and decreased bone turnover markers in postmenopausal women with low or normal BMD. J Bone Min Res 2005; 20: S97.

88. Davidson M, Moffett A, Welty F, et al. Extraskeletal effects of lasofoxifene on postmenopausal women. J Bone Min Res 2005; 20: S173.

89. McClung MR, Siris E, Cummings S, et al. Prevention of bone loss in postmenopausal women treated with lasofoxifene compared with raloxifene. Menopause 2006; 13: 377–86.

90. Goss PE, Ingle JN, Ales-Martinez JE, et al. Exemestane for breast-cancer prevention in postmenopausal women. N Engl J Med 2011; 364: 2381–91.

91. Cuppone F, Bria E, Verma S, et al. Do adjuvant aromatase inhibitors increase the cardiovascular risk in postmenopausal women with early breast cancer? Meta-analysis of randomized trials. Cancer 2008; 112: 260–7.

92. Chlebowski RT, Kuller LH, Prentice RL, et al. Breast cancer after use of estrogen plus progestin in postmenopausal women. N Engl J Med 2009; 360: 573–87.

93. The Women's Health Initiative Steering Committee. Effects of conjugated equine estrogen in postmenopausal women with hysterectomy: the Women's Health Initiative Randomized Control Trial. JAMA 2004; 291: 1701–12.

94. Jordan VC. Selective estrogen receptor modulation: concept and consequences in cancer. Cancer Cell 2004; 5: 207–13.

95. Ellis MJ, Gao F, Dehdashti F, et al. Lower-dose vs high-dose oral estradiol therapy of hormone receptor-positive, aromatase inhibitor-resistant advanced breast cancer: a phase 2 randomized study. JAMA 2009; 302: 774–80.

96. Jordan VC, Ford LG. Paradoxical clinical effect of estrogen on breast cancer risk: a "new" biology of estrogen-induced apoptosis. Cancer Prev Res (Phila) 2011; 4: 633–7.

97. Ariazi EA, Brailoiu E, Yerrum S, et al. The G protein-coupled receptor GPR30 inhibits proliferation of estrogen receptor-positive breast cancer cells. Cancer Res 2010; 70: 1184–94.

6 The biological basis for breast cancer screening and its relevance to treatment

John R. Benson

INTRODUCTION

The principles of screening were enunciated by the World Health Organization (WHO) in 1968 (1) and formed the basis for breast screening programs designed to detect disease before it becomes clinically apparent. The aims of screening are to prevent, delay, or reduce the clinical impact of a target disease. Included among the preconditions for effective population screening was the assumption that the natural history of the disease in question should be "well understood" with a recognizable early stage for which treatment outcome would be enhanced compared with that of later stages. Thus there should be a preclinical phase with a consistent abnormality that is easily detectable with affordable, non-invasive methods. It is implicit that screening programs cannot yield any survival advantage when no effective treatments exist, and conversely no benefit will be apparent in terms of reduction of mortality if the treatments for screen-detected and symptomatic cancers are equally efficacious. Thus the benefits of screening derive from early treatment rather than early detection *per se*. A further consideration with screening programs is the prevalence of a disease which will determine the cost-effectiveness within a particular healthcare system (2). It has also been argued that implementation of a large scale screening program, such as for breast cancer, can only be justified when the cancer in question has serious consequences in terms of mortality and morbidity (3).

Randomized trials of breast screening have now confirmed the efficacy of screening in women over 50 years of age where reductions of breast cancer mortality of between 25 and 30% are attainable (4–7). The World Health Organization in 2002 upheld these conclusions for screening mammography within this age group of women (8). There are clearly trans-Atlantic differences both in philosophy and practice in terms of breast cancer screening. Most of the key trials have been carried out in countries outside the United States and a majority of them are based on European populations. Interpretation of these trial data has varied among experts around the world and indeed within individual countries. Some of this controversy is related to the vagaries of statistical processing and manipulation while other aspects of contention are based on issues of cost-effectiveness and perceived value for money. For example, in 1993 the American Cancer Society and the European Society of Mastology met in New York and Paris respectively to review results of screening trials; they each arrived at opposite conclusions regarding screening of younger women between 40 and 49 years of age (9).

CLINICAL TRIALS OF BREAST CANCER SCREENING

Within the international breast community, it is generally accepted that clinical trials to date support the conclusion that mammographic screening reduces the risk of death from breast cancer in women aged between 50 and 69 years (mortality reduction approximately 20%) (10). Individual trials and limited meta-analyses have reported mortality reductions of up to 30% for postmenopausal women (11). Some of the trials include postmenopausal women up to the age of 75 years, but there are no data assessing the value of screening in women beyond this age (12). Moreover, these trials involved two- or three-yearly mammography and thus the recommendations for biennial screening mammography for women aged 50–74 years seem reasonable and justified on the basis of published data alone (as opposed to patient demand or any emotive/intuitive influences) (13). It must be remembered that false positivity is a potential downside to screening and older patients are at a higher risk from general anesthesia performed for "diagnostic excision biopsies" resulting from indeterminate imaging and percutaneous needle biopsy results.

For women between 40 and 50 years of age, there is evidence for effectiveness of screening in terms of mortality reduction, but it takes rather longer (12–14 years) for that benefit to emerge (14). Moreover, the magnitude of the mortality reduction is only about 15% compared with greater than 20% for women more than 50 years of age. Furthermore, many experts have argued that the "delayed benefit" of screening mammography in younger women can be attributed to screening these women after the age of 50 years! Previous claims for fair evidence that mammographic screening every one to two years significantly reduced the mortality for women aged 40 years and more did not take into account of the potential harms and downside of screening in this age group. Over the past few years, both professionals and the public have become more aware of these concerns about screening (false-positive results, increased anxiety, unnecessary visits, further imaging and biopsy, and false reassurance) and the risk/benefit/(cost) ratio has been shifted such that now some organizations within the United States have recommended against routine screening mammography in women aged 40–49 years in the absence of any known genetic mutation or chest wall irradiation (13). It is essential that women are fully informed and aware of both the benefits and harms of screening, particularly in the younger age group where mortality reductions are more modest. There are issues of overdiagnosis and detection of disease which would not have progressed in a woman's lifetime and which might have led to a surgical recommendation for mastectomy with or without immediate breast reconstruction (which can be associated with complications and long-term adverse sequelae on quality of life).

There is no evidence as yet from clinical trials that breast self-examination is beneficial (15). Once again, though this might seem intuitively beneficial in terms of early cancer detection, overall there is potential to cause harm from false-positive prompts and increased referral to breast specialists for assessment. Many women have a degree of breast lumpiness and it is not surprising that they may find an area which they deem suspicious or worrying!

Likewise, there are currently no data to show any additional benefit from clinical breast examination (CBE) over screening mammography for women either under or over the age of 50 years. Some have suggested that CBE should be carried out at the same time as screening mammography as some cancers are radiologically occult but clinically palpable. Indeed within the Health Insurance Plan trial carried out in the 1960s, a significant proportion of cancers (45%) were detected with this mode of screening. However, methods of mammography have improved enormously since then and in the Edinburgh trial, only 6% of cancers were detected with CBE alone (16).

There is still a powerful patient–consumer-led demand for screening mammography in younger women in the United States, but hopefully a better informed public will lead to attrition of this demand. Health policy must be based on evidence and not emotion, and physicians should abide by these recommendations but respect an individual woman's values and personal perspectives. However, it is incumbent upon them to provide full information for their patients and correct any misguided preconceptions and biases arising from ignorance or misinformation. Some women will insist on screening mammography within the 40–49 year age group despite the most robust reassurance and information on potential harms; it cannot be denied that there is any mortality reduction from screening in this age group. The challenge is to convey the concept of risk–benefit ratio and convince most women that overall the disadvantages outweigh the benefits for most women in this age group. Discretion must be exercised and occasionally biennial mammography offered to these women.

Despite the apparent success of screening as judged by the endpoint of population mortality, it could be argued that the aforementioned screening criteria have not been fully satisfied in relation to breast cancer. For this reason, the underlying mechanism and extent by which advancing the time of diagnosis improves overall survival of a screened population remains unclear and some of the controversy relating to screening trials may emanate from limitations based on disease biology and the natural history of breast cancer. The latter is a heterogeneous disease, in terms both of variation among different tumors and of cellular composition within any individual tumor. This biological heterogeneity confers a variable natural history upon breast cancer, and may ultimately undermine and limit the potential impact not only of screening programs, but also treatment schedules for breast cancer. Conservative estimates reveal a broad range of individual tumor growth rates (17–19), with stochastic models being most applicable to breast cancer growth (20). This limits the breadth of predictions about the growth of mammary tumors and may hinder the design and planning of optimum schedules for breast cancer screening, where there are often "trade-offs" between the generalizability of screening outcomes and the validity of individual trials (7).

BIOLOGICAL MODELS OF BREAST CANCER

The essence of breast cancer screening is to detect malignant lesions at an earlier stage in their natural developmental history for which instigation of appropriate therapies will lead to mortality reduction. Detection of a lesion at a smaller size *per se* will not necessarily impact on mortality; diagnosis of a disease at an earlier chronological stage will only translate into improved outcomes if effective therapies can be instituted at this time. Otherwise, increased survival will be ascribed to "lead time" bias, and individuals merely acquire advance knowledge of their disease, with date of death and mortality remaining unchanged.

For screening to produce a genuine improvement in survival and reduction of cause-specific mortality, there must be an event in the natural history of the disease beyond which prognosis is adversely affected, and for which there is a threshold effect reflected in the size of a detectable lesion. If a lesion progressively increased in size without any such concomitant "event," then it would be of no consequence whether this was excised at size x or x+1 provided that excision was complete.

There are two events which may occur in the natural history and progression of malignant breast lesions which could account for the efficacy of screening and provide a biological rationale for early detection strategies; (*i*) early dissemination and (*ii*) phenotypic progression. Should one or both of these events occur at some stage in neoplastic development which is dependent upon tumor size, then earlier detection and intervention may pre-empt the formation of micrometastases and/or a more biologically aggressive primary tumor and so lead to improved prognosis (21). Stochastic models of tumor growth imply that such an event could occur relatively suddenly during tumor development due to a random growth "spurt" (20). Concepts of orderly progression may be deceptive; tumors can disseminate prior to reaching thresholds of either mammographic detection or clinical presentation (19,22). Screening aims to treat asymptomatic individuals at an early time point in this neoplastic continuum which represents a "window of opportunity" for treatment and can potentially reduce mortality by mechanisms outlined earlier.

There are two dominant paradigms of breast cancer biology which have governed the management of breast cancer over the past century: the Halstedian paradigm and the paradigm of biological predeterminism. Although the latter has become pre-eminent during the past two decades, both are relevant to the philosophy of breast screening and indeed an intermediate paradigm may be most appropriate contemporaneously (Fig. 6.1) (23).

Halstedian Paradigm

Virchow proposed a centrifugal theory for dissemination of breast cancer in which a tumor was considered to initially invade local tissues and to subsequently spread in a progressive,

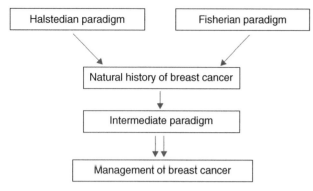

Figure 6.1 Emergence of an intermediate paradigm which incorporates elements of both Fisher and Halsted but is less restrictive than either paradigm in pure form and better informs management decisions.

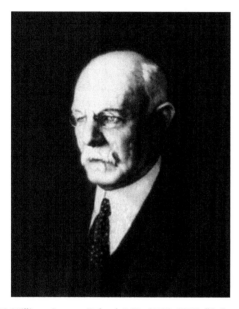

Figure 6.2 William Stewart Halsted MD, (1852–1922) "Father of Breast Surgery," Johns Hopkins Hospital, Baltimore.

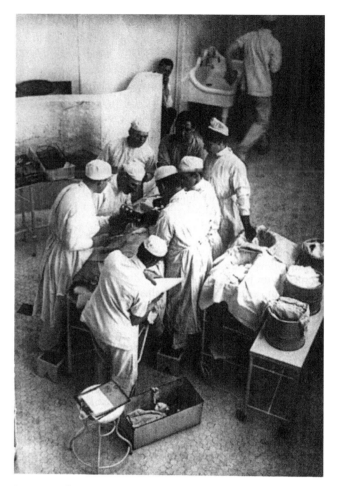

Figure 6.3 William Halsted undertaking surgery at the Johns Hopkins Hospital in Baltimore, Maryland. *Source*: Courtesy of the Alan Chesney Medical Archives, John Hopkins University, Baltimore, Maryland, USA.

sequential, and predictable manner upon ever more distant structures which lay in anatomical continuity (25,26). The lymph nodes were thought to act as mechanical filters that formed a circumferential line of defense against such centrifugal dissemination and temporarily impeded the spread of cancer. However, once this filtration capacity was exhausted, cancer cells would then pass into the efferent lymphatics and thence to more distant sites. This model provided the rationale for the operation of radical mastectomy devised by William Halsted in which an en bloc resection of tumor and locoregional tissues was performed (Figs. 6.2 and 6.3) (27). As a tumor was believed to spread in a sequential manner with successive involvement of structures in anatomical continuity, such en bloc resection was considered to offer the best chance of "cure." Although the operation of radical mastectomy provided high rates of local disease control, there was no evidence for improved survival relative to lesser surgical procedures (28). This implied that some "event" had occurred prior to mastectomy that predetermined survival and was unaffected by surgical intervention *per se*. Analysis of survival data for patients undergoing radical mastectomy revealed that fewer than a quarter of these patients shared a similar hazard ratio as an age-matched control

population (29). Therefore radical mastectomy could not be hailed as a general curative procedure for breast cancer and fostered some doubt in the underlying paradigm.

Biological Predeterminism
An alternative paradigm was proposed by Fisher that challenged the concept of progressive centrifugal spread according to anatomical and mechanical criteria. Instead, breast cancer was considered to be largely a systemic disease at the outset as a consequence of cancer cells entering the bloodstream at an early stage in tumor development (30). In particular, such hematogenous dissemination was not conditional upon lymph node involvement, and regional lymph nodes were not viewed as the instigators of distant metastases. Rather they reflected a tumor–host relationship which favored dissemination and formation of micrometastatic foci of disease. Experimental models were employed to demonstrate the transnodal passage of tumor cells (31) together with destruction of tumor cells by lymph nodes. These findings repudiated the concept of lymph nodes as passive filters (32,33) and showed that cancer cells could pass not only directly into efferent lymphatics, but also into the bloodstream via lymphaticovenous communications. Further, animal models had shown that dormant tumor cells could develop into overt metastases under appropriate conditions. These experimental observations formed the basis for an alternative paradigm of biological predeterminism in which

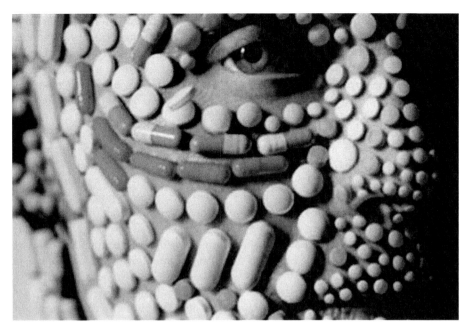

Figure 6.4 Initiation of systemic therapies can destroy these putative micrometastases, which should improve prognosis. These can be administered either as oral (hormonal/chemotherapy) or intravenous (chemotherapy) agents. *Source*: From Breast Cancer Care 2011, http://www.breastcancercare.org.uk.

cancer is viewed as a predominantly systemic disease at inception with clinical outcome predetermined by micrometastases present at the time of diagnosis. Prognosis is ultimately determined by the propensity for these micrometastases to develop into overt metastatic disease—through some process of being "kick started" (34).

There are important consequences of this hypothesis which have implications both for the potential efficacy of any screening program and treatment strategies. In terms of therapeutic sequelae, this paradigm of biological predeterminism will predict that the extent of primary surgery does not influence overall survival, as the latter is dependent upon micrometastases which are present in all patients irrespective of surgical procedure. Trials of breast conservation therapy (BCT) have confirmed that lesser surgical resections do not compromise overall survival, though are associated with higher rates of local recurrence (35–40). A meta-analysis by the Early Breast Cancer Trialists Collaborative Group (EBCTCG) reinforced the link between local failure and survival and underlined how individual BCT trials lack the power to detect any effect of attenuated local control on longer term survival (41). An important reanalysis of the EORTC trial at 20 years' follow-up reaffirmed the equivalence of time to distant metastases and overall survival despite persistent and significant differences in IBTR which could have translated into a survival detriment if IBTR was a potential source for distant metastatic disease (42,43). However, as this group of patients had more advanced stage (II) disease based on tumor size and nodal status, there are competing sources of distant micrometastases at presentation. Thus a significant proportion of patients randomized into each arm will have pre-existent micrometastases which are a principal determinant of distant metastases and driver of mortality. Notably, patients were matched for clinicopathological parameters and by implication the prevalence of micrometastases was similar between the two arms. Therefore individual trials of

BCT have confirmed that overall survival rates are uninfluenced by the extent of primary surgery, and support the notion of predeterminism based on subclinical dissemination of micrometastases (44).

The second therapeutic sequela of this hypothesis is that initiation of systemic therapies which could destroy these putative micrometastases should improve prognosis (Fig. 6.4). This aspect of treatment would therefore be complementary to locoregional therapy (surgery ± radiotherapy). Clinical trials of both adjuvant and neoadjuvant (primary) therapies for breast cancer have provided corroborative evidence for the second prediction of this alternative paradigm (45–47). The third overview by the EBCTCG included 37,000 women from 55 trials of adjuvant tamoxifen and concluded that five years of tamoxifen was better than less than five years with proportional reductions in mortality risk at 1, 2, and 5 years being 14%, 18% and 28% respectively (45). Longer term follow-up confirms that five years of tamoxifen therapy reduces risk of recurrence and contralateral breast cancer for 15 years after starting the treatment (46). This overview by the EBCTCG also included 30,000 women in 69 trials assessing the role of chemotherapy and found that polychemotherapy regimens produced a significant proportional reduction in recurrence of 35% in women <50 years and 20% in women aged 50–69 years. The corresponding proportional mortality reductions for these two groups were 27% and 11% respectively. These proportional effects were similar for node-positive and node-negative women and no survival advantage was seen for treatments longer than three to six months (47). The 2000 overview with 15 years' follow-up reinforced these benefits of tamoxifen and emphasized gradation of benefit based on the strength of estrogen receptor positivity (48). Moreover, a meta-analysis of more mature trials of five years of tamoxifen confirms the benefits of this agent beyond the five-year period. There is a reduction in rates of recurrence throughout the first 10 years, whereas breast cancer mortality is reduced by approximately one-third for each of the follow-up periods, 0–4 years (RR 0.71), 5–9 years (RR 0.66), and 10–14 years (RR 0.68) (49). Randomized controlled trials have shown benefit in disease-free survival in postmenopausal women receiving aromatase inhibitors as adjuvant therapy. These include the oral agents, anastrozole, letrozole, and exemestane, which are of comparable antitumor efficacy and are potentially interchangeable. The most appropriate sequencing with or without tamoxifen and overall survival benefit with aromatase inhibitors are yet to be clearly demonstrated (50–54). A meta-analysis of randomized trials of aromatase inhibitors estimated absolute reductions in recurrence and mortality for aromatase inhibitors as either initial monotherapy or following early switching from two years of tamoxifen therapy compared with five years of tamoxifen. This meta-analysis reported that upfront aromatase inhibitor therapy was associated with an absolute recurrence reduction of 2.9% and a decrease in breast cancer mortality of 1.1% at five years. Similar reductions were found for comparison of an early switch policy with five years of tamoxifen (3.1% and 0.7% for recurrence and mortality respectively). The underlying rationale for neoadjuvant chemotherapy is based on several potential advantages and opportunities. These include improved overall survival, increased chance of breast preservation, and assessment of individual tumor sensitivity to particular chemotherapeutic agents and eventual correlation of tumor response to long-term outcome (55,56). Neoadjuvant approaches have increasingly been advocated for operable breast cancers with the expectation of improved outcomes and possible breast conservation (57,58). Though there is evidence of increased overall survival from preoperative chemotherapy in a rat model of breast cancer, this has not translated into any clinical gains (2). A meta-analysis of neoadjuvant versus adjuvant systemic therapy for early stage breast cancer reveals that overall survival and disease-free survival are comparable for the two schedules (59). If the act of surgery itself causes a systemic perturbation which can be offset by induction chemotherapy, this will provide biological underpinning for neoadjuvant therapy. Nonetheless, it is perhaps naïve to assume that a modest shift in the timing of chemotherapy relative to surgery will have any significant clinical impact from attacking micrometastases slightly sooner (55).

APPLICATION OF MODELS TO BREAST SCREENING
The evidence mentioned earlier together with data on the clinical outcome of stage I and II breast cancer indicates that micrometastases are present in over 50% of cases of "early" breast cancer at the time of clinical diagnosis. If one adopts the philosophy that all breast cancer is systemic at the outset, then any screening program is doomed to failure as earlier detection and treatment of a primary lesion will not reduce mortality if survival has already been predetermined by early dissemination and the presence of micrometastatic disease at the time of preclinical detection of disease.

To date there is no conclusive evidence for any subgroup of breast cancer patients who have been "cured" as defined by either statistical or clinical criteria (60). Statistical cure (61) can only be claimed if after a prolonged follow-up a subgroup of patients are found to have an annual death rate from all causes which is identical to an age-matched control population. Several studies, including that of Brinkley and Haybittle (62) have identified subgroups whose survival approximates to a control group, but in none of these has the ratio of observed deaths to expected deaths been unity (62–64). Similarly, there is no evidence for a clinically cured group who are deemed to have no increased relative risk of subsequently dying from breast cancer. Most studies reveal that all groups of treated patients remain at a relatively increased risk of death from breast cancer and also of developing a contralateral cancer (62–65).

Though "cure" cannot so far be claimed on strict statistical criteria, there are reports that purport to define subgroups with a highly favorable prognosis who may be effectively cured. This particularly applies to small tumors and may have some bearing on screening. Thus, Hayward analyzed the long-term follow-up of stage I and II patients treated at Guy's by mastectomy (66). Some of these have attained hazard ratios very similar to an age-matched control population. Analysis of long-term survival of patients treated for stage I disease prior to the widespread use of adjuvant systemic therapy suggests that breast cancer is a locoregional process in up to 75–80% of node-negative cases who may be considered statistically "cured" (23,67). Siggardson and colleagues analyzed prognostic factors (% S-phase, progesterone receptor, and tumor size) in stage I patients within a screening program and described a subgroup of approximately 30% who would have a calculated relative survival of 100% (68). These data suggest that a subgroup of patients do exist for whom micrometastatic dissemination has not occurred prior to clinical detection.

Notwithstanding the pre-eminence of biological predeterminism, it is implicit from a breast screening program that a substantial proportion of patients are potentially curable by earlier detection. If it is believed that screening can genuinely reduce mortality, then it probably has to be accepted that all breast cancers are not systemic at the outset. Nonetheless, it is assumed that dissemination and establishment of viable micrometastases can occur during the preclinical phase when a breast cancer is mammographically detectable. The crucial question is what proportion of tumors disseminate between the time of radiological detection and clinical presentation. In other words, what proportion of cancers can be successfully detected mammographically *before* any development of micrometastases? Is there a threshold of tumor size above which dissemination occurs? As breast cancer is a heterogeneous disease, the answer to this question is unlikely to be consensual, with a range of sizes rather than a single threshold value. This issue of the stage at which microscopic dissemination occurs is embodied in the emerging concept of an "intermediate" paradigm; some tumors behave in a Halstedian manner and can be "cured" by locoregional treatment. The chances of cure are enhanced by earlier detection, and these tumors will benefit from screening. Other tumors tend to disseminate early and become systemic during either the preclinical or predetection phases of growth. Screening strategies will only be successful if detection occurs prior to the development of micrometastases. A tumor requires a blood supply to grow beyond the size of a million cells (a few cubic millimeters) (69), but it is quite feasible to propose that a tumor can possess an established vasculature without necessarily exhibiting vascular invasion at these early stages of tumor development.

Furthermore, cancer cells could travel to the regional lymph nodes and remain there without entering the circulation via lymphaticovenous communications. In both of these scenarios, cure could theoretically be achieved by excision of tumor and regional nodes. Patients with microscopic nodal deposits on conventional H&E criteria have been reported to have a similar prognosis to node-negative cases, although this remains a controversial area (70–74). An analysis of occult metastases among patients who were initially pathologically sentinel lymph node biopsy negative in the randomized NSABP B-32 trial found occult metastases in 15% of cases. The majority of these were isolated tumor cells only (11%) and an immunohistochemical analysis was performed. The presence of these occult metastases translated into a small, but statistically significant reduction of 1.5% in overall survival. However, this was probably not clinically meaningful. Other studies suggest the presence of microscopic nodal deposits [micrometastases (>0.2 mm to ≤2 mm) or isolated tumor cells (≤0.2 mm)] within sentinel lymph nodes do not impact on longer term survival outcomes (75).

Even if tumor cells gain access to the circulation at a very early stage, these may not necessarily develop into viable micrometastatic foci. The host immune system can destroy rogue cancer cells within the bloodstream and successful establishment of micrometastases will depend upon innate biological properties of the tumor cells as well as local host factors. From a clinical perspective, it is of greater significance to ascertain the earliest stage in tumor development at which viable metastatic foci can form. Screening programs would aim to maximize radiological sensitivity and specificity and hence the capacity to detect lesions before this clinical dissemination occurred. The smallest lesion which can be detected mammographically with state-of-the-art technology is approximately 2–3 mm. By the time a tumor has attained this size, it will probably contain more than 1 million cells and therefore have already entered the vascular phase of growth (76). In experimental models, tumors reach a maximum size of only 1–2 mm in the absence of vascularization, though growth rapidly accelerates upon induction of a vasculature that provides nutritional support for the tumor cells (69). Despite the tendency for new blood vessels to be "leaky" (77), it does not follow that vascular invasion is an obligate phenomenon once neovascularization has occurred. The downregulation of integrin expression and alterations in the cellular profile of other cell adhesion molecules will determine not only the tendency of cells to break away from the tumor bolus and enter the circulation, but also for these self-same cells to harbor at distant sites with formation of micrometastatic foci (78). Therefore detection by screening of smaller tumors that are in the vascular phase of growth could still precede systemic dissemination. Ideally, screening should pick up tumors while they are still in the prevascular phase where growth is relatively slower and there is no opportunity for hematogenous spread. However, such lesions are unlikely to have any radiological "signature," which is dependent upon induction of a stromal response in the vicinity of tumor cells.

It was stated in the introductory section that the efficacy of screening could be accounted for by two possible mechanisms. In addition to detection of tumors prior to any systemic dissemination, screening might also pick up tumors with a more

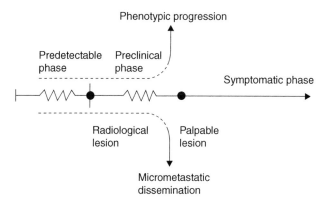

Figure 6.5 Schematic representation of sequential development of a tumor through predetectable, preclinical, and symptomatic phases. Though these are time dependent and a function of absolute tumor size, formation of distant metastases, and phenotypic progression have an unpredictable and non-obligate relationship to size and therefore phase of neoplastic development. When these two processes occur in the preclinical phase (after radiological detection) then screening offers the potential for mortality reduction.

favorable grade and biological credentials. There is some evidence that the malignant phenotype evolves and becomes more "aggressive" as a tumor grows (79), although this remains controversial and unproven (80). If cancers can progress to less differentiated forms, then screening might improve prognosis if it permitted detection and removal of lesions prior to any histological progression (Fig. 6.5).

RELATIONSHIP BETWEEN REDUCTION OF MORTALITY AND CHANGES IN SIZE AND STAGE DISTRIBUTION OF SCREEN-DETECTED TUMORS

So to what extent can screening reduce tumor size, and is such a reduction in tumor size *per se* related to prognosis? Screening is associated with a reduction in the proportion of larger tumors and metastatic lesions (6,81–83). This section examines how improvements in survival among patients with screen-detected cancers can be accounted for by changes in conventional prognostic indices and whether screening can detect lesions prior to any dissemination.

Lymph node status remains the single most important prognostic indicator for breast cancer (84,85), and has yet to be succeeded by newer biological indices such as ploidy, percentage S-phase, and abnormal gene expression (86,87). Survival is closely correlated with the total number of lymph nodes infiltrated by tumor (88); if there is no axillary nodal involvement, then five-year survival rates are of the order of 80–90%, falling to approximately 65% if fewer than four nodes are positive and 30% if four or more nodes are affected. Prognosis is particularly poor if more than 10 nodes are positive. By implication, lymph node status is an indirect indicator of the likelihood of micrometastatic foci pre-existing at the time of primary surgery. Tumor size is related both to lymph node status and the risk of distant metastases (89,90–92), and there is provisional evidence that a similar relationship appertains to screen-detected lesions (82).

In the Swedish Two-County trial, there was a significant reduction in both the size and nodal status of screen-detected invasive cancers. More than half of the tumors were less than 15 mm in diameter and 80% were node negative (93,94). Comparison of tumor size with the control group revealed a

26% reduction in tumors more than 20 mm in size and a 40% reduction in those over 30 mm. The observed incidence of node negativity represented a 24% reduction in proportion of patients with positive nodes. This reduction in tumor size and node positivity was paralleled by an improved survival, presumably reflecting a lower incidence of micrometastases in these screened breast cancer patients.

Hatschek and colleagues reported a highly favorable reduction of node positivity for invasive tumors detected in incidence screens from 40% among controls to 18% in screened patients. There was a corresponding increase in incidence of small tumors (<20 mm) from 59% to 85% (95). Of interest, in the Edinburgh trial, the node positivity rate remained high for the incidence rounds (28%) and only half of invasive tumors detected were 20 mm or smaller. As might be expected, this study found more favorable effects on tumor size, lymph node status, and histology in the prevalence round, but this was not sustained for the incidence round (96). Prevalence screens are innately biased toward tumors with better prognostic indices (97), and there has been some criticism of studies based exclusively on prevalence data (76,77). Crisp and colleagues reported a higher proportion of smaller tumors with less lymph node involvement in a population of 131 screen-detected tumors compared with clinical tumors (7.4 tumors per 1000 women screened) (98). Furthermore, these authors translated these data into predictions of survival using the Nottingham Prognostic Index (NPI) and concluded that screening conferred a survival advantage of 26.5% at five years consistent with the 30% reduction in mortality.

These data suggest that screening can lead to a change in stage distribution of invasive breast cancers. This so-called "stage drift" may represent detection of cancers at an earlier biological stage. However, the relationship between reduction in tumor size and lymph node positivity may be more complex *apropos* screen-detected lesions; an increased proportion of smaller tumors may not necessarily be accompanied by predicted changes in nodal status based on data from clinical tumors. Following introduction of a mass screening program in Colorado involving over 15,000 patients, Abernathy and colleagues reported that there was an increase of approximately 20% in the fraction of tumors smaller than 2 cm (99). However, an interesting finding of this study was an increase in the proportion of tumors between 2 cm and 5 cm with positive lymph nodes. At first, this anomalous result might appear to indicate a reversed stage drift! The authors have suggested that screening detects lesions at a smaller size, and facilitates their removal before they can develop into node-negative tumors within this size range. This implies that increasing tumor size does not invariably lead to a stage shift involving a progression to node positivity. Screening will tend to be biased toward these node-negative tumors because they are likely to be slower growing, that is length-time bias. Therefore the effects of screening on nodal status and hence precise stage distribution may be inherently more complex than previously thought.

Even if there is a genuine stage shift (100), screening methods must ultimately be capable of detecting lesions prior to any hematogenous dissemination; node negativity does not equate with absence of micrometastases, but rather reflects a relationship between tumor and host in which the chances of dissemination are minimized (30). The goal of screening practice is therefore not to achieve stage I status *per se*, but to detect tumors at a size which precedes the threshold for hematogenous dissemination. The fundamental problem is that this threshold size will vary between tumors, and the precise proportion of lesions which are detected at this pre-dissemination stage will be dictated not only by the natural history of individual tumors, but also technical nuances of mammographic screening. There are no specific mammographic features which correlate with the biological behavior of an invasive tumor and its propensity to metastasize, although some correlation between mammographic densities and increased risk of non-invasive proliferative lesions has been reported (101). Screening provides information on size and local extent of a tumor only. Techniques which include genetic expression profiles are currently being developed to extract maximal prognostic information from cytological samples, and these may help predict which screen-detected lesions are likely to have already metastasized (86,102).

The above studies on screen-detected lesions have revealed changes in distribution not only of tumor size and nodal status, but also histological type and grade. Some studies claiming that breast screening detects less aggressive cancers have been confined to prevalence screens only, and should perhaps be interpreted with caution (103). Nonetheless, others have found a persistent change in the histological grade and "malignant potential" of incidence screen-detected tumors (93,96,98,104,105). Indeed, in the Swedish Two-County trial referred earlier, improved survival could not entirely be accounted for by reduction in tumor size and proportion of node-positive tumors. Screen-detected tumors were also of more favorable histological grade, and when taken together with these other two factors, differences in survival between screened and control groups could be fully accounted for (106). However, although any survival advantage from screen detection might intuitively be explained by a stage shift at presentation, evidence has been accumulating which suggests that mode of detection (screen versus symptomatic) *per se* may confer a survival benefit over and above that which is accountable from changes in tumor size, grade, and nodal status (107,107–109). Thus screen detection remains an independent prognostic factor after adjustment for these conventional prognostic parameters (107,108). In a retrospective study examining clinical, histopathological, and biological features of screen-detected cancers compared with symptomatic cancers, screen detection was found to be an independent prognostic variable which reduced the relative hazard ratio for distant recurrence (HR 1.90; 95% CI 1.15 – 3.11; p = 0.01). Moreover, this influence of mode of detection was equal to or even greater than the effect of a 1 cm decrease in tumor size. The risk of distant metastases was therefore overestimated for those women with screen-detected cancers and it is therefore imperative to take mode of detection into account when estimating the risk of recurrence (108). Using a multivariate model, Wishart and colleagues estimated the proportional effect of known prognostic factors on the survival advantage of screen-detected cancers among more than 5000 women in the East of England NHS Breast Screening Programme (110). The combination of age and NPI (which incorporates tumor size, grade, and nodal status) accounted for almost three-quarters (72%) of this survival benefit, but left 28% unexplained. These findings were subsequently confirmed by a study from the Netherlands Cancer Institute involving 2592 screen-detected breast cancers where the hazard ratio for screen-detection (after adjustment for age, tumor grade, nodal status, estrogen receptor (ER) status and adjuvant therapy) was 0.74. Hence smaller, more favorable node-negative tumors account for much, but not all of the mortality reduction in a screened population. This phenomenon relating to mode of detection is not confined to overall survival, but also applies to breast cancer–specific survival which was examined in the Dutch study by Mook and colleagues (109). Indeed, the adjusted hazard ratio for breast cancer specific survival was 0.62 yielding a mortality reduction of 38% compared with a figure of 26% for overall survival.

This theme is further explored in chapter 8 (Survival advantage of screen-detected cancer over stage-matched symptomatic cancer) along with a discussion of possible differences in disease biology which might underpin these effects of mode of detection. Evidence is emerging that screen-detected tumors are more likely to have immunohistochemical positivity for ER, progesterone receptor, and Bcl-2 with a smaller proportion of tumors expressing Ki-67 and epidermal growth factor receptor (111). Indeed, Brown and colleagues have proposed that the biology of breast cancer has changed in a fundamental manner with the advent of screening and urbanized lifestyles. They examined tissue samples from tumors diagnosed over two separate time periods (symptomatic in the 1980s; screen detected in the 1990s) and found an increase in ER positivity over a 10-year period from 64.2% to 71.5%. Moreover, there were more grade 1 tumors among screened patients from the later period and correspondingly fewer grade 3 cancers (112). These findings may partially reflect lead time bias with detection of more indolent, slow growing, and ER-positive tumors with screening. These exist for longer in the preclinical phase and are more likely to be ER positive (113). Nonetheless, though screening may have preferentially benefited ER-positive tumors, lifestyle changes may additionally be increasing the chance of ER-positive, hormone dependent tumors. These include factors such as deferred childbirth, postmenopausal obesity, and use of hormone replacement therapy.

Most studies have revealed a significantly higher proportion of special tumor types among screen-detected lesions compared with symptomatic cancers (96,98,105,114). Approximately 8% of the latter are of special histological type, while these have constituted between 12.5% and 25% of screen-detected invasive lesions. The value of 12.5% reported by Crisp and colleagues (98) is significantly lower than others quoted which are on average approximately 20% (96,115). Of interest, in an analysis of breast cancer histology and age, Wicks and colleagues found the highest incidence of tubular carcinomas in the age group corresponding to the screened population (50–69 years) (115). Anderson and colleagues found a difference in the proportion of special and variant tumors compared with "no special type" tumors in prevalence versus incidence screens, and surmised that this might reflect a natural progression of lesions to less well–differentiated forms (96). In their analysis of the Swedish Two-County trial, Duffy and colleagues noted a much lower

proportion of high-grade (3) tumors among smaller screen-detected lesions (79). By comparing size and grade of malignancy in the control and "unbiased" screen-detected groups, the expected distribution corresponded with the observed, demonstrating that any differences in grade distribution were attributable to size only, an effect therefore independent of length bias. These authors concluded that malignancy grade evolves, that is worsens, as a tumor enlarges. Grade of malignancy was considered to represent an underlying variable which faithfully reflected "malignant potential." However, grade is a surrogate marker for the latter which ideally should be measured by some biological index relating directly to proliferative activity.

The concept of phenotypic progression is supported by the known heterogeneity of tumors. Thus different cell populations within a single tumor would have variable biological behavior and growth characteristics. Up to one-third of breast cancers have foci of more than one histological type (116). Variations in nuclear grade and degrees of pleomorphism are frequently observed within the same tumor. Furthermore, in vitro studies with thymidine labeling have shown a wide variation in indices of proliferative potential between cells derived from a single tumor (117). Curiously, Ponten and colleagues carried out extensive DNA ploidy studies on the incidence of screen-detected cancers and reported no differences in ploidy profiles between screen-detected and clinical cancers (118). However, DNA ploidy has been reported to display less intratumoral variation than these other proliferative indices (119). Hakama and colleagues analyzed the aggressiveness of cancers among a screened population using DNA index (ploidy) and S-phase fraction (80). On these criteria of proliferative indices alone (and not inclusive of histological data), cancers detected in the prevalence round were of lower malignant potential. However, in subsequent incident rounds, the level of aggressiveness was similar between control and screened groups, suggesting that "biological aggressiveness" did not increase during the preclinical phase of tumor development. By contrast, screen-detected lesions in this study were of smaller size and more favorable stage than controls, this being predictive of a future reduction in mortality from population screening (80). Prevalent round cancers generally have a more favorable tumor biology and better prognosis than incident round cancers (120). Further insight into possible biological differences between screen-detected and symptomatic cancers has come from an analysis of copy number imbalances between these two groups of breast cancer. Using a Cox proportional hazards model, approximately 20% of the survival advantage among screen-detected tumors was associated with copy number imbalances involving chromosomes 2p, 3q, 11q, and 20q (121).

PATTERNS OF GROWTH IN THE PRECLINICAL PHASE

The concept of malignant progression during the preclinical phase when lesions are impalpable yet detectable mammographically is attractive, and offers a further explanation for the potential efficacy of breast screening programs in reducing mortality. To some extent, this phenomenon is related to the issue of preclinical dissemination; tumors with a greater malignant potential are more likely to metastasize. The proportion of cells within a tumor with the capacity to invade blood vessels, travel in the circulation and establish viable micrometastases will increase the progression to a more malignant phenotype. The latter may be manifested by enhanced activity at several steps in the process of invasion and metastasis.

Therefore screening could improve prognosis by detecting lesions of smaller size that are better differentiated, of lower metastatic potential, and less likely to have already disseminated. Such lesions could be cured by appropriate locoregional treatment, and systemic therapies would not be indicated, as micrometastases would theoretically be nonexistent.

The issue of whether a subgroup of patients with truly localized breast cancer exists is controversial. Moreover, such a subgroup may only represent a small proportion of all screen-detected lesions and therefore have little impact overall on the screened population as a whole. The locoregional containment of disease in some patients is supported by the results of two randomized trials investigating the value of postoperative radiotherapy in patients undergoing mastectomy and adjuvant chemotherapy. The selective use of radiotherapy in a subgroup of premenopausal node-positive women is associated with proportional gains in overall survival of approximately one-third which compares with the relative benefits of adjuvant systemic therapies and breast cancer screening (122,123). Effective irradiation of locoregional disease at the time of primary treatment may prevent any persistent disease, or oligometastases becoming the source of distant disease (124).

In view of the apparent efficacy of screening programs to date, it might be argued that screening detects not only those lesions that have yet to disseminate, but also some that have already metastasized with a minimal micrometastatic load. Results of adjuvant systemic therapy trials reveal that absolute benefits from such therapies are relatively modest, being of the order of 5–10%. However, in a preclinical setting with a small primary tumor, adjuvant therapies may be much more effective against a lighter micrometastatic burden and a complete elimination of all distant foci of disease may be possible. Thus efficacy of screening may not be confined to strictly "Halstedian" tumors, but may be effective in a subgroup of "Fisherian" tumors that have a minimal micrometastatic component. Micrometastases demonstrate a Gompertzian pattern of growth with an inverse relationship between rates of cell division and size. By virtue of higher rates of cell cycling, these smaller foci of micrometastases are more sensitive to the effects of chemotherapy and total eradication is more likely (20,125). Animal tumor models confirm this quantitative relationship between tumor burden and the efficacy of chemotherapy, with tumor doubling times ranging from 2 to 10 days depending on the size of micrometastases (126). A Gompertzian model appears consistent with the clinical impression that smaller tumors grow more rapidly and rates decrease progressively as a tumor enlarges. Nonetheless, Speer and colleagues have proposed an amended stochastic model for breast cancer growth; tumors are considered to grow in "spurts" with random, spontaneous changes in growth rate from time to time. A series of random episodes of mini-Gompertzian growth results cumulatively in a stepwise pattern of growth with an average predetection growth period of eight years. The random nature of these events accounts for the heterogeneity of breast cancer and a broad spectrum of "sojourn periods." Furthermore, during periods of reduced proliferative activity, tumors would be relatively resistant to adjuvant chemotherapy due to lower rates of cell cycling (20).

As mentioned above, screening is inherently biased toward slow growing, less aggressive tumors. These have a longer sojourn period and hence are less likely to grow to a clinically palpable size prior to screen detection. There is much natural variance in the growth rates of breast cancer within the preclinical phase. Innate rates of growth are a critical aspect of the natural history of this disease and are determined by a combination of time-dependent processes including cell cycle time, nutritional factors (vascular supply), and host immune response. Heuser and colleagues detected a measurable growth in 23 out of 32 primary breast cancers on serial mammograms spaced 88–730 days apart (127). Of interest, the remaining nine tumors showed no measurable growth on the basis of changes in tumor nucleus shadows identified retrospectively. Estimates of tumor volume doubling times calculated from serial mammograms on the assumption that tumors are oblate spheroids, ranged from 109 days to 944 days, with a mean value of 325 days. The authors concluded that tumor growth rates were dichotomized into slowly and rapidly growing subsets, with the latter being more likely to be associated with node-positive disease than slow growing tumors (34% vs. 16% respectively). This difference was statistically significant, suggesting that a more malignant phenotype is ascribable to rapidly growing tumors (127). Within the slowly growing subset, some tumors would grow so slowly that they would never reach a clinically significant size in the patient's lifetime, while a proportion of the rapidly growing lesions would surface within 12 months of a previous negative screening mammogram, that is, present as an interval cancer. Thus screening programs would tend to be skewed in favor of more slowly growing tumors, the so-called length bias. These tumor doubling times were calculated for tumors that were mammographically detectable although still in the preclinical growth phase. The "sojourn period" usually refers to the time interval between a tumor being detected mammographically and its symptomatic presentation. The sojourn period has also been considered to represent the predetectable phase of growth, that is, from tumor induction as a single cell to the point of actual mammographic detection (19). This period is perhaps more appropriately referred to as the "presojourn" period and is a theoretical time interval which cannot be measured for any individual tumor. However, Spratt and colleagues attempted to estimate growth rates within this predetectable phase of growth using a modified definition of sojourn time: the time between a tumor first becoming mammographically visible (assuming a patient to be screened just as a tumor reached a threshold size for detection) and the moment when the tumor was actually detected mammographically (19). These estimates of sojourn times could be derived from the ratio of prevalence to incidence rates within the Breast Cancer Detection and Demonstration Project and values ranged from 365 days to 1383 days within the age group 35–74 years. Tumor doubling times could be calculated by dividing the sojourn times by the number of net cell doublings required for growth from a threshold to size at mammographic detection. Doubling times were variable and dependent upon both stage at detection and age of the patient, with a range from approximately 50 days in the age range 35–39 years and 150 days by age 70 years (19). These tumor doubling times are significantly shorter than estimates for tumors in the preclinical phase (20) and therefore doubling times for tumors that are large enough to be mammographically detectable are longer than those estimated for the predetection phase. Thus many cancers appear to grow more rapidly in the predetectable phase of growth and some will inevitably present clinically as interval cancers between screens. Moreover, these variable rates of growth and proliferative activity in the predetectable phase of breast cancer development portend that some tumors have properties which favor early dissemination and/or phenotypic progression prior to the threshold size for radiological detection.

INTERVAL CANCERS

These variable growth rates for breast cancer are of relevance to interval cancers, which constitute a heterogeneous group of lesions which are diagnosed between screening rounds and generally present as symptomatic cases (128). These cancers are by definition detected within 24 months of a negative mammogram and a distinction must be made between cancers present but missed for whatever reason and rapidly growing cancers that were not mammographically detectable at the time of the last screen. The overall proportion of cancers missed on screening mammograms (total interval cancer rate) ranges from 10% to 30% after the first year of screening (129–131) and within the NHS Breast Screening Programme they represent more than 80% of cancers detected in the third year of screening (132).

There are three reasons why a cancer may not have been evident on a previous mammogram. First, some cancers are missed due to errors of interpretation or suboptimal technical quality (approximately 30%) (133–135). Secondly, there is a group of "masked" cancers that are mammographically occult due either to patient factors such as age or breast density or to tumor characteristics such as particular histological types. Thus lobular tumors spread diffusely and elicit minimal stromal reaction while mucinous tumors contain lakes of mucin that are poorly imaged by mammography (134,136,137). Finally, there are true interval cancers that appear to be rapidly growing and have arisen *de novo* since the last screen (138). These cancers would be expected to be more aggressive and fatal than screen-detected lesions, and their failure to be detected at an earlier stage by screening could undermine the potential for screening programs to reduce mortality. The term "de novo" in this context refers to a tumor that was either non-existent (preinduction) or in a mammographically undetectable phase of growth at the time of a previous screen. In the latter scenario, although tumor induction has occurred and growth rates are relatively high the tumor bolus remains small due to there being few net doublings and there is no radiological correlate. Often masked lesions are classified with true interval cancers as the distinction between these lesions can be blurred. Both lesions are invisible on mammography but true interval cancers are below the threshold size for detection (2 mm) while masked lesions are larger than this. The true interval cancer rate varies from 3% to 17% and is the number of interval cancers expressed as a proportion of the total cancers detected during a screening interval. In their analysis of tumor growth rates, Spratt and colleagues estimated that more than 4% of cancers could grow from a threshold size of 2 mm to a clinically palpable size of 10 mm in a 12-month period and hence present as interval surfacing cancers within a year of a negative mammogram (17). Porter and others (139–141) have concluded that "true" interval lesions represented 65–75% of interval surfacing cancers. Furthermore, there is now evidence that true interval cancers are biologically more aggressive than screen-detected lesions with higher intrinsic growth rates and proliferative indices when adjustments for size and age are made (140,142,143). Thus interval cancers are more likely to be of higher histological (139,144) and nuclear grade (139), to be ER and PgR negative and to be associated with increased proliferative indices such as percentage S-phase fraction (80,139,140,142,145), aneuploidy (80,142,145), Ki-67, (139), and mitotic counts (139). Measurements of proliferative activity *per se* should be interpreted with caution as these only apply to a single time point and rates for any individual tumor are variable (stochastic growth). When time to diagnosis is taken into account and adjustment made for tumor size, interval cancers are more likely to be node positive than their screen-detected counterparts.

The implication of these studies comparing histological and prognostic features of interval and screen-detected lesions is that the former represent a group of biologically aggressive tumors that arise following previous screening and grow rapidly between screens. There is evidence that these histological features *per se* may reduce radiological detectability (146). Thus a proportion of these true interval cancers may indeed be "masked" lesions and may actually be present at the time of previous mammography rather than genuinely arising *de novo*. Nonetheless, they possess the innate properties of rapid growth and propensity to metastasize and tend to be more common in younger women (144). These interval cancers constitute a significant proportion of mammographic failures and the balance of evidence is that they have a poorer outcome (106,128,147). This relatively high frequency coupled with a worse prognosis may limit the impact of screening on mortality reduction (148,149).

CARCINOMA *IN SITU*

Discussion has deliberately been restricted to invasive forms of breast cancer as these are responsible for mortality. However, with the advent of screening, *in situ* disease has acquired increasing prominence with *in situ* change alone or in association with microinvasion now representing approximately 20–25% of all screen-detected cancer (150). By contrast, in the prescreening era, only 2–5% of clinical (symptomatic) cancers were exclusively ductal carcinoma *in situ* (DCIS), while 14% of all new cases of breast cancer are now exclusively in situ disease (151). Although screening is effective at detecting DCIS on account of commonly associated microcalcification, it is currently unknown to what extent this will translate into a reduction of mortality. Not all DCIS will progress to invasive disease, and estimates for this proportion range from 25 to 50%, depending partly on the grade of the lesion (152). Conversely, not all invasive cancers arise from lesions which are recognized histologically as carcinoma *in situ*, though a phase involving some form of increased epithelial proliferation is likely to precede an invasive cancer. Reports on the incidence of DCIS in routine autopsy studies (15–39%) (153,154) suggest that some non-invasive lesions that are detected mammographically and subsequently excised with either complete or partial mastectomy would have been of no clinical consequence to the patient during their lifetime. This raises the issue of "non-obligate progression" and the resulting uncertainties (155) which poses problems both in terms of the biological behavior of non-invasive disease and clinical management. Once detected, clinicians are obliged to treat this disease which usually involves surgical intervention and herein lies the predicament (156). Once DCIS has been detected, treatment must be offered which mandates mastectomy in about 30% of cases and often involves radiotherapy for cases amenable to breast conservation. Undoubtedly some patients with low-grade DCIS undergo surgery for a condition which would never have progressed to life-threatening disease. Indeed, this has been termed "pseudodisease"; it represents overdiagnosis within the NHS Breast Screening Programme and can potentially undermine its benefits (157). The latter is effectively tapping into a reservoir of indolent non-progressive DCIS which partially accounts for failure of the program to reduce the incidence of invasive cancer (158). This concept of pseudodisease applies particularly to women in the age group 40–49 years where DCIS constitutes a higher proportion of all newly diagnosed breast cancers. However, this may result in a delayed mortality reduction in older age groups, in whom there will be a reduction in the number of cases of invasive disease that have progressed from earlier DCIS lesions (higher grade) that have been appropriately treated. By implication, if only 25–50% of DCIS progress to invasive disease, then 50–75% of cases fail to do so and therefore pose no clinical threat to patients. Furthermore, within the older age group, life expectancy is likely to be determined not by a diagnosis of DCIS but by competing causes of death (e.g., atherosclerotic disease) (159).

Evidence to date suggests that screening programs have not encouraged overdiagnosis when analysis is confined to invasive tumors. However, until more is learnt about DCIS and its relationship to the natural history of breast cancer, this claim cannot be extended to non-invasive disease. As DCIS may constitute up to a quarter of all screen-detected lesions, this justifies some concern regarding both overdiagnosis and "excessive" treatment. The potential for overdiagnosis must be weighed against any benefits in terms of lives saved; critics have claimed that the benefits of screening are exaggerated and that 2000 women must be screened for 10 years to save one life and this may overdiagnose up to six cancers (160). An analysis estimates that between 2 and 2.5 lives are saved for every overdiagnosed case of breast cancer within the Swedish Two-County trial and the NHS Breast Screening Programme (161). Overdiagnosis from detection of DCIS, together with inconsistent labeling of proliferative lesions discovered on biopsy after recall, has undermined the net benefits of breast screening. A level of psychosocial morbidity and prognostic liability has been generated which has hitherto been ignored and excluded from information supplied to patients. This must now be incorporated into information leaflets in order to satisfy the basic tenets of informed

consent and conform with the principle of *primum non nocere* (162).

Notwithstanding the above comments on invasive cancers and overdiagnosis, there is limited evidence from screening programs and population-based studies that some occult invasive breast cancers detected by mammographic screening may ultimately have regressed spontaneously and thus may be of no clinical consequence to the patient (163,164). Zhal and colleagues attempted to gain insight into the natural history of small screen-detected invasive tumors in a study which compared cumulative breast cancer incidence for age-matched cohorts before and after introduction of a biennial mammographic screening program. Despite a single prevalence screen at the end of an observation period among control women, the cumulative incidence of invasive breast cancer at six years was 22% higher in the screened group (relative rate 1.22). The implication of this study was that some invasive cancers detected by regular mammographic screening would not have persisted such that they would be detected by a single mammogram at the end of six years (163). Therefore it is possible that some of these small occult lesions might regress spontaneously, but when picked up on screening, treatment is mandatory. The improved prognosis of screen-detected cancers may partially be attributable to detection and treatment of non-lethal invasive breast cancers (164).

PROSPECTS FOR FURTHER REDUCTIONS OF MORTALITY FROM BREAST CANCER SCREENING

More frequent screening could increase the proportion of screen-detected cancers and possibly reduce the number of rapidly growing interval cancers, although of necessity those growing most rapidly will be the last to be detected as the screening interval is reduced. Mortality reductions may therefore be correspondingly limited. Moreover the prognosis of these rapidly growing tumors is probably more dependent upon innate biological parameters than earlier detection at a smaller size. Many of these tumors may indeed be aggressive from the outset, rather than as a consequence of any phenotypic drift. More frequent screening would reduce the average size of screen-detected tumors, which in turn increases the chance of detecting lesions prior to both systemic dissemination and any progression to a more aggressive phenotype. Further clinical trials are required to clarify the relative benefits of reducing the screening interval to establish "clinical equipoise" with maximal sensitivity and specificity of mammography and optimal cost-effectiveness of screening programs (165). Screening schedules and even modality may have to be modified depending on patient characteristics; mammography is of lower sensitivity in younger women and those with a positive family history of breast cancer (166,167). A small study initially suggested that palpable tumors in BRCA-1 mutation carriers are less readily detectable on mammography (168) and this has been subsequently confirmed. This is also likely to apply to impalpable lesions in BRCA-1 carriers and will accord with the lower sensitivity of mammography in patients with a family history of breast cancer. Furthermore, interval cancers share a similar histological phenotype to tumors arising in BRCA-1 and BRCA-2 carriers (169) and these features may render mammographic detection more difficult (170). In recent years, breast MRI screening has been recommended for high risk women with BRCA1/2 gene mutation carriage (171). The sensitivity of breast MRI and cancer detection rates within this group is much improved compared with that of mammography. Nonetheless, the true benefits of screening with MRI are poorly understood with lack of any data from prospective randomized controlled trials assessing the impact on breast cancer mortality. There is indirect evidence that hormone replacement therapy (HRT) usage may reduce the sensitivity of screening mammography with a resultant increase in the numbers of missed cancers (172). A higher proportion of patients developing interval cancers within the first round of screening are reported to be current users of HRT compared with those women with screen-detected cancers and the interval cancer rate is related both to age and HRT usage. Thus within the West of Scotland Breast Screening Programme, the relative risk for a woman using HRT who develops an interval cancer compared with non-users is 1.79 (after adjustment for age, socioeconomic deprivation, and year of screening). HRT increases the risk of an interval cancer in the first year after screening by 2.27 (173). These effects are most likely brought about through changes in breast density which is a documented risk factor for breast cancer. Use of HRT increased rapidly from 1992 until 2000 and almost one-quarter of women aged 45–69 years were taking exogenous hormones at the turn of the millennium. However, this dramatically halved after 2002 following publication of the Women's Health Initiative Study showing increased risk of coronary and cerebrovascular events in addition to breast cancer in women received estrogen plus progesterone HRT (174). This reduction in HRT usage led to a transient decrease in breast cancer incidence after 2002 (175), though a recent analysis of SEER data reveals this decline has not persisted through to 2007 and rates have actually increased for ER-positive cancers in the age group 40–49 years (176). Furthermore, breast cancer incidence rates were stable in some Nordic European countries despite a notable decline in the use of HRT between 2002 and 2004 which was of similar magnitude to that observed in the United States. Hence there is some evidence for proportional discordance between decreases in breast cancer incidence and usage of HRT (177). Indeed, decreases in ER-positive disease began around 2000 and the timing of further reductions after 2002 suggest HRT was stimulating latent cancers rather than inducing *de novo* cancers (178). The use of HRT continues to decline and it seems unlikely that this will impact significantly on the efficacy of screening programs.

Improvements in early detection programs, organization of breast care services, and access to new therapies can potentially reduce mortality in developing countries, but an increasing proportion of ER-negative tumors in poorer countries could adversely affect global breast cancer mortality rates. More than two-thirds of all breast cancer deaths occur in developing countries and simpler screening interventions such as CBE can potentially reduce mortality by decreasing the incidence of more advanced stages of disease (179). This should be part of a combined strategy incorporating public education and increased breast awareness. Mammography screening is logistically complex, resource intensive, and its effectiveness in low resource settings

unproven. Furthermore, enhanced screening technologies offering greater sensitivity cannot yield significant mortality gains in affluent countries where improvements in treatment of early-stage ER-positive disease have diminished both absolute and relative benefits of screening interventions. Since the first randomized trial on breast cancer screening (Health Insurance Plan trial, New York) was undertaken in 1963 (180), there has been an incremental decrease in the initial mortality reduction of 30% attributed to mammographic screening. This has occurred against a background of advances in technology and prompts the question of why the benefits of screening are decreasing in the contemporary era. Jatoi has provocatively suggested two principal reasons for this (181); firstly an increase in public awareness of the disease with better recognition of early signs and symptoms of breast cancer (182). Not only do patients present sooner, but doctors respond more promptly and effectively with instigation of "triple assessment" and performance of percutaneous needle biopsy when indicated. Secondly, with the advent of effective systemic therapies and improvements in locoregional therapy (tumor-free surgical margins, more efficient and accurate radiotherapy techniques) mortality rates for breast cancer have fallen significantly in the past two decades. As previously alluded to in the introductory section of this chapter, treatment of screen-detected cancers must be more effective than symptomatic disease for screening to offer any advantage. With improvements in public awareness and adjuvant therapies, the micrometastatic load at presentation for symptomatic cancers has reduced and/or been more effectively dealt with which has attenuated benefits relative to screen-detected lesions which are hypothesized to have minimal or no micrometastases. Improvements in treatment will reduce both the relative and absolute benefits of screening, the former term expressing benefit as the proportion of patients who would have succumbed from breast cancer in the absence of screening (183). The impact of improvements in treatment of symptomatic disease with adherence to multidisciplinary team working is illustrated by a population-based study which attempted to quantify the contribution of screening *per se* to mortality reductions in a Norwegian breast screening program (184). The staggered introduction of a screening program allowed comparison between groups of women living in counties where screening had been adopted and those where screening had not yet been introduced but where organized multidisciplinary team working had been instituted. These two categories were compared with two historical groups for whom neither screening nor exposure to MDT working applied at the time (1986–1995). For the screened group of women, there was a relative reduction in rate of death of 28% compared with 18% for the nonscreened group (with historical controls the comparator for both these groups). Thus the relative reduction among women in the screened group was (28–18) = 10%. Screening contributed only one-third to the overall estimated reduction in mortality and demonstrates directly how the impact of screening *per se* is limited in the context of modern breast practices. This coupled with the biological uncertainty associated with both carcinoma *in situ* and some smaller invasive tumors indicates that lesion sensitivity alone is an inadequate metric for assessment of how effective new screening technologies are and their potential for ultimately reducing breast cancer mortality (185).

CONCLUSION

This chapter has discussed the scientific rationale for breast screening in the context of proposed paradigms of breast cancer biology. Ironically, the philosophy of screening is an anathema to the paradigm of biological predeterminism in its pure form. A screening program which aims to detect a cancer while it remains localized cannot be applied to a disease which is invariably systemic at the outset. If it is accepted that screening is effective in reducing mortality in certain age groups, then there must be a finite growth period for breast cancers during which disease is localized to the breast (and possibly lymph nodes) with no hematogenous dissemination. A corollary of this is that development of micrometastases can occur between the time of screen detection and clinical presentation of a cancer.

Analysis of survival curves for breast cancer patients with a prolonged follow-up has revealed no evidence for a "cure" in any subgroup according to statistical criteria. However, just as adjuvant treatment can extend life for patients with symptomatic breast cancer, early detection by screening can achieve a "personal cure" whereby disease-free survival is prolonged to a point at which a patient dies of a concomitant condition unrelated to breast cancer. Even if cure is not achieved in the statistical sense, this will be of no consequence to individual patients under these circumstances.

The capacity of any screening modality to reduce mortality is dependent upon the frequency of screening in relation to innate growth characteristics of a tumor and tendency to metastasize. A crucial consideration with breast cancer screening programs is the potential for improving prognosis as the screening interval is contracted. Clearly increased frequency of screening will reduce the average size of tumors, but it is difficult to predict how this will be reflected by further reductions in mortality consequent to removal of a lesion in anticipation of microscopic dissemination and phenotypic progression. Interval cancers can be minimized, although not eliminated from a screening program and those that are refractory to manipulation of screening schedules are likely to have the highest growth rates and worse prognosis. The growth kinetics of indolent tumors is likely to restrict any benefits from mammographic detection at a smaller tumor size. The extreme variability of intrinsic growth rates and metastagenicity among breast cancers, coupled with the stochastic character of tumor growth, is likely to fundamentally limit the maximal efficacy of any screening strategy. Furthermore, any clinical gains must be balanced against adverse effects and the possibility of spontaneous regression of some small invasive cancers. Increased costs associated with more intensive screening and use of sophisticated technologies must be factored into decision making so as to retain cost-effectiveness of any screening program for the population as a whole. Whatever the biological rationale, breast cancer screening remains a contentious issue with the fundamental assertions of screening having been challenged and an enquiry set up in the United Kingdom (160,186). Although some of these criticisms are flawed and based on misinterpretation of data, the case for indefinite mass screening in terms of overall clinical efficacy relative to cost remains unproven (187–189).

REFERENCES

1. Wilson JMG, Junger G. Principles and Practice of Screening for Disease (Public Health Paper No.34). Geneva: World Health Organisation, 1968.
2. Jatoi I, Anderson WF. Cancer screening. Curr Probl Surg 2005; 42: 620–82.
3. Cole P, Morrison AS. Basic issues in population screening for cancer. J Natl Cancer Inst 1980; 64: 1263–72.
4. Shapiro S, Venet W, Strax P, Venet L, Roeser R. Ten- to fourteen-year effect of screening on breast cancer mortality. J Natl Cancer Inst 1982; 69: 349.
5. Tabar L, Fagerberg CJG, Gad A, et al. Reduction in mortality from breast cancer after mass screening with mammography. Lancet 1985; 1: 829–32.
6. Fletcher SW, Black W, Harris R, et al. Report of the international workshop on screening for breast cancer. J Natl Cancer Inst 1993; 85: 1644–56.
7. Nystrom L, Rutqvist LE, Walls S, et al. Breast screening with mammography: overview of Swedish randomised trials. Lancet 1993; 341: 973–8.
8. Vainio H, Bianchini F, eds. IARC Handbook of Cancer Prevention. Breast Cancer Screening. Vol 7 Lyon, France: IARC Press, 2002.
9. NIH Consensus Statement. Breast cancer screening for women ages 40-49. NIH Consensus Statement 1997.
10. Gotzsche PC, Nielsen M. Screening for breast cancer with mammography. Cochrane Database Syst Rev 2006; 3: CD001877.
11. Kerlikowske K, Grady D, Rubin SM, Sandrock C, Ernster VL. Efficacy of screening mammography. A meta-analysis. JAMA 1995; 273: 149–54.
12. Duffy SW, Tabar L, Smith RA. The mammographic screening trials: commentary on the recent work by Olsen and Gotzsche. CA Cancer J Clin 2002; 52: 68–71.
13. US Preventive Services Task Force. Screening for breast cancer: US preventive services task force recommendation statement. Ann Int Med 2009; 151: 716–26.
14. Moss SM, Cuckle H, Evans A, et al. Effect of mammographic screening from age 40 years on breast cancer mortality at 10 years' follow-up: a randomised controlled trial. Lancet 2006; 368: 2053–60.
15. Thomas DB, et al. Randomised trial of breast self-examination in Shanghai: final results. J Natl Cancer Inst 2002; 94: 1445–57.
16. Moss SM. Breast cancer screening. Br J Hosp Med 1992; 48: 178–81.
17. Spratt JA, von Fournier D, Spratt JS, Weber E. Mammographic assessment of human breast cancer growth and duration. Cancer 1993; 71: 2020–6.
18. Wette R, Katz IN, Rodin EY. Stochastic processes for solid tumor kinetics: I. surface regulated growth. Math Biosciences 1974; 19: 231–55.
19. Spratt JS, Greenberg RA, Heuser LS. Geometry, growth rates and duration of cancer and carcinoma in situ of the breast before detection by screening. Cancer Res 1986; 46: 970–4.
20. Speer JF, Petrosky VE, Retsky MW, Wardwell RH. A stochastic numerical model of breast cancer growth that stimulates clinical data. Cancer Res 1984; 44: 4124–30.
21. Holmberg L, Ekbom A, Zack M. Do screen-detected invasive breast cancers have a natural history of their own? Eur J Cancer 1992; 28A: 920–3.
22. Jatoi I. Breast cancer: a systemic or local disease? Am J Clin Oncol 1997; 20: 536–9.
23. Hellman S. Natural history of small breast cancers. J Clin Oncol 1994; 12: 2229–34.
24. Virchow R. Cellular Pathology. Translated from the 2nd German Edition by F. Chance Philadelphia: Lippincott, 1863.
25. Virchow R. Die Krankhaften Geschwulste, 3 volumes Berlin, A. Hirschwald, 1863–1873 Vol, 26–27.
26. Halsted WS. The radical operation for the cure of carcinoma of the breast. Johns Hopkins Hosp Rep 1898; 28: 557.
27. Halsted WS. The results of operations for the cure of cancer of the breast performed at The Johns Hopkins Hospital from June, 1889 to January, 1894. Johns Hopkins Hospital Reports 1894; 5; 4: 297–350.

28. Baum M. The history of breast cancer. In: Forbes JF, ed. Breast Disease. Edinburgh: Churchill Livingston, 1986: 95–105.

29. Brinkley D, Haybittle JL. The curability of breast cancer. Lancet 1973; 2: 95–8.

30. Fisher B. Laboratory and clinical research in breast cancer - a personal adventure: the David A. Karnofsky memorial lecture. Cancer Res 1980; 40: 3863–74.

31. Fisher B, Fisher ER. Transmigration of lymph nodes by tumour cells. Science 1966; 152: 1397–8.

32. Fisher B, Fisher ER. Barrier function of lymph node to tumour cells and erythrocytes I. Normal nodes. Cancer 1967; 20: 1907–13.

33. Fisher B, Fisher ER. Barrier function of lymph node to tumour cells and erythrocytes II. Effect of X-ray, inflammation, sensitisation and tumour growth. Cancer 1967; 20: 1914–19.

34. Baum M, Benson JR. Current and future roles of adjuvant endocrine therapy in management of early carcinoma of the breast. In: Senn H-J, Goldhirsch RD, Gelber RD, Thurlimaan B, eds. Recent Results in Cancer Research 140 -Adjuvant Therapy of Breast Cancer. Berlin: Heidelberg, New York: Springer - Verlag, 1996: 215–26.

35. Atkins H, Hayward JL, Klugman DJ, Wayte AB. Treatment of early breast cancer: a report after 10 years of a clinical trial. Br Med J 1972; 2: 423–9.

36. Fisher B, Redmond C, Poisson R, et al. Eight year results of a randomised clinical trial comparing total mastectomy and lumpectomy with or without irradiation in the treatment of breast cancer. NEJM 1989; 320: 822–7.

37. Veronesi U, Saccozzi R, Del Vecchio M, et al. Comparing radical mastectomy with quadrantectomy, axillary dissection and radiotherapy in patients with small cancers of the breast. NEJM 1981; 305: 6–11.

38. Sarrazin D, Dewar JA, Arriagada R, et al. Conservative management of breast cancer. Br J Surg 1986; 73: 604–6.

39. Fisher B, Anderson S, Bryant J, et al. Twenty-year follow up of a randomized trial comparing total mastectomy, lumpectomy and lumpectomy plus irradiation for the treatment of invasive breast cancer. N Engl J Med 2002; 347: 1233–41.

40. Veronesi U, Cascinelli N, Mariani L, et al. Twenty-year follow up of a randomized study comparing breast conserving surgery with radical mastectomy for early breast cancer. N Engl J Med 2002; 347: 1227–32.

41. Litiere S, Werutsky G, Fentiman IS, et al. Breast-conserving therapy versus mastectomy for stage I-II breast cancer: 20 year follow up of the EORTC 10801 phase 3 randomised trial. Lancet Oncol 2012; 13: 412–19.

42. Early Breast Cancer Trialists Collaborative Group (EBCTCG). Effects of radiotherapy and of differences in the extent of surgery for early breast cancer on local recurrence and 15 year survival: an overview of the randomized trials. Lancet 2005; 366: 2087–106.

43. Benson JR. Long-term outcome of breast conserving surgery. Lancet Oncol 2012; 13: 331–3.

44. Benson JR, Teo K. Breast cancer local therapy: what is it's effect on mortality? World J Surg 2012; 36:1460–74.

45. Early Breast Cancer Trialists Collaborative Group. Tamoxifen for early breast cancer: an overview of the randomized trials. Lancet 1998; 351: 1451–61.

46. Hacksaw A, Roughton M, Forsyth S, et al. Long term benefits of 5 years of tamoxifen: 10 year follow up of a large randomized trial in women at least 50 years of age with early breast cancer. J Clin Oncol 2011; 29: 1657–67.

47. Early Breast Cancer Trialists' Collaborative Group. Polychemotherapy for early breast cancer: an overview of the randomized trials. Lancet 1998; 352: 930–42.

48. Allred DC, Harvey JM, Berardo M, et al. Prognostic and predictive factors in breast cancer by immunohistochemical analysis. Mod Pathol 1998; 11: 155–68.

49. Davies C, Godwin J, Gray R, et al. Early Breast Cancer Trialists' Colloborative Group (EBCTCG). Relevance of breast cancer hormone receptors and other factors to the efficacy of adjuvant tamoxifen: patient-level meta-analysis of randomized trials. Lancet 2011; 378: 771–84.

50. Howell A, Cuzick J, Baum M, et al. Results of the ATAC (Arimidex, Tamoxifen Alone or in Combination. Trial after completion of 5 years adjuvant treatment for breast cancer. Lancet 2011; 378: 771–84.

51. Coombes RC, Hall E, Gibson LJ, et al. A randomized trial of exemestane after two to three years of tamoxifen therapy in postmenopausal women with primary breast cancer. N Engl J Med 2004; 350: 1081–92.

52. Arimidex, Tamoxifen, Alone or in Combination (ATAC) Trialists' Group. Forbes JF, Cuzik J, Buzdar A, et al. Effect of anastrozole and tamoxifen as adjuvant treatment for early-stage breast cancer: a 100-month analysis of the ATAC trial. Lancet Oncol 2008; 9: 45–53.

53. Mourisden H, Giobbie-Hurder A, Goldhirsch A, et al. BIG 1-98 Colloborative Group. Letrozole therapy alone or in sequence with tamoxifen in women with breast cancer. N Engl J Med 2009; 361: 766–76.

54. Goss PE, Ingle JN, Martino S, et al. A randomized trial of letrozole in post-menopausal women after five years of tamoxifen therapy for early-stage breast cancer. N Engl J Med 2003; 349: 1793–802.

55. Davidson NE, Morrow M. Sometimes a great notion – an assessment of neoadjuvant systemic therapy for breast cancer. J Natl Cancer Inst 2005; 97: 159–61.

56. Wolff AC, Davidson NE. Primary systemic therapy in operable breast cancer. J Clin Oncol 2000; 18: 1558–69.

57. Bonadonna G, Valagussa P, Bramnilla C, et al. Primary chemotherapy in operable breast cancer: eight year experience at the Milan Cancer Institute. J Clin Oncol 1998; 16: 93–100.

58. Smith IE, Walsh G, Jones A, et al. High complete remission rates with primary neoadjuvant infusional chemotherapy for large early breast cancer. J Clin Oncol 1995; 13: 424–9.

59. Mauri D, Pavlidis N, Ioannidis JP. Neoadjuvant versus adjuvant systemic treatment for breast cancer: a meta-analyis. J Natl Cancer Inst 2005; 97: 188–94.

60. Haybittle JL. Curability of breast cancer. Br Med Bull 1990; 47: 319–23.

61. Berkson J, Harrington SW, Clagett OT, et al. Mortality and Survival in surgically treated breast caner: a statistical summary of some experience of the Mayo Clinic. Proc Staff Meetings Mayo Clinic 1957; 32: 645.

62. Brinkley D, Haybittle JL. Long-term survival of women with breast cancer. Lancet 1984; 1: 1118.

63. Le MG, Hill C, Rezvani A, et al. Long-term survival of women with breast cancer. Lancet 1984; 2: 922.

64. Langlands AO, Pocock SJ, Kerr GR, Gore SM. Long-term survival of patients with breast cancer: a study of the curability of the disease. Br Med J 1979; 2: 1247–51.

65. Adair F, Berg J, Lourdes J, Robbins GF. Long-term follow up of breast cancer patients: The 30-year report. Cancer 1974; 33: 1145–50.

66. Hayward J, Caleffi M. The significance of local control in the primary treatment of breast cancer. Arch Surg 1987; 122: 1244.

67. Rosen PP, Groshen S, Saigo PE, et al. A long term follow up study of survival in stage I (T1N1M0) and stage II (T1N1M0) breast carcinoma. J Clin Oncol 1989; 7: 355–66.

68. Sigurdsson H, Baldetorp B, Borg A, et al. Indicators of prognosis in node-negative breast cancer. N Engl J Med 1990; 322: 1045–53.

69. Folkman J. What is the evidence that tumours are angiogenesis dependent ? J Natl Cancer Institute 1990; 82: 4–6.

70. Pickren JW. Significance of occult metastases. Cancer 1961; 14: 1266–71.

71. Fisher ER, Swamidoss S, Lee CH, et al. Detection and significance of occult axillary node metastases in patients with invasive breast cancer. Cancer 1978; 45: 2025–31.

72. de Mascerel I, Bonichon F, Coindre JM, Trojani M. Prognostic significance of breast cancer axillary lymph node micro-metastases assessed by two special techniques: re-evaluation with longer follow up. Br J Cancer 1992; 66: 303–6.

73. Trojani M, de Mascarel I, Bonichon F, et al. Micro-metastases to axillary lymph nodes from carcinoma of breast: detection by immunohistochemistry and prognostic significance. Br J Cancer 1987; 55: 303–6.

74. International Ludwig Breast Cancer Study Group. Prognostic importance of occult axillary lymph node micrometastases from breast cancer. Lancet 1990; 335: 1565–8.

75. Hansen NM, Grube B, Ye X, et al. Impact of micrometastases in the sentinel lymph node of patients with invasive breast cancer. J Clin Oncol 2009; 27: 4679–84.

76. Weidner N, Semple JP, Welch WR, Folkman J. Tumour angiogenesis and metastasis - correlation in invasive breast carcinoma. NEJM 1991; 324: 1–8.

77. Liotta L, Kleinerman J, Saidel G. Quantitative relationships of intravascular tumour cells, tumour vessels and pulmonary metastases following tumor implantation. Cancer Res 1974; 34: 997–1004.

78. Rosfjord EC, Dickson RB. Role of integrins in the development and malignancy of the breast. In: Bowcock A, ed. Breast Cancer: Molecular Genetics, Pethogenesis and Therapeutics. Chapter 13 New Jersey: Humana Press, 1999: 285–304.

79. Duffy SW, Tabar L, Fagerberg G, et al. Breast screening, prognostic factors and survival - results from the Swedish two county study. Br J Cancer 1991; 64: 1133–8.

80. Hakama M, Holli K, Isola J, et al. Aggressiveness of screen-detected breast cancer. Lancet 1995; 345: 221–4.

81. Fagerberg CJG, Baldetorp L, Grontoft O, et al. Effects of repeated mammographic screening on breast cancer stage distribution. Acta Radiol Oncol 1985; 24: 465.

82. Tabar L, Duffy SW, Krusemo UB. Detection method, tumour size and node metastases in breast cancers diagnosed during a trial of breast cancer screening. Eur J Cancer 1987; 23: 959–62.

83. Baker LH. Breast cancer detection demonstration project: five-year summary report. CA Cancer J Clin 1982; 32: 194–225.

84. Fisher B, et al. Surgical adjuvant chemotherapy in cancer of the breast. Results of a decade of co-operative investigation. Ann Surg 1968; 168: 337–56.

85. Salvadori B, et al. Prognostic factors in operable breast cancer. Tumori 1983; 69: 477–84.

86. Mamounas EP, Tang G, Fisher B, et al. Association between the 21-gene recurrence score assay and risk of loco-regional recurrence in node negative, estrogen receptor positive breast cancer: results from NSAPBP B-14 and NSABP B-20. J Clin Oncol 2010; 28: 1677–83.

87. Voduc KD, Cheang MCU, Tyldesley S, et al. Breast cancer subtypes and the risk of local and regional relapse. J Clin Oncol 2010; 28: 1684–91.

88. Carter CL, Allen C, Henderson DE. Relation of tumour size, lymph node status and survival in 24, 740 breast cancer cases. Cancer 1989; 73: 505–8.

89. Fisher B, Slack NH, Bross IDJ, et al. Cancer of the breast: size of neoplasm and prognosis. Cancer 1969; 24: 1071–80.

90. Haagensen CD. Diseases of the Breast, 3rd edn. Philapdelphia: Saunders, 1986: 659.

91. Nemoto T, Vanna J, Bedwani RN, et al. Management and survival of female breast cancer: results of a national survey by the American college of surgeons. Cancer 1984; 45: 2917–24.

92. Tabar L, Fagerberg CJG, South MC, Duffy SW, Day NE. The Swedish Two County Trial of mammographic screening for breast cancer: recent results on mortality and tumour characteristics. In: Miller AB, Chamberlain J, Day NE, Hakama M, Prorok P, eds. Screening for Cancer. Bern: Hans Huber, 1991.

93. Tabar L, Duffy SW, Krusemo UB. Detection method, tumour size and node metastases in breast cancers diagnosed during a trial of breast cancer screening. Eur J Cancer Clin Oncol 1987; 23: 959–62.

94. Hatschek T, Fagerberg G, Olle S, et al. Cytometric characterisation and clinical course of breast cancer diagnosed in a population-based screening program. Cancer 1989; 64: 1074–81.

95. Anderson TJ, Lamb J, Donnan P, et al. Comparative pathology of breast cancer in a randomised trial of screening. Br J Cancer 1991; 64: 108–13.

96. Cole P, Morrison AS. Basic issues in population screening for cancer. J Natl Cancer Inst 1980; 64: 1263–72.

97. Crisp WJ, Higgs MJ, Cowan WK, et al. Screening for breast cancer detects tumours at an earlier biological stage. Br J Surg 1993; 80: 863–5.

98. Abernathy CM, Hedegaard H, Weger N. Screening for breast cancer detects tumours at an earlier biological stage (letter). Lancet 1994; 81: 922.

99. Bull A, Mountney L, Sanderson H. Stage distribution of breast cancer: a basis for the evaluation of breast screening programmes. Br J Radiol 1991; 64: 516–19.

100. Boyd NF, Jensen HM, Cooke G, Lee Han H. Relationship between mammographic and histological risk factors for breast cancer. J Natl Cancer Inst 1992; 1170–9.

101. Perou CM, Sorlie T, Eisen MB, et al. Molecular portraits of human breast tumours. Nature 2000; 406: 747–52.

102. Klemi PJ, Joensuu H, Toikkanen J, et al. Aggressiveness of breast cancers found with and without screening. Br Med J 1992; 304: 467–9.

103. Bennet IC, McCaffrey JF, Baker CA, et al. Changing patterns in the presentation of breast cancer over 25 years. Aust NZ J Surg 1990; 60: 665–71.

104. Rajakariar R, Walker RA. The biological nature of screen-detected invasive breast cancer (meeting abstract). J Path 1993; 170(Suppl): 387A.

105. Day NE. Screening for breast cancer. Br Med Bull 1991; 47: 400–15.

106. Shen Y, Yang Y, Innoue LY, et al. Role of detection method in predicting breast cancer survival: analysis of randomized screening trials. J Natl Cancer Inst 2005; 97: 1195–203.

107. Joensuu H, Lehtimaki T, Holli K, et al. Risk for distant recurrence of breast cancer detected by mammography screening or other methods. JAMA 2004; 292. 1064–73.

108. Mook S, Van't Veer LJ, Rutgers E, et al. Independent prognostic value of screen detection in invasive breast cancer. J Natl Cancer Inst 2005; 97: 1195–203.

109. Wishart GC, Greenberg DC, Britton PD, et al. Screen-detected versus asymptomatic breast cancer: is improved survival due to stage migration alone? Br J Cancer 2008; 98: 1741–4.

110. Dawson SJ, Duffy SW, Blows FM, et al. Molecular characteristics of screen-detected versus symptomatic breast cancer and their impact on survival. Br J Cancer 2009; 101: 1338–44.

111. Brown SBF, Mallon EA, Edwards J, et al. Is the biology of breast cancer changing? A study of hormone receptor status1984 – 1986 and 1996 – 1997. Br J Cancer 2009; 100: 807–10.

112. Jatoi I, Anderson WF. Aggressiveness of breast cancers found with and without screening. Br Med J 1992; 304: 467–9.

113. Nicholson S, Webb AJ, Coghlan B, et al. Will screening for breast cancer reduce mortality ? Evidence from the first year of screening in Avon. Ann Roy Coll Surg 1993; 75: 8–12.

114. Wicks K, Fisher CJ, Fentimen IS, Millis RR. Breast cancer histology and age (meeting abstract). J Pathol 1992; 167(Suppl): 139A.

115. Fisher B, Saffer E, Fisher ER, Studies concerning the regional nodes in cancer IV. Tumour inhibition by regional lymph node cells. Cancer 1974; 33: 631–6.

116. Fisher B, Saffer E, Fisher ER, Studies concerning the regional nodes in cancer VII. Thymidine uptake by cells from nodes of breast cancer patients. Cancer 1974; 33: 271–9.

117. Ponten J, Holmberg L, Trichopoulos D. Biology and natural history of breast cancer. Int J Cancer 1990; 5: 1–21.

118. Meyer JS, Witliff JL. Regional heterogeneity in breast carcinoma: thymidine labelling index, steroid hormone receptors, DNA ploidy. Int J Cancer 1991; 47: 213.

119. Anderson TJ, Lamb J, Alexander F, et al. Comparative pathology of prevalent and incident cancer detected by breast screening. Edinburgh Breast Screening Project. Lancet 1986; 1: 519–23.

120. Brewster AM, Thompson P, Sahin AA, et al. Copy number imbalances between screen-detected and symptom-detected breast cancers and impact on disease-free survival. Cancer Prev Res 2011; 4: 1609–16.

121. Ragaz J, Jackson SM, Le N, et al. Adjuvant radiotherapy and chemotherapy in node-positive pre-menopausal women with breast cancer. N Engl J Med 1997; 337: 956–62.

122. Overgaard M, Hansen PS, Overgaard J, et al. Post-operative radiotherapy in high risk pre-menopausal women with breast cancer who receive adjuvant chemotherapy. N Engl J Med 1997; 337: 949–55.

123. Hellman S. Stopping metastases at their source (editorial). N Engl J Med 1997; 337: 996–7.

124. Salmon S. Kinetic rationale for adjuvant chemotherapy of cancer. In: Salmon S, Jones S, eds. Adjuvant Chemotherapy of Cancer. Amsterdam: Elsevier/North-Holland Biomedical Press, 1977: 15–27.

125. Skipper H, Schabel F Jr. Quantitative and cytokinetic studies in experimental tumor systems. In: Holland JF, Frei E III, eds. Cancer Medicine, 2nd edn. Philadelphia: Lea and Febiger, 1982: 636–48.

126. Heuser L, Spratt JS, Polk HC Jr. Growth rates of primary breast cancers. Cancer 1979; 43: 1888–94.

127. Gillilard FD, Joste N, Stauber PM, et al. Biological characteristics of interval and screen-detected cancers. J Natl Cancer Inst 2000; 92: 743–9.

128. Moskowitz M. Breast Cancer: age specific growth rates and screening strategies. Radiology 1986; 161: 37–41.

129. Holland R, Mravunac M, Hendriks JHCL, Bekekr BV. So-called interval cancers of the breasts: pathologic and radiologic analysis of sixty four cases. Cancer 1982; 49: 2527–33.

130. Heuser L, Spratt JS, Polk HC Jr, Buchanan J. Relation between mammary cancer growth kinetics and the intervals between screenings. Cancer 1979; 43: 857–62.

131. Woodman CBJ, Threlfall AG, Boggis CRM, Prior P. Is the three year breast screening interval too long? Occurrence of interval cancers in NHS screening programme's northwestern region. BMJ 1995; 310: 224–6.

132. Martin JE, Moskowitz M, Milbrath JR. Breast cancer missed by mammography. Am J Roentgenol 1979; 132: 737–9.

133. Holland R, Hendriks JH, Mravunac M. Mammographically occult breast cancer. A pathologic and radiologic study. Cancer 1983; 52: 1810–19.

134. Frisell J, Eklund G, Hellstrom L, Somell A. Analysis of interval breast carcinomas in a randomised screening trial in Stockholm. Breast Cancer Res Treat 1987; 9: 219–25.

135. Ma L, Fishell J, Wright B, et al. Case-control study of factors associated with failure to detect breast cancer by mammography. J Natl Cancer Inst 1992; 84: 781–5.

136. Ikeda D, Andersson I, Wattsgard C, Janzon L, Linell F. Interval cancers in the Malmo Mammographic Screening Trial: radiographic appearance and prognostic considerations. Am J Roentgenol 1992; 159: 287–94.

137. Heuser LS, Spratt JS, Kuhns JG, et al. The association of pathologic and mammographic characteristics of primary human breast cancers with "slow" and "fast" growth rates and with axillary lymph node metastases. Cancer 1984; 53: 96–8.

138. Porter PL, El-Bastawissi AY, Mandelson MT, et al. Breast tumor characteristics as predictors of mammographic detection: comparison of interval and screen-detected cancers. J Natl Cancer Inst 1999; 91: 2020–8.

139. Brekelmans CT, van Gorp JM, Peeters PH, Collette HJ. Histopathology and growth rate of interval breast carcinoma. Characterization of different subgroups. Cancer 1996; 78: 1220–8.

140. Frisell J, von Rosen A, Wiege M, Nilsson B, Goldman S. Interval cancer and survival in a randomised breast cancer screening trial in Stockholm. Breast Cancer Res Treat 1992; 24: 11–16.

141. Klemi PJ, Toikkanen S, Rasanen O, Parvinen I, Joensuu H. Mammography screening interval and the frequency of interval cancers in a population-based screening. Br J Cancer 1997; 75: 762–6.

142. Hatschek T, Fagerberg G, Stal O, et al. Cytometric characterization and clinical course of breast cancer diagnosed in a population-based screening program. Cancer 1990; 64: 1074–81.

143. Gilliland FD, Joste N, Stauber PM, et al. Biologic characteristics of interval and screen-detected breast cancers. J Natl Cancer Inst 2000; 92: 743–9.

144. Arnerlov C, Emdin SO, Lundgren B, et al. Breast carcinoma growth rate described by mammographic doubling time and S-phase fraction. Correlations to clinical and histopathologic factors in a screened population. Cancer 1992; 70: 1928–34.

145. Narod SA. Dube M-P Biologic characteristics of interval and screen-detected breast cancers (correspondence). J Natl Cancer Inst 2001; 93: 151.

146. Andersson I, Aspegren K, Janzon L, et al. Effect of mammographic screening on breast cancer mortality in an urban population in Sweden. Results fro the Malmo mammographic screening trial (MMST). Br Med J 1988; 297: 943–8.

147. Vitak B. Invasive interval cancers in the ostergotland mammographic screening programme: radiological analysis. Eur Radiol 1998; 8: 639–46.

148. Day N, McCann J, Camilleri-Ferrante C, et al. Monitoring interval cancers in breast screening programmes: the East Anglian experience. Quality assurance Management Group of the East Anglian Breast Screening Programme. J Med Screen 1995; 2: 180–5.

149. Roberts MM, Alexander FE, Anderson TJ, et al. Edinburgh trial of screening for breast cancer: mortality at seven years. Lancet 1990; 335: 241–6.

150. Surveillance, Epidemiology and End Results (SEER. Program Cancer Statistics Review (1973 – 1995). Bethesda, MD, National Cancer Institute, Division of Cancer Prevention and Control, Surveillance Program, Cancer Statistics Branch, 1998 UPDATED REF.

151. Rosen PP, Braun DW, Kinne DE. The clinical significance of pre-invasive breast cancer. Cancer 1980; 46: 919–25.

152. Anderson J, Nielsen M, Christensen L. New aspects of the natural history of in situ and invasive carcinoma in the female breast: results from autopsy investigations. Verh Dtsch Ges Pathol 1985; 69: 88–95.

153. Welch HG, Black WC. Using autopsy series to estimate the disease "reservoir" for ductal carcinoma in situ of the breast: How much more breast cancer can we find ? Ann Intern Med 1997; 127: 1023–8.

154. Anderson TJ. Genesis and source of breast cancer. Brit Med Bull 1991; 47: 305–18.

155. Kerlikowski K, Salzman P, Philips KA, et al. Continuing screening mammography in women aged 70 – 79 years: impact on life expectancy and cost-effectiveness. JAMA 1999; 282: 2156–63.

156. Satariano WA, Ragland DR. The effect of co-morbidity on 3 year survival of women with primary breast cancer. Ann Intern Med 1994; 120: 104–10.

157. Welch HG, Black WC. Using autopsy series to estimate the disease 'reservoir' for ductal carcinoma in situ of the breast: How much more breast cancer can we find? Ann Int Med 1997; 127: 1023–8.

158. Gotzsche PC, Olsen O. Is screening for breat cancer with mammography justifiable? Lancet 2000; 355: 129–34.

159. Gotzsche PC, Hartling OJ, Nielsen M, Brodersen J, Jorgensen KJ. Breast screening, the facts – or maybe not. BMJ 2009; 338: 446–8.

160. Duffy SW, Tabar L, Olsen A, et al. Absolute numbers of lives saved and overdiagnosis in breast cancer screening, from a randomized trial and from the breast screening programme in England. J Med Screen 2010; 17: 25–30.

161. Benson JR. Will ductal carcinoma in situ defeat breast cancer screening? BMJ 2009; 338: 615.

162. Zahl PH, Maehlen J, Welch HG. The natural history of invasive breast cancers detected by screening mammography. Arch Intern Med 2008; 168:2311–16.

163. Jatoi I, Anderson WF. Breast cancer overdiagnosis with screening mammography. Arch Int Med 2009; 169: 999–1000.

164. Benson JR, Purushotham A, Warren R. Screening and litigation - The rate of interval cancers is too high. BMJ 2000; 321: 760–1.

165. Kerlikowski K, Grady D, Barclay J, Sickles EA, Ernster V. Effect of age, breast density and family history on the sensitivity of first screening mammography. JAMA 1996; 276: 33–8.

166. Tabar L, Fagerberg G, Chen HH, Duffy SW, Gad A. Screening for breast cancer in women aged under 50: mode of detection, incidence, fatality and histology. J Med Screen 1995; 2: 94–8.

167. Chang J, Yang WT, Choo HF. Mammography in Asian patients with BRCA-1 mutations. Lancet 1999; 353: 2070–1.

168. Phillips KA, Andrulis IL, Goodwin PJ. Breast carcinomas arising in carriers of mutations in BRCA-1 and BRCA-2: are they prognostically different ? J Clin Oncol 1999; 17: 3653–63.

169. Phillips KA. Biologic characteristics of interval and screen-detected breast cancers (correspondence). J Natl Cancer Inst 2001; 93: 151–2.

170. Saslow D, Boetes C, Burke W, et al. American cancer society guidelines for breast screening with MRI as an adjunct to mammography. CA Cancer J Clin 2007; 57: 75–89.

171. Sterns EE, Zee B. Mammographic density changes in perimenopausal and postmenopausal women: is effect of hormone replacement therapy predictable? Breast Cancer Res Treat 2000; 59: 125–32.

172. Litherland JC, et al. The effect of hormone replacement therapy in the sensitivity of screening mammography. Clin Radiol 1999; 54: 285–8.

173. Roussouw JE, Anderson GL, Prentice RL, et al. Writing group for the Women's Health Initiative Investigators. Risks and benefits of estrogen plus progestin in healthy postmenopausal women: principal results from the Women's Health Initiative randomized controlled trial. JAMA 2002; 288: 321–33.

174. Ravdin PM, Cronin KA, Howlader N, et al. The decrease in breast cancer incidence in 2003 in the United States. N Engl J Med 2007; 356: 1670–4.

175. Desantis C, Howlader N, Cronin KA, et al. Breast cancer incidence rates in US women are no longer declining. Cancer Epidemiol Biomarkers Prev 2011; 20: 733–9.

176. Zahl PH, Maehlen JA. A decline in breast cancer incidence. N Engl J Med 2007; 357: 509–13.

177. Elfenbein GJ. A decline in breast cancer incidence. N Engl J Med 2007; 357: 509–13.

178. Sankaranarayanan R, Ramadas K, Thara S, et al. Clinical breast examination: preliminary results from a cluster randomized controlled trial in India. J Natl Cancer Inst 2011; 103:1476–80.

179. Shapiro S. Periodic screening for breast cancer: the HIP Randomised Controlled Trial. Health Insurance Plan. J Natl Cancer Inst Monogr 1997; 22: 27–30.

180. Jatoi I. The impact of advances in treatment on the efficacy of mammography screening. Prev Med 2011; 53: 103–4.

181. Rostgaard K, Vaeth M, Rootzen H, et al. Why did the breast cancer lymph node status distribution improve in Denmark in the pre-mammography screening period of. 1978 – 1994? Acta Oncol 2010; 49: 313–21.

182. Jatoi I, Proschan MA. Clinical trial results applied to management of the individual cancer patient. World J Surg 2007; 30: 1184–9.

183. Kalager M, Zelen M, Langmark F, et al. Effect of screening mammography on breast cancer mortality in Norway. N Engl J Med 2010; 363: 1203–10.

184. Lord SJ, Irwig L, Simes RJ. When is measuring sensitivity and specificity sufficient to evaluate a diagnostic test, and when do we need randomized trials? Ann Intern Med 2006; 144: 850–5.

185. Duffy SW. Interpretation of the breast screening trials: a commentary on the recent paper by Gotzsche and Olsen. Breast 2001; 10: 209–12.

186. Baum M. Screening for breast cancer, time to think - and stop ? Lancet 1995; 346: 436.

187. Querci della Rovere G, Benson JR, Warren R. Screening for breast cancer, time to think - and stop? Lancet 1995; 346: 437.

188. Baum M. Commentary: false premises, false promises and false positives – the case against mammographic screening for breast cancer. Int J Epidemiol 2004; 33: 66–7.

189. Gotzsche PC, Hartling OJ, Nielsen M, Brodersen J, Jorgensen KJ. Breast screening, the facts – or may be not. BMJ 2009; 338: 446–8.

7 Interval cancers

Anthony J. Maxwell

INTRODUCTION

Effective mortality reduction in a population-based breast screening programme depends upon maximizing the detection of small cancers through high quality mammography, skilled image interpretation and, where necessary, effective further assessment and histopathological diagnosis. Interval cancers are breast cancers diagnosed in the interval between scheduled screening episodes in women who have been screened and issued with a normal screening result (1). Most interval cancers are diagnosed as a result of the development of symptoms such as a breast lump (2).

Interval cancers are an inevitable consequence of mammographic screening. In some cases they occur because the cancer has been missed or misinterpreted by the film reader(s). In many cases, however, the cancer is not visible on the screening mammograms even in retrospect, either because it was present but not distinguishable from normal breast tissue or because it had not yet developed. Either way, women with interval cancers represent an interesting and important group in which screening has failed to confer a benefit.

IDENTIFICATION OF INTERVAL CANCERS

In most published series interval cancers have been identified through linkage of computerized screening records and cancer registrations at local or national cancer registries (3–9). In the United Kingdom (UK), this process is routinely carried out at a regional level by the Breast Screening Quality Assurance Reference Centres (10–12). It is a time-consuming task, but if done carefully it provides accurate and almost complete ascertainment, particularly if the identified cases are validated by the screening service. Inevitably a few cases will be overlooked in this process, for example where the patient has changed address and the cancer registration has occurred in a different cancer registry. The disadvantage of this system (in the UK at least) is the time taken for new cancer diagnoses to be entered on the cancer registers, with the result that interval cancer data are at least a year (and often much more) out of date. More timely, although generally less complete, ascertainment of cases can be achieved by identification of previously screened women attending symptomatic clinics and being discussed in multidisciplinary team meetings and/or by cross-checking new breast cancer diagnoses on histopathology department databases with screening records. Hospital discharge records may also be useful sources (13,14).

Most programs define interval cancers as any breast cancer diagnosed in the interval after a screen with a normal result. Some published work however excludes women with *in situ* interval cancers. These are relatively uncommon in most programs and are generally asymptomatic. They are usually detected incidentally as a result of interim mammography, either for investigation of (usually unrelated) symptoms or through additional screening outside the organized program, for example because of an increased risk of breast cancer.

INCIDENCE RATES AND TIME SINCE LAST SCREEN

The longer the interval between screens, the greater the number of interval cancers that occur and the lower the proportion of cancers that are detected by screening. The UK, with its three-year screening round, has a higher overall interval cancer rate than other European programs that have two-year screening rounds or the United States (US) where many women are screened annually. It is important, therefore, to ensure that no slippage of the screening interval occurs, particularly in programs with less frequent screening (15). In the UK the round length (the interval between scheduled screens) is rigorously monitored centrally, with a requirement that 90% of eligible women are invited for rescreening within 36 months of the last screen.

Incidence rates for interval cancers are expressed as the number of cases occurring per 1000 (or in some papers per 10,000) women screened and vary widely between reported series. As the number of interval cancers per year varies with time since the last screen it is important to define the period after screening within which the interval cancers are recorded. A number of factors account for the variation in rates, of which, apart from screening round length, the most important is probably the interval cancer ascertainment rate achieved for each series. Older papers in particular are more likely to underestimate the true rates. There are also some differences in the denominator used for defining interval cancer rates. Some papers use cancers per 1000 or 10,000 women screened irrespective of the screening outcome (cancer or no cancer), whereas the European guidelines (9) recommend using the number of negative screening tests (with or without assessment). Given that cancer detection rates are less than 1% in virtually all programs these differences are of minimal significance. A number of European authors express interval cancer rates as a proportion of background cancer incidence. This makes comparison between series difficult, as screening itself increases apparent background incidence, incidence changes over time, and the issue of whether to include *in situ* cancers arises (9).

The risk of an interval cancer occurring increases with the time elapsed since the last screen (16). A pooled analysis of interval cancer rates in six European countries (17) gave a mean incidence of 0.59/1000 women screened negative in the

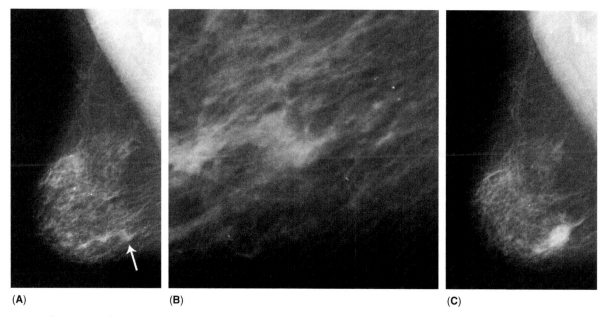

Figure 7.1 Minimal signs interval cancer. (**A**) Right mediolateral oblique screening mammogram which in retrospect shows a small ill-defined soft tissue density in the lower half of the breast (arrow). (**B**) Magnified view of the abnormality on the screening mammogram. (**C**) Right mediolateral oblique mammogram taken at presentation with a breast lump almost 3 years later, showing an ill-defined malignant mass at the same site. The histology was that of a node-negative multifocal grade 2 invasive ductal carcinoma with a main tumor size of 20 mm (estrogen receptor and progesterone receptor positive, HER2 negative).

first year after screening and 1.26 in the second year. Very similar rates were found in an Australian study (6). Three UK studies (12,18,19) quoted figures in the range of 0.48–0.61 in year 1, 0.98–1.21 in year 2, with a rate of 1.21–1.51 in year 3. In the UK NHS Breast Screening Programme (NHSBSP), the "achievable standard" for the interval cancer rate is 1.2/1000 women screened in the first two years and 1.4/1000 in the third year (1).

REVIEW AND CLASSIFICATION OF INTERVAL CANCERS
Review of the screening and subsequent diagnostic mammograms of women with interval cancers should be routine practice in any breast screening program. While the majority of screening examinations can be expected to be normal in retrospect, identification of cases that could have been diagnosed earlier provides valuable educational feedback for film readers and potentially provides opportunities to improve screening processes and detection methods leading to improved program performance.

A number of terms have been used to classify interval cancers, depending on their conspicuity on screening and diagnostic mammograms, but there is no universally recognized system. In the UK the screening mammograms are classified into one of the following three categories (1):

Category 1: Normal/benign. Normal or benign mammographic features.
Category 2: Uncertain. A feature is seen with hindsight on the screening mammogram that is difficult to perceive or does not clearly have either benign or malignant features. All screening film readers may have difficulties with perception or interpretation of such subtle mammographic appearances, for example asymmetric soft tissue density and parenchymal distortion (Fig. 7.1).

Category 3: Suspicious features. An abnormality is seen on the mammogram that has features suspicious of malignancy, for example pleomorphic microcalcification and spiculate mass (Fig. 7.2).

In addition, there is a further category, *unclassified*, which is applied when diagnostic mammograms have not been performed or are not available for review.

Other programs (and previously the UK national program) tend to favor the following terms:

True negative: The cancer is visible on the diagnostic mammogram but the screening mammogram is normal on review.
False negative (also *missed**, *observer error, screening error*): The cancer is visible on both the diagnostic and screening mammograms.
Minimal signs: Subtle signs suggestive of malignancy are visible in hindsight on the screening mammogram at the site of development of the cancer.
Occult† (also *unrecognized*): Cancer is visible on neither the diagnostic mammogram nor the screening mammogram.

The radiological review process can follow a variety of models (8,20–30). Blinded review, where the reviewing film readers are not aware of the site of the subsequently diagnosed cancer, gives a lower rate of false negative classifications than unblinded review, and provides a more realistic measure of the number of cases that could potentially have been diagnosed at

---

* Some authors include both *false-negative* and *minimal sign* cancers under the term *missed*.
† *Occult* may be included in the *true-negative* category.

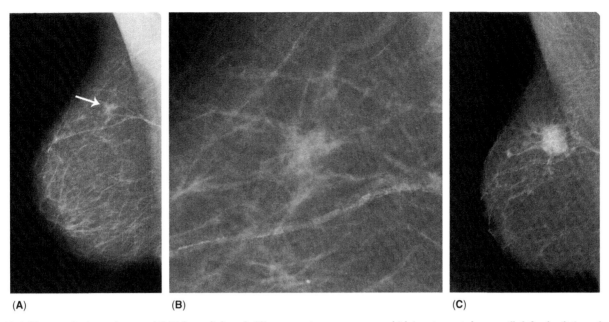

(A)   **(B)**   **(C)**

Figure 7.2 A false-negative interval cancer. (A) Right mediolateral oblique screening mammogram which in retrospect shows an ill-defined soft tissue density in the upper half of the breast with subtle architectural distortion (arrow). (B) Magnified view of the abnormality on the screening mammogram. (C) Right medio-lateral oblique mammogram taken almost 3 years later at presentation with a breast lump, showing a dense ill-defined malignant mass at the same site. The histol-ogy was that of a 22 mm node-negative grade 3 invasive ductal carcinoma (estrogen receptor, progesterone receptor, and HER2 negative—"triple negative"). This is a relatively subtle example of a category 3 interval cancer, but differs from the example of a category 2 case (Fig. 7.1) by the presence of both a soft tissue density and suspicious architectural distortion.

screening. The review process may be performed by several individuals independently and the results then collated, or it can be done in group consensus meetings. The process can be further refined by incorporating a number of normal mam-mograms (26) (preferably with confirmation of normality by normal subsequent round mammograms) although it is argu-able whether this is worthwhile.

This variation in review processes and lack of a standardized classification means that the proportion of interval cancers that fall into each category varies substantially between series. However the false negative rate in most published studies is between 14 and 50%, with a mean of approximately 35% (3,23–25,27–29,31–37). Asbury (38) demonstrated that the proportion of interval cancers that are classified as false nega-tive is higher in the first year after screening than in subse-quent years (60% in year 1, 30% in year 2, and 20% in year 3).

MAMMOGRAPHIC SENSITIVITY
Any factor that reduces the sensitivity of mammographic screening will result in an increase in the interval cancer rate, and indeed most authors define mammographic sensitivity as the number of cancers that are detected by mammography as a percentage of the number diagnosed at mammography plus the number diagnosed within the year following mammogra-phy (year 1 interval cancers). Screening program sensitivity is closely related and is the number of cancers that are detected by mammography as a percentage of the number diagnosed at mammography plus all interval cancers. Programs with long screening intervals can be expected, therefore, to have a lower program sensitivity than those that screen more frequently.

The conspicuity of a cancer on mammography depends upon the quality of the mammogram, the size of the tumor,

the mammographic features that the tumor exhibits, the density of the surrounding breast tissue, and the woman's age. Establishing the diagnosis of cancer then depends upon the reader perceiving and correctly interpreting the mam-mographic abnormality and on the correct procedures being followed when the woman attends for further assessment.

Radiographic Technique
Acceptable levels of sensitivity of screening mammography require a high standard of radiographic technique. Failure to correctly position the breast can result in failure to maximize the volume of breast tissue that is imaged and thereby risk failing to include a cancer (Fig. 7.3) (39–42). This is particu-larly the case for cancers lying posterior in the breast. Expo-sure is an important factor in optimizing cancer detection with film-screen mammography, an optical density of between 1.4 and 1.8 giving the best cancer conspicuity (43,44). Image blurring will of course also reduce cancer con-spicuity, and this is particularly true for microcalcification which can be rendered invisible even by relatively mild blurring.

Most, if not all, organized mammographic screening pro-grams now use two views of each breast (the mediolateral oblique and the craniocaudal). In the first few years of the UK NHS breast screening program only the mediolateral oblique view was employed. A number of studies comparing one- versus two-view mammography have demonstrated a 9–24% increase in cancer detection with two views (44–49). An evaluation of the UK screening program following the introduction of two-view mammography in the incident round showed a 20% increase in incident round cancer detec-tion, particularly for small cancers (50).

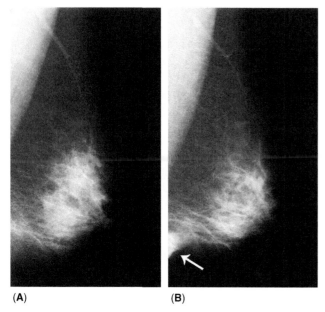

(A) (B)

Figure 7.3 Interval cancer possibly due to technically inadequate mammography. (A) Left mediolateral oblique screening mammogram; normal appearances, although the inframammary fold has not been included on the image. The craniocaudal view was normal (not shown). (B) Left mediolateral oblique mammogram taken following presentation with a lump in the left breast 1 year later. This shows a mass in the inframammary fold (arrow), not visible on the craniocaudal view (not shown). This area has not been fully included on the screening mammogram and emphasizes the importance of high-quality mammography in maximizing cancer detection at screening. The histology showed a node-negative 25 mm grade 2 invasive ductal carcinoma (estrogen receptor and progesterone receptor positive, HER2 negative).

Full-field digital mammography is superior to film-screen mammography for the detection of cancers in young women and those with dense breasts (51) and has now largely replaced it. Exposure is less critical than it is with film-screen mammography but optimal positioning and avoidance of blurring remain essential.

Women with breast implants are increasingly encountered in modern screening practice. In many cases the implants obscure a significant proportion of the breast tissue on the routine mediolateral oblique and craniocaudal views (52). Implant displacement (Eklund) views (53) in either or both of the standard projections are often helpful in increasing the amount of breast tissue demonstrated, but nonetheless women with implants are at an increased risk of interval cancer due to incomplete breast coverage at mammography (54,55).

Tumor Size

In general, the larger a cancer the more likely it is to be detected by mammography. Cancers less than 2 or 3 mm in diameter are seldom diagnosed mammographically, as malignant features in lesions of this size are difficult to distinguish from normal breast tissue. However, much larger cancers may be invisible if they are of certain histological types and/or develop within dense glandular tissue (see the next section).

The Radiological Features of the Cancer

Cancers which form spiculate masses are generally more conspicuous on mammography than those that form ill-defined masses or diffuse asymmetric densities, which may be indistinguishable from normal tissue. Malignant microcalcification

usually shows a high contrast with normal breast tissue and is less likely than other malignant features to be obscured in dense areas.

Breast Density

Breast density is one of the most important factors in determining mammographic sensitivity. Dense glandular tissue may obscure cancers, particularly those that form an ill-defined mass or have a diffuse growth pattern. The overall breast density is related to the relative proportions of epithelial and stromal tissue compared with fat. These epithelial and stromal elements reduce significantly at the menopause in most women, and this is often accompanied by increasing fat deposition in the breast. Mammographic sensitivity has been shown to be inversely related to breast density in both pre- and postmenopausal women (39,56–74). Women with a high body mass index tend to have less dense breasts than thinner women due to their higher volume of breast adipose tissue, and mammographic sensitivity is consequently higher (75).

Hormone replacement therapy (HRT) prevents or reverses the age-related decrease in breast density, and a number of studies have confirmed an associated reduction in mammographic sensitivity in HRT users compared with non-users (58,61,63,74,76–83). The Million Women Study (75) found that mammographic sensitivity was 92.1% in women who had never used HRT compared with 83.0% in current users, and found no difference in sensitivity between current users of estrogen-only HRT compared with those using the combined estrogen-progestogen preparation. Studies that have examined the effect of HRT usage on sensitivity with correction for mammographic density (58,65,69,72,74,84) have produced conflicting findings, although the weight of evidence suggests that HRT usage is an independent predictor of reduced mammographic sensitivity rather than having an effect purely through its influence on breast density. One study (85) found higher levels of breast pain in those women on HRT whose breasts showed an increase in mammographic density compared with those whose breasts did not become denser, and this may limit the amount of compression that can be applied to the breast during mammography, thereby reducing the image quality.

In premenopausal women the breasts change throughout the menstrual cycle, becoming slightly denser in the luteal (premenstrual) phase compared with the follicular phase (86–88). The consequent potential reduction in sensitivity in this phase due to increased density may be compounded by breast tenderness which, as with women on HRT, may limit the amount of mammographic compression that can be applied. A study of women aged 40–44 years in the Canadian National Breast Screening Study (89) suggested that menstruating women who have used hormones (the majority of the women in this study, mostly past users of the oral contraceptive) have an increased risk of interval cancer if the mammogram is performed in the luteal phase of the cycle.

Age

The overall incidence of interval cancers in the population is higher in older women due to increasing breast cancer incidence with age. However, mammographic sensitivity is lower in younger women, and thus a higher proportion of the cancers diagnosed among young screened women are interval cancers (74). Most of this effect is due to the higher mean breast density of younger women. Most (but not all (72)) studies that have examined age as an independent factor have concluded that when corrected for breast density interval cancers are still more likely to occur in younger women (56,64–68). This finding is consistent with the generally higher growth rate of cancers in young women which makes them more likely to present symptomatically before the next screen is due.

Perception or Interpretation Errors

Reading of screening mammograms should aim to maximize the number of cancers detected (and thereby minimize the number of false-negative and minimal signs interval cancers subsequently diagnosed), while minimizing the number of false-positive recalls for further assessment. Errors may arise as a result of failure to identify a suspicious mammographic sign (a perception error) or failure to correctly interpret a mammographic sign as suspicious (an interpretation error) (42).

Double reading of screening examinations is a routine practice in the UK and several other European countries, but is not widely used in the US. It is associated with a 1.5–15% increase in cancer detection compared with single reading, although at the cost of a reduction in specificity (i.e., an increase in recall to assessment rate) (90–96).

Reader experience is an important factor in minimizing "missed" (false-negative and minimal signs) cancers. There is evidence to suggest that high volume readers in general perform better than low volume readers (97–100), although above an average of 5000 mammogram reads per year the differences are minor (101). In the UK NHSBSP 5000 reads per annum has been set as the minimum that film readers are expected to achieve (1). Experimental work on inspection performance (102) suggests that cancer detection is compromised if film readers work for more than 30 minutes at a time without a break.

Other Factors

Incident round examinations have been reported to be less likely to result in interval cancers than prevalent round studies (36). Although this may in part be because of a slightly higher sensitivity for cancer detection in the incident round compared with the prevalent round because of the availability of previous mammograms for comparison, much of the effect (if indeed there is such an effect) is probably due to the lower sensitivity of mammography in younger women. Nonetheless, a Swedish study (103) shows conflicting findings, with a lower interval cancer rate in the prevalent round.

THE CHARACTERISTICS OF INTERVAL CANCERS

Interval cancers differ from screen-detected cancers in a number of important ways.

Size and Mammographic Appearances

As a majority of interval cancers present because of symptoms, they have a larger mean size (around 20 mm) than the mostly asymptomatic screen-detected cancers which average approximately 15 mm (5,31,73,104–108).

There is no real consensus in the literature around the type of lesion most likely to be overlooked or misinterpreted at mammographic screen reading. A study of false-negative interval cancers from Nottingham reported that architectural distortion was the abnormality most commonly overlooked on the screening mammogram, being present on nine (45%) of their 20 false-positive cases (109). Hofvind (105) found that half of their false-negative/minimal sign cancers were visible as poorly defined masses or asymmetric densities on the screening mammograms and 26% had calcifications with or without other features. Amos (24) found that asymmetric densities predominated among interval cancers, whereas screen-detected cancers were more likely to show the features of a spiculate or discrete mass.

Lesion Location

Interval cancers can arise in any part of the breast. Small differences were found in one study between the distribution of interval and screen-detected cancers (110), but these were not considered to be sufficient to be useful in practice. Wang (62) found a higher proportion of false-negative cancers in a deep retroglandular location compared with screen-detected cancers, and Meeson (111) found that false-negative interval cancers were more likely to be close to the chest wall than true-negative interval cases. A review of the previous mammograms of women with cancers detected at incident round screening (112) demonstrated that 25% were visible in retrospect on the previous study, and these were more likely to be in the "review areas" on the mammogram, particularly above the breast disc and in the retroglandular fat.

Biological Features

Some authors have found an excess of invasive lobular, mucinous, and medullary carcinomas among their interval cancers (33,37,104,113,114), and the present author found an excess of invasive lobular carcinomas in a study of screen-detected cancers that were visible retrospectively on the previous round screening films (115). It has been suggested that this is because lobular carcinomas often show a diffuse growth pattern (Fig. 7.4) and mucinous and medullary carcinomas tend to form ill-defined masses (33,116). A further factor is the absence of a significant reaction in the stroma surrounding some of these tumors. Interval lobular carcinomas are more likely than other tumor types to be mammographically occult at diagnosis (117–119).

A number of studies have examined the biological features of interval cancers (68,104–108,113,114,120–124). These cancers tend to show more aggressive features than screen-detected cancers, with a much smaller proportion of *in situ* cancers, a greater tendency to be of high grade, to be estrogen receptor (ER) and progesterone receptor (PR) negative, to have a higher proliferative index such as Ki67 and to have a higher likelihood of expressing p53. They are also more likely to show a basal phenotype (68). Some studies have found overexpression of epidermal growth factor receptor (HER1) (114) and HER2 (c-erbB2) (120) among interval cancers.

Axillary lymph node metastases are found more commonly in association with interval than screen-detected cancers (105–107,123,125). Bucchi (126) compared the nodal status of screen-detected and interval cancers and found that 28% of screen-detected cancers were node positive compared with 38%, 42%, and 44% of the interval cancers diagnosed at 1–12, 13–18, and 19–24 months after screening. Some of these differences are due to the different size and grade distribution

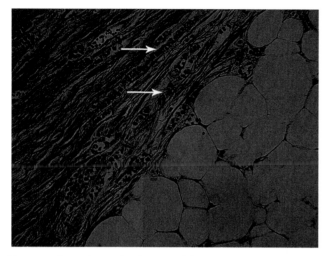

Figure 7.4 Photomicrograph of invasive lobular carcinoma (haematoxylin and eosin stain). Rather than forming a mass, the malignant cells (arrows) diffusely infiltrate along fibrous septa in an "Indian file" pattern. This explains their often subtle or normal mammographic appearances. *Source*: Photograph courtesy of Dr J M Pearson.

found among interval cancers compared with screen-detected cancers (see above). However, correction for these factors gave an odds ratio for nodal positivity of 0.95, 1.34, and 1.37, suggesting that interval cancers presenting in the second year have more aggressive biological features.

These findings are all consistent with the theory that screening has a greater chance of detecting cancers with slower growth rates because of their longer sojourn time (the time between which a tumor becomes potentially mammographically detectable and the point at which the woman would develop symptoms), and conversely that faster growing tumors are more likely to become symptomatic before the next screen is due. This is why women below the age of 50 (who tend to have faster growing tumors than older women) should be screened annually.

True-Negative Vs. False-Negative Interval Cancers
In theory, false-negative interval cancers should be larger than but otherwise resemble screen-detected cancers in their biological features, as these are cancers which could, and arguably should, have been detected at the time of screening. One should therefore expect to find that true-negative interval cancers are more aggressive than false-negative interval cancers. Studies investigating this are limited by relatively small numbers of cases, but several studies have supported this hypothesis (113,118,127–129). One study, however, has found the opposite effect, where true-negative interval cancers appear to be less aggressive than false-negative ones (37). A study from Nottingham found that occult interval cancers, a subtype of type 1, are more often smaller, of lower grade and more likely to have lobular histology compared with other true-negative (category 1) interval cancers (119).

PROGNOSIS OF INTERVAL CANCERS
Relatively little has been published on survival rates for women with interval cancers. A study from the Two Counties trial (130) found that the survival for screened women who developed interval cancers was similar to that of unscreened women with breast cancer. Several subsequent studies have reported

similar findings (106,121,124,131,132), although one study from Sweden suggested that women with interval cancers have a better prognosis than both women uninvited for screening and non-attenders (133).

Vitak (128,134) and Porter (129) found that despite the apparently less aggressive biological features of false-negative interval cancers in their respective series, the survival of women with these tumors was no better than that of women with true-negative interval cancers. They also showed no significant relationship between survival and the interval between the last screen and the cancer diagnosis. However, an earlier Dutch study (127) did report slightly better survival for women with false-negative than those with true-negative interval cancers.

INTERVAL CANCERS FROM HIGHER RISK SCREENING
This group includes women who are on regular mammographic surveillance because of a family history of breast cancer (including those with known gene mutations such as BRCA 1 and 2 and TP53) and those that have previously undergone supradiaphragmatic radiotherapy (e.g., for Hodgkin's lymphoma). These women tend to be younger than those in population-based screening programs and are therefore more likely to have dense breasts. One would therefore expect that this, together with their increased risk, makes the development of interval cancers more likely. These high-risk women are relatively uncommon, and published series have relatively low numbers of cases. A study from the Netherlands (135) found that of nine cancers occurring in BRCA carriers on annual surveillance mammography, four were interval cancers.

INTERVAL CANCERS FROM FOLLOW-UP MAMMOGRAPHY
Regular mammography of women who have undergone treatment for breast cancer is a further category of higher risk screening. Mammography may be accompanied by clinical breast examination, although the trend in the UK is for clinical follow-up to be minimized in view of its low sensitivity. The majority of local recurrences and new cancers occurring in these women are found on mammography, although a significant minority are discovered by the patients themselves between scheduled mammograms, and therefore represent interval cancers.

Mammographic sensitivity for local tumor recurrence and new ipsilateral primary cancers has been reported to be 64–67% (136). This is lower than the sensitivity for primary cancer detection in untreated breasts and is probably due to masking by the effects of surgery and radiotherapy.

The subject of mammographic surveillance following breast cancer treatment is complex and will not be discussed further in this chapter.

INTERVAL CANCERS AFTER SCREENING ASSESSMENT
Cancers developing after discharge from screening assessment where the patient has been given a benign or normal result have received relatively little attention until recently. As a consequence, the literature is rather sparse on this subject. The working assumption has been that if a woman is recalled for further assessment because of a mammographic abnormality which is due to cancer, then that cancer will be diagnosed during the

assessment process. Recent experience in the UK has shown that this is not the case. Failure to diagnose a cancer is often because established assessment processes have not been followed. These include inadequate use of ultrasound to investigate soft tissue masses or asymmetric densities, sometimes because false reassurance has been taken from compression magnification mammograms. These should be interpreted with caution as they sometimes render a cancer less rather than more conspicuous than on the conventional views. Failure to biopsy focal mammographic lesions, particularly clustered microcalcifications (137,138) and ultrasound-negative soft tissue densities (139), is also a common theme found on review of failed assessments. In some cases biopsy has been performed but failed to obtain diagnostic tissue. It is imperative that before a woman is discharged the clinical team should be confident that there is concordance between the radiology and biopsy findings (139,140). This check should normally take place in a multidisciplinary team meeting. If there is not complete concordance then a repeat biopsy should be performed.

Acceptable levels for screening assessment failure have not been established. Sixteen percent of women with interval cancers diagnosed in Scotland after screening between 1991 and 1995 had undergone assessment (19) and a study of interval cancers from East Anglia diagnosed after screening from 1994 to 1999 (117) found that 7% of cases had been previously assessed, higher than the rate in the rest of the screening population of 5%. Warren (138) studied more than half a million women who had been screened in East Anglia between 1989 and 1999. Cancer was diagnosed at assessment in 3689, and a further 193 women subsequently presented with interval cancers at the site of the assessed abnormality, giving a failure rate of 5.0% for cancer diagnosis at assessment. This does not include cancers missed at assessment and diagnosed at the next round of screening. Ciatto (141) in an Italian study of nearly 340,000 women found 57 cancers that were missed at assessment and diagnosed as interval cancers or at the next screening round. Cancer was diagnosed at assessment in 1340, giving a miss rate of 4.1% of all cancers assessed. These figures seem high by modern standards, and work is currently in progress in the UK to more accurately define and quantify the issue of failed screening assessment.

INTERVAL CANCER AS A MEASURE OF SCREENING PERFORMANCE

Given that mammographic screening programs should aim to maximize the number of women with breast cancer who are diagnosed by mammography in order to obtain the greatest survival benefit, the number of screened women who have cancer diagnosed after a supposedly normal screen and before the next screen would seem to be a fundamental measure of the quality of a screening program. The reasons for this not having been the case have already been alluded to and include the variable ascertainment of interval cancers and the delay in cancer registration. This has resulted in data being incomplete and several years out of date. There is an increasing recognition, in the UK at least, that this information should be used and needs to be available in a more accurate and timely manner to assist in the assessment of individual screening unit performance. Work is progressing to ensure that interval cancer data are as complete, accurate, and timely as possible.

In addition, much greater emphasis is being placed upon monitoring interval cancers that occur after screening assessment.

COMMUNICATION WITH THE WOMAN

A woman who has developed breast cancer in the interval following a normal result from screening may at some stage inquire whether the cancer was visible on the screening examination. If this does occur then it is essential that the health care professional who undertakes the discussion has the appropriate knowledge and communication skills to ensure that it is done accurately, openly, and sensitively. Many women, however, do not raise the issue, and it has been recommended that at an appropriate time after the initial treatment the woman should be told that if she wishes to be informed of the result of a review of her previous screening examination then she should say so. In many cases this may be a straightforward discussion in which the woman is informed that even with hindsight the screening mammogram was normal. Women with minimal signs (category 2) and particularly false-negative (category 3) interval cancers may be concerned about a poorer prognosis as a result of the delay in diagnosis, and this should be dealt with in a clear, honest, and empathetic way. Useful guidance on the disclosure of audit results is contained in a UK NHSBSP publication (142).

MEDICOLEGAL ISSUES

It is clear from the foregoing that false-negative (category 3) and perhaps also some minimal signs (category 2) interval cancers are the consequence of a delay in the diagnosis of a cancer that could have been detected at screening, and may therefore have a poorer outcome (143–146). Fortunately, these have not been a major cause of litigation in most European countries (147,148), including the UK. However in the US delay in breast cancer diagnosis has become one of the most common reasons for medical litigation, caused to a large extent by high expectations among the public regarding the sensitivity of mammography (149–151). These unrealistic expectations are often encouraged by health care providers who are keen to promote their screening services (152).

There is controversy over whether a subtle cancer missed on mammography constitutes negligence (150,153), even though it is well recognized that obvious cancers can be missed from time to time by highly competent and conscientious radiologists. Courts view claims for compensation for delayed breast cancer diagnosis in terms of the care of the individual rather than in population terms, and this often results in large awards to the plaintiff. Screening radiologists on the other hand must not only scrutinize large numbers of mammograms for subtle signs of cancer but must also try and serve the interests of the screened population as a whole by maximizing the number of cancers diagnosed at screening and yet minimize the anxiety, discomfort, and inconvenience caused by recalling (and often biopsying) those without cancer.

SUMMARY

Minimizing the number of interval cancers occurring in a mammographic screening program, and thus improving affected women's chance of survival, depends on an appropriate screening interval, high-quality mammography, accurate mammographic interpretation, and skilled further assessment. Interval cancers constitute a higher proportion of cancers diagnosed among younger screened women but overall are more common in older women. They have a greater propensity than screen-detected cancers to occur in those with dense breasts and those on HRT; to be of lobular, mucinous, or medullary subtypes; to be ER and PR negative; to have a high proliferative index; and to be lymph node positive. Their prognosis is intermediate between that of screen-detected cancers and cancers diagnosed in unscreened women. The rate of presentation of interval cancers increases with the time from the last screen. Approximately 0.6 per 1000 women screened are diagnosed with a cancer in the first year after a reportedly normal screen and around a third of interval cancers are due to false-negative screens.

Review and classification of interval cancers is an important exercise, both for the purpose of providing performance feedback to individuals working in the programs and as a means of assessing and improving the program quality. Interval cancers occurring after screening assessment deserve particular attention. Communication with women about interval cancers requires a sensitive approach. Litigation for interval cancers remains relatively uncommon in Europe.

REFERENCES

1. Wilson R, Liston J, eds. Quality Assurance Guidelines for Breast Cancer Screening Radiology. NHSBSP Publication No 59, 2nd edn. Sheffield: NHS Cancer Screening Programmes, 2011: [Available from: http://www.cancerscreening.nhs.uk]
2. Carney PA, Steiner E, Goodrich ME, et al. Discovery of breast cancers within 1 year of a normal screening mammogram: how are they found? Ann Fam Med 2006; 4: 512–18.
3. Burhenne HJ, Burhenne LJW, Goldberg F, et al. Interval breast cancers in the screening mammography program of British Columbia: analysis and classification. AJR Am J Roentgenol 1994; 162: 1067–71.
4. Schouten LJ, de Rijke JM, Schlangen JT, et al. Evaluation of the effect of breast cancer screening by record linkage with the cancer registry, the Netherlands. J Med Screen 1998; 5: 37–41.
5. Fracheboud J, De Koning H, Beemsterboer PMM, et al. Interval cancers in the Dutch breast cancer screening programme. Br J Cancer 1999; 81: 912.
6. Kavanagh AM, Mitchell H, Farrugia H, et al. Monitoring interval cancers in an Australian mammographic screening programme. J Med Screen 1999; 6: 139–43.
7. Törnberg S, Segnan N, Ponti A. Ascertainment and evaluation of interval cancers in population-based mammography screening programmes: a collaborative study in four European centres. J Med Screen 2005; 12: 43–9.
8. Houssami N, Irwig L, Ciatto S. Radiological surveillance of interval breast cancers in screening programmes. Lancet Oncol 2006; 7: 259–65.
9. Perry N, Broeders MJM, De Wolf C, et al. European Guidelines for Quality Assurance in Breast Cancer Screening and Diagnosis, 4th edn. Luxembourg: Office for Official Publications of the European Communities, 2006.
10. Day N, McCann J, Camilleri-Ferrante C, et al. Monitoring interval cancers in breast screening programmes: the East Anglian experience. J Med Screen 1995; 2: 180–5.
11. Lawrence G, Kearins O, O'Sullivan E. The West Midlands breast cancer screening status algorithm–methodology and use as an audit tool. J Med Screen 2005; 12: 179–84.
12. Bennett RL, Sellars SJ, Moss SM. Interval cancers in the NHS breast cancer screening programme in England, Wales and Northern Ireland. Br J Cancer 2011; 104: 571–7.
13. Vettorazzi M, Stocco C, Chirico A, et al. Quality control of mammography screening in the Veneto region. Evaluation of four programs at a local health unit level–analysis of the frequency and diagnostic pattern of interval cancers. Tumori 2006; 92: 1–5.
14. Caumo F, Vecchiato F, Pellegrini M, et al. Analysis of interval cancers observed in an Italian mammography screening programme (2000–2006). Radiol Med 2009; 114: 907–14.
15. Faux A, Lawrence G, Wheaton M, et al. Slippage in the NHS breast screening programme: an assessment of whether a three year screening round is being achieved. J Med Screen 1998; 5: 88–91.
16. Hofvind S, Bjurstam N, Sorum R, et al. Number and characteristics of breast cancer cases diagnosed in four periods in the screening interval of a biennial population-based screening programme. J Med Screen 2006; 13: 192–6.
17. Törnberg S, Kemetli L, Ascunce N, et al. A pooled analysis of interval cancer rates in six European countries. Eur J Cancer Prev 2010; 19: 87–93.
18. Woodman CBJ, Threlfall AG, Boggis CRM, et al. Is the three year breast screening interval too long? Occurrence of interval cancers in NHS breast screening programme's north western region. BMJ 1995; 310: 224–6.
19. Everington D, Gilbert FJ, Tyack C, et al. The Scottish breast screening programme's experience of monitoring interval cancers. J Med Screen 1999; 6: 21–7.
20. Harvey JA, Fajardo LL, Innis CA. Previous mammograms in patients with impalpable breast carcinoma: retrospective vs blinded interpretation. AJR Am J Roentgenol 1993; 161: 1167–72.
21. Duncan A, Wallis MG. Classifying interval cancers. Clin Radiol 1995; 50: 774–7.
22. Simpson W, Neilson F, Young JR. The identification of false negatives in a population of interval cancers: a method for audit of screening mammography. Breast 1995; 4: 183–8.
23. Moberg K, Grundström H, Törnberg S, et al. Two models for radiological reviewing of interval cancers. J Med Screen 1999; 6: 35–9.
24. Amos AF, Kavanagh AM, Cawson J. Radiological review of interval cancers in an Australian mammographic screening programme. J Med Screen 2000; 7: 184–9.
25. Britton PD, McCann J, O'Driscoll D, et al. Interval cancer peer review in East Anglia: implications for monitoring doctors as well as the NHS Breast Screening Programme. Clin Radiol 2000; 56: 44–9.
26. Moberg K, Grundström H, Lundquist H, et al. Radiological review of incidence breast cancers. J Med Screen 2000; 7: 177–83.
27. De Rijke J, Schouten L, Schreutelkamp J, et al. A blind review and an informed review of interval breast cancer cases in the Limburg screening programme, the Netherlands. J Med Screen 2000; 7: 19–23.
28. Hofvind S, Skaane P, Vitak B, et al. Influence of review design on percentages of missed interval breast cancers: retrospective study of interval cancers in a population-based screening program. Radiology 2005; 237: 437–43.
29. Ciatto S, Catarzi S, Lamberini MP, et al. Interval breast cancers in screening: The effect of mammography review method on classification. Breast 2007; 16: 646–52.
30. Gordon PB, Borugian MJ, Burhenne LJW. A true screening environment for review of interval breast cancers: pilot study to reduce bias. Radiology 2007; 245: 411–15.
31. Frisell J, Eklund G, Hellström L, et al. Analysis of interval breast carcinomas in a randomized screening trial in Stockholm. Breast Cancer Res Treat 1987; 9: 219–25.
32. Peeters P, Verbeek ALM, Hendriks JHCL, et al. The occurrence of interval cancers in the Nijmegen screening programme. Br J Cancer 1989; 59: 929–32.
33. Ikeda DM, Andersson I, Wattsgård C, et al. Interval carcinomas in the Malmö Mammographic Screening Trial: radiographic appearance and prognostic considerations. AJR Am J Roentgenol 1992; 159: 287–94.
34. Sylvester PA, Vipond MN, Kutt E, et al. Rate and classification of interval cancers in the breast screening programme. Ann R Coll Surg Engl 1997; 79: 276–7.
35. Yankaskas BC, Schell MJ, Bird RE, et al. Reassessment of breast cancers missed during routine screening mammography. AJR Am J Roentgenol 2001; 177: 535–41.
36. Gower-Thomas K, Fielder HMP, Branston L, et al. Reviewing interval cancers: time well spent? Clin Radiol 2002; 57: 384–8.

37. Hofvind S, Geller B, Skaane P. Mammographic features and histopathological findings of interval breast cancers. Acta Radiol 2008; 49: 975–81.

38. Asbury DL, Boggis CRM, Sheals D, et al. NHS breast screening programme: is the high incidence of interval cancers inevitable? BMJ 1996; 313: 1369–70.

39. Bird R, Wallace T, Yankaskas BC. Analysis of cancers missed at screening mammography. Radiology 1992; 184: 613–17.

40. Huynh PT, Jarolimek AM, Daye S. The false-negative mammogram. Radiographics 1998; 18: 1137–54.

41. Taplin SH, Rutter CM, Finder C, et al. Screening mammography: clinical image quality and the risk of interval breast cancer. AJR Am J Roentgenol 2002; 178: 797–803.

42. Majid AS, de Paredes ES, Doherty RD, et al. Missed breast carcinoma: pitfalls and pearls. Radiographics 2003; 23: 881–95.

43. Young K, Wallis MG, Ramsdale M. Mammographic film density and detection of small breast cancers. Clin Radiol 1994; 49: 461–5.

44. Young K, Wallis MG, Blanks RG. Influence of number of views and mammographic film density on the detection of invasive cancers: results from the NHS Breast Screening Programme. Br J Radiol 1997; 70: 482–8.

45. Wald NJ, Murphy P, Major P, et al. UKCCCR multicentre randomised controlled trial of one and two view mammography in breast cancer screening. BMJ 1995; 311: 1189–93.

46. Blanks RG, Given-Wilson RM, Moss SM. Efficiency of cancer detection during routine repeat (incident) mammographic screening: two versus one view mammography. J Med Screen 1998; 5: 141–5.

47. Blanks RG, Wallis MG, Given-Wilson RM. Observer variability in cancer detection during routine repeat (incident) mammographic screening in a study of two versus one view mammography. J Med Screen 1999; 6: 152–8.

48. Hackshaw AK, Wald N, Michell MJ, et al. An investigation into why two-view mammography is better than one-view in breast cancer screening. Clin Radiol 2000; 55: 454–8.

49. Seigneurin A, Exbrayat C, Labarère J, et al. Comparison of interval breast cancer rates for two-versus single-view screening mammography: a population-based study. Breast 2009; 18: 284–8.

50. Blanks R, Bennett RL, Patnick J, et al. The effect of changing from one to two views at incident (subsequent) screens in the NHS breast screening programme in England: impact on cancer detection and recall rates. Clin Radiol 2005; 60: 674–80.

51. Pisano ED, Gatsonis C, Hendrick E, et al. Diagnostic performance of digital versus film mammography for breast-cancer screening. N Engl J Med 2005; 353: 1773–83.

52. Handel N, Silverstein MJ, Gamagami P, et al. Factors affecting mammographic visualization of the breast after augmentation mammaplasty. JAMA 1992; 268: 1913–17.

53. Eklund GW, Busby RC, Miller SH, et al. Improved imaging of the augmented breast. AJR Am J Roentgenol 1988; 151: 469–73.

54. Miglioretti DL, Rutter CM, Geller BM, et al. Effect of breast augmentation on the accuracy of mammography and cancer characteristics. JAMA 2004; 291: 442–50.

55. Handel N. The effect of silicone implants on the diagnosis, prognosis, and treatment of breast cancer. Plast Reconstr Surg 2007; 120: 81S–93S.

56. Kerlikowske K, Grady D, Barclay J, et al. Effect of age, breast density, and family history on the sensitivity of first screening mammography. JAMA 1996; 276: 33–8.

57. Van Gils CH, Otten JD, Verbeek ALM, et al. Effect of mammographic breast density on breast cancer screening performance: a study in Nijmegen, The Netherlands. J Epidemiol Community Health 1998; 52: 267–71.

58. Rosenberg RD, Hunt WC, Williamson MR, et al. Effects of age, breast density, ethnicity, and estrogen replacement therapy on screening mammographic sensitivity and cancer stage at diagnosis: review of 183,134 screening mammograms in Albuquerque, New Mexico. Radiology 1998; 209: 511–18.

59. Sala E, Warren RML, McCann J, et al. Mammographic parenchymal patterns and mode of detection: implications for the breast screening programme. J Med Screen 1998; 5: 207–12.

60. Foxcroft LM, Evans EB, Joshua HK, et al. Breast cancers invisible on mammography. Aust NZ J Surg 2000; 70: 162–7.

61. Mandelson MT, Oestreicher N, Porter PL, et al. Breast density as a predictor of mammographic detection: comparison of interval-and screen-detected cancers. JNCI J Natl Cancer Inst 2000; 92: 1081–7.

62. Wang J, Shih TT-F, Hsu JC-Y, et al. The evaluation of false negative mammography from malignant and benign breast lesions. J Clin Imaging 2000; 24: 96–103.

63. Wang H, Bjurstam N, Bjorndal H, et al. Interval cancers in the Norwegian breast cancer screening program: frequency, characteristics and use of HRT. Int J Cancer 2001; 94: 594–8.

64. Kolb TM, Lichy J, Newhouse JH. Comparison of the performance of screening mammography, physical examination, and breast US and evaluation of factors that influence them: an analysis of 27,825 patient evaluations. Radiology 2002; 225: 165–75.

65. Carney PA, Miglioretti DL, Yankaskas BC, et al. Individual and combined effects of age, breast density, and hormone replacement therapy use on the accuracy of screening mammography. Ann Intern Med 2003; 138: 168–75.

66. Buist DSM, Porter PL, Lehman C, et al. Factors contributing to mammography failure in women aged 40–49 years. JNCI J Natl Cancer Inst 2004; 96: 1432–40.

67. Ciatto S, Visioli C, Paci E, et al. Breast density as a determinant of interval cancer at mammographic screening. Br J Cancer 2004; 90: 393–6.

68. Collett K, Stefansson IM, Eide J. A basal epithelial phenotype is more frequent in interval breast cancers compared with screen detected tumors. Cancer Epidemiol Biomarkers Prev 2005; 14: 1108–12.

69. Chiarelli AM, Kirsh VA, Shumak RS, et al. Influence of patterns of hormone replacement therapy use and mammographic density on breast cancer detection. Cancer Epidemiol Biomarkers Prev 2006; 15: 1856–62.

70. Boyd NF, Guo H, Martin LJ, et al. Mammographic density and the risk and detection of breast cancer. N Engl J Med 2007; 356: 227–36.

71. Porter GJR, Evans AJ, Cornford EJ, et al. Influence of mammographic parenchymal pattern in screening-detected and interval invasive breast cancers on pathologic features, mammographic features, and patient survival. AJR Am J Roentgenol 2007; 188: 676–83.

72. Kavanagh AM, Byrnes GB, Nickson C, et al. Using mammographic density to improve breast cancer screening outcomes. Cancer Epidemiol Biomarkers Prev 2008; 17: 2818–24.

73. Domingo L, Sala M, Servitja S, et al. Phenotypic characterization and risk factors for interval breast cancers in a population-based breast cancer screening program in Barcelona. Spain. Cancer Causes Control 2010; 21: 1155–64.

74. Lowery JT, Byers T, Hokanson JE, et al. Complementary approaches to assessing risk factors for interval breast cancer. Cancer Causes Control 2011; 22: 23–31.

75. Banks E, Reeves G, Beral V, et al. Influence of personal characteristics of individual women on sensitivity and specificity of mammography in the Million Women Study: cohort study. BMJ 2004; 329: 477–82.

76. Laya MB, Larson EB, Taplin SH, et al. Effect of estrogen replacement therapy on the specificity and sensitivity of screening mammography. JNCI J Natl Cancer Inst 1996; 88: 643–9.

77. Cohen ME. Effect of hormone replacement therapy on cancer detection by mammography. Lancet 1997; 349: 1624.

78. Litherland JC, Stallard S, Hole D, et al. The effect of hormone replacement therapy on the sensitivity of screening mammograms. Clin Radiol 1999; 54: 285–8.

79. Sèradour B, Estève J, Heid P, et al. Hormone replacement therapy and screening mammography: analysis of the results in the Bouches du Rhone programme. J Med Screen 1999; 6: 99–102.

80. Kavanagh AM, Mitchell H, Giles GG. Hormone replacement therapy and accuracy of mammographic screening. Lancet 2000; 355: 270–4.

81. Banks E. Hormone replacement therapy and the sensitivity and specificity of breast cancer screening: a review. J Med Screen 2001; 8: 29–35.

82. Evans AJ. Hormone replacement therapy and mammographic screening. Clin Radiol 2002; 57: 563–4.

83. Crouchley K, Wylie EJ, Khong E. Hormone replacement therapy and mammographic screening outcomes in Western Australia. J Med Screen 2006; 13: 93–7.

84. Kavanagh AM, Cawson J, Byrnes GB, et al. Hormone replacement therapy, percent mammographic density, and sensitivity of mammography. Cancer Epidemiol Biomarkers Prev 2005; 14: 1060–4.

85. McNicholas MMJ, Heneghan JP, Milner MH, et al. Pain and increased mammographic density in women receiving hormone replacement therapy: a prospective study. AJR Am J Roentgenol 1994; 163: 311–15.

86. White E, Velentgas P, Mandelson MT, et al. Variation in mammographic breast density by time in menstrual cycle among women aged 40–49 years. JNCI J Natl Cancer Inst 1998; 90: 906–10.

87. Ursin G, Parisky YR, Pike MC, et al. Mammographic density changes during the menstrual cycle. Cancer Epidemiol Biomarkers Prev 2001; 10: 141–2.

88. Buist DSM, Aiello EJ, Miglioretti DL, et al. Mammographic breast density, dense area, and breast area differences by phase in the menstrual cycle. Cancer Epidemiol Biomarkers Prev 2006; 15: 2303–6.

89. Baines CJ, Vidmar M, McKeown-Eyssen G, et al. Impact of menstrual phase on false negative mammograms in the Canadian National Breast Screening Study. Cancer 1997; 80: 720–4.

90. Anttinen I, Pamilo M, Soiva M, et al. Double reading of mammography screening films–one radiologist or two? Clin Radiol 1993; 48: 414–21.

91. Anderson EDC, Muir BB, Walsh JS, et al. The efficacy of double reading mammograms in breast screening. Clin Radiol 1994; 49: 248–51.

92. Denton ERE, Field S. Just how valuable is double reporting in screening mammography? Clin Radiol 1997; 52: 466–8.

93. Blanks RG, Wallis MG, Moss SM. A comparison of cancer detection rates achieved by breast cancer screening programmes by number of readers, for one and two view mammography: results from the UK National Health Service breast screening programme. J Med Screen 1998; 5: 195–201.

94. Taplin SH, Rutter C, Elmore JG, et al. Accuracy of screening mammography using single versus independent double interpretation. AJR Am J Roentgenol 2000; 174: 1257–62.

95. Liston JC, Dall BJG. Can the NHS Breast Screening Programme afford not to double read screening mammograms? Clin Radiol 2003; 58: 474–7.

96. Hofvind S, Geller BM, Rosenberg RD, et al. Screening-detected breast cancers: Discordant independent double reading in a population-based screening program. Radiology 2009; 253: 652–60.

97. Barlow WE, Chi C, Carney PA, et al. Accuracy of screening mammography interpretation by characteristics of radiologists. JNCI J Natl Cancer Inst 2004; 96: 1840–50.

98. Moss S, Blanks R, Bennett RL. Is radiologists' volume of mammography reading related to accuracy? A critical review of the literature. Clin Radiol 2005; 60: 623–6.

99. Rickard M, Taylor R, Page A, et al. Cancer detection and mammogram volume of radiologists in a population-based screening programme. Breast 2006; 15: 39–43.

100. Cornford EJ, Reed J, Murphy A, et al. Optimal screening mammography reading volumes; evidence from real life in the East Midlands region of the NHS Breast Screening Programme. Clin Radiol 2011; 66: 103–7.

101. Duncan KA, Scott NW. Is film-reading performance related to the number of films read? The Scottish experience. Clin Radiol 2011; 66: 99–102.

102. Laming D, Warren RML. Improving the detection of cancer in the screening of mammograms. J Med Screen 2000; 7: 24–30.

103. Bordas P, Jonsson H, Nystrom L, et al. Interval cancer incidence and episode sensitivity in the Norrbotten Mammography Screening Programme, Sweden. J Med Screen 2009; 16: 39–45.

104. Porter PL, El-Bastawissi AY, Mandelson MT, et al. Breast tumor characteristics as predictors of mammographic detection: comparison of interval- and screen-detected cancers. JNCI J Natl Cancer Inst 1999; 91: 2020–8.

105. Hofvind S, Geller B, Vacek PM, et al. Using the European guidelines to evaluate the Norwegian Breast Cancer Screening Program. Eur J Epidemiol 2007; 22: 447–55.

106. Caumo F, Vecchiato F, Strabbioli M, et al. Interval cancers in breast cancer screening: comparison of stage and biological characteristics with screen-detected cancers or incident cancers in the absence of screening. Tumori 2010; 96: 198–201.

107. Nagtegaal ID, Allgood PC, Duffy SW, et al. Prognosis and pathology of screen detected carcinomas. Cancer 2011; 117: 1360–8.

108. Rayson D, Payne JI, Abdolell M, et al. Comparison of clinical-pathologic characteristics and outcomes of true interval and screen-detected invasive breast cancer among participants of a Canadian breast screening program: a nested case-control study. Clinical Breast Cancer 2011; 11: 27–32.

109. Burrell HC, Sibbering DM, Wilson ARM, et al. Screening interval breast cancers: mammographic features and prognosis factors. Radiology 1996; 199: 811–17.

110. Brown M, Eccles C, Wallis MG. Geographical distribution of breast cancers on the mammogram: an interval cancer database. Br J Radiol 2001; 74: 317.

111. Meeson S, Young KC, Wallis MG, et al. Image features of true positive and false negative cancers in screening mammograms. Br J Radiol 2003; 76: 13–21.

112. Daly CA, Apthorp L, Field S. Second round cancers: how many were visible on the first round of the UK National Breast Screening Programme, three years earlier? Clin Radiol 1998; 53: 25–8.

113. Kirsh VA, Chiarelli AM, Edwards SA, et al. Tumor characteristics associated with mammographic detection of breast cancer in the Ontario Breast Screening Program. JNCI J Natl Cancer Inst 2011; 103: 942–50.

114. Lowery JT, Byers T, Kittelson J, et al. Differential expression of prognostic biomarkers between interval and screen-detected breast cancers: does age or family history matter? Breast Cancer Res Treat 2011; 129: 211–19.

115. Maxwell AJ. Breast cancers missed in the prevalent screening round: effect upon the size distribution of incident round detected cancers. J Med Screen 1999; 6: 28–9.

116. Dershaw DD. Breast disease missed by mammography. Appl Radiol 1997; 26: 24–32.

117. McCann J, Britton PD, Warren RML, et al. Radiological peer review of interval cancers in the East Anglian breast screening programme: what are we missing? J Med Screen 2001; 8: 77–85.

118. Evans AJ, Kutt E, Record C, et al. Radiological and pathological findings of interval cancers in a multi-centre, randomized, controlled trial of mammographic screening in women from age 40–41 years. Clin Radiol 2007; 62: 348–52.

119. Porter GJR, Evans AJ, Burrell HC, et al. NHSBSP type 1 interval cancers: a scientifically valid grouping? Clin Radiol 2007; 62: 262–7.

120. Crosier M, Scott D, Wilson RG, et al. Differences in Ki67 and c-erbB2 expression between screen-detected and true interval breast cancers. Clin Cancer Res 1999; 5: 2682–8.

121. Cowan W, Angus B, Gray J, et al. A study of interval breast cancer within the NHS breast screening programme. J Clin Pathol 2000; 53: 140–6.

122. Gilliland FD, Joste N, Stauber PM, et al. Biologic characteristics of interval and screen-detected breast cancers. JNCI J Natl Cancer Inst 2000; 92: 743–9.

123. Raja MAK, Hubbard A, Salman AR. Interval breast cancer: is it a different type of breast cancer? Breast 2001; 10: 100–8.

124. Groenendijk RPR, Bult P, Noppen CM, et al. Mitotic activity index in interval breast cancers. Eur J Surg Oncol 2003; 29: 29–31.

125. Baré M, Bonfill X, Andreu X. Relationship between the method of detection and prognostic factors for breast cancer in a community with a screening programme. J Med Screen 2006; 13: 183–91.

126. Bucchi L, Puliti D, Ravaioli A, et al. Breast screening: axillary lymph node status of interval cancers by interval year. Breast 2008; 17: 477–83.

127. Brekelmans CT, Peeters PH, Deurenberg JJ. Survival in interval breast cancer in the DOM screening programme. EJC 1995; 31A: 1830–5.

128. Vitak B, Olsen KE, Manson JC, et al. Tumour characteristics and survival in patients with invasive interval breast cancer classified according to mammographic findings at the latest screening: a comparison of true interval and missed interval cancers. Eur Radiol 1999; 9: 460–9.

129. Porter GJR, Evans AJ, Burrell HC, et al. Interval breast cancers: prognostic features and survival by subtype and time since screening. J Med Screen 2006; 13: 115–22.

130. Holmberg LH, Adami HO, Tabar L, et al. Survival in breast cancer diagnosed between mammographic screening examinations. Lancet 1986; 328: 27–30.

131. Collins S, Woodman CBJ, Threlfall A, et al. Survival rates from interval cancer in NHS breast screening programme. BMJ 1998; 316: 832–3.

132. Zackrisson S, Janzon L, Manjer J, et al. Improved survival rate for women with interval breast cancer–results from the breast cancer screening programme in Malmö, Sweden 1976–1999. J Med Screen 2007; 14: 138–43.

133. Bordas P, Jonsson H, Nystrom L, et al. Survival from invasive breast cancer among interval cases in the mammography screening programmes of northern Sweden. Breast 2007; 16: 47–54.

134. Vitak B. Invasive interval cancers in the Ostergötland Mammographic Screening Programme: radiological analysis. Eur Radiol 1998; 8: 639–46.

135. Brekelmans CTM, Seynaeve C, Bartels CCM, et al. Effectiveness of breast cancer surveillance in BRCA1/2 gene mutation carriers and women with high familial risk. J Clin Oncol 2001; 19: 924–30.

136. Robertson C, Arcot Ragupathy SK, Boachie C, et al. The clinical effectiveness and cost-effectiveness of different surveillance mammography regimens after the treatment for primary breast cancer: systematic reviews, registry database analyses and economic evaluation. Health Technol Assess 2011; 15:v–vi, 1–322.

137. Burrell HC, Evans AJ, Wilson RM, et al. False-negative breast screening assessment. What lessons can we learn? Clin Radiol 2001; 56: 385–8.

138. Warren RML, Allgood P, Hunnam G, et al. An audit of assessment procedures in women who develop breast cancer after a negative result. J Med Screen 2004; 11: 180–6.

139. Bennett ML, Welman CJ, Celliers LM. How reassuring is a normal breast ultrasound in assessment of a screen-detected mammographic abnormality? A review of interval cancers after assessment that included ultrasound evaluation. Clin Radiol 2011; 66: 928–39.

140. Youk JH, Kim E-K, Kim MJ, et al. Missed breast cancers at US-guided core needle biopsy: how to reduce them. Radiographics 2007; 27: 79–94.

141. Ciatto S, Houssami N, Ambrogetti D, et al. Minority report – false negative breast assessment in women recalled for suspicious screening mammography: imaging and pathological features, and associated delay in diagnosis. Breast Cancer Res Treat 2006; 105: 37–43.

142. Patnick J, ed. Disclosure of audit results in cancer screening–Advice on best practice. Cancer Screening Series No 3. Sheffield: NHS Cancer Screening Programmes, 2006: [Available from: http://www.cancer-screening.nhs.uk]

143. Richards MA, Smith P, Ramirez AJ, et al. The influence on survival of delay in the presentation and treatment of symptomatic breast cancer. Br J Cancer 1999; 79: 858–64.

144. Richards MA, Westcombe AM, Love SB, et al. Influence of delay on survival in patients with breast cancer: a systematic review. Lancet 1999; 353: 1119–26.

145. Olivotto IA, Gomi A, Bancej C, et al. Influence of delay to diagnosis on prognostic indicators of screen-detected breast carcinoma. Cancer 2002; 94: 2143–50.

146. Barber MD, Jack W, Dixon JM. Diagnostic delay in breast cancer. Br J Surg 2004; 91: 49–53.

147. van Breest Smallenburg V, Setz-Pels W, Groenewoud JH, et al. Malpractice claims following screening mammography in The Netherlands. Int J Cancer 2012; 131: 1360–6.

148. Hafström L, Johansson H, Ahlberg J. Diagnostic delay of breast cancer–an analysis of claims to Swedish Board of Malpractice (LOF). Breast 2011; 20: 539–42.

149. Barratt A, Cockburn J, Furnival C, et al. Perceived sensitivity of mammographic screening: women's views on test accuracy and financial compensation for missed cancers. J Epidemiol Community Health 1999; 53: 716–20.

150. Berlin L. Breast cancer, mammography, and malpractice litigation: the controversies continue. AJR Am J Roentgenol 2003; 180: 1229–37.

151. Mavroforou A, Mavrophoros D, Michalodimitrakis E. Screening mammography, public perceptions, and medical liability. Eur J Radiol 2006; 57: 428–35.

152. Berlin L. Dot size, lead time, fallibility, and impact on survival. AJR Am J Roentgenol 2001; 176: 1123–30.

153. Ikeda DM, Birdwell RL, O'Shaughnessy KF, et al. Analysis of 172 subtle findings on prior normal mammograms in women with breast cancer detected at follow-up screening. Radiology 2003; 226: 494–503.

8 Survival advantage of screen-detected cancer over stage-matched symptomatic cancer

Gordon C. Wishart

INTRODUCTION

Breast cancer remains the most common female cancer in the United Kingdom (UK) with over 47,000 new cases reported per annum and a lifetime risk of 1 in 8 or 12.5%. Following publication of early trials that demonstrated a mortality reduction with screening mammography (1,2), the National Health Service Breast Screening Programme was introduced in 1988 and offered three-yearly screening mammography to women aged 50–65 years in the UK. Since 2004, the upper age limit has been extended to 69 years and current pilot studies are exploring further age extensions to include all women aged 47–73 years. There are currently no plans to decrease the time interval between screening episodes in the UK program.

There is little doubt that widespread introduction of mammographic screening in Europe and North America has made a significant contribution to the reduction in breast cancer mortality that has been observed during the last twenty years. An overview of published breast screening trials in 2002 documented a reduction in breast cancer mortality of 21% in women who attended for mammographic screening (3). The commonly accepted explanation for this survival benefit is that screening picks up breast cancers at an earlier stage in their natural history. This stage shift at diagnosis is a reflection of lead-time bias, which is the time interval between cancer detection by mammography and the time the cancer would have been detected in the absence of screening (4). Another factor that contributes to the improved prognosis of patients with a screen-detected cancer is length bias as screening is more likely to detect slow-growing cancers that are associated with a better survival, as they remain asymptomatic for longer (5).

It is now well documented that screen-detected cancers are usually smaller, of lower grade, and less likely to be lymph node positive (6) when compared with cancers detected outside of screening. Although, until recently, the survival advantage of screen detection has been largely attributed to this shift in stage at presentation, there is an increasing body of evidence to suggest that screen detection remains an independent prognostic factor after adjustment for disease stage at diagnosis (7,8). If the method of detection (screen-detected or symptomatic) does indeed have prognostic value that is independent of known prognostic factors, such as tumor size and lymph node status, then it should be incorporated into current prognostic models that estimate survival following breast cancer treatment. Furthermore, mode of detection should also be incorporated into decision-making tools used to facilitate optimal prescription of adjuvant therapy based on an individual patient's prognostic factors. At present predictive and prognostic models such as the web-based program Adjuvant! (9) and the Nottingham Prognostic Index (NPI) (10), which were developed from a mixture of symptomatic and screen-detected breast cancers, are likely to overestimate treatment benefits for screen-detected cancers leading to potential overtreatment of these patients.

This chapter explores further evidence to support the independent prognostic significance of screen detection, possible reasons to explain the survival advantage beyond stage shift, and how it should be incorporated into current prognostic tools to ensure optimal prescription of adjuvant therapy for patients with screen-detected breast cancer.

STAGE SHIFT WITH SCREEN-DETECTED CANCERS

One way to explore the potential impact of stage shift on the survival advantage of screen-detected breast cancer is to compare the stage distribution between screen-detected and symptomatic breast cancer in a large cohort of patients. In the largest study published to date that examines stage distribution by mode of detection, 5604 patients aged 50–70 years diagnosed with invasive breast cancer in the East of England (UK) between 1998 and 2003 were identified by the Eastern Cancer Registration and Information Centre (ECRIC) and classified as either screen-detected (both prevalent and incident cases) or symptomatic (11). Patients were then allocated to one of six NPI categories (excellent, good, moderate 1, moderate 2, poor, and unknown) according to tumor size, grade, and lymph node status.

The results of this study, presented in Table 8.1, show the percentage of patients by NPI group for symptomatic and screen-detected breast cancer. Patients with screen-detected cancers were significantly more likely to be in an NPI category with a better prognosis (p < 0.001), with 70% of patients allocated to one of the three best prognostic groups compared with only 36% of cases for patients with symptomatic cancers. The same study documented five-year overall survival for all patients, by mode of detection, within each NPI group (Table 8.2). The greatest survival advantage is seen in the two worst prognostic groups, with an absolute 10% benefit for screen detection in the moderate 2 group. These results suggest that the survival advantage of screen-detected breast cancer occurs across all prognostic groups and this was confirmed by survival analysis by continuous NPI where there was a small but systematic overall survival advantage for screen-detected cancers at each NPI value (Fig. 8.1).

Table 8.1 Stage Distribution in Nottingham Prognostic Index (NPI) Groups by Mode of Detection in 5604 Patients Aged 50–70 Diagnosed with Invasive Breast Cancer between 1998 and 2003

NPI Group	Percentage of Patients	
	Symptomatic (%)	Screen-Detected (%)
Excellent	5	19
Good	14	31
Moderate 1	17	20
Moderate 2	18	9
Poor	12	4
Unknown	34	17

Table 8.2 Five-Year Overall Survival Rates for All Patients, and by Mode of Detection, Within Each Nottingham Prognostic Index (NPI) Group

NPI Group	All Patients (%)	Symptomatic (%)	Screen-Detected (%)
Excellent	96	94	98
Good	93	93	94
Moderate 1	90	89	93
Moderate 2	79	78	88
Poor	58	58	65

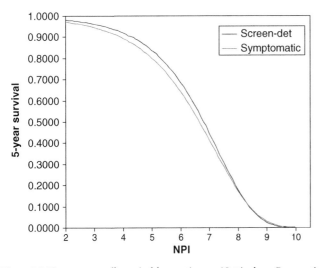

Figure 8.1 Five-year overall survival by continuous Nottingham Prognostic Index (NPI) group. *Source*: Courtesy of British Journal of Cancer (11).

One possible criticism of this study from the Cambridge Breast Unit (UK) is that it may actually *underestimate* the survival benefit associated with screen-detected breast cancer. Although the study contained a large number of cases (n = 5604), the symptomatic control group contained a mixture of patients with very different survival rates including true interval cancers, interval cancers presenting more than three years following the previous screening episode, and patients who had never been screened (11). Furthermore, as reliable information was not available on the cause of death for all patients, all survival analysis in the Cambridge study was based on overall survival rather than breast cancer–specific survival.

Nevertheless, the data presented by Wishart et al. (2008) do support the principle of stage shift due to screen detection; the overall survival analysis, both by NPI groups as well as continuous NPI, supports the contention that even at the same stage patients with screen-detected breast cancer appear to have a better prognosis.

IMPACT OF SCREEN DETECTION ON OVERALL SURVIVAL

An alternative method to examine the effect of screen detection on overall survival is to use a proportional hazards model (12) to estimate the effect of screen detection compared with symptomatic diagnosis unadjusted, then adjusted for age and NPI. By adjusting for NPI, it should be possible to determine the amount of survival advantage with screen detection that is attributable to the stage shift at presentation. In this way the Cambridge group used the method of Freedman (13) to estimate the percentage of the effect of screen detection on survival that can be attributed to known factors in over 5604 women diagnosed with breast cancer in the East of England between 1998 and 2003 (11). In the multivariate model, the effect of screen detection on overall mortality was much attenuated after adjustment for age and NPI, with the relative hazard for the effect of screen detection on overall mortality changing from 0.43 to 0.79.

These earlier results have now been confirmed by a recent study of 2592 patients who were treated at the Netherlands Cancer Institute (NCI) between 1990 and 2000. In this study, screen detection was associated with reduced all-cause mortality, with a hazard ratio (HR) of 0.74 after adjustment for age, tumor size, tumor grade, axillary lymph node status, estrogen receptor (ER) status, and adjuvant systemic therapy (14). The HRs for the effect of screen detection on all-cause mortality from both the Cambridge and NCI studies are almost identical (0.79 *vs.* 0.74 respectively) and this suggests that that the majority of the reduction in all-cause mortality may be due to stage shift and the presence of more favorable prognostic factors in the screen-detected group. This was further examined in the Cambridge study using the method of Freedman (13). Freedman's estimates of the proportion of the effect of screen detection on overall survival accounted for by age and NPI in the Cambridge cohort are presented in Table 8.3. This shows that age and NPI account for 72% of the overall survival advantage leaving 28% unexplained.

Possible explanations for the remaining 28% of the screen-detected overall survival advantage include residual lead-time bias or length bias or perhaps biological differences between screen-detected cancer and symptomatic breast cancer. A tissue microarray study that examined a panel of 13 biomarkers, including ER, PR, and HER2, found that only Bcl-2 retained prognostic significance that was independent of NPI on multivariate analysis (15). This suggests that a number of biomarkers, that on their own are not significant, could contribute to the remaining 28% of the survival advantage and this will be explored later in this chapter.

IMPACT OF SCREEN DETECTION ON BREAST CANCER-SPECIFIC SURVIVAL

Having demonstrated that screen detection confers an overall survival advantage that remains statistically significant after

Table 8.3 Attenuation of Screen Detection Effect on Overall Survival, After Adjustment for Different Factors

Factors	Relative Hazard (95% CI), Screen-Detected *Vs.* Symptomatic	% Screen Detection Effect
None	0.43 (0.34–0.53)	0
Tumor size and node status	0.66 (0.53–0.82)	49
NPI (tumor size, grade and lymph node status)	0.76 (0.60–0.95)	67
NPI and age	0.79 (0.63–0.99)	72

Abbreviations: CI, confidence interval; NPI, Nottingham Prognostic Index.

correction for age and NPI (11), Wishart et al. were unable to confirm a similar pattern for breast cancer–specific survival (BCSS) as exact cause of death was not adequately recorded in their large cohort of patients. However, the recent study by Mook et al. not only analyzed the effect of screen detection on overall survival but also examined the prognostic effect of mode of detection on BCSS (14). Of the 2592 patients diagnosed at the NCI from 1990 to 2000, 958 were screen-detected, 417 were interval cancers, and 1217 were not screening-related. All analyses were adjusted for age, tumor size, tumor grade, axillary lymph node status, ER status, and adjuvant systemic therapy. In an attempt to minimize the effect of lead-time bias, disease outcome was stratified for tumor size and lymph node status across two periods due to changes in the local screening program (1990–1996 and 1997–2000).

The results of Mook's study provide further supporting evidence that screen detection is associated with improved disease outcome, not only for overall survival but for BCSS as well. In this study, screen detection resulted in a reduction in breast cancer–specific mortality with an adjusted HR of 0.62 (95% CI 0.50–0.78). The magnitude of this mortality reduction was greater than for all-cause mortality (38% *vs.* 26%) in the same study and provides further evidence that stage shift is unable to fully explain the survival benefit associated with screen detection. Furthermore, the reduction in breast cancer specific mortality was present across all tumor size categories and was most pronounced in tumors ≤10 mm, where the adjusted HR was 0.35 (95% CI 0.13–0.96) (14). This stratification by tumor size should reduce the proportion of lead-time bias that is caused by stage shift, but may not completely eliminate it as there is still the possibility of stage shift *within* tumor size categories.

The results presented in this chapter to date show that screen detection is independently associated with a better prognosis for both overall survival (13,14) and breast cancer–specific survival (14); also it provides prognostic information over and above stage migration in patients with invasive breast cancer. These findings therefore have clear implications about how to improve the prediction of outcome, and selection of appropriate adjuvant therapy, for patients with screen-detected cancers by taking the mode of detection into account when estimating the prognosis of an individual patient.

MOLECULAR CHARACTERISTICS OF SCREEN-DETECTED CANCERS

As discussed previously in this chapter, approximately 28% of the survival advantage of screen detection remains after adjustment for age and stage shift in NPI (11). One possible explanation for this effect may relate to differences in tumor biology according to mode of detection of the underlying breast cancer. As previously discussed, screening is more likely to detect slow-growing cancers that are associated with a better survival, as they remain asymptomatic for longer due to length bias.

Developments in microarray technology have now revealed five molecular breast cancer subtypes based on gene expression signatures (16,17). These five subtypes (luminal A, luminal B, HER2 overexpressing, basal-like, and normal breast tissue-like) have very different genetic signatures that reflect marked differences in tumor biology and clinical outcome. Luminal A tumors have the best prognosis; HER2 overexpressing and basal-like have worse overall survival (17). In addition, protein expression with immunohistochemistry can also be used to produce a similar classification of breast cancer subtypes (18).

A study from the Cambridge Breast Unit (UK) has examined whether differences in tumor biology may explain some of the survival advantage associated with screen detection (19). In this study a total of 1379 women aged 50–70 years were classified into five groups based on tumor expression of ER, PR, HER2, basal cytokeratins, and EGFR (Table 8.4) measured by immunohistochemistry. Of the 1379 patients, 610 were screen detected and 769 were symptomatic and the mean follow-up was 7 years (range 1–16 years). A summary of the molecular characteristics by mode of detection is shown in Table 8.5. As can be seen in this table, a significantly higher proportion of tumors detected by screening were ER positive, PR positive, and Bcl-2 positive. In addition screen-detected tumors had significantly lower rates of Ki-67 positivity and EGFR expression.

Overall survival at 15 years by molecular subtype is shown in Table 8.6. Although tumors detected by screening had a more favorable outcome regardless of molecular subtype, this difference was only significant in the luminal A subtype (subtype 1) where the 15-year survival was 94% in women with screen-detected cancers compared with 84% in the symptomatic group (p = 0.001).

The effect of screen detection on all-cause mortality was explored in this population after adjustment for NPI, biomarker expression, and molecular subtype. After adjustment for NPI, the HR changed from 0.43 to 0.69. Further adjustment of the model to incorporate individual markers or molecular subtype resulted in minimal change to the underlying HR.

The Freedman estimate (13) of the proportion of survival advantage from screen detection attributable to the NPI was 56% in this study and after adjustment for other molecular characteristics ranged from 59 to 66%. Thus in this study tumor biology only accounted for an additional 3–10% of the screen-detected survival benefit.

A greater percentage of favorable molecular characteristics have previously been described in screen-detected breast cancers including higher expression of ER and PR and lower

Table 8.4 Molecular Subtypes of Breast Cancer Categorized by Protein Expression Using Immunohistochemistry

Subtype	ER	PR	HER2	Basal Markers
1 Luminal A	Pos	Pos	Neg	
2 Luminal B	Pos	Pos	Pos	
3 HER2 overexpressing	Neg	Neg	Pos	
4 Triple negative: No basal markers	Neg	Neg	Neg	Neg
5 Triple negative: With basal markers	Neg	Neg	Neg	Pos

Abbreviations: ER, estrogen receptor; Neg, negative; Pos, positive; PR, progesterone receptor.

Table 8.5 Molecular Characteristics of Screen-Detected *Vs.* Symptomatic Breast Cancer

Characteristic	Mode of Breast Cancer Detection		
	Screen Detected (%)	Symptomatic (%)	P value
ER positive	86	74	<0.0001
PR positive	74	65	0.002
HER2 positive	8	12	0.10
EGFR positive	6	11	0.012
Ki-67 positive	6	15	<0.0001
BCL-2 positive	90	83	0.003

Abbreviations: ER, estrogen receptor; PR, progesterone receptor.

Table 8.6 15-Year Overall Survival Rates by Breast Cancer Molecular Subtypes

Molecular subtype	N	Overall Survival (15 Yrs)		
		Screen Detected (%)	Symptomatic (%)	P Value
1	688	94	84	0.001
2	53	86	78	0.52
3	36	83	54	0.12
4	35	86	64	0.24
5	75	84	79	0.60

expression of Ki-67 and HER2 (8,20). The study by Dawson et al. (19) confirmed these earlier findings but also identified that symptomatic cancers were more likely to be triple negative and EGFR positive and that screen-detected cancers are more likely to show higher expression of Bcl-2, an anti-apoptotic protein whose expression is associated with improved survival from breast cancer (15,21).

In addition, a study from the MD Anderson Cancer Center has explored copy number imbalances (CNIs) to see if any genotypic differences might possibly explain the residual survival difference between screen-detected and symptomatic cancers. In 850 women (screen detected, n = 247; symptomatic, n = 603) diagnosed with stage I–II breast cancer from 1985 to 2000 (22), CNIs were identified using high-density molecular inversion probe arrays. A Cox proportional hazards

model was used to estimate the effect of mode of detection on disease-free survival after adjustment for age, stage at presentation, and CNI. Copy number gains in chromosomes 2p, 3q, 11p, and 20q were significantly associated with mode of detection (p < 0.00001). The authors estimated that 63% of the survival advantage of screen detection was accounted for by age, stage, nuclear grade, and Ki-67 in women aged 40–87 years. Furthermore, an additional 20% of the survival advantage was associated with CNIs associated with the mode of detection. The authors concluded that further interrogation of the tumor genotype may have the potential to improve discrimination between indolent and aggressive screen-detected breast cancer and that this could enhance decision making with regard to surgical and adjuvant therapy. These genotypic differences also appear to contribute to the survival difference between patients with symptomatic and screen-detected breast cancers.

In summary, therefore, about two-thirds of the screen-detected survival advantage can be explained by age and shift in stage at presentation and, despite obvious differences in the molecular characteristics according to the mode of detection of the underlying tumors, until recently these biological differences only seemed to explain some of the residual survival benefit. The paper on CNIs from Brewster et al. (22) suggests however, that genotypic differences might partially account for some of the remaining survival advantage (by as much as 20%). It is possible that this residual gap in unexplained survival benefit with screen detection will gradually reduce with more accurate recording of tumor grade and lymphovascular invasion, greater understanding of the molecular biology of breast cancer, and more accurate methods for adjustment of lead-time and length bias. Nevertheless, the survival advantage associated with screen detection appears consistent across several studies including historical (7,8) and contemporary studies presented in detail in this chapter (11,14,19).

On the basis of these findings, mode of detection should now be included in predictive models of breast cancer survival to help provide more accurate survival estimates as well as treatment benefits for patients with screen-detected breast cancer. This would allow greater individualization of patient treatment and ensure that patients with screen-detected breast cancer are not subjected to toxic and unnecessary treatments such as chemotherapy unless there is a clear survival benefit to be gained.

PREDICTIVE MODELS IN BREAST CANCER

Accurate prediction of survival and treatment benefits is an essential component of the decision-making process following surgery for early breast cancer that allows clinicians to determine those patients who require adjuvant therapy. At present these decisions are based on known pathological prognostic factors that retain independent significance on multivariate analysis including tumor size, tumor grade, and lymph node status. The predicted treatment benefit(s) for an individual patient can be calculated by applying the relative risk reduction for a particular adjuvant therapy to the breast cancer–specific mortality to yield an estimate of absolute survival benefit for that patient.

Nottingham Prognostic Index

The NPI is a UK based prognostic scoring system based on a large cohort of patients with early breast cancer treated in a

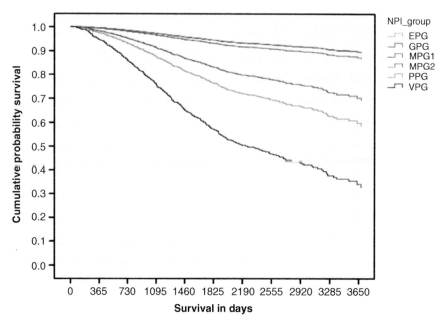

Figure 8.2 Ten-year overall survival according to Nottingham Prognostic Index (NPI) group in women diagnosed in the Cambridge Breast Unit, United Kingdom, from 1998 to 2007. *Abbreviations*: EPG: Excellent Prognosis Group; GPG: Good Prognosis Group; MPG1: Moderate Prognosis Group 1; MPG2: Moderate Prognosis Group 2; PPG: Poor Prognosis Group; VPG: Very Poor Prognosis Group.

single institution. The scoring system is based on the tumor size, grade, and lymph node status and when first described divided patients into three groups with significantly different survival (23). The NPI has been prospectively validated in a second Nottingham dataset (24), as well as in other centers (25), and now allocates patients to one of six prognostic groups (26), with marked differences in survival between individual groups (Fig. 8.2). Subsequently a model was developed to allow prediction of survival based on individual NPI scores rather than the mean survival of the six groups previously described (10). At present the NPI model does not take into account the mode of detection or ER/HER2 receptor status.

Adjuvant!

Adjuvant! is a web-based prognostication and treatment benefit tool for early invasive breast cancer that has been widely used in the UK in recent years to help clinicians and patients make decisions about adjuvant therapy. The mortality estimates used in Adjuvant! were based on 10-year observed overall survival of women aged 36–69 who were diagnosed between 1988 and 1992 and recorded in the Surveillance, Epidemiology and End Results registry (27). BCSS without adjuvant therapy was calculated based on estimates of the number of patients likely to have received systemic therapy and the risk reductions outlined in the Early Breast Cancer Trialists' Collaborative Group (28,29). Although these assumptions have now been validated in a population-based Canadian dataset (30) there has always been some uncertainty about how applicable the Adjuvant! model is to contemporary patients diagnosed and treated in Europe and the UK. In fact, a paper has shown that Adjuvant! overestimated the overall survival by 6% in a UK cohort of 1065 women with early breast cancer treated in Oxford between 1986 and 1996 (31). Furthermore, Adjuvant! does not currently include mode of detection in its model despite the recent study by Mook et al., which demonstrated that Adjuvant! underestimated the BCSS rates in patients with

screen-detected cancers by 3.2% (14). As a result there appears to be a role for a survival prediction and treatment benefit tool based on a group of more contemporary women diagnosed with breast cancer in the UK, and which also includes a mode of detection in the prognostic model.

Following publication of the original paper by Wishart et al. in 2008 (11), confirming the survival advantage associated with screen detection, a group of Cambridge-based clinicians and scientists set out to create a new predictive model for early breast cancer that was based on UK patients and included current known prognostic factors as well as a mode of detection. This UK model, now called Predict, allows the prediction of 5- and 10-year survival as well as treatment benefits with hormone therapy, chemotherapy and trastuzumab and is freely available online at www.predict.nhs.uk.

PREDICT
Dataset

Development of the Predict model was based on a study conducted on 5694 patients diagnosed with invasive breast cancer in East Anglia from 1999 to 2003 using cancer registration and overall survival data recorded by ECRIC including age at diagnosis, number of lymph nodes sampled, number of lymph nodes positive, tumor size, histological grade, ER status, mode of detection (screen detected *vs.* symptomatic), information on local therapy (wide local excision, mastectomy, and radiotherapy), and the type of adjuvant systemic therapy (chemotherapy, endocrine therapy, or both). Patients who did not undergo surgery, patients with incomplete local therapy (wide local excision without radiotherapy), and patients with fewer than four nodes excised with a diagnosis of node-negative disease were excluded. An independent validation dataset comprised 5468 women diagnosed with invasive breast cancer between 1999 and 2003 within the boundaries of the West Midlands Cancer Intelligence Unit (WMCIU).

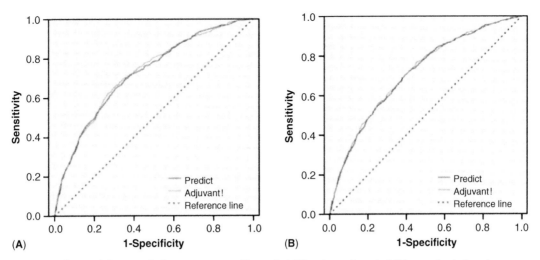

Figure 8.3 Receiver-operator characteristic curves for breast cancer–specific survival (**A**) and overall survival (**B**) according to breast cancer prognostic models: Adjuvant! and Predict.

Model Development

Development of the model was a collaborative project between the Cambridge Breast Unit, University of Cambridge Department of Oncology and ECRIC. In Predict breast cancer–specific mortality and mortality from other causes (competing mortality) are modeled separately. For breast cancer–specific mortality, a Cox proportional hazards model was used to estimate the HR associated with each prognostic factor. As the effect of ER status varies over time (32) ER-negative and ER-positive tumors were modeled separately. For the purposes of this study, screen-detected cancers were those discovered by screening mammography in the NHS Breast Screening Programme, which at the time offered three-yearly mammography to women aged 50–64 years.

Model Validation and Calibration

A paper describing development and initial validation of the Predict model in detail was published by Wishart et al. in 2010 (33). Differences in overall actual and predicted mortality were <1% at 8 years for ECRIC and WMCIU with area under receiver-operator characteristic (ROC) curves (area under the curve) of 0.81 and 0.79 respectively. Differences in breast cancer specific actual and predicted mortality were <1% at 8 years for ECRIC and <1.5% at 8 years for WMCIU with AUC of 0.84 and 0.82, respectively. Model calibration was good for both ER-positive and negative models although the ER-positive model provided better discrimination (AUC 0.82) than ER negative (AUC 0.75). The model performed well across all prognostic groups in the development (ECRIC) dataset except in patients ≥75 years old, where the predicted mortality at year 8 past diagnosis was less than observed (250 predicted *vs.* 276 actual deaths). This was also seen in the validation (WMCIU) data. The model also predicted more favorable outcomes than observed for low-grade tumors and less favorable outcomes than observed for high-grade and ER-negative tumors.

These results confirmed that the Predict model is well calibrated and provides a high degree of discrimination across different prognostic groups and has been validated using data from a second UK registry. A second validation study has now been performed in a British Columbia dataset where it was also compared with Adjuvant! (34). This comparison shows that Predict and Adjuvant! can provide accurate overall survival and BCSS estimates that were comparable. However, the Predict estimates did not include mode of detection, as this information was not available in the Canadian dataset, and as a result this input variable was switched off in the Predict model for the comparison with Adjuvant! Even without this key input variable, Predict was slightly better calibrated for breast cancer specific mortality with predicted deaths being within 3.4% of observed deaths compared with 6.7% for Adjuvant! Both models showed good discrimination with similar AUC for both BCSS (0.723 *vs.* 0.727) and overall survival (0.709 *vs.* 0.712) for Predict and Adjuvant respectively (Fig. 8.3).

PREDICT PLUS: INCLUSION OF HER2

One of the biggest current debates among surgical and medical breast oncologists is how best to treat patients with small, HER2-positive breast cancers that otherwise have very good prognostic features. The Predict model was deliberately developed with 5- and 10-year survival estimates so that new prognostic and predictive factors could be included once validated. As a result the Predict study group initiated a new study to develop version 2 of the model. The aims of this study were to estimate the prognostic effect of HER2 status by ER status over time, include it in a new version of the model (Predict Plus), and to compare the 10-year survival estimates from Predict Plus with the original Predict model, Adjuvant! and the observed 10-year outcome from a British Columbia dataset used previously to validate Adjuvant! and Predict.

Method

Estimates for the prognostic effect of HER2 status were based on an analysis of data for 14,017 breast cancer patients from 15 studies in the Breast Cancer Association Consortium. Estimates of the relative hazard for HER2 positivity over time were obtained separately for ER-positive and ER-negative disease (Fig. 8.4) and these estimates were incorporated into Predict. The validation study was based on 1653 patients with stage I or II invasive breast cancer diagnosed in British Columbia,

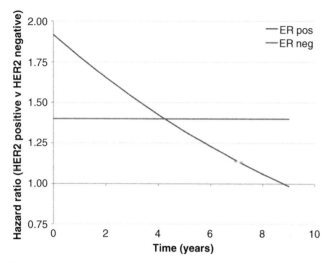

Figure 8.4 Relative hazard estimates for HER2 positivity over time for ER-positive and ER-negative disease (n = 14,017). *Source*: Courtesy of British Journal of Cancer (35).

Canada, from 1989 to 1993 who were identified from the Breast Cancer Outcomes Unit (BCOU) database including demographic, pathological, staging initial treatment data as well as HER2 status. Ten-year predicted overall survival and BCSS were calculated for each patient using Predict Plus, Predict, and Adjuvant! by investigators blinded to the actual outcome data for each patient. Predicted outcomes from all three models were compared with observed outcomes from the dataset.

Results

The total number of deaths predicted by Adjuvant! (n = 492) was within 6.1% of that observed (n = 524) compared with 8.8% for Predict (n = 478) and 8.4% for Predict Plus (n = 8.4) (35). The total number of breast cancer specific deaths predicted by Adjuvant! (n = 311) was within 14% of that observed (n = 360) compared to 3.6% for Predict (n = 347) and 2.5% for Predict Plus (n = 351). In patients with HER2-positive tumors (n = 203), the total number of breast cancer specific deaths predicted by Predict Plus was within 4.0% of observed compared with 20% for Predict and 29% for Adjuvant!.

This study reports the first clinical breast cancer prognostication tool (Predict) based on known clinical and pathological factors that includes HER2 status on tumors. The study has demonstrated a marked improvement in 10-year BCSS estimates using Predict Plus compared with the original Predict model for patients with HER2-positive tumors. Both Predict models provided better BCSS estimates than Adjuvant! in patients with HER2-positive tumors in this dataset.

USING THE PREDICT MODEL

The Predict model is now available online at www.predict .nhs.uk. Key input factors include age at diagnosis, mode of detection, tumor size, tumor grade, ER/HER2 status and the number of positive nodes. By selecting second-generation (anthracycline containing) or third-generation (taxane containing) chemotherapy the 5-year and 10-year survival, with and without trastuzumab, chemotherapy and/or hormone therapy is provided in both graphic and text format allowing a print copy for individual patients (Figs. 8.5 and 8.6). Future versions of the Predict model may be developed to include any additional markers, including the Progesterone receptor and a proliferation marker that may enhance the ability to determine more accurate survival and treatment benefit estimates.

SUMMARY

The data presented in this chapter provide compelling evidence for a survival advantage for screen-detected invasive breast cancer that goes beyond a shift in stage at presentation. This has now been demonstrated in several studies for both overall and BCSS with confirmation that the mode of detection is an independent prognostic factor.

Although most of the improved survival associated with screen detection can be attributed to stage migration, tumor biology also seems to play a role with a greater percentage of favorable molecular characteristics being present in screen-detected breast cancers and differences in genotypic features according to the mode of detection. A proportion of the survival benefit however is at present unexplained and one area that does require further investigation is host immunity and the response of an individual patient to the presence of a breast cancer.

The mammographic features of cancers can reflect the "body's" response to malignancy, for example the scirrhous reaction around a tumor that presents as a spiculate mass on mammography or the presence of malignant microcalcification deposited in necrotic tissue within or around tumors. These mammographic appearances clearly favor screen detection for these relatively good prognosis tumors in contrast to the ill-defined rounded opacities of worse prognosis tumors that are often difficult to detect on mammography.

As a result of these findings it is imperative that the mode of detection is taken into account when estimating the prognosis of an individual patient; otherwise there will be a tendency to underestimate the survival and overestimate treatment benefits for patients with screen-detected breast cancer. Predict, a new breast cancer prognostic model, estimates 5- and 10-year survival after surgery for invasive breast cancer and is the first prognostic model based on clinicopathological features to include both mode of detection as well as HER2 status. Predict also provides estimates of treatment benefits with hormone therapy, chemotherapy, and trastuzumab to facilitate selection of the most appropriate adjuvant systemic therapy.

The inclusion of HER2 status in the Predict model will also help resolve the current clinical dilemma regarding the optimal management of small HER2-positive breast cancers that otherwise have favorable prognostic features such as small tumor size, node negativity, and screen detection. Future prognostic models should incorporate additional prognostic factors as they become validated, including both clinicopathological and molecular factors to ensure that patients receive optimal advice regarding their prognosis and potential treatment benefits.

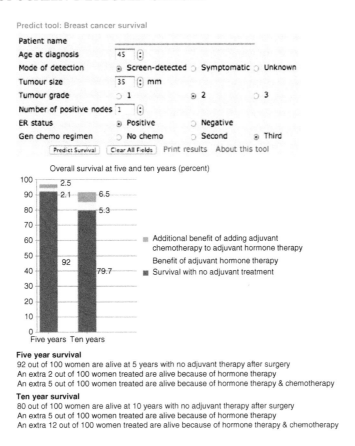

Figure 8.5 Five-year and 10-year survival estimates with additional treatment benefits for adjuvant hormone therapy and chemotherapy in the breast cancer prognostic model Predict.

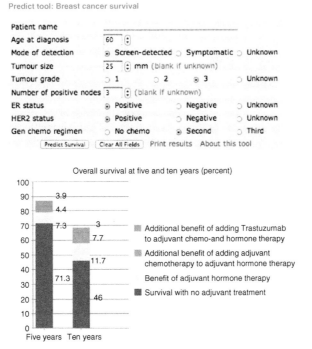

Five year survival

71 out of 100 women are alive at 5 years with no adjuvant therapy after surgery
An extra 7 out of 100 women treated are alive because of hormone therapy
An extra 12 out of 100 women treated are alive because of hormone therapy & chemotherapy
An extra 16 out of 100 women treated are alive because of hormone therapy, chemotherapy & Trastuzumab

Ten year survival

46 out of 100 women are alive at 10 years with no adjuvant therapy after surgery
An extra 12 out of 100 women treated are alive because of hormone therapy
An extra 19 out of 100 women treated are alive because of hormone therapy & chemotherapy
An extra 22 out of 100 women treated are alive because of hormone therapy, chemotherapy & Trastuzumab

Figure 8.6 Five-year survival estimates with benefits of combined trastuzumab/chemotherapy and hormone therapy in breast cancer prognostic model Predict Plus.

ACKNOWLEDGMENTS

1. I thank all my coauthors who have contributed to manuscripts produced by the Cambridge Breast Unit and the University of Cambridge (11,19,33–35) which have made a significant contribution to the content of this chapter.

2. I particularly thank Dr Paul Pharoah from the Department of Oncology, University of Cambridge who had guided me through development of the Predict breast cancer prognostic model from conception to the current model.

REFERENCES

1. Shapiro S, Strax P, Venet L. Periodic breast cancer screening in reducing mortality from breast cancer. JAMA 1971; 215: 1777–85.
2. Tabar L, Fagerberg CJ, Gad A, et al. Reduction in mortality from breast cancer after mass screening with mammography. Randomised trial from the Breast Cancer Screening Working Group of the Swedish National Board of Health and Welfare. Lancet 1985; 1: 829–32.
3. Nystrom L, Andersson I, Bjurstam N, et al. Long term effects of mammography screening: updated overview of the Swedish randomized trials. Lancet 2002; 359: 909–19.
4. Shapiro S, Goldberg JD, Hutchison GB. Lead time bias in breast cancer detection and implications for periodicity of screening. Am J Epidemiol 1974; 100: 357–66.
5. Zahl PH, Strand BH, Maehlen J. Incidence of breast cancer in Norway and Sweden during introduction of nationwide screening: prospective cohort study. BMJ 2004; 328: 921–4.
6. Weaver DL, Rosenberg RD, Barlow WE, et al. Pathologic findings from the Breast Cancer Surveillance Consortium: population-based outcomes in women undergoing biopsy after screening mammography. Cancer 2006; 106: 732–42.
7. Shen Y, Yang Y, Innoue LY, et al. Role of detection method in predicting breast cancer survival: analysis of randomized screening trials. J Natl Cancer Inst 2005; 97: 1195–203.
8. Joensuu H, Lehtimaki T, Holli K, et al. Risk for distant recurrence of breast cancer detected by mammography screening or other methods. JAMA 2004; 292: 1064–73.
9. Olivotto IA, Bajdik CD, Ravdin PM, et al. Population-based validation of the prognostic model ADJUVANT! for early breast cancer. J Clin Oncol 2005; 23: 2716–25.
10. Blamey RW, Pinder SE, Ball GR, et al. Reading the prognosis of the individual with breast cancer. Eur J Cancer 2007; 43: 1498–500.
11. Wishart GC, Greenberg DC, Britton PD, et al. Screen-detected vs symptomatic breast cancer: is improved survival due to stage migration only? Br J Cancer 2008; 98: 1741–4.
12. Cox DR. Regression models and life-tables. J Roy Stat Soc 1972; 34: 187–220.
13. Freedman LS, Graubard BI, Schatzkin A. Statistical validation of intermediate endpoints for chronic diseases. Stat Med 1992; 11: 167–87.
14. Mook S, Van 't Veer LJ, Rutgers EJ, et al. Independent prognostic value of screen detection in invasive breast cancer. J Natl Cancer Inst 2011; 103: 585–97.
15. Callagy GM, Pharoah PD, Pinder SE, et al. BCL-2 is a prognostic marker in breast cancer independently of the Nottingham Prognostic Index. Clin Cancer Res 2006; 12: 2468–75.
16. Perou CM, Sorlie T, Eisen MB, et al. Molecular portraits of human breast tumours. Nature 2000; 406: 747–52.
17. Sorlie T, Tibshirani R, Parker J, et al. Repeated observation of breast tumour subtypes in independent gene expression data sets. Proc Natl Acad Sci USA 2003; 100: 8418–23.
18. Callagy GM, Webber MJ, Daigo Y, et al. Molecular classification of breast carcinomas using tissue microarrays. Diagn Mol Pathol 2003; 12: 27–34.
19. Dawson SJ, Duffy SW, Blows FM, et al. Molecular characteristics of screen-detected vs symptomatic breast cancers and their impact on survival. Br J Cancer 2009; 101: 1338–44.
20. Crosier M, Scott D, Wilson RG, et al. Differeneces in Ki-67 and c-erbB2 expression between screen-detected and true interval breast cancers. Clin Cancer Res 1999; 5: 2682–8.
21. Callagy GM, Webber MJ, Pharoah PD, et al. Meta-analysis confirms BCL2 is an independent prognostic marker in breast cancer. BMC Cancer 2008; 8: 153.
22. Brewster AM, Thompson P, Sahin AA, et al. Copy number imbalances between screen- and symptom-detected breast cancers and impact on disease-free survival. Cancer Prev Res (Phila) 2011; 4: 1609–16.
23. Haybittle JL, Blamey RW, Elston CW, et al. A prognostic index in primary breast cancer. Br J Cancer 1982; 45: 361–6.
24. Todd JH, Dowle C, Williams MR, et al. Confirmation of a prognostic index in primary breast cancer. Br J Cancer 1987; 56: 489–92.
25. D'Eredita G, Giardina C, Martellotta M, et al. Prognostic factors in breast cancer: the predictive value of the Nottingham Prognostic Index in patients with a long term follow-up that were treated in a single institution. Eur J Cancer 2001; 37: 591–6.
26. Blamey RW, Ellis IO, Pinder SE, et al. Survival of invasive breast cancer according to the Nottingham Prognostic Index in cases diagnosed in 1990–1999. Eur J Cancer 2007; 43: 1548–55.
27. Ravdin PM, Siminoff LA, Davis JG, et al. Computer Program to assist in making decisions about adjuvant therapy for women with early breast cancer. J Clin Oncol 2001; 19: 980–91.
28. Early Breast Cancer Trialists' Collaborative Group. Tamoxifen for early breast cancer: an overview of randomized trials. Lancet 1998; 351: 1451–67.
29. Early Breast Cancer Trialists' Collaborative Group. Polychemotherapy for early breast cancer: an overview of randomized trials. Lancet 1998; 352: 930–42.
30. Olivotto IA, Bajdik CD, Ravdin PM, et al. Population-based validation of the prognostic model ADJUVANT! for early breast cancer. J Clin Oncol 2005; 23: 2716–25.
31. Campbell HE, Taylor MA, Harris AL, et al. An investigation into the performance of the Adjuvant! online prognostic programme in early breast cancer for a cohort of patients in the United Kingdom. Br J Cancer 2009; 101: 1074–84.
32. Azzato EM, Greenberg D, Shah M, et al. Prevalent cases in observational studies of cancer survival: do they bias hazard ratio estimates? Br J Cancer 2009; 100: 1806–11.
33. Wishart GC, Azzato EM, Greenberg DC, et al. PREDICT: a new UK prognostic model that predicts survival following surgery for invasive breast cancer. Breast Cancer Res 2010; 12: R1.
34. Wishart GC, Bajdik CD, Azzato EM, et al. A population-based validation of the prognostic model PREDICT for early breast cancer. Eur J Surg Oncol 2011; 37: 411–17.
35. Wishart GC, Bajdik CD, Dicks E, et al. PREDICT Plus: a population based validation of a prognostic model for early breast cancer that includes HER2. Br J Cancer 2012; 107: 800–7.

9   Mammography screening for women under age 50

Ismail Jatoi and Pranjali V. Gadgil

INTRODUCTION

During the last 25 years, mammography screening for women under age 50 has been one of the most intensely debated topics in medicine. American and European perspectives on this issue have differed considerably for many years (1). Historically, after reviewing the same evidence, many experts and medical organizations have often arrived at opposite conclusions concerning its merits. For example, in February 1993, the American Cancer Society (ACS) and the European Society of Mastology (EUSOMA) met in New York and Paris respectively to review the results of mammography screening trials. After reviewing the same data, the two organizations arrived at opposite conclusions: the ACS reaffirmed its long-standing recommendations of screening women starting at age 40, while EUSOMA recommended that screening be reserved for women above age 50 (2).

In light of more data, the US Preventive Services Task Force (USPSTF) updated its recommendations on screening mammography in 2009 (3). In a review undertaken several years prior, the USPSTF had concluded that there was fair evidence that mammography screening every one to two years could significantly reduce breast cancer mortality for women aged 40 and older (4,5). However, in the 2009 updated guidelines, they recommend against routine mammography in women aged 40–49 years, and recommended biennial screening mammography for women aged 50–74 years. The USPSTF argued that the net benefit of screening women between age 40 and 49 years when compared with older women is much smaller, the risk of false positives is greater, and the number needed to screen to prolong one woman's life, is much higher (1339 *vs.* 1904). The USPSTF guidelines have generated considerable controversy, and have been criticized by several scientific organizations. The ACS questioned the quality of evidence used in making these recommendations (6). It also argued that the USPSTF ignored the important concerns of incidence-based mortality and premature mortality. Although the number needed to screen in younger women may be higher, the years of potential life lost (YPLL) saved is high. It criticized that using the number needed to screen is not an appropriate justification to recommend against screening younger women. The ACS continues to recommend annual mammography starting at age 40 years. Other organizations, such as the American College of Radiologists and the American Society of Breast Surgeons, have also refuted these guidelines. Some argue that even if screening does not save a woman's life, it may offer her the option of breast conservation (7) and reduce the need for chemotherapy and so on.

In this chapter, we discuss the ongoing controversy concerning screening in younger women and present our views on this issue.

BIASES OF CLINICAL STUDIES

More is known about screening for breast cancer than screening for any other type of cancer. Over the past four decades, various studies have been undertaken to determine the efficacy of mammography screening: case–control studies, retrospective analyses, and prospective studies. There are three biases pertinent to many of these studies: lead-time, length, and selection (1). An understanding of these biases is necessary before discussing the merits of mammography screening. Ultimately, the success of mammography screening should be measured by its ability to reduce mortality, rather than its ability to improve survival.

Survival refers to the period of time from cancer diagnosis to death. Lead-time bias refers to the interval between diagnosis of cancer by screening and usual clinical detection. Lead-time bias may make it appear that screening prolongs survival, when, in fact, it simply extends the period of time over which the disease is observed. As screening advances the time of breast cancer diagnosis, patients with screen-detected cancers will inevitably have better survival rates than those with clinically detected cancers, even if screening does nothing to delay the time of death. Thus, retrospective studies comparing survival between screened and unscreened populations fail to account for lead-time bias, and are flawed.

Length bias relates to the fact that screening tends to detect tumors with a better prognosis. More slowly growing tumors (those with a better prognosis) exist for a longer period in the preclinical phase and are therefore more likely to be diagnosed by mammography screening. In contrast, more rapidly growing tumors exist for a shorter period of time in the preclinical phase, and are more likely to be detected in the intervals between screening sessions. Thus, length bias invalidates comparisons of tumors detected by screening mammography with those detected by physical examination. The impact of length bias is best seen when cancers detected by screening are compared with interval cancers (cancers detected between screening sessions) (8). Interval cancers generally carry a poorer prognosis than screen-detected cancers (9).

Selection bias refers to the fact that women who volunteer for screening are more likely to be health conscious, and have a lower mortality from all causes. In general, women who volunteer for screening are more likely to eat nutritional foods, exercise regularly, and maintain a healthy lifestyle. This is sometimes also referred to as the "healthy-screenee effect." The impact of selection bias was illustrated in a case–control evaluation of the effect of breast cancer screening in the United Kingdom (UK), comparing attendees and non-attendees for screening (10). By comparing populations from two separate districts (one a breast cancer screening district and the other a comparison district), breast cancer mortality was found to be relatively higher among non-attendees in the screening district. This finding was attributed to selection bias.

RANDOMIZED PROSPECTIVE STUDIES

All of these biases can be excluded by comparing screened and unscreened populations in a randomized study with all-cause mortality as the endpoint and cause-specific mortality as a questionable surrogate endpoint. There have been nine randomized prospective trials designed to evaluate the efficacy of mammography screening, and of these eight have evaluated its impact on mortality reduction in women younger than 50: the Health Insurance Plan (HIP); the Swedish Two-County Trial; the Malmo, Stockholm, Gothenburg, and Edinburgh studies; the first Canadian National Breast Screening Study (CNBSS-I); and the UK Age trial (Table 9.1) (11). Only CNBSS-I and the UK Age trial were specifically designed to evaluate mammography screening in women under age 50, while other trials evaluated the impact of screening in women of a broad age range.

The HIP was the first randomized controlled trial of mammography screening for breast cancer, initiated in 1963 (12). The study involved 62,000 women in the age range of 40–64 years from the HIP medical insurance scheme of New York, who were randomly assigned to either a study or a control group of 31,000 women each. However, the HIP was not designed specifically to assess the potential benefits of screening younger women. Among women aged 40–49 at the start of the study, after a median follow-up of 14 years, there was a non-significant reduction in breast cancer mortality in the screened group, the relative risk being 0.78 [95% confidence interval (CI) 0.56–1.08]. It is also important to note that in the HIP study screening was carried out with clinical breast examinations (CBEs) as well as mammography. Ultimately, only 19% of breast cancers in women of all ages were detected exclusively by mammography, and most of them (57%) were detected by CBE alone. Thus the HIP does not necessarily justify mammography screening for any age group. If anything, it suggests that CBE may have an important role to play as a screening modality.

There have been four screening mammography trials undertaken in Sweden: the Stockholm, Gothenburg, and Malmo studies and the Two-County trial (13,14). For women aged 40–49 at entry, these trials have had median follow-ups of 14.3,

12.7, 13.3, and 13 years, respectively. For each of these trials, the relative risk of breast cancer death in the screened group in comparison with the control group was 1.52 (95% CI 0.8–2.88), 0.58 (95% CI 0.35–0.96), 0.73 (95% CI 0.51–1.04), and 0.87 (95% CI 0.54–1.41) respectively. Each of these trials examined the efficacy of mammography screening alone. CBE was not utilized as a screening modality in any of these trials.

The Edinburgh trial was a randomized clinical trial involving 45,130 women between the age of 45 and 64 years, initiated in 1979 (15). Women in the study group received screening mammography and CBE, while the control group received usual care. Of these only 5913 women were at age below 50 years. After a median follow-up of 13 years, the relative risk of breast cancer death among women below age 50 in the screened group was 0.75 (95% CI 0.48–1.18).

CNBSS-I was the first trial specifically designed to assess the efficacy of screening for women between the age of 40 and 49 years (16). The total number of women enrolled in CNBSS-I was 50,430. It was designed with sufficient statistical power to detect at least a 40% reduction in mortality by screening. The screened group received mammography and CBE on an annual basis for four or five examinations, while the control group received an initial CBE upon entry and thereafter a follow-up by mail. After seven years, there was a non-significant excess in mortality in the screened group, the relative risk in the screened group being 1.36 (95% CI 0.84–2.21). However, after a median follow-up of 13 years, the relative risk of breast cancer deaths in the screened group was 0.97 (95% CI 0.74–1.27).

The CNBSS-I received far greater scrutiny than any of the other mammography screening trials, and it has withstood this scrutiny. Its critics charged that in the first 2 years of the study, over 50% of the mammograms were technically inadequate, and that neither the equipment nor the training of the radiologists was properly standardized (17). However, it should seem apparent that in a large study such as this, total standardization would be impractical and that CNBSS-I represented the true technology and skills of the radiologists of the communities at the time the study was undertaken. It is interesting to note that no such criticisms were leveled against the HIP study, which used techniques and standards now considered obsolete. CNBSS-I was also criticized on the grounds that there was contamination of the control group: about 26% of the unscreened population had 'diagnostic' mammograms to evaluate palpable breast masses (18). The critics argue that mammography is not particularly useful as a "diagnostic" procedure so that in a symptomatic woman, the benefit comes from screening the ipsilateral and contralateral breast for clinically occult cancer. Thus some believe that CNBSS-I in fact compared screened women with other screened women, and that this might account for the lack of mortality reduction in the study group. However, it seems unlikely that such mammograms will change significantly the outcome of such a large study. Given the standard practice of medicine in the world today, it would be impossible to run a trial in which women presenting with palpable breast masses were denied mammography, and had to proceed directly with an excisional biopsy. Finally, there have been charges that CNBSS-I may have failed to demonstrate lower rates of breast cancer deaths among women assigned to the mammography arm because the randomization of enrolled

Table 9.1 The Mammography Screening Trials that Included Women Below Age 50

Screening Trial	Age at Entry (yrs)	Screening Modality
Health Insurance Plan	40–64	MM + CBE
Swedish Two-County	40–74	MM
Malmo	45–69	MM
Stockholm	40–64	MM
Gothenburg	40–59	MM
Edinburgh	45–64	MM + CBE
Canadian (CNBSS-I)	40–49	MM + CBE
UK Age trial	39–41	MM

Abbreviations: CBE, clinical breast examination; CNBSS, Canadian National Breast Screening Study; MM, mammography.

women was compromised (19). These concerns were raised because the mammography group in CNBSS-I contained considerably more women with four or more positive axillary nodes than the control group. Independent reviewers were therefore asked to review the randomization strategy in CNBSS-I, and no subversion of the randomization process was ever found (20). The majority of the trials mentioned above were not designed to study the effect of screening in younger women. One of the reasons for the delayed benefit of screening women below age 50 might actually be attributed to screening these women after age 50.

With this background, the more recent age trial was initiated in UK (21). In this trial, 160,921 women aged 39–41 were randomized to an intervention group of annual mammography to age 48 or to a control group of usual medical care. Screening was by two-view mammography at the first screen and by a single mediolateral oblique view thereafter. At mean follow-up of 10.7 years, there was no statistically significant reduction in breast cancer mortality in women offered screening between the ages 40–48 years. The relative risk of all-cause mortality and breast cancer mortality in the intervention group was 0.97 (95% CI 0.89–1.04) and 0.83 (95% CI 0.66–1.04). The trial was designed to have an 80% power to detect a 20% mortality reduction at 10 years' follow-up. However, the power diminished to 60% by the smaller sample size and lower than expected mortality and the non-significant mortality reduction may be a consequence of this low power. The trial has been criticized for using what is considered "non standard" single-view mammography instead of the standard two-view mammograms.

META-ANALYSES

In addition to the results of the individual trials mentioned earlier, several meta-analyses of mammography screening trials have been published. Many of these indicate that, after a long-term follow-up, a statistically significant benefit to screening women under age 50 does indeed emerge. For example, in their meta-analysis of eight trials, Hendrick et al. (22) and Smart et al. (23) have reported a significant decrease in breast cancer mortality in the screened group after 12.7 years of follow-up, the relative risk being 0.82 (95% CI 0.71–0.95). In a meta-analysis of the eight trials, after a median follow-up of about 12 years, Kerlikowske (24) reported that the relative risk of breast cancer deaths in the screened group was 0.84 (95% CI 0.71–0.99). Humphrey et al. (5) excluded the Edinburgh trial (which they considered of poor quality), and found, after 14 years of follow-up, that the relative risk of death for women under 50, in the screened group, was 0.85 (95% CI 0.73–0.99). However, Olsen and Gotzsche (25) have argued that six of the mammography screening trials are flawed or of poor quality. In their meta-analysis, they included only the Canadian and Malmö trials, and found, after 13 years of follow-up, no benefit to screening women below age 50, the relative risk of breast cancer deaths in the screened group being 1.03 (95% CI 0.77–1.38).

The USPSTF updated its meta-analysis in 2009 (26) to include the UK Age trial and concluded that mammography screening reduces breast cancer mortality by 15% for women aged 39–49 years [relative risk 0.85 (95% CI, 0.75–0.96); 8 trials]. This number is similar to women aged 50–59 years where

the relative risk in favor of screening was 0.86 (CI 0.75–0.99). The number needed to invite for screening to prevent one breast cancer death for women younger than 50 years, was 1904 (CI 929–6378) over several screening rounds that varied by trial (2–9 rounds), and 11–20 years of follow-up. This number is 1339 for women aged 50–59 years and 377 for women aged 60–69 years.

Thus, with the exception of the results of Olsen and Gotzsche (25), the various meta-analyses generally suggest that, after a long-term follow-up, a benefit to mammography screening for younger women does eventually emerge. Overviews of the randomized trials suggest that mammography screening reduces breast cancer mortality by about 25% in women over age 50, and that the benefit emerges after seven to nine years of follow-up. In contrast, mammography screening in women below age 50 reduces breast cancer mortality by only 16–18%, and it takes 12–14 years for that benefit to emerge (27).

BIOLOGICAL CONSIDERATIONS

Why should it take longer to see a benefit for women who are below age 50 at the start of mammography screening trials? This question remains open to speculation, but there are several possible explanations. One possibility is that screening may detect very slowly growing (indolent) tumors in younger women, so that a reduction in breast cancer mortality may take longer to emerge. However, Kerlikowske (24) has argued that if this is indeed the case then detecting these slowly growing tumors after age 50 could perhaps produce the same reduction in risk of breast cancer deaths. Yet another possibility is that mammography screening in younger women is less effective. Thus the delayed benefit of screening women below age 50 might actually be attributed to screening these women after 50 years of age. In their study deKonig et al. (28) addressed this possibility with a computer simulation model known as MISCAN (microsimulation screening analysis). Their study suggested that most of the reduction in breast cancer mortality for women who were between the ages of 40 and 49 at the start of the screening trials was in fact the result of screening these women beyond the age of 50.

Another important question is why the efficacy of mammography screening should abruptly change at age 50. Indeed, some investigators have argued that there is no rational basis for such an abrupt change. Yet, age 50 corresponds approximately to the age at menopause, and the epidemiology and biology of breast cancer differ between pre- and postmenopausal women. There are, for example, changes in the incidence of breast cancer that occur in most populations around the time of the menopause: a steep rise in incidence occurs until about age 45–55 years, followed by a less rapid increase thereafter (29). Changes in tumor characteristics are also apparent, with tumors of younger women having a lower proportion of estrogen receptor (ER)-positive tumors and a higher labeling index (30). There are also differences in risk factors between pre- and postmenopausal women. In many studies, obesity is associated with a higher risk of postmenopausal breast cancer but a lower risk of premenopausal cancer (31). Thus the results of mammography screening trials are consistent with the results of other studies showing differences in the epidemiology and biology of pre- and postmenopausal breast cancer.

Finally, one might ask why mammography screening might be less effective in premenopausal women than in postmenopausal women. Again, there are several possible explanations. It is important to remember that the real benefit of screening is not early detection, but rather early treatment. As screening advances the time of breast cancer diagnosis, it allows for the early initiation of therapy. Thus the results from the screening trials may suggest that premenopausal women benefit less from early therapy than do postmenopausal women. Alternatively, the results of the screening trials may also be largely attributable to the fact that the sensitivity of mammography is lower in premenopausal women, making it a less effective screening test in younger women (32).

However, breast cancer is much less common in women below age 50 than it is in women above that age, and Kopans (33) has argued that there are insufficient numbers of women under the age of 50 in the world's screening trials to show an immediate mortality benefit to screening. Thus one might argue that the delayed benefit of mammography screening in younger women is attributable to the fact that breast cancer is much less common in this age group, and it takes longer to accrue sufficient numbers of deaths in the trials to see a statistically significant benefit to screening younger women. In fact, Kopans (33) had estimated that a trial that could prove a 25% mortality reduction at 5 years for women between the age of 40 and 49 years would require about 500,000 women. It would be very difficult to undertake a screening trial involving such a large number of women. The UK Age trial included 160,921 women and a trial with significantly larger numbers is unlikely to be conducted. Proponents of screening for younger women have argued that technology has improved over the years, and that mammography equipment today is better able to detect earlier breast tumors. Thus the trials of the past would not be indicative of what can be achieved using more modern technology (34). This argument is not supported by the results of the Age trial that was conducted in contemporary settings. As technology is constantly improving, it would be impractical to conduct a new trial every time there is an improvement in mammography equipment.

HAZARDS OF SCREENING

If there is no clear evidence as to the point that mammography screening reduces breast cancer mortality in younger women then is it justifiable to continue to recommend screening for these women? It would seem not, because there are at least five harmful effects of mammography screening: cost, lead time, radiation exposure, false positives, and overdiagnosis (Table 9.2).

Cost

In recent years, healthcare costs have increased dramatically, and governments around the world are attempting to reduce those costs. In the light of these constraints, attention has focused on the cost of mammography screening in younger women, particularly as the efficacy of screening in this age group is not clearly established. Kattlove et al. (35) analyzed the expense and benefits of mammography screening in a hypothetical American healthcare organization in which 360 new cases of breast cancer are diagnosed each year. They

Table 9.2 Hazards of Screening Younger Women

Harmful Effect	Consequences
Cost	Increased expenditure on intervention of no proven value
Lead time	Advanced notice of impending death
Radiation exposure	Increased risk of breast cancer in women who carry the gene for ataxia telangiectasia (ATM)
False positives	Unnecessary breast biopsies
Overdiagnosis	Financial/emotional consequences of being falsely labeled as a cancer patient

concluded that the most cost-effective guideline for such a healthcare organization would be to restrict screening to women aged 50–69. Salzmann et al. (36) have argued that screening mammography is relatively cost-ineffective among women aged 40–49 because mammography is less efficacious in women of this age group, and the incidence of breast cancer is lower than in older age groups.

Lead Time

Mammography screening detects breast cancer earlier, but if this is not accompanied by a reduction in breast cancer mortality then the patient is given advanced notice of impending death, with no tangible gain. This has an adverse effect on the quality of life. This "lead time" is probably in the range of two to four years, meaning that many women will suffer needless worry and anxiety during this period (1).

Radiation Exposure

Mammography screening results in exposure to low-dose radiation, and this may actually induce breast cancer. For most of the average-risk women, the risk for death due to breast cancer from the radiation exposure involved in mammography screening is small and is believed to be outweighed by a reduction in breast cancer mortality rates from early detection (37).

Beemsterboer et al. (38) developed a computer simulation model of a mammography screening program to calculate breast cancer deaths induced by exposure to low-dose radiation and the number of lives saved. Their estimates were based on data from the Swedish screening mammography trials and the Netherlands breast cancer screening program. In their model, they assumed a two-year screening interval and a mean glandular dose of 4 mGy to each breast from a two-view mammogram. They calculated that the ratio between the number of breast cancer deaths prevented and those induced as a result of mammography screening for women aged 50–69 is 242:1. When mammography screening is expanded to include screening women aged 40–49 every two years, the ratio becomes 97:1. Thus their model suggests that the potential hazards of low-dose radiation are greatly increased if screening is initiated before age 50. Additionally, Swift et al. (39) have suggested that heterozygous carriers of the gene for ataxia telangiectasia (ATM) are at increased risk for developing breast cancer after exposure to low-dose radiation. About 1.4% of the general population is estimated to constitute heterozygous carriers of the ATM gene mutations, and they may have a six-fold increased risk of developing breast cancer after exposure to low-dose radiation.

False Positives

Elmore et al. (40) have shown that after 10 screening mammograms, a woman has about a 49% cumulative risk of a false-positive result. Furthermore, the risk of false positives is dependent on age. Thus, for women between the age of 40 and 49, the risk is about 56%, while for women aged 50–79, the cumulative risk of a false-positive result after 10 mammograms is about 47%. It the UK Age trial (21), 23% of the regular attendees had at least one false-positive result compared with 12% of women older than 50 years screened regularly as part of the national program (41). False positives are a valid concern as they can have a detrimental effect on quality of life, resulting in unnecessary anxiety (42,43), unnecessary surgery, and additional costs. The impact of false positives on adherence to subsequent screening mammography is variable across studies and populations with some demonstrating a decreased adherence and others showing little effect (37,43). In the United States, where litigation is of paramount concern, the incidence of false positives has historically been higher than in Europe, probably due to the unwillingness of radiologists to commit themselves to a benign diagnosis. Analysis of data from the American Breast Cancer Detection Demonstration Project (BCDDP) suggested that the positive predictive value of mammography screening was only 10%, meaning that nine women had a false-positive result on screening for every cancer found (44). In contrast, European studies during the same time period indicated positive predictive values ranging from 30% to 60% (45). These figures represent the positive predictive value of screening in all age groups. If women below the age of 50 were considered alone, the incidence of false positives would be higher.

Overdiagnosis

Overdiagnosis of breast cancer is a very serious adverse consequence of mammography screening, and one that profoundly affects quality of life. Peeters et al. (46) define overdiagnosis as "a histologically established diagnosis of invasive or intraductal breast cancer that would never have developed into a clinically manifest tumor during the patient's normal life expectancy if no screening examination had been carried out." Following the introduction of mammography screening, there has been an increase in the incidence of breast cancer, particularly a sharp increase in that of ductal carcinoma *in situ* (DCIS) (47). DCIS is almost exclusively detected by screening mammography, and very rarely by palpation. Prior to screening mammography, DCIS accounted for only 1–2% of all breast cancers, but today accounts for 12% of all such cancers and for 30% of those detected by screening.

There is ample evidence to suggest that most DCIS detected by mammography will not progress to invasive cancer during a woman's lifetime. Several years ago, Nielsen et al. (48) reported the results of 110 medicolegal autopsies of women between the ages of 20 and 54 dying of accidents. DCIS was detected in 15%, a prevalence rate four to five times greater than the number of overt cancers expected to develop over 20 years.

Additionally, in autopsies of women diagnosed with breast cancer, Alpers and Wellings (49) have found DCIS in 48% of the contralateral breasts, even though only 12% of all breast cancer patients develop contralateral breast cancer after 20 years of follow-up. And in two separate studies, Rosen et al. (50) and Page et al. (51) have reviewed benign breast biopsies and found several instances where DCIS has been overlooked by the pathologist. Only a small number of these women developed clinically manifest tumors after 15–18 years of follow-up. All of these studies suggest that not all DCIS progress to invasive cancer and most of the increase in the incidence of DCIS may in fact represent overdiagnosis.

However, the consequences of overdiagnosis can be devastating. Women with DCIS are generally classified as cancer patients, and, in the United States may sometimes face denial of life insurance or dramatically increased health insurance costs (52). In addition, they are subjected to treatments that would have been unnecessary if the lesion had not been detected by screening.

The accurate estimation of overdiagnosis in breast cancer is complicated by the need to account for temporal trends in breast cancer incidence independent of screening and lead time. In Norway where the breast cancer screening program was rolled out over 10 years over different counties, a registry study compared incidence of invasive breast cancer (DCIS was excluded) with and without screening in women aged 50–69 years (53). The percentage of overdiagnosis was calculated by accounting for the expected decrease in incidence following cessation of screening after age 69 years. A second approach compared incidence in the current screening group with incidence among women two and five years older in the historical screening groups, accounting for average lead time. The rate of overdiagnosis was estimated to be at 15–25%. For every 2500 women invited to have mammography screening in the age group of 50–69 years, 6–10 cases were overdiagnosed (20 cases were detected but not overdiagnosed).

ADVANCES IN TREATMENT AND IMPACT ON MAMMOGRAPHY SCREENING

It is interesting to note that although the older mammography trials showed some benefit to mammography screening (30% mortality reduction in HIP trial) the more recent trials (CNBSS I and II and the UK Age trial) have shown no statistically significant benefit. Although screening technology has improved over time, the benefit of mammography appears to be decreasing. This is at least partly related to improvements in treatment, and also an increase in breast cancer awareness, resulting in smaller tumors in the control arms of these trials. Adjuvant treatments were widely available to patients in the CNBSS I and II and the UK Age trial, whereas the patients in the older trials were treated with surgery alone. As cancer treatments continue to improve, both the relative and absolute benefit of screening will diminish (54).

CONCLUSION

Since the 1970s, the United States has been the only major industrialized country to encourage mammography screening for women below the age of 50 years. However, age-adjusted breast cancer mortality rates in the United States continue to mirror those of other Western countries, suggesting that screening younger women has had little effect in altering overall population-based mortality trends (55). Thus any long-term mortality benefits of mammography screening in younger women (as suggested by some of the meta-analyses) do not translate into any real benefits in population-based statistics. Although interpretation of evidence is a scientific exercise, the formation of guidelines is largely a social exercise (56). This process is hence subject to individual biases of professional groups and their conflict of interest (57).

In the debate concerning the efficacy of mammography screening for younger women, the potential harm of screening has largely been ignored. The decision to screen women in this age group should be based on personal risk factors and preferences. Women should be helped to make an informed decision in view of not only the benefits but also the potential risks of screening (58). Given the doubts concerning the efficacy of mammography, screening in younger women and the potential for harm as outlined in Table 9.2, we believe that it is inappropriate to screen women under age 50 without first obtaining a proper informed consent (59). Individualized decision making and informed consent should be viewed as the middle ground in the continuing debate over whether or not to screen women under the age of 50.

REFERENCES

1. Jatoi I, Baum M. American and European recommendations for screening mammography in younger women: a cultural divide? BMJ 1993; 307: 1481–3.
2. Wald NJ, Chamberlain J, Hackshaw A; on behalf of the Evaluation Committee. Report of the European society of mastology breast cancer screening evaluation committee. Breast 1993; 2: 209–16.
3. US Preventive Services Task Force. Screening for Breast Cancer: U.S. Preventive Services Task Force Recommendation Statement. Annals of Internal Medicine 2009; 151:716–26; W-236.
4. US Preventive Services Task Force. Guide to Clinical Preventive Services, 2nd edn. Washington, DC: Office of Disease Prevention and Health Promotion, 1996.
5. Humphrey LL, Helfand M, Chan BKS, Woolf SH. Breast cancer screening: a summary of the evidence for the U.S. Preventive Services Task Force. Ann Intern Med 2002; 137: 347–60.
6. Smith RA, Cokkinides V, Brooks D, Saslow D, Brawley OW. Cancer screening in the United States, 2010: a review of current American Cancer Society guidelines and issues in cancer screening. CA Cancer J Clin 2010; 60: 99–119.
7. Malmgren JA, Parikh J, Atwood MK, Kaplan HG. Impact of mammography detection on the course of breast cancer in women aged 40–49 years. Radiology 2012; 262: 797–806.
8. Miller AB. Mammography in women under 50. Hematol Oncol Clin North Am 1994; 8: 165–77.
9. Domingo L, Blanch J, Servitja S, et al. Aggressiveness features and outcomes of true interval cancers: comparison between screen-detected and symptom-detected cancers. Eur J Cancer Prev 2012; Epub ahead of print.
10. Moss SM, Summerley ME, Thomas BJ, et al. A case–control evaluation of the effect of breast cancer screening in the United Kingdom trial of early detection of breast cancer. J Epidemiol Comm Health 1992; 46: 362–4.
11. Jatoi I. Breast cancer screening. Am J Surg 1999; 177: 518–24.
12. Shapiro S. Periodic screening for breast cancer: the HIP randomized controlled trial. Health Insurance Plan. J Natl Cancer Inst Monogr 1997; 22: 27–30.
13. Nystrom L, Anderson I, Bjurstam N, et al. Long-term effects of mammography screening: updated overview of the Swedish randomized trials. Lancet 2002; 359: 909–19.
14. Tabar L, Vitak B, Chen HH, et al. The Swedish Two-County Trial twenty years later: updated mortality results and new insights from long-term follow-up. Radiol Clin North Am 2000; 38: 625–51.
15. Alexander FE, Anderson TJ, Brown HK, et al. 14 years of follow-up from the Edinburgh randomized trial of breast cancer screening. Lancet 1999; 353: 1903–8.

16. Miller AB, To T, Baines CJ, Wall C. The Canadian National Breast Screening Study-I, breast cancer mortality after 11–16 years of follow-up in women age 40–49. Ann Intern Med 2002; 137: 305–12.
17. Kopans DB. Canadian study of breast screening under 50. Lancet 1992; 339: 1473–4.
18. Kopans DB. Screening for breast cancer and mortality reduction among women 40–49 years of age. Cancer 1994; 74: 311–22.
19. Tarone RE. The excess of patients with advanced breast cancer in young women screened with mammography in the Canadian National Breast Screening Study. Cancer 1995; 75: 997–1003.
20. Bailar JC, MacMahon B, Randomization in the Canadian National Breast Screening Study: a review for evidence of subversion. CMAJ 1997; 156: 193–9.
21. Moss SM, Cuckle H, Evans A, et al. Effect of mammographic screening from age 40 years on breast cancer mortality at 10 years' follow-up: a randomised controlled trial. Lancet 2006; 368: 2053–60.
22. Hendrick RE, Smith RA, Rutledge JH 3rd, Smart CR. Benefit of screening mammography in women aged 40–49: a new meta-analysis of randomized controlled trials. J Natl Cancer Inst Monogr 1997; 22: 87–92.
23. Smart CR, Hendrick RE, Rutledge JH 3rd, Smith RA. Benefit of mammography screening in women ages 40 to 49 years: current evidence from randomized controlled trials. Cancer 1995; 75: 1619–26.
24. Kerlikowske K. Efficacy of screening mammography among women aged 40 to 49 years and 50 to 69 years: comparison of relative and absolute benefit. J Natl Cancer Inst Monogr 1997; 22: 79–86.
25. Olsen O, Gotzsche PC. Cochrane review on screening for breast cancer with mammography. Lancet 2001; 358: 1340–2.
26. Nelson HD, Tyne K, Naik A, et al. Screening for breast cancer: an update for the US Preventive Services Task Force. Ann Intern Med 2009; 151: 727.
27. Kerlikowske K, Grady D, Rubin SM, et al. Efficacy of screening mammography. A meta-analysis. JAMA 1995; 273: 149–54.
28. deKoning HJ, Boer R, Warmerdam PG, et al. Quantitative interpretations of age-specific mortality reductions from the Swedish breast cancer screening trials. J Natl Cancer Inst 1995; 87: 1217–23.
29. Clemmensen J. Carcinoma of the breast. Results from statistical research. Br J Radiol 1948; 21: 583.
30. Henderson IC. Biologic variations of tumors. Cancer 1992; 69: 1888–95.
31. Willett W. Nutritional Epidemiology. New York: Oxford University Press, 1990.
32. Buist DSM, Porter PL, Lehman C, Taplin SH, White E. Factors contributing to mammography failure in women aged 40–49 years. J Natl Cancer Inst 2004; 96: 1432–40.
33. Kopans DB. Screening for breast cancer and mortality reduction among women 40–49 years of age. Cancer 1994; 74: 311–22.
34. Sickles EA, Kopans DB. Deficiencies in the analysis of breast cancer screening data. J Natl Cancer Inst 1993; 85: 1621–4.
35. Kattlove H, Liberati A, Keeler E, Brook RH. Benefits and costs of screening and treatment for early breast cancer. Development of a basic benefit package. JAMA 1995; 273: 142–8.
36. Salzmann P, Kerlikowske K, Phillips K. Cost-effectiveness of extending screening mammography guidelines to include women 40 to 49 years of age. Ann Intern Med 1997; 127: 955–65.
37. Armstrong K, Moye E, Williams S, et al. Screening mammography in women 40 to 49 years of age: a systematic review for the American College of Physicians. Ann Intern Med 2007; 146: 516–26.
38. Beemsterboer PM, Warmerdam PG, Boer R, de Koning HJ. Radiation risk of mammography related to benefit in screening programmes: a favourable balance? J Med Screen 1998; 5: 81–7.
39. Swift M, Morrell D, Massey RB, Chase CL. Incidence of cancer in 161 families affected by ataxia-telangiectasia. N Engl J Med 1991; 325: 1831–6.
40. Elmore JG, Barton MB, Moceri VM, et al. Ten-year risk of false positive screening mammograms and clinical breast examinations. N Engl J Med 1998; 338: 1089–96.
41. Advisory Committee on Breast Cancer Screening. Screening for Breast Cancer in England: Past and Future. NHSBSP Publication no.61. Sheffield, UK: NHS Cancer Screening Programmes, 2006.
42. Jatoi I, Zhu K, Shah M, Lawrence W. Psychological distress in U.S. women who have experienced false-positive mammograms. Breast Cancer Res Treat 2006; 100: 191–200.
43. Brewer NT, Salz T, Lillie SE. Systematic review: the long-term effects of false-positive mammograms. Ann Intern Med 2007; 146: 502–10.

44. Baker LH. Breast cancer detection demonstration project: 5–year summary report. CA Cancer J Clin 1982; 42: 1–35.

45. Reidy J, Hoskins O. Controversy over mammography screening. BMJ 1988; 297: 932.

46. Peeters PHM, Verbeek ALM, Straatman H, et al. Evaluation of overdiagnosis of breast cancer in screening with mammography: results of the Nijmegen programme. Int J Epidemiol 1989; 18: 295–9.

47. Ernster VL, Barclay J, Kerlikowske K, et al. Incidence of and treatment for ductal carcinoma in situ of the breast. JAMA 1996; 275: 913–18.

48. Nielsen M, Thomsen JL, Primdahl S, et al. Breast cancer and atypia among young and middle aged women: a study of 110 medicolegal autopsies. Br J Cancer 1987; 56: 814–19.

49. Alpers CE, Wellings SR. The prevalence of carcinoma in situ in normal and cancer-associated breasts. Hum Pathol 1985; 16: 796–807.

50. Rosen PR, Braum DW Jr, Kinne DE. The clinical significance of pre-invasive breast carcinoma. Cancer 1980; 46: 919–25.

51. Page DL, Dupont WD, Rogers LW, Landenberger M. Intraductal carcinoma of the breast: followup after biopsy only. Cancer 1982; 49: 751–8.

52. Jatoi I, Baum M. Mammographically detected ductal carcinoma in situ: Are we over diagnosing breast cancer? Surgery 1995; 118: 118–20.

53. Kalager M, Adami H-O, Bretthauer M, Tamimi RM. Overdiagnosis of invasive breast cancer due to mammography screening: results from the Norwegian screening program. Ann Intern Med 2012; 156: 491–9.

54. Jatoi I. The impact of advances in treatment on the efficacy of mammography screening. Prev Med 2011; 53: 103–4.

55. Jatoi I, Miller AB. Why is breast cancer mortality declining? Lancet Oncol 2003; 4: 251–4.

56. Quanstrum K, Hayward RA. Lessons from the mammography wars. N Engl J Med 2009; 363: 1076–9.

57. Norris SL, Burda BU, Holmer HK, et al. Author's specialty and conflicts of interest contribute to conflicting guidelines for screening mammography. J Clin Epidemiol 2012; 65: 725–33.

58. Mathieu E, Barratt AL, McGeechan K, et al. Helping women make choices about mammography screening: an online randomized trial of a decision aid for 40-year-old women. Patient Educ Couns 2010; 81: 63–72.

59. Baum M. Commentary: false premises, false promises and false positives – the case against mammographic screening for breast cancer. Int J Epidemiol 2004; 33: 66–7.

10 Mammographic screening in women aged 50 years and above

Chris I. Flowers

INTRODUCTION

The goal of mammographic screening is to detect a cancer before it has the potential to spread. For most breast cancers, smaller tumors are less likely to have local, regional, or systemic metastases at diagnosis than larger lesions. Detecting a cancer when it is small and at an early stage usually means that less aggressive or extensive surgery is possible and there is less likelihood of systemic treatment with chemotherapy.

Mammographic screening for breast cancer is widely accepted as one of the most investigated and validated screening tests, with long-term data now available from service screening throughout Europe. It is often used as an exemplar for other types of cancer screening. Nonetheless, it is also the subject of much controversy and debate, especially with respect to the magnitude of effect upon mortality outcomes for breast cancer along with the potential harms of overdiagnosis.

In most countries, the belief is held that breast screening with mammography carries more benefits than harms thus leading to establishment of National Screening Programs across Europe and promotion of screening in the United States (US) where women are strongly encouraged to have an annual "checkup." Canada also has its own organized screening program but this is based on individual provinces and territories.

This chapter compares and contrasts how breast screening of women above 50 years of age is performed in Europe and North America and considers what lessons may be learned from both sides of the Atlantic.

The debate about breast screening has largely moved on from whether breast screening works (the degree of efficacy being the subject of debate) to one of concern about overdiagnosis and false-positive screening examinations. There have been several overviews of screening trials to which the reader is referred. This chapter focuses on how some of the limitations of mammography screening might be addressed and potential ways for improving screening using newer technologies.

PRINCIPLES OF SCREENING

1. **The cancer needs to be common**
   Breast cancer is the second commonest cancer in women (after lung cancer) Surveillance, Epidemiology and End Results (SEER) data.

2. **Early detection and treatment should improve the eventual outcome of the person being screened**
   Screening advances the stage of breast cancer diagnosis. Most authorities agree that treating breast cancer early before metastasis occurs produces a better outcome for the patient.

3. **Existence of a known precursor lesion or a long preclinical course**
   There are several problems with breast cancer screening, not least of which is the lack of a proven precursor lesion, unlike in colon cancer with the adenoma-carcinoma sequence. In general, noninvasive cancers (*in situ*) disease can potentially progress to invasive cancer. Thus, low-grade ductal carcinoma *in situ* (DCIS) may progress to a low-grade invasive cancer and similarly high grade. However, the data supporting these suppositions are partly based on observational studies of patients who refused treatment for DCIS and were subsequently followed up (1). Indeed, this hypothesis has not been corroborated with more recent studies (2). There is much debate about DCIS in particular, but it is clear that the majority of lesions do not progress to an invasive cancer and the chance of this varies between low and high grades of DCIS (on an average 28%, according to Page (3)). As a result, if all DCIS is lumped together and treated aggressively by surgical excision, then the issue of overtreatment may arise for this pathological group of lesions.

There is a similar group of lesions collectively called lobular neoplasia (4,5), which are considered to be a type of *in situ* disease but are most likely a risk factor for cancer rather than a precursor lesion. Frequently found on core biopsy for investigation of benign calcifications, they are managed currently by initial surgical excision due to concerns about potential undersampling and the risk of an adjacent cancer being missed by initial needle biopsy. However, this is a controversial and developing area and further study of lobular neoplasia needs to be done.

DOES MAMMOGRAPHIC SCREENING WORK FOR ALL WOMEN?

Breast cancer is a heterogeneous disease. Histological tumor grading is based on a combination of factors and a scoring system (e.g., Nottingham modification of the Scarff–Bloom–Richardson grading scheme (6)), which may be subject to reader variation, much like reading a mammogram. Also, the population of estrogen receptor (ER) and progesterone receptor-positive cells within a tumor is measured by a count per field. The ER score is considered positive if there are about 10% of cells staining for ER. The Allred score is used to stratify the positivity of the specimen. Cellular variation within tumors potentially explains some puzzling issues such as why a small grade 1 tumor can metastasize and yet some larger grade 3 tumors do not. Moreover, some slow-growing tumors have been identified using gene arrays which may never become lethal during a patient's lifetime (7). This issue is important in the elderly where comorbidities are more likely to have an effect on mortality than a newly diagnosed breast cancer. This is one of the reasons why many countries cease any recommendation for annual mammography after the age of 70–75 years.

The timing of a screening intervention determines whether a particular patient will benefit from a screening test. Furthermore, the type of a tumor will influence whether it is amenable to early detection by routine screening and therefore whether screening is beneficial.

Screening samples a proportion of the population at a certain point in time. The interval between sampling affects the mix of tumor types detected. If screening is carried out after a long-enough interval, then most of the cancers will present as so-called interval cancers (between screening rounds), leaving slower growing tumors to be picked up by screening.

Ideally, a screening test should detect cancer while it is still localized to the organ of origin before it spreads regionally or systemically. In general, tumors are present and actively growing while not being visible on mammograms for a long preclinical detectable phase, otherwise known as the sojourn time (8,9). Some tumors have a long sojourn time and the patient may die from another cause before it has become visible and been detected radiologically (the fourth curve). Conversely, a rapidly growing tumor may have a short sojourn time and grow so rapidly that the screening test cannot "catch" the cancer before it has spread (the first curve). It follows that this latter type of tumor will never benefit from screening unless there is a very short screening interval.

Tumors that follow a pattern similar to the second and third curves are the ones most likely to benefit from screening mammography. With a three-year screening interval, a cancer following the growth pattern shown in curve 2 will have spread regionally before it has been detected. If the screening interval is shorter (say two years), the ratio of moderate growth tumors will increase and the outcome will be more beneficial.

The more frequently screening is undertaken, the more likely is the chance of "catching" a cancer in the detectable range before it starts to spread. If screening is too frequent, apart from any increase in false-positive examinations and the associated deployment costs there is the issue of detecting the change. There needs to be significant-enough change between two separate images to detect that something is growing and therefore likely to be suspicious.

Both cancer detection and recall rates depend on whether it is the first screening round or a subsequent screening round though this is not always true in practice according to Wallis (10). The *prevalent* round of a screening program is the first sampling of the screened population and essentially picks up all visible cancers at that time and therefore this tends to be an enriched population at screening. Subsequent rounds are termed *incident* screens and represent cancers that have occurred since the last screening examination. These serial incident screening rounds are important, as reductions in breast cancer mortality which are evident from screening trials require that mammographic screening be routinely repeated over a sustained period of time (11).

TRADE-OFF BETWEEN SENSITIVITY AND SPECIFICITY

A perfect screening tool will have 100% sensitivity and never miss a cancer, while 100% specificity will permit only cancers to be treated and nothing else. However, in achieving a high sensitivity there is a trade-off with lower specificity. Mammography has a reported sensitivity rate of between 80 and 89%, but also has a relatively high specificity. There are variations in the diagnostic accuracy of mammography with differences in sensitivity according to changes in breast density and age group (12).

THE HISTORY OF MAMMOGRAPHIC SCREENING: EARLY TRIALS

Critical appraisal of various mammographic screening trials has been thoroughly reviewed by several authors; therefore this chapter only sums up those trials which were responsible for the introduction of breast screening in Europe. These inform and help understand why mammographic screening services were structured in the way they are.

The introduction of mammographic screening in the United Kingdom (UK) was largely predicated on a small number of trials which showed significant potential for mortality reduction by the use of mammography. The rationale for providing a national screening program was contained in the 1986 Forrest Report, which reported to the UK government (13). There was relatively little data originally available at the time, including the Health Insurance Plan study (14) plus early results of the Swedish (15) and Edinburgh (16) studies with publication of the latter following the Forrest report.

The first breast screening randomized controlled trial (RCT) from the Health Insurance Plan of New York was started in 1963 by Shapiro and colleagues (14). This recruited 62,000 women aged 40–64 years inviting them to a special clinic where they had a physical examination and bilateral mammograms. They were invited annually for three years when the trial stopped. The uptake was approximately 65% in the first round but eventually dropped off to 45% in the third round. Analysis of the data showed a reduction in breast cancer mortality after five years which was maximal in the above-50 age group. At 18 years, the published data showed a relative risk reduction of 0.80 in the above-50 age group (95% CI 0.59–1.08).

In the late 1970s, the Swedish Two-County trial started and was a mammogram-only trial of a single mediolateral oblique (MLO) examination with no physical examination on women aged 40–74 years. The nine-year follow-up which was used in the Forrest Report showed that there was a significant effect on mortality with reduction concentrated in those women aged above 50 years. The Edinburgh trial started in 1979 with a cohort of 45,000 women being randomized to either a control or intervention group. The intervention group had both mammography and physical examination. The data showed only a small benefit for the screened group with a lower relative risk of death from breast cancer.

Many countries have published data from their own screening programs, including Norway, Denmark, and Canada among others. The largest of these trials (The Swedish two-county trial) has regularly produced results over many years with data published on outcomes for up to 27 years of follow-up and has become the gold standard RCT used for evaluation of screening (17).

BEYOND RCTs: THE DEVELOPMENT OF "SERVICE SCREENING" IN EUROPE

The UK rolled out its screening program over a period of years from the late 1980s, until complete geographical coverage was achieved in the mid-1990s with invitations being sent to women every three years for a screening appointment. Early concerns about compliance were largely dispelled as the uptake was standardized at around 70%, and eventually was closer to 75%. Localized iterations of screening were introduced in both Scotland and Wales following publication of their own reports in 1993 and 1990 respectively, but Northern Ireland had introduced screening in 1989 (shortly after England).

Although the standard age for screening invitation in the UK was set at 50–64 years, the UK government extended the program up to 70 years of age in 2007 and later following a pilot study, extended the program further; there is now a standardized upper age limit of 73 years and the program has been extended to some younger women under age 50 years (47 years) starting in 2012. The Netherlands introduced their national screening program in a manner similar to the UK, but chose to screen every two years and provided the "nationalized" service in a decentralized manner using mobile screening vans. In the Netherlands model, the reading, assessment, and treatment of screen-detected abnormalities is dealt with at a local hospital or at a regional level.

Other European countries have also developed their own screening programs with assistance from the European Union (EU). Each country's program is managed differently but they all follow common European Guidelines which were originally formulated by Kirkpatrick in 1993. These were developed from the National Health Service Breast Screening Programme (NHSBSP) guidelines, covered diagnosis through cancer surgery, and provided the framework for organization of breast screening services throughout Europe (18). According to the EU Report in 2007, 59 million women were within the target age of 50–69 years as specified in the Council Recommendation and 47% of these women could be screened by the 11 member states which have used a population-based approach to breast cancer screening. By contrast, non-population-based screening was continuing to be practiced in five other member states. A 70% screening uptake was calculated as the required standard to give an expected benefit of a 30% mortality reduction. A screening interval of two years was harmonized across the EU with the notable exception of the UK and Malta who opted for a three-yearly screening interval.

The drivers of mammographic screening in Europe were primarily programs from the UK, Sweden, and the Netherlands but arguably some of the most important developments came from the practice of screening in the UK. These included the national quality assurance (QA) and multidisciplinary teams. Although not unique to the UK, QA was developed in such a way that there were national coordinating committees for each branch of the multidisciplinary service. This set new standards for improving the quality of screening with a minimum baseline standard and also to apply new targets to aim for. These guidelines fostered a mentality of striving for continuous improvement in standards of screening.

QA AND THE RIPPLE EFFECT PRODUCING DEVELOPMENTS IN THE SYMPTOMATIC SERVICES

QA Guidelines for Breast Cancer Screening were produced for individual disciplinary groups, and these were documented and published by the NHSBSP screening office, where the latest versions are available online. In addition, each region in the UK has its own QA reference centre (QARC), with a director who is responsible to the Regional Director of Public Health. The performance of breast screening programs is carefully monitored against NHSBSP standards, and regular reports are produced. Eighteen big committees (representing the 18 regions of the UK) were set up around the subspecialties, which allowed each specialty to ensure compliance with UK standards and targets.

MULTIDISCIPLINARY TEAM WORKING

In the UK, the development of specialized surgical, radiology, and pathology teams for screening led to extension of expertise to symptomatic women attending hospital services, who up till then were mainly being seen by general surgeons, where the standard of care was typically "lumpectomy with frozen section query proceed to mastectomy." The Association of Breast Surgeons (ABS) at the British Association of Surgical Oncology (BASO) produced guidelines on running a symptomatic breast clinic, which was then followed by the BASO surgical guidelines, published as a supplement to the European Journal of Surgical Oncology. The ABS at BASO was instrumental in the monumental changes in providing symptomatic breast services in the UK, which now closely mirror the service given to screened patients. BASO produces an annual report with QA data on symptomatic clinics (19).

TECHNICAL IMPROVEMENTS IN SCREENING

Over successive years, there have been major developments and step-wise improvements in the quality of mammography with the introduction of optimal optical density for mammography film, high-contrast film/screens and processing with the eventual transition to digital with computed radiography and then full-field digital mammography.

One of the most important quality improvements in UK screening was the change in funding to allow for two-view mammography for all screening examinations. Till then, many centers had only two-view mammography available for the prevalent round (initial) screen, before reverting to a single MLO view for incident (subsequent) round screens. Approximately 25% more cancers were identified using two view mammography compared with a single MLO view which was the earlier practice. This change occurred during a time when there was pressure to extend the program from 64 to 70, and the move to two-view mammography was considered mandatory before any expansion of the program.

The UK decided to extend the screening program both upward to 73 years and downward to 47 years with implementation starting in 2012. A recent update (20) to the NHSBSP Quality Assurance Guidelines for Breast Cancer Screening Radiology has stated that the current "achievable" standards (previously termed targets) are only applicable to women aged between 50 and 70 at the time of their screening invitation. New and adjusted standards may be required for women outside of this age range. Despite apparently having increased manpower to extend the program, the UK still lags behind the European standard of two-yearly mammograms (Table 10.1). There is no indication that the UK will move to two-yearly screening due to the additional costs and workforce required. Moreover, the additional benefits to screened women may be insufficient compared with the costs of implementation to justify a shortened screening interval.

SKILL MIX
There have been several challenges to expanding the screening program relating to both personnel and equipment. This has been resolved mainly by the training and tiered advanced practice structure of the College of Radiographers and also by employing breast clinicians. The latter employ a mix of skills and can function as part of the surgical or radiological team, thereby increasing the breadth of professionals involved in breast care in the UK. The Department of Health has labeled this as skill mix (21). The development of a diploma for radiographers, who undergo training as part of the advanced practice infrastructure has assisted this move with the emergence of advanced practitioners who primarily assist with film reading and stereotactic biopsy and consultant radiographers.

At the same time, the College of Radiographers introduced a fourth tier with a new role of assistant practitioners. This allowed the profession to increase both numbers and influence and facilitated the move to digital mammography with its attendant increased rate of detection of microcalcifications. A report in 2010 (22) to the Society and College of Radiographers showed that consultant radiographers have had a significant impact on throughput in those sites where they were employed and this new grade permitted radiologists to use their time more effectively.

A COMPARISON WITH NORTH AMERICA
In North America, there are both similarities with and differences to the European approach. The approach in the US is totally different to that of Canada which has always closely followed the UK healthcare system. The Canadian organization that has provided the lead is known as Health Canada which unites the various provinces and territories to provide a nationwide service. The Canadian government established a working group in 1995 which produced their first "Quality Determinants of Organized Breast Cancer Screening Programs'" report in 1998 and emphasized a client-based and team approach to the service. Canada also chose to initially target the 50–69 year age range and recognized that success and effectiveness of a population screening program is dependent on obtaining high participation rates. As a result, they recommended that screening women aged below 50 and above 70 should only take place if the target population was achieving an uptake of 70%. An important quality measure emphasized by Health Canada was that programs had a responsibility to ensure equitable access for all women in the target age group and some funding was allocated to assist with recruitment of women for screening thereby helping to ensure that targets were met.

Canada sends out letters of invitation to schedule a screening mammogram, but this does not include an appointment date and time in contrast to the UK. Health Canada has expressed a desire to match the UK program with scheduled appointment times, as this intervention has been shown to improve compliance (23,24).

The goals of both Canadian and European screening programs include giving patients full information about the

Table 10.1 A Comparison of Screening Policies Across North America and Europe

Country	Starting Age	Ending Age	Frequency	Uptake
US	40 (ACS, ACR, ACOG) 50 (USPSTF) 50 (shared decision making 40–50)	No upper limit given 74 (USPSTF)	Q1 yr Q2 yr (USPSTF)	n/a
Canada	50	69	Q2 yr	15–54%[a] (historic data)
UK	47 (from 2012)	73 (from 2012)	Q3 yrs	75 %
Sweden	40	74	<50 18 months >50 Q2 yr	81 %
Netherlands	50	75	Q2 yr	78 %
France	50	74	Q2 yr	70 %
Spain	50	70	Q2 yr	70 %
Germany	50	69	Q2 yr	70 %
Austria	50	69	Q2 yr	70 %

[a]Data from Health Canada. *Organized Breast Cancer Screening Programs in Canada 1997 and 1998 Report.* Ottawa: Minister of Public Works and Government Services Canada, 2001.
Abbreviations: ACOG, The American College of Obstetricians and Gynecologists; ACS, The American Cancer Society; ACR, The American College of Radiology; USPSTF, US Preventive Services Task Force.

risks and benefits of screening together with the following factors:

- Quality of mammography
- Reporting
- Communicating results
- Follow-up and diagnostic workup
- Program evaluation

These programs are in stark contrast to the US program, where the majority of women either have to remember to schedule a screening mammogram or are to be encouraged to undergo a screening mammogram when they attend for an annual checkup with a primary care doctor or gynecologist. Provision for mammographic screening is mainly the responsibility of local hospitals, doctors' offices, or imaging centers offering mammography. There is no regional or statewide service apart from those for the underserved, such as local programs funded through the National Breast and Cervical Cancer Early Detection Program which have provided free or low-cost mammograms for more than 20 years (25). The majority of mammographic screening in the US tends to be undertaken on those with medical insurance (employer-based insurance plans are being downgraded or abolished with the economic downturn) with smaller numbers receiving screening via Medicare or State-funded initiatives.

When a patient is given an abnormal screening result, she is notified along with her primary care doctor and the onus is upon the woman to schedule her workup. Unlike the UK screening program, there is no call and recall system, and therefore it is potentially easier for patients to slip through the cracks and fail to be diagnosed in a timely manner. The Mammographic Quality Standards Act mandates that radiologists follow up women who have been assessed as "BIRADS 0: further workup is required." However, after writing to the physician to ascertain whether a woman has been worked up elsewhere, there is no specific follow-up. The lack of central coordination or even oversight at city or state level illustrates how this type of screening is vastly different from what is practiced in Europe.

There is no national breast cancer database in the US which is once again in contrast with the UK, for example. There is a National Mammography Database that has recently been set up by the American College of Radiology as part of the National Radiology Data Registry. However, participation in this scheme is voluntary and it aims to leverage data that radiology practices are already collecting and provide them with comparative information for national and regional benchmarking (such as true positive rates, positive predictive values, and recall rates). There is no mechanism in place to collect all the data captured in the National Breast Screening System. It is not just the issue of radiology; most pathologists in the US still use narrative reporting and as a result there is no state or national database which documents types of tumor or biomarker expression profiles. Other problems relate to independence of the cancer registries which precludes benefits of sharing knowledge about breast cancers at a national level which has contributed much to knowledge of the disease as witnessed in the UK. There is a North American Association of Central Cancer Registries (which includes Canada and the US) which works to promote uniform data standards across the various registries within each country. However, this is restricted to incidence and mortality data.

The nearest the US gets to the European style of a comprehensive data set is provided by the Breast Cancer Surveillance Consortium (BCSC) (26) which is a composite database comprising seven designated cancer registries in the US:

- Carolina Mammography Registry
- San Francisco Mammography Registry
- Vermont Breast Cancer Surveillance System
- New Hampshire Mammography Network
- Colorado Mammography Project
- New Mexico Mammography Project
- Group Health in Washington State

This consortium has been highly influential and provided longitudinal data that have spawned multiple publications over the last 10–15 years. For example, there were 33 collaborative papers using BCSC data in 2011 which included subjects such as "changes in invasive breast cancer and DCIS rates in relation to the decline in hormone therapy use."

For breast teams practicing in the US, apart from institutional databases, there is a general lack of data on the work actually undertaken, including patient outcomes. Nonetheless, women who are screened and subsequently diagnosed with breast cancer tend to get the best treatment available, without the vagaries of "postcode prescribing" which characterizes some aspects of cancer drug provision in the UK. However, there has been a review of healthcare policy in the US due to the need for cost savings and cuts in reimbursement made by both insurance companies and proposed cuts by the Centers for Medicare and Medicare Services. This may ultimately reduce the number of physicians who care for Medicare patients as costs will be more aligned with income received. Attempts to reform Medicare seem doomed and have proved difficult to implement due to opposing political influences. With a higher incidence of cancer in an aging population, cancer treatment costs continue to rise. This trend will be apparent on both sides of the Atlantic and is likely to be a persistent challenge for years to come.

US CANCER SCREENING GUIDELINES

The American Cancer Society, the American College of Radiology, and the American College of Obstetricians and Gynecologists recommend annual screening for average-risk women, starting at age 40 years. The US Preventive Services Task Force guidelines which are followed mainly by family physicians in the US were changed in November 2009 amid much controversy. These limited routine screenings were more in line with European models and recommended biennial mammograms between 50 and 74 years of age. Both younger and older women were advised to discuss personal risk with their physician prior to being screened.

OVERDIAGNOSIS AND FALSE POSITIVES FROM SCREENING

It is well documented that the US has a recall rate between two and five times higher than most European countries (27–29). This has been attributed mainly to medicolegal concerns but some consider that this could be due to differences in reading procedures; single reading with or without computer-aided diagnosis is commonly used in the US while independent

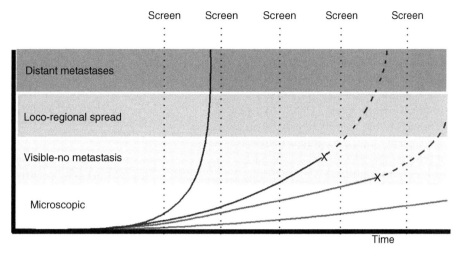

Figure 10.1 Representation of a tumor lifecycle from the microscopic phase to metastasis, superimposed with timelines of sampling with screening.

double-reading with consensus or arbitration is preferred in Europe (30). This higher false-positive rate triggered concerns about the potential for overdiagnosis which has come to the fore in recent debate about the effectiveness of mammographic screening.

The issues of overdiagnosis and false-positive examinations tend to be linked together in any discussion about potential "harms of screening." The latter are a mixture of concerns about patient anxiety, pain, and discomfort associated with mammography, false-positive recall, benign biopsies, borderline histopathological lesions, and the possibility of overtreatment of a lesion that may never progress to a lethal cancer. Several authors have included low-grade DCIS in this discussion, in a manner analogous to low-grade tumors in prostate cancer (31) (Figure 10.1).

Anxiety is an inevitable aspect of a screening test for most individuals but this usually subsides shortly after a negative result is obtained (within several months). However, the effect can last for a longer period in those women recalled with an abnormal screening mammogram. Indeed, 18 months after a screening mammogram, those women with false-positive results have greater anxiety about breast cancer than women with negative screening mammograms (32). In retrospect, most women with false-positive results regard this as one of several minor stressful experiences in their lives. They generally attend for further screening and report similar quality-of-life scores 18 months later as women with negative screening results. Therefore, from an anxiety point of view a false-positive screening examination is a minor harm and does not constitute a significant problem for most women. An example of a strategy used in the UK to reduce anxiety is to minimize the time between receipt of an "abnormal mammogram report" and the diagnostic workup (33). A short turn-around time significantly reduces the impact of anxiety following a call back from screening.

OVERTREATMENT

Following a diagnostic workup and biopsy, some women may go on to have surgery for a non-life-threatening condition. This includes a range of treatments from surgical excision biopsy for suspicious core biopsy findings of atypical ductal hyperplasia, radial scar, or lobular neoplasia to definitive surgical treatment of low-grade DCIS. For those women who have

had surgery, up to one-third may suffer from pain or reduced sensitivity of the breast (34) and a concern which should stimulate trials to determine whether continued surgical excision of these lesions is necessary. It may be possible to identify some types which can be followed with *active surveillance*, such as occurs for some types of prostate cancer. The National Comprehensive Cancer Network's practice guidelines for prostate cancer (35) recommend the use of active surveillance as the sole initial treatment—not just an option—for many men with prostate cancer. The same approach may be appropriate for some borderline lesions of the breast.

Nowadays, DCIS is almost always detected during mammographic screening, rather than as a symptomatic presentation such as Paget's disease of the nipple or a palpable mass. In the UK, screening data have revealed that most of the cases of DCIS detected are of high grade (36), which is also the case in Australia (37). By contrast, in the US, it is much more common to detect low-grade DCIS (38) thereby providing a greater opportunity for overdiagnosis and treatment. However, DCIS is a spectrum of noninvasive disease and therapy remains a controversial topic. Depending on the disease extent, there is a range of treatment options from breast conservation to mastectomy, with the possibility of adjuvant radiation treatment when the breast is conserved (39). As a result, it is possible to have a mastectomy for what otherwise may represent indolent disease.

DEVELOPMENTS THAT MAY REDUCE FALSE-POSITIVE EXAMINATIONS

Apart from the switchover analog to digital mammography over the last decade, there have been few developments which have improved the accuracy of screening mammography and thus reduced the recall rate for false-positive examinations in the US and Europe. The most recent development is the use of tomosynthesis (a type of three-dimensional examination of the breast) which has been approved by the Food and Drug Administration (FDA letter, February 2011). Although the technique has yet to find a place in routine screening and diagnostic workup, there is much potential based on early work with this technology. Poplack reported in 2007 reduced rates of call back from the use of tomosynthesis (40). There are also unpublished reports of significantly improved cancer detection rates using this technique (based on the so-called Reader Study 2). If more cancers can be detected and there are fewer unnecessary call-backs due to superimposition of normal tissue, then some of the harms of false-positive recall will be ameliorated. The downside with current techniques of tomosynthesis is the radiation dose, which can be 1.6–3 times higher than for a conventional mammogram. This is partly due to insistence from the FDA that tomosynthesis be an adjunct, rather than a replacement, to mammography thereby mandating that a regular mammogram be undertaken as part of the examination. This is currently automated on the same system so that a patient is unaware of any additional imaging.

Other developments include the use of two different x-ray energies (Dual Energy Mammography) and contrast injection. This is facilitating development of new tools such as spectral imaging, which may help characterize the breast tissue more accurately and lead to detection of more breast cancers by separating glandular tissue, fat, and calcifications. The procedure known as contrast-enhanced spectral mammography has been approved by the FDA and is now available from vendors.

CONCLUSION

Despite the continuing controversy, mammographic screening remains the gold standard for breast cancer screening, though overall efficacy is open to debate. The screening interval used by most countries is biennial, with notable outliers being the UK (triennial) and the US (annual). Future innovations in technology may improve diagnostic accuracy by eliminating some false-positive examinations. Further significant developments in the field of breast cancer screening may result from controlled trials evaluating management of less aggressive disease by the use of active surveillance, as pioneered for prostate screening.

ACKNOWLEDGEMENTS

The author is thankful to Nick Perry, St Barts Breast Care Centre, London UK and Chris de Wolf, Fribourg Breast Cancer Screening Centre, Switzerland for their assistance with European Screening information.

REFERENCES

1. Sanders ME, Schuyler PA, Dupont WD, Page DL. The natural history of low-grade ductal carcinoma in situ of the breast in women treated by biopsy only revealed over 30 years of long-term follow-up. Cancer 2005; 103: 2481–4.
2. King TA, Sakr RA, Muhsen S, et al. Is there a low-grade precursor pathway in breast cancer? Ann Surg Oncol 2012; 19: 1115–21.
3. Page DL, Dupont WD, Rogers LW, Landenberger M. Intraductal carcinoma of the breast: follow-up after biopsy only. Cancer 1982; 49: 751–8.
4. Purdie CA, McLean D, Stormonth E, et al. Management of in situ lobular neoplasia detected on needle core biopsy of breast. J Clin Pathol 2010; 63: 987–93.
5. Crisi GM, Mandavilli S, Cronin E, Ricci A Jr. Invasive mammary carcinoma after immediate and short-term follow-up for lobular neoplasia on core biopsy. Am J Surg Pathol 2003; 27: 325–33.
6. Dalton LW, Pinder SE, Elston CE, et al. Histologic grading of breast cancer: linkage of patient outcome with level of pathologist agreement. Mod Pathol 2000; 13: 730–5.
7. van't Veer LJ, Bernards R. Enabling personalized cancer medicine through analysis of gene-expression patterns. Nature 2008; 452: 564–70.
8. Duffy SW, Chen HH, Tabar L, Day NE. Estimation of mean sojourn time in breast cancer screening using a Markov chain model of both entry to and exit from the preclinical detectable phase. Stat Med 1995; 14: 1531–43.
9. Shen Y, Zelen M. Screening sensitivity and sojourn time from breast cancer early detection clinical trials: mammograms and physical examinations. J Clin Oncol 2001; 19: 3490–9.
10. Wallis M, Neilson F, Hogarth H, Whitaker C, Faulkner K. Cumulative attendance, assessment and cancer detection rate over four screening rounds in five English breast-screening programmes: a retrospective study. J Public Health (Oxford, England) 2007; 29: 275–80.
11. Scaf-Klomp W, van Sonderen FL, Stewart R, van Dijck JA, van den Heuvel WJ. Compliance after 17 years of breast cancer screening. J Med Screen 1995; 2: 195–9.
12. Kerlikowske K, Hubbard RA, Miglioretti DL, et al. Comparative effectiveness of digital versus film-screen mammography in community practice in the United States: a cohort study. Ann Intern Med 2011; 155: 493–502.
13. Forrest AP. Breast Cancer Screening: Report to the Health Minister of England, Wales, Scotland and Northern Ireland. London: HMSO, 1986.
14. Shapiro S VW, Strax P, et al. Periodic Screening for Breast Cancer. The Health Insurance Plan Project and its Sequelae, 1963–1986. Baltimore: Johns Hopkins, 1988.
15. Tabar L, Fagerberg CJ, Gad A, et al. Reduction in mortality from breast cancer after mass screening with mammography. Randomised trial from the Breast Cancer Screening Working Group of the Swedish National Board of Health and Welfare. Lancet 1985; 1: 829–32.
16. Roberts MM, Alexander FE, Anderson TJ, et al. Edinburgh trial of screening for breast cancer: mortality at seven years. Lancet 1990; 335: 241–6.
17. Tabar L, Vitak B, Chen TH, et al. Swedish two-county trial: impact of mammographic screening on breast cancer mortality during 3 decades. Radiology 2011; 260: 658–63.
18. Perry N, Broeders M, de Wolf C, et al. European guidelines for quality assurance in breast cancer screening and diagnosis. Fourth edition–summary document. Ann Oncol 2008; 19: 614–22.
19. Association of Breast Surgery at BASO 2009. Surgical guidelines for the management of breast cancer. Eur J Surg Oncol 2009; 35: 1–22.
20. NHSBSP. Quality Assurance Guidelines for Breast Cancer Screening Radiology. 2011.
21. DOH. Radiography Skills Mix - A Report on the Four-tier Service Delivery Model. 2003.
22. Price R. An Evaluation of the Impact of Implementation of Consultant Practitioners in Clinical Imaging: Report to the Society and College of Radiographers. London: The Society and College of Radiographers, 2010.
23. Williams EM, Vessey MP. Randomised trial of two strategies offering women mobile screening for breast cancer. BMJ (Clinical research ed.) 1989; 299: 158–9.
24. Jepson R, Clegg A, Forbes C, et al. The determinants of screening uptake and interventions for increasing uptake: a systematic review. Health Technology Assess (Winchester, England) 2000; 4: i–vii, 1-133.
25. Hoerger TJ, Ekwueme DU, Miller JW, et al. Estimated effects of the National Breast and Cervical Cancer Early Detection Program on breast cancer mortality. Am J Prev Med 2011; 40: 397–404.
26. BCSC. [Available from: http://breastscreening.cancer.gov/] [Accessed February 27, 2012].
27. Elmore JG, Barton MB, Moceri VM, et al. Ten-year risk of false positive screening mammograms and clinical breast examinations. N Engl J Med 1998; 338: 1089–96.
28. Hubbard RA, Kerlikowske K, Flowers CI, et al. Cumulative probability of false-positive recall or biopsy recommendation after 10 years of screening mammography: a cohort study. Ann Intern Med 2011; 155: 481–92.
29. Yankaskas BC, Klabunde CN, Ancelle-Park R, et al. International comparison of performance measures for screening mammography: can it be done? J Med Screen 2004; 11: 187–93.
30. Roman R, Sala M, Salas D, et al. Effect of protocol-related variables and women's characteristics on the cumulative false-positive risk in breast cancer screening. Ann Oncol 2012; 23: 104–11.
31. Esserman L, Thompson I. Solving the overdiagnosis dilemma. J Natl Cancer Inst 2010; 102: 582–3.
32. Gram IT, Lund E, Slenker SE. Quality of life following a false positive mammogram. Br J Cancer 1990; 62: 1018–22.
33. Lebel S, Jakubovits G, Rosberger Z, et al. Waiting for a breast biopsy. Psychosocial consequences and coping strategies. J Psychosom Res 2003; 55: 437–43.
34. Baines CJ, To T, Wall C. Women's attitudes to screening after participation in the National Breast Screening Study. A questionnaire survey. Cancer 1990; 65: 1663–9.

35. NCCN. Practice Guidelines. 2012.[Available from: http://www.nccn.org/professionals/physician_gls/f_guidelines.asp] [Accessed 2/27/12].

36. BASO. An Audit of Screen Detected Breast Cancers for the Year of Screening April 2001 - March 2002. Association of Breast Surgeons at BASO. UK: NHSBSP, 2003.

37. Farshid G, Sullivan T, Downey P, Gill PG, Pieterse S. Independent predictors of breast malignancy in screen-detected microcalcifications: biopsy results in 2545 cases. Br J Cancer 2011; 105: 1669–75.

38. Baxter NN, Virnig BA, Durham SB, Tuttle TM. Trends in the treatment of ductal carcinoma in situ of the breast. J Natl Cancer Inst 2004; 96: 443–8.

39. Moran MS, Bai HX, Harris EE, et al. ACR appropriateness criteria((R)) ductal carcinoma in situ. Breast J 2012; 18: 8–15.

40. Poplack SP, Tosteson TD, Kogel CA, Nagy HM. Digital breast tomosynthesis: initial experience in 98 women with abnormal digital screening mammography. AJR Am J Roentgenol 2007; 189: 616–23.

11 The organization of breast screening

Julietta Patnick

INTRODUCTION

The value of breast screening in preventing deaths from breast cancer was first investigated by the Health Insurance Plan of Greater New York in the early 1960s, using annual mammography and clinical breast examination. This study showed benefit to women, with a 30% reduction in mortality from breast cancer (1,2). It was followed in the 1970s by the Swedish Two-County study, which used mammography only and showed comparable results (3). This trial has now reported a 29-year follow-up and continues to show an approximate 30% reduction in mortality in women screened (4). Several other studies investigating the value of breast cancer screening were subsequently initiated in Sweden and in Canada which have now also reported long-term follow-up (5–7). By the late 1980s, mammographically based breast screening programs were being introduced in many European countries and opportunistic breast screening was becoming part of routine health care for women in other developed countries. According to a 2008 report on the implementation of cancer screening in Europe, over 64 million women were targeted each year by breast cancer screening programs (8).

With passage of time, concerns have arisen about the efficacy of breast screening with the Danish Cochrane Centre having published a highly critical review which suggests breast screening saves few lives in relation to the heavy costs of screening (9). In response to the first of these Cochrane reviews, the International Agency for Research on Cancer examined the evidence and concluded that for women aged 50–69, "there is sufficient evidence from randomized trials that inviting women 50–69 years of age to screening with mammography reduces their mortality from breast cancer." There is inadequate evidence on the value of screening beyond age 69, but there is some belief that it may benefit women who are otherwise well and have a life expectancy of 10 years or more (10). A major trial is now underway in the United Kingdom evaluating screening in older women. As for the harms of screening, longer term follow-up of the Two-County study concluded that between 400 and 500 women needed to be screened for seven years to save one life which is consistent with reviews by the United States Preventive Services Task Force (which worked on the basis of number needed to invite) and in Canada (11,12). Overdiagnosis is a major cause of debate, but can only be estimated statistically and never proven. Most estimates are about 10% (13–15) although they can reach up to 30% (9). Another potential accusation made against screening is that it increases the mastectomy rate (16). However, data from England show a mastectomy rate in screened women of around half that of women who present outside screening (17) and in the Netherlands a case–control study demonstrating a 49% reduction in mortality showed comparable mastectomy rates (18).

Screening within an organized, quality-assured program appears to improve the prognosis for women diagnosed with breast cancer. An analysis of the 50,286 cases of breast cancer diagnosed in 2007 in England showed that most breast cancers are detected by means other than screening, even among those women in the screening age group (50–69 years). However, when they are detected through the screening program, treatments are on average less severe. Among women with screen-detected invasive breast cancer or *in situ* disease, 27% and 28% underwent a mastectomy compared with figures of 53% and 48% respectively for women presenting symptomatically. Screen-detected tumors were more likely to be smaller in size, of lower grade, and node negative with less likelihood of vascular invasion. These characteristics were found across all age groups and deprivation quintiles; indeed, screening appears to reduce observed inequalities in one-year and five-year survival which are associated with deprivation (17).

When assessing the effectiveness of mammographic screening, it should be emphasized that its impact will be dependent upon the quality of the service delivered. This variation in effectiveness due to quality issues may be considered a weakness of screening programs. Furthermore, the effects of quality variation will become apparent only after several years have elapsed. In the earlier trials of breast screening, benefits emerged after four years and the full impact was seen only with a more prolonged follow-up. In service screening, even longer periods are necessary, because populations targeted for service screening (unlike "clean" trial populations), include many women with a pre-existent breast cancer diagnosis. In addition, women are now living longer due to improvements in treatment, particularly introduction of hormonal therapy, and improved use of chemotherapy. Thus when considering the effectiveness of screening, a follow-up over several decades is necessary. Furthermore, assiduous attention to quality is vital when planning and executing operational issues.

The initial impact of screening interventions has been demonstrated in Finland (19), the Netherlands (20), and the United Kingdom (21). However, it becomes more difficult to estimate the effect of screening with increasing years that pass since introduction of screening into a population. As cohort effects come into play, changes in the environment, such as the introduction of hormone replacement therapy, better understanding of the disease and improvements in treatment collectively render it difficult to quantify the contribution of breast screening to reductions in breast cancer deaths in developed countries over the last 20 years. Nevertheless, case–control studies have claimed reductions in mortality of about 48% in the age group 50–69 in both the Netherlands and the East Anglia region in the United Kingdom (18,22).

Many breast screening programs have now been in operation for around 20 years and it is a challenge for those involved in the organization of such programs to remain as committed today as the early enthusiasts to the delivery of high-quality programs to women in the local population. While the trials are based on the treatment regimens of earlier decades, they nevertheless demonstrate that screening confers real benefits and current service programs must still deliver on the expectation of trial results. This chapter discusses the organization of screening programs for defined populations of women at average risk. It does not consider women with a family history or screening for known breast cancer genes (see chap. 10). However, many of the principles outlined for population screening will have general application.

ESSENTIAL COMPONENTS OF A BREAST SCREENING PROGRAM

Breast screening takes place within a range of different healthcare systems. At one extreme, screening may be at the complete discretion of an individual woman and her clinician. Breast cancer mortality rates are highest in the developed world, where most countries have screening policies, reflecting a professional consensus about age, frequency, and quality of mammography. In Europe these are enshrined in the Council of Europe declaration (23) which has been followed up by the publication of quality assurance guidelines for breast screening in Europe (24). Organized population breast screening is considered to be more efficient than opportunistic screening, and is particularly appropriate where a suitable population can be defined and targeted. Under these circumstances, there are several essential components of a screening program including:

- support for a screening service within the population as a whole;
- resources;
- clear protocols underpinned by training and quality assurance;
- evaluation;
- information systems and database;
- public information and recruitment.

SUPPORT WITHIN THE POPULATION AS A WHOLE

Wilson and Jungner (25), on behalf of the World Health Organization stipulated that a disease for which population screening takes place should be recognized as "an important public health problem." In the absence of such recognition, there will be no financial support from funders, clinicians will neither recommend nor participate in a screening program and attendance is likely to be poor among the target population.

Breast cancer is a leading cause of cancer death in developed countries, second only to lung cancer. However, it is the commonest malignancy among women, and in recognition of this significant health problem there is both political and financial support for management of this disease, with funding coming from central government and insurance companies. It is essential that these sources of funding incorporate provision for treatment of cancers detected at screening. Screening without appropriate follow-up treatment will be unethical.

Professional support for a breast screening program is crucial in order that clinicians will encourage women to participate and to enable the recruitment and retention of staff. Breast screening can sometimes be perceived as a repetitive and rather tedious activity. However, the many subtle radiological signs present a considerable challenge and film reading demands constant vigilance if abnormalities are not to be missed. Finally, there must be support from the population targeted for screening. Strategies to maximize recruitment of women will be discussed later in this chapter, but it is important that women within the target population recognize screening to be an effective tool in the fight against breast cancer, as this will help engage the population.

RESOURCES
Staff

Breast screening is an image-driven program, so a major resource is the image reader and his or her visual skills. Computer-aided devices (CAD) for the reading of mammograms are coming into use, but have yet to supplant the interpretational ability of the human brain, generally due to limited specificity. However, they can offer support to the individual reader (26). Double reading of films is generally preferred and CAD could act as a second reader. A minimum amount of regular mammogram reporting is needed to develop and maintain expertise (27,28). Thus many countries set a minimum number of mammograms to be reported; in the United Kingdom, a radiologist must report at least 5000 sets of films per year (29). In addition, obtaining good-quality images requires a level of skill that should not be underestimated. The requisite qualifications to undertake this task vary around the world. Mammography has traditionally been undertaken in the United Kingdom by state-registered radiographers, but a program to train lay women, without a background in imaging, to take mammograms has proven very successful. It is one of a number of areas where clinical imaging is using these "assistant practitioners" (30).

By employing non-state-registered practitioners to carry out mammography, radiographers have been released to undertake advanced tasks previously undertaken by medical staff. These include mammography reading and interpretation, ultrasound examinations, and image-guided biopsies. Breast clinicians who are neither specialist surgeons nor radiologists are also a valuable component of the screening scene, with their role varying according to their skills and abilities and with local service requirements.

Following initial imaging, further investigation may be required to make a complete diagnostic assessment. Women should undergo triple assessment (clinical, radiological, and pathological), although for screen-detected lesions there is often no clinical correlate to the radiological abnormality. This involves a multidisciplinary team composed not only of imaging staff, but also of a pathologist with a special interest in breast disease, a breast surgeon, and a breast care nurse trained in counseling. The precise role of the surgeon in the diagnostic workup of screen-detected lesions is often debated, but while the majority of these can now be diagnosed nonoperatively with percutaneous biopsy techniques (96% in the National

Health Service Breast Screening Programme, NHSBSP) (31), there remains a proportion of women who require a surgical opinion and will proceed to an open surgical biopsy to establish a definitive diagnosis.

Many women value and appreciate the support of a breast care nurse along the screening pathway. This might involve discussion of possible procedures prior to attending the assessment clinic or further explanation and clarification following diagnosis of cancer. Although breast care nurses are accustomed to dealing with newly diagnosed breast cancer patients and explaining treatment options, a woman diagnosed through screening presents additional challenges, having been previously asymptomatic. She has had little time to contemplate the possibility of having cancer, which can prove to be an additional burden when coping initially with a diagnosis of breast cancer. Under these circumstances, an experienced and understanding nurse can be of great assistance. Close teamwork between the various professional disciplines is essential.

Facilities

The quality of X-ray imaging equipment is of primary importance to a screening program. Full-field digital mammography is now well established and must be regarded as the standard of care for women going for mammography generally. It has been shown to be more sensitive for premenopausal women with denser breasts (32) and most equipment delivers a lower dose of radiation than old analog equipment. It tends to show calcifications particularly well and the reader's eye must be retrained to interpret the images with appropriate sensitivity and also specificity. A setup that permits full diagnostic workup will have facilities for magnification and stereotaxis. All equipment should enable both 18 mm × 24 mm and 24 mm × 30 mm images to be taken, which will ensure that larger breasts can be encompassed in a single exposure, thus minimizing the radiation dose. Ultrasound has been shown to be beneficial in providing additional information in the denser breast; tomosynthesis which combines both techniques is increasingly being considered for service use. However, it is at the moment thought more suitable for diagnostic than screening work due to the expense. Specimen radiography equipment should also be available and within easy reach of the theater to ensure that excised lesions can be imaged to check that the identified radiological abnormality is contained within the specimen.

Ultrasound equipment for use in the diagnostic process has always been an integral component of a full breast screening service and as technology develops its usefulness also grows (33). It reliably distinguishes between solid and cystic lesions, and permits aspiration of cysts and biopsy of solid masses under image guidance. A range of equipment and needles are available for percutaneous biopsy procedures, and although these may appear expensive, these costs should be considered in comparison with the physical, psychological, and financial costs of an open surgical biopsy. The ready availability of these techniques compared with operative biopsy may have contributed to the improvements in the cancer detection rate within the NHSBSP and have certainly contributed to the high rate of a nonoperative diagnosis.

Breast screening is carried out on well women, and the general atmosphere and physical ambience of a screening unit is important. When women attend for screening, they should find themselves in as pleasant and relaxing an environment as possible. Mobile screening units have proved very popular in many countries, although they are only suitable for basic screening activity and a more comprehensive diagnostic workup must be undertaken in a hospital setting. It must be remembered that most of the women do not have breast cancer and care should be taken to ensure they are kept separated from cancer patients or from women presenting symptomatically. In effect, they should be treated as well women, as the majority are just this.

Finance

The finance required to operate a breast screening service will clearly vary with context. Different countries in the developed world have adopted different approaches to the funding of national screening programs, which generally depend on central funding or reimbursement or a combination. The cost-effectiveness evidence supporting the use of breast screening is dependent on studies that have examined not only the overall cost-effectiveness of screening, but also aspects of screening technique such as the number of views, reports, frequency, and the age band exposed to screening.

The above comments on the multifactorial nature for attainment of high quality and effectiveness in breast screening illustrate why it is essential that the funding be sufficient to support the chosen regimen. Moreover, a screening program should not be embarked upon where women who are diagnosed with cancer are unable to access appropriate treatment. This is true across any particular health system as a whole and for individual women.

PROTOCOLS, TRAINING, AND QUALITY ASSURANCE

Population screening for breast cancer has certain parallels with a production line, whereby a single hospital clinic or doctor is capable of screening thousands of women per year, the vast majority of whom will not have cancer. In order to cope with the volume of work and minimize psychological distress to the majority of women without cancer, standard protocols must be developed and adhered to. These should encompass a broad remit, including the administrative aspects of dealing with large numbers of women, the optimum methods for imaging women in different circumstances and how radiologically suspicious abnormalities should be assessed to obtain diagnostic clarification. In the latter situation, the screening process becomes more focused, with women receiving more individual attention.

Clinical protocols are outlined in medical texts and often discussed at scientific meetings. With experience, a multidisciplinary team will derive its own detailed protocols, reflecting the skill mix and knowledge available locally, and reach a consensus on which protocols should be applied to women under their care. These days many colleges and associations produce professional guidelines (34), as do national institutions established to develop evidence-based guidelines (35). Once this point is reached, professional training programs can be set up to ensure that minimum standards of practice are guaranteed for that community and to encourage inflow of skilled personnel into the community with dissemination of knowledge and skills relating to new techniques.

Breast screening is a high-risk activity in a medicolegal context and, from a clinical perspective, has the potential to cause harm to women. Screening involves large numbers of healthy women, and relatively minor aberrations can affect large numbers of women in a very short space of time. Quality assurance measures must be applied to every step of the process to ensure that any minor faults or problems are quickly identified and promptly corrected. All units should have written protocols and audits undertaken to ensure that protocols are adhered to. Protocols should be regularly reviewed and updated in the light of changes in hospital procedures and advances in knowledge and techniques. Audits and quality assurance may expose an area where further training is needed or where the protocols need amending. The audit loop involves constant monitoring and quality improvement. Protocols, training, and quality assurance are important elements of all aspects of breast screening and increase the chances that women participating in screening will ultimately derive more benefit than harm.

EVALUATION

Evaluation of screening is most conveniently considered within two timescales: the short term, which deals with the process of screening, and the long term, where the outcome of screening is examined. Long-term outcomes inevitably reflect screening practices and activity dating back several years when they may have been suboptimal compared with current practice. Short-term indicators of performance are therefore important in the early identification of problems and minimizing the chance of doing harm rather than good.

Short-term process indicators will reflect current screening practice. They will include the uptake and cancer detection rates, the proportion of women found to have a radiological abnormality requiring further assessment, and the positive predictive value of these investigations. The histopathological features of individual tumors detected will be predictive of the future outcome of current screening methods and practice. In addition to overall program indicators, each speciality within breast screening will have its own criteria for assessment of current professional practice. Radiographers, for example, will be particularly interested in the technical repeat rate and the pathologist in the predictive values of reports issued.

The ultimate long-term outcome indicator for a breast screening program is the mortality rate. As mentioned above, breast cancer mortality is falling worldwide, which is partly due to improvements in adjuvant therapy in recent years and the precise proportion of the mortality reduction attributable to screening *per se* is difficult to determine.

Measurements of survival might provide another potential long-term outcome indicator, with improved survival among screen-detected compared with symptomatic cancers. However, these data can be difficult to interpret because of the phenomena of lead-time and selection biases. More favourable tumors may be overdiagnosed in a screening program. It is essential therefore that any studies of survival look at extremely long-term follow-up. In the United Kingdom this has now extended to 15 years, and the relative survival for women with breast cancers detected by the screening program in 1990/91 stands at 86% (36). This compares with estimates of around 67% 10-year survival for women diagnosed symptomatically at around the same time (37).

The interval cancer rate can be useful for longer-term evaluation of a breast screening program. There is no evidence to suggest that women who develop interval cancers have a worse prognosis than women who present symptomatically. In particular, there is no evidence that presentation is delayed as a consequence of "false reassurance" from a negative screen. Nonetheless, much can be learned from the occurrence of interval cancers, as they represent an element of failure and are by definition "the ones that got away." Comparison of current with previous screening films can be instructive, with some interval cancers being apparent in retrospect on the previous screen. The proportion of cancers that present as interval cases compared with the underlying incidence should be minimal in order to maximize the effectiveness of the screening program.

Interval cancers can be notoriously difficult to monitor and obtain information about. Screening programs that have low rates of interval cases must ensure that appropriate efforts have been made to identify all such cases and thus for the quoted rates to be accurate rather than there existing much missing data with a resultant overoptimistic impression of efficacy.

INFORMATION SYSTEMS AND DATABASE

A robust and reliable information system is essential for any screening service, whether this is run by an individual clinician or is a formal population screening program. With regular screening, serial films are built up and provide a useful documentation of personal screening history. The timing and results of previous episodes should be available at the time of the current screen and previous films available for comparison.

When screening is adopted as a public health policy, the service must be accessible to the entire population. If this is to be achieved then a reliable database of the population providing a minimum of age, sex, and address is mandatory. This facilitates the process of sending invitations: the proportion of women in the population who have recently been screened (the coverage rate) can be calculated; those women who have not been screened can be identified and targeted, and population demographics can be kept under review for planning purposes.

How these population databases or registers are compiled varies from one health system to another. The United Kingdom has almost complete registration of the population with the NHS, which has allowed a universal invitation system to be introduced relatively easily. Other countries have been able to use the electoral or fiscal registers as a starting point. In some countries, there has been no access to any kind of pre-existing database, which has led to registers being built up as women are recruited. The variations between systems often reflect the data protection legislation pertaining to each country.

Information systems should ideally hold or have access to all relevant data about an individual woman within a screening program. Recorded information should include if and when a woman was invited for screening, and her acceptance or otherwise. In addition, the outcome of an attendance should be clearly documented. If cancer is detected, information relevant to referral for further investigation and management should be recorded, together with the prognostic details about the cancer, such as size, grade, and lymph node status. Collating data for each individual screened will provide an overall picture of the effectiveness of the screening program and its effect in the screened population.

Information systems such as this are complicated in design, but they should be as easy to use as possible for doctors, nurses, radiographers, and administrative staff in order for that data to be as accurate and complete as possible. It is essential that all users of the system be well trained and comfortable with its use. It is advantageous for staff to be able to enter the data for which they are directly responsible themselves, and thus transcription, with its attendant faults, is avoided.

PUBLIC INFORMATION AND RECRUITMENT

Hand in hand with the introduction of a screening program is the provision of information to the public. This should include basic information such as for whom the program is intended and how women may access its services. Various strategies can be employed to encourage general awareness of the program and raise the public profile. These include contact with local and national print and broadcast media, liaison with charities and other women's organizations, and advertising campaigns. When a woman is invited for screening, she needs more specific information. She not only needs to know where and when to go for screening, but must also have some understanding of the process involved and the likely benefits and potential harms from screening. In the early days of breast cancer screening, there was a tendency to underplay the disadvantages and potential adverse effects of screening. For example, women were often not informed that mammography might be uncomfortable or that screening is not guaranteed to identify all cancers present at the time of screening. Today, however, women are encouraged to make an informed choice about whether or not to attend for screening, rather than being persuaded to attend even if they have an element of doubt or reluctance. It is quite unacceptable to attempt to convince non-attenders that they have made an unwise or even foolish decision and try to persuade them to attend after all.

There are always some women who are difficult to reach with invitations and information. These are often women without a fixed address who relocate regularly and/or who are without a "usual care provider" (e.g., a general practitioner). In addition, this group of women are likely to have poor literary skills and may find it difficult to grasp the issues presented with the intention of helping them make an "informed choice." Immigrants whose command of the host language and culture is weak present a particular challenge, as do women who have disabilities. Socioeconomic factors have been shown to be very influential in affecting a woman's ability to access breast screening even when there is no charge for the service itself (38). Several strategies have been adopted to improve uptake of screening among these "hard to reach" groups of women. Community health educators have worked successfully with women from ethnic minority groups (39), and special materials are available for women with learning disabilities (40). Opening screening clinics in the evenings and weekends have not proved successful in raising the rates of attendance, although many women appreciate the convenience of attending out of working hours. Studies are regularly undertaken to examine the reasons for non-attendance, but this is a heterogeneous group of women and the development of a range of novel strategies is required to ensure that these individuals have access to and can make an informed choice about whether to attend for screening or not.

CONCLUSION

Mammographic screening of women aged 50–69 has been shown to reduce mortality from breast cancer. There may be benefits from screening women outside this age group, although this remains unproven. The success and effectiveness of a screening program depends on a combination of organization, ability to recruit women from the target population, and the quality of the mammography and diagnostic processes. Successful screening programs can play a significant part in the continued reduction in the mortality rates from breast cancer.

REFERENCES

1. Shapiro S, Strax P, Venet L, et al. Periodic breast cancer screening in reducing mortality from breast cancer. JAMA 1971; 215: 1777–85.
2. Shapiro S, Venet W, Strax P, et al. 10 to 14 year effect of breast cancer screening on mortality. J Natl Cancer Inst 1982; 69: 349–55.
3. Tabar L, Fagerberg CJG, Gad A, et al. Reduction in mortality from breast cancer after mass screening with mammography. Randomised trial from the Breast Cancer Screening Working Group of the Swedish National Board of Health and Welfare. Lancet 1985; 1: 829–32.
4. Tabár L, Vitak B, Chen TH, et al. Swedish two-county trial: impact of mammographic screening on breast cancer mortality during 3 decades. Radiology 2011; 260: 658–63.
5. Nystrom L, Rutqvist L E, Wall S, et al. Breast cancer screening with mammography: overview of Swedish randomised studies. Lancet 1993; 341: 973–8.
6. Miller AB, To T, Baines CJ, Wall C. The Canadian National Breast Screening Study-1: breast cancer mortality after 11 to 16 years of follow-up. A randomized screening trial of mammography in women age 40 to 49 years. Ann Intern Med 2002; 137: 305–12.
7. Miller AB, To T, Baines CJ, Wall C. Canadian National Breast Screening Study-2: 13-year results of a randomized trial in women aged 50-59 years. J Natl Cancer Inst 2000; 92: 1490–9.
8. von Karsa L, Anttila A, Ronco G, et al. Cancer Screening in the European Union Report on the Implementation of the Council Recommendation on Cancer Screening. Lyon: IARC, 2008.
9. Gøtzsche PC, Nielsen M. Screening for breast cancer with mammography. Cochrane Database Syst Rev 2011: CD001877.
10. International Agency for Research on Cancer. Handbook of Cancer Protection no 7: Breast Cancer Screening. Lyon: IARC, 2002.
11. USPSTF. Screening for Breast Cancer: U.S. Preventive Services Task Force recommendation statement. Ann Intern Med 2009; 151: 716–26.
12. The Canadian Task Force on Preventive Health Care. Recommendations on screening for breast cancer in average-risk women aged 40–74 years. CMAJ 2011; 183: 1991–2001.
13. Advisory Committee on Breast Cancer Screening. Screening for Breast Cancer in England: Past and Future. NHSBSP 61 Sheffield, UK, 2006.
14. Duffy SW, Tabar L, Olsen AH, et al. Absolute numbers of lives saved and overdiagnosis in breast cancer screening, from a randomized trial and from the Breast Screening Programme in England. J Med Screen 2010; 17: 25–30.
15. Puliti D, Zappa M, Miccinesi G, et al. An estimate of overdiagnosis 15 years after the start of mammographic screening in Florence. Eur J Cancer 2009; 45: 3166–71.
16. Suhrke P, Mæhlen J, Schlichting E, et al. Effect of mammography screening on surgical treatment for breast cancer in Norway: comparative analysis of cancer registry data. BMJ 2011; 343: d4692.
17. The Second All Breast Cancer Report. London: NCIN 2011.[Available from: http://www.cancerscreening.nhs.uk/breastscreen/second-all-breast-cancer-report.pdf] [Last accessed 26 February 2012].
18. Otto SJ, Fracheboud J, Verbeek AL, et al. National Evaluation Team for Breast Cancer Screening. Mammography screening and risk of breast cancer death: a population-based case-control study. Cancer Epidemiol Biomarkers Prev 2012; 21: 66–73.

19. Hakama M, Pukkala E, Kallio M, Heikkila M. Effectiveness of the public health policy for breast cancer screening in Finland: population based cohort study. BMJ 1997; 314: 864–7.

20. van den Akker-van Marle E, de Koning H, Boer R, van der Maas T. Reduction in breast cancer mortality due to the introduction of mass screening in the Netherlands: comparison with the United Kingdom. J Med Screen 1999; 6: 30–4.

21. Blanks RG, Moss SM, McGahan CE, et al. Effect of the breast screening programme on mortality from breast cancer in England and Wales, 1990–98. Comparison of observed with predictive mortality. BMJ 2000; 321: 663–9.

22. Allgood PC, Warwick J, Warren RML, Day NE, Duffy SW. A case-control study of the impact of the East Anglian breast screening programme on breast cancer mortality. Br J Cancer 2008; 98: 206–9.

23. Council of Europe Recommendation of 2 December 2003 on Cancer Screening (2003/878/EC). [Available from: http://eur-lex.europa.eu/LexUriServ/LexUriServ.do?uri=OJ:L:2003:327:0034:0038:EN:PDF] [Last accessed 22 January 2012].

24. Perry N, Broeders M, de Wolf C, et al. European guidelines for quality assurance in breast cancer screening and diagnosis. Fourth edition–summary document. Ann Oncol 2008; 19: 614–22.

25. Wilson JMG, Jungner G. Principles and Practice of Screening for Disease. WHO Public Health Paper 34. Geneva: World Health Organisation, 1968.

26. Gilbert FJ, Astley SM, Gillan MG, et al. CADET II Group. Single reading with computer-aided detection for screening mammography. N Engl J Med 2008; 359: 1675–84.

27. Buist DS, Anderson ML, Haneuse SJ, et al. Influence of annual interpretive volume on screening mammography performance in the United States. Radiology 2011; 259: 72–84.

28. Kan L, Olivotto IA, Warren Burhenne LJ, Sickles EA, Coldman AJ. Standardized abnormal interpretation and cancer detection ratios to assess reading volume and reader performance in a breast screening program. Radiology 2000; 215: 563–7.

29. Quality assurance guidelines for breast cancer screening radiology. NHSBSP Publication No. 59: Mar 2011.

30. Shaw A. The Scope of Practice of Assistant Practitioners in Clinical Imaging Society of Radiographers 2007. [Available from: http://www.improvement.nhs.uk/documents/18weeks/Scope-practical-assistance-of-assistant-practitioner.pdf] [Last accessed 26 February 2012].

31. NHS Breast Screening Programme and Association of Breast Surgery an Audit of Screen Detected Breast Cancers for the Year of Screening, April 2009–March 2010. [Available from: http://www.cancerscreening.nhs.uk/breastscreen/publications/baso2009-2010.pdf] [Last accessed 17 February 2012].

32. Pisano ED, Gatsonis C, Hendrick E, et al. Digital Mammographic Imaging Screening Trial (DMIST) Investigators Group. Diagnostic performance of digital versus film mammography for breast-cancer screening. N Engl J Med 2005; 353: 1773–83.

33. Corsetti V, Houssami N, Ferrari A, et al. Breast screening with ultrasound in women with mammography-negative dense breasts: evidence on incremental cancer detection and false positives, and associated cost. Eur J Cancer 2008; 44: 539–44.

34. Newell MS, Birdwell RL, D'Orsi CJ, et al. Expert Panel on Breast Imaging. Guideline Summary NGC-7916 ACR Appropriateness Criteria® Nonpalpable Mammographic Findings (Excluding Calcifications). Reston (VA): American College of Radiology (ACR), 2010.

35. National Collaborating Centre for Cancer. Early and Locally Advanced Breast Cancer: Diagnosis and Treatment (CG80). London: National Institute for Health and Clinical Excellence, 2009.

36. NHSBSP and ABS at BASO. An audit of screen detected breast cancers for the year of screening April 2006 to March 2007. Sheffield, 2008.

37. Breast cancer–survival statistics. [Available from: http://info.cancerresearchuk.org/cancerstats/types/breast/survival/breast-cancer-survival-statistics#Trends CRUK] [Last accessed 26 February 2012].

38. Moser K, Patnick J, Beral V. Inequalities in reported use of breast and cervical screening in Great Britain: analysis of cross sectional survey data. BMJ 2009; 338: b2025.

39. Chiu LF. Straight Talking: Communicating Breast Screening Information in Primary Care. Training Pack for Hard to Reach Groups. Nuffield Institute for Health, University of Leeds, 2002.

40. Good Practice in Breast and Cervical Screening for Women with Learning Difficulties. NHSBSP Publication 46. Sheffield: NHS Breast Screening Programme, 2000.

12 Quality assurance and evaluation of outcomes in the NHS breast screening programme

Gill Lawrence

INTRODUCTION

The United Kingdom (UK) National Health Service Breast Screening Programme (NHSBSP) was set up in 1988 in response to the recommendations of the Forrest Report published in 1986 (1). Based on the results of the Swedish Two-County Randomized Controlled trial (2), it was anticipated that the introduction of organized breast cancer screening should lead to a significant reduction in mortality from breast cancer in the UK. This belief was further reinforced by the specific inclusion in the 1992 *The Health of the Nation* white paper (3) of a target to reduce by 25% breast cancer mortality in women aged 50–69 years by the year 2000. This target was subsequently amended to apply to women aged 55–69 years. When the NHSBSP began, women aged 50–64 years were invited every three years for two-view (craniocaudal and mediolateral oblique) screening at the initial screen, and single-view (mediolateral oblique) screening at subsequent screens. In 2000, two-view screening was introduced for all screens; in 2002, the NHSBSP was extended to invite women aged 50–70 years for screening in England and Wales. In Scotland the 50–70 year age extension began in 2008. More recently, a randomized controlled trial evaluating the effects of extending the age range for breast screening to women aged 47–49 years and 71–73 years has been instituted (4). Randomization will be run over two three-year screening rounds and should be complete by 2016. If the proposed age extension is found to be effective, full roll-out will mean that all women will receive their first invitation for screening before their 50th birthday, and that all women will potentially receive two additional invitations to screening in their lifetime.

Given the long-term nature of improvements expected to result from screening, it was necessary to identify a number of key proxy measures against which standards of performance could be monitored in order to gauge progress toward the NHSBSP's ultimate aim of reducing breast cancer mortality. One of the prime purposes of quality assurance (QA), which has been an integral part of the NHSBSP since its inception, is to monitor performance against these key national standards and to work with screening programs to identify and address the reasons for underperformance.

KEY ELEMENTS OF BREAST SCREENING QUALITY ASSURANCE

QA Structures, Policies, and Standards

The key elements of the breast screening QA program are summarized in Table 12.1. Policies and standards are set by the National Coordination Team with advice from national coordinating groups for each of the professions involved in the NHSBSP. These are published by the NHSBSP in a series of guidelines which are regularly reviewed and updated (5–12) and can be downloaded from the NHS Cancer Screening website (www.cancerscreening.nhs.uk). At regional level, the cornerstones of the QA service are the QA teams and the analytical and administrative support staff in the Quality Assurance Reference Centres (QARCs). Each regional QA team is composed of professional QA coordinators for each of the areas covered by the screening program and is led by a Regional Director of Breast Screening Quality Assurance who is currently directly accountable to the Regional Director of Public Health (13). The areas covered by the professional QA coordinators include screening office management (in the screening unit and at the primary care trust (PCT) where call/recall registers are usually held), radiography, medical physics, radiology, pathology, surgery, and breast care nursing. Each QA coordinator is nominated by their peers and is formally appointed to their role. Service level agreements with the QARC specify the service that will be provided in return for payments received by the QA coordinators' employers. The regional QA coordinators meet regularly with their professional counterparts at the national level and with their professional colleagues at regional level, forming an important communication channel between the NHSBSP's National Office and local professionals.

Data Collection, Audit, and Dissemination of Results

Data concerning the performance of individual screening services are collected each year via standard contract data set returns submitted to the NHS Health and Social Care Information Centre (NHSIC) by screening services (KC62 reports) and PCTs running call/recall registers (KC63 returns). These data are published each year by the NHSBSP in an annual review of the program (14) and by the Department of Health in an NHSBSP statistical bulletin (15). Selected data concerned with radiological performance are analyzed each year by the NHSBSP Radiology Coordinating Group and are disseminated at regional level via regional radiology QA coordinators. Since 1997, surgical performance data have been collected and analyzed at the national level through a joint NHSBSP/Association of Breast Surgery (ABS) audit. These data are published each year (16) and presented for discussion at the annual meeting of the ABS. In each region the Surgical QA Coordinator, QA Director, and QA Coordinator work together to ensure that the data are collected from their breast screening services.

Table 12.1 The Key Elements of a Successful QA Programme

Key Element	Detail
Set up a structure within which to carry out quality assurance	• Establish multidisciplinary professional quality assurance (QA) teams at the national and regional level • Establish regional QA reference centers to provide administrative and analytical support for the QA teams • Provide funding to pump prime regional and local QA initiatives that can be disseminated more widely if they are successful
Set policies and standards	• Set policies and standards against which to judge performance • Ensure that standards are consistent across the program being monitored and preferably also in different countries offering similar programs to facilitate evaluation of outcomes • Involve professional groups in the development of policies and standards to ensure ownership
Implementation	• Use a multidisciplinary team approach • Set up standard data collection and analysis procedures, emphasizing structured reporting and data quality • Seek out champions to win the hearts and minds of peer groups to provide pressure for change
Audit the process	• Establish local audit to encourage critical analysis of the service by those who provide it • Carry out national and regional comparative audits to demonstrate performance relative to other services • Undertake peer review via QA team visits to individual services using standardized proforma for each professional area and supported by routine performance data for each aspect of the service
Disseminate the results	• Provide services and host trust management with detailed QA team visit reports containing clear recommendations with deadlines for completion • Inform commissioners of services, cancer networks, and the national office of the recommendations made at QA team visits and the points of good practice noted • Organize workshops at cancer network, regional, and national level to discuss performance against standards and to share good practice
Encourage improvements in performance	• Work with each professional group and each screening service to look for the reasons for poor performance against standards • Ensure that QA team visit reports are considered by host trust and service commissioner executive teams and clinical governance committees • Follow-up recommendations at regular intervals, involving service commissioners and performance management staff as necessary
Target investment	• Work with clinicians and commissioners of services to ensure that limited resources are targeted at areas of most clinical need using evidence collected during the QA process
All important overall approach	• Carry out QA in a non-confrontational environment • Develop a climate of mutual trust and honesty • Look for the reasons for failure rather than apportioning blame

Lead surgeons in each breast screening unit are responsible for making sure that the data are made available and are complete. The identification of people responsible for ensuring that data are gathered and are a true reflection of surgical work is intended to encourage ownership of the information for this audit. As with the radiology outcome data distributed by the NHSBSP Radiology Coordinating Group, ownership of the information is essential if a need for change is highlighted, which must be accepted and implemented.

One of the key functions of the QARCs is to pre-process KC62, KC63, and NHSBSP/ABS audit data and to liaise with their local screening services and PCTs to resolve data quality problems. QARCs can then combine these data with information obtained from the computer systems in their screening units using standard co-writer reports (e.g., round length, screen to results and screen to assessment times, cytology and histology data) or other sources (e.g., medical physics external survey data and customer satisfaction surveys) to produce regional outcome data summarizing the overall performance of their screening units. These data can then be disseminated locally in an annual outcomes booklet (in paper and electronic form). In addition, key outcome data for each screening service are presented at an annual regional breast screening QA study day and more detailed analyses at workshops for each professional group. In the West Midlands, surgical and pathological outcome data for the NHSBSP are presented alongside and compared with data for symptomatic women obtained via the Breast Cancer Clinical Outcome Measures audit of symptomatic breast cancers (17).

QA Team Visits, Recommendations, and Performance Management

Peer review QA team visits to NHSBSP breast screening services and to the PCTs providing the call/recall service are carried out by the regional QA team each year (12). Every screening service is visited at least once every three years. Additional visits, either by the whole QA team or by selected professional QA coordinators may be instituted if a formal review of the annual outcome data identifies areas of concern for a particular screening service. QA team visits provide an opportunity for the QA team to look at the whole screening service, to visit the facilities in the organizations that host the screening service, and to meet with all the screening staff. Prior to a QA team visit, the QA team reviews the outcome data for each component of the service to identify areas of concern. Standardized proformas are completed in advance of the QA team visit by staff leading each element of the screening service. The proforma, which covers outcome data, policies, procedures, qualifications, and training, together with participation in external quality assurance (EQA) schemes, is discussed with the professional QA coordinators at the QA visit during one to one discussions with their counterparts. Because, the QA team does not formally audit the everyday use of systems of work, policies, and procedures during a QA visit, the effectiveness of a QA team visit is dependent on the screening service's willingness to share all relevant information in a frank and complete manner with the professional QA coordinators.

The QA team visit also provides an opportunity for formal reviews of interval cancers by the Radiology QA Coordinator, of selected slides by the Pathology QA Coordinator and of internal radiographic quality control data and external survey results by the Medical Physics QA Coordinator. A formal audit by the Administrative and Clerical QA Coordinator of the patient records maintained in the screening office is generally included in the QA team visit, and the Radiography QA Coordinator may also take this opportunity to lead a formal review of film quality by carrying out a PGMI (perfect, good, moderate, and inadequate) assessment exercise with the radiographers.

Most QA teams send members to observe a routine multidisciplinary meeting shortly before the QA team visit, and many QA teams include a multidisciplinary case review session at the QA team visit. In the West Midlands region, cases for discussion at these sessions are selected jointly by the QARC and the screening service. All benign open biopsies are included, as are selected interval cancers and early recall cases. Other interesting or discordant cases are chosen by the QARC on the basis of data submitted to the annual NHSBSP/ABS audit and the annual KC62 returns. All of the cases are reviewed by the Pathology QA Coordinator as part of the slide review and by the Radiology QA Coordinator as part of the film review. Another feature which may form part of a QA team visit is a "patient journey" during which a member of the QA team attempts to find and attend the screening service's assessment clinic in response to a standard recall to assessment letter.

One of the key features of a QA team visit is the feedback of the findings to the screening service, the host organization, and other interested parties. This process generally begins with a verbal feedback session to which all screening staff and the representatives from the host management, commissioners, and cancer network(s) are invited. In this session, feedback is provided on each aspect of the screening service, either by each professional QA coordinator or by the QA Director, and areas of good practice and recommendations for improvement are identified. QA team visit recommendations are classified as for immediate action, for action with a three-month deadline and for longer-term action. The latter are followed up at six-monthly intervals. The three-month recommendations are confirmed in writing to the screening service and its commissioners within one week of the QA team visit. Details of the longer-term recommendations are provided in a full report which is available within one month of the QA team visit. Importantly, this report also highlights areas of good practice which can be disseminated to other services.

At the end of or shortly after the QA team visit, it is helpful to include a management meeting where the recommendations can be discussed and action plans initiated. Experience has demonstrated that, if the host organization's chief executive or another member of the host organization's senior management team is present at the verbal feedback session and the management meeting, more progress tends to be made in achieving the recommendations from the QA team visit. It is also beneficial if service commissioners are present so that they can appreciate the context in which recommendations have been made with cost implications, as this greater understanding often results in appropriate investments being made.

Local ownership is further increased if the report of the QA team visit is considered formally by the executive boards and clinical governance committees of the host organization and the service commissioner, as recommended by the Commission for Health Improvement's report on the West of London Breast Screening Service (18). The importance of engaging host management in the QA process cannot be overemphasized, as the implementation and maintenance of reliable internal quality management systems must be the major means by which service quality is assured rather than through the external QA provided by the regional QA team. The QA team for its part must ensure that recommendations from QA team visits are followed up tenaciously and that appropriate measures are taken if difficulties arise. These may initially take the form of further meetings with screening staff and/or host chief executives, but may eventually require the involvement of service commissioners, cancer networks, or performance management/clinical governance leads at the Strategic Health Authority.

QUALITY ASSURANCE STANDARDS

QA standards for each professional area contributing to the NHSBSP are published in a series of NHSBSP guidelines (5–12). Of these, a smaller number of key standards have been identified to monitor the performance of the NHSBSP (19). These key standards are listed in Table 12.2 where they have been divided into those that are designed to minimize risk and

Table 12.2 Key NHSBSP Quality Assurance Standards

Objective	Criteria	Minimum Standard	Target
(A) Standards designed to minimize risk			
1. To achieve optimum image quality	a) High contrast spatial resolution	≥12 1p/mm	
	b) Minimal detectable contrast	≤1.2%	≤0.8%
	5–6 mm detail	≤5%	≤3%
	0.5 mm detail	≤8%	≤5%
	0.25 mm detail		
	c) Standard film density	1.5–1.9	
2. To limit radiation dose	Mean glandular dose per film to standard breast using a grid	≤2.5 mGy	
3. To minimize anxiety for women who are awaiting the results of screening	The percentage of women who are sent their result within 2 wks	≥90%	100%
4. To minimize the interval from the screening mammogram to assessment	The percentage of women who attend an assessment centre within 3 wks of attendance for the screening mammogram	≥90%	100%
5. To minimize the number of women screened who are referred for further tests	a) The percentage of women who are referred for assessment	Prevalent screen <10% Incident screen <7%	Prevalent screen <7% Incident screen <5%
	b) The percentage of women screened who are placed on short-term recall	<0.25%	≤0.12%
6. To minimize the number of women undergoing repeat examinations	The number of repeat examinations	<3% of total examinations	<2% of total examinations
7. To ensure that the majority of cancers, both palpable and impalpable, receive a non-operative tissue diagnosis of cancer	The percentage of women who have a non-operative diagnosis of by needle histology after a maximum of two attempts		
	a) Invasive cancers	≥90%	≥95%
	b) Non-invasive cancers	>85%	>90%
8. To minimize diagnostic delay for women who are diagnosed non-operatively	Proportion of women for whom the time interval between non-operative biopsy and result is 1 wk or less	≥90%	100%
9. To minimize the number of unnecessary operative procedures	The rate of benign biopsies	Prevalent round <1.5/1000 Incident round <1.0/1000	Prevalent round <1.0/1000 Incident round <0.75/1000
10. To minimize the delay for women who require surgical assessment	Proportion of women for whom the time interval between the decision to refer to a surgeon and surgical assessment is a wk or less	≥90%	100%
11. To minimize any delay for women who require treatment for screen-detected breast cancer	The percentage of women who are admitted for treatment within 2 months of their first assessment visit	≥90%	100%

(Continued)

Table 12.2 Key NHSBSP Quality Assurance Standards (*Continued*)

Objective	Criteria	Minimum Standard	Target
(B) Standards designed to maximize benefit			
12. To maximize the number of eligible women who attend for screening	The percentage of eligible women who attend for screening	≥70% of invited women attend for screening	80% of invited women attend for screening
13. To ensure that women are recalled for screening at appropriate intervals	The percentage of eligible women whose first offered appointment is within 36 months of their previous screen	≥90%	100%
14. To maximize the number of cancers detected	a) The rate of invasive cancers detected in eligible women invited and screened.	Prevalent screen ≥3.6/1000 Incident screen ≥4.1/1000	Prevalent screen ≥5.1/1000 Incident screen ≥5.7/1000
	b) The rate of cancers detected which are *in situ* carcinoma	Prevalent screen ≥0.5/1000 Incident screen ≥0.6/1000	
	c) Standardized detection ratio (SDR) for invasive cancers	≥1.0	≥1.4
15. To maximize the number of small invasive cancers detected	The rate of invasive cancers <15 mm in diameter detected in eligible women invited and screened	Prevalent screen ≥2.0/1000 Incident screen ≥2.3 /1000	Prevalent screen ≥2.8/1000 Incident screen ≥3.1/1000
16. To minimize the number of cancers in the women screened presenting between screening episodes	The rate of cancers presenting in screened women a) In the 2 yrs following a normal screening episode	Expected Standard 1.2/1000 women screened in the first 2 yrs	
	b) In the 3rd yr following a normal screening episode	1.3 women/1000 women screened in the 3rd yr	

those that are designed to maximize benefit. Together with the installation of at least one digital mammography unit and the need for all film readers to have a minimum annual workload of 5000 films, four of these standards (round length, time from screen to results, recall to assessment rate, and repeat examination rate) have in turn been selected for additional attention by the NHSBSP's National Office in connection with the roll-out of the most recent age expansion.

Minimizing Risk

The importance of minimizing unnecessary risk is an important feature of screening QA as the majority of those invited for screening will be free from disease and will thus receive little benefit (other than reassurance) from the screening process. It is also important in this context to find the right balance of sensitivity (i.e., maximizing the identification of women who have cancer in the population invited for screening) and specificity (i.e., ensuring that women without cancer are not invited back for further investigations). This inevitably means that the screening process cannot be "perfect," and that unnecessary stress is caused to some women who are recalled to assessment only to be placed on normal recall.

One major area of risk is the danger from excess radiation exposure due to faulty equipment. This is minimized through routine quality control measurements undertaken by radiographers, and regular surveys carried out by external medical physics services which can lead to equipment being suspended from use. Excess radiation exposure is also minimized by setting a standard limiting the number of women who have to have additional mammograms because of technical errors. A second area of concern is the frequency of unnecessary surgical treatment and the risks associated with general anesthesia. This is minimized by monitoring non-operative diagnosis and benign open biopsy rates. Finally, it is important to take into account the stress that may be caused to women as a result of the screening process. Upper limits on the proportion of women recalled for assessment or placed on early recall, and process standards measuring time to results, time to assessment, time between the first assessment appointment and surgical assessment, and waiting times for therapeutic surgery are designed to minimize this type of risk.

Maximizing Benefit

Of the standards included to maximize the benefits of screening, the most important are cancer detection rates (particularly for small cancers less than 15 mm in diameter), uptake rates, screening round length, and interval cancer rates. Cancer detection rates are now usually expressed as age-standardized detection ratios (SDRs) which compare the sensitivity for the detection of invasive cancers with the equivalent that would have been achieved by the Swedish Two-County Randomized Controlled Trial (2,20). Detection of small early-stage cancers is vital. Initially, the minimum standards set for the SDRs for all cancers and small cancers were that they should be greater than or equal to 0.75 (i.e., cancer detection rates should be at least three-quarters of those achieved by the Swedish Two-County Randomized Controlled trial) with target SDRs of greater than or equal to 1.0. In 2011, with the increasing baseline incidence of breast cancer in the UK and the expansion of the NHSBSP to include women aged 65–70 years, the minimum standards for the SDRs

of all cancers and small cancers were increased to greater than or equal to 1.0 and the targets to greater than or equal to 1.4 (item 14 in Table 12.2). In 2009–2010, the overall SDR for the NHSBSP in women aged 50–70 years was 1.44 (15).

Uptake (attendance) rates are important because, if only a small proportion of eligible women attend for screening, high cancer detection rates will have little influence on overall cancer mortality and survival of women in the screening age band. As underlying breast cancer incidence is higher in the most affluent women who are the most likely to attend for screening (21,22), breast screening services in areas with relatively low uptake rates may need to take uptake and socioeconomic status into account when using SDRs to monitor performance. Joint studies with the local cancer registry to determine screening histories for all women in the screening age band diagnosed with breast cancer may provide additional insights into the efficacy of the screening program through the calculation of mortality and survival rates in non-attenders and lapsed attenders, and in women with screen-detected breast cancer (23).

The screening round length standard monitors the proportion of women who receive a subsequent appointment for screening within 36 months of their last screen, and gives an indication of whether or not the screening program is running on schedule. If the screening round length is too long, more cancers may develop between screens and the cancers detected may be of a later stage and may therefore require more radical treatment. Interval cancer rates are important because they measure the number of cancers that are diagnosed symptomatically between screens and hence give an indication of the total number of cancers that might have been detected had the NHSBSP been more effective. However, with the current technology and screening round length, some interval cancers are inevitable. Thus, some cancers are radiologically occult and as such are not visible on mammograms, and "true" interval cancers are not visible on previous screens having developed between three-year screening rounds. The roll-out of digital mammography that is currently taking place across the UK NHSBSP may improve the sensitivity of the screening process.

USING QA TO ENCOURAGE IMPROVED PERFORMANCE AND CHANGES IN PRACTICE

Key features of QA include peer review breast screening QA visits and the sharing of comparative outcome data to enable professionals to see and discuss their performance relative to that of their peers coupled with constructive discussion concerning the reasons for poor outcomes. These processes must be carried out in a non-confrontational environment, and a climate of mutual trust and honesty is essential if service improvement is to be achieved. The main purpose of QA should not be to allocate blame, but to work with service providers to find the reasons for failure to meet national standards and to agree on mechanisms for improvement. The success of this approach is illustrated by the improvements in outcome measures that have been recorded since the introduction of the NHSBSP.

Improved Data Quality

If meaningful outcome measures are to be calculated, data quality is of paramount importance. The data collected by the NHSBSP are now recognized to be amongst the most complete and most accurate in the world. This has been achieved by having a single standardized computer software system on which to collect the data, and by ensuring that the screening office staff members are fully trained in its use. In addition, the introduction of standard reporting forms for pathology and surgery has markedly enhanced the quality of the diagnostic and treatment data. Further improvements have resulted from the involvement of regional QARCs in the pre-processing of KC62 and KC63 returns prior to their submission to the NHSIC to ensure that the information on screening unit computer systems is accurately and completely recorded. By feeding these collated comparative data back to screening services, QARCs can stimulate local discussion about the efficacy of data transfer to the screening office computer system and highlight deficiencies in the recording of clinical details in patient notes or on the NHSBSP's structured reporting forms. The improvements in data quality that these processes have brought about are particularly well illustrated by the completeness of nodal status data for invasive breast cancers which has increased from only 58% in 1992–1993 to 99% in 2009–2010.

Round Length

Monthly round length data are now collected on a routine basis by each QARC for submission to the NHSBSP's National Office. The data are obtained directly from screening office computer systems which are accessed via the NHS Net. Comparative data for the region and for each service are fed back to the QARC and to screening services each month. If a screening service has failed to meet the 90% minimum standard (item 14 in Table 12.2), an explanation is requested by the QARC. Breast screening services which have consistently failed to meet this minimum standard are not able to roll out the most recent age extension.

Non-Operative Diagnosis

Besides having a significant impact at the local and regional level, screening QA initiatives have brought about changes in practice at the national level. One of the best examples of this is the increase in the non-operative diagnosis rate for screen-detected breast cancers that has been demonstrated by the NHSBSP/ABS audit. Between 1996–1997 and 2010–2011, the overall non-operative diagnosis rate increased from 63% to 96%, largely because of the introduction of wide bore needle or tru-cut biopsy (core biopsy) as a non-operative diagnosis technique.

As the non-operative diagnosis rate for invasive breast cancers has leveled off at 98%, attention has turned to the lower non-operative diagnosis rate achieved for non-invasive breast cancers and the method by which a non-operative diagnosis was obtained. In 2009 (10), separate targets and standards were introduced for non-operative diagnosis of invasive and non-invasive breast cancers (item 7 in Table 12.2), and more detailed analyses of individual screening unit performance have been introduced into the NHSBSP/ABS audit. Figure 12.1 shows the variations between screening units in the proportion of non-invasive breast cancers with a non-operative diagnosis in the screening year 2010–2011. As part of the QA audit cycle, each year following the publication of such audit data, QARCs and Surgical QA Coordinators investigate why screening units in their region fail to meet the 85% minimum standard. Examples of unusual diagnostic practice highlighted by the NHSBSP/ABS audit are also investigated. For example, in 2010–11, although only 54 breast cancers were diagnosed by cytology alone compared with 1934 in 2000–2001, in five screening units more than 40% of breast cancers were diagnosed using both cytology and core biopsy. More detailed local audits are used by QARCs and their Radiology QA Coordinators to ascertain the reasons for such atypical practice.

Open Biopsies

As routine audit has developed to become a key component of screening QA, more sophisticated methods of examining the performance of individual screening services have been introduced. For example, as the non-operative diagnosis rate has increased from 63% in 1996–1997 to 96% in 2010–2011, the

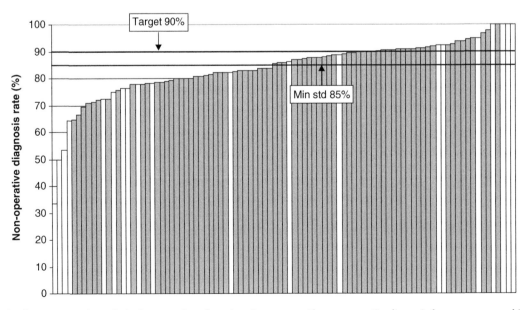

Figure 12.1 Variation between screening units in the proportion of non-invasive cancers with a non-operative diagnosis for women screened in 2010–2011. The 20 smallest units are highlighted in white.

malignant open biopsy rate has decreased from 2.04 to 0.32 per 1000 women screened. These results suggest that the majority of malignant cases are being picked up non-operatively leaving behind a residue of difficult cases where a definitive diagnosis can only be obtained from a surgical excision specimen. However, more detailed analyses using control charts to examine variations in practice between screening units in 2010–2011 identified four units with significantly higher numbers of invasive cancers where the worst non-operative result was C4/B4 (suspicious of malignancy) during the three-year period 2008–2009 to 2010–2011. It is possible, therefore, that more cancers could have been picked up by these units prior to open biopsy, and more detailed local audits can again be used by QARCs and their Radiology and Pathology QA Co-ordinators to ascertain if this is indeed the case.

Surgical Practice

Control charts can also be used to examine differences in surgical practice between screening units and individual surgeons. This approach is illustrated in Figures 12.2 and 12.3 which show the variation between screening units and surgeons respectively in the proportion of cancers in the three-year period 2008–2009 to 2010–2011 which were initially treated with breast conserving surgery and then patients underwent re-excision to clear margins. In these charts, the dashed lines are the upper and lower control limits which

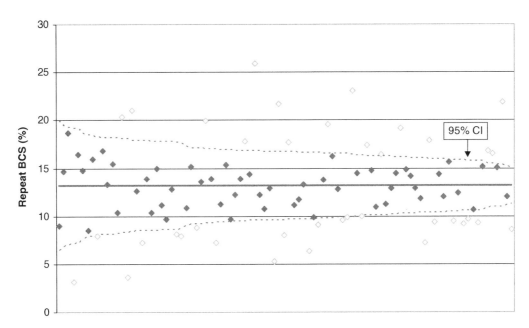

Figure 12.2 Variation between screening units in the proportion of cancers which were initially treated with a breast conserving surgery (BCS) and had a repeat BCS to clear margins in the 3-year period 2008–2009 to 2010–2011.

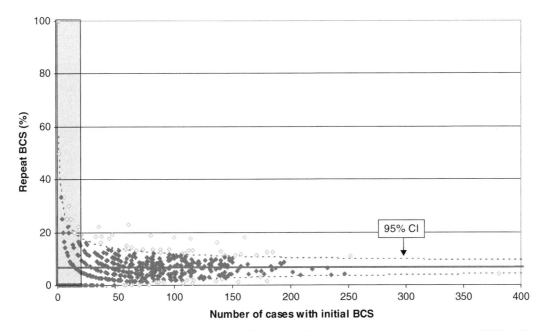

Figure 12.3 Variation between surgeons in the proportions of cancers which were initially treated with breast conserving surgery (BCS) and had re-excisions to clear margins in the 3-year period 2008–2009 to 2010–2011. Surgeons who initially treated fewer than 20 cases with breast conserving surgery in the 3-year period are shaded.

approximate to the 95% confidence intervals of the average rates (13.2% and 6.7%, respectively) depicted by the solid line. Sixteen screening units and 34 of the 440 surgeons who had 20 or more cases with initial breast conserving surgery had repeat operation rates above the upper control limits. Twenty two screening units and 19 surgeons had repeat rates below the lower control limits. Sophisticated analyses such as these allow QARCs and Surgical QA Coordinators to investigate the reasons for unusual practice by some of their screening units and surgeons. It is important to remember when examining control charts, that "outliers" above and/or below the control limits may represent practices that are potentially beneficial or potentially detrimental to the women treated. If the data demonstrate evidence of good clinical practice, these results should be disseminated more widely to encourage take-up by others and to improve the outcomes for more women. On the other hand, evidence of poor clinical practice must be raised with the appropriate authorities, generally the screening unit director in the first instance, with escalation to the host organization's medical director and/or clinical governance lead, if necessary.

Adjuvant Therapy

Although oncologists are not included in regional QA teams, they are important members of the multidisciplinary teams in each screening unit. Therefore, audits of oncologic practice should be included in the QA audit portfolio. Figures 12.4 and 12.5 illustrate the type of information that has been obtained through the inclusion since 2002 of a retrospective adjuvant therapy component to the NHSBSP/ABS audit. It is generally recognized that invasive breast cancers treated with breast conserving surgery should receive adjuvant radiotherapy to

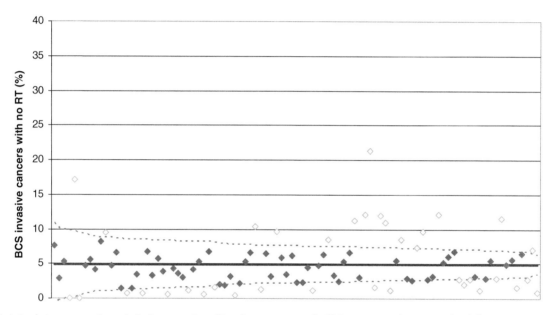

Figure 12.4 Variation between screening units in the proportion of invasive cancers treated with breast conserving surgery that did not receive radiotherapy in the 3-year period 2007–2008 to 2009–2010. Open diamonds represent units which lie outside the control limits.

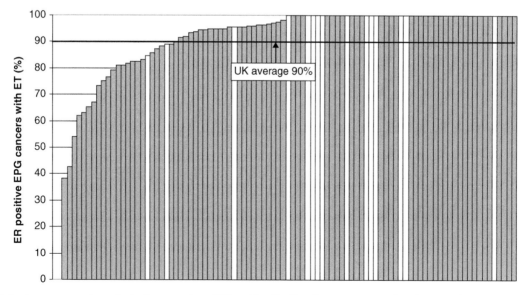

Figure 12.5 Variation between screening units in the proportion of ER-positive, Excellent Prognostic Group (EPG) cancers that had endocrine therapy (ET) recorded in 2010–2011. The 20 smallest units are highlighted in white.

the breast (24). In 2009–2010, of the 9829 invasive cancers treated with breast conserving surgery, 384 (4%) did not have adjuvant radiotherapy recorded. Of these, 16% were larger than 20 mm in diameter, 13% were grade 3 and 14% were node positive. The proportion of conservatively treated invasive breast cancers that did not have adjuvant radiotherapy varied from none in 15 screening units to more than 21% in one screening unit and more than 15% in two other units.

The significance of the variation between screening units in the proportion of invasive breast cancers treated with breast conserving surgery without radiation therapy over the three-year period 2007–2008 to 2009–2010 is examined in the control chart in Figure 12.4 in which the dashed lines are the upper and lower control limits which approximate to the 95% confidence intervals of the average rate (solid line). Sixteen units lie above the upper control limit and have significantly lower rates of radiotherapy. Eight of these units are in two regions of England. The two regional QARCs and their Surgical QA Coordinators are carrying out further work with these screening units in order to understand the reasons for this unusual clinical practice.

It is generally recognized that endocrine therapy is beneficial to women diagnosed with estrogen receptor (ER) positive invasive breast cancers (24). In 2010–2011, in the UK as a whole, 499 (4%) of ER-positive invasive cancers had no endocrine therapy recorded. Fifty-six (11%) of these cancers were grade 3, 45 (9%) were node positive, and 47 (9%) were larger than 20 mm in diameter. The proportion of ER-positive invasive breast cancers which did not have endocrine therapy recorded varied from none in 22 screening units to more than 20% in three units.

One reason for not treating ER-positive breast cancers with endocrine therapy could be when the risk–benefit balance is less clear cut, as might be the case for very early-stage breast cancers. Figure 12.5 shows how the proportion of ER-positive cancers in the Nottingham Prognostic Index (25) Excellent Prognostic Group (EPG) that were treated with endocrine therapy varied between screening units. In the UK as a whole, 90% of these cancers did receive endocrine therapy, but in 25 screening units, the rate fell below the 90% UK average. When the significance of the variation between screening units in the proportion of ER positive invasive breast cancers in the EPG which did not have endocrine therapy over the three-year period 2007–2008 to 2009–2010 is examined in a control chart (not shown), 15 units are low outliers. Seven of these screening units are in two regions of England. Once again, QARCs and Surgical QA Coordinators are working with these 15 units to establish the reason for their unusual clinical practice.

CONCLUSION

There is considerable evidence that breast cancer screening (26) and the NHSBSP in particular (27) can significantly affect breast cancer mortality in women in the screening age band. Steadily improving SDRs suggest that the influence of the NHSBSP on breast cancer mortality rates should increase in the future. QA has contributed to this success by encouraging improvements in performance and changes in practice through peer review and the sharing of comparative outcome data between the professional groups providing the screening service. Many of the principles of breast screening QA are now

being adopted in policies designed to improve the general quality of the UK's health services. The introduction of the concept of clinical governance in the *NHS Cancer Plan* in 2000 (28) and the encouragement of the development of a "no blame culture" in which organizations can learn from their experiences (29,30) are both extensions of these principles. It will be important to ensure that these similarities are recognized and that the wealth of expertise developed by those working within breast screening QA is shared with and built upon by those in the wider health service community.

ACKNOWLEDGMENTS

The author thanks all the staff members working in NHS Breast Screening Programme screening units and QA reference centres, and Surgical QA Coordinators for ensuring that the routine data used to monitor the performance of the UK NHSBSP are of the highest quality. Also, the author is grateful to the NHSBSP and the Association of Breast Surgery (ABS) for giving their permission for reproducing some of the results and figures from the 2011 NHSBSP/ABS audit of screen-detected cancers in this chapter.

REFERENCES

1. Breast Cancer Screening: Report to the Health Ministers of England, Wales, Scotland and Northern Ireland by a working group chaired by Professor Sir Patrick Forrest. London: Department of Health and Social Security, 1986.
2. Tabar L, Fagerberg CJ, Gad A, et al. Reduction in mortality from breast cancer after mass screening with mammography. Randomised trial from the breast cancer screening working group of the Swedish National Board of Health and Welfare. Lancet 1985; 1: 829–32.
3. The Health of the Nation: a Strategy for Health in England. Department of Health London: HMSO, 1992.
4. Evaluating the age extension of the NHS Breast Screening Programme. [Available from: www.controlled-trials.com/ISRCTN33292440].
5. Quality Assurance Guidelines for Administrative and Clerical Staff. NHSBSP Publication No. 47 Sheffield: NHS Cancer Screening Programmes, 2000.
6. Quality Assurance Guidelines for Mammography: Including Radiographic Quality Control. NHSBSP Publication No. 30 Sheffield: NHS Cancer Screening Programmes, 2006.
7. Quality Assurance Guidelines for Medical Physics Services. NHSBSP Publication No. 33 2nd edn. Sheffield: NHS Cancer Screening Programmes, 2005.
8. Quality Assurance Guidelines for Breast Screening Radiology. NHSBSP Publication No. 59 2nd edn. Sheffield: NHS Cancer Screening Programmes, 2011.
9. Quality Assurance Guidelines for Breast Pathology Services. NHSBSP Publication No. 2 2nd edn. Sheffield: NHS Cancer Screening Programmes, 2011.
10. Quality Assurance Guidelines for Surgeons in Breast Cancer Screening. NHSBSP Publication No. 20 4th edn. Sheffield: NHS Cancer Screening Programmes, 2009.
11. Quality Assurance Guidelines for Nurses in Breast Cancer Screening. NHSBSP Publication No. 29 4th edn. Sheffield: NHS Cancer Screening Programmes, 2008.
12. NHSBSP Guidelines on Quality Assurance Visits. NHSBSP Publication No. 40 2nd edn. Sheffield: NHS Cancer Screening Programmes, 2000.
13. EL(97)67. Cancer Screening: Quality Assurance and Management. London: NHS Executive, 1997.
14. NHS Breast Screening Programme Annual Review 2011. Sheffield: NHS Cancer Screening Programmes, 2011.
15. Breast Screening Programme - England, 2010–11. London: NHS Health and Social Care Information Centre, 2012.
16. An Audit of Screen Detected Breast Cancers for the Year of Screening April 2010 to March 2011. London: NHS Breast Screening Programme and Association of Breast Surgery, 2012.

17. Breast Cancer Clinical Outcome Measures (BCCOM Project: Analysis of the Management of Symptomatic Breast Cancers Diagnosed in 2004. 3rd Year Report. Birmingham: West Midlands Cancer Intelligence Unit and Breakthrough Breast Cancer, 2007.

18. Investigation into the West of London Breast Screening Service at Hammersmith Hospitals NHS Trust. London: Commission for Health Improvement, 2002.

19. Consolidated Guidance on Standards for the NHSBSP. NHSBSP Publication No. 60 2nd edn. Sheffield: NHS Cancer Screening Programmes, 2005.

20. Blanks RG, Day NE, Moss SM. Monitoring the performance of breast screening programmes: use of indirect standardisation in evaluating the invasive cancer detection rate. J Med Screen 1996; 3: 79–81.

21. Chiu LF. Inequalities of Access to Cancer Screening: A Literature Review. Cancer Screening Series No. 1. Sheffield: NHS cancer Screening Programmes, 2003.

22. The Second All Breast Cancer Report: Focussing on Inequalities: Variation in Breast Cancer Outcomes with Age and Deprivation. Birmingham: West Midlands Cancer Intelligence Unit, 2011.

23. Lawrence GM, Kearins O, O'Sullivan E, et al. The West Midlands Breast Cancer Screening Status Algorithm – Methodology and Use as an Audit Tool. J Med Screen 2005; 12: 179–84.

24. Breast Cancer (Early and Locally Advanced): Diagnosis and Treatment. Clinical Guideline 80. London: National Institute for Health and Clinical Excellence, 2009.

25. Galea MH, Blamey RW, Elston CE, et al. The Nottingham prognostic index in primary breast cancer. Breast Cancer Res Treat 1992; 22: 207–19.

26. Nystrom L, Andersson I, Bjurstam N, et al. Long-term effects of mammography screening: updated overview of the swedish randomised trials. Lancet 2002; 359: 909–19.

27. Blanks RG, Moss SM, McGahan CE, et al. Effect of NHS breast screening programme on mortality from breast cancer in England and Wales, 1990–8: comparison of observed with predicted mortality. Br Med J 2000; 321: 665–9.

28. The NHS Cancer Plan: A Plan for Investment, a Plan for Reform. London: Department of Health, 2000.

29. An Organisation with a Memory: Report of an Expert Group on Learning from Adverse Events in the NHS Chaired by the Chief Medical Officer. London: Department of Health, 2000.

30. Building a Safer NHS for Patients: Implementing an Organisation with a Memory. London: Department of Health, 2001.

13 Clinical assessment of symptomatic patients

J. Mathew and K.L. Cheung

INTRODUCTION

Breast cancer presents either symptomatically or through screening. Depending on the local healthcare system, symptomatic patients may first be assessed by their family physicians (otherwise known as general practitioners) who then decide whether a specialist referral to a breast unit is required. The logical approach to a patient presenting to a symptomatic breast clinic is clinical evaluation of the presenting problem. Radiology also plays an important role in accurate and timely diagnosis of breast pathology in these patients, and some centers undertake radiological imaging before clinical assessment in patients presenting to symptomatic breast clinics. In contrast, with a screening program, the starting point is always radiological imaging, although patients are called back on occasions for radiological or clinical reasons, and at this point clinical assessment is performed in most cases.

This chapter focuses on the clinical assessment of breast symptoms as a possible presentation of breast cancer. Occasionally breast cancer may present symptomatically with features of local and/or regional recurrence, or metastatic disease, rather than with a symptom in the breast (e.g., breast lump) which are aspects beyond the scope of this chapter.

TRIPLE ASSESSMENT

Before the advent of triple assessment, all breast lumps were removed by surgical excision as there was no other reliable way to establish a diagnosis. Triple assessment allows us to make an accurate diagnosis in almost all cases without resorting to surgical biopsy. Triple assessment is a combination of (*i*) clinical assessment (dominated by clinical breast examination); (*ii*) radiological assessment (normally ultrasonography and/or mammography); and (*iii*) pathological assessment [normally needle core biopsy and/or fine needle aspiration cytology (FNAC)]. Conclusions are drawn following each assessment as follows: normal, benign, indeterminate, suspicious, or malignant. The result of pathological assessment is interpreted according to the "worse" conclusion of the clinical and radiological assessments. In other words, in order to safely arrive at a final diagnosis, the result of the biopsy (or cytology as appropriate) must concur with the "worse" assessment outcome; neither clinical nor radiological assessment can override one another. Otherwise, further investigation will need to be carried out, as explained in the coming sections.

Since the introduction of FNAC to the breast clinic in the early 1980s, the rate of surgical excision biopsy has significantly decreased. However, even in combination with mammography FNAC is not always sufficiently sensitive to exclude malignancy, particularly in younger women (1). The overall false negative rate of triple assessment in the breast clinic is between 1.4% (2) and 4% (3). There must be consistency between each component; otherwise further investigations (e.g., repeat needle biopsy, surgical excision biopsy etc.) must be carried out. There are some features of these individual assessments that overlap in terms of benign and malignant breast disease and combination of the three significantly improves the diagnostic accuracy. The sensitivity of clinical examination and mammography varies with age. One-third of the cancers identified in patients less than 50 years are deemed not to be suspicious or malignant on clinical examination or mammography (4).

Breast cancer in young women is a particular problem as it often presents with asymmetrical nodularity or thickening rather than a discrete lump.

Sensitivity of clinical examination varies among clinicians and may lie somewhere between 45% and 65% (5). Mammogram and ultrasound have a sensitivity of 86% and 90% respectively (4). In spite of the diagnostic accuracy of radiological assessment, there are situations where clinical assessment is crucial. This is especially true when there is discrepancy between radiological and clinical assessment, that is, clinically suspicious or malignant while radiologically benign, and also in some radiologically occult tumors. These patients need further evaluation and may require repeat needle biopsies or even surgical excision biopsy if the core biopsies are inconclusive.

Over the last decade, core biopsy has replaced FNAC and has several distinctive advantages (6). FNAC has a false-positive rate of 0.2–0.5% (4) and a small number will have C3 (atypia of uncertain significance) lesions. In a study by Bak and colleagues on more than 1300 women undergoing FNAC for over 47,000 mammographically non-negative lesions, approximately 7.8% had C3 lesions (7). Lesions most likely to be misinterpreted are fibroadenomas, papillary lesions, and areas of breast tissue that have been irradiated. FNAC also has a false negative rate of 4–5% (4) and a proportion of samples are interpreted to have inadequate amounts of material to produce an accurate diagnosis (the "C1" category). Core biopsies on the other hand allow multiple cores of tissue to be sampled from the area of abnormality providing a histological diagnosis and in particular can differentiate between invasive and *in situ* carcinoma. Other information about the tumor (e.g., grade, type, lymphovascular permeation, estrogen receptor (ER), and human epidermal receptor 2 (HER2) status) may be obtained which potentially benefits treatment planning. The use of image-guided (generally using ultrasound) biopsies which is the gold standard now, allows multiple cores of tissue to be sampled accurately from the area of concern and is almost 100% accurate (8). However in certain situations where the lesion is clinically suspicious or malignant and the biopsy is benign, a repeat core biopsy or an ultrasound guided vacuum-assisted biopsy of the lesion is done. Vacuum-assisted biopsy allows more tissue or even the entire lesion to be biopsied and/or removed. In benign conditions like fibroadenoma, the vacuum-assisted biopsy could be therapeutic as well as diagnostic (9). If malignancy is proven, further excision needs to be planned following vacuum-assisted biopsy. In certain situations where repeat core biopsies are suspicious but not malignant, a diagnostic surgical excision biopsy is indicated.

CLINICAL ASSESSMENT
History
A brief history is taken in every patient before clinical examination and it is also an opportunity to develop a rapport with the patient. The commonest presenting complaint is a breast lump and the required history to be taken is shown in Table 13.1. The duration of symptoms often provides a clue to likely diagnosis as cysts may appear overnight compared with solid lesions which are slower growing. Some benign breast lumps have a cyclical pattern to them.

There are numerous risk factors for breast cancer, the history of which may not influence the clinician in terms of reaching a diagnosis in patients presenting to a symptomatic breast clinic. However it is valuable to know the probable risk factors for cancer, which will help alleviate some of the concerns raised by patients and guide provision of appropriate advice to those making informed decisions about management of their risk. Most importantly, the symptomatic breast clinic serves as an opportunity to identify patients who are at a significantly higher risk of developing breast cancer so that they may be referred for further detailed risk assessment, including genetic counseling as appropriate.

In this section, history which is generally applicable to all breast patients is discussed while specific questions related to presenting symptoms (e.g., inflammation) will be dealt with later in the chapter.

Age
Age is one of the most important risk factors for breast cancer. Breast cancer is uncommon before the age of 30 years but rises rapidly until 40 years and thereafter continues to increase in

prevalence at a slower rate (10). Age also influences the appropriate choice of radiological and pathological assessment. For instance, mammography is seldom considered in women younger than 35 years due to the density of the breast tissue. The value of screening mammography (which is often carried out in a symptomatic breast clinic if the patient falls within the appropriate age range) is debatable in women under the age of 40 and in their 70s and beyond (11,12). Pathological assessment may be omitted in very young women (e.g., late teens and early 20s) if the presenting lump has clinical and ultrasonographic features which are typical for a fibroadenoma.

Family History
Hereditary is probably one of the most important risk factors for breast cancer, with up to 10% of breast cancers having a strong genetic predisposition. Patients with bilateral breast cancer, those with family members (especially multiple members on the same side of the family) who develop a combination of breast cancer and another epithelial cancer (e.g., ovarian) or breast cancer in an "unusual" manner (e.g., in a man), and women who get the disease at an early age are most likely to be carrying a genetic mutation that has predisposed them to developing breast cancer. Susceptibility to breast cancer is generally inherited as an autosomal dominant trait with limited penetrance. Many genes are known to be involved in the development of breast cancer. Deleterious mutations in BRCA1 (13,14), and BRCA2 (15) are well known for conferring an increased lifetime risk of breast and ovarian cancer. BRCA1 and BRCA2 are located on the long arms of chromosomes 17 and 13, respectively. The prevalence of a BRCA1/2 mutation is estimated to be 1/800 in the general population. The lifetime risk of breast cancer in women with BRCA1 and BRCA2 mutations varies from 56% to as high as 80–85% (16–18). The probability of detecting a deleterious mutation in BRCA1 or BRCA2 is higher when there is a family history of both breast and ovarian cancer compared with either breast or ovarian cancer alone (17). Of note, BRCA 1 mutations are found in 75% of families with both breast and ovarian cancers in a single individual.

Age of onset of breast cancer is also important as early age of onset (diagnosed at the age of 40 years or younger) of breast cancer is more likely to be associated with a deleterious mutation (19). Women with inherited susceptibility generally have breast cancer at a younger age. As cancer evolves from a multistep process with several mutations rather than one, a smaller number of genetic changes are required in those patients with an inherited genetic predisposition to reach the threshold for malignancy. Thus the inherited form of breast cancer is likely to occur earlier, and among women with sporadic breast cancer the incidence peaks one or two decades later than those who have detectable mutations.

Women who carry an abnormal ataxia telangiectasia (AT) gene have an increased risk of breast cancer (20,21). Inherited mutations in two other genes, p53 and PTEN, are associated with familial syndromes (Li-Fraumeni and Cowden's, respectively) that include a high risk for breast cancer but both syndromes are rare.

Lastly, the age of the patient in the symptomatic breast clinic is also relevant. Despite a potentially significant family history, the chance of the patient having a genetic predisposition herself depends on her age and relationship with the affected

---

Table 13.1 History of Patients Presenting with a Breast Lump

History
General
  Age
  Duration
Risk Factors
Family history
Previous breast disease
  Exposure to radiation
  Drugs: OCP/HRT
Other relevant history
  Comorbidities
  Anticoagulants

Abbreviations: HRT, hormone replacement therapy; OCP, oral contraceptive pill.

relatives. For instance, an elderly patient is likely to have "escaped" the influence and a patient with a cluster of breast cancer cases in a few very distant relatives is less likely to belong to a high risk group.

As a "rule of thumb," having a first-degree relative with unilateral breast cancer at the age of 40, in the absence of any other known factors, yields an approximate relative risk of four times (borderline moderate risk category) (22). Therefore, the presence of any scenario "worse" than this would justify referral to a local family history service for more formal evaluation of risk.

Previous Breast Disease
Patients who have had previous breast cancer are at a higher risk for development of breast cancer in the opposite (contralateral) breast. Those patients with atypical ductal hyperplasia, lobular hyperplasia, and lobular carcinoma *in situ* are at high risk for development of breast cancer. Women with severe atypical epithelial hyperplasia have over five times the risk of developing breast cancer than women who do not have any proliferative changes in their breasts (23). Women with palpable cysts, complex fibroadenomas, duct papillomas, sclerosing adenosis, and moderate or florid epithelial hyperplasia have a slightly higher risk of breast cancer (1.5–3 times) than women without these changes, but this increase (less than four times relative risk) is not clinically important to warrant any intervention (4).

Knowing that there is a past history of breast surgery allows the clinician to consider possible recurrence of a previously treated or inadequately treated condition (e.g., benign phyllodes tumor excised with involved margins). It should also be borne in mind that scar tissue from previous surgery can affect the interpretation of clinical (e.g., skin tethering) and/or radiological (e.g., distortion seen on mammogram) signs.

Radiation
The relationship between ionizing radiation and the risk of breast cancer is well established (24,25). Increased risk has been observed in patients receiving fluoroscopy for tuberculosis and radiation treatment for medical conditions. The risk is inversely associated with age at exposure. Women treated for Hodgkin's disease by the age of 16 have a subsequent risk of developing breast cancer as high as 35% by the age of 40 years (26,27). Higher dose of radiation and treatment between the ages of 10 and 16 are associated with a higher risk. The risk of breast cancer is also raised when radiation therapy was administered in the late teens and 20s, but to a lesser degree. With these studies, the majority of breast cancers (85–100%) developed either within the field of radiation or at the margin (28).

Oral Contraceptives and Hormone Replacement Therapy
Meta-analysis of data from 54 epidemiological studies (53,000 women) on oral contraceptive use and a risk of breast cancer showed that subjects taking oral contraceptives have a slightly increased risk of breast cancer compared with the risk in non-users (29). The risk decreased with increasing years after stopping the oral contraceptives and there was no evidence of increased risk for a breast cancer diagnosis 10 years or more after stopping the use of oral contraceptives. Moreover, breast cancers diagnosed in users of oral contraceptives were less advanced than in never users.

The data linking hormone replacement therapy (HRT) to the risk of breast cancer are extensive (30). Among current users and those who used HRT within 1–4 years previously, the risk of having breast cancer diagnosed increases by 2.3% for each year of usage and the relative risk is 1.35 for women who used HRT for five or more years. However this elevated risk disappears five years after stopping HRT. A randomized controlled primary prevention trial involving over 16,000 postmenopausal women aged 50–79 years receiving combined hormone preparation showed an increased risk of breast cancer in the users of 26%. Data from the Women's Health Initiative study, however, have shown that breast cancers diagnosed in women taking HRT were more likely to be node positive and associated with a higher mortality rate (30). This is contradictory to the previous belief that HRT is associated with cancers of better prognosis. Regardless of the above, the increased risk of breast cancer, following the use of oral contraceptives and/or HRT is low to moderate and currently does not justify further evaluation and additional surveillance as compared with a significant family history as described earlier. The above information serves as a reference guide to inform patients. On the other hand, as will be explained in later sections, the use of HRT may impact on the differential diagnosis of a breast symptom.

Other Relevant History
Some patients diagnosed with cancer are old and frail with multiple comorbid conditions and may not be fit for surgery. They may be eligible for alternative modes of treatment, that is, primary endocrine therapy or radiation treatment. In the setting of the symptomatic breast clinic, obtaining some basic information about general health and support is helpful to guide subsequent decision making, though further detailed assessment is still required, which can be carried out upon confirmation of a breast cancer diagnosis. History of any medication especially anticoagulant (e.g., warfarin) or antiplatelet agents (e.g., clopidogrel) should also be noted as they may influence the appropriateness and/or timing of core biopsy and/or surgical treatment.

Physical Examination
When compared with history, physical examination of the breast has an extremely important role in the diagnostic assessment process. In almost all cases, the conclusion (as part of triple assessment) as to whether a lump is clinically benign or not is based on physical findings rather than history which, as explained earlier, plays a more important role in identifying an at risk population.

Although there may be some variation in the precise techniques (including the order of examining different anatomical areas), the principles of physical examination remain the same and should cover (*i*) introduction [consideration of consent, chaperone, infection control (e.g., use of antiseptic gel) and appropriate exposure]; (*ii*) inspection (sitting position); (*iii*) palpation (lying down position); and (*iv*) examination of other areas [e.g., abdomen, chest, spine, and testes (in a male patient)] as appropriate.

All patients should have both their breasts exposed down to the waist and inspection should take place with the patient's arms by their side, above their head, then pressing on their

Table 13.2 Mandatory Assessment of Core Clinical Skills

Step	Detail
Exposure	Removal of clothing while maintaining patient dignity to expose all of chest including both breasts and arms
Position	Initially standing or sitting upright, then lying at 45 degrees
Inspection at rest	Inspects for skin color and texture, breast shape and symmetry, areolae and nipples with subject at rest
Inspection with arms elevated	Inspects for changes
Inspects with hands on hips	Inspects for changes on pressing hands against hips
Breast palpation	Palpates both breasts gently in all four quadrants using an appropriate technique with the flat of fingers
Axillary palpation	Palpates both axillae in all five areas
Lymph node palpation	Palpates infra/supraclavicular nodes bilaterally
Scope for further examination	Proposes palpating the spine, auscultating the chest, and palpating the liver

hips as shown in Table 13.2 (Mandatory Assessment of Core Clinical Skills used for training and assessing clinical medical students at the University of Nottingham).

The focus of evaluation should be on the presence of asymmetry which could be due to the presence of a mass or a focal area of glandular nodularity, inflammation, or skin changes. Any changes in contour of the breast or any skin dimpling should be carefully looked for. Although usually associated with an underlying malignancy, skin dimpling can follow surgery or trauma, be associated with benign conditions (breast infection), or occur as part of breast involution.

Patients should be lying comfortably on the bed, with one or two pillows to support the head and neck. The arm should initially be placed above the patient's head on the side to be examined (so that the breasts become "flatter," reducing the distance between the skin and the chest wall to allow more accurate palpation of masses) before palpation. Breast tissue is examined with the flat part of the fingers (not the tips). All palpable lesions should be measured with calipers and assigned to a particular quadrant of the breast with relation to the nipple specifically noted. Also the contour and consistency should be assessed along with any fixity to deep structures by asking the patient to press their hands on their hips.

Benign lesions are often smooth and mobile. Subtle signs of cancer include an irregular surface and tethering to the surrounding tissue. Some patients may present with obvious signs of cancer with a hard fixed mass with or without skin involvement or chest wall fixity. Some patients with cancer may present with nipple retraction or inflammatory changes in the breast. However these features are not exclusive to malignancy as some of them overlap with benign disease. For example cysts may feel firm or hard in consistency and patients with benign conditions like periductal mastitis or duct ectasia may present with nipple retraction.

Lymph nodes in the axillary and supraclavicular regions are checked on both sides. Palpation of the axilla is carried out feeling for enlarged nodes in the anterior (behind the edge of the pectoralis major), posterior (in front of the edge of the latissimus dorsi), medial (on the chest wall), lateral (along the proximal humerus), and apical ("deep" down in the high axilla) areas. Once an enlarged axillary lymph node is identified, its size, consistency, and mobility need to be assessed as these features may point to different diagnoses (e.g., reactive lymphadenopathy, lymphoma, metastatic carcinoma) and stage (e.g., fixed lymph nodes imply locally advanced disease).

This part of the examination can often be done relatively easily when the patient is lying down, after completion of breast palpation, but if necessary the patient can be sat up with palpation performed from the front.

SPECIFIC SCENARIOS
Lump
Introduction
The detection of a breast lump in women often causes considerable fear because of a possible breast cancer diagnosis. A methodical and meticulous examination will help ensure that a correct diagnosis is ultimately made.

Clinical Assessment
A young adolescent girl presenting with a breast lump is likely to turn out to have a fibroadenoma which is often slow growing. Breast cysts on the other hand are commonly seen in premenopausal women in their 30s–40s and may appear quite suddenly with patients often complaining of associated pain. Fibroadenomas are freely mobile within the breast tissue ("breast mouse"), multilobulated, and rubbery to touch. Cysts can be discrete and tender, but their consistency is variable and sometimes they are even felt as a hard lump. However they are more likely smooth when compared with cancers which classically have an irregular surface.

Phyllodes tumors are rare and represent only 2.5% of all fibroepithelial lesions (24). They tend to occur 15–20 years later than fibroadenomas and are uncommon in the teenage years. They often grow rapidly and have a high chance of local recurrence after excision (in the region of 20%), which often tends to be incomplete or have close margins. Fewer than 5% of phyllodes tumors metastasize; those which do so behave rather like sarcomas with blood borne metastasis being most common.

Further Diagnostic Assessment
Longstanding fibroadenomas have classical radiological features on both ultrasound and mammography, especially when calcified. Ultrasound-guided biopsy is often done to confirm the diagnosis. However, when diagnosis is in doubt, sometimes ultrasound-guided vacuum-assisted biopsy is employed which can also be a therapeutic option for small fibroadenomas (9). Breast cysts often have characteristic halos on mammography, and ultrasound is diagnostic (anechoic mass with through transmission).

Management

Over a two-year period of observation on patients less than 40 years of age with fibroadenomas, approximately 55% remained the same, 37% decreased in size or disappeared, and 8% increased in size (31). Honest discussion of all three treatment options [no treatment, or excision either surgically or by ultrasound-guided vacuum-assisted technique (mammotome)] is required. Management depends on age, patient preference, and outcome of triple assessment (32). Small to moderate sized (less than 3 cm) fibroadenomas diagnosed on core biopsy can be left alone and reassurance is all that is required. For those patients presenting with multiple fibroadenomas, core biopsies should be taken from the largest lump. Excision is recommended for those fibro-adenomas which are rapidly increasing in size, those which are large (>3–4 cm in size), those that cause significant distortion of the breast profile or when there is an element of histological concern. Excision using a vacuum-assisted biopsy technique is an alternative to open surgery but can be difficult technically if lesions are large, and/or located in "difficult" positions (e.g., very close to the chest wall skin or nipple).

Painful cysts are aspirated and only bloodstained fluid is sent for cytology. After aspiration the breast should be re-examined for any residual mass which requires full assessment as shown in Figure 13.1.

Those patients diagnosed with a phyllodes tumor need surgical excision in the form of breast conserving surgery or mastectomy depending on the size and site of the lesion and patient choice. Despite being the preferred choice of treatment, breast conservation surgery can yield a high percentage of cases with incomplete excision margins that require revisional surgery (33). Radiation treatment has been evaluated in a recent report by Barth and colleagues and found to significantly reduce the local recurrence rate for borderline and malignant tumors after breast conservation surgery with negative margins (34). Nonetheless, the role of radiation treatment in the management of phyllodes tumors remains to be established.

Asymmetrical Thickening

Introduction

Some patients especially those in their 30s and 40s may present with a thickening rather than a true discrete lump. Approximately 10% of all breast cancers present as asymmetrical nodularity rather than a discrete mass and these patients pose a particular challenge to clinicians.

Clinical Assessment

The clinician needs to differentiate between whether the nodularity is asymmetrical or is part of generalized nodularity. Generalized nodularity is ill-defined, often bilateral, and tends to fluctuate with the menstrual cycle; further investigations are generally not required. Asymmetrical thickening could be due to an underlying sinister condition, and must be fully investigated.

One other differential diagnosis is traumatic fat necrosis, although a history of trauma is present in a minority of cases. Seat belt trauma to the breast following a road traffic accident is one of the common causes. The mass may be similar on palpation and imaging to that of breast cancer which it typically mimics. Sometimes bruising is evident in cases of fat necrosis,

although some patients with an underlying cancer may have bruising which becomes apparent only following trauma.

Further Diagnostic Assessment

Mammography is often not useful for assessment of these young groups of patients and an ultrasound scan may or may not identify a lump. Mammography should nonetheless still be performed except in very young patients (namely <35 years) where increased breast density renders it generally insensitive. Mammography may also detect suspicious microcalcifications associated with ductal carcinoma *in situ* which can present as asymmetrical thickening. If an abnormality (e.g., a mass lesion) is identified on ultrasound and/or a mammogram, this should be further investigated with an image-guided needle biopsy. If not, a clinical core biopsy should be undertaken.

Management

In most cases, normal breast tissue or benign fibrocystic change is found on histology in the absence of any focal mass lesion or other radiological abnormality; important potentially sinister conditions to exclude are invasive lobular carcinoma and ductal carcinoma *in situ*. The incidence of cancer in these patients is around 8% and is mostly seen in patients over the age of 35 years (35). In a study reported by one of the authors involving 116 women with asymmetrical thickening, a total of nine (7.8%) cancers were found. The chance of cancer was more likely when the patient was older than 43 years or when thickening was particularly marked ($p < 0.04$) (35).

Inflammatory Conditions

Introduction

Breast infection is a relatively common problem and can be broadly divided into lactational and non-lactational cases (36).

Lactational

Patients presenting with an inflammatory condition during breast feeding, are likely to have a lactational breast infection (37). These patients present with a painful lump or inflammatory changes involving the affected breast. The most common organism isolated is *Staphylococcus aureus*, but *Staphylococcus epidermidis* and streptococci are occasionally implicated. Most of the organisms involved produce penicillinase (38) and an appropriate antibiotic should be started as soon as possible. If inflammation or an associated mass lesion persists after completing the course, further investigation is required to exclude an underlying carcinoma. Breast cancer should also be suspected in patients with an inflammatory lesion that is solid on ultrasonography or to aspiration. Most abscesses should be treated with antibiotics and aspiration (normally done under ultrasound guidance) which can be repeated two to three times. Occasionally it may be necessary to resort to surgical incision and drainage particularly when the abscess is "pointing" with very thin and distended overlying skin. This may follow failed ultrasound aspiration with little response to a conservative approach (e.g., multiloculated abscesses with very thick pus and debris). Sometimes a punch biopsy needle can be used to drain the abscess.

Breast cancer incidence during pregnancy and lactation is assumed to be the same as for non-pregnant women and

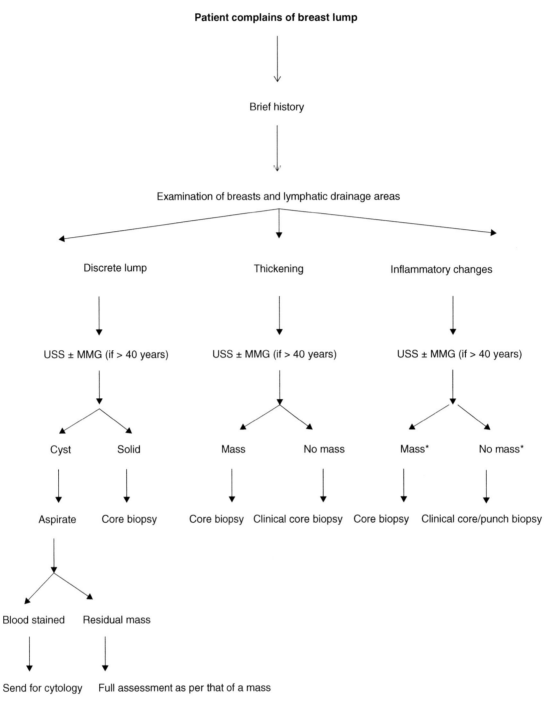

Figure 13.1 A flowchart showing the management of a patient presenting with a breast lump. *Abbreviations*: MMG, mammography, USS, ultrasound scan. *Observation and a short-term follow-up are indicated if obvious infections are identified.

prognosis is similar to age-matched controls (39,40). However diagnosis during lactation can be particularly problematic, often leading to delayed diagnosis and treatment.

Non-Lactational

Periareolar inflammation is most commonly seen in young women and in most cases it is secondary to periductal mastitis. Smoking is an important factor in the etiology of this condition (41). Patients with periductal mastitis may present with either periareolar inflammation, or a well-formed abscess. There may be associated nipple discharge or retraction. Ultrasound should be undertaken and any abscess treated by aspiration. Appropriate antibiotics should be commenced and the causative organisms are usually a mixture of aerobic and anaerobic species. Incision and drainage is rarely required for periareolar sepsis. If the mass is solid on ultrasonography or inflammation fails to resolve after appropriate treatment, care should be taken to exclude an underlying neoplasm. Recurrence is common, and a third of patients may develop formation of a duct fistula after drainage of a non-lactating periareolar abscess. Mammary duct fistulas and recurrent infections need a more radical approach by excision of the fistula or diseased ducts under antibiotic cover.

Peripheral mastitis is less common than periareolar sepsis. The etiology of this condition is unknown and may not necessarily be infective, but can be associated with an underlying condition such as diabetes, rheumatoid arthritis, steroid treatment, granulomatous lobular mastitis, and trauma (42). These conditions may require specific treatment e.g., a course of steroids. Unusual infections such as tuberculosis should also be considered under these circumstances and likewise require specific anti-tuberculosis medication.

Nipple Discharge

Introduction
Important factors determining treatment in patients presenting with nipple discharge are whether the discharge is spontaneous, blood-stained, or from a single duct (43). Most cases of nipple discharge are either physiological or due to benign disease (e.g., duct papilloma), though the significance of this presenting symptom is that it could represent the only clinical manifestation of an underlying malignancy (e.g., ductal carcinoma *in situ*).

Clinical Assessment
The main goal of assessment is to identify the group of patients who require further investigations. This will include those with persistent and spontaneous discharge (in contrast to intermittent discharge provoked by stimuli e.g., midcycle and sex), together with unilateral and single-duct discharge which is neither milky (see the next paragraph) nor purulent (see above under periductal mastitis). The color and consistency of the discharge should be noted. It is normal to express discharge with pressure and since this is physiological, no treatment is required. This physiological discharge varies in color from white, yellow to green/blue or even black. Galactorrhea is copious bilateral milky discharge not associated with pregnancy or breastfeeding. Prolactin levels are usually but not always raised in women with galactorrhea. A careful drug history should be taken, particularly focusing on psychotropic agents which can cause increased prolactin secretion. In the absence of relevant drugs, a search for a pituitary tumor should be instituted in a patient with a raised prolactin level of >1000 IU/L.

Duct ectasia is a common cause of nipple discharge and its incidence increases with age. The discharge is often creamy or cheesy in nature. It may also present as nipple retraction or a mass around the nipple.

Further Diagnostic Assessment
Some clinicians test all cases of single duct discharge for hemoglobin. Most blood-stained discharges are due to simple papillomas or other benign conditions. Only about 5–10% of patients will be found to have an underlying malignancy, most often ductal carcinoma *in situ*, and age is an important predictor of cancer (44). It should be noted that a negative hemoccult test does not exclude cancer as its sensitivity is only 50% (45). Similarly, nipple discharge cytology is also of limited clinical utility because of its low sensitivity (46,47).

All patients with nipple discharge should have clinical examination and any associated mass identified and evaluated as for any breast lump. In patients over 35 years with spontaneous discharge a mammogram should be done and ultrasound is useful at any age for identifying any periductal abnormality.

In an attempt to avoid unnecessary surgery, a number of investigational techniques have been used including ductoscopy, ductal lavage, and ductography. There are encouraging reports with ductoscopy, especially as an adjuvant to surgery in directing duct excision (48). Similarly, ductography may help to localize a lesion and confine excision to the lesion only, thus retaining the ducts which are not affected and can be used for future lactation (49,50). However this is a painful procedure and is not widely used. Ductal lavage is another technique in which a duct is cannulated and irrigated with saline as a method for improving the yield several times compared with simple discharge cytology (51). However, the above three techniques are still under evaluation and not routinely used in most centers.

Management
All patients with spontaneous single duct discharge should normally undergo surgery to establish the cause of discharge. In young women only the affected duct is removed (microdochectomy) which thus maintains the capacity to breast feed. However in patients who have completed their family, total duct excision is the preferred treatment, and is especially the case when the discharge is copious and distressing to the patient.

Mastalgia

Introduction
Most women at some point in their life are likely to suffer from breast pain and up to 70% have symptoms severe enough to seek medical attention. Some may not have true mastalgia, and may have referred pain emanating from the chest wall; these patients classically have tenderness over the ribcage.

Clinical Assessment
True mastalgia is often cyclical and is associated with swollen and tender breasts. It is worse before menstruation and often relieved following it. It is often aggravated by exogenous hormones like oral contraceptive pills or HRT. As for every patient presenting with a breast complaint, a full clinical examination of the breast and axilla is carefully carried out. Should a discrete lump be identified, then investigation proceeds as for any breast lump (see the earlier section, "Lump").

Further Diagnostic Assessment
Symptoms of breast pain alone are seldom due to breast cancer and therefore if clinical examination is normal, no imaging is generally required. However, patients over the age of 35 years should be considered for opportunistic mammographic assessment as 5% of women diagnosed with breast cancer complain of breast pain (52) and 2.7% of women presenting with breast pain are diagnosed with breast cancer (53). Mammographic screening also has some proven value for women between 40 and 50 years, though is not necessarily cost-effective.

Management
Reassurance that the pain is not due to cancer is all that is required in most cases. A pain chart allows confirmation that pain is cyclical, and also indicates the effect of any treatment intervention on the patient. Simple analgesics and a supportive bra are the only measures required in many patients with persistent pain. Some lifestyle changes (e.g., cessation of caffeine intake and reduced smoking) may be of clinical benefit though firm evidence is lacking. Evening primrose oil has been used

traditionally for managing patients with mastalgia (54). However it is now considered to have only a placebo effect and two double-blind placebo-controlled randomized trials have failed to demonstrate the effectiveness of this agent (55,56). If the above measures fail, danazol (an androgen analog) has been used in cases of severe mastalgia. However, side effects (including weight gain, acne, and hirsutism) are generally not tolerated by women and hence its use has been restricted to severe cases of breast pain only. Tamoxifen has been found to be useful in the treatment of mastalgia and clinical benefit has been confirmed in double-blind placebo controlled trials (57). Theoretically ovarian function suppression using a luteinizing hormone releasing hormone agonist (e.g., goserelin) can effectively treat cyclical mastalgia but once again potential adverse consequences of treatment are significant especially when used long term. Furthermore, these treatments are not licensed for the management of mastalgia.

Changes in Skin Contour
Introduction and Clinical Assessment
Patients may present with changes of skin contour including skin dimpling, puckering, or thickening of the skin. All these changes need to be fully investigated as they may represent an underlying malignancy. However, a number of benign conditions can have a similar clinical presentation. Patients with either fat necrosis or breast infection may each present with the above changes. It is also important to ascertain any history of previous breast cancer treatment with radiotherapy as this can lead to similar skin changes.

A rare presentation has been reported termed Mondor's disease and is a consequence of thrombosis involving superficial veins of the breast and chest wall (58). It is often seen following breast surgery or trauma and patients typically complain of breast pain which may be associated with localized swelling and redness. Clinically a linear abnormality which resembles a gutter in the skin is seen, and "a chain of beads" can be felt underneath the "line." The condition is often self-limiting and settles spontaneously with time.

Further Diagnostic Assessment and Management
All patients should have an ultrasound scan and those above the age of 35 years should also have mammography. Any abnormality needs further evaluation including core biopsy. If there is any discordance between the above tests, patients may need subsequent clinical or radiological follow-up. Mondor's disease is self-limiting and provided that no significant radiological abnormality is identified, no further tests are required. For patients with an isolated skin dimple in the absence of any palpable or radiological abnormality, a short-term follow-up (e.g., 2–3 months) is acceptable. A clinical hand-guided core biopsy of the breast tissue lying beneath the area of tethering can also be performed, if considered appropriate.

Nipple Changes
Patients may present with a variety of nipple changes which may be benign or represent a manifestation of an underlying cancer. Nipple retraction or inversion can be attributed to either physiological or pathological causes. Physiological retraction is not permanent and the nipple can be re-everted with manipulation using the finger tips. True pathological inversion of the nipple

may be due to benign conditions such as breast infection (periductal mastitis) or duct ectasia. Thus a history of smoking, recurrent breast infections, or associated nipple discharge is important. However, malignancy may present with nipple inversion and therefore all patients require imaging with either ultrasound or mammography (above 35 years).

Once malignancy has been excluded, reassurance, and appropriate treatment of the benign condition is often all that is required. For cases of unsightly retraction and those that do not respond to conservative measures (including use of a nipple shield), surgery involving duct division or excision can be contemplated and may be successful at everting the nipple. Nonetheless, women need to be informed that duct excision can preclude subsequent breast feeding and result in loss or reduction of nipple sensation (and in some cases nipple hypersensitivity).

Some patients may present with skin changes involving the nipple. These are usually eczematous changes which can extend beyond the areola. It is useful to identify whether patients have similar changes elsewhere in the body, as the nipple changes may be part of a more widespread skin condition. However, if the condition is unilateral, it may represent Paget's disease of the nipple (which classically involves the skin of the nipple only). Paget's disease is of uncertain pathology but is due to intraepidermal infiltration of the nipple with large "Pagetoid" cells which have a high cytoplasmic to nuclear ratio (59). It represents an underlying invasive or *in situ* cancer and needs urgent investigation. Mammogram and ultrasound of the nipple-areola region may identify any underlying cancer but 50% of patients with Paget's disease have a normal mammogram. If there is no obvious lesion on imaging, a punch biopsy of the involved area of skin will usually establish the diagnosis. The treatment and prognosis of Paget's disease depend on the pathological characteristics of the underlying cancer and the stage of disease.

Nipple adenoma is one of the differential diagnoses of Paget's disease of the nipple (60). This is a palpable papillary growth of the nipple seen in women in their 40s. They may cause erosion of the nipple tip with surface bleeding. It is difficult to image these lesions and the only treatment option is complete excision (61).

The Male Patient
Introduction and Clinical Assessment
A proportion of patients presenting to the breast clinic are male patients with breast complaints and approximately 1% of all breast cancers are diagnosed in men (25).

Gynecomastia is the commonest condition affecting the breast in men and can occur at any age. The condition is broadly divided into two groups, pubertal gynecomastia (occurring in the teenage years and early 20s), and an older group in whom there is often an obvious underlying cause such as drugs, alcohol, or liver disease. Clinical assessment of the breast itself is similar in men as their female counterparts. However, gynecomastia is the commonest presentation and all male patients should be examined to look for stigmata of liver disease which also includes palpation of the liver. In particular, both testes should be examined to determine the presence of any abnormal lumps or atrophy (62).

Further Diagnostic Assessment and Management

Imaging is less useful in male patients though ultrasound could be performed to exclude any underlying mass lesions when there is doubt clinically. If there is a suspicion of breast cancer, core biopsy should be performed. Blood tests [e.g., hormone profile, tumor markers (such as alpha fetal protein, beta human chorionic gonadotropin, and lactic dehydrogenase)] should be performed to exclude any rare but potentially sinister conditions (such as endocrine secreting conditions or testicular tumors) if the cause of gynecomastia is not clinically obvious. The approach for management of breast cancer is similar to that in women, but men usually require mastectomy (rather than wide local excision) and sentinel lymph node biopsy can be undertaken when there is no clinical or sonographic evidence of involved axillary lymph nodes.

REFERENCES

1. Bates AT, Bates T, Hastrich DJ, et al. Delay in the diagnosis of breast cancer: the effect of the introduction of fine needle aspiration cytology to a breast clinic. Eur J Surg Oncol 1992; 18: 433–7.
2. Barber MD, Jack W, Dixon JM. Diagnostic delay in breast cancer. Br J Surg 2004; 91:49–53.
3. Jenner DC, Middleton A, Webb WM, Oommen R, Bates T. In-hospital delay in the diagnosis of breast cancer. Br J Surg 2000; 87: 914–19.
4. Dixon JM, Thomas J. ABC of Breast Disease. London: Blackwell Publishing Ltd, 2006: 1–7.
5. Wishart GC, Warwick J, Pitsinis V, Duffy S, Britton PD. Measuring performance in clinical breast examination. Br J Surg 2010; 97: 1246–52.
6. NHS cancer screening programmes. [Available from: http://www.cancer-screening.nhs.uk/breast screening/index.html].
7. Bak M, Konyár E, Schneider F, et al. The "gray zone" in organized mammography screening: histocytological correlations. Orv Hetil 2011; 152: 292–5.
8. Garg S, Mohan H, Bal A, Attri AK, Kochhar S. A comparative analysis of core needle biopsy and fine-needle aspiration cytology in the evaluation of palpable and mammographically detected suspicious breast lesions. Diagn Cytopathol 2007; 35: 681–9.
9. Mathew J, Crawford D, Lwin M, Barwick C, Gash A. Ultrasound guided vacuum assisted excision in the diagnosis and treatment of clinically benign breast lesions. Ann R Coll Surg Engl 2007; 89: 494–6.
10. McKinnell RG, Parchment RE, Perantoni AO, Pierce GB. The Biological Basis of Cancer. New York: Cambridge university press, 1998: 189–92.
11. A comprehensive review of all the available data on the effectiveness of breast cancer screening in reducing breast cancer mortality. WHO Handbook of Cancer Prevention, 7th edn. Lyons: IARC press, 2002.
12. Nystrom L, Andesson I, Bjurstam N, et al. Long term effects of mammographic screening: update overview of Swedish randomised trials. Lancet 2002; 359: 909–19.
13. Miki Y, Swensen J, Shattuck-Eidens D, et al. A strong candidate for the breast and ovarian cancer susceptibility gene BRCA1. Science 1994; 266:66–71.
14. Futreal PA, Liu Q, Shattuck-Eidens D, et al. BRCA1 mutations in primary breast and ovarian carcinomas. Science 1994; 266: 120–2.
15. Wooster R, Neuhausen SL, Mangion J, et al. Localization of a breast cancer susceptibility gene, BRCA2, to chromosome 13q12-13. Science 1994; 265: 2088–90.
16. Easton DF, Ford D, Bishop DT. Breast and ovarian cancer incidence in BRCA1-mutation carriers. Breast Cancer Linkage Consortium. Am J Hum Genet 1995; 56: 265–71.
17. Struewing JP, Hartge P, Wacholder S, et al. The risk of cancer associated with specific mutations of BRCA1 and BRCA2 among Ashkenazi Jews. N Engl J Med 1997; 336: 1401–8.
18. Easton DF, Bishop DT, Ford D, Crockford GP. Genetic linkage analysis in familial breast and ovarian cancer: results from 214 families. The Breast Cancer Linkage Consortium. Am J Hum Genet 1993; 52: 678–701.
19. Berry DA, Parmigiani G, Sanchez J, Schildkraut J, Winer E. Probability of carrying a mutation of breast-ovarian cancer gene BRCA1 based on family history. J Natl Cancer Inst 1997; 89: 227–38.
20. Athma P, Rappaport R, Swift M. Molecular genotyping shows that ataxia-telangiectasia heterozygotes are predisposed to breast cancer. Cancer Genet Cytogenet 1996; 92: 130–4.
21. FitzGerald MG, Bean JM, Hegde SR, et al. Heterozygous ATM mutations do not contribute to early onset of breast cancer. Nat Genet 1997; 15: 307–10.
22. Blamey RW. The British Association of Surgical Oncology Guidelines for surgeons in the management of symptomatic breast disease in the UK (1998 revision). BASO Breast Specialty Group. Eur J Surg Oncol 1998; 24: 464–76.
23. Dupont WD, Page DL. Risk factors for breast cancer in women with proliferative breast disease. N Engl J Med 1985; 312: 146–51.
24. John EM, Kelsey JL. Radiation and other environmental exposures and breast cancer. Epidemiol Rev 1993; 15: 157–62.
25. Evans JS, Wennberg JE, McNeil BJ. The influence of diagnostic radiography on the incidence of breast cancer and leukemia. N Engl J Med 1986; 315: 810–15.
26. Bhatia S, Robison LL, Oberlin O, et al. Breast cancer and other second neoplasms after childhood Hodgkin's disease. N Engl J Med 1996; 334: 745–51.
27. Hancock SL, Tucker MA, Hoppe RT. Breast cancer after treatment of Hodgkin's disease. J Natl Cancer Inst 1993; 85: 25–31.
28. Sankila R, Garwicz S, Olsen JH, et al. Association of the Nordic Cancer Registries and the Nordic Society of Pediatric Hematology and Oncology. J Clin Oncol 1996; 14: 1442–6.
29. Collaborative Group on Hormonal Factors in Breast Cancer. Breast cancer and hormonal contraceptives: collaborative reanalysis of individual data on 53 297 women with breast cancer and 100 239 women without breast cancer from 54 epidemiological studies. Lancet 1996; 347: 1713–27.
30. Beral V. Breast cancer and hormone-replacement therapy in the Million Women Study. Lancet 2003; 362: 419–27.
31. Dixon Jm, Dobie V, Lamp J, et al. Assessment of acceptability of conservative management of fibroadenoma of the breast. Br J Surg 1996; 83: 264–5.
32. Dixon JM, ed. Breast Surgery- A Companion to Specialist Surgical Practice, 4th edn. 2009: 260–2.
33. Guillot E, Couturaud B, Reyal F, et al. Management of phyllodes breast tumors. Breast J 2011; 17: 129–37.
34. Barth RJ Jr, Wells WA, Mitchell SE, Cole BF. A prospective, multi-institutional study of adjuvant radiotherapy after resection of malignant phyllodes tumors. Ann Surg Oncol 2009; 16: 2288–94.
35. Cheung KL, Ho LW, Leung EY, Khoo US. Palpable asymmetrical thickening of the breast: a clinical, radiological and pathological study. Br J Radiol 2001; 74: 402–6.
36. Thursh S, Banergee S, Sayer G, et al. Breast sepsis: a unit's experience. Br J Surg 2002; 89: 75–6.
37. Boutet G. Breast inflammation: clinical examination, aetiological pointers. Diagn Interv Imaging 2012; 93: 78–84.
38. Goodman MA, Benson EA. An evaluation of the current trends in the management of breast abscesses. Med J Aust 1970; 1: 1034–9.
39. Middleton LP, Amin M, Gwyn K, Theriault R, Sahin A. Breast carcinoma in pregnant women: assessment of clinicopathologic and immunohistochemical features. Cancer 2003; 98: 1055–60.
40. Shousha S. Breast carcinoma presenting during or shortly after pregnancy and lactation. Arch Pathol Lab Med 2003; 124: 1053–60.
41. Sahafer P, Furrec C, Merillod B. An association between smoking with recurrent subareolar breast abscess. Int J Epidemiol 1998; 17: 810–13.
42. Rogers K. Breast abscess and problems with lactation. In: Smallwood JA, Talor L, eds. Menign Breast Disease. London: Edward Arnold, 1990: 96.
43. Alexis MW, Michael JM, Martin JRL. Best Practice Diagnostic Guidelines for Patients Presenting with Breast Symptoms. 2010: 1–43.
44. Selzer MH, Perloff LJ, Kelley RI, et al. Significance of age in patients with nipple discharge. Surg Gynecol Obstet 1970; 131: 519.
45. Snadison AT. An Autopsy of the Human Breast. National Cancer Institute Monograph. No: 8. Bethesda, MD: US dept of health, education and welfare, 1962: 1–145.
46. Simmons R, Adamovich T, Brennan M, et al. Non surgical evaluation of pathologic nipple discharge. Ann Surg Oncol 2003; 10: 113–16.
47. Groves AM, Carr M, Wadhera V, et al. An audit of cytology in the evaluation of nipple discharge: a retrospective study of 10 years experience. Breast 1995; 5: 96.
48. Dooley WS. Routine operative breast endoscopy for blood nipple discharge. Ann Surg Oncol 2002; 9: 920–3.

49. King BL, Love SM, Rochman S, et al. The fourth international symposium on the intraductal approach to breast cancer, Santa Barbara, California, 10-13 March 2005. Breast Cancer Res 2005; 7: 198–204.

50. Ambrogetti D, Berni D, Catarzi S, et al. The role of ductal galactography in the differential diagnosis of breast carcinoma. Radiol Med 1996; 91: 198.

51. Shen KW, Wu J, Lu JS, et al. Fibroptic ductoscopy for breast cancer patients with nipple discharge. Surg Endosc 2001; 15: 1340–5.

52. Haagenson CD. Diseases of the Breast, 3rd edn. Philidelphia: WB Saunders, 1986.

53. Mansel RE. ABC of breast disease: breast pain. Br Med J 1994; 309: 866–8.

54. Cheung KL. Management of cyclical mastalgia in oriental women: pioneer experience of using gamolenic acid (Efamast) in Asia. Aust NZ Surg 1999; 69: 492–4.

55. Khoo SK, Munro C, Battistutta D. Evening primrose oil and treatment of premenopausal syndrome. Med J Aust 1990; 153: 189–92.

56. Blommer J, delange-De Klerk ES, Kurk DJ, et al. Evening primrose oil and fish oil for severe chonic mastalgia: a randomised, double blind controlled trial. Am J Obstet Gynaecol 2002; 187: 1389–94.

57. Fentiman IS, Caleffi M, Brame K, et al. Double blind controlled trial of tamoxifen therapy for mastalgia. Lancet 1986; 1: 287–8.

58. Shetty M, Watson A. Mondor's disease of the breast: sonographic and mammographic findings. AJR 2001; 177: 893–6.

59. Dalberg K, Hellborg H, Wärnberg F. Paget's disease of the nipple in a population based cohort. Breast Cancer Res Treat 2008; 111: 313–19.

60. Healy CE, Dijkstra B, Walsh M, Hill AD, Murphy J. Nippleadenoma: a differential diagnosis for Paget's disease. Breast J 2003; 9: 325–6.

61. Tuveri M, Calò PG, Mocci C, Nicolosi A. Florid papillomatosis of the male nipple. Am J Surg 2010; 200: e39–40.

62. White J, Kearins O, Dodwell D, et al. Male breast carcinoma: increased awareness needed. Breast Cancer Res 2011; 13: 219.

14 Film reading and recall from screening mammography

Sabrina Rajan, Susan J. Barter, and Erika Denton

BACKGROUND

The National Health Service Breast Screening Programme (NHSBSP) was implemented in 1988 following publication of the Forrest report (1) and was gradually rolled out across the United Kingdom (UK) in the subsequent few years. The latest statistics published by the National Screening Office show that from April 2010 to March 2011, over 2.4 million women were invited to attend for breast screening and almost three-quarters of women accepted their invitation. Approximately 75,000 women were recalled for assessment and more than 14,725 cancers were diagnosed in women aged 45 and over (2).

The vast majority of women attending breast screening do not have breast cancer and the screening program is organized to rapidly reassure these women. A small proportion of women who attend screening will have a cancer and the aim is to promptly diagnose and refer these women for treatment. There are four stages that complete a screening episode:

- Invitation and attendance for screening
- Interpretation of the screening mammogram
- Assessment of a potential abnormality
- Surgery and further treatment or discharge back to routine screening

INVITATION AND ATTENDANCE FOR SCREENING

At present, women are called for their first NHSBSP mammograms between their 50th and 53rd birthday and thereafter every three years until they are 70. Currently the screening range is being extended from age 47 to 73, which means that all women will potentially get two extra screening invitations in their lifetime. The evidence base behind this decision was limited and there is an ongoing centrally funded trial of the women in the upper and lower age bands of the proposed age extension to try to establish best practice in these groups. In total, 1.88 million women aged 45 and over were screened within the programme in 2010–11, compared with 1.79 million in 2009–10 (2).

Only women registered with a General Practitioner (GP) are invited for screening as the invitation lists are derived from GP registers. For any population-based screening to be successful the investigation of choice needs to be acceptable to the general population (3) and ideally easily accessible for the target population. In the UK, many women are screened on mobile vans that move from area to area often parking in supermarkets or GP surgery car parks to improve accessibility.

Screening Mammography

The success of cancer detection by screening is dependent on high-quality mammography underpinned by rigorous quality assurance. When the screening program was first introduced, only a single view mammogram was performed. A randomized control trial conducted with the support of the UK Coordinating Committee on Cancer Research demonstrated major gains could be made by introducing two views at the prevalent screen while remaining financially cost-effective (4). Two-view mammography increased the detection of breast cancer by 24% and reduced the number of women recalled for assessment by 15% at the first screening examination. Subsequently, it was shown that two-view mammography was particularly effective at detecting small invasive breast cancers and therefore should also increase breast cancer detection at subsequent screens (5,6).

Since 2003, two mammographic views are taken of each breast at each attendance for screening mammograms in the NHSBSP. The standard views are the mediolateral oblique (MLO) and craniocaudal (CC) projections (Fig. 14.1). A satisfactory MLO view will fulfill the following criteria:

- Lower edge of the pectoral muscle should reach the nipple level to ensure that the posterior aspect of the breast is satisfactorily included on the image.
- Inframammary angle should be clearly demonstrated.
- Nipple in profile to allow the retroareolar region to be adequately assessed.

A satisfactory CC view will show virtually all except the most lateral and axillary part of the breast, fulfilling the following criteria:

- Clear demonstration of the medial border of the breast
- Pectoral muscle may be seen on the posterior edge of the image depending on anatomical characteristics
- Nipple in profile

Image Acquisition

Traditionally, screening mammography was performed using a film–screen combination with the films brought back to a central office for processing and interpretation. All modern mammography equipment now uses digital image acquisition and the NHSBSP is in the process of replacing analog film–screen equipment with digital mammography. Conventional processing and digital acquisition both require robust quality assurance to ensure optimal diagnostic images are available for interpretation while keeping radiation doses as low as reasonably practicable.

INTERPRETATION OF THE SCREENING MAMMOGRAM

Very low ambient light levels are required for both analog and digital mammography reporting. Windows in reporting rooms

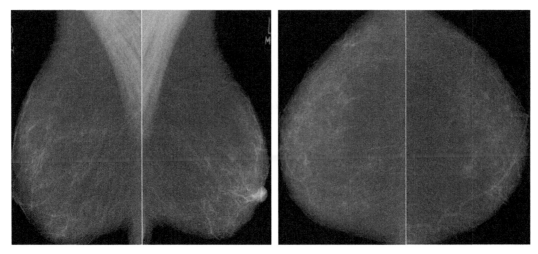

Figure 14.1 Normal mediolateral oblique and craniocaudal views. These are the standard views taken at screening mammography.

should be fitted with blinds to exclude any background light and reporting workstations placed such that glare from other equipment does not compromise viewing conditions. Analog films are loaded onto mammographic roller viewers and for incident examinations, the previous screening mammograms also mounted on the viewer to allow direct comparison by the reader (7). This is a time-consuming and labor intensive process that is now being replaced by full-field digital mammography, which results in images being sent directly to picture archiving and communication system (PACS) workstations for viewing and interpretation.

Digital mammography has a similar sensitivity and higher specificity when compared with conventional film mammography (8–10). The benefits of digital mammography include reduced radiation doses, reduction in the need for repeat images, and the ability to manipulate the image on a workstation. Other benefits include instant transfer of information electronically across single or multiple organizations and reduction in physical storage space required.

Mammographic readers include trained radiologists, advanced practitioner radiographers, and breast clinicians. Readers must be involved in breast screening assessment and participate in multidisciplinary team meetings that provide each member of the team with information on their diagnostic accuracy. To achieve NHSBSP quality standards, each mammographic reader should undertake a minimum of 5000 screening and/or symptomatic cases per year and participate in an approved radiology performance quality assurance scheme for mammography. Readers involved in breast cancer screening are encouraged to participate in the voluntary PERsonal perFORmance in Mammographic Screening (PERFORMS) self-assessment program that is distributed to all national screening centers biannually (11).

Mammographic abnormalities that require further assessment include an asymmetric density, mass, architectural distortion, microcalcification, and enlarged axillary lymph nodes. In the majority of UK screening centers, two trained mammographic readers double read all screening mammograms as this has been shown to improve sensitivity (12,13). The decision of the individual reader is recorded on the NHSBSP computer system. If the decision of the two readers is unanimous, the outcome is considered concordant. Local protocols are used regarding discordant decisions. Some units recall every

query raised but others reach a consensus or have arbitration by a third reader. These different strategies can give rise to very different recall rates and it is essential that the benefit in improved sensitivity is achieved without a reduction in specificity. The highest rate of age standardized cancer detection without inappropriately high recall rates is achieved by programs using double reading with arbitration (14).

To improve the efficiency of breast screening, trials have been conducted to evaluate the accuracy of computer-aided detection (CAD). CAD uses a sophisticated software system that highlights abnormalities that can then be analyzed by a mammographic reader who decides whether the prompt is highlighting an area of genuine concern. The CADET II prospective study showed that one radiologist plus CAD are just as effective as two radiologists when identifying potential cancers (15). However, the main drawback of the technology is that it is too sensitive, generating two or three prompts for each mammogram, many of which are normal or benign. CAD may have a role within the NHSBSP to ease the pressure on busy breast screening services or help where services are understaffed. This is especially relevant in the context of increasing workload volume with age extension and the incorporation of screening high-risk women from the age of 40 within the NHSBSP.

Outcome Following Interpretation of Screening Mammogram

There are four main outcomes following mammography reporting:

- Normal mammogram with return to routine screening
- Technical recall
- Clinical recall
- Mammographic abnormality requiring further assessment

A majority of women do not have breast cancer and are reassured that their mammograms are normal. A small number of women are recalled because of a technical problem with their images, usually relating to exposure factors or a movement-related blur that render the images nondiagnostic. The NHSBSP set strict criteria stipulating that the minimum standard for the number of repeat examinations should be <3% of total

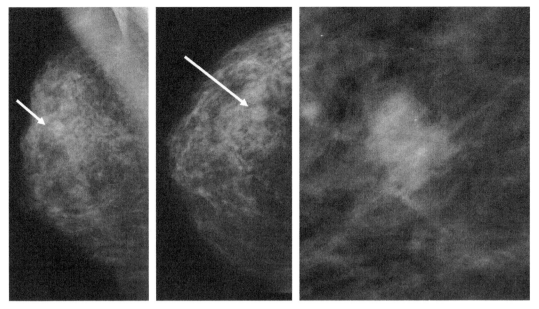

Figure 14.2 Standard screening mammograms (mediolateral oblique and craniocaudal views) and a magnification/paddle view taken at assessment. Note how the small mass becomes much more conspicuous and the irregularity of its borders can be readily seen on the magnification view.

examinations (16). There are mechanisms in place to identify and record significant symptoms and signs of potential breast problems in women attending for screening. This information is made available to the readers at the time of mammography reporting. Clinical recall for assessment of these symptoms and signs may be appropriate even if the screening mammograms are normal.

The expectations and needs of "well women" recalled for assessment of a screen-detected abnormality are very different from those of symptomatic women attending one-stop clinics. In order to reduce the period of uncertainty following the screening attendance, the aim is that ≥90% of women who require assessment should be seen within three weeks (17). Ideally, the time between the receipt of the appointment for the assessment clinic and actual attendance should be as short as practically possible. There is a delicate balance between reducing the recall rates so far that cancers are missed and calling back too many women, which causes anxiety and may reduce reattendance for subsequent screening episodes. The minimum NHSBSP standard is that <10% of women screened for the first time and <7% of women who have been screened before should be recalled for assessment (17).

ASSESSMENT VISIT
Triple Assessment
About one in eight women screened regularly by the NHSBSP will be recalled for assessment at least once over a 10-year period (18). Triple assessment is the gold standard for non-operative diagnosis of breast disease, which involves clinical examination, imaging, and pathology. When the results of all three arms of assessment agree, the level of diagnostic accuracy exceeds 95% (19).

The radiologist or advanced practitioner radiographer running the assessment clinic usually performs the clinical examination. Alternatively, a breast care nurse or breast clinician working alongside the radiology team may undertake the clinical examination. The majority of women have no palpable

clinical abnormality. Some women may have a palpable abnormality corresponding to the mammographic area of concern, while others rarely may have a mammographically occult cancer that is detected clinically.

Further mammographic views are performed if needed to establish whether a mammographic abnormality is real or a composite of overlapping shadows casting an apparent mammographic density. Magnification and paddle views are useful for evaluating the borders of masses, architectural distortion, and to examine the morphology of microcalcification (Fig. 14.2). Targeted breast ultrasound is performed of the mammographically detected abnormality to aid lesion characterization and distinguish between solid and cystic lesions. If a solid mass is identified, image-guided core biopsy is performed to secure a definitive histological diagnosis. If the breast mass has features suspicious for malignancy, ipsilateral axillary ultrasound is performed with needle sampling of morphologically abnormal lymph nodes for preoperative regional staging.

Biopsies can be performed under ultrasound or stereotactic guidance. If the lesion is visualized under ultrasound, this is the preferred modality for image-guided biopsy, as it is quicker and easier to perform and is more comfortable for the patient. Stereotactic guided biopsy can be performed with the patient in an upright or prone position and requires the patient to tolerate mammographic compression for the duration of the procedure. This is usually reserved for biopsy of microcalcifications that are best appreciated on mammography and for lesions occult on ultrasound.

Currently it is standard practice in the UK to perform a core biopsy (14G) of a breast abnormality rather than fine needle aspiration for cytology due to the higher sensitivity and specificity (20). Core biopsy histology is able to differentiate between in situ and invasive carcinoma while providing additional information regarding tumor grade, type, and hormone receptor status to inform management decisions (21). Vacuum-assisted core biopsy is a relatively new technique that

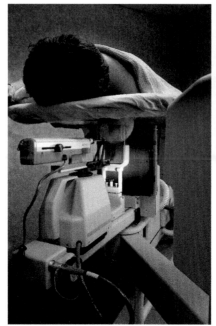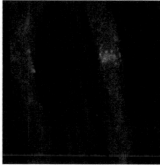

Figure 14.3 Vacuum-assisted core biopsy performed on a prone table. The cores are x-rayed to ensure representative calcium retrieval.

permits large-volume non-operative sampling. The device is equipped with a large-caliber needle (8 gauge or 11 gauge) that procures a larger volume of tissue in comparison with a standard automated core biopsy device (22). It is increasingly used as a first line sampling method for mammographically detected microcalcification due to higher rates of calcium retrieval and lower rates of underdiagnosis of in situ and invasive cancer (Fig. 14.3). With regards to axillary sampling, the practice is more variable across the country. Ultrasound-guided core biopsy is the sampling method of choice for morphologically abnormal lymph nodes in many centers. However, some centers with good access to cytology services perform fine needle aspiration for axillary lymph nodes with good reported results.

Outcome Following Assessment Visit

For those women who have a breast biopsy, their results are discussed in a multidisciplinary team meeting with breast radiologists, pathologists, surgeons, oncologists, and breast care nurses present. Women with a cancer diagnosis are referred to a breast surgeon for treatment. All women assessed without a diagnosis of cancer are returned to routine screening and should receive written confirmation of the outcome of their assessment. Short term or "early" recall for repeat assessment usually at one year is reserved for those women with a low risk of malignancy, but whose assessment has not given a definitive answer. Short-term recall should not be considered a routine outcome of assessment and should be kept to a minimum (target ≤0.25% of women screened). The adverse psychological consequences of being placed on short-term recall because of a diagnostic uncertainty were significantly higher than those women who turned out to have a false-positive mammographic result and were returned to routine screening after assessment (23).

Numerous studies have investigated the experience of "false-positive" women, that is, those who have undergone

further investigations following routine breast screening and received a final clear result. These women were found to experience significantly greater adverse psychological consequences at one month and five months after assessment compared with women who received a clear result after the initial screening mammogram (23,24). Despite having received a final clear result at the previous screening episode three years ago, women who had undergone further investigation at assessment including fine needle aspiration or referral for surgical biopsy suffered significantly greater adverse psychological consequences at one month before their next routine breast screening appointment than women who received a clear result after the initial screening mammogram. Women who were recalled for further investigation that confirmed false positivity were not necessarily more motivated to attend for their next routine appointment, with 15% of these women not returning for subsequent routine screening three years later (25).

SURGERY AND FURTHER TREATMENT

Women with a cancer diagnosis should receive their results in the presence of a clinician and specialist breast care nurse with sufficient time allocated to provide the necessary counseling and support. The NHS Cancer plan in England has set a maximum one month wait from the date of diagnosis to the date of first definitive treatment (26). A care plan is specifically tailored to each patient taking into consideration tumor biology, age at diagnosis, general health, social circumstances, and personal preferences (27). Women must be given adequate information to make a fully informed decision regarding their treatment. Screen-detected breast cancers generally present with earlier stage disease and surgery with curative intent is usually the first stage of treatment. Treatment planning should allow sufficient time for discussion of oncoplastic and reconstructive surgery for those women who wish to consider these options. Close communication is maintained between surgeons and oncologists at multidisciplinary team meetings to plan subsequent adjuvant therapy once primary treatment is complete.

EMERGING STRATEGIES

There has been widespread publicity of several emerging technologies in the field of breast imaging, but none of these have been validated by large scale trials in the screening setting. They are briefly discussed in the coming sections as they may become relevant in the future with regard to population-based breast screening.

Tomosynthesis

In standard two-dimensional film or full-field digital mammography, overlapping dense fibroglandular breast tissue can reduce visibility of malignant abnormalities or simulate the appearance of an abnormality. This can lead to unnecessary recalls for assessment, biopsies, and unnecessary psychological stress for the women concerned. Digital breast tomosynthesis is a new form of three-dimensional imaging, in which multiple projection images of the breast are acquired from different angulations of the x-ray tube (28). The images are then processed using reconstruction algorithms to produce tomographic sections through the breast. By minimizing the superimposition of overlying breast tissue, tomosynthesis has the potential to reduce false-positive recalls for assessment, improve lesion conspicuity, and depth localization. A multicenter trial is currently underway to compare the sensitivity and specificity of tomosynthesis in relation to digital mammography and this will hopefully provide useful information with regards to the role of tomosynthesis within the context of breast screening (29).

Whole-Breast Ultrasound

Whole-breast ultrasound is a time-consuming process that is difficult to standardize or reproduce for population-based screening. Although ultrasound has the benefit of no radiation and may improve cancer detection rates in dense breasts, it has a poor sensitivity for DCIS and has high false-positive rates (30). It is best utilized when targeted to a palpable or mammographic abnormality and has not proven to be an effective screening test at any age (31).

Magnetic Resonance Imaging

Dedicated contrast-enhanced breast MRI has the highest sensitivity for invasive breast cancer of all currently available imaging techniques (32,33). While the sensitivity of mammography decreases from 100% in low density fatty breasts to 45% in extremely dense breasts (34), MRI maintains its advantage even in women with dense breast tissue (35). However, it is an expensive, time-consuming technique that requires the injection of intravenous contrast. In addition, a major disadvantage is a high proportion of false-positive findings in comparison with mammography. These factors make MRI unsuitable for population-based screening targeted at women at average risk of developing breast cancer. It is however the technique of choice for screening younger women who are at an extremely high risk of breast cancer, as recommended by National Institute for Health and Clinical Excellence (NICE) (36–38).

REFERENCES

1. Department of Health and Social Security. Breast Cancer Screening: Report to Health Ministers of England, Wales, Scotland and Northern Ireland by a working group chaired by Professor Sir Patrick Forrest. London: HMSO, 1987.
2. Breast Screening Programme, England 2010–11. The NHS Information Centre for Health and Social Care. [Available from www.ic.nhs.uk/pubs/brstscreen1011].
3. Wilson JMG, Jungner G. Principles and Practice of Screening for Disease. Geneva: World Health Organisation, 1968.
4. Wald NJ, Murphy P, Major P, et al. UKCCCR multicentre randomised controlled trial of one and two view mammography in breast cancer screening. BMJ 1995; 311: 1189–93.
5. Blanks RG, Moss SM, Wallis MG. Use of two view mammography compared with one view in the detection of small invasive cancers: further results from the National Health Service breast screening programme. J Med Screen 1997; 4: 98–101.
6. Given-Wilson RM, Blanks RG. Incident screening cancers detected with a second mammographic view: pathological and radiological features. Clin Radiol 1999; 54: 724–35.
7. Callaway MP, Boggis CR, Astley SA, et al. The influence of previous films on screening mammographic interpretation and detection of breast carcinoma. Clin Radiol 1997; 52: 527–9.
8. Lewin JM, Hendrick RE, D'Orsi CJ, et al. Comparison of full-field digital mammography with screen-film mammography for cancer detection: results of 4,945 paired examinations. Radiology 2001; 218: 873–80.
9. Lewin JM, D'Orsi CJ, Hendrick RE, et al. Clinical comparison of full-field digital mammography and screen-film mammography for detection of breast cancer. AJR 2002; 179: 671–7.
10. Skaane P, Skjennald A. Screen-film mammography versus full-field digital mammography with soft-copy reading: randomized trial in a population-based screening program - the Oslo II Study. Radiology 2004; 232: 197–204.
11. Quality assurance guidelines for breast cancer screening radiology. NHSBSP Publication No 59. NHS Cancer Screening Programmes 2005. [Available from: www.cancerscreening.nhs.uk].
12. Seradour B, Wait S, Jacquemier J, et al. Modalities of reading of detection mammographies of the programme in the Bouches-du-Rhone. Results and costs 1990–1995. J Radiol 1997; 78: 49–54.
13. Warren RM, Duffy SW. Comparison of single reading with double reading of mammograms, and change in effectiveness with experience. Br J Radiol 1995; 68: 958–62.
14. Blanks RG, Wallis MG, Moss SM. A comparison of cancer detection rates achieved by breast cancer screening programmes by number of readers, for one and two view mammography: results from the UK National Health Service breast screening programme. J Med Screen 1998; 5: 195–201.
15. James JJ, Gilbert FJ, Wallis MG, et al. Mammographic features of breast cancers at single reading with computer-aided detection and at double reading in a large multicenter prospective trial of computer-aided detection: CADET II. Radiology 2010; 256: 379–86.
16. Quality assurance guidelines for mammography including radiographic quality control. NHSBSP Publication Number 63. NHS Cancer Screening Programmes 2006. [Available from: www.cancerscreening.nhs.uk].
17. Consolidated guidance on standards for the NHS breast screening programme. NHSBSP Publication No 60 (version 2). NHS Cancer Screening Programmes 2005. [Available from: www.cancerscreening.nhs.uk].
18. Screening for breast cancer in England: past and future. NHSBSP Publication No 61. NHS Cancer Screening Programmes 2006. [Available from: www.cancerscreening.nhs.uk].
19. Willett AM, Michell MJ, Lee MJR. Best practice diagnostic guidelines for patients presenting with breast symptoms. Department of Health 2010, Gateway reference 13737. [Available from: www.dh.gov.uk/publications].
20. Britton PD. Fine needle aspiration or core biopsy. Breast 1999; 8: 1–4.
21. Guidelines for non-operative diagnostic procedures and reporting in breast cancer screening. NHSBSP Publication No. 50. NHS Cancer Screening Programmes 2001. [Available from: www.cancerscreening.nhs.uk].
22. Burbank F, Parker SH, Fogarty TJ. Stereotactic breast biopsy: improved tissue harvesting with the Mammotome. Am Surg 1996; 62: 738–44.
23. Ong G, Austoker J, Brett J. Breast screening: adverse psychological consequences one month after placing women on early recall because of a diagnostic uncertainty. A multicentre study. J Med Screen 1997; 4: 158–68.

24. Brett J, Austoker J, Ong G. Do women who undergo further investigation for breast screening suffer adverse psychological consequences? A multi-centre follow-up study comparing different breast screening result groups five months after their last breast screening appointment. J Public Health Med 1998; 20: 396–403.

25. Brett J, Austoker J. Women who are recalled for further investigation for breast screening: psychological consequences 3 years after recall and factors affecting re-attendance. J Public Health Med 2001; 23: 292–300.

26. NHS Cancer Plan: a plan for investment, a plan for reform. Department of Health 2000, Gateway reference 2000. [Available from: www.dh.gov.uk/publications].

27. Bishop H, Chan C, Monypenny I, et al. Surgical guidelines for the management of breast cancer. Eur J Surg Oncol 2009; 35:1–22.

28. Dobbins JT 3rd. Tomosynthesis imaging: at a translational crossroads. Med Phys 2009; 36: 1956–67.

29. TOMMY trial: a comparison of tomosynthesis with digital mammography in the UK NHS Breast Screening Programme. NIHR Health Technology Assessment project in progress. [Available from: http://www.hta.ac.uk/2296].

30. Warner E, Plewes DB, Hill KA, et al. Surveillance of BRCA1 and BRCA2 mutation carriers with magnetic resonance imaging, ultrasound, mammography, and clinical breast examination. JAMA 2004; 292: 1317–25.

31. Teh W, Wilson AR. The role of ultrasound in breast cancer screening. A consensus statement by the European Group for Breast Cancer Screening. Eur J Cancer 1998; 34: 449–50.

32. Biglia N, Bounous VE, Martincich L, et al. Role of MRI versus conventional imaging for breast cancer presurgical staging in young women or with dense breast. Eur J Surg Oncol 2011; 37: 199–204.

33. Liberman L, Morris EA, Dershaw DD, et al. MR imaging of the ipsilateral breast in women with percutaneously proven breast cancer. AJR 2003; 180: 901–10.

34. Berg WA, Gutierrez L, NessAiver MS, et al. Diagnostic accuracy of mammography, clinical examination, US, and MR imaging in preoperative assessment of breast cancer. Radiology 2004; 233: 830–49.

35. Sardanelli F, Giuseppetti GM, Panizza P, et al. Sensitivity of MRI versus mammography for detecting foci of multifocal, multicentric breast cancer in fatty and dense breasts using the whole-breast pathologic examination as a gold standard. AJR 2004; 183: 1149–57.

36. Kriege M, Brekelmans CT, Boetes C, et al. Efficacy of MRI and mammography for breast-cancer screening in women with a familial or genetic predisposition. N Engl J Med 2004; 351: 427–37.

37. Leach MO, Boggis CR, Dixon AK, et al. Screening with magnetic resonance imaging and mammography of a UK population at high familial risk of breast cancer: a prospective multicentre cohort study (MARIBS). Lancet 2005; 365: 1769–78.

38. Familial breast cancer: the classification and care of women at risk of familial breast cancer in primary, secondary and tertiary care. NICE Clinical Guideline 41. Issue date: October 2006. [Available from: www.nice.org.uk].

15 Radiology of the normal breast and differential diagnosis of benign breast lesions

Jessica Kuehn-Hajder, Claudia Engeler, and Tim Emory

INTRODUCTION

Radiologic findings of the normal breast are dependent on normal breast anatomy, its variations, and the imaging technique used. Benign breast lesions have their origins in normal anatomic structures. Assessing a lesion's location in reference to the normal surrounding structures helps in determining its origin. In this chapter, we concentrate on imaging findings of normal structures and benign breast lesions with mammography, ultrasound, and MRI.

The vast majority of available information related to imaging findings of benign breast lesions is derived from patients undergoing biopsy for suspected breast cancer. So, it should not be surprising that there is considerable overlap between imaging characteristics of benign breast lesions and breast cancer.

Certain benign breast lesions diagnosed on core needle biopsy have been reported to be associated with underdiagnosis of malignancy, and excision biopsy is often necessary in such cases. These include: atypical ductal hyperplasia, atypical lobular hyperplasia (ALH), pseudoangiomatous stromal hyperplasia (PASH) with atypia, flat epithelial atypia, as well as lobular carcinoma in situ (LCIS), radial scar, complex sclerosing lesions, papillary lesions with or without atypia (1), and mucocele-like lesions (2). The finding of a benign diagnosis on breast biopsy, whether core needle or excisional biopsy, always needs to be assessed for concordance with imaging and clinical findings in order to obtain optimal accuracy.

NORMAL BREAST

Anatomically, breasts are bilateral collections of modified sweat glands that are located around the nipple. The breast can be divided into three zones: (*i*) mammary zone central, containing the fibroglandular tissue, (*ii*) the fatty predominant premammary zone anteriorly, and (*iii*) the retromammary zone posteriorly (3). Fat, blood vessels, and lymphatic channels are distributed throughout the adult breast, which varies in its relative composition of fibrous, glandular, and fatty elements. Mammographically dense or fatty breasts can be seen at any age even though dense fibroglandular tissue occurs most frequently in younger patients and breast fibroglandular tissue tends to involute with age.

Imaging of the breast with any modality depends upon contrast in order to discriminate between different adjacent structures. On mammography, fat appears dark while fibrous and glandular elements look white. Most lesions in the breast are also white. Therefore, the more "dense" a mammogram is,

meaning that more fibrous and glandular tissue is present, the less easy it is to identify other benign or malignant lesions.

In the white-on-black format of standard ultrasound, fat is set to a midlevel gray and fibroglandular tissue is most commonly white or light gray (hyperechoic) with a repetitive pattern of ducts and terminal ductal lobular units (TDLUs) coursing through. Masses can be any shade of gray, usually darker than the fat, creating the contrast necessary for detection. Occasionally masses can be isoechoic to the adjacent fat or glandular tissue, creating a potential pitfall for detection.

On MRI, most of the contrast in the breast is provided by administering intravenous gadolinium. The normal background tissue usually enhances minimally, while both benign and malignant processes enhance to a greater extent, thus providing contrast with normal tissue. However, in some patients background tissue enhances avidly which makes masses more difficult to visualize. MRI is sometimes performed at a defined time in the patient's menstrual cycle in an effort to minimize background fibroglandular enhancement and to maximize contrast.

BREAST MATURATION MISTAKEN FOR PATHOLOGY

The milk line develops during the fourth week of gestation, in utero, as a curvilinear ectodermal thickening which extends from the axilla to the groin. Most of this thickening regresses with the exception of the tissue at the fourth costal interspace where the breast will subsequently develop. Where regression fails, individuals may develop supernumerary nipples and/or accessory breast tissue (4).

In the prepubertal period the breasts are composed of epithelialized ducts surrounded by connective tissue. Thelarche is the term given to the second stage of normal breast development in girls between age 8 and 13 years (5). During this stage the ducts, approximately 12 in number, lengthen and branch posteriorly and radially leading to lobular differentiation and formation of TDLUs. Breast development occurring earlier than 8 years of age has been termed *precocious thelarche* (Fig. 15.1), although it has been proposed that African-American girls may demonstrate normal breast development as early as 6 years old and in some Caucasian girls thelarche can be as early as 7 years old (6).

In the developing breast, ultrasound is the preferred initial method of imaging to avoid ionizing radiation exposure in this susceptible population. Since breast cancer is a rare condition in the pediatric population, ultrasound allows accurate assessment of the breast, with mammography reserved

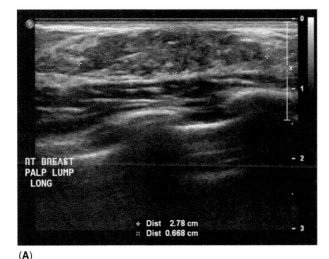

(A)

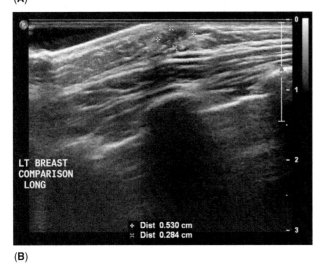

(B)

Figure 15.1 Premature thelarche. A 2-year-old female with breast bud development. Ultrasound demonstrates mixed but mostly hypoechoic tissue behind both nipples, right (A) greater than left (B).

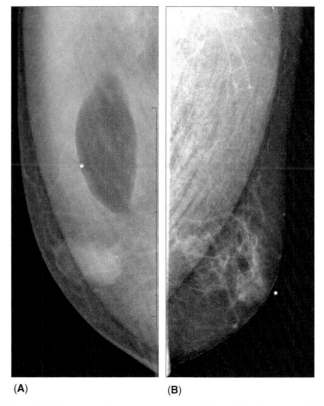

(A)   **(B)**

Figure 15.2 Gynecomastia on mammography. (A) Incidental characteristic flame-shaped retroareolar tissue of mild gynecomastia with small metallic marker indicating a palpable intramuscular lipoma in the pectoralis muscle. (B) More extensive branching tissue involving a greater extent of the breast.

for the rare case in the older adolescent which is worrisome for cancer. Breast development has been divided into five distinct stages (Tanner classification (7)) leading to the mature breast composed of fatty tissue, glandular elements, and supporting fibrous connective tissue. On ultrasound, the Tanner stage 1 breast appears as a small retroareolar focus of echogenic tissue. As the adolescent matures, a hypoechoic nodule develops within the echogenic tissue behind the nipple (Tanner stages 2–4). This central hypoechoic focus gradually becomes less evident as the TDLUs develop and is replaced by a more diffuse pattern of heterogeneous echogenicity (Tanner stage 5) (5). Furthermore, as the breast matures, there is a gradual increase in premammary and retromammary breast fat.

Most conditions that result in breast masses in adolescents and children are benign. In utero hormone stimulation of the retroareolar ducts from maternal sources can result in physiological subareolar lumps in both male and female infants which may persist into the twelfth month of life (5). *Thelarche* can be mistaken for disease because it may present as a unilateral tender lump beneath the nipple and lead to asymmetry in development between the two breasts. This is more likely when thelarche is precocious. *Supernumerary nipples and accessory*

breast tissue can be a cause of symptoms anywhere along the milk line (4).

Gynecomastia is excessive development of the male breast resulting from a relative imbalance of testosterone in relation to estrogen. Gynecomastia presents both in boys during puberty and grown men as a firm subareolar mass which may or may not be tender. On mammography, gynecomastia is often asymmetric and appears as a retroareolar, flame-shaped density with concave margins (Fig. 15.2). Gynecomastia tends to have the same features sonographically as thelarche (Fig. 15.3). Most boys experience breast enlargement during puberty, peaking at 13–14 years and typically resolving within two years (5). A second peak occurs at age between 50–80 years with an incidence of approximately 25%. Most often gynecomastia is idiopathic and the result of normal physiologic change. Medication and recreational drug use (particularly marijuana) are also implicated etiologically. Medical conditions which may also be associated with gynecomastia include liver failure secondary to chronic alcohol abuse (cirrhosis), kidney disease, liver tumors such as hepatoblastoma, or fibrolamellar carcinoma, feminizing adrenal cortical tumors or testicular Sertoli and Leydig cell tumors (7).

Recognizing these normal stages and variants is important to avoid unnecessary biopsies that may cause patient discomfort, increased costs, and negative long-term consequences. Care must be taken not to damage the developing breast bud in females by surgical intervention or large caliber needle biopsy because the breast may subsequently fail to develop normally.

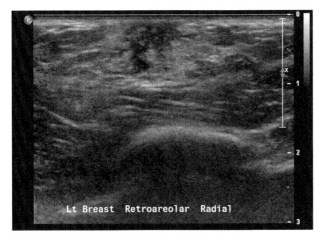

Figure 15.3 Gynecomastia on ultrasound. Ultrasound of a 13-year-old male with tender retroareolar lump demonstrates hyperechoic tissue behind the nipple with a central branching area of hypoechogenicity.

AXILLA AND BENIGN CAUSES
OF LYMPHADENOPATHY

The axilla is often included in breast evaluation for several reasons: (*i*) normal breast tissue can be found under the arm, (*ii*) breast cancer can sometimes present with an axillary lump or axillary mammographic abnormality, and (*iii*) the breast lymphatics drain preferentially to the ipsilateral axilla. While part of the axilla is included on routine mammogram views, ultrasound and MRI provide a more direct interrogation of the axilla. Ultrasound has limited value higher up toward the axillary apex, and MRI is limited posteriorly, especially in the obese patient.

Breast tissue can extend into the axilla along the *axillary tail (of Spence)* or as an island of *accessory breast tissue* left as a remnant along the milk line during embryogenesis. Imaging characteristics of axillary breast tissue accord with those of normally positioned breast tissue and axillary breast tissue can be especially symptomatic during pregnancy and lactation.

Lymph nodes in the axilla are divided into surgical levels with the pectoralis minor muscle as the defining landmark. Level I lymph nodes are located inferior and lateral to the pectoralis minor muscle and extend caudad along the anterior axillary line as far as the nipple. The axillary tail of the breast may overlap with the most inferior level I lymph nodes in some patients; indeed, intramammary lymph nodes are part of the normal breast anatomy. Level II lymph nodes are located deep to the pectoralis minor muscle, and level III lymph nodes are located medial and superior to the pectoralis minor muscle (3). Lymph nodes between the pectoralis major and minor are referred to as interpectoral or Rotter's nodes.

On mammography, lymph nodes are isodense to breast tissue and usually described as having a reniform shape with a fatty hilum, a smooth circumscribed margin and a short transverse axis that measures less than 1 cm. Nonetheless in practice, lymph nodes vary considerably in overall shape and size (Fig. 15.4). On ultrasound, lymph nodes have a typically hypoechoic cortex and a hyperechoic fatty hilum. The vascular pedicle in the lymph node hilum can be detected by color flow Doppler imaging which is useful in distinguishing a lymph node from other similarly shaped masses (especially intramammary lymph nodes). Lymph nodes demonstrate bright

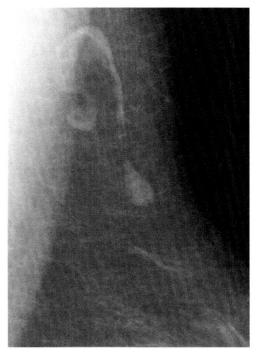

Figure 15.4 Normal variations in the appearance of axillary lymph nodes. Serpiginous-appearing lymph node with a thin cortex demonstrating no eccentric nodularity and prominent fatty hilum.

T2 signal and intermediate T1 signal on MRI with rapid enhancement and washout.

The axillary artery, axillary vein, and brachiocephalic nerve travel in a neurovascular bundle in the apical region of the axilla and pass laterally along the posterior aspect of the pectoralis minor muscle in close proximity to the axillary lymph nodes. These structures must be identified and avoided during axillary lymph node biopsy.

A variety of both benign and malignant disorders can lead to *axillary adenopathy*. Benign causes include collagen vascular diseases, cat scratch fever, tuberculosis, granulomatous mastitis, sarcoidosis, Castleman's disease, and various acute and chronic infections involving the upper extremities or breasts (8). Silicone adenopathy from ruptured or even nonruptured silicone breast implants, or other silicone devices (e.g., joint replacement) may cause a characteristic "snowstorm" posterior acoustic shadowing on ultrasound examination.

BENIGN LESIONS OF THE NIPPLE–AREOLA
COMPLEX AND SKIN

The nipple is surrounded by the similarly pigmented areola, which is 3–5 mm in thickness. *Areolar thickening* is a nonspecific finding which can be seen in both benign and malignant conditions, and is often associated with adjacent skin thickening. The areola contains Montgomery glands, which open on the skin as Morgagni tubercles. These can occasionally become obstructed, accumulate secretions, and develop inflammation or present as a lump. Both *benign and malignant calcifications* can occur within the nipple (9). *Cutaneous horns* can occasionally arise off the nipple. *Adenoma, papilloma, and leiomyoma* can all involve the nipple–areola complex and are usually seen on ultrasound as circumscribed oval solid masses (9). An abscess can also involve the nipple–areola complex and

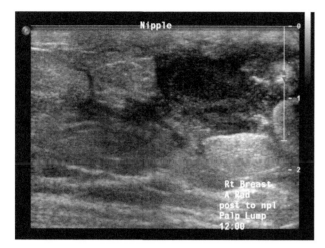

Figure 15.5 Breast abscess. Ultrasound demonstrates an irregular fluid collection with debris and increased through transmission. Note breast edema as characterized by fluid separating fat lobules.

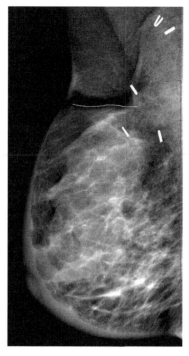

Figure 15.6 Skin thickening on mammogram after breast conservation therapy for breast cancer. Surgical clips and linear skin marker denote the area of prior lumpectomy. Breast skin is thicker than normal especially centrally, near the nipple. Also note the increased trabeculation of the subcutaneous fat from breast edema.

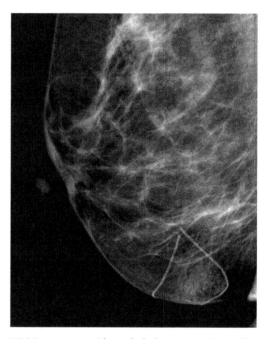

Figure 15.7 Mammogram with marked skin nevus. Linear skin markers placed by the technologist outline a skin lesion on the lower inner quadrant of the right breast. Note the air outlining the crevices of the lesion.

presents as a complicated, irregular fluid collection with an avid surrounding blood flow (Fig. 15.5).

Both papillomas and adenomas are found in true ducts and have a fibrovascular stalk covered by epithelium (4). Papillomas are benign lesions, but excision is recommended after needle biopsy because of difficulties in pathological interpretation, potential sampling errors (papillomas may contain areas of atypia or carcinoma), and the premalignant potential of these lesions (10). Nipple adenomas are also known as florid papillomatosis, papillomatosis of the nipple, subareolar duct papillomatosis, or erosive adenomatosis. A nipple adenoma can erode the nipple and in these cases surgical excision is mandatory (4).

The skin is composed of the epidermis, dermis, and fatty hypodermis and has a normal thickness of approximately 1–3 mm; the epidermis and dermis are readily distinguished from underlying fat by ultrasound and digital mammography. Central lucencies measuring 2–3 mm visible on mammography in the skin are cutaneous caves on the underside of the dermis that have columns of fat projecting up into them (11). Importantly, a large number of both benign and malignant processes, including primary breast cancer, can be associated with focal or diffuse unilateral breast *skin thickening*, with or without associated erythema and tenderness (Fig. 15.6) (12). A negative punch biopsy of thickened skin does not exclude the presence of underlying cancer involving the breast or axilla, even when inflammatory breast cancer is present.

Skin surface lesions such as nevi can simulate masses on mammography and are thus marked by technicians so patients are not unnecessarily called back for additional imaging (Fig. 15.7). *Sebaceous or epidermal inclusion cysts* developing in the skin may present as palpable lumps, and can be characterized most accurately by ultrasound which confirms their location in the skin when there is uncertainty on clinical examination. They are seen on ultrasound as complicated cysts with uniform echogenicity, and occasionally a pore connecting to the skin surface is visualized as a punctum clinically (Fig. 15.8). *Steatocystomas* are related to sebaceous cysts, and when multiple may be part of an autosomal dominant disorder, termed *steatocystoma multiplex*. *Hidradenitis* and *hidradenitis suppurativa* involving the axillary skin can be

symptomatic or may be seen at the time of mammographic screening. The ultrasound appearances of hidradenitis suppurativa are characterized by a complicated fluid collection within the thickened dermis (13).

Skin calcifications typically have a rounded shape with lucent centers and most commonly are encountered over the upper inner quadrants of the breasts with a bilateral distribution. They are much more easily identified within the skin when

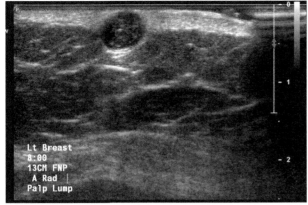

(A)

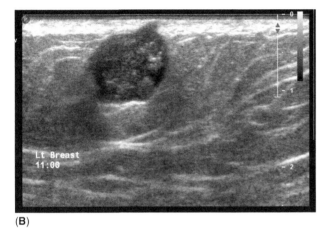

(B)

Figure 15.8 Ultrasound of sebaceous cysts. (**A**) Complex cystic lesion with increased through transmission located in the skin. There is a "claw sign," with the dermis coursing deep to the cyst. (**B**) Complex cyst is located deep to the skin with a pore extending to the skin surface.

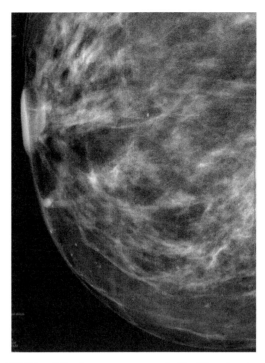

Figure 15.9 Skin calcifications on mammography. Small lucent centered calcifications confirmed to be within the skin inferior to the nipple where the x-ray beam travels through the skin of the breast tangentially. This patient has a history of prior reduction mammoplasty.

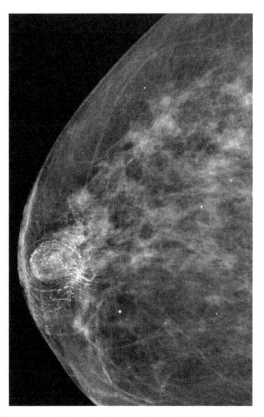

Figure 15.10 Zinc oxide on the skin, mimicking calcifications. Delicate linear radiodensities are seen surrounding the nipple and along the upper aspect of the image, collecting in folds.

captured tangentially on digital mammography (Fig. 15.9). Occasionally, when localized into a cluster mimicking the microcalcifications of ductal carcinoma in situ (DCIS), special techniques may be required to demonstrate them to be within the skin on a tangential view (14,15). *Tattoos*, baby powder, and some creams/ointments on the breast can occasionally present as radio-opacities which can mimic breast calcifications on mammography (Fig. 15.10) (16).

BENIGN LESIONS OF THE NON-TERMINAL DUCTS

During puberty, the ductal system progressively elongates and branches within the layer of fat beneath the skin. The ducts are widest in diameter immediately posterior to the nipple where these segments are termed lactiferous sinuses. The size and length of these lactiferous sinuses vary widely between patients. The description of a duct as an *ectatic duct* indicates the presence of a duct that is larger than the others rather than exceeding a certain minimum size; these lesions are rarely found on mammography, but may be associated with breast cancer.

The ducts progressively divide beyond the lactiferous sinuses in a roughly conical configuration, each supplying a breast segment, and the duct branches terminate within numerous roughly spherical structures called lobules, where milk production occurs. The lobules consist of acini that vary in number during the menstrual cycle, with proliferation being the greatest in the secretory phase. Lobules and acini atrophy and

decrease in number and size after the menopause (unless supported by estrogen replacement therapy), and these changes in the postmenopausal breast correspond to decreased breast density on mammography. Concomitant increased blood flow

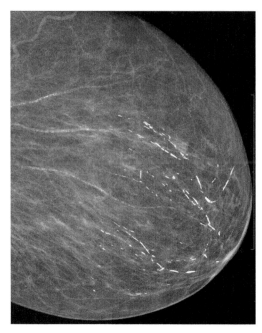

Figure 15.11 Mammogram with secretory and arterial calcifications. Linearly oriented, thick, rod-like, or cigar-shaped calcifications of plasma cell mastitis are seen radiating into the mid breast from the nipple. There are also arterial calcifications more posteriorly in the breast.

and fluid retention in the breast during the secretory phase of the menstrual cycle may also be reflected on breast imaging with increased density on mammography due to a variety of factors including decreased breast compression. Increased parenchymal enhancement may also be found on MRI during the secretory phase leading some to recommend MRI screening during the proliferative phase; however, the benefit of this strategy appears to be marginal.

A common mammographic finding within the ducts is *plasma cell mastitis*, also known as benign secretory disease, and duct ectasia. Plasma cell mastitis presents as large smooth rod-like calcifications (in comparison with the smaller and rougher microcalcifications of malignancy), and is typically bilateral, although commonly greater in extent in one breast (Fig. 15.11). The calcifications of plasma cell mastitis can occasionally branch though these rarely resemble the linear branching appearance of calcifications seen in DCIS.

The most common benign neoplasm affecting the lactiferous sinuses and segmental ducts proximal to the terminal ducts is a *papilloma*, discussed above in reference to the nipple. Papillomas can present clinically as unilateral single duct fluid discharge (often bloody or clear and watery), a palpable lump, be incidental on ultrasound, or be detected during breast cancer mammographic screening in asymptomatic patients. Papillomas have been classified as a solitary central or multiple peripheral lesions. As previously discussed, papillomas are usually benign but can be associated with atypia or malignancy. Furthermore, papillomas may be linked to subsequent development of malignancy following excision, especially when atypia is present in multiple peripheral papillomas (1). Papilloma morphology varies from a spherical focal dilatation of the duct containing a mass with a vascular pedicle on Doppler, to a more serpiginous soft tissue lesion filling a variable portion of a nondilated duct. There is controversy as to whether papillomas can be reliably diagnosed on core needle

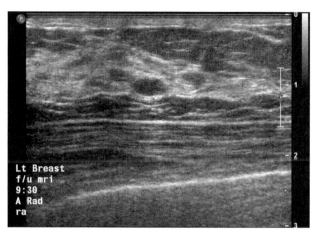

Figure 15.12 Sclerosing adenosis on ultrasound. Sclerosing adenosis has a variety of nonspecific appearances on ultrasound including the small elliptical mass with increased posterior through transmission within the mammary zone on this image.

biopsy alone because of potential sampling errors related to areas of focal malignant involvement within a papilloma.

BENIGN LESIONS OF THE TERMINAL DUCTAL LOBULAR UNIT

The termination of a duct within a lobule is collectively referred to as the terminal ductal lobular unit (TDLU) which is the site of origin of most breast cancers and many benign breast lesions. Cystic dilatation of a lobule may initially form a *cluster of microcysts*, which may be seen on ultrasound and mammography. The microcysts may contain milk of calcium that can be reliably detected on mammography. Calcium aggregates in microcysts may present as a cluster of pleomorphic calcifications which may mimic DCIS mammographically; when these findings are associated with sclerosis within the lobule, the lesion is then termed *sclerosing adenosis* (Fig. 15.12). Progressive cystic dilation of the lobule can result in the formation of a larger cyst which then more commonly presents clinically as a palpable lump. Cysts present mammographically as solitary unilateral, or multiple unilateral or bilateral masses, typically round and circumscribed but variably obscured by adjacent glandular tissue and stromal collagen. Fluid within cysts may be watery or thick and range in color from clear, yellow, bloodstained, or frankly purulent (even when the patient is asymptomatic). The sonographic appearance of cysts can appear simple, complicated, or complex. Cysts are typically bright on T2-weighted images and dark on T1-weighted images with the absence of enhancement on MRI. However, inflamed cysts may enhance peripherally which differs from the characteristic ringed enhancement of malignancy.

Fibroadenomas are the commonest benign breast neoplasm. Though generally solitary, they are multiple in 15% of cases. Fibroadenomas have a natural history, beginning as a cellular smooth soft tissue mass containing variable amounts of stromal and epithelial elements that develop within the lobule, eventually becoming sclerotic, with characteristic "popcorn" calcifications most commonly seen on a mammogram after the menopause (Fig. 15.13). Although fibroadenomas can grow rapidly, most lesions remain smaller than 3 cm in diameter. Rapidly growing fibroadenomas in adolescents and

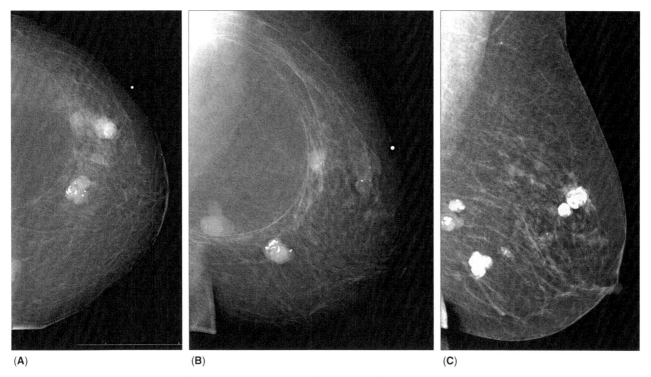

(A)   **(B)**   **(C)**

Figure 15.13 Mammographic appearances of fibroadenomas. (A and B) Multiple, round, elliptical, and lobulated masses with circumscribed margins scattered throughout the breast with a few nonspecific calcifications. Incidental large fat density lipoma involving the posterior upper outer quadrant of the breast is also seen. (C) Mammogram performed seven years later demonstrates the progression of calcifications to the typical "popcorn calcification" appearance pathognomonic for fibroadenomas. Incidental lipoma on prior mammogram has been resected.

young women are labeled *juvenile fibroadenoma* or *giant juvenile fibroadenoma*. The juvenile fibroadenoma is histologically similar to a regular fibroadenoma but tends to have a more cellular stroma (4). Fibroadenomas may have regressed to a size which is not detectable clinically and present as indeterminant calcifications without an associated mass on mammography (3,4,17).

Fibroadenomas usually present on imaging as solitary unilateral, multiple unilateral, or bilateral masses. The typical appearance of a fibroadenoma on ultrasound is a circumscribed, ellipsoid mass with a thin echogenic capsule. The long axis of the fibroadenoma is typically parallel to the skin ("wider than tall") and the echogenicity is similar to fat or slightly darker (Fig. 15.14) (3,17). Whenever a solid mass shows features suspicious for malignancy, it should be biopsied. However, those solid masses with imaging characteristics as described above may be confidently followed up with less than a 2% chance of malignancy *when no suspicions are present radiologically*. Such masses are considered benign when stable for at least two years (3). When solitary fibroadenomas continue to grow and exceed 3 cm in their longest diameter, it is the authors' practice to recommend surgical consultation to discuss possible excision, even when a previous needle biopsy is benign. Fibroadenomas and juvenile fibroadenomas typically demonstrate long T2 and intermediate T1 relaxation times on MRI and have progressive enhancement on dynamic postcontrast acquisitions. As fibroadenomas become progressively sclerotic and calcified, their appearances may more readily be diagnostic on mammography as opposed to ultrasound and MRI, where the heterogeneity of cellular, sclerotic, and calcified elements may mimic malignancy.

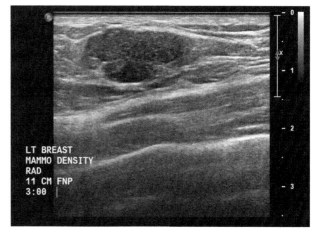

Figure 15.14 Fibroadenoma on ultrasound. Elliptical mass oriented parallel to the skin surface, slightly hypoechoic to fat with at least three lobulations. This lesion was biopsied due to multiple lobulations and found to represent a fibroadenoma.

A tubular adenoma is considered by many to be a variant of a fibroadenoma (4) from which these lesions are indistinguishable on imaging. Histologically, tubular adenomas are composed of small ductal structures embedded within a stromal background (4).

Phyllodes tumors are relatively rare lesions that also develop from the TDLU. They are considered to be neoplastic radiologically in contrast to the fibroadenomas which can appear similar but are hyperplastic lesions. Phyllodes tumors can occur at any age, but are most common in the sixth decade and rarely occur in young women and teenage girls. While most of them are benign, they can be malignant and sometimes metastasize to distant sites such as the lungs (4). The appearance of a phyllodes tumor may overlap with that of a benign fibroad-enoma; however, phyllodes tumors may be distinguished clini-cally by their rapid growth, which may be confirmed at six-month follow-up ultrasound. Theoretically, benign phyl-lodes with infiltrative rather than circumscribed margins are more likely to recur following excision and must be resected with a narrow rim of normal surrounding breast tissue (Fig. 15.15).

Lobular neoplasia includes ALH and LCIS. ALH and LCIS have traditionally been considered a benign incidental finding at pathology unassociated with imaging findings. However, reports indicate both classic and pleomorphic LCIS can pres-ent as indeterminate calcifications on mammography, and approximately half of lobular neoplasia diagnosed on core needle biopsy is prompted by stereotactic biopsy of calcifica-tions (18,19).

A spectrum of benign *columnar cell changes* involving the TDLU have been found on pathological evaluation after biopsy of indeterminate calcifications. These changes include a lesion now termed *flat epithelial atypia*, which is often associated with underdiagnosis of malignancy on core needle biopsy (1).

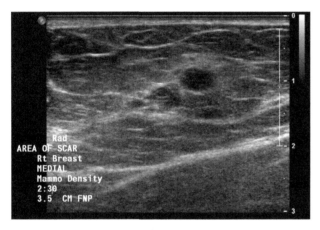

Figure 15.15 Recurrent benign phyllodes tumor on ultrasound. Two larger homogeneous hypoechoic masses surrounded by multiple smaller satellite nodules at the site of previously resected benign phyllodes tumor. Core needle biopsy confirmed recurrence.

BENIGN LESIONS OF FAT

Subcutaneous fat is widely distributed throughout the breast envelope except beneath the nipple, and is a common site for *lipomas*. The latter typically present as soft palpable subcuta-neous lumps, are often indistinguishable from adjacent subcu-taneous fat on mammography, and have a typical homogeneous but slightly hyperechoic appearance compared with adjacent fat sonographically (Figs. 15.2, 15.13, 15.16). A combination of mammography and ultrasound can usually diagnose lipomas with a high degree of accuracy.

Fat necrosis may result from either non-iatrogenic or iatro-genic trauma. Fat necrosis from non-iatrogenic trauma is most often blunt trauma that occurs superficially. Clinically, patients most commonly present with palpable lumps, but other findings may include bruising, tenderness, skin thicken-ing, skin tethering, and nipple retraction in a minority of cases (20). Patients may not volunteer a history of trauma and bruising at the site of the lump until specifically asked since the injury may have occurred several months ago. Typically an episode of trauma is followed by immediate bruising and sub-sequent development of a lump six to eight weeks later. Mam-mographically, fat necrosis may be invisible or seen as faint hazy density in the subcutaneous fat at the site of the palpable lump. However, there may be a more dramatic appearance with a definite mass of mixed echogenicity on ultrasound, especially in the subacute phase. The ultrasound appearance often overlaps that of malignancy and a short-term follow-up is frequently necessary—even after core biopsy.

Oil cysts, calcifications, and architectural distortion can be seen mammographically. Oil cysts can mimic simple cysts on ultrasound except for the absence of posterior acoustic enhancement. Oil cysts may also be seen as complex cystic and solid masses, sometimes with curvilinear rim calcifications which are seen mammographically resulting in shadowing on ultrasound. Fat necrosis causing architectural distortion on mammography and irregularly shaped masses with indistinct margins can mimic malignancy on ultrasonography (2,20). An oblique pattern of fat necrosis across the superior aspect of the breast is commonly seen after a seat belt injury associated with a motor vehicle accident.

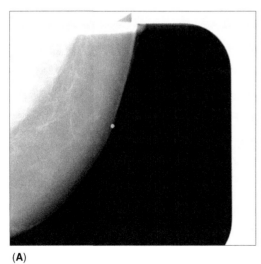
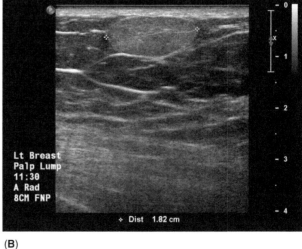

(A)   **(B)**

Figure 15.16 Lipoma. (**A**) Mammogram. BB marks a palpable lump in a patient with only fat density seen, indistinguishable from the normal breast fat. (**B**) Ultra-sound. An elliptical circumscribed hyperechoic mass is present at the site of the lump, correlating with only fat density on the mammogram.

Iatrogenic fat necrosis should be suspected in patients with a history of breast reduction or cancer surgery. Less commonly fat necrosis can follow thoracotomy, or fat injections for cosmetic surgery. Iatrogenic fat necrosis may either be located superficially as for non-iatrogenic disease or lie deep within the breast parenchyma (Fig. 15.17). Fat necrosis can result in small dystrophic calcifications near surgical scars that can be confused with residual or recurrent malignancy on mammography, especially when the cancer initially presented with mammographic calcifications (Fig. 15.18). Comparison of calcifications with the original appearances of malignancy prior to treatment may be helpful in excluding the need for biopsy. For patients treated with breast conservation therapy, an MRI may occasionally demonstrate fat necrosis with ring-shaped enhancement surrounding fat on the post contrast T1-weighted imaging. This finding must be distinguished from ring enhancement of malignancy which doesn't surround fat (20). Edema within the necrotic fat may be seen at T2-weighted imaging.

BENIGN LESIONS ASSOCIATED WITH THE STROMA
The stroma surrounds the breast lobules and ducts and is composed of mostly fat and collagen. Condensations of stromal collagen surrounding the radially oriented ductal system are known as Cooper's ligaments. Breast density on mammography is principally determined by the relative proportion of more dense fat and less dense collagen, ducts, and lobules. Greater breast density on analog mammography has been associated with both increased risk of developing breast cancer and delayed cancer detection with mammography.

Stromal fibrosis, also known as focal fibrosis, focal fibrous disease of the breast, fibrous mastopathy, fibrous tumor, and chronic indurative mastitis, is characterized pathologically by focal fibrosis with either complete absence or hypoplasia of lobules and ducts. Stromal fibrosis is associated with a wide spectrum of imaging findings, but most frequently appears as a mass or focal asymmetry on mammography, and as a hypoechoic mass with rather indistinct margins on ultrasound (Fig. 15.19) (17,21).

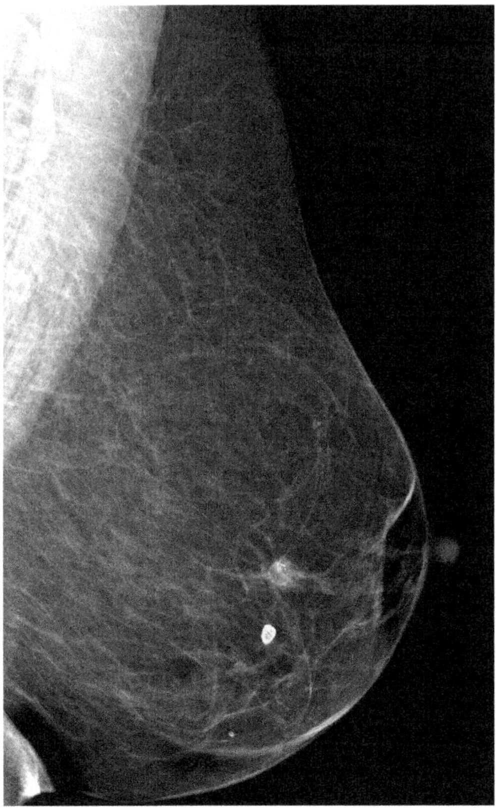

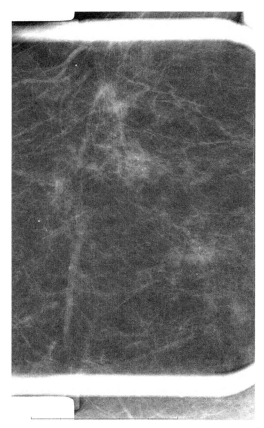

Figure 15.18 Spot magnification mammographic views of fat necrosis with calcifications. Subtle pleomorphic calcifications located within areas of architectural distortion, surrounding central lucent oil cysts.

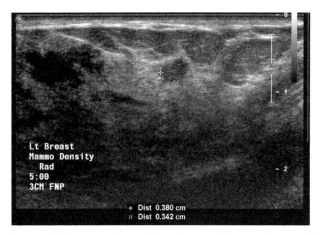

Figure 15.19 Ultrasound of stromal fibrosis. A round hypoechoic mass with irregular margins. Imaging characteristics are very similar to multiple other entities such as fibroadenoma, malignancy, sclerosing adenosis, and proliferative fibrocystic change.

Figure 15.17 Mammogram of a patient with a history of reduction mammoplasty. Three round and elliptical rim calcified structures are diagnostic for oil cysts years postoperatively.

PASH (17,22) is a benign lesion characterized by slit-like spaces lined by spindle cells within stromal fibrosis, which may be mistaken pathologically for a low-grade angiosarcoma (4,17). About one-quarter of breast specimens contain PASH on microscopic examination, but tumoral forms presenting as palpable lumps are rare. Mammographic findings of tumoral forms typically are either a mass with sharp or indistinct margins or focal asymmetry and are usually uncalcified. Similarly, ultrasound findings vary from the more common circumscribed solid hypoechoic mass to a more poorly defined area of heterogeneous echogenicity (Fig. 15.20). Limited experience with MRI in cases of PASH detected incidentally when imaging a newly diagnosed breast cancer has mainly demonstrated a persistent or plateau area of segmental or clumped enhancement (22).

Radial scar, also known as a complex sclerosing lesion, is characterized histologically by a fibroelastic core with entrapped ducts surrounded by radiating ducts and lobules. It has also been referred to as sclerosing papillary proliferation, infiltrating epitheliosis, indurative mastopathy, benign sclerosing ductal proliferation, and nonencapsulated sclerosing lesion. Mammographically, it is characterized by the absence of a central opacity, the presence of multiple elongated thin spicules radiating from the center of the lesion, and infrequency of any palpable correlate, even for superficial lesions of relatively large size. Nonspecific microcalcifications are found mammographically in about one-third of cases (23).

Lymphocytic mastitis, also known as diabetic mastopathy, and sclerosing lymphocytic lobulitis, is characterized by aggregates of lymphocytes around lobules, ducts, and vessels with associated fibrotic stroma. It usually presents as a palpable breast lump in long standing type 1 diabetics but may occasionally be seen in nondiabetic patients as well. It is usually not identified on mammography but is more often seen as an indistinctly marginated hypoechoic mass on ultrasound (Fig. 15.21) (24).

Mammary fibrosis is a rare, benign, nonmetastasizing stromal tumor presenting clinically as a palpable mass which appears as a spiculated and locally invasive tumor radiologically. MRI has been found useful for evaluation of potential chest wall involvement (25).

BENIGN LESIONS AND CONDITIONS OF PREGNANCY AND OF THE LACTATING BREAST

The influence of circulating hormones during lactation and pregnancy are evident on mammography, ultrasound, and MRI (26). Breast MRI is rarely used in the setting of pregnancy or lactation, because enhancement of background tissue is so intense that it obscures specific enhancement of breast pathology. Furthermore, the contrast material used for MRI is not approved in pregnancy. On mammography, breasts of pregnant women appear more dense, heterogeneous, and nodular with a prominent ductal pattern and loss of fatty tissue due to proliferation of ductal and lobular growth and also increased vascularity. These features collectively hinder detection of breast cancer, though in some

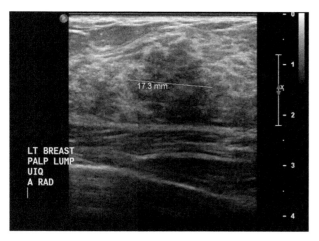

Figure 15.20 Pseudoangiomatous stromal hyperplasia on ultrasound. A round hypoechoic mass with multilobulated margins is seen within the echogenic fibroglandular tissue.

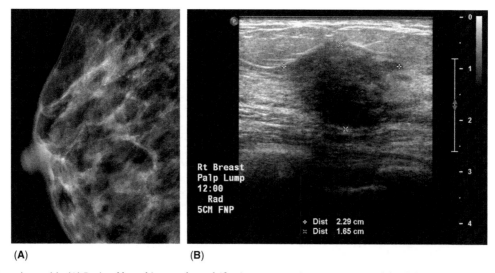

Figure 15.21 Lymphocytic mastitis. (**A**) Regional branching powdery calcifications on screening mammogram of this diabetic patient. More often, mammogram is normal in lymphocytic mastitis. (**B**) Ultrasound in the same patient demonstrates a hypoechoic mass with shadowing and angulated margins. Both the mammogram and ultrasound demonstrate imaging characteristics which overlap with malignancy.

women breast density does not change significantly with pregnancy (27). If mammography is necessary in the lactational state then images are ideally obtained immediately following feeding/milk expression when the breasts are less dense (26). Breast tissue is diffusely more hypoechoic on ultrasound during pregnancy but with onset of lactation, the breast parenchyma becomes diffusely hyperechogenic (due to the production of fat rich milk) with prominent ducts and an increased blood flow.

In the context of pregnancy or lactation, most women come to the attention of their physician because of a palpable mass; for this group of patients, ultrasound is the preferred first choice of imaging (26). Mammography can be performed secondarily if suspicious sonographic or clinical findings are present, though preferably this should be performed after the first trimester, with lead shielding of the abdomen (26,28–30). The principle benefit of mammography in this setting is detection of microcalcifications in the same or opposite breast or other signs of malignancy which are only visible on mammography (26).

Gestational (during pregnancy) *and secretory* (during lactation) *hyperplasia* can be manifest as microcalcifications on mammography which are often rounded in shape due to lobular hyperplasia and may be focal or diffuse. These calcifications can also be pleomorphic in nature due to ductal hyperplasia and be correspondingly ductal in distribution (26). If bloody nipple discharge is present and limited to one duct, further evaluation with ultrasound and galactography are recommended to search for a possible *papilloma* or invasive/noninvasive malignancy (26).

Galactoceles are found as painless lumps in women of childbearing age with a history of recent childbirth and lactation. They are best evaluated with ultrasound and appear as well-circumscribed masses with increased through transmission, but variable appearances of internal echoes are thought to be related to the age of their milk contents. Characteristic sonographic features include a complicated cystic appearance with diffuse internal echoes, fluid–fluid levels, and heterogeneous echogenic shadowing foci attributable to inspissation of internal contents. Needle aspiration and/or short-term follow-up with clinical examination and imaging are usually sufficient for diagnosis in the appropriate clinical setting (26).

Gigantomastia is a rare condition which presents as excessive enlargement of the breasts with subsequent ulceration, necrosis, hemorrhage, and infection which can be life threatening. Both breasts can become grossly enlarged with each breast individually weighing several kilograms. No imaging is specifically required as this is a clinical diagnosis. If a needle biopsy is performed, then the pathological features are similar to a fibroadenoma (26).

Mastitis usually occurs once breast feeding has started and is most often due to *Staphylococcus aureus* or streptococcal infections but also can be caused by anaerobic or mycobacterial organisms. For uncomplicated mastitis no imaging is usually indicated unless one suspects an abscess or inflammatory breast cancer. The ultrasound appearances of mastitis are an ill-defined region of heterogeneous (increased and decreased) echogenicity without a distinct fluid collection. Mammography is only performed if the clinical course is

protracted, mastitis occurs outside of the peripartum period and or when the patient is older than 30 years (31). Combinations of skin thickening, focal asymmetry, and architectural distortion may be seen with mastitis which can resemble carcinoma. When these findings are also associated with microcalcifications, biopsy should be considered. An *abscess* may be palpable as a painful fluctuant mass, present as a focal area of tenderness, or may be too small to be clinically detectable. Puerperal abscesses occur most commonly within the first 12 weeks after birth or during weaning in primiparous mothers (31). Ultrasound is the imaging test of choice, which can show an irregular hypoechoic to anechoic mass. Currently, the preferred method of treatment is initial ultrasound-guided drainage using a 14- or 16-gauge needle with culture and sensitivities to guide antibiotic therapy. Indwelling catheters and surgical drainage can usually be avoided and the success rate with repeated aspirations every 7–14 days is high with a lower risk of cutaneous fistula and less patient discomfort. Following abscess drainage, patients should be advised to continue breast feeding, unless the antibiotic regimen employed is contraindicated in newborns (31). With complete clinical resolution, no follow-up imaging is needed.

Granulomatous mastitis is uncommon and typically presents in young women within a few years of pregnancy, most often with a palpable mass (26). Histologically this condition is a non-caseating, nonvasculitic granulomatous inflammatory process of lobules and must be differentiated from other granulomatous diseases such as tuberculosis and sarcoidosis (26,32). In the majority of cases, the infectious agent *Corynebacterium* can be isolated (26). Clinically a firm mass is felt which spares the subareolar region; reactive lymphadenopathy may also be evident. Mammographic appearances are nonspecific and range from invisibility to focal asymmetry to features of benign or malignant breast masses (26,33). Ultrasonography may show an irregular hypoechoic mass associated with tubular finger-like extensions (32,34), clustered tubular hypoechoic areas (34), or a hypoechoic irregular mass lesion characteristic of malignancy. Treatment includes antibiotics and steroids with rarely any need for surgical intervention.

Juvenile papillomatosis is probably caused by hormonal stimulation and is infrequently seen in mainly younger patients. There may be an association with pregnancy and lactation (26). Noncircumscribed hypoechoic masses with multiple cystic spaces have been reported on ultrasound examination. Mammography may be unremarkable or show microcalcifications or focal asymmetry. On histological examination, cystic changes and ductal or papillary hyperplasia involving cyst walls are seen (26). The condition is associated with carcinoma in about 15% of patients and there is increased risk of recurrence of carcinoma in female relatives.

Lactating adenoma is a more common mass found during pregnancy and the puerperium, and can sometimes resemble fibroadenomas on imaging, being a well-circumscribed oval homogenous solid mass. Hyperechoic areas due to milk fat can be seen sonographically and radiolucent regions can be identified with mammography. Some lesions, however, have a more ominous appearance (Fig. 15.22). These lesions

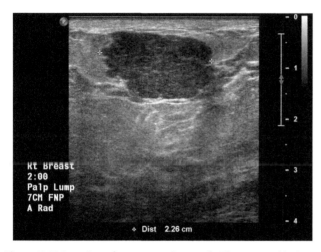

Figure 15.22 Lactating adenoma on ultrasound. Ultrasonographic image shows a homogeneous elliptical mass with microlobulated margins and increased through transmission. The margins of this mass necessitated a core needle biopsy performed without complication.

may have a rapid growth phase with subsequent infarction and typically regress spontaneously after pregnancy and lactation (26).

SELECTED DIFFERENTIAL DIAGNOSES
Cystic Breast Lesions
Complicated or complex cysts may be attributable to any of the following: (*i*) galactocele, (*ii*) hematoma, (*iii*) fat necrosis or oil cyst, (*iv*) abscess, (*v*) intracystic papilloma or carcinoma, and (*vi*) necrotizing neoplasm.

T2 Hyperintense Masses on MRI
The following lesions can exhibit enhancement on T2-weighted images: (*i*) simple cyst, (*ii*) lymph node, (*iii*) fibroadenoma, (*iv*) papilloma, (*v*) seroma, (*vi*) hematoma, (*vii*) phyllodes (benign or malignant), (*viii*) fibrosarcoma, and (*ix*) myelofibroblastoma and cavernous hemangioma. In addition, the following carcinomas show hyperintense images on MRI: mucinous, invasive ductal, intracystic papillary, intraductal papillary, invasive lobular, and adenoid cystic.

Well-Circumscribed Breast Malignancies
Intracystic (encapsulated) papillary cancer, invasive papillary cancer, mucinous carcinoma, medullary carcinoma, and malignant phyllodes.

REFERENCES
1. Georgian-Smith D, Lawton TJ. Controversies on the management of high-risk lesions at core biopsy from a radiology/pathology perspective. Radiol Clin North Am 2010; 48: 999–1012.
2. Shaheen R, Schimmelpenninck CA, Stoddart L, et al. Spectrum of diseases presenting as architectural distortion on mammography: multimodality radiologic imaging with pathologic correlation. Semin Ultrasound CT MR 2011; 32: 351–62.
3. Stavros A. Breast Ultrasound. Philadelphia: Lippincott, Williams and Wilkins, 2004.
4. O'Malley P, Pinder S, Goldblum J, eds. Breast Pathology, 1st edn. Philadelphia: Elsevier, 2006.
5. Chung EM, Cube R, Hall GJ, et al. Breast masses in children and adolescents: radiologic-pathologic correlation. Radiographics 2009; 29: 907–31.
6. Kaplowitz PB, Oberfield SE. Reexamination of the age limit for defining when puberty is precocious in girls in the United States: implications for evaluation and treatment. Drug and Therapeutics and Executive Committees of the Lawson Wilkins Pediatric Endocrine Society. Pediatrics 1999; 104: 936–41.
7. Greydanus DE, Matytsina L, Gains M. Breast disorders in children and adolescents. Prim Care 2006; 33: 455–502.
8. Murray ME, Given-Wilson RM. The clinical importance of axillary lymphadenopathy detected on screening mammography. Clin Radiol 1997; 52: 458–61.
9. Nicholson BT, Harvey JA, Cohen MA. Nipple-areolar complex: normal anatomy and benign and malignant processes. Radiographics 2009; 29. 509–23.
10. Shin HJ, Kim HH, Kim SM, et al. Papillary lesions of the breast diagnosed at percutaneous sonographically guided biopsy: comparison of sonographic features and biopsy methods. AJR Am J Roentgenol 2008; 190: 630–6.
11. Kopans DB, Rusby JE. Cutaneous caves and subcutaneous adipose columns in the breast: radiologic-pathologic correlation. Radiology 2008; 249: 779–84.
12. Pope TL Jr, Read ME, Medsker T, et al. Breast skin thickness: normal range and causes of thickening shown on film-screen mammography. J Can Assoc Radiol 1984; 35: 365–8.
13. Kelekis NL, Efstathopoulos E, Balanika A, et al. Ultrasound aids in diagnosis and severity assessment of hidradenitis suppurativa. Br J Dermatol 2010; 162: 1400–2.
14. Cao MM, Hoyt AC, Bassett LW. Mammographic signs of systemic disease. Radiographics 2011; 31: 1085–100.
15. Giess CS, Raza S, Birdwell RL. Distinguishing breast skin lesions from superficial breast parenchymal lesions: diagnostic criteria, imaging characteristics, and pitfalls. Radiographics 2011; 31: 1959–72.
16. Honegger MM, Hesseltine SM, Gross JD, et al. Tattoo pigment mimicking axillary lymph node calcifications on mammography. AJR Am J Roentgenol 2004; 183: 831–2.
17. Goel NB, Knight TE, Pandey S, et al. Fibrous lesions of the breast: imaging-pathologic correlation. Radiographics 2005; 25: 1547–59.
18. Brem RF, Lechner MC, Jackman RJ, et al. Lobular neoplasia at percutaneous breast biopsy: variables associated with carcinoma at surgical excision. AJR Am J Roentgenol 2008; 190: 637–41.
19. Hanby AM, Hughes TA. In situ and invasive lobular neoplasia of the breast. Histopathology 2008; 52: 58–66.
20. Taboada JL, Stephens TW, Krishnamurthy S, et al. The many faces of fat necrosis in the breast. AJR Am J Roentgenol 2009; 192: 815–25.
21. Revelon G, Sherman ME, Gatewood OM, et al. Focal fibrosis of the breast: imaging characteristics and histopathologic correlation. Radiology 2000; 216: 255–9.
22. Jones KN, Glazebrook KN, Reynolds C. Pseudoangiomatous stromal hyperplasia: imaging findings with pathologic and clinical correlation. AJR Am J Roentgenol 2010; 195: 1036–42.
23. Kennedy M, Masterson AV, Kerin M, et al. Pathology and clinical relevance of radial scars: a review. J Clin Pathol 2003; 56: 721–4.
24. Ely KA, Tse G, Simpson JF, et al. Diabetic mastopathy. A clinicopathologic review. Am J Clin Pathol 2000; 113: 541–5.
25. Glazebrook KN, Reynolds CA. Mammary fibromatosis. AJR Am J Roentgenol 2009; 193: 856–60.
26. Sabate JM, Clotet M, Torrubia S, et al. Radiologic Evaluation of breast disorders related to pregnancy and lactation. Radiographics 2007; 27: S101–24.
27. Swinford AE, Adler DD, Garver KA. Mammographic appearance of the breasts during pregnancy and lactation: false assumptions. Acad Radiol 1998; 5: 467–72.
28. Bevers TB, Anderson BO, Bonaccio E, et al. NCCN clinical practice guidelines in oncology: breast cancer screening and diagnosis. J Natl Compr Cancer Netw 2009; 7: 1060–96.
29. Robbins J, Jeffries D, Roubidoux M, et al. Accuracy of diagnostic mammography and breast ultrasound during pregnancy and lactation. AJR Am J Roentgenol 2011; 196: 716–22.
30. Sechopoulos I, Suryanarayanan S, Vedantham S, et al. Radiation dose to organs and tissues from mammography: Monte Carlo and Phantom study. Radiology 2008; 246: 434–43.

31. Trop I, Dugas A, David J, et al. Breast abscesses: evidence-based algorithms for diagnosis, management, and follow-up. Radiographics 2011; 31: 1683–99.

32. Hovanessian Larsen LJ, Peyvandi B, Klipfel N, et al. Granulomatous lobular mastitis: imaging, diagnosis, and treatment. AJR Am J Roentgenol 2009; 193: 574–81.

33. Sabate JM, Clotet M, Gomez A, et al. Radiologic evaluation of uncommon inflammatory and reactive breast disorders. Radiographics 2005; 25: 411–24.

34. Han BK, Choe YH, Park JM, et al. Granulomatous mastitis: mammographic and sonographic appearances. AJR Am J Roentgenol 1999; 173: 317–20.

16 Breast masses

A. Robin M. Wilson

INTRODUCTION

Masses are the commonest abnormality seen in the breast on screening mammograms and a lump is the commonest presenting symptom in symptomatic breast clinics. Breast masses are defined as circumscribed lesions and these may be well defined, ill defined, or spiculated. A mass that is palpable on clinical examination is often referred to as a "lump." Imaging plays a vital role in the diagnostic assessment and management of both palpable and impalpable breast masses.

Ultrasound and mammography are the standard imaging techniques used for detecting and assessing breast masses. The method of imaging used depends on the age of the patient. Below age 40 ultrasound alone is the imaging technique of first choice, whereas above the age of 40 both mammography and ultrasound are usually indicated (1). Mammography is used at all ages where there is a strong suspicion of breast cancer. Magnetic resonance imaging (MRI) is used as an adjunct to mammography and ultrasound when these standard imaging techniques show equivocal or contradictory results (2,3).

Mammography is the technique of choice for screening women for breast cancer (4). Screening is routinely offered to women at normal risk of breast cancer from age 50 to 70, but in some countries routine screening is offered from the age of 40. For women with dense breasts on mammography, ultrasound may also be offered as an adjunct to improve the chances of cancer detection (5). MRI is also used as the primary screening technique (usually with mammography) for women at a very high risk of breast cancer (e.g., BRCA1/2 gene carriers) (6).

BREAST MASSES: CHARACTERISTICS

A circumscribed mass demonstrated on mammography is defined as a localized rounded lesion of predominantly homogeneous density with convex margins (Fig. 16.1), in contrast to an asymmetric density (Fig. 16.2), which is made up of tissue of mixed density and has predominantly concave margins (Fig. 16.2) (7). The characteristics of the margin of a breast mass constitute the most important diagnostic feature. Well-defined masses are likely to be benign while ill-defined and spiculated masses are more likely to be malignant.

Ill-defined and spiculated masses are the commonest feature of breast cancer detected by screening mammography. The vast majority of well-defined masses are benign (8–10). It is often possible to distinguish benign masses from malignant ones on the basis of their mammographic features alone, but all masses require careful evaluation (11,12). The mammographic features

that assist in differentiation of normal, benign, and malignant masses are as follows:

- number
- size
- density
- composition
- position
- morphology
  - character of margin (well defined, ill defined, or spiculated)
  - contour (oval or round, lobulated, notched)
- associated features (e.g., calcifications and ductal prominence)
- patient age

Each of these is described separately, but it should be stressed that all these features need to be considered together when weighing up the probabilities of a mammographic mass representing malignancy and no single characteristic should be regarded as diagnostic.

A comprehensive list of the differential diagnosis of breast masses is given in Table 16.1.

On ultrasound additional features that help to differentiate normal, benign, and malignant masses include thin echogenic halo (benign), ill-defined thick echogenic halo (malignant), height/width orientation (wider than tall— benignity; taller than wide—malignancy), internal echo pattern (absent—cyst; heterogeneous reduced—malignant; homogeneous reduced– benign) and distal acoustic pattern (bright up–benign; shadow–suspicious) (13–16).

Similarly on MRI it is the same morphological features that are used for mammography that are most important for defining the nature of breast masses (17,18). However, MRI has the additional advantage of providing functional information in the form of dynamic contrast enhancement characteristics with a rapid take-up of contrast and a wash-out pattern (type 3 curve) being suspicious of malignancy, while slow take-up and a persistent pattern (type 1 curve) is highly predictive of a benign cause. Rapid or moderate early enhancement with a persistent enhancement curve (plateau–type 2) is indeterminate and occurs with both benign and malignant masses.

Further assessment of those that do not fulfill the imaging criteria for being definitively benign should include imaging (initially with mammography and ultrasound) clinical examination, and core needle biopsy where indicated (this combination of investigations being known as "triple assessment") (19,20). It is

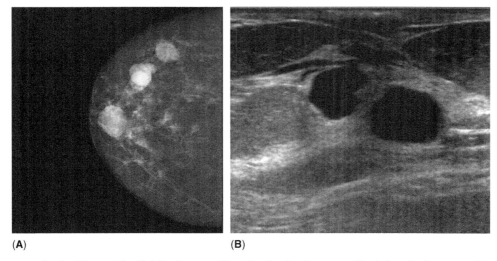

(A)   **(B)**

Figure 16.1 (**A**) Mammography showing several well-defined masses of varying size showing surrounding halos; simple cysts are the most likely diagnosis. (**B**) Cysts confirmed on ultrasound showing well-defined anechoic masses with distal acoustic enhancement.

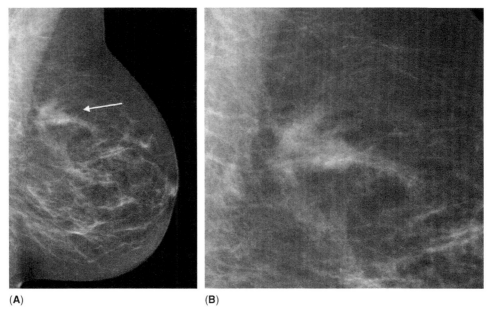

(A)   **(B)**

Figure 16.2 (**A** and **B**) Mammography showing an asymmetric density with amorphous mixed density and convex margins.

only by doing so that unnecessary open surgical biopsy can be avoided for what prove to be benign abnormalities. This approach to assessment also has the advantage of providing a definitive preoperative diagnosis of malignancy, allowing the breast team to plan treatment and the patient to make informed decisions about their treatment options.

Single or Multiple Masses

The differential diagnosis of single and multiple circumscribed masses is shown in Table 16.1; malignancy is more likely with a solitary lesion than with multiple lesions. However, before dismissing multiple masses as benign, they must all be seen to have similar features and a careful search made for a mass with significantly different characteristics that may warrant further assessment. Figure 16.1 shows the typical mammographic and ultrasound features of multiple benign circumscribed masses.

Size

On its own, the size of an abnormality is not of particular importance, as malignant tumors may be identified at any stage in

their development. However, as a general rule, a well-defined mass that is less than 1 cm in diameter is unlikely to be malignant but any solitary well-defined mass over 1 cm in diameter warrants further assessment (Fig. 16.3). All ill-defined and partially well-defined masses of any size need to be further investigated (Fig. 16.4).

Density and Composition

Density and composition are important in assessing the nature of a mass found on mammography. Masses of reduced density compared with normal adjacent tissue (radiolucent) are very likely to be benign (Fig. 16.5). The commonest causes of radiolucent masses are oil cysts, lipomas, and galactoceles; these rarely cause any diagnostic difficulty.

Masses of mixed density containing tissue of fat density are also highly likely to be benign. The differential diagnosis includes normal lymph nodes, fibroadenoma (Fig. 16.6), galactocele, and hematoma.

Masses showing increased density require careful evaluation, as most malignant circumscribed lesions are radio-opaque

Table 16.1 The Differential diagnosis of Masses on Mammography

Multiple masses
- Cysts
- Fibroadenomas
- Papillomas
- Multifocal carcinoma
- Galactocele
- Metastasis:
  - Carcinoma
  - Melanoma
- Lymphoma

Solitary masses
- Normal structures:
  - Nipple
  - Normal breast lobule
  - Intramammary lymph node
  - Vascular structures
  - Skin lesion (mole, sebaceous cyst, nevus)
- Common pathological causes:
  - Cyst
  - Fibroadenoma
  - Carcinoma
  - Abscess
  - Hematoma
  - Galactocele
  - Papilloma
- Uncommon pathological causes:
  - Phyllodes tumor
  - Hamartoma
  - Metastasis (contralateral breast, melanoma, lung, ovary)
  - Adenoma
- Rare causes:
  - Sarcoma
  - Fibromatosis
  - Tuberculosis
  - Sarcoid
  - Hemangioma
  - Neurofibroma
  - Leiomyoma
  - Granular cell tumor

(Fig. 16.7). However, increased density is a non-specific feature, with many benign lesions (e.g., cysts and fibroadenomas) often showing significantly increased density when compared with the adjacent normal breast tissue (11).

Position

A circumscribed mass can occur in any part of the breast. However, masses demonstrated in certain areas deserve special attention. These areas are often referred to as the "review areas," and include the retroareolar area, the retroglandular space on the mediolateral oblique projection, the medial aspect of the breast and the inframammary angle. The majority of circumscribed masses in the axillary tail of the breast are normal lymph glands, but all such masses should be carefully reviewed and further assessment arranged if there is any doubt about their nature.

Margin

The nature of the margin of a mass is the most important single feature in deciding the need for further assessment. A well-defined mass with clearly circumscribed margins, where there is a sharp differentiation between the tumor edge and normal breast tissue is unlikely to represent malignant disease (Fig. 16.1); the risk of malignancy in a solitary well-defined mass is reported to be between 0.5% and 2%. Benign circumscribed masses often show a surrounding halo that is either partial or complete (Figs. 16.1 and 16.3), a feature that is rarely seen in malignant lesions.

However, if the margins of the circumscribed lesion are ill defined, such that there is no clear distinction between the margin of the mass and adjacent normal breast tissue (Figs. 16.7 and 16.8), then the risk of malignancy is significant; all poorly defined circumscribed masses require further assessment. Virtually all circumscribed masses that represent invasive carcinoma will have ill-defined margins; only a few benign lesions will show this feature. Circumscribed masses with margins that are mostly well-defined but with a portion that is ill-defined

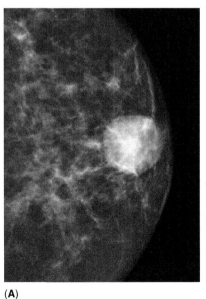

(A)

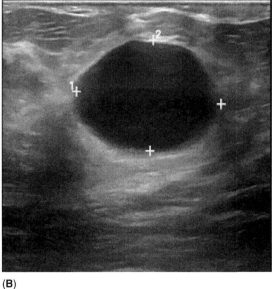

(B)

Figure 16.3 (**A**) Mammography showing a solitary well-defined mass behind the nipple. The appearances strongly favour a benign lesion; (**B**) a corresponding cyst is shown on ultrasound.

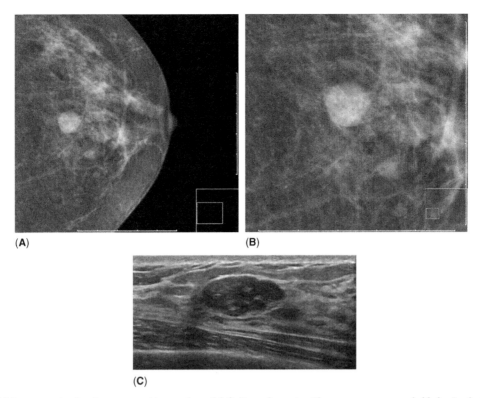

(A)   (B)

(C)

Figure 16.4 (**A** and **B**) Mammography showing a mass with some loss of definition of margins. The appearances are probably benign but further assessment is required. (**C**) Ultrasound showing a well-defined solid mass with features consistent with those of a fibroadenoma.

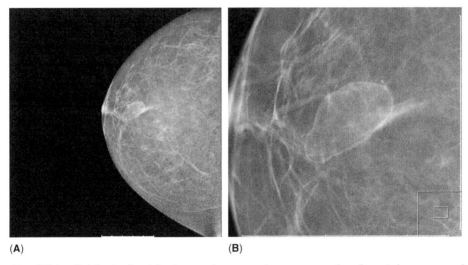

(A)   (B)

Figure 16.5 (**A** and **B**) A well-defined reduced-density mass demonstrated on mammography—the typical appearances of an oil cyst.

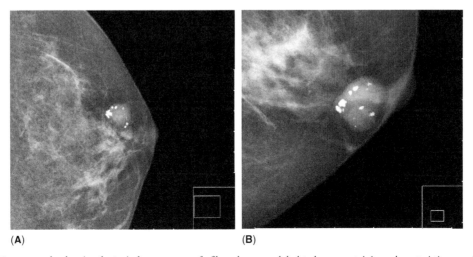

(A)   (B)

Figure 16.6 (**A** and **B**) Mammography showing the typical appearances of a fibroadenoma; a lobulated mass containing a characteristic coarse "popcorn" calcification.

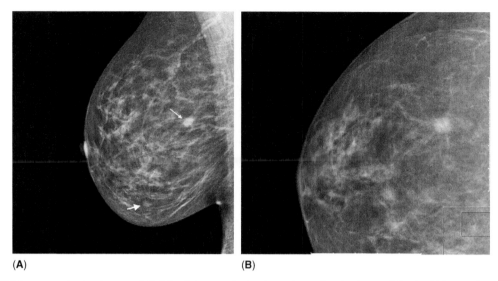

Figure 16.7 (**A** and **B**) Mammography showing a small ill-defined circumscribed malignant mass showing increased density (thin arrow) compared with a similar benign isodense mass (thick arrow) (Fig. 16.2). Histology confirmed as an invasive ductal carcinoma.

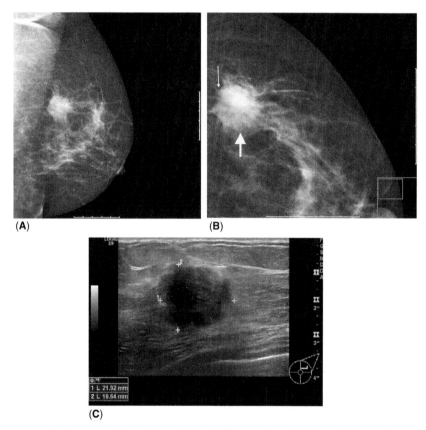

Figure 16.8 (**A** and **B**) Mammography showing a mass with partially well-defined (thin arrow) and ill-defined (thick arrow) margins. (**C**) Ultrasound of the same mass showing features suspicious of carcinoma.

(Fig. 16.9) should be managed in the same way as other ill-defined masses. Most of these will prove to be benign, the ill-defined portion of their margin being caused by overlying normal breast parenchyma (Fig. 16.9), but the risk of malignancy is such that at least further imaging is required.

Masses with a spiculated margin should always be considered malignant until proven otherwise (Fig. 16.10). The risk of a spiculated mass being malignant is in excess of 80%.

Contour

Benign masses are almost always circular or oval and often show one or two smooth shallow lobulations (Fig. 16.6). The exceptions are hematoma and infection (abscess), but the history usually points to the diagnosis in these cases. However, masses that show multiple irregular lobulations must be considered to be malignant and until proven otherwise (Fig. 16.11). Most malignant lesions show some degree of

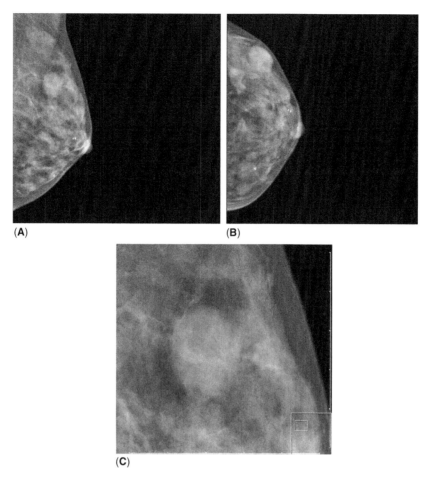

Figure 16.9 (A–C) Mammography in a dense breast showing a mass with margins partly obscured by the surrounding dense breast tissue.

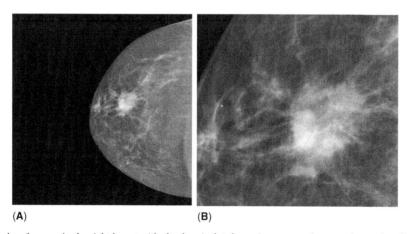

Figure 16.10 (A and B) Mammography of a mass in the right breast with clearly spiculated margins representing a carcinoma invading the surrounding breast tissue and producing reactive changes.

irregularity to their contour; some circumscribed malignancies also show lobulations, particularly papillary and medullary carcinomas (21,22). A few carcinomas may show what appear to be smooth margins, particularly mucinous carcinoma.

Palpability
Another feature, of less importance, is whether or not the abnormality is palpable. A mass that is palpable at small size on imaging (approximately 1 cm or less in diameter) is more likely to be malignant than one that is not. This is true because the desmoplastic reaction induced in the surrounding breast tissue is often palpable around the tumor mass, exaggerating the true size of the lesion. However, this is not a reliable means of differentiation between benign and malignant lesions; small benign inflammatory lesions may be easily palpable while small invasive carcinomas very often are not.

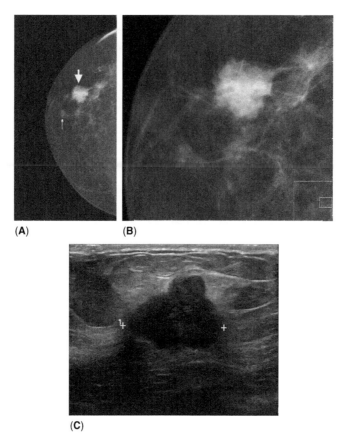

Figure 16.11 (**A** and **B**) Mammography showing a multilobulated irregular mass with features suspicious of malignancy (thick arrow). A second smaller mass (thin arrow) is a satellite lesion. (**C**) Ultrasound of the larger mass showing the lobulated margin; biopsy confirmed grade 3 invasive ductal carcinoma.

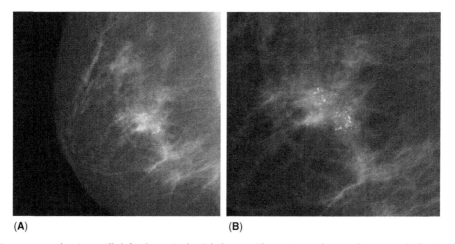

Figure 16.12 (**A** and **B**) Mammograms showing an ill-defined mass in the right breast with prominent pleomorphic microcalcifications both within and adjacent to the mass. The calcifications represent high-grade ductal carcinoma *in situ* both within and adjacent to invasive carcinoma.

Associated Features

The presence of calcification in and around a mass is often a helpful feature in deciding its nature. Macrocalcification within a mass can be characteristic of a fibroadenoma that has undergone partial hyaline degeneration (Fig. 16.6). This appearance is diagnostic and a needle biopsy is unnecessary; malignant change within a fibroadenoma is rare.

On the other hand, pleomorphic calcifications in or around a mass are of much more significance and should suggest a diagnosis of ductal carcinoma in situ (Fig. 16.12); the soft tissue mass in these circumstances does not necessarily indicate the presence of invasive malignant disease, as, not infrequently, the mass represents a localized non-malignant inflammatory response to the in situ disease.

PATIENT AGE

The differential diagnosis of masses is influenced by the age of the patient. Those presenting in women aged below 40 are very likely to be benign, fibroadenoma being the most likely diagnosis. Between the age of 40 and 50 years, cysts are common, but after age 40, all circumscribed masses should be assessed fully if they show equivocal features on imaging.

HISTOLOGICAL CORRELATION

Circumscribed breast carcinomas without evidence of adjacent desmoplastic reaction to produce architectural distortion are considered more likely to be of high histological grade as the tumor grows rapidly without the stimulation of a response from the adjacent breast tissue. The most likely diagnosis of a poorly defined circumscribed mass in the breast that is malignant is invasive ductal carcinoma of no specific type. However, any type of breast cancer can give this appearance, including lobular carcinoma. Mucinous and medullary carcinomas typically produce a circumscribed mass in the breast as opposed to a stellate lesion or a spiculate mass.

ASSESSMENT OF BREAST MASSES

If there is any doubt in the mind of the mammogram film reader about the nature of a mass, then further imaging and clinical assessment are mandatory (23–25). The assessment process for circumscribed masses is straightforward. The single most useful complementary imaging tool is ultrasound, which, using frequencies of at least 10 MHz, should be the routine initial imaging investigation for circumscribed masses detected on routine mammography. The majority of breast masses are demonstrable on ultrasound. Ultrasound will readily differentiate solid lesions from the cystic ones (Figures 16.3B and 16.4C); where there is doubt, needle aspiration should be attempted. All solid lesions deemed worthy of further assessment should undergo core needle biopsy for histology. Fine needle aspiration is not recommended for routine assessment of breast masses. Ultrasound-guided breast biopsy is the method of choice for any abnormality visible on ultrasound.

If a circumscribed lesion is not visible on ultrasound then further mammography is indicated. It should not be assumed that a mass that is not seen on ultrasound either does not exist as a true mass or is benign. Paddle compression is particularly useful in confirming the presence of a circumscribed mass, and will often give more information about the contour and margins. Stereotactic (x-ray) guided core biopsy or vacuum-assisted biopsy should be performed if the mass is not clearly benign.

SUMMARY

Masses are common findings on both screening mammography and in the symptomatic breast clinic the majority of which are benign. Differentiation between definitively benign from possibly malignant circumscribed masses is usually straightforward, with mass margin and density being the most important mammographic features. Ultrasound is the most useful imaging tool for further assessment of circumscribed masses.

REFERENCES

1. Willett AM, Michell MJ, Lee JR, eds. Best practice guideline for patients presenting with breast Symptom 2010. [Available from: www.associationofbreastsurgery.org.uk/media/4585/best practice diagnostic guidelines for patients presenting with breast symptoms.pdf].
2. National Institute for Clinical Excellence. CG 80 early and locally advance breast cancer: NICE guideline 2009. [Available from: http://guidance.nice.org.uk/CG80/NICEGuidance/pdf/English]
3. Sardanelli F, Boetes C, Borisch B, et al. Magnetic resonance imaging of the breast: recommendations from the EUSOMA working group. Eur J Cancer 2010; 46: 1296–316.
4. Smith RA, Duffy SW, Tabár L. Breast cancer screening: the evolving evidence. Oncology (Williston Park) 2012; 26: 471–5; 479-81, 485-6.
5. Berg WA, Blume JD, Cormack JB, et al. Combined screening with ultrasound and mammography vs mammography alone in women at elevated risk of breast cancer. JAMA 2008; 299: 2151–63.
6. Kuhl CK, Schmutzler RK, Leutner CC, et al. Mammography, breast ultrasound and magnetic resonance imaging for surveillance of women at high familial risk for breast cancer. J Clin Oncol 2005; 23: 8469–76.
7. Kopans DB, Swann CA, White GW, et al. Asymmetric breast tissue. Radiology 1989; 171: 639–43.
8. Stomper P, Leibowich S, Meyer J. The prevalence and distribution of well circumscribed nodules on screening mammography: analysis of 1500 mammograms. Breast Dis 1991; 4: 197–203.
9. Sickles E. Nonpalpable, circumscribed, noncalcified, solid breast masses: likelihood of malignancy based on lesion size and age of patient. Radiology 1994; 192: 439–42.
10. Feig S. Breast masses: mammographic and sonographic evaluation. Radiol Clin North Am 1992; 30: 67–92.
11. Tabar L, Dean P. Teaching Atlas of Mammography. Stuttgart: Georg Thieme Verlag, 1985.
12. Klein S. Evaluation of palpable breast masses. Am Fam Physician 2005; 71: 731–8.
13. Stavros AT. Ultrasound of solid breast nodules: distinguishing benign from malignant. In: Stavros AT, Rapp CL, Parker S, eds. Breast Ultrasound. Lipincott: Williams and Wilkins, 2004.
14. Lister D, Evans AJ, Burrell HC, et al. The accuracy of breast ultrasound in the evaluation of clinically benign discrete breast lumps. Clin Radiol 1998; 53: 490–2.
15. Rinaldi P, Ierardi C, Costantini M, et al. Cystic breast lesions: sonographic findings and clinical management. J Ultrasound Med 2010; 29: 1617–26.
16. Raza S, Goldkamp AL, Chikarmane SA, et al. US of breast masses categorized as BI-RADS 3, 4, and 5: pictorial review of factors influencing clinical management. Radiographics 2010; 30: 1199–213.
17. Uematsu T, Kasami M. MR imaging findings of benign and malignant circumscribed breast masses: part 1. Solid circumscribed masses. Jpn J Radiol 2009; 27: 395–404.
18. Schnall M, Orel S. Breast MR imaging in the diagnostic setting. Magn Reson Imaging Clin N Am 2006; 14: 329–37.
19. Teh W, Evans AJ, Wilson ARM. Definitive non-surgical breast diagnosis: the role of the radiologist. Editorial Clin Radiol 1998; 53: 81–4.
20. O'Flynn EAM, Wilson ARM, Michell MJ. Breast biopsy: state of the art. Clin Radiol 2010; 65: 259–70.
21. Meyer JE, Amin E, Lindfors KK, et al. Medullary carcinoma of the breast: mammographic and US appearance. Radiology 1989; 170: 79–82.
22. Karan B, Pourbagher A, Bolat FA. Unusual malignant breast lesions: imaging-pathological correlations. Diagn Interv Radiol 2012; 18: 270–6.
23. Harvey JA, Nicholson BT, Cohen MA. Finding early invasive breast cancers: a practical approach. Radiology 2008; 248: 61–76.
24. Jackson VP. Diagnostic mammography. Radiol Clin North Am 2004; 42: 853–70.
25. Mendelson EB. Problem-solving ultrasound. Radiol Clin North Am 2004; 42: 909–18.

17 Asymmetry and architectural distortion

Michael J. Michell

INTRODUCTION

Asymmetry or distortion of architecture of the breast tissue may be the only sign of malignancy on x-ray mammography. These signs account for up to 1.6% and 4.9% of small screen-detected invasive cancers measuring less than 15 mm in diameter respectively (1), and a small proportion of cases of in situ carcinoma. Both signs may cause difficulties for the mammography film reader—asymmetry is a common appearance in the normal glandular or involuting breast (2), and areas of architectural distortion may show only subtle mammographic features and be difficult to perceive. Assessment, diagnosis, and management of cases in which either of these signs is the principal abnormality may be challenging because of the complex and varied pathology which may be associated particularly with architectural distortion. Furthermore, lack of concordance may occur between the mammographic features and other elements of the triple diagnostic workup. A thorough knowledge of mammographic features, differential diagnosis, and appropriate assessment pathways as well as an integrated multidisciplinary approach is necessary to achieve an accurate diagnosis and correct management (3,4).

ASYMMETRY

Mammographic Features

Mammograms are routinely viewed with right and left mediolateral oblique (MLO) views and right and left craniocaudal (CC) views positioned "back to back" so that the pattern and distribution of the glandular tissue may be compared between the two sides and any asymmetry identified. A classification of asymmetry on mammography is described in the American College of Radiologists BI-RADS system (5,6). In clinical practice, asymmetry on mammography may be classified as follows:

1. Focal
2. Segmental
3. Diffuse

Focal Asymmetry

The only mammographic sign of a small invasive cancer may be a non-specific asymmetric soft tissue density opacity measuring up to 2 cm diameter and displaying none of the classic signs of malignancy such as spiculation or margin irregularity (7) (Fig. 17.1). A focal asymmetry on standard mammography views is distinguished from a mass lesion because of the absence of definite convex outward boarders, usually evident on two orthogonal views. Film readers should pay special attention to the review areas on both the MLO and CC views

in order to perceive such abnormalities (8). The review areas are as follows:

1. A 3–4 cm wide area anterior to the edge of the pectoralis muscle on the lateral oblique view
2. The retro glandular clear space between the posterior margin of the parenchyma and the chest wall on both the MLO and CC projections
3. The medial half of the breast on the CC views
4. The retroareolar area: perception of carcinomas in this site may be difficult because of superimposition of ductal structures and stroma
5. The inferior part of the breast

Having identified a focal asymmetric density, the reader should analyze the following features to decide whether recall for further assessment is indicated.

1. Density: is density the same or greater than the glandular tissue? Malignant lesions often have a density which is greater than the glandular tissue and greater than might be expected for the size of the lesion.
2. Interval change: is the asymmetric density a new finding or has it increased in size since previous examinations?
3. Margin: does the margin between the asymmetric density and the surrounding tissue show smooth, curved concave contours, usually associated with an area of normal glandular tissue, or is there evidence of irregularity or spiculation raising the suspicion for malignancy?
4. Associated signs: are there any other features such as microcalcification, skin thickening, retraction of the subcutaneous connective tissue, or distortion of the surrounding parenchyma in the area of the asymmetric density? (Fig. 17.2)

Segmental Asymmetry

Segmental asymmetry is characterized by an asymmetric area of soft tissue density usually measuring 2–10 cm in extent. It may be a normal finding but may be the only mammography feature of either in situ or invasive cancer.

Causes of segmental asymmetry:

1. Normal/physiological
2. Invasive cancer
3. Ductal carcinoma in situ

Both invasive ductal and lobular carcinomas may cause asymmetry on mammography. Invasive lobular carcinomas, however,

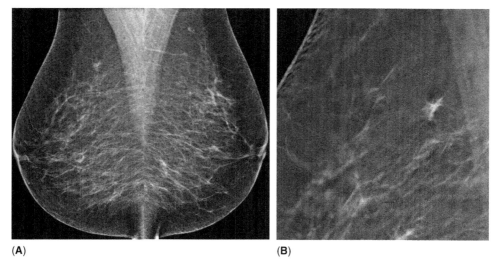

(A)   **(B)**

Figure 17.1 Invasive duct carcinoma. MLO views (A) show a small asymmetric soft tissue density in the upper right breast. Tomosynthesis view (B) shows a spiculated tumor. *Abbreviation*: MLO, mediolateral oblique.

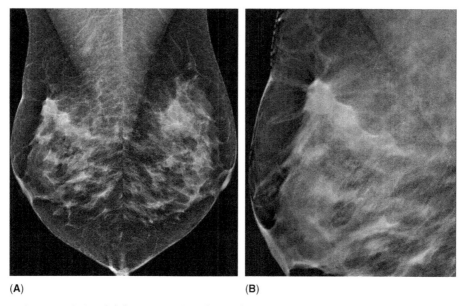

(A)   **(B)**

Figure 17.2 Invasive duct carcinoma. MLO views (A) show an irregular soft tissue density in the upper right breast with retraction of the overlying skin. Tomosynthesis view (B) shows spiculation. *Abbreviation*: MLO, mediolateral oblique.

account for a larger proportion of carcinomas when asymmetry is the primary abnormality because of their histological growth pattern (9–13). Ductal carcinoma in situ may appear as asymmetric soft tissue opacity with no evidence of microcalcification (14).

The mammographic features which should be analyzed on the basic standard mammograms to decide whether further assessment is required are as follows:

1. The appearance on two views
2. Interval change
3. Associated signs

The appearance on two views: a normal asymmetric density is often seen as a localized opacity in one view but "spreads" out and is recognized as normal glandular tissue in the orthogonal view (Fig. 17.3). If the asymmetry is due to underlying pathology, the same asymmetric density is often seen in both views.

Interval change: comparison with previous films will show whether the asymmetry is a new finding and may be due to

pathology or is a stable appearance and due to normal asymmetry (15).

Associated signs: the asymmetric tissue and the tissue surrounding it should be carefully inspected for any evidence of other signs of malignancy such as distortion, retraction, skin change, or microcalcification (Fig. 17.4).

Assessment and Diagnosis of Focal and Segmental Asymmetry

Cases recalled following routine screening should be assessed using the triple diagnostic method—clinical assessment, imaging, and needle biopsy for a persistent abnormality (Fig. 17.5) (16). The clinical and imaging assessment should be completed before any needle biopsy is performed.

Comparison of areas of asymmetry with appearances on previous mammograms may be very helpful and such examinations should be obtained if possible. Further imaging should include both mammography and ultrasound. The mammography workup may include further views in different

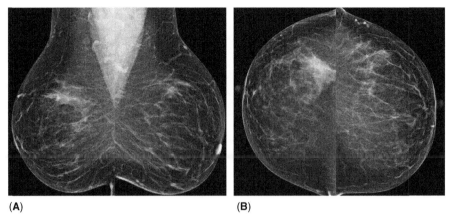

Figure 17.3 Normal glandular asymmetry. MLO views (A) and CC views (B) show asymmetric glandular tissue in the right upper outer quadrant. *Abbreviations*: CC, craniocaudal; MLO, mediolateral oblique.

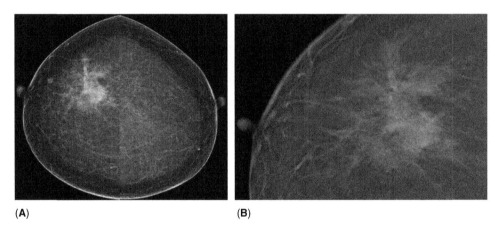

Figure 17.4 Complex sclerosing lesion with *in situ* carcinoma. CC views (A) show asymmetric tissue in the lateral right breast. Tomosynthesis view (B) shows associated distortion. *Abbreviation*: CC, craniocaudal.

projections according to the site and extent of the suspicious area—lateral and extended craniocaudal views, spot compression with magnification, and tomosynthesis (17,18) may help in characterizing the mammographic appearances. Further mammography may result in a change in mammographic features; a localized non-specific soft tissue density may show spiculation on spot compression or tomosynthesis (Fig. 17.6). The additional information provided by the mammographic workup allows the radiologist to define the site, extent, and level of suspicion for any persisting abnormality.

Ultrasound should also be carried out and may show a definite mass or an area of abnormal reflectivity in cases of in situ or invasive malignancy. In those cases, where malignancy is thought to be due to normal asymmetric glandular tissue on the basis of clinical and mammography work-up, ultrasound may help confirm this diagnosis by demonstrating normal parenchyma which correlates with mammography appearances. In most cases of localized or segmental asymmetry, a combination of clinical assessment, mammography workup, and ultrasound will confirm or exclude significant pathology. In those cases considered to be normal, the patient is subsequently discharged. In cases where there is a persistently abnormal area, a 14 gauge core needle biopsy should be carried out to establish a

histological diagnosis. The biopsy is performed under image guidance—ultrasound is the preferred method and stereotaxis employed for cases where the abnormality is not visible on ultrasound.

In a small number of cases, there may be uncertainty about the significance of a focal or segmental area of asymmetry on mammography following initial clinical and imaging assessment. Such cases should be discussed in the multidisciplinary meeting. Breast MRI, with its high negative predictive value or multiple image-guided core biopsies may be helpful in confirming or excluding malignant disease.

Diffuse Asymmetry

Diffuse asymmetry is characterized by an increase in the density of the majority of the glandular tissue of one breast compared with the other. The causes are as listed below:

1. Normal/physiological
2. Congenital
3. Acute inflammation
4. Inflammatory carcinoma
5. Postradiotherapy treatment
6. Other causes of edema: cardiac failure and renal failure.

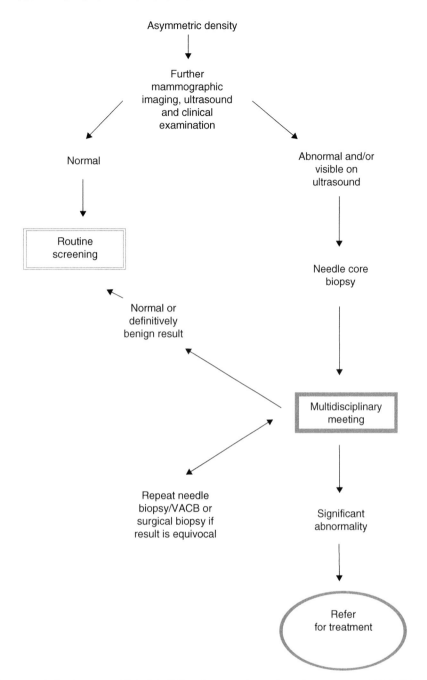

Figure 17.5 Investigation of asymmetric density. *Source*: Clinical Guidelines for Breast Cancer Screening Assessment, Third edition. NHSBSP Publication No 49, June 2010. Editors Liston J, Wilson R.

The mammographic features of edema which may accompany diffuse asymmetry are:

1. Generalized increase in the density of the parenchyma
2. Thickening of the trabeculae
3. Skin thickening

Assessment and Diagnosis of Diffuse Asymmetry

Normal physiological and congenital causes of diffuse asymmetry are readily diagnosed from the absence of any associated mammographic features of edema and from the clinical history and examination. Congenital hypoplasia of one breast may be associated with the absence of the ipsilateral pectoralis major muscle in Poland's syndrome (19). Women with involuted breasts may develop asymmetric increased density of the glandular parenchyma following commencement of HRT (20–22).

Inflammatory cancer may be difficult to differentiate from severe acute inflammation. In both conditions there is swelling, redness, and skin thickening or *peau d'orange*. Imaging may show evidence of edema only, or may show a mass or malignant microcalcification in inflammatory cancer (23,24). In both conditions, there may be a cavity or cavitating mass seen on ultrasound and axillary lymphadenopathy may be a common feature. In most cases, a tissue diagnosis can be made by carrying out a needle biopsy on a mass or cavity, or punch biopsy of the skin.

Clinical history and comparison with previous examinations will enable a diagnosis of post radiotherapy change to be made. Clinical history and associated clinical signs will

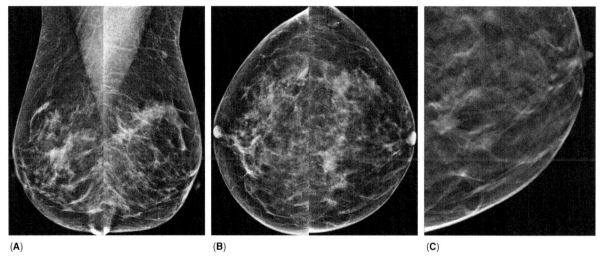

Figure 17.6 Invasive lobular carcinoma. MLO views (**A**) and CC views (**B**) show a focal asymmetric density in the upper inner quadrant of the left breast. Tomosynthesis (**C**) in the CC projection demonstrates a spiculated tumor medially.

distinguish a diagnosis of edema from general medical causes such as cardiac or renal failure.

ARCHITECTURAL DISTORTION
Mammographic Features
An area of architectural distortion of the breast is seen mammographically as numerous thin straight lines measuring from a few millimeters to 4–5 cm in length radiating toward a central area–similar in distribution to the spokes of a wheel. The central part of the lesion typically shows either no central soft tissue mass, or a central soft tissue density which is small in relation to the length of the radiating lines or spicules (8). Localized distortion may be difficult to perceive on standard MLO and CC views, and may only be visible in one projection. The mammography film reader should carefully inspect both the anterior and posterior margins of the glandular tissue on the MLO and CC projections for any signs of retraction, as well as the pattern of the glandular tissue for any evidence of disruption of the normal pattern and appearance.

Conversely, overlying normal structures may mimic an area of distortion on standard two-dimensional mammography. The structures are carefully analyzed and the trained experienced film reader is able to identify many of these cases as normal. Some cases, however, will require further assessment to exclude a mammographic abnormality.

Differential diagnosis of architectural distortion: (25)

1. Surgical scar
2. Carcinoma
3. Complex sclerosing lesion (CSL)/radial scar
4. Sclerosing adenosis

Assessment and Management of Architectural Distortion
A surgical scar can be confidently diagnosed from the appropriate clinical history and physical examination which should indicate that the position of the radiological scar corresponds to the position of the scar on the breast (Fig. 17.7). If there is doubt, a mammogram can be performed with a radio-opaque marker at the site of the dermal scar. Surgical scars will often

show a difference in appearance between the MLO and CC views because of their discoid shape.

The initial clinical and imaging assessment of a possible area of distortion, having excluded those cases due to previous surgery, is to establish whether a lesion is present. Clinical examination may confirm a palpable abnormality in cases of malignancy, but may also be abnormal in some cases of a benign radial scar (26). Further mammography with spot compression and magnification views is used to spread the parenchyma in the area of interest resulting in normal appearances in those cases of composite shadowing, and accentuation of abnormal features in those cases in which a true distortion is present. Recent evidence has shown that digital breast tomosynthesis is as effective as spot compression views in these cases.

Further assessment of a localized parenchymal distortion is aimed at identifying those cases which are due to malignancy and require treatment, and those cases due to benign causes such as CSL or sclerosing adenosis. Cases of localized parenchymal distortion, about 50–60%, are due to carcinoma, often of special type, for example tubular and grade 1 invasive ductal cancers. It is not possible to use clinical and imaging features alone to distinguish benign from malignant cases (Figs. 17.8–17.10). Some features, however, may strongly suggest the diagnosis–a palpable mass is more commonly associated with malignancy; very long spicules and absence of a central mass are more commonly associated with a benign CSL. Ultrasound may show a localized abnormality and this may be helpful in directing the needle biopsy but the imaging features are not specific (27). MRI has been used by some groups but the features are not specific and cannot be used to exclude malignancy. Both benign and malignant cases of distortion may be associated with microcalcification.

Any persistent localized area of parenchymal distortion, except those due to a surgical scar, requires a histological diagnosis (16). At initial assessment, 14 gauge needle core biopsy samples can be obtained under either ultrasound or stereotactic guidance–ultrasound is preferred if the lesion is sufficiently well visualized. Multiple samples should be obtained to achieve the greatest accuracy (28,29). The imaging and needle

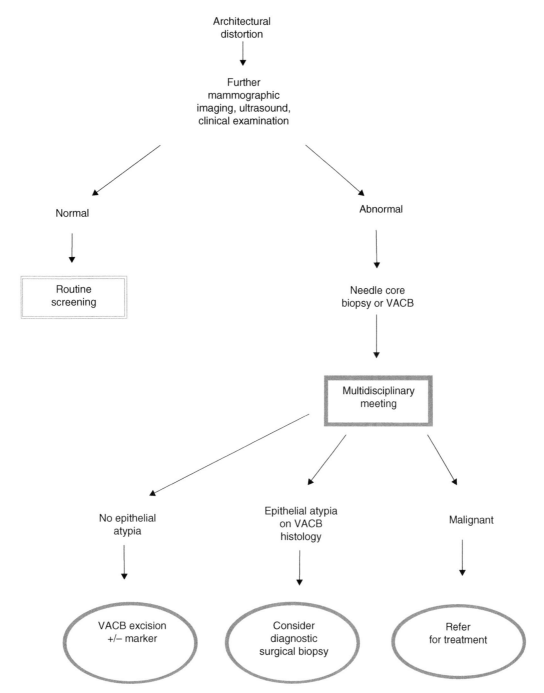

Figure 17.7 Investigation of architectural distortion. *Source*: Clinical Guidelines for Breast Cancer Screening Assessment, third edition. NHSBSP Publication No 49, June 2010. Editors Liston J, Wilson R.

biopsy findings should be discussed in a multidisciplinary meeting to ensure there is concordance between the findings before reaching a diagnosis. If invasive or in situ malignancy is confirmed, treatment is planned accordingly. If the histology shows features of a CSL with any evidence of atypical ductal epithelial proliferation, diagnostic surgical excision should be carried out because of the risk of coexistent malignant disease (30). The excised specimen is x-rayed to ensure that the mammographic lesion has been removed. The surgical histology is then considered in the multidisciplinary meeting in order to reach a final diagnosis and decide on further management.

If initial core biopsy shows evidence of a CSL with no evidence of atypia, further tissue should be obtained to verify the diagnosis and to exclude significant coexistent pathology. This can be achieved either by diagnostic surgical excision or by image-guided vacuum-assisted core biopsy acquiring twelve 11 gauge samples or the equivalent (16). The core biopsy histology is reviewed in the multidisciplinary meeting to ensure concordance between the imaging and histology findings. If there is no evidence of atypia or malignancy, the patient is discharged back to routine screening. If any atypia is diagnosed, diagnostic surgical excision is usually recommended.

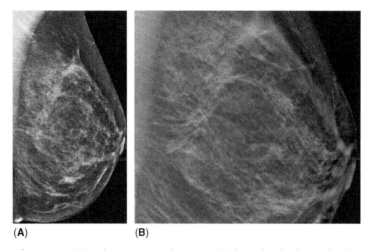

(A)   (B)

Figure 17.8 Invasive duct carcinoma. Left MLO view (**A**) and MLO tomosynthesis view (**B**) show a localized area of architectural distortion.

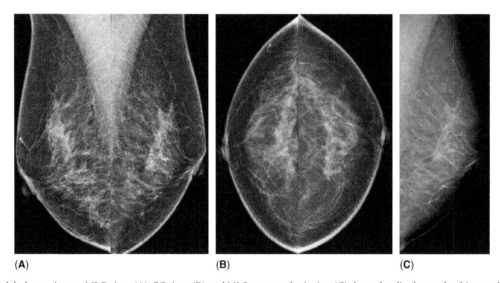

(A)   (B)   (C)

Figure 17.9 Invasive lobular carcinoma. MLO views (**A**), CC views (**B**), and MLO tomosynthesis view (**C**) show a localized area of architectural distortion posterior and medial to the nipple.

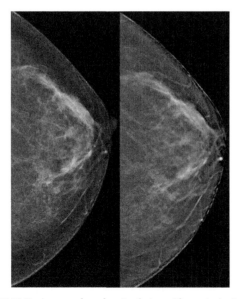

Figure 17.10 Benign complex sclerosing lesion with no atypia. Left standard CC view and left CC tomosynthesis view show a localized area of architectural distortion medial to the nipple.

REFERENCES

1. Michell MJ, Wasan R. The detection of small invasive breast cancers by mammography. In: Michell MJ, ed. Breast Cancer. Contemporary Issues in Cancer Imaging. London: Cambridge University, 2010: 6: 99–112.
2. Kopans DB, Swann CA, White G, et al. Asymmetric breast tissue. Radiology 1989; 171: 639–43.
3. Sickles EA. The spectrum of breast asymmetries: imaging features, work-up, management. Radiol Clin North Am 2007; 45: 765–71, v.
4. Brenner RJ. Asymmetric densities of the breast: strategies for imaging evaluation. Semin Roentgenol 2001; 36: 201–16.
5. American College of Radiology. ACR BI-RADS: mammography. In: ACR Breast Imaging Reporting and Data System, Breast Imaging Atlas, 4th edn. Reston, VA: American College of Radiology, 2003.
6. Youk JH, Kim EK, Ko KH, Kim MJ. Asymmetric mammographic findings on the fourth edition of BI-RADS: types, evaluation and management. Radiographics 2009; 29: e33.
7. Samardar P, Shaw de Paredes E, Grimes MM, Wilson JD. Focal asymmetric densities seen at mammography: US and pathological correlation. Radiographics 2002; 22: 19–33.
8. Michell MJ. The breast. In: Sutton D, ed. Textbook of Radiology and Imaging. London, UK: Churchill Livingstone, 2003; 45: 1462.
9. Newstead GM, Baute PB, Toth HK. Invasive lobular and ductal carcinoma: mammographic findings and stage at diagnosis. Radiology 1992; 184: 623–7.

10. Evans WP, Burhenne LJW, Laurie L et al. Invasive lobular carcinoma of the breast: mammographic characteristics and computer aided detection. Radiology 2002; 225: 182–189.

11. Krecke K, Gisvold J. Invasive lobular carcinoma of the breast: mammographic findings and extent of disease. AJR 1993; 161: 957–60.

12. Sickles EA. The subtle and atypical mammographic features of invasive lobular carcinoma. Radiology 1991; 178: 25–6.

13. Cornford EJ, Wilson AR, Athanassiou E, et al. Mammographic features of invasive lobular and invasive ductal carcinoma of the breast: a comparative analysis. Br J Radiol 1995; 68: 450–3.

14. Ikeda DM, Andersson I. Ductal carcinoma in situ: atypical mammographic appearances. Radiology 1989; 172: 661–6.

15. Leung JWT Sickles EA. Developing asymmetry identified on mammography: correlation with imaging and pathologic findings. AJR 2007; 188: 667–75.

16. NHS Cancer Screening Programmes. Clinical Guidelines for Breast Cancer Screening Assessment, 3rd edn. Sheffield, UK: NHSBSP publication No 49, 2010.

17. Tagliafico A, Astengo D, Cavagnetto F, et al. One to one comparison between digital spot compression view and digital breast tomosynthesis. Eur Radiol 2012; 22: 539–44.

18. Noroozian M, Hadjiiski L, Rahnama-Moghadam S, et al. Digital breast tomosynthesis is comparable to mammographic spot views for mass characterization. Radiology 2012; 262: 61–8.

19. Samuels TH, Haider MA, Kirkbride P. Poland's syndrome: a mammographic presentation. AJR AM J Roentgenol 1996; 166: 347–8.

20. Persson I, Thurtjell E, Holber L. Effect of estrogen and estrogen-progestin replacement regimes on mammographic breast parenchyma density. J Clin Oncol 1997; 15: 3201–7.

21. Cylak D, Wong CH. Mammographic changes in postmenopausal women undergoing hormonal replacement therapy. AJR 1993; 161: 1177–83.

22. Stomper PC, Van Woorhis BJ, Ravnikar VA, Meyer JE. Mammographic changes associated with post-menopausal hormone replacement therapy: a longitudinal study. Radiology 1990; 174: 487–90.

23. Kushwaha AC, Whitman GJ, Stelling CB, et al. Primary inflammatory carcinoma of the breast. AJR 2000; 174: 535–8.

24. Dershaw DD, Moore MP, Liberman L, Deutch BM. Inflammatory breast carcinoma: mammographic findings. Radiology 1994; 190: 831–4.

25. Tabar L, Dean PB. Teaching Atlas of Mammography. New York: Thieme, 2001.

26. Wallis MG, Devakumar R, Hosie KB, et al. Complex sclerosing lesions (radial scars) of the breast can be palpable. Clin Radiol 1993; 48: 319–20.

27. Cohen MA, Sferlazza SJ. Role of sonography in evaluation of radial scars of the breast. AJR 2000; 174: 1075–8.

28. Kirwan SEM, Denton ERE, Nash RM, Humphreys S, Michell MJ. Multiple 14G stereotactic core biopsies in the diagnosis of mammographically detected stellate lesions of the breast. Clin Radiol 2000; 55: 763–6.

29. Brenner RJ, Jackman RJ, Parker SH, et al. Percutaneous core needle biopsy of radial scars of the breast: when is excision necessary? AJR 2002; 179: 1179–84.

30. Mayers MM, Sloane JP. Carcinoma and atypical hyperplasia in radial scars and complex sclerosing lesions: importance of lesion size and patient age. Histopathology 1993; 23: 225–31.

18 The radial scar

Sabrina Rajan and Pauline J. Carder

INTRODUCTION

The term radial scar or *Strahlige Narben* was first introduced by the Austrian pathologist Herwig Hamperl in 1975 (1). Radial scars are benign foci of proliferative breast disease giving rise to stellate distortions of the tissue architecture. The pathogenesis of radial scars is uncertain; they may be part of the spectrum of benign fibrocystic change or secondary to an injury that obliterates ducts and results in fibrosis, elastosis, ductal proliferation and contraction of adjacent tissue (2). There is no known association with parity, menopausal status or exposure to hormonal agents such as the oral contraceptive.

Current National Health Service Breast Screening Programme pathology guidelines recommend the term radial scar for lesions less than 10 mm in size, with larger lesions of otherwise similar appearance designated as complex sclerosing lesions (3). Lesions of either size rarely present with a breast lump and are usually picked up incidentally; either by the radiologist through identification of a mammographic abnormality or by the pathologist while examining the breast tissue removed for other reasons. The significance of radial scars stems from their potential to mimic malignancy both radiologically and histologically, and from the possibility that they may be associated with malignant and premalignant lesions.

INCIDENCE

Radial scars are relatively common breast lesions which have been reported to be present in 28% of unselected autopsies if the tissue is sampled extensively and are multicentric in 67% and bilateral in 43% of cases (4). The incidence is higher in cancer bearing breasts and in the contralateral breasts of women with a history of breast cancer. Moreover, there is an increased risk of finding multiple lesions in these patients (5,6). The high incidence of lesions reported in autopsy studies relates to large numbers of radial scars identified microscopically that are not clinically or radiologically detectable.

With the advent of population-based screening programs, radial scars may be seen with increased frequency in the clinical setting and the current incidence is 0.6 to 0.9 per 1000 women screened (7–9). Data from the East Midlands region in the United Kingdom report a doubling in incidence over the decade from 1998 to 2008 (10). This may reflect detection of more subtle radiological abnormalities following the introduction of digital mammography and improvements in the resolution of ultrasound. Most of the radial scars are not associated with concurrent malignancy and there is a risk that this increased rate of detection may increase the number of unnecessary benign diagnostic surgical biopsies. In a retrospective audit of benign surgical biopsies performed in the screening population, we have previously demonstrated that referral for diagnostic surgery may rest on radiological and/or pathological suspicion of a radial scar in up to one-third of cases (11).

HISTOPATHOLOGY

Radial scars may be seen on gross inspection of cut tissue as a small stellate "star- shaped" lesion. Microscopically, the typical radial scar is characterized by a central fibroelastotic core with a peripheral corona of radiating parenchymal structures, often showing cyst formation and proliferative epithelial changes (Fig. 18.1) (12). The histological appearances have been likened to a daisy head. The central scarred area often contains entrapped, distorted tubules that may create difficulties in histological interpretation and confusion with invasive malignancy, especially tubular carcinoma.

IMAGING TECHNIQUES
Mammography

The classical appearance as described by Tabar and Dean (9) is an area of architectural distortion with radiating thin spicules that may aggregate centrally creating a "sheaf of wheat" appearance. There are radiolucent linear structures parallel to the spicules that represent entrapped fat and create a "black star" appearance (Fig. 18.2). There is a central radiolucency with no solid central mass commensurate in size to the length of the spicules. In comparison, a typical carcinoma has a distinct central tumor mass from which dense spicules radiate in all directions. The growth pattern of the radial scar is typically uniplanar with a plate-like rather than spherical configuration (13). This may contribute to the marked variation in appearance of the radial scar in different mammographic projections, although this is by no means pathognomonic (14).

Radiologically visible microcalcification is reported in association with radial scars in 25–59% of cases (15–17). The presence of microcalcification in the context of a mammographically detected stellate lesion was initially considered to be suspicious for malignancy (18). However, subsequent studies with careful radiological-pathological correlation have demonstrated that microcalcification can be associated with benign changes within radial scars and is usually localized to areas of adenosis or cysts adjacent to the central fibroelastotic core (15,19). Therefore the presence or absence of associated mammographic microcalcification is not helpful in differentiating between benign and malignant disease unless there is characteristic pleomorphic, linear and branching calcification reflecting the presence of ductal carcinoma in situ (DCIS) (20).

Ultrasound

At least two-thirds of mammographically detected radial scars are visible on ultrasound (21). Findings include an irregular hypoechoic mass associated with posterior acoustic shadowing, often indistinguishable from the features of an invasive cancer (Fig. 18.3) (22,23). More subtle ultrasound features consist of parenchymal distortion with an apparent disruption in normal tissue planes appearing as an abrupt transition between normal lobules of fat and fibrous tissue. In a review of 75 consecutive screen-detected radial scars and invasive cancers, Cawson (24) identified certain ultrasound features that may help to discriminate between the two entities. An echogenic halo was present in 58% of breast cancers but was not seen in any of the 22 radial scars reviewed. Invasion at the peripheral margin of invasive tumors creates a band of echoes but radial scars distort rather than invade breast tissue, hence the absence of a halo. In addition, tiny cysts may be present in the periphery of radial scars but this feature has never been described in cancers.

Although there are no features specific to radial scars that allow confident exclusion of malignancy (25,26), ultrasound assessment is useful to confirm the presence and location of a lesion that may be mammographically subtle or equivocal. If a lesion is seen only on one mammographic projection, ultrasound may localize it with greater accuracy than stereotactic guided biopsy. In addition, ultrasound-guided biopsy is quicker and easier to perform under direct visualization and is more comfortable for the patient.

Magnetic Resonance Imaging

On MRI, contrast-enhanced T1-weighted sequences often demonstrate an irregular or spiculate mass that is indistinguishable from carcinoma (27). Recent data have suggested that enhancement characteristics may be useful in detecting malignant disease associated with radial scars (28). Pediconi et al. (29) evaluated the role of contrast-enhanced breast MRI in 30 patients with suspected radial scars at mammography. The mammographic lesion was subsequently confirmed to be due to invasive malignancy in eight patients. The remaining 22 patients were diagnosed with radial scars of which only four exhibited enhancement and were found to have associated DCIS at final surgical histology. The radial scars in all 18 patients without enhancement had no associated malignancy. The authors postulated that the lack of enhancement reflects the relatively avascular nature of the central fibroelastotic core, but were cautious not to advocate that MRI could reliably exclude malignant change associated with a radial scar. With an overall specificity of 89% and a sensitivity of 83%,

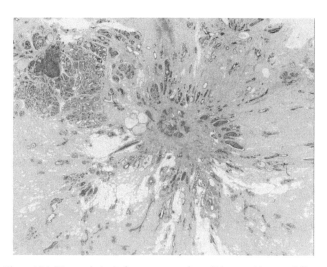

Figure 18.1 Histopathological appearance of a radial scar with central fibroelastotic core and peripheral radiating spicules showing benign changes including cyst formation.

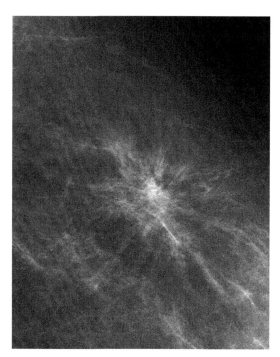

Figure 18.2 Mammogram demonstrating the classical "black star" appearance of a radial scar with radiolucent linear structures parallel to long thin spicules and a central radiolucency with no solid mass commensurate in size to the length of the spicules.

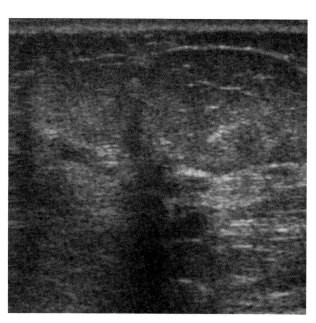

Figure 18.3 Ultrasound of a radial scar revealing a hypoechoic mass with ill-defined borders and posterior acoustic shadowing due to the high fibrous content of the lesion.

MRI is not routinely used in the diagnostic workup of radial scars, as it cannot reliably demonstrate the presence of associated atypia or malignancy.

BIOLOGICAL SIGNIFICANCE
Risk of Developing Malignancy
Early studies suggested radial scars may confer an increased risk of developing malignancy (30,31). Jacobs et al. (32) reviewed 1396 women with benign open biopsies in the Nurses' Health study and found an almost doubling of the risk of developing malignancy, with the risk increasing with lesion size and number. The relative risk was 1.8 although this increased to 3.5 for radial scars >4 mm in size. However, follow-up studies have failed to reveal an increased risk of malignancy following local excision (33,34). More recent studies have demonstrated that the increased risk associated with radial scars could be largely attributed to the presence of coexistent proliferative breast disease and there was no difference in risk if the proliferative changes were found within or outside the radial scar (35,36).

Association with Concurrent Malignancy
Radial scars may be associated with concurrent malignancy in a significant number of cases although the reported incidence varies. Mokbel et al. (37) reviewed 32 cases of histologically confirmed radial scars in breast excision specimens and found 31% contained malignancy; six with invasive carcinoma and four with DCIS. In a review of 125 surgically excised radial scars from the Irish screening population, Doyle et al. (38) found malignancy in 25% cases, with a third of cases proving invasive. Douglas-Jones and Pace (39) reviewed the histological findings in 46 screen-detected radial scars undergoing open diagnostic biopsy and found malignancy in 20%; one with invasive carcinoma and eight containing only DCIS. A more recent report from the Irish group (40) and a prospective study from an Australian population-based screening program (8) however have reported lower incidences of 12% and 7% respectively with all malignancies in these two series present only as DCIS.

In a retrospective review of their routine surgical practice, the pathologists Sloane and Mayers (41) found malignancy in seven of 74 (9.5%) radial scars; of which six cases were DCIS. However, these included both symptomatic and screening cases, as well as lesions detected incidentally in pathology specimens. Of note, a significantly higher incidence of carcinoma and atypical hyperplasia was found in mammographically detected lesions compared with those discovered incidentally in breast specimens removed for other benign or malignant changes. There was also a clear relationship between the presence of carcinoma in relation to the size of the radial scar and patient age; with carcinoma very uncommon in radial scars <7 mm and patients <50 years.

Association with Atypia
Radial scars are commonly associated with atypical epithelial proliferations such as atypical ductal hyperplasia or lobular neoplasia (LN) – a term which incorporates both atypical lobular hyperplasia (ALH) and lobular carcinoma in situ. A similar variation in the frequency of these lesions exists with the likelihood of finding associated atypia ranging from 22% (38) to 57% (8). The recognized inter-observer variation in the diagnosis of atypical epithelial proliferations and the inconsistent use of confirmatory immunohistochemistry could well contribute to variation in reported incidence. Immunohistochemistry for CK5/6 and estrogen receptor may be of value in distinguishing between the epithelial hyperplasia of usual type and atypia, especially when assessing the limited tissue samples present in needle core biopsies (42). Immunohistochemistry demonstrating areas with reduced or absent staining for E-cadherin may highlight small foci of LN (43) and may also help distinguish LN from areas of artifactual dyscohesion. Previous studies have demonstrated the usefulness of the myoepithelial markers CK14 and p63 in papillary lesions (44,45) and these markers can also be helpful in highlighting the background architecture of radial scars. The judicious use of these immunohistochemical markers may play an important role in achieving an accurate diagnosis and informing subsequent management decisions.

MANAGEMENT
Traditionally, almost all radial scars diagnosed on needle core biopsy have been surgically excised due to the potential risk of associated malignancy. Exceptions include incidental small radial scars reported on core biopsies of microcalcification or clinical thickening with no true radiological correlate; following multidisciplinary team discussion these are often not subjected to further biopsy or surgical excision. Brenner et al. (46) reviewed 157 patients with core biopsy–diagnosed radial scars undergoing either surgical excision or mammographic surveillance and reported malignancy at excision in 8% of cases. In biopsies with associated atypia on the core, the risk of malignancy was 28%, but in biopsies without atypia the risk was only 4%. However, no malignant lesions were missed if 12 or more cores were taken or if the lesions were biopsied using a directional vacuum-assisted device. Two other groups reported that 44% (47) and 37% (48) of radial scars with atypia on core biopsy harbored malignancy, but the rate in both series following biopsies without atypia was only 6%.

Breast screening aims to reduce deaths due to breast cancer through early detection and management while avoiding unnecessary interventions for benign disease in asymptomatic women (49). The general consensus is that radial scars with atypia on core biopsy should be surgically excised due to the higher risk of associated malignancy. However, there is increasing evidence, that if the radiological findings suggest a radial scar and the core biopsy confirms a radial scar with no atypia, then surgical excision may be unnecessary (50–52). The introduction of large-volume vacuum-assisted excision (VAE) provides an opportunity to sample small screen-detected lesions more extensively such that malignancy may be more confidently excluded (53). Used in this way, VAE offers an alternative to surgery and if the lesion has been entirely removed, effectively becomes a therapeutic procedure.

We recently published our clinical experience with the use of VAE in the management of radial scars (54). We reviewed all screen-detected radial scars diagnosed on needle core biopsy (14-gauge) from July 2004 to September 2008. Prior to the introduction of VAE in our institution, all patients underwent diagnostic surgery in accordance with local guidelines. From January 2006 onwards, all patients with non-atypical radial scars on core biopsy were offered VAE as an alternative to surgery. Exceptions due to technical limitations of the device include

Table 18.1 Data from Patients with Non-Atypical Radial Scars on NCB

Case	Age (yrs)	Screen Round	Size (mm)	NCB Histology	Mammotome Histology	Surgical Histology
1	53	1	12	RS	RS	–
2	66	6	4	RS	RS	–
3	53	2	10	RS	RS	–
4	57	2	20	RS	RS	–
5	53	2	15	RS	RS	–
6	70	4	15	RS	RS	–
7	52	1	7	RS	RS	–
8	63	6	7	RS	RS	–
9	62	5	6	RS	RS	–
10	54	2	25	RS	RS	–
11	52	2	10	RS	RS	–
12	50	1	25	RS	RS + LN	RS + ALH
13	49	1	15	RS	Failure	RS + ALH
14	56	2	15	RS	Failure	RS
15	61	4	17	RS	–	RS
16	58	3	6	RS	–	RS
17	62	5	9	RS	–	RS
18	66	5	10	RS	–	RS
19	51	1	15	RS	–	RS
20	59	4	7	RS	–	RS
21	68	5	6	RS	–	RS + DCIS
22	64	5	7	RS	–	Declined

Abbreviations: ALH, atypical lobular hyperplasia; DCIS, ductal carcinoma in situ; LN, lobular in situ neoplasia; NCB, needle core biopsy; RS, radial scar; Failure, failure of mammotome to localize or adequately sample the lesion; Declined, surgery declined by patient.

lesions abutting the skin or areola and lesions exceeding 25 mm. VAE was performed under stereotactic or ultrasound guidance with 8- or 11-gauge needles. All procedures were performed under local anesthetic in an outpatient setting.

Our series included 22 core biopsies containing radial scars without atypia (Table 18.1). Eleven of 14 (78%) patients with non-atypical radial scars had concordant benign histology following VAE and thus avoided surgery. No cases managed in this way subsequently developed malignancy, with a mean mammographic follow-up of 23 months. One patient demonstrated atypia in the form of LN associated with the radial scar on VAE cores, prompting surgical excision at this point. The final surgical histology demonstrated a radial scar and associated LN amounting to ALH. Two further patients proceeded to surgery as it was not possible to localize the lesion under stereotactic guidance or to adequately sample the mammographic abnormality; both these patients had no in situ or invasive malignancy associated with the radial scar on excision.

In our series, DCIS was found at subsequent excision in only 1 of 22 (4.5%) cases identified as non-atypical radial scars on initial sampling with core biopsy. This case was exceptional in that there was radiological-pathological discordance with malignant imaging features and the multidisciplinary team recommendation was therefore to proceed directly to surgical excision rather than VAE. The DCIS in this case was found at the edge of the lesion and was not sampled on the initial needle core biopsy. This highlights an inherent limitation of core biopsy sampling, which is the potential for missing a malignant or atypical component to the radial scar. Foci of malignant change within radial scars are often small and can comprise as little as 5% of the lesion (55). In addition, atypical

hyperplasia and malignancy, while usually confined to the lesion, are thought to occur most frequently at the periphery (41). Our conservative approach is supported by Tennant et al. (56) who reported their experience of VAE in the management of lesions of uncertain malignant potential. Reassuringly, none of their 18 patients with non-atypical radial scars managed in this way have subsequently developed malignancy.

CONCLUSION

The diagnosis of a radial scar can be suggested by certain imaging characteristics but the radiological appearances are not sufficiently distinctive to permit reliable differentiation from cancer, thus core biopsy is essential to secure a definitive diagnosis. Further pathological evaluation subsequent to core biopsy diagnosis is important due to the known association with concurrent malignancy. However, the selection of patients suitable for VAE rather than surgical excision requires careful histological evaluation and meticulous multidisciplinary team discussion to ensure radiological-pathological concordance. In our experience, the selective use of VAE in the management of non-atypical radial scars has significantly reduced the need for diagnostic surgery in the asymptomatic screening population.

REFERENCES

1. Hamperl H. Radial scars and obliterating mastopathy. Virchows Arch A Pathol Anat Histol 1975; 369: 55–68.
2. Elston CW, Ellis IO. The Breast. Edinburgh: Churchill-Livingstone, 1998.
3. Royal College of Pathologists Working Group. Pathology reporting in breast cancer screening. J Clin Pathol 1991; 44: 710–25.
4. Nielsen M, Jensen J, Andersen JA. An autopsy study of radial scar in the female breast. Histopathology 1985; 9: 287–95.
5. Wellings SR, Alpers CE. Subgross pathologic features and incidence of radial scars in the breast. Hum Pathol 1984; 15: 475–9.

6. Nielsen M, Christensen L, Andersen J. Radial scars in women with breast cancer. Cancer 1987; 59: 1019–25.

7. Burnett SJ, Ng YY, Perry NM, et al. Benign biopsies in the prevalent round of breast screening: a review of 137 cases. Clin Radiol 1995; 50: 254–8.

8. Cawson JN, Malara F, Kavanagh A, et al. Fourteen-gauge needle core biopsy of mammographically evident radial scars: is excision necessary? Cancer 2003; 97: 345–51.

9. Tabar L, Dean PB. Teaching Atlas of Mammography. New York: Thieme-Stratton Inc, 1985.

10. Rakha EA, Ho BC, Naik V, et al. Outcome of breast lesions diagnosed as lesion of uncertain malignant potential (B3) or suspicious of malignancy (B4) on needle core biopsy, including detailed review of epithelial atypia. Histopathology 2011; 58: 626–32.

11. Carder PJ, Liston JC. Will the spectrum of lesions prompting a "B3" breast core biopsy increase the benign biopsy rate? J Clin Pathol 2003; 56: 133–8.

12. Hayes BD, Quinn CM. Pathology of B3 lesions of the breast. Diagn Histopathol 2009; 15: 459–69.

13. Alleva DQ, Smetherman DH, Farr GH, et al. Radial scar of the breast: radiologic-pathologic correlation in 22 cases. Radiographics 1999; 19: S27–35.

14. Cawson JN, Nickson C, Evans J, et al. Variation in mammographic appearance between projections of small breast cancers compared with radial scars. J Med Imaging Radiat Oncol 2010; 54: 415–20.

15. Frouge C, Tristant H, Guinebretiere JM, et al. Mammographic lesions suggestive of radial scars: microscopic findings in 40 cases. Radiology 1995; 195: 623–5.

16. Ciatto S, Morrone D, Catarzi S, et al. Radial scars of the breast: review of 38 consecutive mammographic diagnoses. Radiology 1993; 187: 757–60.

17. Boute V, Goyat I, Denoux Y, et al. Are the criteria of Tabar and Dean still relevant to radial scar? Eur J Radiol 2006; 60: 243–9.

18. Mitnick JS, Vazquez MF, Harris MN, et al. Differentiation of radial scar from scirrhous carcinoma of the breast: mammographic-pathologic correlation. Radiology 1989; 173: 697–700.

19. Adler DD, Helvie MA, Oberman HA, et al. Radial sclerosing lesion of the breast: mammographic features. Radiology 1990; 176: 737–40.

20. Demirkazik FB, Gulsun M, Firat P. Mammographic features of nonpalpable spiculated lesions. Clin Imaging 2003; 27: 293–7.

21. Lee E, Wylie E, Metcalf C. Ultrasound imaging features of radial scars of the breast. Australas Radiol 2007; 51: 240–5.

22. Vega A, Garijo F. Radial scar and tubular carcinoma. Mammographic and sonographic findings. Acta Radiol 1993; 34: 43–7.

23. Cohen MA, Sferlazza SJ. Role of sonography in evaluation of radial scars of the breast. AJR Am J Roentgenol 2000; 174: 1075–8.

24. Cawson JN. Can sonography be used to help differentiate between radial scars and breast cancers? Breast 2005; 14: 352–9.

25. Finlay ME, Liston JE, Lunt LG, et al. Assessment of the role of ultrasound in the differentiation of radial scars and stellate carcinomas of the breast. Clin Radiol 1994; 49: 52–5.

26. Linda A, Zuiani C, Furlan A, et al. Radial scars without atypia diagnosed at imaging-guided needle biopsy: how often is associated malignancy found at subsequent surgical excision, and do mammography and sonography predict which lesions are malignant? AJR Am J Roentgenol 2010; 194: 1146–51.

27. Morris E, Liberman L. Breast MRI. New York: Springer, 2005.

28. Perfetto F, Fiorentino F, Urbano F, et al. Adjunctive diagnostic value of MRI in the breast radial scar. Radiol Med 2009; 114: 757–70.

29. Pediconi F, Occhiato R, Venditti F, et al. Radial scars of the breast: contrast-enhanced magnetic resonance mammography appearance. Breast J 2005; 11: 23–8.

30. Fisher ER, Palekar AS, Kotwal N, et al. A nonencapsulated sclerosing lesion of the breast. Am J Clin Pathol 1979; 71: 240–6.

31. Linell F, Ljungberg O, Andersson I. Breast carcinoma. Aspects of early stages, progression and related problems. Acta Pathol Microbiol Scand Suppl 1980; 272: 14–62.

32. Jacobs TW, Byrne C, Colditz G, et al. Radial scars in benign breast-biopsy specimens and the risk of breast cancer. N Engl J Med 1999; 340: 430–6.

33. Andersen JA, Gram JB. Radial scar in the female breast. A long-term follow-up study of 32 cases. Cancer 1984; 53: 2557–60.

34. Fenoglio C, Lattes R. Sclerosing papillary proliferations in the female breast. A benign lesion often mistaken for carcinoma. Cancer 1974; 33: 691–700.

35. Sanders ME, Page DL, Simpson JF, et al. Interdependence of radial scar and proliferative disease with respect to invasive breast carcinoma risk in patients with benign breast biopsies. Cancer 2006; 106: 1453–61.

36. Berg JC, Visscher DW, Vierkant RA, et al. Breast cancer risk in women with radial scars in benign breast biopsies. Breast Cancer Res Treat 2008; 108: 167–74.

37. Mokbel K, Price RK, Mostafa A, et al. Radial scar and carcinoma of the breast: microscopic findings in 32 cases. Breast 1999; 8: 339–42.

38. Doyle EM, Banville N, Quinn CM, et al. Radial scars/complex sclerosing lesions and malignancy in a screening programme: incidence and histological features revisited. Histopathology 2007; 50: 607–14.

39. Douglas-Jones AG, Pace DP. Pathology of R4 spiculated lesions in the breast screening programme. Histopathology 1997; 30: 214–20.

40. Hayes BD, O'Doherty A, Quinn CM. Correlation of needle core biopsy with excision histology in screen-detected B3 lesions: the Merrion breast screening unit experience. J Clin Pathol 2009; 62: 1136–40.

41. Sloane JP, Mayers MM. Carcinoma and atypical hyperplasia in radial scars and complex sclerosing lesions: importance of lesion size and patient age. Histopathology 1993; 23: 225–31.

42. Graesslin O, Antoine M, Chopier J, et al. Histology after lumpectomy in women with epithelial atypia on stereotactic vacuum-assisted breast biopsy. Eur J Surg Oncol 2010; 36: 170–5.

43. O'Malley FP. Lobular neoplasia: morphology, biological potential and management in core biopsies. Mod Pathol 2010; 23: S14–25.

44. Tse GM, Tan PH, Lacambra MD, et al. Papillary lesions of the breast - accuracy of core biopsy. Histopathology 2010; 56: 481–8.

45. Carder PJ, Garvican J, Haigh I, et al. Needle core biopsy can reliably distinguish between benign and malignant papillary lesions of the breast. Histopathology 2005; 46: 320–7.

46. Brenner RJ, Jackman RJ, Parker SH, et al. Percutaneous core needle biopsy of radial scars of the breast: when is excision necessary? AJR Am J Roentgenol 2002; 179: 1179–84.

47. Lee AH, Denley HE, Pinder SE, et al. Excision biopsy findings of patients with breast needle core biopsies reported as suspicious of malignancy (B4) or lesion of uncertain malignant potential (B3). Histopathology 2003; 42: 331–6.

48. Dillon MF, McDermott EW, Hill AD, et al. Predictive value of breast lesions of "uncertain malignant potential" and "suspicious for malignancy" determined by needle core biopsy. Ann Surg Oncol 2007; 14: 704–11.

49. Department of Health and Social Security. Breast Cancer Screening: Report to Health Ministers of England, Wales, Scotland and Northern Ireland by a working group chaired by Professor Sir Patrick Forrest. London: HMSO, 1987.

50. Kirwan SE, Denton ER, Nash RM, et al. Multiple 14G stereotactic core biopsies in the diagnosis of mammographically detected stellate lesions of the breast. Clin Radiol 2000; 55: 763–6.

51. El-Sayed ME, Rakha EA, Reed J, et al. Predictive value of needle core biopsy diagnoses of lesions of uncertain malignant potential (B3) in abnormalities detected by mammographic screening. Histopathology 2008; 53: 650–7.

52. Morel J, Michell M. Therapeutic mammotome excisions: radial scars. Breast Cancer Online 2008; 11: e6.

53. Carder PJ, Khan T, Burrows P, et al. Large volume "mammotome" biopsy may reduce the need for diagnostic surgery in papillary lesions of the breast. J Clin Pathol 2008; 61: 928–33.

54. Rajan S, Wason AM, Carder PJ. Conservative management of screen-detected radial scars: role of mammotome excision. J Clin Pathol 2011; 64: 65–8.

55. Farshid G, Rush G. Assessment of 142 stellate lesions with imaging features suggestive of radial scar discovered during population-based screening for breast cancer. Am J Surg Pathol 2004; 28: 1626–31.

56. Tennant SL, Evans A, Hamilton LJ, et al. Vacuum-assisted excision of breast lesions of uncertain malignant potential (B3) - an alternative to surgery in selected cases. Breast 2008; 17: 546–9.

19 Role of ultrasound in the diagnosis of breast cancer

Hannah Gay and Steven D. Allen

INTRODUCTION

Breast ultrasound has long been performed in an attempt to diagnose and characterize primary breast cancer. While mammography remains the modality of choice for breast screening for the majority of women, ultrasound has found an increasing role in many aspects of breast imaging. The practical advantages of ultrasound include speed, ease of use, patient safety and cost effectiveness. When utilized alongside other breast imaging modalities such as mammography and MRI, ultrasound represents a key component of the diagnostic workup (1–3). Ultrasound continues to be the investigation of choice to guide tissue biopsy as part of "triple assessment" of breast lesions (4). Newer investigational aspects of ultrasound application are also discussed in this chapter, such as ultrasound screening and fusion imaging.

TECHNICAL ASPECTS AND EQUIPMENT

Sound waves travel at frequencies higher than the upper limit for audibility (>20 kHz), hence prompting the term "ultrasound." The spatial resolution of ultrasound images is proportional to the frequency of sound waves employed and high frequencies are preferred in order to maximize image quality. However, attenuation (absorption) of the ultrasound beam as it passes through tissues increases in proportion to frequency. Therefore for optimal imaging a balance has to be reached between frequency and penetration capacity of sound waves. In practice, with new ultrasound technology, frequencies between 12 and 15 MHz are typically used for breast examination with the facility for reduction of frequency down to 8 MHz for larger breasted patients or those with particularly dense breast tissue. Following application of acoustic coupling gel on the breast skin to reduce impedance created by intervening air, a hand-held transducer continuously emitting high-frequency sound waves is placed on the skin surface. These sound waves pass through the breast and bounce off progressively the deeper layers of soft tissue. Reflected sound waves are received back by the transducer at varying frequencies according to the reflectivity or echogenicity of the tissues through which they pass. A computer assigns a visual gray scale to the collection of frequencies and constructs a "real-time" picture, thus providing a moving image on the ultrasound screen as the transducer is moved over the skin. As previously indicated, probe frequencies of 12–18 MHz are now used for breast work, allowing good tissue penetration to a depth of approximately 7–10 cm from the skin surface (which is adequate for most breast and small part work). At the same time these frequencies provide excellent spatial resolution in the near field (5). By exploiting the Doppler shift effect, blood flow in small vessels within soft tissues can be detected using ultrasound and the vascularity of breast masses can be assessed based on flow velocity.

BI-RADS AND STAVROS CRITERIA

The use of ultrasound for breast imaging is highly operator dependent and its effectiveness relies on obtaining technically high quality images, correct interpretation of these, and a clear reporting procedure. In order to establish standards for reporting and reduce inter-observer variability in assessment and description of solid breast masses, the American College of Radiology published the Breast Imaging Reporting and Data System (BI-RADS) Atlas which has mammography, ultrasound, and MRI components (6). This system created a standardized breast ultrasound lexicon for reporting.

The lexicon provides terms that describe features or findings on breast ultrasound including shape, orientation, margin, lesion boundary, echopattern, posterior acoustic features, surrounding tissue changes, calcification, and vascularity (7). Several of these terms are described in more detail below. The BI-RADS system also incorporates a section for special cases such as: clustered microcysts, complicated cysts and masses in the skin, foreign bodies, or lymph nodes that may be either intramammary or axillary. The BI-RADS ultrasound lexicon has seven separate assessment categories into which each lesion is placed. This categorization subsequently determines the follow-up or a specific management modality (Table 19.1) (7).

Ultrasound was originally used primarily to distinguish simple cysts (which did not require sampling) from solid masses that might require biopsy, many of which turned out to have benign histological features. In 1995, Stavros et al. published a landmark study that described a classification system which could more definitively differentiate benign from malignant nodules on ultrasound and thus obviate the need for biopsy of certain lesions (8). In this study, 750 solid breast nodules were examined over a four-year period and were prospectively classified as benign, malignant, or indeterminate according to their sonographic characteristics (Table 19.2). These nodules were subsequently biopsied and the results showed a negative predictive value of 99.5% for benign lesions and a 98.4% sensitivity for correctly identifying malignant lesions using this classification scheme (8).

Strict criteria were used to categorize individual lesions. First, features suggestive or indicative of malignancy were identified. Even when a single malignant feature was present, the nodule was excluded from benign classification (8). Second, benignity demanded a combination of specific findings: (*i*) lack of any malignant characteristics, (*ii*) intense and uniform hyperechogenicity, (*iii*) an ellipsoid shape plus a thin

Table 19.1 The American College of Radiology BI-RADS Ultrasound Lexicon (7)

Category	Description
Category 0 - Incomplete	Additional imaging evaluation required before final assessment
Category 1 - Negative	No lesion found (routine follow-up)
Category 2 - Benign finding	No malignant features (routine follow-up for age/clinical management)
Category 3 - Probably benign finding	Malignancy is highly unlikely e.g., fibroadenoma (initial short interval follow-up)
Category 4 - Suspicious abnormality	Low to moderate probability of cancer, biopsy should be considered
Category 5 - Highly suggestive of malignancy	Almost certainly cancer, appropriate action should be taken
Category 6 - Known cancer	Biopsy proven malignancy, prior to institution of therapy

Table 19.2 Individual Sonographic Characteristics of Solid Breast Nodules

Malignant	Benign	Indeterminate
Spiculation	Absent malignant	Maximum diameter
Angular margin	findings	Isoechogenicity
Marked	Intense	Mild
hypoechogenicity	hyperechogenicity	hypoechogenicity
Shadowing	Ellipsoid shape	Normal sound
Calcification	Gentle bi- or	transmission
Duct extension	trilobulations	Enhanced
Branch pattern	Thin, echogenic	transmission
Microlobulation	pseudocapsule	Heterogeneous texture
		Homogeneous texture

Source: Adapted from Ref. (8).

echogenic pseudocapsule or (*iv*) two or three gentle lobulations plus a thin echogenic pseudocapsule. If this combination of factors was not identified, the lesion was by default classified as indeterminate (8). This schematic was designed to minimize the risk of false-negative findings. Using these criteria in conjunction with a robust sonographic technique, the authors have concluded that ultrasound can accurately define a subgroup of solid lesions with a low probability of malignancy such that a biopsy is not required (8).

Malignant Characteristics
Spiculations
These are linear bands that radiate perpendicularly from the margin of a solid lesion. These can also been seen as a thick, echogenic halo around the peripheral edge of a nodule (8).

Angular Margins
Angular margins are sharp corners to the margins of the mass. Can be obtuse, acute, or at 90 degrees (7).

Non-Parallel (Taller than Wide)
Part or all of the nodule measures greater in AP dimension than its transverse or longitudinal diameter.

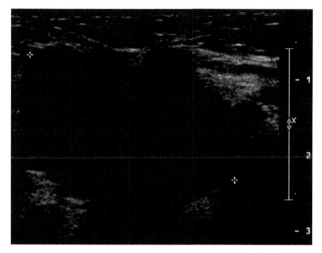

Figure 19.1 Sonographic image of a large irregular hypoechoic mass that was proven on biopsy to represent an invasive ductal carcinoma. It is ill marginated, heterogeneous in echotexture, and distorts the surrounding normal tissues. A thick echogenic halo is often present (not shown).

Markedly Hypoechoic
Appears very "black" when compared with the surrounding tissue. Defined relative to fat (8).

Shadowing
Part or all of the solid nodule demonstrates decreased posterior echoes when compared with the adjacent tissue.

Calcifications
These are foci of echogenicity within a lesion. Can be macro, >0.5 mm (which can cast a posterior acoustic shadow) or micro, <0.5 mm. May be benign (7).

Duct Extension
A hypoechoic projection from a nodule within or around a duct that extends toward the nipple.

Branch Pattern
As for duct extension but usually multiple and extends away from the nipple (8).

Microlobulations
Multiple tiny (1–2 mm) undulations along the surface margin of a nodule. (Fig. 19.1)

Benign Characteristics
Markedly Hyperechoic
Pertains to a lesion of uniformly increased echogenicity akin to that of fat and usually represents fibrous tissue. Any heterogeneity of the lesion excludes it from this category (8).

Ellipsoid Shape
The longitudinal and transverse diameters are greater than the anteroposterior dimension.

Gentle Lobulations
Undulations in the contour of a nodule that are gentle and smooth, numbering less than three (8).

Thin Echogenic Pseudocapsule
Narrow hyperechoic rim around a lesion. May only be identified on part of the nodule (8).

COMPLEX CYSTIC MASSES

One of the chief roles of ultrasound in the diagnosis of breast disease is to identify and characterize cystic masses. Cystic lesions can be categorized into three subtypes: simple, complicated, and complex (9). A simple cyst appears as a well-defined, thin-walled, anechoic mass and is round or ovoid demonstrating posterior acoustic enhancement. Management of these cystic lesions is dependent on symptoms; painful cysts can be aspirated but simple cysts are not associated with any increased risk of malignancy and therefore, do not require intervention unless symptomatic. (Fig. 19.2)

Complicated cysts contain low level internal echoes or debris that may layer or be mobile within the cyst. This internal component can sometimes be very prominent and mimic the appearance of a solid lesion making interpretation more difficult. It should be noted that complicated cysts do not have thick walls, internal septae, or discrete solid components and the risk of malignancy is <2% for these lesions (10). Nonetheless, aspiration is usually attempted; if the aspirate is non-blood stained and the cyst completely collapses as for a simple cyst, then it is discarded. By contrast, if the aspirate is blood-stained, the sample should be sent for cytological analysis.

Complex cysts are characterized by thick walls, thickened septae, and internal solid components or masses and can be subdivided into four types. Type 1 masses have thickened walls or septae; type 2 masses contain internal solid masses; type 3 masses have mixed cystic/solid internal components but are at least 50% cystic; and type 4 masses have mixed cystic/solid internal components but are at least 50% solid (10). Unlike complicated cysts, complex cysts have a significant chance of being malignant, (11) and therefore tissue sampling is generally advised unless there is a recent history suggesting trauma (including needle biopsy). In the latter circumstances, a short-interval follow-up may suffice if a hematoma is suspected (10).

Percutaneous sampling of complex cystic lesions can be performed by fine needle aspiration (FNA), core biopsy, or surgical biopsy. The technique used takes into consideration the need to obtain sufficient material for accurate diagnosis.

Fine needle aspiration cytology (FNAC) should be undertaken as the initial diagnostic investigation if the mass is predominantly cystic or if the nature of the solid component is indeterminate. Thus, FNAC should be performed if echogenic material within the cyst is mobile and avascular which is suggestive of the presence of debris, pus, or hematoma. If a true solid component remains identifiable on ultrasound after FNAC, then an immediate core biopsy is advised as the remaining mass could be malignant despite the cytology of the aspirate being benign (10). Occasionally, FNAC of the cystic component of a complex mass may render the solid component more difficult to visualize. If this occurs, insertion of a marker clip at the site of aspiration aids future radiological identification.

Percutaneous core biopsy is the primary diagnostic method if there is a definite solid component to a mass or if the lesion has any suspicious features such as calcifications on mammography. Core biopsy is also indicated if there is concern that the solid component cannot be accurately targeted after FNAC. Core biopsy can be undertaken using a spring loaded or vacuum-assisted device. The latter is preferable when the solid component is small (10) as the cystic component may decompress after an initial core biopsy making the solid component impossible to visualize. If the initial core biopsy has missed the solid component, any subsequent tissue acquisition is extremely difficult. Once again, a clip should be deployed at the biopsy site if there is any concern regarding future identification of the area.

Biopsy of complex cystic masses yields a wide variety of benign, atypical, and malignant diagnoses. Benign pathological findings include fibrocystic change, intraductal or intracystic papillomas without atypia, and rarely fibroadenomas. Lesions demonstrating cellular or architectural atypia include atypical papilloma, atypical ductal hyperplasia, atypical lobular hyperplasia, and lobular carcinoma *in situ* (lobular neoplasia) (10).

UNCOMMON AND RARE BREAST LESIONS

A small number of less common breast lesions possess distinctive imaging features and many cannot be readily differentiated radiologically from breast carcinomas. Though these lesions are only occasionally encountered in clinical practice, it is important for radiologists to be familiar with the imaging characteristics of these unusual breast lesions to confidently determine whether pathological results of needle core biopsy concur with radiological findings. When there is lack of concordance surgical excision is usually indicated (12). The World Health Organization classifies rare breast lesions according to cell lineage (13). However, for the purposes of this chapter, we will concentrate on the ultrasound features of these lesions.

Lymphoma and Leukemia

Breast lymphomas are more prevalent in perimenopausal women, can be primary or metastatic, and account for 0.4–0.7% of breast cancers (14). The sonographic features of both primary and secondary lymphoma include a predominantly hypoechoic, solid mass (with occasional mixed internal echogenicity). The margins of the mass may be well-circumscribed or irregular and the lesion may also exhibit a fine echogenic rim, together with posterior acoustic enhancement (15).

Leukemic deposits within the breast are rare and usually present as a breast mass or masses in the context of hematogenous spread from an already established systemic disease. Ultrasound findings are those of mixed echogenicity, singular or multiple masses with lobulated or irregular margins that demonstrate central anechogenicity, and peripheral hyperechoic components (12). Increased Doppler vascularity has been reported in some leukemic masses (16).

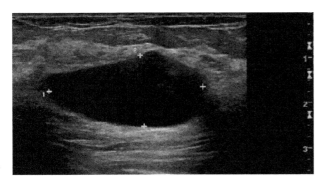

Figure 19.2 Sonographic image depicting a large simple cyst: well-defined, anechoic, thin-walled and demonstrating increased through transmission.

Granular Cell Tumor

These rare tumors are thought to be neurogenic in origin and are more frequent in African-American women. Although these lesions are usually benign, cases of malignant granular cell tumors with nodal spread have been reported (12). Ultrasound features include a hypoechoic mass with a modest propensity for inner breast quadrants, indistinct margins, posterior acoustic shadowing or enhancement (12). One study describing the sonographic features of seven granular cell tumors found that some of these tumors demonstrate an echogenic halo and can appear partially hyperechoic (17).

Plasmacytoma

Plasmacytomas are rare extramedullary tumors that usually are present in patients with a previous diagnosis of multiple myeloma or very rarely as a primary isolated tumor. Ultrasound features include a hypoechoic mass, with posterior acoustic enhancement (12).

Phyllodes Tumors

Phyllodes tumors can develop *de novo* or rarely from a pre-existing fibroadenoma. Their morphological features range from those resembling fibroadenomas to stromal sarcomas (13). Although the majority (60%) of these lesions are benign, about 20% are malignant and a further 20% demonstrate borderline features (18). Ultrasound features are similar to those of a fibroadenoma, although they can be more heterogeneous in appearance, have cystic components and can rapidly grow to a large size which may exceed 10 cm (12).

Pseudoangiomatous Stromal Hyperplasia

Pseudoangiomatous stromal hyperplasia (PASH) is a benign mesenchymal breast tumor that is often manifest as an incidental histological finding, and can present as palpable or non-palpable nodular forms or diffuse breast involvement (12). PASH is usually diagnosed in premenopausal women or those on hormone replacement therapy. Ultrasound features are those of a well-circumscribed, hypoechoic, sometimes heterogeneous solid mass. However, reticular lace-like areas can be observed internally with scattered cystic foci. Moreover, these lesions can be associated with posterior acoustic enhancement or shadowing (12,19).

Adenomyoepithelioma

Adenomyoepithelioma is a predominantly benign myoepithelioid breast lesion, although occasionally can be malignant. Ultrasound features are those of a hypoechoic solid mass which may have a lobulated margin and demonstrate posterior acoustic enhancement (benign lesion) or posterior acoustic shadowing (malignant lesion) (12).

Tubular Adenoma

Tubular adenomas are benign, usually encapsulated, epithelioid lesions, with 90% being found in patients below 40 years of age. On ultrasound, they exhibit features similar to fibroadenomas and represent a hypoechoic solid mass that can be associated with posterior acoustic enhancement (20). In older patients, tubular adenomas can contain punctate or irregular calcifications (12).

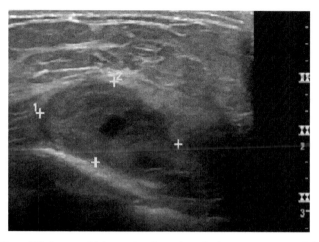

Figure 19.3 Sonographic image showing an irregular heterogeneous mass. It is partly hyperechoic, has mixed cystic and solid components, posterior enhancement, and has microlobulated margins typical of features commonly found in mucinous carcinomas.

Mucinous Tumors

Mucinous tumors account for 2% of all breast cancers and are more common in older women. Sonographically, they typically appear as masses with mixed solid and cystic components and microlobulated margins. These tumors may demonstrate posterior acoustic enhancement but this is not an invariable feature (21). A homogeneous mass is more likely to represent a pure histological type of mucinous carcinoma which is associated with a more favorable prognosis (Fig. 19.3) (21).

PREGNANCY AND LACTATION

Pregnancy and lactation induce distinct hormonal changes within the breast that give rise to a collection of disorders that are either unique to pregnancy and lactation or are more likely to be associated with these physiological states. Benign disorders include galactoceles, lactational adenomas, and mastitis. Furthermore, fibroadenomas may increase in size or undergo infarction. Malignant lesions include Burkitt's lymphoma and pregnancy-associated breast cancer (see chapter 48 breast cancer and pregnancy) (PABC) (22).

Radiological evaluation of the breast during pregnancy and lactation is more challenging as sensitivity of mammography is reduced secondary to increased breast parenchymal density. Ultrasound is therefore the most appropriate tool for assessment of breast problems in pregnant and lactating women (23). Pregnancy-associated physiological changes of the breast lead to an increase in fibroglandular tissue that often appears as a subtle generalized hypoechogenicity on ultrasound. Conversely, during lactation the parenchyma is often diffusely echogenic with a prominent ductal pattern and increased vascularity (22).

Galactoceles are the most frequent benign breast lesion in lactating women. On ultrasound, they appear as complicated cysts that vary in appearance according to their fat and/or water content (22). Those lesions composed entirely of milk appear as benign solid tumors with well-defined internal echogenicity and posterior acoustic enhancement (22). Hyperechoic and hypoechoic fat–fluid levels can be identified when the galactocoele contains fresh milk. Increasing water content produces mixed hypo- and hyperechoic internal components (22,24). Ultrasound-guided aspiration confirms the diagnosis.

Puerperal mastitis occurs not infrequently during breast-feeding and is most often caused by *Staphylococcus*. Ultrasound is the investigation of choice if an associated abscess is suspected (22). The affected breast parenchyma appears ill-defined with a concurrent abscess manifesting as a thick-walled hypoechoic mass with posterior acoustic enhancement and containing debris. This can be aspirated or drained under ultrasound guidance (22). An abscess is usually avascular in its necrotic centre which is a useful application of Doppler imaging in distinguishing between such lesions and a hypoechoic tumor.

Lactational Adenoma

Lactational adenomas histologically resemble both tubular adenomas and fibroadenomas and occur in pregnant or lactating patients. On ultrasound, they usually demonstrate similar characteristics to fibroadenomas although their echotexture can be heterogeneous and iso- or hyperechoic depending on the fat content of the milk (25). Rarely, the margins have been described as irregular and/or lobulated, and these lesions can show posterior acoustic shadowing instead of enhancement (25). Furthermore, some reports have described lactational adenomas as possessing an echogenic pseudocapsule. The majority of these lesions regress spontaneously (22).

Pregnancy Associated Breast Cancer (PABC)

Patients with PABC have a significantly worse prognosis compared with those with breast carcinoma that is not associated with pregnancy and poorer outcomes are probably secondary to delays in diagnosis (22). Over 90% of women with PABC present with palpable breast masses, and several studies have now confirmed that ultrasound has a much greater sensitivity than mammography in detecting cancer in these patients (26). Ultrasound can also help differentiate between a discrete focal mass lesion and normal parenchyma or widespread fibrocystic changes. Sonographic features of PABC are the same as breast carcinomas in non-pregnant women.

LYMPH NODES

For accurate staging and appropriate treatment of breast cancer, the status of the ipsilateral axillary lymph nodes must be established. Pretreatment ultrasound evaluation of the axilla should be performed for all patients with early invasive breast cancer and when morphologically abnormal lymph nodes are found, some form of ultrasound-guided needle sampling should be undertaken (27). The latter can be either a core needle biopsy or an FNAC.

If there is no evidence of lymph node involvement on ultrasound or the results of needle biopsy of a lymph node are negative, a limited staging surgery of the axilla (rather than lymph node clearance) should be performed for patients with early invasive breast cancer as up to one third of benign-appearing lymph nodes on ultrasound may harbor metastases. Sentinel lymph node biopsy is the procedure of choice for surgical staging of the axilla (27).

The location of axillary lymph nodes are anatomically defined by their relationship to the pectoralis minor muscle (28). Level I lymph nodes, where most sentinel nodes are located, lie below the lateral border of the muscle. Level II lymph nodes are situated behind the muscle and level III lymph nodes are positioned above the medial border of the muscle (28). Ultrasound is most

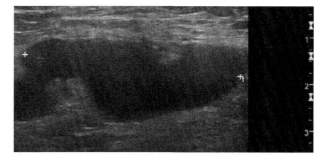

Figure 19.4 Sonographic image demonstrates an axillary lymph node of abnormal morphology in a woman with breast cancer. It is markedly enlarged, non–lobulated; note the loss of the central fatty hilum.

likely to demonstrate nodes in level I, with some level II nodes being visualised, while level III nodes are unlikely to be seen due to their extreme cranial location.

Axillary nodal disease is subdivided into three categories, N1, N2, and N3. These are distinguished by the absolute number of metastatic nodes in the axilla. N1 disease is defined as one to three involved axillary nodes. N2 disease is characterized by four to nine metastatic nodes and N3 disease is associated with metastases in at least 10 lymph nodes.

Benign lymph nodes appear ovoid in shape on ultrasound; have a relatively large fatty hilum and a central feeding artery and draining vein with bidirectional flow on color Doppler imaging. The cortex of a normal node is thin and smooth although may be gently lobulated. The absolute size of a lymph node is not a good indicator of malignancy as lymph nodes as small as 5 mm may contain metastatic deposits (30).

An abnormal lymph node usually has a thickened or eccentrically bulging cortex which should be targeted during needle sampling (30). The involved cortex is usually markedly hypoechoic and their is loss of the central fatty hilum. Measurements for cortical thickness are not set standards but a reasonable limit is a cortical thickness of >2.5 mm (31) or cortical thickening pertaining to over half the thickness of the lymph node in the short axis (30). Doppler flow of abnormal nodes demonstrates increased hilar vascularity or a peripheral (cortical), rather than a central flow (Fig. 19.4) (32).

If an abnormal lymph node is detected, ultrasound-guided FNAC is routinely used. Clear diagnostic results from FNAC can be variable as it is operator dependent. In the event of cytology being inconclusive, core biopsy can produce a higher diagnostic yield and can avoid unnecessary surgery (30). Some units routinely perform core biopsy of lymph nodes in preference to initial FNAC.

MALE BREAST LESIONS

Almost 99% of masses involving the male breast are benign (33). The small size of the male breast facilitates effective assessment with both clinical examination and imaging. Ultrasonography with a high frequency probe can identify deeper structures than is generally possible on mammography and is especially useful in determining the relationship of a lesion to the nipple and guiding biopsy (34).

Gynecomastia is caused by ductal and stromal proliferation of breast tissue and is the most common benign condition affecting the male breast (35). It can be subdivided into three types: early nodular, chronic dendritic, and diffuse glandular (33).

Mammography has been shown to be effective in distinguishing between gynecomastia and breast cancer, but this is rarely required in practice. The, ultrasound appearances of early nodular gynecomastia are that of a central, retroareolar hypoechoic nodular area which may have a lobular margin, be hypervascular, and may have an ill-defined transitional zone (33). Chronic dendritic gynecomastia characteristically demonstrates multiple hypoechoic linear projections from a central anechoic nodule. The diffuse glandular subtype combines the ultrasound features of the other two (33).

Conditions associated with gynecomastia include PASH which can be identified as multiple well-defined hyperechoic nodules and intraductal papillomas which appear on ultrasound as hypoechoic elongated retroareolar masses within enlarged central ducts (33). Other benign conditions affecting the male breast include lipomas which appear as well-defined homogeneous, avascular echogenic masses and epidermal inclusion cysts which have features of a hypoechoic nodule contiguous with the epidermis and posterior acoustic enhancement (33).

Primary breast cancer in men accounts for 0.7% of all breast cancers (36). As the incidence of male breast cancer is extremely low, screening is not appropriate and the diagnosis is based on symptomatic presentation. The latter is most commonly as a painless breast lump. Other malignant conditions affecting the breast in men include lymphoma and dermatofibrosarcoma.

Ultrasound findings of breast cancer in men have similar appearances to those in women, namely a hypoechoic mass lesion with angulated or spiculated margins, which is taller than wide and may show increased through transmission or posterior acoustic shadowing (33). The mass may also contain small echogenic foci representing microcalcifications. A lesion that lies eccentric in relation to the nipple is more likely to be suspicious for malignancy (33). Complex cysts or masses which are easily evaluated on ultrasound frequently prove to be malignant in men, so they should be investigated with ultrasound (37). The axilla should also be evaluated carefully when malignancy is suspected as 50% of men with breast cancer present with involved axillary nodes (33).

ULTRASOUND-GUIDED INTERVENTION

Many diagnostic and some therapeutic procedures of the breast are performed under direct ultrasound visualization. Sonographic techniques have the advantage of real-time imaging to allow for safe and accurate placement of needles and wires. Procedures include core biopsy, FNAC, vacuum-assisted biopsy, and wire localization. Individual practices and technical equipment vary to some degree, and as such each operator and unit may develop a technique with which they are most comfortable.

Core Biopsy

This is now the standard technique for obtaining tissue samples and provides a much higher diagnostic yield than FNAC. Biopsy is performed using automatic spring-loaded 14-gauge devices which allow fine cylindrical pieces of tissue to be extracted and collected within the notch of the needle. After locating the lesion under ultrasound, verbal consent is obtained following explanation of the procedure. The patient is appropriately positioned, usually lying obliquely with the

ipsilateral arm raised above the head. The skin at the site of insertion of the biopsy needle is aseptically prepared. The transducer (a high frequency linear array probe) is also cleaned with solution and covered. Cleaning solution is usually sufficient to use as the acoustic coupling medium. The skin and subcutaneous tissues at the site of the needle insertion (usually at least a couple of centimeters away from the lesion itself) are infiltrated with lignocaine. The transducer is positioned over the lesion on the skin surface, and a further local anesthetic is injected along the path of the beam down to and just beyond the level of the lesion. A small skin incision is made with a scalpel in the anesthetized area. The biopsy needle is primed so that the spring-loaded device will fire when required. The transducer is again positioned over the lesion. The biopsy needle is inserted through the incision and guided under direct vision into or adjacent to the mass, usually in a plane oblique to the chest wall. The exact positioning of the needle depends on the size of the lesion to be biopsied and its relationship to the chest wall. Care must be taken to ensure that the chest wall is not breached by aligning the needle track as parallel to the chest wall as possible. The device is then fired through the mass and a tissue sample obtained. Between two and four cores are usually sufficient. If the lesion contains calcifications on mammography, then specimen radiography is done to confirm that the cores are representative and contain calcifications. The cores are then fixed in formalin and sent for histological assessment. Post procedure, there is a risk of bruising and discomfort which the patient should be forewarned about and extra care should be taken with those patients on anticoagulants; a pressure dressing can be applied if required. Current guidelines suggest that only those patients with an international normalized ratio (INR) of more than 4 should stop warfarin prior to biopsy but ultimately the decision whether to proceed or not with biopsy in warfarinized patients is at the discretion of the clinician (38).

Core biopsy of axillary lymph nodes is sometimes undertaken if FNAC fails to yield a diagnosis. Often abnormal lymph nodes identified in the region of the axillary tail provide a relatively safe area to perform core biopsy (30). However, biopsy technique and approach should always be carefully planned in order to avoid major vessels and nerves within the axilla. An inferolateral to superomedial approach often provides the safest option (30). Patient positioning is also important, and the use of a wedge pillow can help to even out the axilla when raising the patient's arm (30). Using a biopsy device that has the option not to fire the stylet further than its initial placement can also help in sampling lesions in difficult locations (e.g., adjacent to a vessel). The core biopsy specimen should have a white (usually pathological) or brown (lymph node tissue) component while any associated fatty components are yellow in color (30). Two good samples are usually sufficient for accurate tissue diagnosis.

Fine Needle Aspiration Cytology

FNAC is no longer used for the standard evaluation of breast masses because the cytology findings are not concordant with examination and imaging in up to 40% of cases (39). However, it is still sometimes used in the assessment of cystic lesions and does confer a few advantages because it is relatively inexpensive, quick to perform and results are rapidly available in some

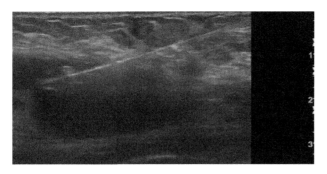

Figure 19.5 Sonographic image shows fine needle aspiration of the pathological lymph node. As the needle and transducer are well aligned, the entirety of the needle can be visualized. The needle is moved gently back and forth while aspirating to withdraw a sample of cells.

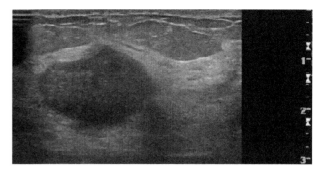

Figure 19.6 Sonographic image demonstrating a well-circumscribed, homogeneous, oval, hypoechoic mass with a smooth, thin, echogenic capsule and posterior acoustic enhancement in keeping with a fibroadenoma.

centers, allowing a one-stop diagnosis. If the contents of a cystic lesion are bloody or complex or if the cavity does not completely collapse post-aspiration, material is sent for cytological analysis on the basis of suspicion of malignancy.

Verbal consent is again obtained following explanation, and the lesion located. The transducer is prepared, and the skin cleaned and anesthetized as for a core biopsy. A 21-gauge needle is used and guided into the lesion under direct visualization. Some operators prefer to add a connecting tube to the needle to allow an assistant to provide suction while the operator directs the needle and passes it through the lesion a number of times. To facilitate expulsion of contents from the syringe post aspiration, it can be helpful to withdraw the plunger by 1 mL prior to the start of the procedure. The aspirate is then smeared thinly onto slides and fixed as per local laboratory protocols. Simple pressure and a small dressing applied to the aspiration site is all that is required post procedure (Fig. 19.5).

Vacuum-Assisted Core Biopsy

Although core biopsy has improved accuracy in the diagnosis of breast lesions, problems remain with underestimation and sampling error which have led to the development of larger-volume vacuum-assisted biopsy devices. There are now several commercially available devices which allow larger-volume samples to be taken without the discomfort and costs of an open surgical biopsy. They are commonly used in cases where histology findings are inconclusive or borderline lesions have been diagnosed on core biopsy and more tissue is required for confident diagnosis. The vacuum-assisted biopsy has also been shown to be more accurate in diagnosing both ductal carcinoma *in situ* and atypical ductal hyperplasia (40,41) than the 14-gauge core biopsy and is increasingly being used as first-line choice in the assessment of microcalcifications. Vacuum-assisted core biopsy devices have also been used to remove smaller benign lesions such as fibroadenomas (42).

These devices are each unique in design but generally employ 11 gauge needles or larger with vacuum suction to pull a sample of tissue through the probe into the sampling chamber. The rotating cutter element then removes the tissue sample which is collected into a receptacle by suction. The rotating device can then be moved into a different position to take a further sample. This process can be repeated in a 360-degree rotational fashion around the lesion until all suspicious areas have been adequately sampled or the whole lesion has been removed via a single insertion of the biopsy device. A marker

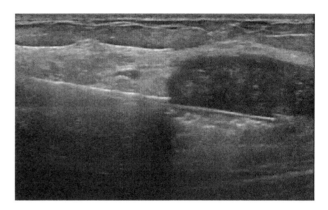

Figure 19.7 Sonographic image showing a vacuum-assisted removal of fibroadenoma. The needle is passed beneath the lesion under direct ultrasound visualization following local anesthesia. The rotating cutting device then removes tissue that is sucked into a collecting chamber.

clip is often inserted into the area (post biopsy) so it can be identified on subsequent imaging if required (written consent is required for this procedure in many institutions). Skin preparation, administration of local anesthetic, and image identification of the lesion and use of ultrasound to guide the biopsy needle is the same as previously described for core biopsy. However, larger amounts of anesthetic may be required to minimize patient discomfort. A pressure dressing is often used post procedure to minimize bleeding and bruising. Patients on warfarin with an INR of more than 2.5 should stop anticoagulation for three days prior to biopsy if this has been agreed by their clinician (Figs. 19.6 and 19.7) (38).

Wire Localization

Wire localization is performed for nonpalpable breast lesions that require surgical excision and can be undertaken either sonographically or stereotactically depending on whether the lesion can be visualized on ultrasound. A hook wire is used to transfix the lesion and therefore guide the surgeon to the area that requires excision. A variety of wire localization devices are employed depending on local practice and expertise. Most are coaxial systems with a stiffer outer component which is subsequently removed after placement leaving the wire *in situ* although some systems do require the outer cannula to be left *in situ*. The needle tip is placed through and just beyond the lesion which ideally should be transfixed by the wire. Confirmation of satisfactory wire position can be done with post-localization mammography.

SECOND-LOOK ULTRASOUND POST MRI

Ultrasound is also routinely used as a "second-look" investigation for further interrogation of MRI-detected lesions. This is primarily indicated for incidentally enhancing lesions identified on MRI that have not been identified on initial conventional imaging assessment (or possibly following screening breast MRI). A limited number of small studies have demonstrated that a targeted ultrasound of the enhancing area depicted on MRI is successful in over 70% of cases (43,44). This procedure can help to further characterize the lesion as benign or suspicious, provide guidance for preoperative localization and percutaneous biopsy, and reduce the numbers of MRI-guided biopsies which are more expensive and time consuming than ultrasound-guided biopsy (43). Malignant lesions are especially likely to be identified on second-look ultrasound especially when seen as masses on MRI (45). However, other lesions may be subtly depicted on ultrasound and require careful and skilled scanning techniques for successful identification of these small MRI-defined lesions (often while simultaneously reviewing the MRI scan) (45).

ULTRASOUND SCREENING

Mammography is an effective screening tool and is the only modality shown to reduce breast cancer mortality. However, despite its proven benefits in mass screening programs, mammography is less sensitive for detecting lesions in dense breasts (46). Ultrasound has never been considered as a comparative screening modality, although several smaller studies have shown that whole bilateral breast ultrasound may identify small, non-palpable, mammographically occult invasive breast cancers, especially in denser breasts (47–49). Ultrasound breast screening has major drawbacks including being highly operator dependent, having significant intra- and inter-observer variability, coupled with low specificity and unknown sensitivity. These limitations can lead to unnecessary biopsies and ultimately unacceptably high false-positive and false-negative outcomes in detecting malignant lesions. A large, prospective multicenter study is currently in progress to define the use of ultrasound as a screening tool (50). Currently, ultrasound is only recommended as an adjuvant tool for screening mammography and clinical examination. Ultrasound should not be used for population screening but may have a limited role in specific patient subgroups. Potential applications include screening patients who have a history of occult carcinoma which was not originally identified on mammography and for lactating women.

DOPPLER IMAGING OF BREAST LESIONS

Malignant breast lesions and axillary nodes usually display altered vascularity when compared with benign lesions (51). However, there is so much overlap in patterns of vascularity between the two so that Doppler imaging may hinder rather than help in determining a diagnosis. Malignant axillary nodes demonstrate an increased peripheral flow when compared with the normal central and perihilar flow characteristic of benign lesions (52). Malignant breast masses can be associated with both penetrating intratumoral vascularity as well as increased numbers of peripheral vessels when compared with

benign lesions and normal breast tissue (53). However, some benign lesions such as fibroadenomas can also demonstrate lesional blood flow (53) and conversely some malignant breast lesions can appear avascular. Therefore, color doppler ultrasound alone cannot be used to accurately depict malignant characteristics. Studies have examined whether color Doppler increases the accuracy of BI-RADS categorization but results have shown that even though evaluation with color Doppler increases detection rates for malignancy, specificity and diagnostic accuracy are reduced and biopsy rates increased (54). Thus, assessment of Doppler flow within breast lesions and axillary nodes remains an adjunct rather than a primary diagnostic tool.

ELASTOGRAPHY

Ultrasound elastography is a tool used to measure the stiffness of tissues (55) and has been extensively researched in many different organs and tissues, but particularly breast and prostate imaging. Elastography is not currently employed in a routine capacity for investigation of breast lesions. However, several studies (56) have now shown that this modality can be useful in distinguishing benign masses from malignant masses, with breast cancers having different tissue characteristics compared with those of normal tissue.

Many sonoelastographic techniques have been developed including compression elastography, vibration elastography, shear velocity imaging, and acoustic radiation forces produced by the ultrasound pulse (57). The type most commonly employed in imaging breast lesions is compression elastography. This method involves calculating the stiffness of a lesion (strain) after an external compression force is applied to it in a perpendicular direction (57). Stiff tissues deform less and therefore exhibit less strain than compliant tissues. The difference between the ultrasound radiofrequencies of a region of interest is calculated and the strain data projected as color scale images are superimposed onto B mode images. Red color represents zones of greatest strain (softest tissue); green color zones of average strain; and blue color depicts the least strain (hardest tissue) (58). The data can also be demonstrated in gray scale with stiffer areas being darker and softer tissues, lighter and brighter (57). Lesions that are stiffer than their surrounding tissue appear larger on the elastogram than the corresponding B mode images. This characteristic can be used to help clarify the likelihood of a lesion being malignant (57).

Despite studies showing that elastography may provide a useful contribution in assessing breast lesions, it does have substantial drawbacks. It is extremely operator dependent, and studies have shown significant inter-observer variability in both the technique of acquiring and interpreting data (58). Other mechanical variables affecting elastographic performance include force of applied strain, transducer frequency, bandwidth, and radiofrequency sampling rate (58). The majority of elastography machines also rely on qualitative rather than quantitative assessment of the data obtained. However, advances in software have allowed quantitative assessment of image quality that hopefully will reduce operator dependence (59). Patient factors affecting performance include breast thickness at the site of the lesion, lesion size, and lesion depth (58).

Normal Breast Tissue

Fibroglandular tissue is far stiffer than the fatty components of breast tissue (60). Therefore, fatty tissue appears lighter (or red on color scale mapping) when compared with the darker (or green) fibroglandular parenchyma (57). A normal lymph node with its large central fatty hilum is also depicted as relatively light (or red) (57).

Cystic Lesions

Simple cysts are best assessed with B-mode imaging. On elastography, they most conventionally appear as a "target sign" with a bright center and a dark surrounding rim. Often, a further bright focus can be identified deep to the cyst (57). Complex cysts containing septae and internal debris often appear solid on conventional ultrasound and may warrant biopsy. However, on elastography they still have cystic characteristics, which help clarify the nature of the lesion and theoretically obviate the need for core biopsy (57).

Fibroadenomas

Fibroadenomas are identified on conventional ultrasound as well-defined hypoechoic, parallel lesions that may contain coarse calcifications. However, occasionally they can show unusual features such as being taller than wide (non parallel). In such cases, elastography may help confirm the benign nature of a fibroadenoma as they project brighter than malignant lesions and also appear smaller on the elastogram than on B-mode imaging. (57). Malignant lesions appear larger on elastography compared with conventional ultrasound. It should be noted that elastography can sometimes be a hindrance as some fibroadenomas demonstrate elastographic features more usually associated with malignancy, especially larger lesions or those containing calcifications (61).

Invasive Ductal Carcinomas

Invasive ductal carcinomas demonstrate characteristic malignant elastographic features of a dark (or blue) lesion that appears significantly larger than it does on B-mode imaging. An echogenic halo is often not fully quantified on conventional imaging though elastography may more clearly depict tumor extension as this area is also stiff. This feature may allow better quantification of the tumor size (57).

CONTRAST-ENHANCED ULTRASOUND

Contrast-enhanced ultrasound is a technique undergoing active research which potentially allows more intricate assessment of the enhancement and vascular characteristics of breast lesions. This involves injection of tiny microbubbles into the venous system that then expand and can be identified when exposed to a sonographic beam. Over a short period, the enhancement, wash out, and pooling characteristics of a lesion can be observed which may help delineate the nature of a lesion. Multiple studies have evaluated whether contrast-enhanced ultrasound can distinguish between benign and malignant masses with variable results (51,62). Malignant masses and lymph nodes tend to exhibit an increased number of vessels and different enhancement characteristics compared with benign lesions (51,63). Benign lesions may enhance homogeneously, while malignant lesions may demonstrate a claw-like pattern with prolonged enhancement times compared with benign masses (51,63).

Further studies have examined whether contrast-enhanced sonography is useful in determining the preoperative size of a cancer, aiding the surgeon in decisions regarding the size of lumpectomy, thus potentially reducing positive margins thus ultimately recurrence rates (64,65). Two feasibility studies have looked at the use of contrast enhancement in identifying the sentinel node prior to surgery via intradermal injection and drainage via the lymphatics. A guide wire was then inserted to localize the sentinel node before operative intervention (66,67). This remains an area of active investigation and research.

FOUR-DIMENSIONAL ULTRASOUND

In the past 5 years conventional ultrasound technology has advanced considerably and with the advent of 3-D and 4-D images it is now possible to analyze and present data based on acquired ultrasound volumes (68). Four-D imaging provides continuously updated real-time 3-D images and permits imaging in the coronal plane (c-mode). In this plane, benign lesions exhibit a compression pattern, displacing the tissue surrounding it which is compressed into a thin echogenic pseudocapsule. Malignant lesions incite a fibroblastic reaction which creates a retraction pattern (69). Indeterminate lesions demonstrate a combination of both. Thus, 4-D ultrasound has a use in helping to differentiate between benign and malignant lesions. In addition, it may assist in the biopsy of breast lesions by showing needle placement in all three planes, (70), although this feature is unlikely to be of much clinical use. It also has potential applications in accurately evaluating tumor volume changes in response to chemotherapy (71). Some studies have suggested that 4-D ultrasound has a place alongside conventional 2-D imaging in a routine clinical setting (68). However, other studies suggest that it confers no significant advantage over conventional 2-D imaging in the diagnostic work up of breast lesions (72). Further research is, therefore, needed in order to ascertain the future of this modality in clinical practice.

AUTOMATED SYSTEMS

Automated breast ultrasound is another new development in ultrasound imaging. The automated machine acquires data in a volume format by taking images in all three planes including coronal. The data is then rendered and viewed as a 3-D data set. The procedure involves a larger-than-usual ultrasound probe (approximately 14 cm in diameter) which provides a better spectral resolution. This probe is positioned over and secured on the breast. The transducer then performs a sweeping scan to acquire a preview image before automatically acquiring multiple images of the entire breast that are then reconstructed. This application has potential use as an adjuvant to mammographic screening of women with dense breast tissue in whom mammograms are less sensitive (73,74). It is also potentially useful in women with breast implants and is currently being piloted in some leading United Kingdom (UK) centers.

OTHER RECENT ADVANCES

Computer-Aided Diagnosis Systems

Computer-aided diagnosis (CAD) technology for ultrasound has been difficult to develop as it uses static images rather than real-time data. However, studies have shown that using CAD in breast ultrasound screening/diagnostics may reduce intra-observer variability and improve the performance of junior readers (75). It also may assist in quality improvement and research.

When using CAD, the operator identifies an area of concern on ultrasound which CAD then outlines, measures, and provides descriptive terms, based on the BI-RADS ultrasound lexicon (7). It also generates a BI-RADS score based on the descriptive terms used. Improved diagnostic accuracy by standardizing descriptive terms and thus reducing intra-observer variability will likely minimize the number of negative biopsies (76). However, although CAD is very sensitive in identifying breast cancers, some studies have shown that it reduces the specificity of the radiologist's interpretation which may ironically increase the number of negative biopsies (77). Research in this area is ongoing and will determine whether it should be incorporated into routine clinical practice.

Fusion Imaging

The advent of fusion PET/CT over the last decade which provides simultaneous anatomic and physiological data, has paved the way for the development of fusion technology using other imaging modalities. Ultrasound fusion is still largely in the research setting but may combine real-time imaging with previously acquired CT or MRI dicom data providing radiologists with high-resolution images. In breast imaging, ultrasound may be fused with MRI as CT is not routinely used in the assessment of breast lesions. The cross-sectional data are sent to an ultrasound machine and viewed adjacent to or superimposed upon the real-time sonogram to assist in accurately identifying and characterizing lesions as well as providing high-quality images for biopsy. Very limited studies suggest that this type of fusion imaging may well be more sensitive than any other single modality in identifying breast cancers (78). However, this exciting technological advance is in its infancy and whether it will ever be used routinely remains uncertain.

CONCLUSION

This chapter has discussed the wide diagnostic spectrum of ultrasound and its application in early breast cancer imaging including technical aspects, its current application in assessing different pathologies, as well as developing research areas.

REFERENCES

1. Zonderland HM, Coerkamp EG, Hermans J, et al. Diagnosis of breast cancer: contribution of US as an adjunct to mammography. Radiology 1999; 213: 413–22.
2. Baker JA, Soo MS. The evolving role of sonography in evaluating solid breast masses. Semin Ultrasound CT MR 2000; 21: 286–96.
3. Rizzatto G, Chersevani R. Breast ultrasound and new technologies. Eur J Radiol 1998; 27: S242–9; Review.
4. Liberman L. Percutaneous image-guided core breast biopsy. Radiol Clin North Am 2002; 40: 483–500.
5. Harvey CJ, Pilcher JM, Eckersley RJ, et al. Advances in ultrasound: review article. Clin Radiol 2002; 57: 157–77.
6. D'Orsi CJ, Mendelson EB, Ikeda DM, et al. Breast Imaging Reporting and Data System: ACR BI-RADS – Breast Imaging Atlas. Reston, VA: American College of Radiology, 2003.
7. Mendelson EB, Baum JK, Berg WA, et al. BI-RADS: ultrasound. In: D'Orsi CJ, Mendelson EB, Ikeda DM, et al. eds. Breast Imaging Reporting and Data System: ACR BI- RADS – Breast Imaging Atlas, 1st edn. Reston, VA: American College of Radiology, 2003.

8. Stavros AT, Thickman D, Rapp CL, et al. Solid breast nodules: use of sonography to distinguish between benign and malignant lesions. Radiology 1995; 196: 123–34.
9. Mendelson EB, Berg WA, Merritt CR. Toward a standardized breast ultrasound lexicon, BI-RADS: ultrasound. Semin Roentgenol 2001; 36: 217–25.
10. Doshi DJ, March DE, Crisi GM, et al. Complex cystic breast masses: diagnostic approach and imaging- pathologic correlation. Radiographics 2007; 27: S53–64.
11. Doshi DJ, March DE, Coughlin BF, Crisi GM. Accuracy of ultrasound-guided percutaneous biopsy of complex cystic breast masses (abstract). In: Radiological Society of North America Scientific Assembly and Annual Meeting Program. Oak Brook, ILL: Radiological Society of North America, 2006: 655.
12. Irshad A, Ackerman SJ, Pope TL, et al. Rare Breast Lesions: Correlation of Imaging and Histologic Features with WHO Classification. Radiographics 2008; 28: 1399–414.
13. Tavassoli FA, Devilee P, eds. Tumours of the breast. In: Pathology and Genetics of Tumours of the Breast and Female Genital Organs. World Health Organization Classification of Tumours. Lyon, France: IARC, 2003: 9–112.
14. Arber DA, Simpson JF, Weiss LM, Rappaport H. Non-Hodgkin's lymphoma involving the breast. Am J Surg Pathol 1994; 18: 288–95.
15. Lyou CY, Yang SK, Choe DH, Lee BH, Kim KH. Mammographic and sonographic findings of primary breast lymphoma. Clin Imaging 2007; 31: 234–8.
16. Memis A, Killi R, Orguc S, Ustün EE. Bilateral breast involvement in acute lymphoblastic leukemia: color Doppler sonography findings. AJR Am J Roentgenol 1995; 165: 1011.
17. Yang WT, Edeiken-Monroe B, Sneige N, Fornage BD. Sonographic and mammographic appearances of granular cell tumors of the breast with pathological correlation. J Clin Ultrasound 2006; 34: 153–60.
18. Moffat CJ, Pinder SE, Dixon AR, et al. Phyllodes tumours of the breast: a clinicopathological review of thirty-two cases. Histopathology 1995; 27: 205–18.
19. Cohen MA, Morris EA, Rosen PP, et al. Pseudoangiomatous stromal hyperplasia: mammographic, sonographic and clinical patterns. Radiology 1996; 198: 117–20.
20. Soo MS, Dash N, Bentley R, Lee LH, Nathan G. Tubular adenomas of the breast: imaging findings with histologic correlation. AJR Am J Roentgenol 2000; 174: 757–61.
21. Lam WW, Chu WC, Tse GM, et al. Sonographic appearance of mucinous carcinoma of the breast. AJR Am J Roentgenol 2004; 182: 1069–74.
22. Sabate JM, Clotet M, Torrubia S, et al. Radiologic evaluation of breast disorders related to pregnancy and lactation. Radiographics 2007; 27: S101–24.
23. Ring AE, Smith IE, Ellis PA. Breast cancer and pregnancy. Ann Oncol 2005; 16: 1855–60.
24. Son EJ, Oh KK, Kim EK. Pregnancy-associated breast disease: radiologic features and diagnostic dilemmas. Yonsei Med J 2006; 47: 34–42.
25. Sumkin JH, Perrone AM, Harris KM, et al. Lactating adenoma: US features and literature review. Radiology 1998; 206: 271–4.
26. Liberman L, Giess CS, Dershaw DD, Deutch BM, Petrek JA. Imaging of pregnancy-associated breast cancer. Radiology 1994; 191: 245–8.
27. Early and locally advanced breast cancer, Diagnosis and treatment. NICE clinical guideline 80. February 2009.
28. Berg JW. The significance of axillary node levels in the study of breast carcinoma. Cancer 1955; 8: 776–8.
29. Neal CH, Daly CP, Nees AV, Helvie MA. Can preoperative axillary US help exclude N2 and N3 metastatic breast cancer? Radiology 2010; 257: 335–41.
30. Abe H, Schmidt RA, Sennett CA, et al. US-guided core needle biopsy of axillary lymph nodes in patients with breast cancer: why and how to do it. Radiographics 2007; 27: S91–9.
31. Damera A, Evans AJ, Cornford EJ, et al. Diagnosis of axillary nodal metastases by ultrasound-guided core biopsy in primary operable breast cancer. Br J Cancer 2003; 89: 1310–13.
32. Yang WT, Chang J, Metreweli C. Patients with breast cancer: differences in color Doppler flow and gray-scale US features of benign and malignant axillary lymph nodes. Radiology 2000; 215: 568–73.
33. Chen L, Chantra PK, Larsen LH, et al. Imaging characteristics of malignant lesions of the male breast. Radiographics 2006; 26: 993–1006.

34. Stavros AT. Breast Ultrasound. Philadelphia, Pa: Lippincott Williams & Wilkins, 2004: 712–14.
35. Braunstein GD. Gynecomastia. N Engl J Med 1993; 328: 490–5.
36. Jaiyesimi IA, Buzdar AU, Sahin AA, et al. Carcinoma of the male breast. Ann Intern Med 1992; 117: 771–7.
37. Yang WT, Whitman GJ, Yuen EH, et al. Sonographic features of primary breast cancer in men. AJR Am J Roentgenol 2001; 176: 413–16.
38. Pritchard JN, Townend JN, Lester WA et al. Management of patients taking antiplatelet or anticoagulant medication requiring invasive breast procedures: United Kingdom survey of radiologists' and surgeons' current practice. Clin Radiol 2008 63; 3: 305–311.
39. Salami N, Hirschowitz SL, Nieberg RK et al. Triple test approach to inadequate fine needle aspiration biopsies of palpable breast lesions. Acta Cytol. May-Jun 1999; 43: 339–43.
40. Jackman RJ, Burbank FH, Parker SH, et al. Accuracy of sampling ductal carcinoma in situ by three stereotactic breast biopsy methods. Radiology. 1998; 209: 197–8.
41. Jackman RJ, Burbank FH, Parker SH, et al. Atypical ductal hyperplasia diagnosed at stereotactic breast biopsy: improved reliability with 14-gauge, directional, vacuum-assisted biopsy. Radiology. Aug 1997; 204: 485–8.
42. Thurley P, Evans A, Hamilton L, James J, et al. Patient satisfaction and efficacy of vacuum-assisted excision biopsy of fibroadenomas. Clin Radiol. 2009; 64: 381–385.
43. Carbognin G, Girardi V, Calciolari C, et al. Utility of second-look ultrasound in the management of incidental enhancing lesions detected by breast MR imaging. Radiol Med 2010; 115: 1234–45.
44. Luciani ML, Pediconi F, Telesca M. Incidental enhancing lesions found on preoperative breast MRI: management and role of second-look ultrasound. Radiol Med 2011; 116: 886–904.
45. Abe H, Schmidt RA, Shah RN, et al. MR-Directed ("Second-Look") ultrasound examination for breast lesions detected initially on MRI: MR and sonographic findings. AJR Am J Roentgenol 2010; 194: 370–7.
46. Kerlikowske K, Grady D, Barclay J, Sickles EA, Ernster V. Effect of age, breast density, and family history on the sensitivity of first screening mammography. JAMA 1996; 276: 33–8.
47. Kaplan SS. Clinical utility of bilateral whole-breast US in the evaluation of women with dense breast tissue. Radiology 2001; 221: 641–9.
48. Kolb TM, Lichy J, Newhouse JH. Comparison of the performance of screening mammography, physical examination, and breast US and evaluation of factors that influence them: an analysis of 27,825 patient evaluations. Radiology 2002; 225: 165–75.
49. Buchberger W, Niehoff A, Obrist P, et al. Clinically and mammographically occult breast lesions: detection and classification with high-resolution sonography. Semin Ultrasound CT MR 2000; 21: 325–36.
50. Berg WA. Rationale for a trial of screening breast ultrasound: American College of Radiology Imaging Network (ACRIN) 6666. AJR Am J Roentgenol 2003; 180: 1225–8.
51. Yang WT, Metreweli C, Lam PK, Chang J. Benign and malignant breast masses and axillary nodes: evaluation with echo-enhanced color power Doppler US. Radiology 2001; 220: 795–802.
52. Yang WT, Chang J, Metreweli C. Patients with breast cancer: differences in color doppler flow and gray-scale US features of benign and malignant axillary lymph nodes. Radiology 2000; 215: 568–73.
53. Raza S, Baum JK. Solid breast lesions: evaluation with power Doppler US. Radiology 1997; 203: 164–8.
54. Tozaki M and Fukuma E. Does power doppler ultrasonography improve the BI-RADS category assessment and diagnostic accuracy of solid breast lesions? Acta Radiol 2011; 52: 706–10.
55. Lerner RM, Huang SR, Parker KJ. "Sonoelasticity" images derived from ultrasound signals in mechanically vibrated tissues. Ultrasound Med Biol 1990; 16: 231–9.
56. Itoh A, Ueno E, Tohno E, et al. Breast disease: clinical application of US elastography for diagnosis. Radiology 2006; 239: 341–50.
57. Ginat DT, Destounis SV, Barr RG, et al. US elastography of breast and prostate lesions. Radiographics 2009; 29: 2007–16.
58. Chang JM, Moon WK, Cho N, et al. Breast mass evaluation: factors influencing the quality of US elastography. Radiology 2011; 259: 59–64.
59. Jiang J, Hall TJ, Sommer AM. A novel performance descriptor for ultrasonic strain imaging: a preliminary study. IEEE Trans Ultrason Ferroelectr Freq Control 2006; 53: 1088–102.
60. Krouskop TA, Wheeler TM, Kallel F, et al. Elastic moduli of breast and prostate tissues under compression. Ultrason Imaging 1998; 20: 260–74.
61. Giuseppetti GM, Martegani A, Di Cioccio B, et al. Elastosonography in the diagnosis of the nodular breast lesions: preliminary report. Radiol Med 2005; 110: 1–69–76.
62. Sorelli PG, Cosgrove DO, Svensson WE, et al. Can contrast-enhanced sonography distinguish benign from malignant breast masses? J Clin Ultrasound 2010; 38: 177–81.
63. Zhao H, Xu R, Ouyang Q, et al. Contrast-enhanced ultrasound is helpful in the differentiation of malignant and benign breast lesions. Eur J Radiol 2010; 73: 288–93.
64. Balleyguier C, Opolon P, Mathieu MC, et al. New potential and applications of contrast-enhanced ultrasound of the breast: Own investigations and review of the literature. Eur J Radiol 2009; 69: 14–23.
65. Van Esser S, Veldhuis WB, van Hillegersberg R, et al. Accuracy of contrast-enhanced breast ultrasound for pre-operative tumor size assessment in patients diagnosed with invasive ductal carcinoma of the breast. Cancer Imaging 2007; 7: 63–8.
66. Sever AR, Mills P, Jones SE, et al. Preoperative sentinel node identification with ultrasound using microbubbles in patients with breast cancer. AJR Am J Roentgenol 2011; 196: 251.
67. Sever A, Jones S, Cox K, et al. Preoperative localization of sentinel lymph nodes using intradermal microbubbles and contrast-enhanced ultrasonography in patients with breast cancer. Br J Surg 2009; 96: 1295–9.
68. Weissman C, Hergan K. Current status of 3D/4D volume ultrasound of the breast. Ultraschall Med 2007; 28: 273–82.
69. Eberhard M. Ultrasound in obstetrics and gynaecology. Gynaecology, 2nd edn. Vol 2. New York, NY: Thieme, 2007: 273.
70. Weismann CF, Forstner R, Prokop E, Rettenbacher T. Three-dimensional targeting: a new three-dimensional ultrasound technique to evaluate needle position during breast biopsy. Ultrasound Obstet Gynecol 2000; 16: 359–64.
71. Warm M, Duda V, Eichler C, et al. 3D breast ultrasound: a significant predictor in breast cancer reduction under pre-operative chemotherapy. Anticancer Res 2011; 31: 4039–42.
72. Cho N, Moon WK, Cha JH, et al. Differentiating benign from malignant solid breast masses: comparison of two-dimensional and three-dimensional US. Radiology 2006; 240: 26–32.
73. Kelly KM, Dean J, Lee SJ, et al. Breast cancer detection: radiologists' performance using mammography with and without automated whole-breast ultrasound. Eur Radiol 2010; 20: 2557–64.
74. Kelly KM, Richwald GA. Automated whole-breast ultrasound: advancing the performance of breast cancer screening. Semin Ultrasound CT MR 2011; 32: 273–80.
75. Wang Y, Jiang S, Wang H. CAD algorithms for solid breast masses discrimination: evaluation of the accuracy and interobserver variability. Ultrasound Med Biol 2010; 36: 1273–81.
76. Baker JA, Kornguth PJ, Soo MS, et al. Sonography of solid breast lesions: observer variability of lesion description and assessment. AJR Am J Roentgenol 1999; 172: 1621–5.
77. Chabi ML, Borget I, Ardiles R, et al. Evaluation of the accuracy of a computer-aided diagnosis (CAD) system in breast ultrasound according to the radiologist's experience. Acad Radiol 2012; 19: 311–19.
78. Nakano S, Yoshida M, Fujii K, et al. Fusion of MRI and sonography image for breast cancer evaluation using real-time virtual sonography with magnetic navigation: first experience. Jpn J Clin Oncol 2009; 39: 552–9.

20 The role of MRI in preoperative evaluation and postoperative follow-up of breast cancer patients

Richard J. Bleicher

INTRODUCTION

The role of MRI has been in evolution since it was first assessed for breast abnormalities back in 1984 (1,2). For some aspects of care, breast MRI has become a standard part of imaging (3); but for other aspects, even if it is routinely used, there has been debate which at times has become contentious (4). This controversy stems from 20 years of data that, in some cases, appear contradictory on face value.

Great enthusiasm has naturally developed as breast MRI has repeatedly been shown to detect foci of cancer in 8–40% of patients, which other imaging modalities do not reveal (5). The use of MRI has been further promoted by consistent and reproducible demonstration that the measurement of a primary tumor size with breast MRI is more accurate when compared with other methods of assessment including mammogram, ultrasound, and physical examination (Table 20.1). Even though greater sensitivity cannot be linked directly to an improvement in outcomes, MRI has been assumed to do this for many aspects of care. Therefore, very broad guidelines and consensus statements have been developed for various clinical scenarios related to breast cancer and screening (Table 20.2).

Rates of MRI usage in the United States have markedly increased by two- to three-fold since its introduction, according to some studies (6–10). While some clinical indications included in MRI guidelines are supported by the medical literature, others are not. In evaluating breast MRI, the question is not whether the modality is valuable per se but whether the data support its use in a particular clinical setting when considering the potential disadvantages.

ROUTINE PREOPERATIVE EVALUATION

The most controversial aspect of breast MRI is its role in the routine preoperative evaluation of patients with a newly diagnosed cancer. Since breast MRI is more sensitive and has greater accuracy for estimating tumor size as compared with mammography and ultrasound, it may be advantageous in guiding surgical options and determining whether a patient is a candidate for breast conservation as opposed to mastectomy.

Moreover, another proposed benefit of MRI is to lower the close or positive margin rate and to decrease the re-excision rate when attempting breast conservation surgery. This is based on its greater correlation to pathological tumor size relative to other imaging modalities. Moreover, MRI may be useful in this setting for lobular carcinomas, whose mammographic presentation and findings on physical examination are less sensitive than for ductal tumors (11,12). In consequence, guidelines specifically mention the use of breast MRI for the assessment of lobular cancer (13,14). The published medical literature has largely concluded that routine preoperative MRI is not associated with improvements in assessment of candidacy for breast conservation, increased chance of obtaining negative margins, nor in decreased rates of re-excision even for lobular carcinoma.

Breast Conservation Candidacy and Achieving Negative Margins

Historically, assessment of patients for breast conservation has been satisfactory prior to the availability of breast MRI. In 1985, the National Surgical Adjuvant Breast and Bowel Project (NSABP) B-06 trial demonstrated that among 1257 patients, 90% were found to be suitable for breast conservation, with the majority of these having a successful first attempt at achieving negative margins (15). The following year, the Danish Breast Cancer Cooperative Group published a randomized breast conservation trial showing that patients in the breast conservation arm of the trial were found to have uninvolved margins after segmental mastectomy in 93% of 407 patients (16).

Retrospective non-randomized series have also confirmed a high degree of success in choosing patients for breast conservation using mammography alone. In a series by Morrow and colleagues of 263 women with early-stage breast cancer, 97.2% of women were successfully chosen for breast conservation. In a separate study from the H. Lee Moffitt Cancer Center with over 900 patients, breast conservation was successful in 92% of cases (12). As such, the data suggest that the margin of benefit for improvement by MRI may be approximately 10% at most.

Retrospective and prospective contemporary studies have directly compared the outcomes of patients with and without preoperative MRI. In a series of 577 stage I, II, and III patients, Bleicher and colleagues (6) reported that MRI was not associated with increased rates of breast conserving surgery; breast conservation was successful in 94.1% of those having no preoperative MRI, and in 90.2% of those having a preoperative MRI ($p = 0.35$). In a series of 349 women, Pengel and colleagues (17) found that the margin positivity rate in patients having breast MRI was 13.8% as compared with a 19.4% positive margin rate in the non-MRI group ($p = 0.17$). A similar lack of benefit on the margin status and re-excision rate has also been found for preoperative breast MRI performed for pure ductal cell carcinoma *in situ* (DCIS) (18). Furthermore, it has been suggested that this lack of improvement of margin status in the context of invasive tumors may result, in part, from underestimation of DCIS at the periphery of an invasive tumor (19).

Table 20.1 Correlation Between Sizes Seen by Detection Method as Vs. Histological Size

Study	n	Histology	Correlation (MRI)	Correlation (US)	Correlation (MMG)	Correlation (PE)	Lesion Over-/ Underestimation by MRI
Davis, 1996 (167)	14	All invasive types	$r = 0.98$	$r = 0.45$	$r = 0.46$	–	–
Mumtaz, 1997 (168)	53	All invasive types and DCIS	$r^2 = 0.93$	–	$r^2 = 0.59$	–	–
Amano, 2000 (74)	58	All invasive types and DCIS	$r = 0.78$	$r = 0.55$	$r = 0.63$	–	–
Munot, 2002 (71)	20	Lobular	$r = 0.97$	$r = 0.67$	$r = 0.66$	–	–
Boetes, 2004 (72)	36	Lobular	$r = 0.81$	$r = 0.24$	$r = 0.34, 0.27$[a]	–	50%, 56% underestimated; 11%,17% overestimated[a]
Bazzocchi, 2006 (169)	112	All invasive types having calcifications	$r = 0.75$	–	$r = 0.80$	–	–
Schouten van der Velden, 2006 (170)	66	All invasive types <10 mm and DCIS	$r = 0.49$	–	$r = 0.44$	–	47% underestimated; 38% overestimated
Kim, 2007 (171)	72	DCIS	$r = 0.79$	–	$r = 0.63$	–	17% underestimated; 11% overestimated
Caramella, 2007 (73)	57	Lobular	$r = 0.87$	$r = 0.57$	$r = 0.40$	$r = 0.53$	7% underestimated; 12% overestimated
Mann, 2008 (75)	67	Lobular	$r = 0.85$	–	$r = 0.27$	–	16% underestimated; 10% overestimated
Onesti, 2008 (76)	10	Lobular	$r = 0.65$	–	–	–	10% underestimated; 50% overestimated
Turnbull, 2010 (20)	1623	All invasive types	$r = 0.53$	$r = 0.29$	$r = 0.37$	–	–
McGhan, 2010 (77)	70	Lobular	$r = 0.75$	$r = 0.45$	$r = 0.65$	$r = 0.63$	14% underestimated; 31% overestimated
Behjatnia, 2010 (172)	10	All invasive types	–	–	–	–	27% underestimated; 70% overestimated

[a]This study separately reported these values for each radiologist.
Abbreviations: DCIS, ductal cell carcinoma in situ; MMG, mammogram; PE, physical examination; US, ultrasound.

Table 20.2 Summary of Guidelines for the Use of Breast MRI

	American College of Radiology, 2004 (13)	European Society of Breast Imaging, 2008 (64)	American Society of Breast Surgeons, 2005 (14)	Society of Breast Imaging and Breast Imaging Commission of the American College of Radiology, 2010 (175)[a]
High-risk surveillance	√	√	√	√
Inconclusive/conflicting information	√	√	√	–
Pre-/during/post-neoadjuvant chemotherapy	√	√	√	–
Search for an occult primary	√	√	√	–
Check for contralateral cancer	√	√	√	√
Preoperative evaluation of extent of disease	√ (IDC and ILC)	√	√ (especially ILC)	–
Evaluate post-implant reconstruction	√	√	–	–
Check for post-lumpectomy residual disease	√	√	–	–
Dense breasts	–	√	√	–
Evaluate recurrence post-tissue reconstruction	√	–	–	–
Evaluate any suspected recurrence	√	–	–	–
"Lesion characterization"	√	–	–	–
Evaluate for chest wall invasion	√	–	–	–

[a]This statement was restricted to screening recommendations only.
Abbreviations: IDC, Infiltrating ductal carcinoma; ILC, Infiltrating lobular carcinoma.

Two completed prospective randomized trials (the Comparative Effectiveness of Magnetic Resonance Imaging in Breast Cancer (COMICE) trial (20) from the United Kingdom (UK) and the Dutch MR Mammography of Nonpalpable Breast Tumors (MONET) trial (21)) evaluated women felt to be eligible for breast conservation by mammographic and/or ultrasound imaging and physical examination. These trials randomized women to preoperative breast MRI or no MRI. Both the COMICE and MONET trials had primary endpoints of reoperation rates including re-excision or conversion to mastectomy. Neither trial demonstrated a benefit for MRI in terms of achieving clean margins. In the COMICE trial, the positive margin rates for patients having an MRI were 16% and 13% for patients with DCIS and invasive cancer respectively, as compared with 15% for both groups of patients not having an MRI. The MONET trial paradoxically noted a significantly lower positive margin rate in the non-MRI (12%) compared with the MRI group (34%) ($p = 0.008$). Reoperation rates were similar in each arm of the COMICE trial (MRI, 18.8%; no MRI 19.3%; $p = 0.77$) and in the MONET trial, there were 78 and 76 surgical procedures in the MRI and non-MRI groups respectively ($p = 0.78$).

False Positives and Associated Mastectomy Rates

Breast MRI has been associated with a significant elevation in the rate of unnecessary mastectomy based on pathological correlation, thus countering claims for theoretical benefit when MRI is used in the routine preoperative setting. Rates of mastectomy associated with routine performance of breast MRI vary widely, with many series demonstrating about 20–30% unnecessary mastectomy rates (22–24) or a stage-specific likelihood of undergoing a mastectomy which is approximately 1.8-fold higher than for those patients not having an MRI (6,7,25). In the COMICE trial, pathologically avoidable intent-to-treat mastectomy rate was 4.6 times higher for patients who underwent preoperative breast MRI (20) while for patients whose initial decision was for mastectomy, the mastectomy rate was seven-fold higher in the MRI group (26).

Several studies have correlated the choice of mastectomy with MRI use. In one series of 267 patients undergoing an MRI prior to definitive surgery, the surgical plan was altered in 69 patients with 16.5% converting from breast conservation to mastectomy; 29% of these additional excisions or conversions to mastectomy were found to be unnecessary when the MRI findings were correlated with the pathological specimens (22). In another series of 111 breast cancer patients who underwent preoperative MRI, 24 patients were advised to undergo mastectomy based upon the MRI and 21% of these ($n = 5$) were altered unnecessarily (23). In a smaller study of 73 patients, surgical treatment was altered by breast MRI in 36 patients; 20% of conversions from breast conservation to mastectomy were considered unnecessary based on pathology. Furthermore, 52% of wider excisions were unnecessary; and 40% of contralateral procedures were unnecessary. In a recent series of 71 patients having an MRI after an excisional biopsy, 19 patients were found to have MRI findings suspicious for multifocal or multicentric disease, five patients had a mastectomy based upon the MRI alone without further evaluation (27), and three patients (16%) had unicentric disease on pathology (and therefore, underwent unnecessary mastectomy).

It is perhaps ironic that the reason for the higher associated mastectomy rate in patients having breast MRI stems from the exact benefit that MRI confers: visualization of more detailed findings in the breast by its significantly greater sensitivity. With this greater sensitivity comes a lower specificity and higher false-positive rate (28), as demonstrated in the COMICE trial where the latter was 38% (26). False positives on MRI can represent a variety of benign findings, including fibrocystic change, fibroadenomas, benign intramammary lymph nodes, sclerosing adenosis, hyperplasia without atypia, atypical hyperplasia, papillomas, lobular carcinoma *in situ*, fat necrosis, and inflammatory lesions (21,29,30). A substantial false-positive rate is demonstrable even in screening trials of high risk women (31–35) where standard imaging is particularly difficult because of intrinsic tumor biology (36,37).

These false-positive results prompt additional imaging and biopsies to rule out malignancy. In the American College of Radiology Imaging Network (ACRIN) study, MRI detected occult contralateral breast cancer in 3.1% of patients undergoing breast MRI (38). However, 121 additional biopsies for suspicious MRI findings were performed among 969 women; malignant pathology was identified in only 30 cases (24.8%) from these 121 biopsies. In another major trial assessing MRI and mammography for women with a familial or genetic predisposition to breast cancer, screening by MRI led to twice as many additional examinations compared with mammography and three times as many biopsies for benign conditions (31).

A targeted "second look" ultrasound is the preferred method by over 85% of breast radiologists to assess suspicious or indeterminant MRI lesions (39). Nonetheless, ultrasound visualizes such lesions in only 47% of cases and obviates biopsy in 10%, thus leaving 37% to be biopsied under ultrasound guidance (40). MRI-guided core biopsy is therefore, subsequently required in 53% of cases, to detect cancers in only 12% of cases (40). A comprehensive review of studies involving breast cancer patients found that MRI was associated with frequent false positives and identified additional disease in only 16% of cases (28).

The elevated mastectomy rate is thought to result from patients or physicians deciding to proceed to mastectomy without sampling the additional foci (27). For example, in a series of 441 patients (41) with newly diagnosed cancer undergoing MRI, targeted "second look" ultrasound was recommended for suspicious MRI findings in 200 patients. However, one-third of patients chose to proceed with the treatment decision based upon the MRI result alone instead of undergoing targeted ultrasound. Unfortunately, breast MRI cannot substitute for pathological evaluation, because of limited specificity (5,28,31,42), and therefore omission of additional investigation results in inappropriate changes in the surgical plan with unnecessary conversion to mastectomy. A meta-analysis of 19 studies among 2610 women (28) revealed that the surgical plan changed in 7.8–33.3% of patients because of MRI, while additional surgery was specifically attributed to false-positive outcomes in 5.5% of cases.

Accelerated Partial Breast Irradiation

Although there is a significant false-positive rate, it should be restated that breast MRI may detect cancer that is multifocal or multicentric but occult on standard imaging. Although true positive results have been shown to change management plan, the presence of these occult foci of disease on MRI have long been recognized from studies of mastectomy specimens (43–46). The whole-breast radiotherapy component of breast conservation therapy significantly decreases the risk of locoregional or distant recurrence and even death (35,47). These foci explain why whole-breast radiotherapy is an essential part of the breast conservation paradigm, which provides similar overall survival outcomes to mastectomy (48). The need to excise foci of tumor seen only on MRI is therefore questionable when the breast is to be radiated. Until the advent of breast MRI, these foci had just not been visible on preoperative imaging, but long been known to exist.

When breast MRI is not performed, local recurrence rates after breast conserving surgery plus whole-breast radiation are only of the order 0.5–1.0% per breast per year (49) and the addition of breast MRI does not improve these recurrence rates. Accelerated partial breast irradiation (APBI) is currently undergoing investigation as an alternative to whole-breast radiotherapy and shows promise as an alternative option (50,51). MRI has been used, and currently remains a reasonable adjunct to detect other foci of malignancy for APBI candidates, as current recommendations regarding APBI candidacy primarily consider only those with unicentric disease (52,53). In one study, MRI detected foci of ipsilateral disease in 7.1% of patients initially felt to be eligible for APBI, suggesting a significant impact on patient selection (54). It is consequently conceivable that MRI may eventually not be required for all patients receiving APBI if equivalent local recurrence rates in such patients are maintained. For now, however, in an attempt to continue assessment of APBI under the most conservative and safe conditions, use of MRI is warranted while patient selection is refined.

Invasive Lobular Carcinoma

Invasive lobular carcinoma may be difficult to detect on conventional mammographic imaging (11,12) and more elusive on physical examination than ductal cancers with only half of patients having a suspicious physical examination finding (11,55). Still, recurrence rates for lobular cancers have been similar to ductal cancers, even before the advent of breast MRI (56–62).

Nonetheless, concerns about difficulties in visualizing the extent of lesions and a higher chance of multifocality and multicentricity with lobular cancers have persisted (45,63). As a result, several societies have supported the routine use of MRI for preoperative evaluation of invasive lobular carcinoma even though data do not suggest that breast MRI improves outcome (13,14,64). Breast MRI techniques have been refined for identification and assessment of lobular carcinoma for which MRI measurements have a higher correlation to the final pathological tumor size than those of mammography, ultrasound, or physical examination (65–70). Correlation coefficients to pathological size for MRI range from 0.53 to 0.98 while coefficients for mammography range from 0.3 to 0.66. For ultrasound and physical examination, these coefficients range from 0.24 to 0.67 and 0.53 to 0.63 respectively (20,71–77).

Some published studies noted "beneficial" management changes in 9–42% of cases as a result of information provided by breast MRI although conversion to mastectomy without pathological correlation (to confirm necessity for any change in management plan) are included among these cases (73,78,79). The reoperation rate for patients undergoing breast MRI is not significantly lower in most series of patients with lobular cancers, including the prospective randomized COMICE trial.

Re-excision rates vary widely across these series from 7% to 38% (26,77,80). However, one study of 267 patients reported that MRI was associated with a lower risk of reoperation (MRI, 5%; no MRI, 15%; $p = 0.01$) (81). Moreover, this study demonstrated no difference in mastectomy rates for those patients with lobular cancer irrespective of whether they received an MRI which is consistent with other studies (77,80).

In a single-institutional analysis from Germany (80), 178 patients with infiltrating lobular cancer diagnosed between 2007 and 2009 were reviewed to assess the impact of breast MRI on the primary surgery and the number of secondary surgical interventions. MRI was significantly associated with a greater probability of bilateral procedures. However, MRI was not significantly associated with increased primary or secondary mastectomy rates (8% vs. 9% $p = 0.401$), or with increased re-excision rates (19% in the MRI group vs. 18% in the non-MRI group $p = 0.429$).

In a study by McGhan and colleagues (77) 70 patients with invasive lobular carcinoma underwent clinical breast examination, mammography, ultrasound, and MRI. The mean tumor size was 0.94 cm with a maximum size of 5.2 cm. MRI correctly estimated the size to be within 0.5 cm of the true pathological size in 56% of cases, overestimated the size by >0.5 cm in 31% of cases, but there was a significantly improved correlation coefficient for tumor size compared with mammography, breast examination, and ultrasound. The only local recurrence in the 10-year study period was in the MRI group, and there were no significant differences in re-excision rates or breast conservation failures (need for mastectomy) between MRI and non-MRI patients.

In summary, evidence to date overwhelmingly suggests that MRI does not improve outcomes for lobular cancer, which is consistent with other histological types. The ability of MRI to confer improvement in local recurrence seems limited and recurrence rates are similar for ductal and lobular cancers irrespective of MRI imaging (56,59,61).

Recurrence Rates and Survival

Even if one remains skeptical about data on margin status and surgical treatment, the preponderance of data on local recurrence corroborate the notion that routine preoperative MRI has little impact overall. The exception to this is a study comparing outcomes of patients with (121 patients) and without (225 patients) preoperative MRI (82). Although recurrence rates were significantly decreased in the MRI group (MRI, 1.2%; non-MRI, 6.8%; $p < 0.001$), the non-MRI group had more T3/4 tumors and a higher frequency of lymph node metastasis (45.8% vs. 38.8%). In addition, adjuvant chemotherapy use was greater in the MRI group with omission of chemotherapy for node-positive disease in 14% of patients in the non-MRI group compared with 6% in the MRI group. The conclusion of this study was that preoperative MRI was beneficial in terms of local recurrence rates, but the greater proportion of advanced disease and the less aggressive systemic treatment in the non-MRI group render the interpretation difficult and higher recurrence cannot necessarily be attributed to lack of MRI.

In other series, decreased local recurrence rates have not been associated with MRI use. The only prospective randomized data available are from the COMICE trial, in which 99.9% of MRI patients and 99.7% of non-MRI patients remained recurrence free, with no statistical difference between the two groups (20). However, follow-up was limited to one year only and therefore inferences cannot yet be drawn. Two retrospective series with a much longer follow-up specifically evaluated breast conservation and also showed no difference between patients receiving and not receiving MRI. In a study of 756 women with stages 0, I, and II breast cancer undergoing breast conservation, no differences were observed in the T or N stage, receptor status, systemic therapy, or tamoxifen between the MRI and non-MRI groups (8). At eight years, this study demonstrated similar local recurrence, disease-specific survival, and overall survival rates between the two groups. Likewise, in another study of 463 women who had breast conservation, the actuarial eight-year in-breast tumor recurrence rates were similar for MRI and non-MRI groups.

In the absence of clear evidence that MRI confers a recurrence benefit, it is even less likely that a survival benefit will ensue from the use of MRI. Currently, the only imaging modality associated with a survival benefit in women with breast cancer is mammography (83). A review of prospective randomized screening trials, even with elimination of those biased toward mammography, demonstrates a relative risk reduction in breast cancer mortality of 15% or greater (84). Although these data refer to mammographic screening for primary breast cancer, survival benefits have also been attributed to mammography for the detection of asymptomatic second breast cancers (85). There are no corresponding data demonstrating a survival benefit for routine preoperative breast MRI.

Contralateral Breast Cancer

One of the most common arguments made for use of breast MRI is that it detects contralateral breast cancer, and therefore has a beneficial effect on operative planning. In the ACRIN trial, MRI was used to stage 969 asymptomatic women with breast cancer; occult contralateral disease undetected by standard imaging and physical examination was identified in 3.1% of cases (38). A meta-analysis of contralateral cancer detection in 22 screening MRI studies encompassing 3253 women demonstrated suspicious findings in 9.3% of patients with a positive predictive value of only 47.9% (86). The effect on surgical treatment was inconsistently reported, and a rate could not be accurately inferred.

The risk of metachronous contralateral breast cancer remains low at 2–4% over five years (87–90) with a detection rate of about 3% by MRI. This observation suggests that many of the foci detected by MRI are clinically insignificant as new breast cancers also develop during that time. Some studies suggest that the incidence of contralateral breast cancer is declining (91,92), which controversially may be due to the use of systemic therapies over the past 20 years (93–97). Such a decline in contralateral cancers will minimize any potential impact of MRI on this particular outcome. Hence, the proportion of contralateral surgeries performed unnecessarily because of false positives or malignant foci that will clinically be insignificant remains uncertain. Consequently, the precise benefit of MRI in terms of detection of occult foci of contralateral breast cancer has yet to be determined.

Occult Cancer

Although routine use of MRI in the preoperative, previously diagnosed breast cancer patient has not been shown to be beneficial, MRI does have a role in clinical circumstances when standard imaging is insufficient or contradictory, whereby additional information provided by MRI can be of critical importance in determining treatments or expanding treatment options.

In spite of accounting for less than 1% of breast cancer cases, patients having occult primary tumors may benefit from the routine use of breast MRI. These patients typically present with axillary lymphadenopathy, which is confirmed upon nodal biopsy, despite unremarkable mammography and physical examination. Mastectomy provides reasonable local control, but a primary tumor fails to be identified in up to 92% of specimens (98–101). Alternatively, whole-breast radiotherapy without excision of the breast affords similar local control rates to mastectomy (102,103). However, observation of the breast alone leaves patients with an eventual breast tumor growth in up to 60% of cases (104), suggesting that a tumor is usually present, but simply not visible.

Occult tumors have identical overall and disease-specific survival to primary breast cancers which are mammographically visible (105) and breast conservation should be feasible if the primary tumor can be localized. Although historically breast conservation was not recommended because the primary could not be seen mammographically, breast MRI can identify the primary in 25–100% of cases, thus providing an alternative surgical option for some patients (Table 20.3). Preoperative breast MRI consequently provides these patients with an equivalent surgical option that is precluded when standard imaging alone is employed. MRI is therefore clearly indicated and potentially beneficial in the setting of occult disease.

Paget's Disease

Paget's disease is an uncommon entity, representing less than 5% of all diagnosed breast cancers (106). The disease is associated with underlying noncontiguous *in situ* or invasive parenchymal carcinoma in up to 53% of cases (107–109). About 29–100% of Paget's disease and concurrent underlying parenchymal pathology is occult on mammogram (108,110–112).

Table 20.3 Series Demonstrating Performance of MRI for Identifying Occult Primary Tumors. True Positives are Defined as MRIs Demonstrating a Pathologically Confirmed Malignancy in the Breast over All MRIs Performed

Study	*n*	True Positives (%)	False Negatives (%)
Morris, 1997 (174)	12	75	0
Tilanus-Linthorst, 1997 (175)	4	100	0
Henry-Tillman, 1999 (176)	10	100	0
Orel, 1999 (177)	22	85	66
Stomper, 1999 (178)	8	25	N/P
Olson, 2000 (179)	40	N/P	20
Obdeijn, 2000 (180)	20	40	0
Chen, 2002 (181)	3	0	N/P
McMahon, 2005 (182)	18	67	0
Buchanan, 2005 (183)	55	47	15
Ko, 2007 (184)	12	83	N/P
Barton, 2011 (102)	20	35	N/P

Abbreviation: N/P, data not provided.

Table 20.4 Sensitivity of MRI in Paget's Disease for Underlying Parenchymal Disease

Study	Sensitivity (%)	n
Eccevaria, 2004 (112)	100	3
Morrogh, 2008 (185)	54	7
Siponen, 2010 (109)	100 – Invasive 44 – DCIS	14
Kim, 2010 (186)	100	8
Schilling, 2011 (187)	100	3

The results of studies evaluating use of MRI for Paget's disease are summarized in Table 20.4.

The principles of surgical excision are similar to occult cancers, and breast conservation is feasible for Paget's disease when the underlying malignancy can be identified and resection undertaken with low local recurrence rates (109,113). MRI is a valuable adjunct in the routine preoperative evaluation of Paget's disease, and potentially allows the option of breast conservation to be considered by patients should this be desired.

Neoadjuvant Chemotherapy Response Assessment

Neoadjuvant chemotherapy benefits patients by allowing breast conservation for those who were solely candidates for mastectomy at diagnosis and by downstaging unresectable tumors (defined as those involving skin or chest wall) to resectable tumors. It does not change overall survival relative to adjuvant therapy. Some measurable response is evident in 80% of patients, with a complete pathological response in 6–19% of patients (114–117). Traditionally, responses were assessed by physical examination and mammogram, but more recently by ultrasound and now breast MRI.

MRI has been demonstrated in several series to be more sensitive and accurate than standard imaging to evaluate response to neoadjuvant chemotherapy as well as having a higher correlation with the final pathological tumor size (Table 20.5). This observation is plausible because enhancement on MRI is related to blood flow, while mammographic visualization cannot readily distinguish increased density that occurs from post-treatment scar as opposed to viable tumor.

Some data suggest that the accuracy of MRI for detection of complete response in the neoadjuvant setting is tumor phenotype-dependent. McGuire and colleagues (118) reviewed 203 patients and the predictive value of several factors for complete pathological response. The positive predictive value of MRI for triple-negative tumors was 73.6% compared with 27.3% for hormone receptor-positive/HER2/*neu*-negative luminal tumors. A similar evaluation by De Los Santos (119) found that the predictive value of MRI for triple negative tumors was 100%, and only 62% for receptor-positive/HER2/*neu*-negative luminal tumors.

Furthermore, some data suggest that the accuracy of MRI in the neoadjuvant setting varies depending on the type of treatment given. In a series of 40 patients with locally advanced breast cancer, the extent of residual tumor after treatment with taxane was found to be frequently underestimated by in excess of 15 mm with MRI (120). In another study which compared MRI with ultrasound and final pathology, MRI and ultrasound demonstrated comparable accuracy in predicting residual disease after neoadjuvant chemotherapy (121). The linear correlation between imaging and pathological tumor size was *r* = 0.53 for MRI and *r* = 0.66 for ultrasound. Although not significantly different, ultrasound also fared minimally but not significantly better. The mean of the deltas between imaging and pathological size was 0.16 cm for MRI and 0.06 cm for ultrasound, with no discrepancy between imaging and pathological size for 20.3% of the MRI patients and 15.2% of the ultrasound patients. This study is notable in that it found a lower correlation between MRI and pathology than most other series, and the authors suggest that taxanes may have modulated the accuracy of MRI (120). Utilization of contrast-enhanced MRI to assess post-neoadjuvant surgical treatment is associated with an acceptable level of local recurrence and permits more widespread and accurate use of breast conservation (122).

High-Risk Patients

Perhaps the least controversial benefit of breast MRI relates to patients who are considered to be at high risk, either from the carriage of a deleterious genetic mutation, or a significant family history. The benefits of MRI have only been established in the screening setting, although some of the benefits may apply to the preoperative use of MRI to evaluate high-risk patients recently diagnosed with breast cancer. Further evaluation in this area is needed, especially as development of breast cancer at an early age often prompts high risk and genetic assessment. Therefore, many of these patients will not have had an MRI previously, and the benefit of adding such a modality to a standard diagnostic workup remains uncertain.

The main advantage for patients at high risk, especially those with deleterious BRCA mutations, is improved sensitivity of MRI over mammography in detecting breast cancer (31–34,123). Although there is a slight fall in specificity for MRI relative to mammography, MRI has greater utility in the assessment of cancers in high risk patients because of intrinsic differences in tumor biology. Compared with non–high risk patients, these tumors are of a higher grade, more frequently estrogen receptor-negative, have higher mitotic counts, more frequent necrotic elements, and shorter tumor doubling times. These differences are more pronounced for BRCA1 than for BRCA2 mutation carriers (36,37,124–127). These differences are further underlined by the mammographic appearance of these lesions. Tumors in patients with BRCA2 and especially BRCA1 mutations have pushing margins, fewer spiculations, and can appear as well-defined masses more frequently than controls (36,37,127). These appearances make imaging with standard methods less accurate, and as there are no data on additional benefits of MRI in high-risk women with a confirmed cancer diagnosis, further data are needed.

There are well-documented differences in the sensitivity of breast MRI for the screening of high-risk patients. Published data suggest a greater sensitivity compared with mammography for those with a BRCA1 mutation versus those with a BRCA2 mutation (33,128). When evaluating relative benefits between these two modalities one study has applied a well-established model to breast MRI in BRCA carriers (129). The estimated life expectancy in BRCA1 carriers was increased with addition of MRI by 2.1 years, versus 1.2 years for BRCA2 carriers. Cost analysis calculations reinforce this further and show a cost of $88,651 per quality-adjusted life year for MRI in

Table 20.5 MRI Assessment after Neoadjuvant Chemotherapy

Study	*n*	Endpoint	MRI Accuracy	MRI Sensitivity	Correlation Coefficients as *Vs.* Pathology			
					MRI	Mammo	Ultrasound	Physical Exam
Gilles, 1994 (188)	25	Residual Disease	96%	94%	–	–	–	–
Abraham, 1996 (189)	39	Correlation with MRI Assessment	–	–	–	($\kappa = 0.32$)[a]	–	($\kappa = 0.15$)[a]
Drew, 2001 (190)	17	Residual Disease	100%	–	–	–	–	–
Esserman, 2001 (191)	33	Residual Disease	–	–	0.92	–	–	–
Weatherall, 2001 (192)	20	Residual Disease	–	–	0.93	0.63	–	0.72
Partridge, 2002 (193)	52	Residual Disease	–	–	0.89	–	–	0.60
Balu-Maestro, 2002 (194)	60	Complete Response	100%	100%	–	–	–	–
Cheung, 2003 (195)	33	Residual Disease	–	–	0.98	–	–	0.64
Rosen, 2003 (196)	21	Residual Disease	90%	95%	0.75	–	–	0.61
Wasser, 2003 (197)	31	Residual Disease	–	–	0.74	–	–	–
Martincich, 2004 (198)	30	Complete Response	–	93%	0.72	–	–	–
Denis, 2004 (120)	40	Residual Disease	–	–	0.89	–	–	–
Londero, 2004 (199)	15	Complete Response	80%	83%	0.70	0.67	0.57	–
Schott, 2005 (200)	41	Complete Response	89%	25%	–	–	–	–
Belli, 2006 (201)	45	Residual Disease	91%	91%	0.97	–	–	–
Kim, 2007 (202)	50	Residual Disease	–	–	0.65	–	–	–
Segara, 2007 (203)	68	Complete Response	72%	–	0.75	–	0.61	0.44
Yu, 2007 (204)	29	Residual Disease	–	–	0.49	–	–	–
Straver, 2010 (205)	208	Residual Disease	76%	78%	–	–	–	–
Croshaw, 2011 (206)	61	Residual Disease	70%	85%	–	–	–	–
De Los Santos, 2011 (119)	81	Complete Response	75%	92%	–	–	–	–
Guarneri, 2011 (121)	157	Residual Disease	–	–	0.53	–	0.66	–
Loo, 2011 (207)	188	Residual Disease	–	–	0.074–0.61[b]	–	–	–

Endpoint refers primarily to accuracy and sensitivity data here, if available.
[a]These are kappa values; correlations to MRI as versus to pathology.
[b]Multiple values ranging by tumor phenotype.

BRCA1 carriers versus \$188,034 in BRCA2 carriers. The Magnetic Resonance Imaging Breast Screening (MARIBS) trial reported similar findings, with greater costs per cancer detected for BRCA2 patients versus BRCA1 (130).

The benefit of adding MRI to the preoperative evaluation of high-risk women already diagnosed with a breast cancer remains uncertain. Any benefit will primarily be limited to potential alteration in the initial surgical plan, but there are few data examining whether there are quantitative or qualitative differences in disease detected solely by MRI in high-risk patients than when a primary tumor is detected by other means in this group of patients. Additionally, although mutation carriers have an elevated risk of developing contralateral disease over 15 years (131), it appears that the incidence of synchronous bilateral tumors (which would otherwise be another reason to use MRI) is not significantly elevated (132). So although MRI is beneficial for routine screening of high-risk patients, the precise role of breast MRI, after a cancer has been diagnosed by other methods in such patients, remains uncertain. Nevertheless, screening with MRI as an adjunct to mammography for high-risk patients remains standard practice at this time.

POSTOPERATIVE EVALUATION
Postoperative Assessment of a Prior Excision
There is little published data on the frequency of MRI use following a primary tumor excision associated with close or positive margins. Nonetheless, MRI is sometimes useful in this setting (133). MRI enhancement is related to blood flow and water content (134), which are often increased secondary to neovascularization of malignant tumors. This causes them to enhance in a similar fashion to areas of inflammation and other phenomena linked to increased vascular permeability (65). Postoperative surgical sites therefore enhance significantly (135,136) and can be a challenge for the radiologist to interpret (137). In addition, there are a wide range of benign entities that may also be seen and can represent false positives (29).

Several studies have evaluated the utility of MRI to detect additional disease after a wide local excision. It is perhaps intuitive that MRI may have a role in the assessment of the surrounding cavity after excision with compromised margins. Values for sensitivity range from 57% to 92%, and for specificity range from 29% to 76%. Moreover, the positive predictive value for MRI in this context ranges from 75% to 90%, and the negative predictive value ranges from 19% to 65% (22,27,133,135,138). Re-excision remains standard for pathologically positive margins and cannot be obviated based upon MRI findings. Thus, performance of MRI following wide local excision to assess residual disease is unlikely to be of any practical value.

Postoperative Assessment of Breast Implants
Prior to MRI, ultrasound was considered the modality of choice for detection of implant rupture (139). In the earliest published comparison between imaging modalities and their

efficacy to evaluate silicone breast implants, Steinbach et al. (140) utilized gelatin cubes in which fat or silicone was suspended and compared these with a control cube. In the same study, breast of veal with its fat, muscle, cartilage, and bone also underwent silicone breast implant insertion for imaging. The authors found that xeromammography demonstrated the implant, but fat and muscle could not be well defined; mammography had difficulty with the assessment of the posterior implant margin; ultrasound was only useful to assess the anterior and posterior implant. CT had difficulty with implant margins but was better for bone and soft tissue, whereas MRI showed the anatomy and the implant border clearly including small quantities of silicone. That same year, the first published cases of MR detection of breast implant rupture in patients were performed (141,142), while shortly thereafter a study using a rabbit animal model to assess imaging for implant rupture demonstrated greater accuracy by MRI and CT than for mammogram and ultrasound (143). Further evaluation noted that MRI body coils are not superior to ultrasound in the assessment of implant rupture, having a sensitivity of approximately 58% and a specificity of 88%, while surface coils better demonstrated findings indicative of rupture (144). Internal implant membranes ("linguine sign") or fluid droplets on MRI strongly suggest rupture, versus echoes on ultrasound that can be confused with hemorrhage.

In an early series of breast MRI using an adaptation of two shoulder coils, 70 symptomatic patients having removal of their silicone implants were evaluated. Even before a dedicated breast coil existed at this early stage of assessment, MRI already had a sensitivity and specificity for intracapsular and extracapsular rupture of 76% and 97%, respectively with an accuracy of 94% (142).

In another series of 82 implants in 63 patients where MRI, ultrasound, and mammography were compared with surgical pathology (145) the sensitivity of MRI for rupture was 93% versus 68% for mammography and 77% for ultrasound. The specificity was the highest for mammogram at 81% with MRI at 73% and ultrasound at 69% while the accuracy was the highest for MRI at 85%, 71% for ultrasound, and 68% for mammography. The authors therefore recommended that mammogram and ultrasound be employed first, prior to selectively employing MRI for further assessment.

Even modern MRI techniques may have difficulty with siliconomas, which can appear identical to a malignancy in the breast (146). The diagnostic advantage of MRI also remains important in light of the limited efficacy of clinical examination for the diagnosis of implant rupture, which only has a sensitivity of 30%, specificity of 88%, and a negative predictive value of 49% (147). The most widely known finding on MRI that is representative of capsular rupture is the linguine sign, thought to be an artifact of the implant capsule after rupture (148). The presence of a linguine sign has been found to be 87% sensitive and 100% specific for intracapsular rupture, and 67% sensitive and 75% specific for extracapsular rupture (149). Other radiological signs exist to assist with assessment, but are not as diagnostic (149).

In short, breast MRI has slightly higher performance than other imaging modalities for breast implant rupture. If standard assessments demonstrate such rupture, then MRI becomes superfluous in light of its expense (129), but in cases where the diagnosis on imaging is suspected but remains uncertain, MRI is a valuable tool to assess breast prostheses.

Assessment of Local Recurrence

Breast MRI has been used in conjunction with physical examination and mammography to detect local recurrences after breast conserving surgery which can be difficult to distinguish from scar tissue. A series of 40 women having breast conservation surgery for whom clinical and mammographic or ultrasound features of local recurrence were nonspecific or suspicious at least one year after radiotherapy were evaluated by Belli et al. Amongst these 40 patients, 22 were found to have a recurrence, there were two false-positive results (5%) but no false-negative results and MRI detected all cases of recurrence (150). In a review of 2061 studies evaluating mammography, ultrasound, MRI, and clinical examination for surveillance of ipsilateral breast tumor recurrence and contralateral metachronous breast cancer, mammography was found to have a sensitivity and specificity as high as 83% and 75% respectively. However, these metrics were surpassed by MRI having a sensitivity rate as high as 100% and specificity of up to 96% (151). By contrast, clinical examination in this study had the lowest sensitivity ranging from 43 to 62% with ultrasound being marginally superior at 43–87%. Even for those primary tumors that are occult on mammography initially, local recurrence within the breast is detectable on mammography in 68–77% of cases (105,152). Whether MRI provides a survival improvement or even lead-time bias for mammographically occult recurrences or for any postoperative screening remains unclear.

Nonetheless, MRI may present difficulties in assessing recurrence as demonstrated by a study evaluating ipsilateral and contralateral findings in 248 women with breast cancer who underwent breast conservation and one MRI prior to radiotherapy and at least two postoperatively (153). Features such as edema, skin thickening, seroma, and surgical site enhancement can be seen within the treated breast for at least six years after surgery and thus make MRI more difficult to interpret.

The clinical assessment of breast reconstruction using autogenous tissue can be particularly problematic. Fat necrosis and scarring can cause nodularity in such reconstructions, making physical examination difficult in a clinical setting where mammography has no role because there is no breast tissue. MRI utility in autogenous tissue reconstruction has been well described and represents a setting where other imaging techniques currently have a limited role (154,155).

There has been at least one dedicated attempt to assess the benefit of MRI in screening for breast cancer survivors. A competing risk model was created at Brigham and Women's Hospital for patients with a prior breast cancer to determine which women would have at least a 20–25% risk of developing another breast cancer over their lifetime (156). At this threshold, they would fall within American Cancer Society recommendations for MRI screening (3). This model assumed that the risk of a second breast cancer developing was constant over time, was not related to the patient's age, that risk was equivalent in the ipsilateral and contralateral breasts, and that the calculated risk should be the cumulative sum of annual risk up to an age of 99 years. Based upon these assumptions, the authors found that women having mastectomy would only reach the 25% threshold or above when screening began at 31–33 years of age. In contrast, they found that a 45-year-old woman having breast conserving therapy for a receptor-positive tumor fell into the lower 20% or greater threshold until age 66, and that all women developing primary breast cancer with conservation surgery before age 51 met this threshold. The authors have concluded that MRI should not be routinely recommended for screening in this group. They have noted an absence of evidence for any benefit within this population at the present time and the performance characteristics of MRI within the subset of women who have had prior surgery remain unclear. The authors have also noted that there may be benefit among some subsets of women with a risk of developing breast cancer which is estimated to be less than 20%, but this requires further study.

While the risk of relapse is one factor in determining the utility of any type of postoperative screening, the benefit conferred relates to the threat posed by such a relapse, which may be variable. This is evident from a series evaluating the importance of time to relapse and distinction between breast cancer recurrences and new primary tumors (157). This series showed at least one major histological characteristic differing between the primary tumor and relapse in 89% of cases and two or more characteristics varying in 60% of cases, suggesting that the risk posed from any relapse episode may be highly variable and therefore difficult to predict.

OTHER ROUTINE CONSIDERATIONS
Cost Effectiveness in the Postoperative Period
In a study by Zendejas and colleagues (158), contralateral prophylactic mastectomy in women with a diagnosed breast cancer was found to be more cost effective than surveillance for women who are younger than 70 years of age, with declining benefit from age 45 upward. The cost effectiveness and quality-adjusted-life-year benefit of contralateral prophylactic mastectomy were more pronounced in women of high risk, where a benefit existed in all ages. In this Markov model, patients were assumed to be seen at six-month intervals for five years and annually thereafter until recurrence. In addition to the physician visits, surveillance patients and those having a local recurrence were modeled as having annual mammography alone, while patients who developed a suspected contralateral breast cancer were then assumed to undergo mammography, ultrasound with biopsy, and breast MRI for confirmation and diagnosis. Although this model did not consider potential surgical complications and lost wages in its cost analysis, it also did not utilize MRI (and thus its associated costs) for routine screening in the postoperative period. The authors suggested that breast MRI is not a cost-effective routine screening tool when compared with contralateral prophylactic mastectomy in both the high-risk and non–high risk settings.

Breast MRI and the Cost of Care
The cost of health care has been a highly debated topic due in part to the current worldwide economic downturn. This topic has become a focus recently in the United States (US) in particular, where the cost of care has been demonstrated to be rising significantly as a whole and within mainstream US healthcare

markets (159). Because there is a desire to slow down the rising cost of healthcare, use of healthcare resources and the benefits they confer are likely to be given a much greater scrutiny in future in order to justify individual costs.

The rising cost of care may partly be due to an increase in the number of institutions offering specialized services, and MRI of all anatomic regions increased from 50% in 1998 to 58% in 2003 (160). Data also show that the cost of care has markedly increased for Medicare patients; for breast cancer patients specifically, there has been an annual increase in the total cost of care of 4.1%, but an annual increase in imaging costs of 9.9%. This has resulted in an overall rise in imaging costs as a percentage of total cost of care for the breast cancer patient, with a documented increase from 3.6% in 1999 to 5.0% in 2006 (161).

The reason for overall cost increases is undoubtedly multifactorial, but higher radiological costs are presumably due to greater utilization of various modalities of imaging, including breast MRI. In a recent series evaluating Surveillance, Epidemiology, and End Results (SEER)-Medicare data for 67,751 Medicare patients (10), a significant increase was noted in the number of days individual patients underwent mammograms, ultrasounds, and breast MRI in the preoperative period. This also included those patients, who were undergoing simultaneously more than one imaging type on any given day. This large increase in the volume of imaging per patient is strongly echoed by individual series where the percentages of patients receiving a breast MRI have shot up exponentially for those presenting with breast cancer (Table 20.6).

Rising imaging costs are not merely related to the cost of the test itself (which for MRI vs. mammogram has been estimated at $1038 vs. $86) but also to the issue of workflow resulting from this investigation. Were the costs simply due to a more expensive test, one solution might be to simply charge less for the test. Unfortunately, previously occult findings on breast MRI often require further evaluation with additional imaging and biopsy (see the section "Medicolegal Aspects"). Current standard workflow entails review of the MRI for new suspicious lesions not previously seen on mammography or ultrasound, and then performance of a targeted ultrasound (formerly known as a "second-look" ultrasound) to see whether the lesion can be visualized. If it is detected by ultrasound, an ultrasound-guided core biopsy is performed. However, these incidental lesions are only seen by a targeted ultrasound in 47% of cases, requiring a second MRI with an MRI-guided biopsy in 53% of cases to determine those 12% of foci that are malignant (40).

Callbacks and short-term follow-up studies for equivocal findings are required in nearly twice as many cases of MRI as mammography, even for women with a familial risk, where the likelihood of having a malignancy is elevated (162). In a modeling study of imaging costs, MRI was found to have 10 times the diagnostic cost after the initial MRI ($336) versus the diagnostic cost following mammographic screening ($28) (129). Prospective data further reinforce these cost concerns. In the COMICE trial, MRI did not save resources (including overall costs, cost of surgery, complications, hospital stay, follow-up, and other components), but insignificantly increased costs at £236.45 per patient (20).

Table 20.6 Institutional Series Noting Rates of Breast MRI Usage

Study	Institution	Cohort	n MRI	Overall MRI %	Periodic Proportion of Patients Having Breast MRI	
Solin, 2008 (8)	University of Pennsylvania, Philadelphia, Pennsylvania, USA	756	215	28.4	1992–1995	14%
					1996–1998	35%
					1999–2001	42%
Bleicher, 2009 (6)	Fox Chase Cancer Center, Philadelphia, Pennsylvania, USA	577	133	23.1	2004	13%
					2005	24%
					2006	27%
Katipamula, 2009 (7)	Mayo Clinic, Rochester, Minnesota, USA	5,405	337	15.7 (after 2002)	2002 or prior	0%
					2003	10%
					2004	12%
					2005	19%
					2006	23%
Hwang, 2009 (9)	Princess Margaret Hospital, Ontario, Canada	463	127	27.4	2000	1%
					2001	5%
					2002	16%
					2003	18%
					2004	41%
					2005	46%

A test such as MRI should not be discarded simply because it is costly. The value of MRI must be carefully assessed in a clinical scenario where demonstrable benefit is questionable. The resource implications are significant, especially when considered in aggregate for a population receiving healthcare.

Medicolegal Aspects

Another aspect related to MRI use in the perioperative period is the medicolegal pressures that can exist even when use of the study may not be indicated. Such pressure can come from the patient herself or from recommendations or documentation by another clinician. There is considerable enthusiasm for use of MRI both on the part of radiologists and also by physicians generally. In a web-based survey of the Society of Breast Imaging, 8.5% noted that MRI is frequently performed in their practice for an abnormal screening mammogram when no other workup has yet been attempted (39). In the same study, only 10.6% of radiologists felt that the requests they received for breast MRI were "always" appropriate. Meanwhile in a series of 577 patients referred to the multidisciplinary clinic of a comprehensive cancer center, among whom 130 underwent breast MRI, 30.8% of the MRI studies were ordered simply for "breast cancer," while 12.3% were performed for a yet-undiagnosed palpable abnormality prior to any biopsy, and 3.1% were performed for an abnormal mammogram. The general use of this modality has become widespread, perhaps in part due to breast radiologists having the perception that they are at risk from a lawsuit (163–165).

Delays

Several series have evaluated the timing of care and potential for delays related to requests for preoperative breast MRI and report waiting times of up to 19 days (6,25,164–166). Delay associated with MRI is consistent with findings from a series evaluating the number of imaging dates required in Medicare patients between 1992 and 2005 (10). Although multiple imaging modalities were noted to be increasingly consolidated for patients on one date and mammography accounted for 71.9% of dates where one imaging modality was done alone, MRI was the only imaging modality performed on a given day more than 90% of the time. These findings suggest that scheduling logistics for breast MRIs may contribute to the delays seen in these studies. In contrast, a study from Canada reported that the lengths of time between core biopsy result and surgery date were no different between those who underwent MRI as compared with those who did not (166); likewise, the time between the proposed surgery date and the executed surgery date was not significantly increased with breast MRI examination.

CONCLUSION

Breast MRI can be a valuable tool for clinicians, but has some associated disadvantages. There are several clinical scenarios where breast MRI is of benefit, such as for high risk screening and assessment, and in cases where other imaging information either conflicts or is insufficient. As there are high costs and other disadvantages associated with this modality, the use of breast MRI should be confined to those areas where a benefit has been consistently demonstrated in published literature. Conversely it should be used more judiciously where clear benefits are not evident.

REFERENCES

1. El Yousef SJ, Duchesneau RH. Magnetic resonance imaging of the human breast: a Phase I trial. Radiol Clin North Am 1984; 22: 859–68.
2. El Yousef SJ, Duchesneau RH, Alfidi RJ, et al. Magnetic resonance imaging of the breast. Work in progress. Radiology 1984; 150: 761–6.
3. Saslow D, Boetes C, Burke W, et al. American cancer society guidelines for breast screening with MRI as an adjunct to mammography. CA Cancer J Clin 2007; 57: 75–89.
4. Hede K. Preoperative MRI in breast cancer grows contentious. J Natl Cancer Inst 2009; 101: 1667–9.
5. Houssami N, Hayes DF. Review of preoperative magnetic resonance imaging (MRI) in breast cancer: should MRI be performed on all women with newly diagnosed, early stage breast cancer? CA Cancer J Clin 2009; 59: 290–302.

6. Bleicher RJ, Ciocca RM, Egleston BL, et al. Association of routine pretreatment magnetic resonance imaging with time to surgery, mastectomy rate, and margin status. J Am Coll Surg 2009; 209: 180–7; quiz 294-5.

7. Katipamula R, Degnim AC, Hoskin T, et al. Trends in mastectomy rates at the Mayo Clinic Rochester: effect of surgical year and preoperative magnetic resonance imaging. J Clin Oncol 2009; 27: 4082–8.

8. Solin LJ, Orel SG, Hwang WT, Harris EE, Schnall MD. Relationship of breast magnetic resonance imaging to outcome after breast-conservation treatment with radiation for women with early-stage invasive breast carcinoma or ductal carcinoma in situ. J Clin Oncol 2008; 26: 386–91.

9. Hwang N, Schiller DE, Crystal P, Maki E, McCready DR. Magnetic resonance imaging in the planning of initial lumpectomy for invasive breast carcinoma: its effect on ipsilateral breast tumor recurrence after breast-conservation therapy. Ann Surg Oncol 2009; 16: 3000–9.

10. Bleicher RJ, Ruth K, Sigurdson ER, et al. (In-)Efficiencies in the preoperative imaging evaluation of the medicare breast cancer patient. Cancer Res 2011; 71: 549s.

11. Hilleren DJ, Andersson IT, Lindholm K, Linnell FS. Invasive lobular carcinoma: mammographic findings in a 10-year experience. Radiology 1991; 178: 149–54.

12. Yeatman TJ, Cantor AB, Smith TJ, et al. Tumor biology of infiltrating lobular carcinoma. Implications for management. Ann Surg 1995; 222: 549–59; discussion 59-61.

13. ACR Practice Guideline for the Performance of Magnetic Resonance Imaging (MRI) of the Breast. 2004. [Available from: http://www.green-emedicalimaging.com/services/BreastMRI.htm].

14. Consensus Statement: The Use of Magnetic Resonance Imaging in Breast Oncology. Newsletter of the American Society of Breast Surgeons 2005;Winter: 7.

15. Fisher B, Bauer M, Margolese R, et al. Five-year results of a randomized clinical trial comparing total mastectomy and segmental mastectomy with or without radiation in the treatment of breast cancer. N Engl J Med 1985; 312: 665–73.

16. Blichert-Toft M, Rose C, Andersen JA, et al. Danish randomized trial comparing breast conservation therapy with mastectomy: six years of life-table analysis. Danish Breast Cancer Cooperative Group. J Natl Cancer Inst Monogr 1992: 19–25.

17. Pengel KE, Loo CE, Teertstra HJ, et al. The impact of preoperative MRI on breast-conserving surgery of invasive cancer: a comparative cohort study. Breast Cancer Res Treat 2009; 116: 161–9.

18. Itakura K, Lessing J, Sakata T, et al. The impact of preoperative magnetic resonance imaging on surgical treatment and outcomes for ductal carcinoma in situ. Clin Breast Cancer 2011; 11: 33–8.

19. Vanderwalde LH, Dang CM, Bresee C, Phillips EH. Discordance between pathologic and radiologic tumor size on breast MRI may contribute to increased re-excision rates. Am Surg 2011; 77: 1361–3.

20. Turnbull LW, Brown SR, Olivier C, et al. Multicentre randomised controlled trial examining the cost-effectiveness of contrast-enhanced high field magnetic resonance imaging in women with primary breast cancer scheduled for wide local excision (COMICE). Health Technol Assess 2010; 14: 1–182.

21. Peters NH, van Esser S, van den Bosch MA, et al. Preoperative MRI and surgical management in patients with nonpalpable breast cancer: the MONET - randomised controlled trial. Eur J Cancer 2011; 47: 879–86.

22. Bedrosian I, Mick R, Orel SG, et al. Changes in the surgical management of patients with breast carcinoma based on preoperative magnetic resonance imaging. Cancer 2003; 98: 468–73.

23. Berg WA, Gutierrez L, NessAiver MS, et al. Diagnostic accuracy of mammography, clinical examination, US, and MR imaging in preoperative assessment of breast cancer. Radiology 2004; 233: 830–49.

24. Bilimoria KY, Cambic A, Hansen NM, Bethke KP. Evaluating the impact of preoperative breast magnetic resonance imaging on the surgical management of newly diagnosed breast cancers. Arch Surg 2007; 142: 441–5; discussion 5–7.

25. Hulvat M, Sandalow N, Rademaker A, Helenowski I, Hansen NM. Time from diagnosis to definitive operative treatment of operable breast cancer in the era of multimodal imaging. Surgery 2010; 148: 746–51.

26. Turnbull L, Brown S, Harvey I, et al. Comparative effectiveness of MRI in breast cancer (COMICE) trial: a randomised controlled trial. Lancet 2010; 375: 563–71.

27. Wilkinson J, Appleton CM, Margenthaler JA. Utility of breast MRI for evaluation of residual disease following excisional biopsy. J Surg Res 2011; 170: 233–9.

28. Houssami N, Ciatto S, Macaskill P, et al. Accuracy and surgical impact of magnetic resonance imaging in breast cancer staging: systematic review and meta-analysis in detection of multifocal and multicentric cancer. J Clin Oncol 2008; 26: 3248–58.

29. Harms SE, Flamig DP, Hesley KL, et al. MR imaging of the breast with rotating delivery of excitation off resonance: clinical experience with pathologic correlation. Radiology 1993; 187: 493–501.

30. Fornasa F, Pinali L, Gasparini A, Toniolli E, Montemezzi S. Diffusion-weighted magnetic resonance imaging in focal breast lesions: analysis of 78 cases with pathological correlation. Radiol Med (Torino) 2011; 116: 264–75.

31. Kriege M, Brekelmans CT, Boetes C, et al. Efficacy of MRI and mammography for breast-cancer screening in women with a familial or genetic predisposition. N Engl J Med 2004; 351: 427–37.

32. Warner E, Plewes DB, Hill KA, et al. Surveillance of BRCA1 and BRCA2 mutation carriers with magnetic resonance imaging, ultrasound, mammography, and clinical breast examination. JAMA 2004; 292: 1317–25.

33. Leach MO, Boggis CR, Dixon AK, et al. Screening with magnetic resonance imaging and mammography of a UK population at high familial risk of breast cancer: a prospective multicentre cohort study (MARIBS). Lancet 2005; 365: 1769–78.

34. Kuhl CK, Schrading S, Leutner CC, et al. Mammography, breast ultrasound, and magnetic resonance imaging for surveillance of women at high familial risk for breast cancer. J Clin Oncol 2005; 23: 8469–76.

35. Early Breast Cancer Trialists' Collaborative Group. Darby S, McGale P, Correa C, et al. Effect of radiotherapy after breast-conserving surgery on 10-year recurrence and 15-year breast cancer death: meta-analysis of individual patient data for 10,801 women in 17 randomised trials. Lancet 2011; 378: 1707–16.

36. Kaas R, Kroger R, Peterse JL, Hart AA, Muller SH. The correlation of mammographic-and histologic patterns of breast cancers in BRCA1 gene mutation carriers, compared to age-matched sporadic controls. Eur Radiol 2006; 16: 2842–8.

37. Hamilton LJ, Evans AJ, Wilson AR, et al. Breast imaging findings in women with BRCA1- and BRCA2-associated breast carcinoma. Clin Radiol 2004; 59: 895–902.

38. Lehman CD, Gatsonis C, Kuhl CK, et al. MRI evaluation of the contralateral breast in women with recently diagnosed breast cancer. N Engl J Med 2007; 356: 1295–303.

39. Bassett LW, Dhaliwal SG, Eradat J, et al. National trends and practices in breast MRI. AJR Am J Roentgenol 2008; 191: 332–9.

40. Wiratkapun C, Duke D, Nordmann AS, et al. Indeterminate or suspicious breast lesions detected initially with MR imaging: value of MRI-directed breast ultrasound. Acad Radiol 2008; 15: 618–25.

41. Pettit K, Swatske ME, Gao F, et al. The impact of breast MRI on surgical decision-making: are patients at risk for mastectomy? J Surg Oncol 2009; 100: 553–8.

42. Bluemke DA, Gatsonis CA, Chen MH, et al. Magnetic resonance imaging of the breast prior to biopsy. JAMA 2004; 292: 2735–42.

43. Holland R, Veling SH, Mravunac M, Hendriks JH. Histologic multifocality of Tis, T1-2 breast carcinomas. Implications for clinical trials of breast-conserving surgery. Cancer 1985; 56: 979–90.

44. Fisher ER, Sass R, Fisher B, et al. Pathologic findings from the National Surgical Adjuvant Breast Project (protocol 6). II. Relation of local breast recurrence to multicentricity. Cancer 1986; 57: 1717–24.

45. Gump FE, Shikora S, Habif DV, et al. The extent and distribution of cancer in breasts with palpable primary tumors. Ann Surg 1986; 204: 384–90.

46. Sarnelli R, Squartini F. Multicentricity in breast cancer: a submacroscopic study. Pathol Annu 1986; 21: 143–58.

47. Clarke M, Collins R, Darby S, et al. Effects of radiotherapy and of differences in the extent of surgery for early breast cancer on local recurrence and 15-year survival: an overview of the randomised trials. Lancet 2005; 366: 2087–106.

48. Fisher B, Jeong JH, Anderson S, et al. Twenty-five-year follow-up of a randomized trial comparing radical mastectomy, total mastectomy,

and total mastectomy followed by irradiation. N Engl J Med 2002; 347: 567–75.

49. Whelan TJ, Pignol JP, Levine MN, et al. Long-term results of hypofractionated radiation therapy for breast cancer. N Engl J Med 2010; 362: 513–20.

50. Shaitelman SF, Vicini FA, Beitsch P, et al. Five-year outcome of patients classified using the American Society for Radiation Oncology consensus statement guidelines for the application of accelerated partial breast irradiation: an analysis of patients treated on the American Society of Breast Surgeons MammoSite Registry Trial. Cancer 2010; 116: 4677–85.

51. Beitsch P, Vicini F, Keisch M, et al. Five-year outcome of patients classified in the "unsuitable" category using the American Society of Therapeutic Radiology and Oncology (ASTRO) Consensus Panel guidelines for the application of accelerated partial breast irradiation: an analysis of patients treated on the American Society of Breast Surgeons MammoSite(R) Registry trial. Ann Surg Oncol 2010; 17: 219–25.

52. Polgar C, Van Limbergen E, Potter R, et al. Patient selection for accelerated partial-breast irradiation (APBI) after breast-conserving surgery: recommendations of the Groupe Europeen de Curietherapie-European Society for Therapeutic Radiology and Oncology (GEC-ESTRO) breast cancer working group based on clinical evidence (2009). Radiother Oncol 2010; 94: 264–73.

53. Vicini F, Arthur D, Wazer D, et al. Limitations of the American Society of Therapeutic Radiology and Oncology Consensus Panel guidelines on the use of accelerated partial breast irradiation. Int J Radiat Oncol Biol Phys 2011; 79: 977–84.

54. Kuhr M, Wolfgarten M, Stolze M, et al. Potential impact of preoperative magnetic resonance imaging of the breast on patient selection for accelerated partial breast irradiation. Int J Radiat Oncol Biol Phys 2011; 81: e541–6.

55. Mendelson EB, Harris KM, Doshi N, Tobon H. Infiltrating lobular carcinoma: mammographic patterns with pathologic correlation. AJR Am J Roentgenol 1989; 153: 265–71.

56. Schnitt SJ, Connolly JL, Recht A, Silver B, Harris JR. Influence of infiltrating lobular histology on local tumor control in breast cancer patients treated with conservative surgery and radiotherapy. Cancer 1989; 64: 448–54.

57. Weiss MC, Fowble BL, Solin LJ, Yeh IT, Schultz DJ. Outcome of conservative therapy for invasive breast cancer by histologic subtype. Int J Radiat Oncol Biol Phys 1992; 23: 941–7.

58. White JR, Gustafson GS, Wimbish K, et al. Conservative surgery and radiation therapy for infiltrating lobular carcinoma of the breast. The role of preoperative mammograms in guiding treatment. Cancer 1994; 74: 640–7.

59. Winchester DJ, Chang HR, Graves TA, et al. A comparative analysis of lobular and ductal carcinoma of the breast: presentation, treatment, and outcomes. J Am Coll Surg 1998; 186: 416–22.

60. Peiro G, Bornstein BA, Connolly JL, et al. The influence of infiltrating lobular carcinoma on the outcome of patients treated with breast-conserving surgery and radiation therapy. Breast Cancer Res Treat 2000; 59: 49–54.

61. Molland JG, Donnellan M, Janu NC, et al. Infiltrating lobular carcinoma—a comparison of diagnosis, management and outcome with infiltrating duct carcinoma. Breast 2004; 13: 389–96.

62. Santiago RJ, Harris EE, Qin L, Hwang WT, Solin LJ. Similar long-term results of breast-conservation treatment for Stage I and II invasive lobular carcinoma compared with invasive ductal carcinoma of the breast: the University of Pennsylvania experience. Cancer 2005; 103: 2447–54.

63. Fisher ER, Gregorio R, Redmond C, et al. Pathologic findings from the National Surgical Adjuvant Breast Project (protocol no. 4). I. Observations concerning the multicentricity of mammary cancer. Cancer 1975; 35: 247–54.

64. Mann RM, Kuhl CK, Kinkel K, Boetes C. Breast MRI: guidelines from the European society of breast imaging. Eur Radiol 2008; 18: 1307–18.

65. Knopp MV, Weiss E, Sinn HP, et al. Pathophysiologic basis of contrast enhancement in breast tumors. J Magn Reson Imaging 1999; 10: 260–6.

66. Yeh ED, Slanetz PJ, Edmister WB, et al. Invasive lobular carcinoma: spectrum of enhancement and morphology on magnetic resonance imaging. Breast J 2003; 9: 13–18.

67. Kusama R, Takayama F, Tsuchiya S. MRI of the breast: comparison of MRI signals and histological characteristics of the same slices. Med Mol Morphol 2005; 38: 204–15.

68. Leinsinger G, Schlossbauer T, Scherr M, et al. Cluster analysis of signal-intensity time course in dynamic breast MRI: does unsupervised vector quantization help to evaluate small mammographic lesions? Eur Radiol 2006; 16: 1138–46.

69. Mann RM, Veltman J, Huisman H, Boetes C. Comparison of enhancement characteristics between invasive lobular carcinoma and invasive ductal carcinoma. J Magn Reson Imaging 2011; 34: 293–300.

70. Kim SH, Cha ES, Park CS, et al. Imaging features of invasive lobular carcinoma: comparison with invasive ductal carcinoma. Jpn J Radiol 2011; 29: 475–82.

71. Munot K, Dall B, Achuthan R, et al. Role of magnetic resonance imaging in the diagnosis and single-stage surgical resection of invasive lobular carcinoma of the breast. Br J Surg 2002; 89: 1296–301.

72. Boetes C, Veltman J, van Die L, et al. The role of MRI in invasive lobular carcinoma. Breast Cancer Res Treat 2004; 86: 31–7.

73. Caramella T, Chapellier C, Ettore F, et al. Value of MRI in the surgical planning of invasive lobular breast carcinoma: a prospective and a retrospective study of 57 cases: comparison with physical examination, conventional imaging, and histology. Clin Imaging 2007; 31: 155–61.

74. Amano G, Ohuchi N, Ishibashi T, et al. Correlation of three-dimensional magnetic resonance imaging with precise histopathological map concerning carcinoma extension in the breast. Breast Cancer Res Treat 2000; 60: 43–55.

75. Mann RM, Hoogeveen YL, Blickman JG, Boetes C. MRI compared to conventional diagnostic work-up in the detection and evaluation of invasive lobular carcinoma of the breast: a review of existing literature. Breast Cancer Res Treat 2008; 107: 1–14.

76. Onesti JK, Mangus BE, Helmer SD, Osland JS. Breast cancer tumor size: correlation between magnetic resonance imaging and pathology measurements. Am J Surg 2008; 196: 844–8; discussion 9-50.

77. McGhan LJ, Wasif N, Gray RJ, et al. Use of preoperative magnetic resonance imaging for invasive lobular cancer: good, better, but maybe not the best? Ann Surg Oncol 2010; 17: 255–62.

78. Teller P, Jefford VJ, Gabram SG, Newell M, Carlson GW. The utility of breast MRI in the management of breast cancer. Breast J 2010; 16: 394–403.

79. Lau B, Romero LM. Does preoperative magnetic resonance imaging beneficially alter surgical management of invasive lobular carcinoma? Am Surg 2011; 77: 1368–71.

80. Heil J, Buhler A, Golatta M, et al. Does a supplementary preoperative breast MRI in patients with invasive lobular breast cancer change primary and secondary surgical interventions? Ann Surg Oncol 2011; 18: 2143–9.

81. Mann RM, Loo CE, Wobbes T, et al. The impact of preoperative breast MRI on the re-excision rate in invasive lobular carcinoma of the breast. Breast Cancer Res Treat 2010; 119: 415–22.

82. Fischer U, Zachariae O, Baum F, et al. The influence of preoperative MRI of the breasts on recurrence rate in patients with breast cancer. Eur Radiol 2004; 14: 1725–31.

83. Berry DA, Cronin KA, Plevritis SK, et al. Effect of screening and adjuvant therapy on mortality from breast cancer. N Engl J Med 2005; 353: 1784–92.

84. Gotzsche PC, Nielsen M. Screening for breast cancer with mammography. Cochrane Database Syst Rev 2006; CD001877.

85. Houssami N, Ciatto S, Martinelli F, Bonardi R, Duffy SW. Early detection of second breast cancers improves prognosis in breast cancer survivors. Ann Oncol 2009; 20: 1505–10.

86. Brennan ME, Houssami N, Lord S, et al. Magnetic resonance imaging screening of the contralateral breast in women with newly diagnosed breast cancer: systematic review and meta-analysis of incremental cancer detection and impact on surgical management. J Clin Oncol 2009; 27: 5640–9.

87. Rutqvist LE, Cedermark B, Glas U, et al. Contralateral primary tumors in breast cancer patients in a randomized trial of adjuvant tamoxifen therapy. J Natl Cancer Inst 1991; 83: 1299–306.

88. Gao X, Fisher SG, Emami B. Risk of second primary cancer in the contralateral breast in women treated for early-stage breast cancer: a population-based study. Int J Radiat Oncol Biol Phys 2003; 56: 1038–45.

89. Schaapveld M, Visser O, Louwman WJ, et al. The impact of adjuvant therapy on contralateral breast cancer risk and the prognostic significance of contralateral breast cancer: a population based study in the Netherlands. Breast Cancer Res Treat 2008; 110: 189–97.

90. Montgomery DA, Krupa K, Jack WJ, et al. Changing pattern of the detection of locoregional relapse in breast cancer: the Edinburgh experience. Br J Cancer 2007; 96: 1802–7.

91. Bernstein JL, Lapinski RH, Thakore SS, Doucette JT, Thompson WD. The descriptive epidemiology of second primary breast cancer. Epidemiology 2003; 14: 552–8.

92. Nichols HB, Berrington de Gonzalez A, Lacey JV Jr, Rosenberg PS, Anderson WF. Declining incidence of contralateral breast cancer in the United States from 1975 to 2006. J Clin Oncol 2011; 29: 1564–9.

93. Kurian AW, McClure LA, John EM, et al. Second primary breast cancer occurrence according to hormone receptor status. J Natl Cancer Inst 2009; 101: 1058–65.

94. Interim analysis at four years by Nolvadex Adjuvant Trial Organisation. Controlled trial of tamoxifen as adjuvant agent in management of early breast cancer. Lancet 1983; 1: 257–61.

95. Howell A, Cuzick J, Baum M, et al. Results of the ATAC (Arimidex, Tamoxifen, Alone or in Combination) trial after completion of 5 years' adjuvant treatment for breast cancer. Lancet 2005; 365: 60–2.

96. Bonadonna G, Valagussa P, Moliterni A, Zambetti M, Brambilla C. Adjuvant cyclophosphamide, methotrexate, and fluorouracil in node-positive breast cancer: the results of 20 years of follow-up. N Engl J Med 1995; 332: 901–6.

97. Romond EH, Perez EA, Bryant J, et al. Trastuzumab plus adjuvant chemotherapy for operable HER2-positive breast cancer. N Engl J Med 2005; 353: 1673–84.

98. Ellerbroek N, Holmes F, Singletary E, et al. Treatment of patients with isolated axillary nodal metastases from an occult primary carcinoma consistent with breast origin. Cancer 1990; 66: 1461–7.

99. Kemeny MM, Rivera DE, Terz JJ, Benfield JR. Occult primary adenocarcinoma with axillary metastases. Am J Surg 1986; 152: 43–7.

100. Patel J, Nemoto T, Rosner D, Dao TL, Pickren JW. Axillary lymph node metastasis from an occult breast cancer. Cancer 1981; 47: 2923–7.

101. Ashikari R, Rosen PP, Urban JA, Senoo T. Breast cancer presenting as an axillary mass. Ann Surg 1976; 183: 415–17.

102. Barton SR, Smith IE, Kirby AM, et al. The role of ipsilateral breast radiotherapy in management of occult primary breast cancer presenting as axillary lymphadenopathy. Eur J Cancer 2011; 47: 2099–106.

103. Walker GV, Smith GL, Perkins GH, et al. Population-based analysis of occult primary breast cancer with axillary lymph node metastasis. Cancer 2010; 116: 4000–6.

104. Fourquet A, Kirova YM, Campana F. Occult primary cancer with axillary metastases. In: Harris JR, Lippman ME, Morrow M, Osborne CK, eds. Diseases of the Breast, 4th edn. Philadelphia: Lippincott Williams & Wilkins, 2009: 817–21.

105. Yang TJ, Yang Q, Haffty BG, Moran MS. Prognosis for mammographically occult, early-stage breast cancer patients treated with breast-conservation therapy. Int J Radiat Oncol Biol Phys 2010; 76: 79–84.

106. Jamali FR, Ricci A Jr, Deckers PJ. Paget's disease of the nipple-areola complex. Surg Clin North Am 1996; 76: 365–81.

107. Paone JF, Baker RR. Pathogenesis and treatment of Paget's disease of the breast. Cancer 1981; 48: 825–9.

108. Ikeda DM, Helvie MA, Frank TS, Chapel KL, Andersson IT. Paget disease of the nipple: radiologic-pathologic correlation. Radiology 1993; 189: 89–94.

109. Siponen E, Hukkinen K, Heikkila P, Joensuu H, Leidenius M. Surgical treatment in Paget's disease of the breast. Am J Surg 2010; 200: 241–6.

110. Sawyer RH, Asbury DL. Mammographic appearances in Paget's disease of the breast. Clin Radiol 1994; 49: 185–8.

111. Fu W, Mittel VK, Young SC. Paget disease of the breast: analysis of 41 patients. Am J Clin Oncol 2001; 24: 397–400.

112. Echevarria JJ, Lopez-Ruiz JA, Martin D, Imaz I, Martin M. Usefulness of MRI in detecting occult breast cancer associated with Paget's disease of the nipple-areolar complex. Br J Radiol 2004; 77: 1036–9.

113. Bijker N, Rutgers EJ, Duchateau L, et al. Breast-conserving therapy for Paget disease of the nipple: a prospective European Organization for Research and Treatment of Cancer study of 61 patients. Cancer 2001; 91: 472–7.

114. Fisher B, Brown A, Mamounas E, et al. Effect of preoperative chemotherapy on local-regional disease in women with operable breast cancer: findings from National Surgical Adjuvant Breast and Bowel Project B-18. J Clin Oncol 1997; 15: 2483–93.

115. Bear HD, Anderson S, Brown A, et al. The effect on tumor response of adding sequential preoperative docetaxel to preoperative doxorubicin and cyclophosphamide: preliminary results from National Surgical Adjuvant Breast and Bowel Project Protocol B-27. J Clin Oncol 2003; 21: 4165–74.

116. Bear HD, Anderson S, Smith RE, et al. Sequential preoperative or postoperative docetaxel added to preoperative doxorubicin plus cyclophosphamide for operable breast cancer: National Surgical Adjuvant Breast and Bowel Project Protocol B-27. J Clin Oncol 2006; 24: 2019–27.

117. Rastogi P, Anderson SJ, Bear HD, et al. Preoperative chemotherapy: updates of National Surgical Adjuvant Breast and Bowel Project Protocols B-18 and B-27. J Clin Oncol 2008; 26: 778–85.

118. McGuire KP, Toro-Burguete J, Dang H, et al. MRI staging after neoadjuvant chemotherapy for breast cancer: does tumor biology affect accuracy? Ann Surg Oncol 2011; 18: 3149–54.

119. De Los Santos J, Bernreuter W, Keene K, et al. Accuracy of breast magnetic resonance imaging in predicting pathologic response in patients treated with neoadjuvant chemotherapy. Clin Breast Cancer 2011; 11: 312–19.

120. Denis F, Desbiez-Bourcier AV, Chapiron C, et al. Contrast enhanced magnetic resonance imaging underestimates residual disease following neoadjuvant docetaxel based chemotherapy for breast cancer. Eur J Surg Oncol 2004; 30: 1069–76.

121. Guarneri V, Pecchi A, Piacentini F, et al. Magnetic resonance imaging and ultrasonography in predicting infiltrating residual disease after preoperative chemotherapy in stage II-III breast cancer. Ann Surg Oncol 2011; 18: 2150–7.

122. Garimella V, Qutob O, Fox JN, et al. Recurrence rates after DCE-MRI image guided planning for breast-conserving surgery following neoadjuvant chemotherapy for locally advanced breast cancer patients. Eur J Surg Oncol 2007; 33: 157–61.

123. Lehman CD, Blume JD, Weatherall P, et al. Screening women at high risk for breast cancer with mammography and magnetic resonance imaging. Cancer 2005; 103: 1898–905.

124. Tilanus-Linthorst MM, Obdeijn IM, Hop WC, et al. BRCA1 mutation and young age predict fast breast cancer growth in the Dutch, United Kingdom, and Canadian magnetic resonance imaging screening trials. Clin Cancer Res 2007; 13: 7357–62.

125. Brekelmans CT, Tilanus-Linthorst MM, Seynaeve C, et al. Tumour characteristics, survival and prognostic factors of hereditary breast cancer from BRCA2-, BRCA1- and non-BRCA1/2 families as compared to sporadic breast cancer cases. Eur J Cancer 2007; 43: 867–76.

126. Lakhani SR, Reis-Filho JS, Fulford L, et al. Prediction of BRCA1 status in patients with breast cancer using estrogen receptor and basal phenotype. Clin Cancer Res 2005; 11: 5175–80.

127. Lakhani SR, Jacquemier J, Sloane JP, et al. Multifactorial analysis of differences between sporadic breast cancers and cancers involving BRCA1 and BRCA2 mutations. J Natl Cancer Inst 1998; 90: 1138–45.

128. Rijnsburger AJ, Obdeijn IM, Kaas R, et al. BRCA1-associated breast cancers present differently from BRCA2-associated and familial cases: long-term follow-up of the Dutch MRISC Screening Study. J Clin Oncol 2010; 28: 5265–73.

129. Plevritis SK, Kurian AW, Sigal BM, et al. Cost-effectiveness of screening BRCA1/2 mutation carriers with breast magnetic resonance imaging. JAMA 2006; 295: 2374–84.

130. Griebsch I, Brown J, Boggis C, et al. Cost-effectiveness of screening with contrast enhanced magnetic resonance imaging vs X-ray mammography of women at a high familial risk of breast cancer. Br J Cancer 2006; 95: 801–10.

131. Metcalfe K, Gershman S, Lynch HT, et al. Predictors of contralateral breast cancer in BRCA1 and BRCA2 mutation carriers. Br J Cancer 2011; 104: 1384–92.

132. Rogozinska-Szczepka J, Utracka-Hutka B, Grzybowska E, et al. BRCA1 and BRCA2 mutations as prognostic factors in bilateral breast cancer patients. Ann Oncol 2004; 15: 1373–6.

133. Kim JA, Son EJ, Kim EK, et al. Postexcisional breast magnetic resonance imaging in patients with breast cancer: predictable findings of residual cancer. J Comput Assist Tomogr 2009; 33: 940–5.

134. Sinha S, Sinha U. Functional magnetic resonance of human breast tumors: diffusion and perfusion imaging. Ann NY Acad Sci 2002; 980: 95–115.

135. Lee JM, Orel SG, Czerniecki BJ, Solin LJ, Schnall MD. MRI before reexcision surgery in patients with breast cancer. AJR Am J Roentgenol 2004; 182: 473–80.

136. Warren R, Hayes C, Pointon L, et al. A test of performance of breast MRI interpretation in a multicentre screening study. Magn Reson Imaging 2006; 24: 917–29.

137. Kinkel K, Hylton NM. Challenges to interpretation of breast MRI. J Magn Reson Imaging 2001; 13: 821–9.

138. Hollingsworth AB, Stough RG, O'Dell CA, Brekke CE. Breast magnetic resonance imaging for preoperative locoregional staging. Am J Surg 2008; 196: 389–97.

139. van Wingerden JJ, van Staden MM. Ultrasound mammography in prosthesis-related breast augmentation complications. Ann Plast Surg 1989; 22: 32–5.

140. Steinbach BG, Hiskes SK 2nd, Fitzsimmons JR, Lanier L. Phantom evaluation of imaging modalities for silicone breast implants. Invest Radiol 1992; 27: 841–6.

141. Brem RF, Tempany CM, Zerhouni EA. MR detection of breast implant rupture. J Comput Assist Tomogr 1992; 16: 157–9.

142. Gorczyca DP, Sinha S, Ahn CY, et al. Silicone breast implants in vivo: MR imaging. Radiology 1992; 185: 407–10.

143. Gorczyca DP, DeBruhl ND, Ahn CY, et al. Silicone breast implant ruptures in an animal model: comparison of mammography, MR imaging, US, and CT. Radiology 1994; 190: 227–32.

144. Berg WA, Caskey CI, Hamper UM, et al. Diagnosing breast implant rupture with MR imaging, US, and mammography. Radiographics 1993; 13: 1323–36.

145. Di Benedetto G, Cecchini S, Grassetti L, et al. Comparative study of breast implant rupture using mammography, sonography, and magnetic resonance imaging: correlation with surgical findings. Breast J 2008; 14: 532–7.

146. Grubstein A, Cohen M, Steinmetz A, Cohen D. Siliconomas mimicking cancer. Clin Imaging 2011; 35: 228–31.

147. Holmich LR, Fryzek JP, Kjoller K, et al. The diagnosis of silicone breast-implant rupture: clinical findings compared with findings at magnetic resonance imaging. Ann Plast Surg 2005; 54: 583–9.

148. Gorczyca DP, DeBruhl ND, Mund DF, Bassett LW. Linguine sign at MR imaging: does it represent the collapsed silicone implant shell? Radiology 1994; 191: 576–7.

149. Tark KC, Jeong HS, Roh TS, Choi JW. Analysis of 30 breast implant rupture cases. Aesthetic Plast Surg 2005; 29: 460–9; discussion 70-1.

150. Belli P, Costantini M, Romani M, Marano P, Pastore G. Magnetic resonance imaging in breast cancer recurrence. Breast Cancer Res Treat 2002; 73: 223–35.

151. Robertson C, Ragupathy SK, Boachie C, et al. Surveillance mammography for detecting ipsilateral breast tumour recurrence and metachronous contralateral breast cancer: a systematic review. Eur Radiol 2011; 21: 2484–91.

152. Weinstein SP, Orel SG, Pinnamaneni N, et al. Mammographic appearance of recurrent breast cancer after breast conservation therapy. Acad Radiol 2008; 15: 240–4.

153. Li J, Dershaw DD, Lee CH, Joo S, Morris EA. Breast MRI after conservation therapy: usual findings in routine follow-up examinations. AJR Am J Roentgenol 2010; 195: 799–807.

154. Peng C, Chang CB, Tso HH, et al. MRI appearance of tumor recurrence in myocutaneous flap reconstruction after mastectomy. AJR Am J Roentgenol 2011; 196: W471–5.

155. Shaikh N, LaTrenta G, Swistel A, Osborne FM. Detection of recurrent breast cancer after TRAM flap reconstruction. Ann Plast Surg 2001; 47: 602–7.

156. Punglia RS, Hassett MJ. Using lifetime risk estimates to recommend magnetic resonance imaging screening for breast cancer survivors. J Clin Oncol 2010; 28: 4108–10.

157. Patt A, Li T, Cristofanilli M, et al. Clinical significance of time to relapse and the distinction between breast cancer recurrences and new primary tumors. J Clin Oncol 2011; 29: 97s.

158. Zendejas B, Moriarty JP, O'Byrne J, et al. Cost-effectiveness of contralateral prophylactic mastectomy versus routine surveillance in patients with unilateral breast cancer. J Clin Oncol 2011; 29: 2993–3000.

159. Fisher ES, Bynum JP, Skinner JS. Slowing the growth of health care costs–lessons from regional variation. N Engl J Med 2009; 360: 849–52.

160. Medicare Payment Advisory Commission (U.S.). Report to the Congress, Medicare Payment Policy. Washington, D.C: Medicare Payment Advisory Commission, 2006: 261.

161. Dinan MA, Curtis LH, Hammill BG, et al. Changes in the use and costs of diagnostic imaging among Medicare beneficiaries with cancer, 1999–2006. JAMA 2010; 303: 1625–31.

162. Kuhl C, Weigel S, Schrading S, et al. Prospective multicenter cohort study to refine management recommendations for women at elevated familial risk of breast cancer: the EVA trial. J Clin Oncol 2010; 28: 1450–7.

163. Dick JF 3rd, Gallagher TH, Brenner RJ, et al. Predictors of radiologists' perceived risk of malpractice lawsuits in breast imaging. AJR Am J Roentgenol 2009; 192: 327–33.

164. Krishnan M, Thorsteinsson D, Horowitz N, et al. The influence of preoperative MRI in the timing and type of therapy in women newly diagnosed with breast cancer. AJR Am J Roentgenol 2008; 190: A31–4.

165. Landercasper J, Linebarger JH, Ellis RL, et al. A quality review of the timeliness of breast cancer diagnosis and treatment in an integrated breast center. J Am Coll Surg 2010; 210: 449–55.

166. Angarita FA, Acuna SA, Fonseca A, Crystal P, Escallon J. Impact of preoperative breast MRIs on timing of surgery and type of intervention in newly diagnosed breast cancer patients. Ann Surg Oncol 2010; 17: 273–9.

167. Davis PL, Staiger MJ, Harris KB, et al. Breast cancer measurements with magnetic resonance imaging, ultrasonography, and mammography. Breast Cancer Res Treat 1996; 37: 1–9.

168. Mumtaz H, Hall-Craggs MA, Davidson T, et al. Staging of symptomatic primary breast cancer with MR imaging. AJR Am J Roentgenol 1997; 169: 417–24.

169. Bazzocchi M, Zuiani C, Panizza P, et al. Contrast-enhanced breast MRI in patients with suspicious microcalcifications on mammography: results of a multicenter trial. AJR Am J Roentgenol 2006; 186: 1723–32.

170. Schouten van der Velden AP, Boetes C, Bult P, Wobbes T. The value of magnetic resonance imaging in diagnosis and size assessment of in situ and small invasive breast carcinoma. Am J Surg 2006; 192: 172–8.

171. Kim do Y, Moon WK, Cho N, et al. MRI of the breast for the detection and assessment of the size of ductal carcinoma in situ. Korean J Radiol 2007; 8: 32–9.

172. Behjatnia B, Sim J, Bassett LW, Moatamed NA, Apple SK. Does size matter? Comparison study between MRI, gross, and microscopic tumor sizes in breast cancer in lumpectomy specimens. Int J Clin Exp Pathol 2010; 3: 303–9.

173. Lee CH, Dershaw DD, Kopans D, et al. Breast cancer screening with imaging: recommendations from the Society of Breast Imaging and the ACR on the use of mammography, breast MRI, breast ultrasound, and other technologies for the detection of clinically occult breast cancer. J Am Coll Radiol 2010; 7: 18–27.

174. Morris EA, Schwartz LH, Dershaw DD, et al. MR imaging of the breast in patients with occult primary breast carcinoma. Radiology 1997; 205: 437–40.

175. Tilanus-Linthorst MM, Obdeijn AI, Bontenbal M, Oudkerk M. MRI in patients with axillary metastases of occult breast carcinoma. Breast Cancer Res Treat 1997; 44: 179–82.

176. Henry-Tillman RS, Harms SE, Westbrook KC, Korourian S, Klimberg VS. Role of breast magnetic resonance imaging in determining breast as a source of unknown metastatic lymphadenopathy. Am J Surg 1999; 178: 496–500.

177. Orel SG, Weinstein SP, Schnall MD, et al. Breast MR imaging in patients with axillary node metastases and unknown primary malignancy. Radiology 1999; 212: 543–9.

178. Stomper PC, Waddell BE, Edge SB, Klippenstein DL. Breast MRI in the evaluation of patients with occult primary breast carcinoma. Breast J 1999; 5: 230–4.

179. Olson JA Jr, Morris EA, Van Zee KJ, Linehan DC, Borgen PI. Magnetic resonance imaging facilitates breast conservation for occult breast cancer. Ann Surg Oncol 2000; 7: 411–15.

180. Obdeijn IM, Brouwers-Kuyper EM, Tilanus-Linthorst MM, Wiggers T, Oudkerk M. MR imaging-guided sonography followed by fine-needle aspiration cytology in occult carcinoma of the breast. AJR Am J Roentgenol 2000; 174: 1079–84.

181. Chen C, Orel SG, Schnall MD, Harris E, Solin LJ. Breast conservation treatment for patients presenting with axillary lymphadenopathy from presumed primary breast cancer: the role of breast magnetic resonance imaging for staging. Clin Breast Cancer 2002; 3: 219–22.

182. McMahon K, Medoro L, Kennedy D. Breast magnetic resonance imaging: an essential role in malignant axillary lymphadenopathy of unknown origin. Australas Radiol 2005; 49: 382–9.

183. Buchanan CL, Morris EA, Dorn PL, Borgen PI, Van Zee KJ. Utility of breast magnetic resonance imaging in patients with occult primary breast cancer. Ann Surg Oncol 2005; 12: 1045–53.

184. Ko EY, Han BK, Shin JH, Kang SS. Breast MRI for evaluating patients with metastatic axillary lymph node and initially negative mammography and sonography. Korean J Radiol 2007; 8: 382–9.

185. Morrogh M, Morris EA, Liberman L, et al. MRI identifies otherwise occult disease in select patients with Paget disease of the nipple. J Am Coll Surg 2008; 206: 316–21.

186. Kim HS, Seok JH, Cha ES, et al. Significance of nipple enhancement of Paget's disease in contrast enhanced breast MRI. Arch Gynecol Obstet 2010; 282: 157–62.

187. Schilling K, Narayanan D, Kalinyak JE, et al. Positron emission mammography in breast cancer presurgical planning: comparisons with magnetic resonance imaging. Eur J Nucl Med Mol Imaging 2011; 38: 23–36.

188. Gilles R, Guinebretiere JM, Toussaint C, et al. Locally advanced breast cancer: contrast-enhanced subtraction MR imaging of response to preoperative chemotherapy. Radiology 1994; 191: 633–8.

189. Abraham DC, Jones RC, Jones SE, et al. Evaluation of neoadjuvant chemotherapeutic response of locally advanced breast cancer by magnetic resonance imaging. Cancer 1996; 78: 91–100.

190. Drew PJ, Kerin MJ, Mahapatra T, et al. Evaluation of response to neoadjuvant chemoradiotherapy for locally advanced breast cancer with dynamic contrast-enhanced MRI of the breast. Eur J Surg Oncol 2001; 27: 617–20.

191. Esserman L, Kaplan E, Partridge S, et al. MRI phenotype is associated with response to doxorubicin and cyclophosphamide neoadjuvant chemotherapy in stage III breast cancer. Ann Surg Oncol 2001; 8: 549–59.

192. Weatherall PT, Evans GF, Metzger GJ, Saborrian MH, Leitch AM. MRI vs. histologic measurement of breast cancer following chemotherapy: comparison with x-ray mammography and palpation. J Magn Reson Imaging 2001; 13: 868–75.

193. Partridge SC, Gibbs JE, Lu Y, et al. Accuracy of MR imaging for revealing residual breast cancer in patients who have undergone neoadjuvant chemotherapy. AJR Am J Roentgenol 2002; 179: 1193–9.

194. Balu-Maestro C, Chapellier C, Bleuse A, et al. Imaging in evaluation of response to neoadjuvant breast cancer treatment benefits of MRI. Breast Cancer Res Treat 2002; 72: 145–52.

195. Cheung YC, Chen SC, Su MY, et al. Monitoring the size and response of locally advanced breast cancers to neoadjuvant chemotherapy (weekly paclitaxel and epirubicin) with serial enhanced MRI. Breast Cancer Res Treat 2003; 78: 51–8.

196. Rosen EL, Blackwell KL, Baker JA, et al. Accuracy of MRI in the detection of residual breast cancer after neoadjuvant chemotherapy. AJR Am J Roentgenol 2003; 181: 1275–82.

197. Wasser K, Sinn HP, Fink C, et al. Accuracy of tumor size measurement in breast cancer using MRI is influenced by histological regression induced by neoadjuvant chemotherapy. Eur Radiol 2003; 13: 1213–23.

198. Martincich L, Montemurro F, De Rosa G, et al. Monitoring response to primary chemotherapy in breast cancer using dynamic contrast-enhanced magnetic resonance imaging. Breast Cancer Res Treat 2004; 83: 67–76.

199. Londero V, Bazzocchi M, Del Frate C, et al. Locally advanced breast cancer: comparison of mammography, sonography and MR imaging in evaluation of residual disease in women receiving neoadjuvant chemotherapy. Eur Radiol 2004; 14: 1371–9.

200. Schott AF, Roubidoux MA, Helvie MA, et al. Clinical and radiologic assessments to predict breast cancer pathologic complete response to neoadjuvant chemotherapy. Breast Cancer Res Treat 2005; 92: 231–8.

201. Belli P, Costantini M, Malaspina C, et al. MRI accuracy in residual disease evaluation in breast cancer patients treated with neoadjuvant chemotherapy. Clin Radiol 2006; 61: 946–53.

202. Kim HJ, Im YH, Han BK, et al. Accuracy of MRI for estimating residual tumor size after neoadjuvant chemotherapy in locally advanced breast cancer: relation to response patterns on MRI. Acta Oncol 2007; 46: 996–1003.

203. Segara D, Krop IE, Garber JE, et al. Does MRI predict pathologic tumor response in women with breast cancer undergoing preoperative chemotherapy? J Surg Oncol 2007; 96: 474–80.

204. Yu HJ, Chen JH, Mehta RS, Nalcioglu O, Su MY. MRI measurements of tumor size and pharmacokinetic parameters as early predictors of response in breast cancer patients undergoing neoadjuvant anthracycline chemotherapy. J Magn Reson Imaging 2007; 26: 615–23.

205. Straver ME, Loo CE, Rutgers EJ, et al. MRI-model to guide the surgical treatment in breast cancer patients after neoadjuvant chemotherapy. Ann Surg 2010; 251: 701–7.

206. Croshaw R, Shapiro-Wright H, Svensson E, Erb K, Julian T. Accuracy of clinical examination, digital mammogram, ultrasound, and MRI in determining postneoadjuvant pathologic tumor response in operable breast cancer patients. Ann Surg Oncol 2011; 18: 3160–3.

207. Loo CE, Straver ME, Rodenhuis S, et al. Magnetic resonance imaging response monitoring of breast cancer during neoadjuvant chemotherapy: relevance of breast cancer subtype. J Clin Oncol 2011; 29: 660–6.

21 PET scanning and breast cancer management

Rebecca Wight and Patrick Borgen

INTRODUCTION

Positron emission tomography with ^{18}F-fluorodeoxyglucose (FDG-PET) has become a widely accepted imaging tool in oncology. Although this technology is not routinely used in breast cancer management, there is a large body of research examining its utility in breast cancer screening, diagnosis, preoperative evaluation, and monitoring of recurrence and response to chemotherapy (1–4). The advantage of FDG-PET over conventional imaging modalities, such as mammography, ultrasonography, computer tomography (CT), and magnetic resonance imaging (MRI), is its ability to provide functional tumor information. The technology exploits the "Warburg effect" first described by Warburg et al. in the 1920s, in that tumor cells have a higher metabolic rate than normal tissue with higher glucose avidity and increased glucose utilization (5).

The most commonly used radiotracer in PET technology, ^{18}F-fluorodeoxyglucose (FDG), is a glucose analog which is taken up by cells following the same initial metabolic pathway as glucose. After phosphorylation, given the lack of an oxygen atom at its C-2 position, the tracer molecule is unable to undergo further catabolism, thereby allowing accumulation of FDG within the cell. A subsequent decay of radioisotope occurs, during which positrons travel approximately 1 mm and collide with electrons in an annihilation reaction which produces two high-energy photons. These photons are emitted in opposite directions and can be detected during the whole-body scanning process as 3-D images representing the distribution of the radiotracer (6,7). Images also denote the intensity of FDG uptake and are reported as a standardized uptake value (SUV) representing metabolic data corresponding to both local and regional disease. Combining this process with CT (Fig. 21.1) allows correlation with anatomical data and increased accuracy of tumor detection. Indeed many studies have shown the combination of both the PET and CT modalities to have a higher sensitivity and specificity than either modality alone (4,8,9). In breast cancer management FDG-PET can be used in initial staging, follow-up staging, assessment of locoregional disease, and response to therapy.

INITIAL STAGING

Controversy exists with regards to the use of FDG-PET imaging for detection of systemic diseases and postoperative surveillance of primary operable breast cancer (Fig. 21.2). As per the American Society of Clinical Oncology (ASCO) 2006 guidelines, regularly performed history and physical examination, self breast examinations and mammography are recommended for routine breast cancer surveillance while PET scanning is discouraged (10). For the initial detection and diagnosis of primary lesions, studies have shown the utility of FDG-PET to be variable, largely due to the heterogeneity of the disease and variations in tumor size (11). PET is often unable to detect small (<10 mm) or low-grade lesions and it has consistently demonstrated a low sensitivity for the detection of axillary disease in cases of limited spread (12). Despite the ability of FDG-PET scanning to reliably detect recurrent and metastatic disease with fairly high sensitivity and specificity, many studies evaluated by the ASCO panel have shown no correlation between "early" diagnosis of stage IV disease and improved outcomes such as increased survival, better quality of life, or cost effectiveness. Additionally, PET has the propensity to produce false-positive results leading to a higher incidence of invasive procedures, such as ultrasound-guided biopsy and needle localization excisional biopsies, with their associated risk of complications. Additionally, the high cost of performing and interpreting the test has limited its use in screening and the routine evaluation of suspected breast cancer.

However, consideration may be given to applying this technology in subsets of high-risk patients in whom the results could substantially change the clinical management. This has been examined by Seagert et al. who suggested that some stage IIb and III breast cancer patients may have preclinical metastatic disease despite a normal conventional workup (13). In this retrospective study of 70 patients, seven (10%) were found to be in this group causing tumor staging to be changed from M0 to M1 with a shift from adjuvant to palliative therapy.

Additionally, a prospective analysis by Heudel et al. involving 45 women with biopsy-proven breast cancer showed that FDG-PET/CT played an important role in the preoperative staging of patients with triple-negative breast tumors (ER-PR-HER2) (14). Basu et al. reported that triple negative disease was correlated with a higher SUV_{max} on PET/CT regardless of the tumor size (15). These studies also demonstrated an increased uptake in primary lesions with a higher histological grade. Given that patients who present with triple-negative or high-grade breast lesions tend to have a worse prognosis, it is reasonable to consider histopathological and immunohistochemical analysis of biopsy specimens of primary lesions in considering whether to perform a further workup with a staging PET/CT (16).

In the workup of primary invasive breast cancer, an evaluation of the axilla is important for planning treatment strategies that may or may not involve surgical excision. Obtaining control of disease in the axilla is valuable. It is well accepted that axillary nodal status remains the most reliable prognostic indicator for recurrence and survival (12,17). However, axillary dissection carries risks of co-morbid conditions including infection, seroma, lymphedema, pain, and limitation of motion of the arm. Theoretically, an imaging strategy that will obviate the need for axillary dissection is ideal. Patients with negative imaging result can be spared an axillary dissection while a positive result will indicate further treatment.

The role of PET in evaluating axillary disease during initial workup is unclear. In a 360-patient multicenter study using PET-CT to evaluate the axilla, Wahl et al. demonstrated a sensitivity and specificity of 61% and 80% respectively in detecting nodal metastases, indicating that PET can often be unreliable (12). Better results were seen in a smaller study by Fuster et al. when examining 60 patients with large primary tumors (>3 cm), with the sensitivity and specificity for PET/CT to detect axillary lymph node metastasis of 70% and 100%, respectively (18). Many studies have demonstrated similar results (12).

As it currently stands, given its low sensitivity, a negative PET scan cannot rule out minimally or microscopically involved axillary nodes or the need for sentinel lymph node biopsy. In positive studies, however, metastasis is highly likely.

With regards to evaluating internal mammary and supraclavicular nodal status, at least one study, examining the stage IIb and stage III breast cancer, demonstrated a 100% sensitivity with the implication that these patients tend to have a worse prognosis than patients with axillary disease alone (13). This study indicates that, in patients with clinically positive axillary nodes, PET can play a role in examining distal lymphatic drainage as well as metastatic disease.

FOLLOW-UP STAGING

Compared with the initial workup of breast cancer, the use of FDG-PET scanning in re-staging patients after treatment has been more promising. However, current ASCO guidelines about initial staging do not recommend routine PET scanning for this purpose, for a number of reasons. First, PET has an average specificity of approximately 71–77% in screening the whole body for disease (19–21). This can lead to false-positive results mandating invasive procedures such as US-, CT- or MR-guided biopsies as well as surgical excision to confirm a recurrence, leading to morbidity. This problem may be overcome in part by utilizing combined anatomical-molecular imaging techniques, such as PET/CT or PET with MRI to increase specificity, increasing the likelihood of a true positive result.

Secondly, PET has consistently been found to have low sensitivity in detecting metastatic lesions less than 10 mm in size. These lesions are at the limit of current scanner resolution which may be as low as 6 mm in some newer systems. Radiation exposure during a PET scan is not trivial, especially when combining PET with CT. This combined procedure can increase the radiation dose from 8 to 30 millisieverts (mSv) possibly increasing the risk for future malignancy. Finally, the timing of discovery of stage IV disease has been found to play no role in improving the overall survival of breast cancer, suggesting no advantage to the routine use of PET without a clinical suspicion of recurrence. Given these points, current guidelines continue to advise against the use of routine PET for follow-up evaluation.

Exceptions are often made, however. For example, PET is increasingly used to evaluate lesions that have progressed despite treatment as well as lesions that may mandate immediate intervention. PET/CT may be helpful for assessing bony metastases seen in the femoral head or lumbar spine that may portend impending fracture, requiring local radiation therapy, hip replacement, or spinal fusion to avoid catastrophe.

In studying PET as a re-staging tool, Yap et al. found that the clinical stage was altered in over one-third (36%) of the 50 breast cancer patients evaluated and lead to a change in the clinical management of 60% of the total group (3). It was suggested in this study that physicians consider FDG-PET as a re-staging tool despite current ASCO recommendations.

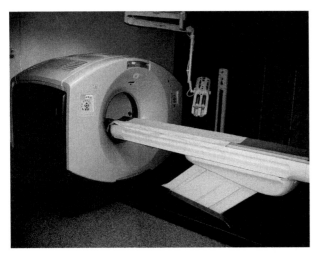

Figure 21.1 A PET/CT system with a 16-slice CT capability.

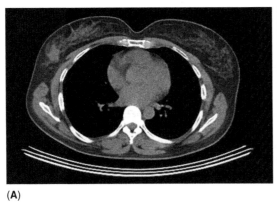

(A)

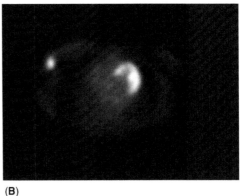

(B)

Figure 21.2 A transaxial CT image (**A**) and a corresponding ^{18}F-fluorodeoxyglucose-PET image (**B**), demonstrating a right primary breast lesion.

Given the high number of patients requesting this procedure it is important to acknowledge and understand the patients' concerns and desires in terms of further management of their disease. Importantly, in deciding whether to perform a re-staging PET, it is essential to educate the patient about its advantages, disadvantages, risks, limitations, and implications of any results.

ASSESSMENT OF LOCOREGIONAL DISEASE

Locoregional recurrence of disease occurs in approximately 7–30% of previously treated breast cancer patients and is associated with decreased survival (approximately 21–36% at five years) (22,23). In a meta-analysis including 42,000 women, the Early Breast Cancer Trialists' Collaborative Group demonstrated that treatment to successfully avoid a local recurrence would prevent one breast cancer death for every four local recurrences avoided, as well as reduce the 15-year overall mortality (24). This study illuminated the importance of local control in breast disease. If one interprets these data as suggesting that the locoregional recurrence is a cause of systemic disease, then it is reasonable to postulate that the timing of diagnosis and intervention in patients with recurrent disease may be important.

PET scanning has been shown to be especially useful in detecting locally recurrent disease and differentiating this from scarring and fibrosis (Fig. 21.3). Suarez et al. demonstrated the ability of PET to detect recurrence when used alone over a combination of conventional imaging modalities in a study of 45 patients with known complete remission who presented with elevated tumor markers (19). PET performed with a sensitivity of 92% (24/26), specificity of 75% (9/12), and 87% accuracy in this group of patients. In a similarly designed study that investigated the use of PET in patients with elevated tumor markers by Radat et al., comparable values were found for sensitivity, specificity, and accuracy. In addition, the discovery of recurrence on PET/CT led to a change in clinical management in half (51%) of the patients evaluated (20). Alternatively, some groups have suggested combining PET data with data from MRI rather than CT. Hathaway et al. (22) found this approach was also useful in defining the anatomy of recurrent disease for possible surgical resection, especially when involving brachial plexus invasion.

DISTANT DISEASE

Apart from locoregional disease, FDG-PET has the ability to evaluate distant recurrent disease (Fig. 21.4). In a study by Fuster et al. examining patients with large T3 (>5 cm) primary breast cancers, PET/CT was compared with conventional imaging; the overall sensitivity and specificity of PET in detecting distant metastases of 100% and 98%, respectively (18). Other studies report similar results as illustrated in Table 21.1.

In patients who present with distant metastases, 70% have involvement of the skeleton. The current standard of evaluating bony metastases is bone scintigraphy, which uses nuclear imaging to detect areas of increased bone turnover. Predominantly osteolytic lesions, however, are not visualized well and so FDG-PET scanning has become an alternative modality for this purpose. PET has been studied against scintigraphy in patients with bony metastases with mixed results. A study by Cook and colleagues found that FDG-PET was able to detect more lesions overall compared with bone scintigraphy; however, PET was inferior in a subgroup of patients with predominantly osteoblastic lesions (25). In detecting osteolytic lesions, however, PET outperformed bone scintigraphy, findings confirmed by other studies (26). Thus, PET can be used as a complimentary study, not a replacement, to bone scintigraphy in evaluating for bone metastases.

RESPONSE TO THERAPY

Management of locally advanced breast cancer often involves neoadjuvant chemotherapy followed by surgical excision. PET has become especially useful in evaluating and monitoring response to chemotherapeutic treatments in a variety of cancers.

The ability to detect alterations in tissue glucose metabolic rate allows for assessment of tumor dynamics during chemotherapy. Numerous studies have confirmed the utility of PET for monitoring such response, particularly in locally advanced or metastatic breast disease (1,27) as seen in Figure 21.5.

Given that SUV measurements change as tumor biology is altered, Schelling et al. found that treatment non-responders may be identified early on after one cycle of chemotherapy as evidenced by minimal variation in SUV level (27). In this prospective study of 22 patients with locally advanced breast cancer, PET images were compared with histopathological

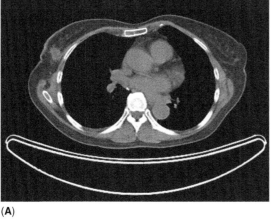
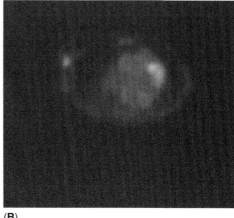

(A)   **(B)**

Figure 21.3 Irregular nodular density in the upper outer quadrant of right breast on CT (**A**), 2 months status post lumpectomy associated with a moderate ¹⁸F-fluorodeoxyglucose uptake on PET (**B**) representing recurrent local disease.

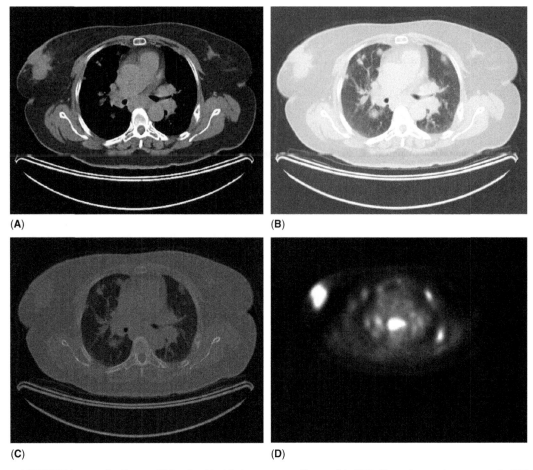

Figure 21.4 Transaxial PET/CT images of a 67-year-old female with right breast cancer diagnosed in 2000. She underwent lumpectomy in 2008 with subsequent recurrence. Soft tissue window demonstrating a large, lobulated heterogeneously enhancing, centrally necrotic mass within the right retroareolar region (**A**); lung window demonstrating extensive pulmonary metastases (**B**); bone window demonstrating multiple bony rib metastases (**C**); a corresponding transaxial ¹⁸F-fluorodeoxyglucose-PET image showing an extensive uptake in these areas (**D**).

specimens to determine response to the first round of chemotherapy. A decrease in SUV to <55% below baseline with a sensitivity and specificity of 100% and 85% respectively was found. Similarly, in a smaller study of 11 patients using conventional imaging for assessment of clinical response, Schwarz et al. found a decrease in SUV to 72% ± 21% of baseline after the first cycle of chemotherapy and a 54% ± 16% decrease after the second cycle indicating responding lesions. By contrast, non-responding metastases were found to decrease only to 94% ± 19% and 79% ± 9% after the first and second cycles respectively, suggesting a need for change in chemotherapeutic agent (1).

These findings demonstrate that PET scanning performed early in the course of treatment may allow for identification of non-responders and for medication adjustments to be made if necessary. Early modifications permit reduction in exposure to ineffective drugs and unnecessary morbidity such as nausea, vomiting, alopecia, as well as more serious adverse effects such as hematologic toxicity, infections, neurotoxicity, and cardiotoxicity (1). At the same time, the maximum potential for therapeutic success may be achieved ensuring that patients are being treated with effective medications. In comparing PET with ultrasound, CT, or MRI for this purpose, PET is frequently found to be superior as many cycles of treatment are commonly required before producing an anatomic change in tumor size, thus making these modalities less reliable when

used alone. Additionally, conventional imaging is limited in differentiating active tumor from necrotic or residual fibrous scar tissue left after tumor treatment.

Alternatively, serial dynamic contrast-enhanced MRI has been developed as a predictor of tumor vascularity and functional tumor volume in considering response to chemotherapy. A study by Partridge et al. investigated the association between dynamic contrast-enhanced MRI and PET and concluded that using the two technologies together may optimize sensitivity for measuring treatment response by providing details regarding change in tumor perfusion, size, and metabolism (28).

DISCUSSION
With regard to the extent of disease workup, generally CT of the chest, abdomen, and pelvis is performed in conjunction with bone scintigraphy for detection of metastases. Port et al. compared this conventional strategy to whole-body PET scanning for 80 patients with high-risk operable breast cancer; the sensitivity was 80% for both approaches; however, the specificity of PET in detecting metastatic disease was significantly higher than conventional imaging (PET, 94%; conventional imaging, 74%; p = 0.01) (29). Further, comparisons of the two strategies reveal other important differences, notably a higher radiation exposure with PET. The total effective dose to the patient due to the ¹⁸F-FDG tracer is approximately 6–7 mSv which increases to

Table 21.1 Evidence on Comparative Imaging Accuracy Sensitivity and Specificity for Studies Reporting on the Detection of Distant Metastases in Breast Cancer

Author (Year)	Test	n (total)	n (any mets)	Sensitivity	Specificity	Positive Predictive Value	Negative Predictive Value
Heusner (2008)	FDG-PET/CT	40	10	10/10	Nr, nr	Nr, nr	Nr, nr
				100.0%	nr , nr	Nr, nr	Nr, nr
	Conventional Imaging (BS, CXR, LUS)			7/10 70.0%			
Segaert (2010)	FDG-PET	70	23	18/23	Nr, nr	Nr, nr	nr , nr
	FDG-PET/CT			78.0%	Nr, nr	Nr, nr	nr, nr
	Conventional imaging (BS, CXR, LUS)			22/23 95.7%	46/47 97.9%	16/17 94.1%	46/53 86.8%
				16/23 69.6%			
Fuster (2008)	FDG-PET/CT	60	8	8/8 100.0%	51/52 98.1%	8/9 88.9%	51/51 100.0%
			Lung 2	2/2 100.0%	57/58 98.3%	2/3 66.7%	57/57 100.0%
			Liver 2	2/2 100.0%	58/58 100.0%	2/2 100.0%	58/58 100.0%
			Bone 6	6/6 100.0%	54/54 100.0%	6/6 100.0%	54/54 100.0%
	Conventional imaging (BS, chest CT, LUS)		8	3/8 37.5%	45/52 86.5%	3/10 30.0%	45/50 90.0%
			Lung (CT) 2	2/2 100.0%	54/58 93.1%	2/6 33.3%	54/54 100.0%
			Liver (US) 2	½ 50.0%	53/58 91.4%	1/6 16.7%	53/54 98.1%
			Bone (BS) 6	2/6 33.3%	47/54 87.0%	2/9 22.2%	47/51 92.2%
Niikura (2001)	FDG-PET/CT	225	67	76/78 97.4%	134/147 91.2%	76/89 85.4%	134/136 98.5%
	Conventional imaging (BS, CXR, CT)			67/68 85.9%	99/147 67.3%	67/115 58.3%	99/110 90.0%
Abe (2005)	FDG-PET	44	14	14/14 100.0%	29/30 96.7%	14/15 93.3%	29/29 100.0%
	Conventional imaging BS (bone mets only)			11/14 78.6%	30/30 100.0%	11/14 78.6%	30/30 100.0%

Abbreviations: nr, not recorded; BS, bone scan; CXR, chest x-ray; LUS, liver ultrasound; mets, metastases.
Source: From Ref. (37).

>10 mSv when a combined PET/CT is used, more than three times the dose of using diagnostic CT alone (30). The additional effect of bone scintigraphy in conventional imaging is minimal (0.008 mSv) in comparison (31).

The cost of PET is also substantially higher with scans costing approximately £1006 (€1256; US$1605) and up to £1236 (€1543; $1972) for combined PET/CT; in contrast, a conventional workup (£485/€605/$774) and bone scanning (£164/€204/$261) are less expensive, based on recent data (32). Additionally, Depending on the model of healthcare and insurance limitations, some patients may not be offered a PET for evaluation.

In addition to the high cost, FDG-PET has other limitations as discussed earlier, including the consistent inability to detect small lesions and minimal axillary nodal disease (13). This inadequacy is due mostly to the limited spatial resolution of current PET scanners which is only partly overcome by correlating with anatomical data from CT (33). Additionally, PET scanning does not include evaluation of the head, allowing for missed skull and brain metastasis. Hence, it is impossible to rely solely on PET-CT for staging, and therefore, it is often used in conjunction with other imaging tools. PET also suffers from many false positives due to background signal from metabolically active normal tissues, thus prompting invasive interventions which otherwise may not be indicated. Finally, performing a PET scan may take from 30 to 45 minutes and may cause patient discomfort and claustrophobia.

New tracers are being developed for PET imaging which may allow the study of various aspects of tumor biology including proliferation, angiogenesis, apoptosis, hypoxia, and receptor expression (34,35). By developing radioactively tagged molecules which act as markers for these cell processes, follow-up examinations allow assessment of whether chosen chemotherapeutic agents interact with target molecules and are in effect causing a specific change.

Conceptually it may also be possible to develop chemotherapeutic agents that in themselves can be radiolabeled and thus permit concentration of these agents to predetermined tumor locations.

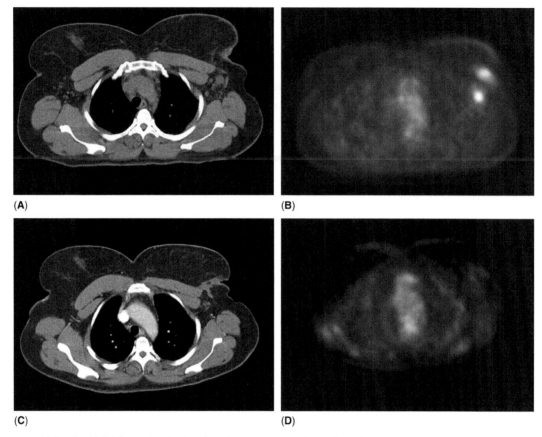

(A)

(B)

(C)

(D)

Figure 21.5 A 47-year-old female with left breast invasive ductal carcinoma prior to and post chemotherapy (CT and corresponding PET images). Note on pre-treatment images: a 1.2-cm left axillary lymph node, with a mild ^{18}F-fluorodeoxyglucose (FDG) uptake and a 1.3-cm left axillary lymph node, with an intense FDG uptake suspicious for malignancy (**A** and **B**). On post-treatment images (**C** and **D**) previously noted enlarged left axillary lymph nodes are significantly improved in size with decreased FDG activity.

Additionally, dedicated breast PET/CT scanners as well as positron emission mammography which have a higher spatial resolution and photon sensitivity than whole body scanners are being developed which may allow more accurate detection of primary disease as well as axillary involvement (36). This targeted imaging tool may increase PET sensitivity, reduce false-negative rates, and allow expansion of the use of PET to routine workup.

In the past, physicians have been largely nihilistic about stage IV breast disease, primarily due to the unavailability of effective therapeutic agents. This paradigm is slowly changing in favor of investigating improved imaging modalities and better targeted therapeutic agents to detect, treat, and follow disease progress. A "cure" for breast cancer today is largely the ability to achieve long-term remission in certain subsets of patients. For this reason as technology improves, with the development of dedicated, higher resolution scanners, and new radiotracer molecules, the role of PET scanning is likely to expand to become a routine part of the breast cancer management algorithm and we are likely to use the technology throughout all stages of breast cancer.

REFERENCES
1. Schwarz JD, Bader M, Jenicke L, et al. Early prediction of response to chemotherapy in metastatic breast cancer using sequential 18F-FDG PET. J Nucl Med 2005; 46: 1144–50.
2. Fleming IN, Gilbert FJ, Miles KA, Cameron D. Opportunities for PET to deliver clinical benefit in cancer: breast cancer as a paradigm. Cancer Imaging 2010; 10: 144–52.
3. Yap CS, Seltzer MA, Schiepers C, et al. Impact of whole-body 18F-FDG PET on staging and managing patients with breast cancer: the referring physician's perspective. J Nucl Med 2001; 42: 1334–7.
4. Pan L, Han Y, Sun X, Liu J, Gang H. FDG-PET and other imaging modalities for the evaluation of breast cancer recurrence and metastases: a meta-analysis. J Cancer Res Clin Oncol 2010; 136: 1007–22.
5. Warburg OH, Posener K, Negelein E. Über den Stoffwechsel der Karzinomzelle. Biochem Zeitschr 1924; 152: 309–52.
6. Kelloff GJ, Hoffman JM, Johnson B, et al. Progress and promise of FDG-PET imaging for cancer patient management and oncologic drug development. Clin Cancer Res 2005; 11: 2785–808.
7. Gennari A, Piccardo A, Altrinetti V, et al. Whither the PET scan? The role of PET imaging in the staging and treatment of breast cancer. Curr Oncol Rep 2012; 14: 20–6.
8. Townsend DW. Dual-modality imaging: combining anatomy and function. J Nucl Med 2008; 49: 938–55.
9. Bar-Shalom R, Yefremov N, Guralnik L, et al. Clinical performance of PET-CTin evaluation of cancer: additional value for diagnostic imaging and patient management. J Nucl Med 2003; 44: 1200–9.
10. Khatcheressian JL, Wolff AC, Smith TJ, et al. American society of clinical oncology 2006 update of the breast cancer follow-up and management guidelines in the adjuvant setting. J Clin Oncol 2006; 24: 5091–7.
11. Quon A, Gambhir SS. FDG-PET and beyond: molecular breast cancer imaging. J Clin Oncol 2005; 23: 1664–73.
12. Wahl RL, Siegel BA, Coleman RE, Gatsonis CG. Prospective multicenter study of axillary nodal staging by positron emission tomography in breast cancer: a report of the staging of breast cancer with PET study group. J Clin Oncol 2004; 22: 277–85.
13. Segaert I, Mottaghy F, Ceyssens S, et al. Additional value of PET-CT in staging of clinical stage IIB and III breast cancer. Breast J 2010; 16: 617–24.
14. Heudel P, Cimarelli S, Montella A, Bouteille C, Mognetti T. Value of PET-FDG in primary breast cancer based on histological and immunohistochemical prognostic factors. Int J Clin Oncol 2010; 15: 588–93.

15. Basu S, Chen T, Tchou J, et al. Comparison of triple-negative and estrogen receptor-positive/progesterone receptor positive/HER2-negative breast carcinoma using quantitative fluorine-18 fluorodeoxyglucose/positron emission tomography imaging parameters: a potentially useful method for disease characterization. Cancer 2008; 112: 995–1000.

16. Kim BS, Sung SH. Usefulness of (18)F-FDG uptake with clinicopathologic and immunohistochemical prognostic factors in breast cancer. Ann Nucl Med 2012; 26: 175–83.

17. Meng Y, Ward S, Cooper K, Harnan S, Wyld L. Cost-effectiveness of MRI and PET imaging for the evaluation of axillary lymph node metastases in early stage breast cancer. Eur J Surg Oncol 2011; 37: 40–6.

18. Fuster D, Duch J, Paredes P, et al. Preoperative staging of large primary breast cancer with [18F] fluorodeoxyglucose positron emission tomography/computed tomography compared with conventional imaging procedures. J Clin Oncol 2008; 26: 4746–51.

19. Suárez M, Pérez-Castejón MJ, Jiménez A, et al. Early diagnosis of recurrent breast cancer with FDG-PET in patients with progressive elevation of serum tumor parkers. Q J Nucl Med 2002; 46: 113–21.

20. Radan L, Ben-Haim S, Bar-Shalom R, Guralnik L, Israel O. The role of FDG-PET/CT in suspected recurrence of breast cancer. Cancer 2006; 107: 2545–51.

21. Lind P, Igerc I, Beyer T, Reinprecht P, Hausegger K. Advantages and limitations of FDG PET in the follow-up of breast cancer. Eur J Nucl Med Mol Imaging 2004; 31(Suppl 1): S125–34.

22. Hathaway PB, Mankoff DA, Maravilla KR, et al. Value of combined FDG PET and MR imaging in the evaluation of suspected recurrent local-regional breast cancer: preliminary experience. Radiology 1999; 210: 807–14.

23. Bongers V, Perre C, de Hooge P. The use of scintimammography for detecting the recurrence of loco-regional breast cancer: histopathologically proven results. Nucl Med Commun 2004; 25: 145–9.

24. Clarke M, Collins R, Darby S, et al. Effects of radiotherapy and of differences in the extent of surgery for early breast cancer on local recurrence and 15-year survival: an overview of the randomized trials. Lancet 2005; 366: 2087–106.

25. Cook GJ, Houston S, Rubens R, Maisey MN, Fogelman I. Detection of bony metastases in breast cancer by 18FDG-PET: differing metabolic activity in osteoblastic and osteolytic lesions. J Clin Oncol 1998; 16: 3375–9.

26. Constantinidou A, Martin A, Sharma B, Johnston SRD. Positron emission tomography/computed tomography in the management of recurrent/metastatic breast cancer: a large retrospective study from the Royal Marsden Hospital. Ann Oncol 2011; 22: 307–14.

27. Schelling M, Avril N, Nährig J, et al. Positron emission tomography using [(18)F] Fluorodeoxyglucose for monitoring primary chemotherapy in breast cancer. J Clin Oncol 2000; 18: 1689–95.

28. Partridge SC, Vanantwerp RK, Doot RK, et al. Association between serial dynamic contrast-enhanced MRI and dynamic 18F-FDG PET measures in patients undergoing neoadjuvant chemotherapy for locally advanced breast cancer. J Magn Reson Imaging 2010; 32: 1124–31.

29. Port ER, Yeung H, Gonen M, et al. 18F-2-fluoro-2-deoxy-D-glucose positron emission tomography scanning affects surgical management in selected patients with high-risk, operable breast carcinoma. Ann Surg Oncol 2006; 13: 677–84.

30. Leide-Svegborn S. Radiation exposure of patients and personnel from a PET/CT procedure with 18F-FDG. Radiat Prot Dosimetry 2010; 139: 208–13.

31. Weber DA, Makler PTJ, Watson EE, et al. Radiation absorbed dose from technetium-99m-labeled bone imaging agents. Task Group of the Medical Internal Radiation Dose Committee, The Society of Nuclear Medicine. J Nucl Med 1989; 30: 1117–22.

32. Auguste P, Barton P, Hyde C, Roberts TE. An economic evaluation of positron emission tomography (PET) and positron emission tomography/computed tomography (PET/CT) for the diagnosis of breast cancer recurrence. Health Technol Assess 2011; 15: 1–54.

33. Kurata A, Murata Y, Kubota K, Osanai T, Shibuya H. Multiple 18F-FDG, PET-CT for postoperative monitoring of breast cancer patients. Acta Radiol 2009; 50: 979–83.

34. Groheux D, Giacchetti S, Rubello D, et al. The evolving role of PET/CT in breast cancer. Nucl Med Commun 2010; 31: 271–3.

35. Cochet A, Generali D, Fox SB, Ferrozzi F, Hicks RJ. Positron emission tomography and neoadjuvant therapy of breast cancer. J Natl Cancer Inst Monogr 2011: 111–15.

36. Narayanan D, Madsen KS, Kalinyak JE, Berg WA. Interpretation of positron emission mammography: feature analysis and rates of malignancy. AJR Am J Roentgenol 2011; 196: 956–70.

37. Brennan ME, Houssami N. Evaluation of the evidence on staging imaging for detection of asymptomatic distant metastases in newly diagnosed breast cancer. Breast 2012; 21: 112–23.

22 Core biopsy of breast lesions

Kathryn Taylor and Peter D. Britton

INTRODUCTION

Accurate preoperative cancer diagnosis is essential to ensure appropriate patient counseling and tailored treatment plans. This is currently undertaken in the form of "triple assessment," incorporating clinical examination, imaging, and needle biopsy. Needle core biopsy (CB) has become the mainstay of breast cancer diagnosis largely replacing fine needle aspiration cytology (FNAC) (1). CB is quick, inexpensive, well tolerated and reliably distinguishes benign from malignant breast lesions in the vast majority of patients. In the past 5 years, ultrasound-guided CB has also been used to diagnose axillary lymph node metastases to more accurately stage patients with newly diagnosed breast cancer (2).

Clearly, no diagnostic test is 100% accurate; therefore, clinical, imaging, and biopsy findings should be discussed in a multidisciplinary setting to ensure safe patient care. Occasionally, some patients will still require surgical excision to reach a definitive diagnosis.

HISTORY

Initial experience with needle biopsy in the breast was with FNAC which was widely performed in Europe and especially Scandinavia where excellent results were reported (3). To achieve reliable results, however, the services of an experienced and dedicated breast cytopathologist are required. Such expertise was not always widely available and radiologists required alternative techniques to produce reliable high-standard results. In 1990, Parker published his results combining an automated biopsy device produced in Sweden with stereotactic guidance to perform a large-gauge core needle biopsy of the breast (4). Shortly thereafter, ultrasound guidance was utilized for CB, and a multicenter trial demonstrated that it could be introduced reliably on a large scale (5,6). CB represented a reliable, cost effective alternative to diagnostic surgical excision and did not require such expert pathological interpretation required of FNAC. Following its initial introduction, CB was rapidly adopted as the first-line technique for most diagnostic procedures in the breast.

CORE BIOPSY VS. FINE NEEDLE ASPIRATION CYTOLOGY

FNAC is a very simple procedure with no local anesthetic required and can be performed in as little as 30 seconds; the interpretation of a cellular smear can be available within a few minutes. When a dedicated and skilled team is assembled, a truly "one stop" diagnostic service is feasible with results available during the same clinic. A substantial number of benign and malignant abnormalities can be confidently diagnosed on FNAC alone. Although CB takes substantially longer to process, the procedure is associated with higher diagnostic accuracy and is often needed as a supplementary test when FNAC has failed to yield a definitive result. Comparison of the scoring criteria for FNAC and CB is shown in Table 22.1.

In the event of a malignant result, CB will also provide additional information about the presence or absence of invasion, tumor type, grade, and receptor status (ER PgR and HER2). Lesions with a paucity of cells, such as hyalinized fibroadenomas and some lobular carcinomas, make accurate diagnosis with FNAC difficult. False-negative results are also possible with FNAC in well-differentiated tumors, such as tubular and mucinous carcinomas, and low-grade ductal types. The categories C3 and C4 are perhaps the most difficult lesions to assess with FNAC because of the lack of full cytological features to define either a benign or unequivocally malignant diagnosis. FNAC cannot reliably distinguish atypia from low-grade ductal carcinoma in situ (DCIS) or indeed in situ from invasive carcinoma. In addition, the tumor hormone receptor status cannot be assessed. These lesions will necessitate a CB or a diagnostic excision biopsy for definitive diagnosis or to determine hormone receptor status. CB takes solid cores of breast tissue sufficient for paraffin-embedded histological examination allowing assessment of both breast architecture and cellular morphology; in consequence, CB has improved sensitivity and specificity compared with FNAC.

The high inadequacy rates in some centers coupled with inability to clearly distinguish in situ carcinoma from invasive disease have led to the increasing use of CB (in preference to FNAC) during the last decade. In the United Kingdom (UK) NHS Breast Screening Programme (NHSBSP) the number of breast cancers diagnosed solely by FNAC fell from 19% in 2000–2001 to 3% in 2008–2009 (7).

GUIDELINES

In the UK NHSBSP, latest guidelines stipulate CB as the expected standard for sampling in the breast (8). In the symptomatic population, CB is advocated, but guidelines acknowledge situations where FNAC is possible (1). Importantly, preoperative breast cancer diagnosis should be achieved by correlation of clinical and radiological assessment with decisions made in a multidisciplinary setting. Minimum and target standards expected for the preoperative diagnosis of non-invasive and invasive cancers are shown in Table 22.2.

Ultrasound examination of the axilla and needle biopsy of potentially abnormal axillary nodes has become a routine practice in the preliminary staging of patients with suspected breast cancer and is recommended in National Institute for

Table 22.1 FNAC and CB Diagnostic Categories

Fine needle aspiration cytology (FNAC)
C1 – Inadequate material for diagnosis
C2 – Benign lesions
C3 – Atypical features but probably benign
C4 – Atypical features but suspicious of malignancy
C5 – Unequivocal malignant cells

Core biopsy (CB)
B1 – Normal tissue or inadequate material
B2 – Benign lesions
B3 – Lesion of uncertain malignant potential
B4 – Suspicious of malignancy. Not fully diagnostic due to either the sample being too small, crushed or poorly preserved.
B5 – Malignant
  a) in situ carcinoma
  b) invasive disease

Table 22.2 Minimum and Target Standards for the Non-Operative Diagnosis Rate for Breast Cancer

	Minimum Standard (%)	Target (%)
Invasive disease	90	95
Non-invasive disease	85	90

Table 22.3 Upgrade Rates of ADH to DCIS and DCIS to Invasive Carcinoma for 14-gauge (G) Stereo CB and 11-G VAB

	Stereo CB, 14 G (%)	VAB, 11 G (%)
Upgrade of atypical ductal hyperplasia (ADH) to ductal carcinoma in situ (DCIS)	48	17
Upgrade of DCIS to invasive carcinoma	25	11

surgical drainage is only about 0.2% (15). A pneumothorax can rarely occur during either procedure if the needle is pushed in too deeply and is more likely in women with small breasts.

TECHNIQUE
Ultrasound-Guided Core Biopsy
Although breast lumps can be biopsied using manual palpation, image guidance does allow for more accurate needle placement. The vast majority of breast lesions are now sampled under ultrasound guidance by taking core biopsies (16). This method is quick, comparatively inexpensive, and does not involve any radiation exposure. It is particularly useful for impalpable sonographically visible lesions (17). Standard practices utilize a 14-gauge needle which is known to yield good results; however, a smaller 16- or even 18-gauge needle should be considered where the superior maneuverability of a smaller needle can assist in traversing either the dense breast tissue or the limited space available within the axilla (18,19). Standard needle throw is 2 cm which allows the acquisition of 20–25 mg strips of tissue (20). The procedure is performed under local anesthetic, and the needle is introduced usually at least two or three times through a single 2–3 mm skin incision. The needle needs to be withdrawn from the patient to obtain the sample from the needle, and care must be taken when doing this to avoid disruption of tissue architecture. Two accurately placed needle passes are usually sufficient to achieve a reliable diagnosis although the size and type of lesion and compliance of the patient must be taken into consideration. The false-negative rate of FNAC is about 2–3% which is much higher than with CB and likely represents incomplete sampling of the lesions rather than pathological misinterpretation (Figs. 22.1–22.3) (21,22).

Stereotactic Guided Core Biopsy
The majority of stereotactic biopsies are performed for mammographic microcalcifications which are frequently not visible on ultrasound. Stereotactic equipment is designed to calculate the position of a designated site within the breast by localizing its position in the x, y, and z axes from the surface of the breast. Routine imaging at the beginning of the procedure enables calculation of the x and y axes, and two-angled images allow calculation of the depth of the lesion (z axis) within the breast. When sampling microcalcification, multiple cores should be obtained and a specimen radiograph be taken to confirm adequate sampling of the cluster. Although highly acceptable results can be obtained using stereotactic CB, the

Health and Clinical Excellence (NICE) guidelines (9). The performance of FNAC compared with CB is less clear in the axilla than in the breast. Reported sensitivities of FNAC vary greatly from 21% to 63% and the sensitivity of CB is approximately 40% (10–12). A recent meta-analysis found no significant difference in the diagnostic performance between FNAC and CB for biopsy of axillary nodes (13). The outcomes depend on the expertise and preference within each center as to the technique chosen, and neither method is specifically recommended in any national or international guidance.

VACUUM-ASSISTED BIOPSY
In a breast care program, the number of benign excisional surgical breast biopsies should be minimized. The vast majority of breast lesions which are visible on ultrasound can be adequately assessed by ultrasound-guided 14-gauge core needle biopsy. However, in some cases this technique may not appear to be sufficiently reliable, and 11-gauge vacuum-assisted biopsy (VAB) may be considered either at the outset or as an alternative to diagnostic surgical biopsy in the event of either discrepant or inconclusive 14-gauge histology results. The increased yield afforded with VAB also reduces the frequency of histological underestimation found with conventional CB as demonstrated in Table 22.3.

In some cases VAB enables the removal of the entire lesion without an increase in the complication rate. VAB is also more successful than CB at sampling microcalcification (14). VAB is discussed fully in the next section.

COMPLICATIONS
Both CB and FNAC are operator dependent and serious complications are rare with either procedure. CB can cause more trauma; ecchymosis of a varying degree is common with this technique, although the risk of hematoma formation requiring

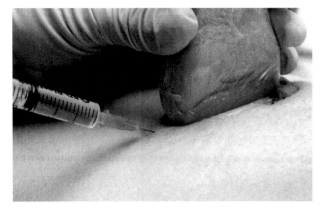

Figure 22.1 Administration of local anesthesia prior to an ultrasound-guided core biopsy.

operator tissue yield with VAB makes this the preferred technique for microcalcification. However, improved diagnostic performance needs to be offset against a substantial increase in cost (23).

Biopsy with Magnetic Resonance Imaging

With the increased use of dynamic contrast-enhanced magnetic resonance imaging (MRI) of the breast, the number of MRI-detected abnormalities has increased. If such lesions are suspicious of malignancy and warrant further investigation, then a "second-look" ultrasound examination of the area in question is performed. If no lesion is identified by ultrasound and the suspicion for malignancy persists, then an MRI-guided biopsy is indicated (24). As with stereotactic guided biopsy, use of vacuum-assisted sampling, 11-gauge MR VAB is recommended over standard 14-gauge core needle biopsy. Although it is feasible to perform 14-gauge core needle biopsy under MRI guidance, the greater volume of tissue retrieved using VAB allows a more extensive biopsy, a lower false-negative rate and easier appreciation that a lesion has been adequately sampled or even removed (25).

REPORTING CATEGORIES

All aspects of triple assessment are categorized using a similar five-point scoring system. The imaging component (UK Five-Point Breast Imaging Classification) has been formalized but does not specify the percentage likelihood of malignancy for each category (26). The Breast Imaging Reporting and Data System (BI-RADS) is used in North America and most of Europe and, unlike the UK system, it encompasses a lexicon of descriptors for each category and the likelihood of malignancy within each category. BI-RADS allows standardization and uniformity of reporting; UK scoring can be mapped to parallel BI-RADS categories with equivalent cancer risks (Table 22.4) (27).

INDICATIONS

Ultrasound-Guided Core Biopsy

Ultrasound-guided CB is indicated for most focal solid lesions visible by ultrasound whether palpable or not. This method is recognized as a quick, inexpensive, and accurate method of sampling which is well tolerated by patients (28). The maneuverability of a small hand-held device imaged

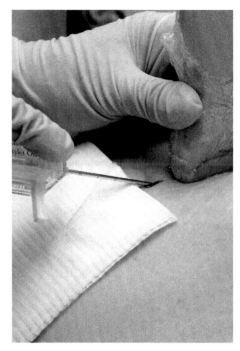

Figure 22.2 Insertion of a 14 gauge needle through a scalpel blade nick in the skin during an ultrasound-guided core biopsy.

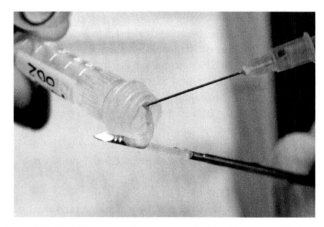

Figure 22.3 A 20–25 mg strip of tissue removed with a 14-gauge needle during a core biopsy.

under real time is particularly useful for patients with small breasts or lesions deep in the breast and is the method of choice for biopsy of axillary nodes. Unequivocally benign lesions containing fat, such as hamartomas, lipomas, and fat necrosis do not require sampling. There is also evidence that lesions with the appearance of fibroadenomas in women under the age of 25 years do not require biopsy as malignancy is rare in this age group (29). However, management of these lesions varies. UK Five-Point Breast Imaging Classification scores fibroadenomas as 2-benign, and the patient under 25 years of age may be discharged. Using the BI-RADS system, fibroadenomas score as category 3-probably benign and undergo short-term imaging follow-up at 6–12 months. In all cases of non-biopsy, there must be typical benign imaging features and concordance with clinical findings. Any atypical features should precipitate a biopsy, and results should be discussed within a multidisciplinary setting.

Table 22.4 UK Scorings Linked to the Parallel BI-RADS Category with the Equivalent Cancer Risk

UK Category	Likelihood of Malignancy (%)	BI-RADS Category
1– Normal	0	1–2
2– Benign	<2	3
3– Indeterminate/probably benign findings	2–95	4a–4b
4– Findings suspicious of malignancy	2–95	4
5– Findings highly suspicious of malignancy	>95	5

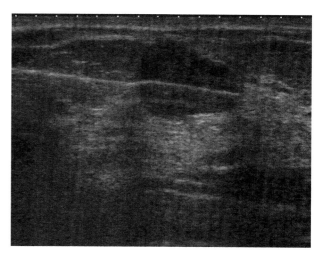

Figure 22.4 Documentation of the needle in the lesion in one of two orthogonal planes during an ultrasound-guided core biopsy.

Stereotactic Core Biopsy

Stereotactic CB is indicated for mammographic abnormalities which are often sonographically occult, predominantly microcalcification. The widespread availability of 11-gauge VAB has largely superseded the initial use of 14-gauge core needle biopsy under stereotactic guidance. Lesions such as radial scars and complex sclerosing lesions without atypia that have been diagnosed at stereotactic CB can be completely removed with the addition of VAB without the need for surgical intervention.

MRI-Guided Biopsy

MRI-guided biopsy is increasingly needed to obtain histological examination of suspicious lesions detected on MRI that are occult on mammography and ultrasound. Breast MRI may identify cancers not visualized on mammography in 33% of breast cancer patients, while up to 10% of patients will have another malignant lesion seen on MRI that is not detected by mammography or sonography (30,31).

EQUIPMENT AND TECHNIQUE

The earlier reusable biopsy devices have given way to lighter disposable models which allow for a variety of gauges. Whichever method of image guidance is used, the sampling technique is similar. Approximately 2–5 mL of local anesthetic is administered enabling a small scalpel blade nick to be made in the skin. Breast biopsy with a 14-gauge needle necessitates repeated entries into the breast as samples are taken, and the needle withdrawn each time for tissue removal. In contrast, during VAB the needle remains in the breast as tissue is sucked into the sampling window and removed with the needle in situ.

Accurate sampling is documented with images of the needle in the lesion in two orthogonal planes and post-procedure imaging of stereotactic and MRI-VAB confirms that the correct area has been sampled. When microcalcification or a small lesion is sampled an imaging compatible marker clip can be deployed and imaged to mark the biopsy site in case there is a need for further intervention (Fig. 22.4).

RESULTS

CB histology results should always be correlated with imaging and clinical findings in the interests of safe practice and optimum patient management. Histology results which can be accepted for each histology classification score are shown in Table 22.5.

Table 22.5 Showing Examples of Pathology for Each Histology Category and Suggested Management

CB Result Category	Example of Pathology	Management
B1	Lipoma, hamartoma, dense breast tissue	Discharge if there is clinical and imaging correlation
B2	Benign focal solid lesions	Discharge if there is clinical and imaging correlation
B3	Papilloma, sclerosing lesions, lobular neoplasia. ADH	VAB or diagnostic surgical excision
B4	ADH, insufficient or crushed tissue	Surgical excision
B5a	DCIS	Therapeutic surgery
B5b	Invasive malignancy	Therapeutic surgery

Abbreviations: ADH, atypical ductal hyperplasia; CB, core biopsy; DCIS, ductal carcinoma *in situ*; VAB, vacuum-assisted biopsy.

Repeat biopsy, VAB, or surgical excision should be considered if the safety of a diagnosis is doubted, in particular with scores B3 and B4 which are associated with finite upgrade rates to malignancy following subsequent surgical excision.

B3 Unknown Malignant Potential

Radial Scars

Radial scars and complex sclerosing lesions (radial scars >1 cm in diameter) are benign lesions which are usually impalpable and are frequently screen detected as areas of parenchymal distortion or spiculation (often mimicking a carcinoma). Although CB can suggest a diagnosis of radial scar, it may fail to diagnose areas of atypia or malignancy (typically low-grade DCIS or low-grade invasive cancers) that can be associated with these lesions in 0–43% of cases (32). The histological appearances of radial scars and tubular carcinomas overlap to some degree and care is required to avoid a false-positive CB result. A B3 benign radial scar result at CB, particularly with cytological atypia, should be regarded with caution and warrants surgical excision. If CB reveals no atypia, then either a surgical or a therapeutic VAB excision is still warranted (33).

Atypical Ductal Hyperplasia

Atypical ductal hyperplasia (ADH) is also more frequently detected in asymptomatic patients or following mammographic screening and is often diagnosed following a biopsy of mammographic microcalcification. ADH demonstrates all the morphological features but in insufficient quantity to make a definitive diagnosis of DCIS, with up to two duct spaces involved in ADH and more than two duct spaces in DCIS (34). As a result, CB may underestimate the presence of DCIS due to an inadequate amount of tissue being sampled. The transition from ADH to DCIS sometimes warrants a B4 (suspicious for malignancy) result at CB rather than B3 (uncertain malignant potential). Up to 50% of cases where ADH is diagnosed on a 14-gauge core needle biopsy are subsequently upgraded to DCIS at surgical excision (35). A B3/B4 ADH result at 14-gauge core needle biopsy should therefore always be followed by a diagnostic surgical excision.

Lobular Neoplasia

Lobular carcinoma in situ and atypical lobular hyperplasia (ALH) are pathological entities that are occasionally diagnosed on CB and are collectively referred to as "lobular neoplasia." They have similar morphology and are usually diagnosed incidentally, although occasionally it may present as clustered mammographic microcalcification. As with ADH and low-grade DCIS, these processes are distinguished according to the degree of involvement, but here in terms of lobular units rather than duct spaces. In lobular carcinoma in situ more than half the acini in a lobular unit are involved; whereas in ALH less than half the acini show proliferative changes. Importantly, the basement membrane is not breached, hence the term in situ and its distinction from invasive disease.

Reported incidence of lobular neoplasia in CBs varies greatly from 0.02% to 2%. It has been described as a biological marker of increased risk of breast cancer. There is more recent evidence to suggest that like DCIS, lobular neoplasia can act as a precursor for invasive disease with lobular carcinoma being the most common malignant outcome. The overall rate for upstaging lobular neoplasia at surgical excision is not clear as reported series are often small and only selected patients have undergone surgical excision. About 20% of patients diagnosed with lobular neoplasia on CB will have DCIS or invasive disease at subsequent surgical excision. Consequently, surgical excision is frequently advocated when lobular neoplasia is diagnosed on CB.

Papilloma

Intraductal papillary lesions of the breast are most commonly benign; however, papillary lesions may show atypical or malignant histological features. The distinction between benign, atypical, and even malignant papillary lesions is difficult using the limited tissue supplied by CB. These lesions can present either as an asymptomatic opacity apparent on screening mammograms or symptomatically as a palpable lump and/or nipple discharge. Papillary lesions are composed of fibrovascular cores supporting a variable degree of epithelial proliferation. Distinction between benign and more suspicious forms requires assessment of both cytological and architectural features. Although the majority of these lesions are benign, malignancy on subsequent excisional biopsy is present in up to 25% of cases (36) and when atypia is present on CB, the rate of upstaging ranges from 20% to 75% (37). Consequently, excision by VAB (when there is no atypia on CB) or by excisional surgery is generally recommended for all papillary lesions to establish a definitive diagnosis.

B4 Suspicious, Probably Malignant

As the distinction between both ADH and DCIS and types of lobular neoplasia relies on the amount of tissue sampled, accurate categorization at CB can be difficult. Occasionally when severity and extent of the lesion are captured with more certainty, a B4 score (suspicious probably malignant) is justified over a B3 score. Crushed, damaged, or poorly fixed cores that contain probable carcinoma but cannot provide the definitive diagnosis are also categorized as B4.

B5a DCIS

DCIS arises in the epithelial cells of the terminal duct lobular unit with the myoepithelial basement membrane remaining intact. DCIS arises in the ductal portion of the terminal duct lobular unit and is morphologically, biologically, and clinically different from lobular neoplasia. DCIS is usually unifocal, following a single duct system; however, because of the highly variable lobular anatomy of the breast, it may be apparent in more than one quadrant of the breast. DCIS is classified as low, intermediate, and high grade, the latter being most likely to progress to invasive disease. High-grade DCIS has large, malignant cells and is often visible on mammograms as rod-shaped calcification arising from comedo-type necrosis in the ductal lumen. DCIS accounts for 20% of screen-detected carcinomas, whereas it has a frequency of about 5% in the symptomatic setting (38–40). The upstage rate for DCIS diagnosed on 14gauge core needle biopsy to invasive disease at surgery is 20–50%, with low-grade DCIS accounting for a very small proportion of these cases (41,42). Using VAB, the upstage rate is lower at about 5–15% which emphasizes the advantage of VAB over 14-gauge core needle biopsy for the investigation of microcalcification (43,44).

For patients diagnosed with DCIS, the extent of the in situ component, architectural type (e.g., cribriform and comedo), nuclear grade, and the presence of necrosis and micro invasion should be available at histology. This information can assist in treatment planning and prognostic assessment.

B5b Invasive Carcinoma

Any CB histology report should comment on the presence of specialized breast tissue, epithelial hyperplasia (usual and atypical), and calcification (including relationship with benign or malignant lesions). When invasive disease is diagnosed on CB there is the potential for additional histological information. This can provide detailed information on the prediction of outcome and response to therapy of an individual patient as a basis for accurate pretreatment planning of preoperative, surgical, and postoperative therapy.

The histology report should include the type and grade of infiltrating or in situ carcinoma and the relative amount of each component. Estrogen receptor (ER), progesterone receptor, and HER2 status should be reported. The presence of lymphovascular invasion and necrosis should also be noted.

Tumors can be typed at CB according to the most common categories, such as ductal/no specific type or classical lobular carcinoma. In such cases, the rate of concordance with the full surgical specimen is in the range from 93% to 100% (45). Invasive carcinoma of special type, however, cannot be accurately predicted until the resection specimen is available. Grading on CB is reasonably accurate with current evidence suggesting that concordance between grade on CB and that in the definitive excision specimen can be achieved in approximately 75% of cases (46). Highest concordance is achieved in grade 3 carcinomas. When the grade differs on the subsequent resection specimen, it is usually by one grade category only. Mitotic count in particular may be lower in the CB than excision specimen, therefore leading to lower grading on CB. ER assessment on CB has been shown to correlate with the subsequent surgical excision specimen and also to predict response to hormone therapy. An ER-positive tumor can be treated with hormone therapy and has a more favorable prognosis than ER-negative tumors. Lymphovascular invasion is another important prognostic factor in breast cancer. However, the presence of histologically confirmed lymphovascular invasion is better assessed on final surgical histology.

In addition to histological information, CB can be used to evaluate the status of molecular markers with prognostic and predictive value that can contribute to the selection of an optimum treatment regimen, especially for patients who may undergo neoadjuvant therapy. Assessment of hormone receptors on CB correlates well with subsequent surgical excision specimens, although slightly higher for ER than progesterone receptor. HER2 status is recognized in breast carcinoma as a prognostic marker; overexpression being associated with a worse prognosis. More importantly, testing is now required as a prerequisite to predict drug response and to select patients for trastuzumab treatment. Assessment of HER2 status on CB in breast cancer is accurate and reliable. When initial testing is equivocal, accuracy can be increased further by using fluorescence in situ hybridization analysis.

THE AXILLA
Axillary lymph node status is the single most important prognostic factor in patients with breast cancer. During the last decade, sentinel lymph node biopsy has largely replaced routine axillary node dissection to reduce unnecessary surgery and its attendant morbidity. Increasingly, axillary lymph nodes are assessed preoperatively by ultrasound of the ipsilateral axilla at the same time as performing CB of a suspicious breast lesion. This practice is now recommended in NICE guidelines and allows patients found to have metastatic disease on needle biopsy to proceed directly to axillary node dissection without initial sentinel lymph node biopsy (9). Superior diagnostic performance of CB or FNAC in the axilla is much less clear cut than in the breast and literature reports similar accuracy using either technique (13). The sensitivity of preoperative axillary staging is related to the proportion of node-positive patients in the population being evaluated. Emphasis should be placed on the ultrasound evaluation of axillary nodes and morphological criteria employed when assessing the need for needle biopsy. Size and morphology of the nodes have been shown to be important with cortical thickening the most consistently

important morphological criterion in determining the likelihood of malignancy. The decision whether to use FNAC or CB in the axilla ultimately rests within each unit and depends upon the level of expertise available.

The place for preoperative axillary node sampling in the routine workup of suspected breast cancer will undoubtedly change but at the present time it remains an important part of modern triple assessment (47).

CONCLUSION
In a breast care program, it is imperative to maximize the accurate diagnosis of malignancy while keeping the number of benign surgical breast biopsies to a minimum. This is achieved by accurate evaluation of potential breast abnormalities using triple assessment incorporating clinical, imaging, and histological evaluation with CB as the mainstay of modern breast diagnosis. There should be correlation between all aspects and any discrepancies discussed in a multidisciplinary setting. Further imaging and sampling techniques should be employed as appropriate to achieve a definitive diagnosis. Meticulous technique and multidisciplinary team working will result in a highly accurate diagnostic service that is essential for safe patient care.

REFERENCES
1. Surgical guidelines for the management of breast cancer. Association of Breast Surgery at BASO 2009. Eur J Surg Oncol 2009; 35: 1–22.
2. Britton PD, Goud A, Godward S, et al. Use of ultrasound-guided axillary node core biopsy in staging of early breast cancer. EurRadiol 2009; 19: 561–9.
3. Azavedo E, Svane G, Auer G. Stereotactic fine-needle biopsy in 2594 mammographically detected non-palpable lesions. Lancet 1989; 1: 1033–6.
4. Parker SH, Lovin JD, Jobe WE, et al. Stereotactic breast biopsy with a biopsy gun. Radiology 1990; 176: 741–7.
5. Parker SH, Jobe WE, Dennis MA, et al. US-guided automated large-core breast biopsy. Radiology 1993; 187: 507–11.
6. Parker SH, Burbank F, Jackman RJ, et al. Percutaneous large-core breast biopsy: a multi-institutional study. Radiology 1994; 193: 359–64.
7. An audit of screen detected breast cancer for the year of screening April 2008 to March 2009. NHS Breast Screening Programme and Association of Breast Surgery at BASO 2009.
8. Clinical Guidelines for Breast Screening Assessment. NHS Cancer Screening Programmes 3rd edn. NHSBSP Publication No 49, 2010.
9. National Institute for Health and Clinical Excellence. CG80 early and locally advanced breast cancer, full guideline. 2009. [Available from: http://www.nice.org.uk/guidance/index.jsp?action=byid &o=12132].
10. van Rijk MC, Deurloo EE, Nieweg OE, et al. Ultrasonography and fine-needle aspiration cytology can spare breast cancer patients unnecessary sentinel lymph node biopsy. Ann Surg Oncol 2005; 13: 31–5.
11. Bonnema J, van Geel AN, van Ooijen B, et al. Ultrasound-guided aspiration biopsy for detection of nonpalpable axillary node metastases in breast cancer patients: new diagnostic method. World J Surg 1997; 21: 270–4.
12. Damera A, Evans AJ, Cornford EJ, et al. Diagnosis of axillary nodal metastases by ultrasound-guided core biopsy in primary operable breast cancer. Br J Cancer 2003; 89: 1310–13.
13. Houssami N, Ciatto S, Turner R, et al. Preoperative ultrasound-guided needle biopsy of axillary nodes in invasive breast cancer: meta-analysis of its accuracy and utility in staging the axilla. Ann Surg 2011; 2: 243–51.
14. Al-Attar MA, Michell MJ, Ralleigh G, et al. The impact of image guided needle biopsy on the outcome of mammographically detected indeterminate microcalcification. Breast 2006; 15: 635–9.
15. Harvey J, Moran R, DeAngelis G. Technique and pitfalls of ultrasound-guided core-needle biopsy of the breast. Semin Ultrasound CTMR 2000; 21: 362–74.
16. Ciatto S, Houssami N, Ambrogetti D, et al. Accuracy and underestimation of malignancy of breast core needle biopsy: the florence experience of over 4000 consecutive biopsies. Breast Cancer Res Treat 2007; 101: 291–7.

17. Liberman L. Clinical management issues in percutaneous core breast biopsy. Radiol Clin North Am 2000; 38: 791–807.

18. Nath M, Robinson T, Tobon H, et al. Automated large core needle biopsy of surgically removed breast lesions : comparison of samples obtained with 14, 16 and 18 gauge needles. Radiology 1995; 197: 739–42.

19. Margolin F, Leung J, Jacobs R, et al. Percutaneous image-guided core breast biopsy: 5 yrs experience in a community hospital. Am J Roentgenol 2001; 177: 559–64.

20. Sittek H, Schneider P, Perlet C, et al. Minimally invasive surgical procedures of the breast: comparison of different biopsy systems in a breast parenchymal model. Radiologe 2002; 42: 6–10.

21. Britton P, McCann MJ. Needle biopsy in the NHS breast screening programme 1996/97: how much and how accurate? Breast 1999; 8: 5–11.

22. Kuo YL, Chang T. Can concurrent core biopsy and fine needle aspiration biopsy improve the false negative rate of sonographically detectable breast lesions? BMC Cancer 2010; 10: 371.

23. Kettritz U, Rotter K, Schreer I, et al. Stereotactic vacuum-assisted breast biopsy in 2874 patients: a multicenter study. Cancer 2004; 100: 245–51.

24. Orel SG, Rosen M, Mies C, et al. MR imaging–guided 9-gauge vacuum-assisted core needle breast biopsy: initial experience. Radiology 2006; 238: 54–61.

25. Heywang-Köbrunner SH, Sinnatamby R, Lebeau A, et al. Interdisciplinary consensus on the uses and technique of MR-guided vacuum-assisted breast biopsy (VAB): results of a European consensus meeting. Eur J Radiol 2009; 72: 289–94.

26. Maxwell AJ, Ridley NT, Rubin G, et al. The royal college of radiologists breast group breast imaging classification. Clin Radiol 2009; 64: 624–7.

27. Taylor K, Britton P, O'Keeffe S, et al. Quantification of the UK 5-point breast imaging classification and mapping to BI-RADS to facilitate comparison with international literature. Br J Radiol 2011; 84: 1005–10.

28. Crystal P, Koretz M, Shcharynsky S, et al. Accuracy of sonographically guided 14-gauge core-needle biopsy: results of 715 consecutive breast biopsies with at least two-year follow-up of benign lesions. J Clin Ultrasound 2005; 33: 47–52.

29. Smith GEC, Burrows P. Ultrasound diagnosis of fibroadenoma – is biopsy always necessary? Clin Radiol 2008; 63: 511e5.

30. Weiss CR, Nour SG, Lewin JS. MR-guided biopsy: a review of current techniques and applications. J Magn Reson Imaging 2008; 27: 311–25.

31. Schneider E, Rohling KW, Schnall MD, et al. An apparatus for MR-guided breast lesion localization and core biopsy: design and preliminary results. J Magn Reson Imaging 2001; 14: 243–53.

32. Cawson J, Malara F, Kavanagh A, et al. 14-gauge needle core biopsy of mammographically evident radial scars: is excision necessary? Cancer 2003; 97: 345–51.

33. Brenner R, Jackman R, Parker S, et al. Percutaneous core needle biopsy of radial scars of the breast: when is excision necessary? Am J Roentgenol 2002; 179: 1179–84.

34. Pinder SE, Ellis IO. The diagnosis and management of pre invasive breast disease: ductal carcinoma in situ (DCIS) and atypical ductal hyperplasia (ADH) – current definitions and classification. Breast Cancer Res 2003; 5: 254–7.

35. Houssami N, Ciatto S, Ellis I, et al. Underestimation of malignancy of breast core needle biopsy: concepts and precise overall and category-specific estimates. Cancer 2007; 109: 487–95.

36. Rizzo M, Lund MJ, Oprea G, et al. Surgical follow-up and clinical presentation of 142 breast papillary lesions diagnosed by ultrasound-guided core-needle biopsy. Ann Surg Oncol 2008; 15: 1040–7.

37. Agoff SN, Lawton TJ. Papillary lesions of the breast with and without atypical ductal hyperplasia: can we accurately predict benign behaviour from needle core biopsy? Am J Clin Pathol 2004; 122: 440–3.

38. National Health Service Breast Screening Programme. Annual Review. Sheffield: NHSBSP publications, 2011.

39. Veldkamp W, Karssemeijer N, Otten J, Hendricks J. Automated classification of clustered microcalcifications into malignant and benign types. Med Phys 2000; 27: 2600–8.

40. Yang W, Tse G. Sonographic, Mammographic, and histopathologic correlation of symptomatic ductal carcinoma in situ. Am J Roentgenol 2004; 182: 101–10.

41. Brem RF, Schoonjans JM, Sanow L, et al. Reliability of histologic diagnosis of breast cancer with stereotactic vacuum-assisted biopsy. Am Surg 2001; 67: 388–92.

42. Jackman RJ, Burbank F, Parker SH, et al. Stereotactic breast biopsy of nonpalpable lesions: determinants of ductal carcinoma in situ underestimation rates. Radiology 2001; 218: 497–502.

43. Darling ML, Smith DN, Lester SC, et al. Atypical ductal hyperplasia and ductal carcinoma in situ as revealed by large-core needle breast biopsy: results of surgical excision. Am J Roentgenol 2000; 175: 1341–6.

44. Meyer JE, Smith DN, DiPiro PJ, et al. Stereotactic breast biopsy of clustered microcalcifications with a directional, vacuum-assisted device. Radiology 1997; 204: 575–6.

45. Rakha EA, Ellis IO. An overview of assessment of prognostic and predictive factors in breast cancer needle core biopsy specimens. J Clin Pathol 2007; 60: 1300–6.

46. Astall EC, Bobrow LG. Assessment of the accuracy of diagnostic and prognostic information provided by core biopsy in breast cancer. J Pathol 1998; 186: 6.

47. Giuliano AE, Hunt KK, Ballman KV, et al. Axillary dissection vs no axillary dissection in women with invasive breast cancer and sentinel node metastasis: a randomized clinical trial. J Am Med Assoc 2011; 305: 569–75.

23 Vacuum-assisted breast biopsy

Thomas Conner and William Teh

INTRODUCTION

Vacuum-assisted biopsy (VAB) is a wide bore percutaneous needle biopsy device that has been developed to allow larger volumes of tissue to be obtained with vacuum assistance. The ability to obtain larger volumes of tissue under image guidance allows greater accuracy by reducing sampling error and the chance of "underdiagnosis." The use of vacuum assistance also allows for the possibility of therapeutic intervention in the breast which is precluded with conventional spring-loaded biopsy devices.

PRINCIPLES OF PREOPERATIVE NEEDLE BIOPSY

Mammography has been used as the initial imaging investigation in the United Kingdom (UK) NHS Breast Screening Programme since its introduction in the late 1980s. This modality was shown to have a high sensitivity for detection of cancer but a much lower specificity (1–4). However, use of the triple assessment principle (clinical examination, imaging, and tissue sampling) has increased overall diagnostic accuracy with a low incidence of false-negative cases.

A high proportion of definitive tissue diagnosis was originally performed by open surgical techniques following wire localization. This inevitably is associated with a relatively high rate of unnecessary benign surgical excisions with consequent physical and psychological morbidity (5). Improvements in breast imaging as an interventional and diagnostic tool together with advances in percutaneous biopsy techniques have led to a gradual increase in preoperative image-guided tissue diagnosis. The audit data of the UK NHS Breast Screening Programme from 2009 to 2010 show that 96% of cancers detected were diagnosed non-operatively compared with 63% in 1996–1997 and 49% in 1994–1995. The malignant open biopsy rate has also significantly decreased to 0.35 per 1000 women in 2009–2010 compared to 2.04 per 1000 women in 1996–1997 (6).

There are multifold advantages from an accurate preoperative tissue diagnosis of malignancy. In particular, it allows for a planned definitive therapeutic operation rather than an initial diagnostic surgical excision followed by a second procedure in a proportion of patients to obtain clear surgical margins involving either re-excision of the tumor bed or completion mastectomy. The ability to diagnose invasive cancer preoperatively helps the surgeon to determine those patients who require sentinel lymph node biopsy. Additionally, if a diagnosis of lobular cancer is made on a core biopsy, then a preoperative MRI is usually recommended to determine the multifocal disease or clarify the extent of disease which can be difficult to assess accurately using mammography and ultrasound. A preoperative tissue diagnosis may thus reduce the number of surgical episodes which in turn will minimize both morbidity and cost. The effect of increased preoperative diagnosis on repeat operation rates in the UK Breast Screening Programme was examined in a publication by Wallis and colleagues (7). In 2000–2001 when the non-operative diagnosis was only 87% the number of women requiring more than one operation was 24%. This contrasts with a preoperative diagnosis of 94% in 2005–2006 when 18% of women required more than one operation. Using a linear model to extrapolate data back to 1994–1995 when the pre-operative diagnosis rate was 49%, it was estimated that 58% of women would have had more than one operation. A further advantage of a preoperative tissue diagnosis is that hormonal and biological markers such as estrogen receptor, progesterone receptor, and HER2 can be determined from the needle biopsy specimens, together with histological grade. These factors are crucial in the early planning of medical therapies in either the neoadjuvant or adjuvant setting. A comprehensive surgical and medical treatment strategy for the patient can thus be planned at a multidisciplinary meeting following which a clear decision-making process can be undertaken with the patient at an early stage.

METHODS OF OBTAINING PREOPERATIVE DIAGNOSIS

Fine needle aspiration cytology (FNAC) was the conventional image-guided sampling technique employed at the start of the UK Breast Screening Programme and has the advantages of being inexpensive, quick, and relatively less traumatic to tissues. Nonetheless, it has several disadvantages in terms of assessment of malignant lesions, and cannot distinguish between invasive and non-invasive disease. Furthermore, FNAC is less reliable for the diagnosis of invasive lobular cancer and cannot readily provide important information on hormone receptor status of the tumor. Additionally, FNAC is associated with a variable rate of inadequate sampling for reliable analysis which ranges from 8.5% to 46% (8,9). This leads to a high rate of follow-up as well as diagnostic excisional surgery with a resultant low rate of accurate preoperative diagnosis.

Core biopsy techniques were developed in the 1990s to obtain larger tissue samples suitable for histological examination. Their use for breast sampling was popularized following a seminal publication on its application in the breast in 1991 (10). A histological, rather than a cytological, diagnosis reduced the number of insufficient samples for analysis and provided information on tumor pathology including grade and receptor status. Biopsies are obtained using a spring-loaded system available in a range of different sized needles which can be suited to local practice, though 14-gauge needles are the most commonly used with 16-gauge needles sometimes being used for women with a denser glandular tissue. The mean false-negative rate of breast core biopsy has been reported to be as low as 0.4 % from assessment of 3380 biopsies (11) in comparison with a mean false-negative rate of 2.5% from assessment of 280 needle localized open surgical biopsies of impalpable lesions (12).

Core biopsy has now replaced fine needle aspiration as the percutaneous biopsy technique of choice for assessment of breast lesions. Moreover, it is the introduction of core biopsy which has led to the dramatic improvement in preoperative diagnosis over the past 20 years. Fine needle aspiration continues to be used in many centers as a first-line imaging-guided technique for biopsy of axillary lymph nodes.

Core biopsy as a preoperative assessment tool has its limitations; underestimation of disease extent with respect to micro-calcifications or asymmetric densities is well reported. Histological underestimation is also reported in high-risk lesions such as phyllodes tumors, atypical ductal hyperplasia (ADH), lobular carcinoma in situ (LCIS), radial scars, and papillary lesions. In a retrospective study of 1352 cases by Schueller et al. (13) ADH on core biopsy was reported as being associated with either invasive or non-invasive cancer in 39.7% of cases at surgical excision, while a finding of ductal carcinoma in situ (DCIS) on core biopsy was associated with a histological upgrade to invasive cancer at open surgery in 36.5% of cases. The tendency of core biopsy to underestimate the true extent of malignant disease in the assessment of high-risk lesions has led to a low threshold for repeat biopsy and/or surgical diagnostic excision if there remains uncertainty as to whether adequate sampling has been obtained. The aim of improving preoperative diagnostic accuracy has led to the development of VAB techniques.

PRINCIPLE OF MAMMOTOMY/VACUUM-ASSISTED BIOPSY

Mammotomy or a VAB system was developed to obtain a larger volume of biopsy tissue to help reduce the problems of underestimation. The first vacuum-assisted device (VAD) for biopsy was the Mammotome which became available in 1995. This utilizes the suction technique to allow multiple contiguous samples to be taken during a single needle insertion. Once the sampling aperture is open, the vacuum draws tissue into the aperture which is excised by the rotating cutter. Vacuum is used to transport the tissue to the specimen chamber for retrieval, without removing the needle from the biopsy site (Fig. 23.1). This results in a technique to remove a larger volume of tissue through a relatively small incision in the skin.

A number of different-gauge needles are available, but generally a VAD has a size range of 10–12 gauges that is commonly used for diagnostic biopsies, whereas larger 7- to 9-gauge needles are used for therapeutic biopsies. The use of vacuum has the advantage that an adjacent tissue can be sampled and up to 2 cm of the surrounding breast tissue can be fully excised without repositioning the needle. The needle of the vacuum biopsy system can be positioned adjacent to the target lesion, thereby allowing biopsy of breast lesions that are not easily accessible due to their anatomical position (e.g., adjacent to chest wall). Vacuum devices also permit sampling of larger tissue volumes which enable a more accurate histological assessment to be made by minimizing sampling errors due to more tissue being obtained for analysis (14–16). Evidence shows that the number of preoperative VAB sample upgrades to malignancy from high-risk lesions such as ADH and papillary lesions were significantly lower for VAD compared with a standard image-guided core biopsy (17–24). In particular, for

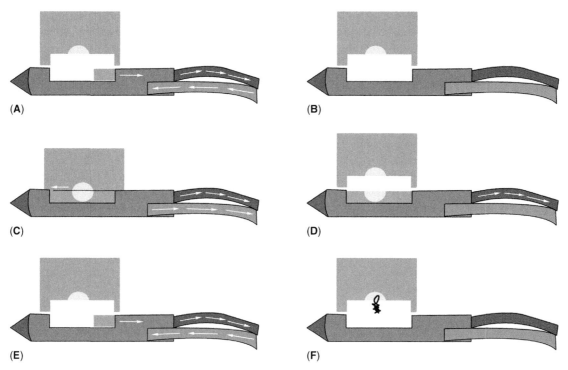

Figure 23.1 Basic principles of a vacuum biopsy device. (**A**) Position probe under lesion. (**B**) Vacuum tissue into aperture. (**C**) Transect tissue. (**D**) Trans-section completed. (**E**) Transport tissue and repeat as necessary. (**F**) Insert marker clip.

microcalcifications, the resultant higher calcification retrieval rate increases the chance of a more definitive diagnosis, especially when all mammographically visible microcalcification has been excised (18,25–28). Other advantages of VAD include fewer targeting errors and facilitation of marker clip placement. Sampling errors are reduced compared with standard 14-gauge ultrasound core biopsy with false-negative rates of 0.6–5.2% cited for ultrasound-guided VAB (29–32).

VAB techniques have been adapted for use as a method for excision of benign lesions and share common benefits of minimally invasive techniques over conventional open surgery including decreased morbidity, better cosmetic results, a shorter recovery time, and a shorter hospital stay. Their use for removal of benign breast lesions such as fibroadenomas has been supported by the UK National Institute of Clinical Excellence. Removal of these benign lesions by VAB techniques achieves varying degrees of complete resection ranging between 22% and 98%, depending on the size of lesion, the gauge of the probe, and the quality of imaging used (33). VAB techniques may also be used as an alternative to surgical duct excision in the management of single duct discharge (34) and as a minimally invasive technique to excise gynecomastia (35). Vacuum-assisted excision of benign breast lesions have higher levels of patient acceptance and satisfaction and are more cost effective with minimal complications compared with surgical excisions (36). A recent study suggests that less pain was experienced with the use of an 11-gauge hand-held VAB device, compared with an automated 14-gauge core needle biopsy (37).

COMPARISON OF DIFFERENT VACUUM-ASSISTED BIOPSY DEVICES

The first VAD to be developed was the Mammotome™ (Devicor Medical Products, Inc., Cincinnati, Ohio, USA) in 1995 which has subsequently been followed by other VADs (38). These included portable devices such as the Vacora™ (Bard Biopsy Systems, Tempe, Arizona, USA) which have to be inserted each time a biopsy is performed and has limited self-contained vacuum. A more recent portable device, the Finesse™ (Bard Biopsy Systems) has a sample retrieval system which necessitates only a single insertion of the VAD. Other devices are available and include the Atec™ (Hologic, Inc. Bedford, Massachusetts, USA), Eviva™ (Hologic, Inc.), and EnCor™ (Bard Biopsy Systems) and the main technical differences among these are outlined in Table 23.1. These devices have been developed to be used in conjunction with a range of imaging modalities dependent on a specific manufacture. Of particular interest is the development of "closed" tissue collection systems. Earlier systems required each individual core biopsy to be manually removed after biopsy. However, with the development of a closed system the biopsy cores can be collected in a mesh-like container and removed en-masse after multiple biopsies have been taken which allows for a quicker sampling time. Also of note is that certain systems have a lavage system which can help reduce hematoma formation. These lavage systems allow additional top-up doses of local anesthetic without needle reinsertion. Some of the different vacuum biopsy systems available are shown in figure 23.2.

Table 23.1 Comparison of Vacuum-Assisted Mammotomy Devices

Attributes	Mammotome™ (Devicor)	Finesse™ (Bard)	Vacora™ (Bard)	Atec™ (Hologic)	Eviva™ (Hologic)	Senorx™ (EnCor)
Compatibility	US, stereotactic and MRI (specific compatible driver required)	US	US, stereotactic	US, stereotactic and MRI	Stereotactic	US, stereotactic and MRI
Probe offset	Yes	No	Yes	No	Yes	Yes
Needle gauge	11 and 8	14 and 10	14 and 10	12 and 9	12 and 9	10 and 7
Manual vacuum control	Yes	No	No	Yes	Yes	Yes
Multiple core retrieval	Yes	Yes	No	Yes	Yes	Yes
Cutting method	Rotating	Rotating	Rotating	Rotating	Rotating	Scissor
Volume of tissue per minute	++	+	+	++	++	++
Open or closed tissue collection	Open	Closed	Open	Closed	Closed	Closed
Speed of tissue removal	++	++	+	+++	+++	+++
Needle rotation	Manual	Manual	Manual	Manual	Manual	Manual or automated
Lavage	No	No	No	Full	Full	Sample chamber
Programmable functions	Yes	No	No	No	No	Yes
Biopsy site marker insertion	Yes	Yes	No	Yes	Yes	Yes
Local anesthetic function	Not dedicated	No	No	Yes	Yes	Yes

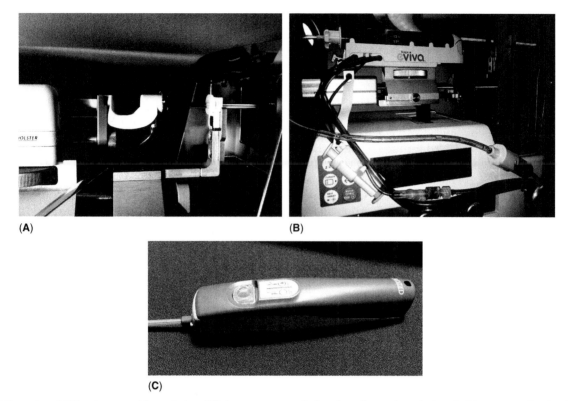

Figure 23.2 Examples of different vacuum biopsy devices. (A) An open vacuum device where the specimen is deposited in an open chamber for retrieval. (B) A "closed system" where irrigation with saline occurs and tissue is collected in a collection basket and retrieved en masse. (C) A portable single insertion hand-held device used under ultrasound guidance.

CURRENT INDICATIONS

VADs can be used for either diagnostic or therapeutic purposes and tissue is acquired under ultrasound, stereotactic, or magnetic resonance imaging (MRI) guidance.

Diagnostic

- Microcalcifications: Usually performed under stereotactic guidance though high-resolution ultrasound enables ultrasound-guided VAB when sonographically visualized.
- High-risk lesions (diagnosed on core biopsy): Including ADH, epithelial proliferation with or without atypia, lobular neoplasia, papillary lesions, papillomas, radial scars, phyllodes lesions and complex sclerosing lesions (39). Where ADH is diagnosed on 14-gauge core biopsy, upgrade to malignancy after surgical excision, occurs in 40–50% of cases and is reduced to 20–25% with mammotomy (40,41).
- Suspicious enhancing lesions on MRI (morphologically suspicious or type 2/3 enhancing lesions).
- Small sonographically visible lesions when ultrasound-guided core biopsy may be difficult (42).
- Ultrasound occult mammographic abnormalities (42).

Therapeutic (43)

- Excision of benign breast lesions, for example, fibroadenomas. These procedures are usually performed under ultrasound guidance (43–46).
- Irrigation and drainage of breast abscesses and seromas resistant to conventional needle aspiration.

CONTRAINDICATIONS

There are no absolute contraindications to VAB techniques. Relative contraindications include current use of anticoagulants (especially warfarin) and low-molecular-weight heparin preparations (clopidogrel).

ANESTHESIA

The procedure is performed using a local anesthetic, which is usually 2% lidocaine for subdermal injection (maximum of 4 mg/kg) and 2% lidocaine with 1 in 100,000 epinephrine (adrenaline), for deeper infiltration (maximum of 7 mg/kg). The addition of epinephrine reduces bleeding by causing vasoconstriction but must not be used for more superficial lesions due to the risk of skin necrosis.

EQUIPMENT

- Vacuum device: Hand held or mounted depending on the imaging modality.
- Ultrasound: High-frequency linear array transducer >7.5 MHz.
- Magnetic Resonance (MR): MR localizer and biopsy coil. MR-compatible consumables and vacuum drivers. This can be used with or without dedicated computer-aided detection workstations.
- Stereotactic: Upright, recumbent, or prone positions with a digital stereotactic device.
- Other consumables and local anesthetic: 25-gauge (orange), 23-gauge (blue) needles and 5 mL syringe for 1–2% lidocaine.
  - A 21-gauge (green) needle and 10 mL syringe for 1 in 100,000 epinephrine (adrenaline)

- ○ Spinal needle if it is a deep lesion
- ○ Scalpel
- ○ Chlorhexidine
- ○ Gauze squares
- ○ Probe cover
- ○ Sterile drapes
- ○ Sterile gloves
- ○ Specimen pot
- ○ Marker clip

POSITIONING

- Ultrasound-guided procedures: For lateral lesions the patient should be positioned in the oblique supine turning to the opposite side with the ipsilateral arm overhead. For medially placed lesions, the patient can be positioned supine.
- Stereotactic procedures:
  - ○ Upright or recumbent position—with or without lateral arm dedicated chair or couch.
  - ○ Prone position—dedicated prone table.
  - ○ MR-guided procedures: Prone position.

TECHNIQUE

Written informed consent is obtained. Common complications are bleeding and bruising though patients should also be informed about risks of infection, post-procedure pain/discomfort, and allergy to local anesthetic. The patient should also be aware that surgery may be required on the rare occasion when bleeding is excessive and hemostasis cannot be achieved. For those patients with a prosthesis the risk of implant rupture should also be mentioned. As for any procedure involving needle biopsy of the breast, pneumothorax is a potential complication. Where a fibroadenoma is being excised, incomplete removal of the lesion can occur. The diagnostic benefits of VAB include a more accurate preoperative histological label, which may obviate the need for diagnostic surgery or enable definitive therapeutic surgery to be done at the outset. Symptomatic benefits include excision of any palpable benign mass (e.g., fibroadenoma and gynecomastia) or relief of pain associated with breast abscesses or seromas without the need for surgical intervention. The patient should also be consented for insertion of a marker clip following a VAB procedure which is diagnostic and may be followed by surgical excision.

The patient is positioned as mentioned earlier and the procedure is performed with an aseptic technique. The skin is cleaned with chlorhexidine solution and the area is appropriately draped. Five milliliter of 1–2% lidocaine is injected to form a subdermal bleb and then infiltrated deeper toward the lesion. Approximately 10 mL of lidocaine and epinephrine (adrenaline) is then infiltrated deeply around the lesion. For ultrasound-guided procedures, if the lesion is close to the chest wall, then the local anesthetic can be infiltrated deep to the lesion to elevate it from the chest wall and similarly if the lesion is close to the skin, local anesthetic (without adrenaline) infiltrated superficially between the lesion and skin to create a safe zone. Sterile saline can be used in addition should a larger volume be required. A small (5–10 mm) incision is made in the skin and the probe inserted. The probe should be positioned along the posterior/deep margin of the lesion in ultrasound procedures.

Ensure that the tip of the needle is beyond the lesion so that the trough encompasses the lesion. Sampling then starts with the rotation of the needle to ensure the entire lesion is excised. If microcalcification is being biopsied, specimen radiography must be undertaken to ensure that there is representative calcification present in the samples (Fig. 23.3). A marker clip is inserted at the end of the procedure.

The vacuum component can be used to suction blood out of the biopsy cavity during and after the procedure. Post procedure, sustained pressure is applied for about 10–15 minutes over the biopsy area and not the skin incision to reduce hematoma formation. Once hemostasis is achieved, adhesive strips are applied to the incision and a sterile dressing applied. A pressure dressing may be required if the wound is still oozing. Written after-care instructions are given regarding wound care and pain relief and patients are advised to avoid strenuous exercise. Aspirin and ibuprofen should be avoided as they may increase bruising. Ice packs can also be used to reduce post-procedure swelling. Advice about signs of infection and a possible expanding hematoma should also be included.

COMPLICATIONS

Significant bleeding occurs in between 1% and 3.9% of cases (24,47). Hematoma formation is the main complication and may require an open surgical procedure to achieve hemostasis and evacuate any hematoma. Infection is rare, with reported rates of 0.01% (24). Recurrence of benign lesions, such as fibroadenomas and papillomas following VAD excision, has been reported as 15%. However, fibroadenomas in all these studies were larger than 2 cm at presentation (48,49). Another potential complication is clip migration which has been reported to be as high as 20% with stereotactic procedures (50).

CONCORDANCE OF BIOPSY OUTCOMES

Though VAB procedures have been reported to significantly reduce the number of cases with underestimation of malignant disease and to improve the accuracy of preoperative diagnosis, careful correlation between VAB pathology results and radiology is required. For microcalcifications, it is mandatory to ensure that there is adequate and representative calcification retrieved using specimen radiography. Where ADH is diagnosed on vacuum biopsy, the presence of residual microcalcification is associated with an upgrade rate to malignancy in 20% of cases compared with a rate of between 1.6% and 3% when there is no residual microcalcification or at least 95% has been removed (51,52). The presence of significant cytological atypia on vacuum biopsy also significantly correlates with the presence of malignancy and therefore should prompt a recommendation for surgical excision. It has recently been suggested that flat epithelial atypia or ADH in conjunction with complete excision of microcalcification by vacuum biopsy may be managed conservatively by surveillance mammography (51–53). There are variable reports on rates of upgrade to malignancy associated with LCIS or atypical lobular hyperplasia on vacuum biopsy ranging from 17 to 33% (53–56). In view of these figures, surgical excision should be undertaken for the majority of these lobular neoplastic (LCIS or atypical lobular hyperplasia) lesions.

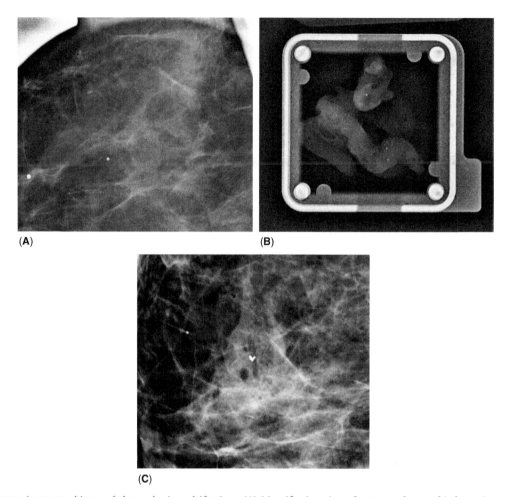

(A)   (B)

(C)

Figure 23.3 A stereotactic vacuum biopsy of clustered microcalcifications. (A) Magnification view of a 4 mm cluster of indeterminate microcalcifications. (B) Specimen radiograph of retrieved samples showing representative microcalcification. (C) Post-biopsy mammogram showing a marker clip in situ and no residual microcalcification.

CONCLUSION

As a diagnostic tool, VADs have proven to be a useful adjunct in the assessment of breast lesions by improving the rate of preoperative diagnosis of malignant lesions secondary to more tissue being sampled percutaneously. It can also be utilized effectively as an alternative to diagnostic surgery and can permit ultimate conservative management of some high-risk lesions. Radiological–pathological concordance is essential and a multidisciplinary team discussion of vacuum biopsy results is essential for management of these borderline-type lesions. New vacuum devices are also effective in offering a minimally invasive approach for the excision of benign lesions such as fibroadenomas as well as effective treatment of complex breast abscesses and seromas.

REFERENCES

1. Harvey JA, Fajardo LL, Innis CA. Previous mammograms in patients with impalpable breast carcinoma: retrospective vs. blinded interpretation. AJR Am J Roentgenol 1993; 161: 1167–72.
2. Linden SS, Sickles EA. Sedimented calcium in benign breast cysts: the full spectrum of mammographic presentations. AJR Am J Roentgenol 1989; 152: 967–71.
3. Sickles EA. Mammographic features of "early" breast cancer. AJR Am J Roentgenol 1984; 143: 461–4.
4. Heywang-Kobrunner SH, Schreer I, Dershaw DD. Diagnostic Breast Imaging. Stuttgart: Thieme, 1997: 209–20.
5. Cowley G, Rosenburg D. A needle instead of a knife. Newsweek 1992; 119: 62.
6. NHS. [Available from: http://www.cancerscreening.nhs.uk/breastscreen/publications/baso2009-2010.pdf].
7. Wallis MG, Cheung S, Kearins O, Lawrence GM. Non-operative diagnosis – effect on repeat-operation rates in the UK breast screening programme. Eur Radiol 2009; 19: 318–23.
8. Pisano ED, Fajardo LL, Tsimikas J, et al. Rate of insufficient samples for fine needle aspiration for nonpalpable breast lesions in a multicenter clinical trial: the radiologic diagnostic oncology group 5 study. Cancer 1998; 82: 678–88.
9. Perry NM. Quality assurance in the diagnosis of breast disease. EUSOMA working party. Eur J Cancer 2001; 37: 159–219.
10. Parker SH, Jobe WE, Dennis MA, et al. Ultrasound guided automated large-core breast biopsy. Radiology 1991; 180: 403–7.
11. Pijnappel RM, van den Donk M, Holland E, et al. Diagnostic accuracy for different strategies of image guided breast intervention in cases of non-palpable breast lesions. Br J Cancer 2004; 90: 595–600.
12. Jackman RJ, Marzoni FA Jr. Needle-localised breast biopsy: why do we fail? Radiology 1997; 204: 677–84.
13. Schuller G, Jaromi S, Ponhold L, et al. US-guided 14 gauge core-needle breast biopsy: results of a validation study in 1352 cases. Radiology 2008; 248: 406–13.
14. Kettritz U, Rotter K, Schreer I, et al. Stereotactic vacuum-assisted breast biopsy in 2874 patients. a multicenter study. Cancer 2004; 100: 245–51.
15. Jackman RJ, Marzoni FA, Rosenberg J. False-negative diagnoses at stereotactic vacuum-assisted needle breast biopsy: long-term follow-up of 1,280 lesions and review of the literature. AJR Am J Roentgenol 2009; 192: 341–51.
16. Jackman RJ, Rodriguez-Soto J. Breast microcalcifications: retrieval failure at prone stereotactic core and vacuum breast biopsy—frequency, causes, and outcome. Radiology 2006; 239: 61–70.

17. Kim MJ, Kim SI, Youk JH, et al. The diagnosis of non-malignant papillary lesions of the breast: comparison of ultrasound-guided automated gun biopsy and vacuum-assisted removal. Clin Radiol 2011; 66: 530–5.

18. Meyer JE, Smith DN, DiPiro PJ, et al. Stereotactic breast biopsy of clustered microcalcifications with a directional, vacuum-assisted device. Radiology 1997; 204: 575–6.

19. Darling ML, Smith DN, Lester SC, et al. Atypical ductal hyperplasia and ductal carcinoma in situ as revealed by large-core needle breast biopsy: results of surgical excision. AJR Am J Roentgenol 2000; 175: 1341–446.

20. Harvey JM, Sterrett GF, Frost FA. Atypical ductal hyperplasia and atypia of uncertain significance in core biopsies from mammographically detected lesions: correlation with excision diagnosis. Pathology 2002; 34: 410–16.

21. Jackman RJ, Birdwell RL, Ikeda DM. Atypical ductal hyperplasia: can some lesions be defined as probably benign after stereotactic 11-gauge vacuum-assisted biopsy, eliminating the recommendation for surgical excision? Radiology 2002; 224: 548–54.

22. Rao A, Parker S, Ratzer E, Stephens J, Fenoglio M. Atypical ductal hyperplasia of the breast diagnosed by 11-gauge directional vacuum-assisted biopsy. Am J Surg 2002; 184: 534–7.

23. Darling ML, Smith DN, Lester SC, et al. Atypical ductal hyperplasia and ductal carcinoma in situ as revealed by large-core needle breast biopsy: results of surgical excision. AJR Am J Roentgenol 2000; 175: 1341–6.

24. Burbank F. Stereotactic breast biopsy: comparison of 14- and 11-gauge Mammotome probe performance and complication rate. Am Surg 1997; 63: 998–5.

25. Brennan ME, Turner RM, Ciatto S, et al. Ductal carcinoma in situ at core-needle biopsy: meta-analysis of underestimation and predictors of invasive breast cancer. Radiology 2011; 260: 199–28.

26. Liberman L, Giess CS, Dershaw DD, Deutch BM, Petrek JA. Imaging of pregnancy-associated breast cancer. Radiology 1994; 191: 245–8.

27. Philpotts LE, Shaheen NA, Carter D, Lange RC, Lee CH. Comparison of rebiopsy rates after stereotactic core needle biopsy of the breast 11-gauge vacuum suction probe versus 14-gauge needle and automatic gun. AJR Am J Roentgenol 1999; 172: 683–7.

28. Penco S, Rizzo S, Bozzini AC, et al. Stereotactic vacuum-assisted breast biopsy is not a therapeutic procedure even when all mammographically found calcifications are removed: analysis of 4,086 procedures. AJR Am J Roentgenol 2010; 195: 1255–60.

29. Pijnappel RM, van den Donk M, Holland R, et al. Diagnostic accuracy for different strategies of image-guided breast intervention in cases of non-palpable breast lesions. Br J Cancer 2004; 90: 595–600.

30. Simon JR, Kalbhen CL, Cooper RA, et al. Accuracy and complication rates of US-guided vacuum-assisted core biopsy: initial results. Radiology 2000; 215: 694–7.

31. Grady I, Gorsuch H, Wilburn-Bailey S. Ultrasound-guided, vacuum-assisted, percutaneous excision of breast lesions: an accurate technique in the diagnosis of atypical ductal hyperplasia. J Am Coll Surg 2005; 201: 14–17.

32. Cassano E, Urban LA, Pizzamiglio M, et al. Ultrasound-guided vacuum-assisted core breast biopsy: experience with 406 cases. Breast Cancer Res Treat 2007; 102: 103–10.

33. NHS. [Available from: http://www.nice.org.uk/nicemedia/live/11210/31511/31511.pdf].

34. Govindarajulu S, Narreddy SR, Shere MH, et al. Sonographically guided mammtome excision of ducts in the diagnosis and management of single duct nipple discharge. Eur J Surg Oncol 2006; 32: 725–8.

35. Qutob O, Elahi B, Garimella V, et al. Minimally invasive excision of gynaecomastia – a novel and effective surgical technique. Ann R Coll Surg Engl 2010; 92: 198–200.

36. Kim MJ, Kim EK, Lee JY, et al. Breast lesions with imaging-histologic discordance during US-guided 14 G automated core biopsy: can the directional vacuum-assisted removal replace the surgical excision? Initial findings. Eur Radiol 2007; 17: 2376–83.

37. Szynglarewicz B, Matkowski R, Kasprzak P, et al. Pain experienced by patients during minimal-invasive ultrasound-guided breast biopsy: Vacuum-assisted vs core-needle procedure. Eur J Surg Oncol 2011; 37: 398–403.

38. O'Flynn EAM, Wilson ARM, Michell MJ. Image-guided breast biopsy: state-of-the-art. Clin Radiol 2010; 65: 259–70.

39. Bianchi S, Caini S, Renne G, et al. On behalf of VANCB Study Group. Positive predictive value for malignancy on surgical excision of breast lesions of uncertain malignant potential (B3) diagnosed by stereotactic vacuum-assisted needle core biopsy (VANCB): a large multi-institutional study in Italy. Breast 2011; 20: 264–70.

40. Linda A, Zuiani C, Furlan A, et al. Radial scars without atypia diagnosed at imaging-guided needle biopsy: how often is associated malignancy found at subsequent surgical excision, and do mammography and sonography predict which lesions are malignant? AJR Am J Roentgenol 2010; 194: 1146–51.

41. Rajan S, Wason AM, Carder P. Conservative management of screen-detected radial scars: role of mammotome excision. J Clin Pathol 2011; 64: 65–8.

42. Heywang-Köbrunner SH, Heinig A, Hellerhoff K, Holzhausen HJ, Nährig J. Use of ultrasound-guided percutaneous vacuum-assisted breast biopsy for selected difficult indications. Breast J 2009; 15: 348–56.

43. Alonso-Bartolome P, Vega-Bolivar A, Torres-Tabanera M, et al. Sonographically guided 11-G directional vacuum-assisted breast biopsy as an alternative to surgical excision: utility and cost study in probably benign lesions. Acta Radiol 2004; 45: 390–6.

44. Slanetz PJ, Wu SP, Mendel JB. Percutaneous excision: a viable alternative to manage benign breast lesions. Can Assoc Radiol J 2011; 62: 265–71.

45. Mathew J, Crawford DJ, Lwin M, Barwick C, Gash A. Ultrasound-guided, vacuum-assisted excision in the diagnosis and treatment of clinically benign breast lesions. Ann R Coll Surg Engl 2007; 89: 494–6.

46. Sperber F, Blank A, Metser U, et al. Diagnosis and treatment of breast fibroadenomas by ultrasound-guided vacuum-assisted biopsy. Arch Surg 2003; 138: 796–800.

47. Parker SH, Klaus AJ. Performing breast biopsy with a directional, vacuum-assisted biopsy instrument. Radiographics 1997; 17: 1233–52.

48. Grady I, Gorsuch H, Wilburn-Bailey S. Long-term outcome of benign fibroadenomas treated by ultrasound-guided percutaneous excision. Breast 2008; 14: 275–8.

49. Bonaventure T, Cormier B, Lebas P, et al. Benign papilloma: is US-guided vacuum-assisted breast biopsy an alternative to surgical biopsy? J Radiol 2007; 88: 1165–8.

50. Chaveron C, Bachelle F, Fauquet I, et al. Clip migration after stereotactic macrobiopsy and presurgical localization: technical considerations and tricks. J Radiol 2009; 90: 31–6.

51. Villa A, Tagliafico A, Chiesa F, et al. Atypical ductal hyperplasia diagnosed at 11 gauge vacuum assisted breast biopsy performed on suspicious clustered microcalcifications: could patients without residual micro-calcification be managed conservatively? AJR Am J Roentgenol 2011; 197: 1012–18.

52. Nguyen CV, Albarracin CT, Whitma GJ, et al. Atypical ductal hyperplasia in directional vacuum-assisted biopsy of breast microcalcifications considerations for surgical excision. Ann Surg Oncol 2011; 18: 752–61.

53. Krishnamurthy S, Bevers T, Kuerer H, Yang WT. Multidisciplinary considerations in the management of hig risj breast lesions. AJR Am J Roentgenol 2012; 198: W132–40.

54. Brem RF, Lecher MC, Jackman MC, et al. Lobular neoplasia at percutaneous breast biopsy: variables associated with carcinoma at surgical excision. AJR Am J Roentgenol 2008; 190: 637–41.

55. Ibrahim N, Bessissow A, Lalonde L, et al. Surgical outcome of biopsy-proven lobular neoplasia: is there any difference between lobular carcinoma in situ and atypical lobular hyperplasia? AJR Am J Roentgenol 2012; 198: 288–91.

56. Destounis SV, Murphy PF, Seifert PJ. Management of patients diagnosed with lobular carcinoma in situ at needle core biopsy at a community-based outpatient facility. AJR Am J Roentgenol 2012; 198: 281–7.

24 Preoperative localization of impalpable breast lesions

Sabrina Rajan, Erika Denton, and Susan J. Barter

BACKGROUND

The National Health Service Breast Screening Programme (NHSBSP) has detected an increasing number of mammographic abnormalities including clustered microcalcifications, stromal deformities, and masses that are impalpable because of their nature, small size, or position within the breast. Following triple assessment, comprising clinical examination, imaging, and biopsy, a proportion of these lesions require surgical excision. Preoperative image-guided localization is used for diagnostic surgical biopsies where a larger volume of tissue is required to reach a definitive histopathological diagnosis and for therapeutic wide local excisions for treatment of clinically occult breast carcinomas.

Increasingly, neoadjuvant chemotherapy is used in patients with large, biologically aggressive, node-positive tumors. A proportion of these tumors show an excellent response to chemotherapy with almost no visible residual disease on final imaging. Unfortunately, this does not always correlate with a complete pathological response and patients still require local surgery to the tumor site. Such patients benefit from early marker clip placement to localize the site of the primary tumor. The clip then subsequently acts as a guide for localization prior to surgery if the tumor is no longer evident on imaging following neoadjuvant treatment.

Lesions should be localized using the imaging modality that best depicts the abnormality. Standard imaging techniques utilized for preoperative lesion localization include ultrasound and mammographic guidance. Specialist breast units also offer MRI-guided localization for lesions occult on conventional imaging. CT is not the primary imaging modality for breast disease and carries a significantly higher radiation dose. Although it is possible to perform CT-guided localization, this is not standard practice.

PURPOSE

Preoperative localization ensures that impalpable lesions are accurately identified enabling complete surgical excision with the required margin of surrounding breast tissue. The aim is to keep the volume of tissue removed to a minimum in order to reduce unnecessary breast deformity and ensure an optimal cosmetic result. The NHSBSP quality assurance standards for surgery stipulate that 90% of screen-detected cancers should be completely excised at first therapeutic operation and >80% of benign diagnostic biopsies should weigh <20 g (1). Localization methods have been continually updated and improved to meet and surpass these standards.

LOCALIZATION METHODS

Skin Marking

This method is best reserved for superficial lesions. The lesion is identified under ultrasound guidance with the patient in the supine position and the arm abducted to mimic the position in theater. An indelible marker pen is used to mark the skin directly overlying the lesion and a record is made of the depth of the lesion from the skin surface.

Needle and Wire Localization

Most of the lesions are deeper in the breast and require the use of an internal marker for localization. In 1976, Frank et al. (2) first proposed the use of a needle and hook wire for localization, and this method remains the most commonly used localization technique for impalpable lesions. In a series of 665 guide-wire localized biopsies, excision of the radiological lesion was achieved with a single procedure in 99% of cases. In only 4% of cases was repositioning of the wire required (3). The needle and wire system used varies between different manufacturers and different units, but the principles remain the same. For example, an Accura spring-hook wire has a thickened segment that begins 2 cm from the wire tip to act as a palpable landmark for the surgeon to gauge distance to the tip and therefore the lesion. Alternatively, the Reidy wire has an X-shaped hook that provides secure fixation and limits wire migration once deployed (Fig. 24.1).

Following infiltration of local anesthetic, the needle containing the wire is inserted under imaging guidance, proceeding along the shortest and most direct course toward the lesion (preferably with consideration of the position of the skin entry site in relation to the operative field). Once the needle tip is seen to traverse the lesion, the inner wire is advanced and the hook or other anchoring mechanism forms fixing the wire in the breast tissue (Fig. 24.1).

The NHSBSP quality assurance standards for surgery state that >95% of marker wires should be within 10 mm of the lesion in any plane (1). Abrahamson et al. reported that being within 5 mm of the lesion was a significant predictor of successful lesion removal (4). Gallagher et al. have suggested that being within 2 mm of the lesion allows accurate lesion retrieval combined with minimal volume of tissue excised (5). Jackman found that traversing the lesion in both mammographic planes was the factor most likely to lead to successful excisional surgery (6). In addition to traversing the lesion, the distance from the wire tip is also a consideration since a lesion traversed but with the tip well beyond the lesion may mislead the surgeon (7).

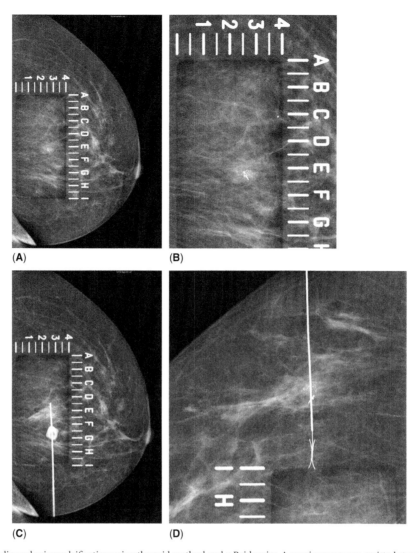

Figure 24.1 Localization of a clip and microcalcification using the grid method and a Reidy wire. A previous vacuum-assisted stereotactic biopsy of small cluster of microcalcification had shown high-grade ductal carcinoma in situ. A clip had been placed at the site of the microcalcification at the time of the procedure. (**A** and **B**) A craniocaudal (CC) and magnified CC view showing microcalcification and clip. (**C**) The introducer needle is deployed, and its position checked. (**D**) Following deployment of the localization wire a check view in the orthogonal plane confirms the Reidy wire transfixes the lesion.

Ideally, the tip of the wire should be placed approximately 1 cm beyond the lesion. This allows the lesion itself to act as an anchor ensuring the wire tip will not be inadvertently withdrawn proximal to the lesion following insertion and prior to surgery. The exposed end of the wire is gently taped to the skin with enough slack to allow the patient to move without displacing the wire. Check mammograms are performed in the craniocaudal and lateral positions to confirm that the correct area has been localized prior to surgery and to guide the surgical team (Fig. 24.2 B,C).

Traditionally, surgeons have followed the wire from its skin entry site down to the lesion and then removed a cylinder of tissue around the wire tip as indicated by the post-localization images. This ensures complete removal of the wire as well as the lesion. However, often the skin entry site of the wire lies some distance from the site of projection of the lesion on the skin, which can cause unnecessary trauma to tissue and less satisfactory cosmesis. This technique has been refined with the additional localization of the tip of the wire and lesion under ultrasound guidance. The patient is scanned in the surgical position, the skin mark is made directly over the lesion, and

the depth of the lesion from the skin surface is conveyed to the surgeon. This allows the surgical incision to be made over the site of the lesion; the wire is found in the subcutaneous tissue and brought into the incision allowing the surgeon to dissect down along the length of the wire to reach the lesion. This has been shown to increase the accuracy of lesion localization, reduce the weight of diagnostic biopsy specimens, and reduce operation time (8,9).

Wire localization of breast lesions is a safe technique that is well tolerated by patients, and severe complications are uncommon. Perception of pain varies between patients and a local anesthetic is routinely used prior to insertion of the needle through the skin. Bleeding is rarely a problem unless an artery is inadvertently punctured during localization; firm compression is usually sufficient to stop any bleeding. In dense breast tissue, the insertion and positioning of the wire can be difficult. Following wire insertion, displacement of the wire can occur during confirmatory mammograms or patient transfers. There have been reports of wire migration into the supraclavicular fossa and pleural space potentially causing a pneumothorax (10–12). The wire itself is fine and care must

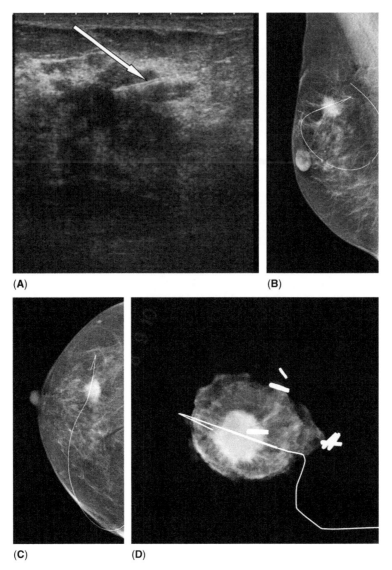

Figure 24.2 Ultrasound localization of a mass lesion. (**A**) Ultrasound image showing the introducer needle (arrow) traversing the mass. (**B** and **C**) Right lateral and craniocaudal views following deployment of the hook wire confirm the mass is transfixed. (**D**) A specimen radiograph of the same patient shows the mass lying in the center of the resection with the inferior margin appearing inadequate. This was communicated to the surgeon who performed a cavity shave inferiorly.

be taken to ensure that the wire is not transected during surgery, as guidance to the lesion is lost and foreign bodies can be left within the breast (13). Unsuccessful localization and excision are uncommon but reported to be more likely with microcalcifications, small lesions, two lesions per breast and small excision specimens (6).

Injection of Carbon Suspension

Carbon localization was first described by Svane (14) in 1983, and numerous studies have subsequently confirmed its advantages (15–18). In a consecutive case series of 511 procedures comparing carbon localization with hook-wire localization, Rose et al. demonstrated that carbon localization was an accurate alternative with better logistics and favorable costs (19). This technique involves the placement of a carbon tract (1–2 mL of sterile 4% carbon suspension), which stains the tissues black in color and does not diffuse into the surrounding tissues. The shortest track for best visibility and cosmesis is chosen, leaving a small skin tattoo.

Due to its inert nature, carbon localization can be performed at the time of initial needle core biopsy and still be safely used by the surgeons to locate the lesion days or weeks later. Therefore, the need for an additional localization immediately prior to surgery is eliminated, and patients are spared an additional invasive procedure. Importantly, as it is performed concurrently with core biopsy, carbon localization ensures that the biopsied lesion is correctly identified for the surgeon and pathologist. The main advantage for the pathologist is that the carbon track can be used to locate the lesion in the specimen. However, carbon tracks may distort or obscure the lesion.

Radioguided Occult Lesion Localization

Radioguided occult lesion localization (ROLL) is a relatively new technique first described by Luini et al. in 1996 (20). This procedure uses a small quantity (0.2–0.3 mL) of ^{99m}Tc-labeled colloid particles of human serum albumin (10–150 μm in diameter), which is injected directly into the lesion under imaging guidance. Originally the technique was described using stereotactic guidance, but of late, the use of ultrasound guidance has become popular.

For stereotactic ROLL, accurate lesion localization is confirmed by planar scintigraphy and the scintigraphic images then compared with the initial mammogram. However, frontal and lateral view planar scintigraphy is time consuming and costly. Instead, the radioisotope can be combined with 0.2 mL water-soluble non-ionic iodinated contrast medium, allowing mammography to be used to check the accuracy of radioisotope injection (21). Although rare, a potential pitfall is the intraductal injection of radioisotope that may result in failed localization of the lesion with migration of radioisotope away from the injection site (22). Check mammography allows early recognition and timely intervention including alternative methods of lesion localization.

When localization is performed under ultrasound guidance, real-time scanning shows an alteration in the echogenicity of the lesion when the radioisotope is injected, reflecting accurate targeting. A bolus of air can be injected after the radioisotope as a "chaser" and marker. The skin is then marked to indicate the position of the lesion with the patient in the surgical position.

At the time of surgery, a gamma ray probe is used to locate the lesion. The intensity and frequency of the auditory signal are directly proportional to the level of radioactivity detected. The "hot spot" is defined as the area of maximum radioactivity corresponding to the site of the lesion. The edges of the excision are defined as the locus of points surrounding the hot spot where radioactivity falls off sharply. After excising the specimen, the probe is used to check for residual radioactivity at the excision site. Complete excision is confirmed by no residual activity while the excision is enlarged if activity is still detected. The mean absorbed dose to the inoculated area is negligible, as only a small quantity of radioactive material is injected and it is concentrated in tissue that is to be removed. These radiation doses are well below the United Kingdom (UK) dose limit and no additional radiation protection measures are required (23,24).

ROLL is rapidly gaining recognition as a technique that allows accurate localization and removal of impalpable lesions, ranging from 98% to 100% (25–29). Importantly, ROLL has several benefits when compared with wire-guided localization including reduced time required for localization and smaller excision volumes allowing better cosmetic results to be achieved (30–34). For patients with a malignant diagnosis, ROLL has been associated with a significantly higher rate of clear margins and fewer re-excisions in comparison with wire-guided excision (33,35,36). However, ROLL is a more expensive technique when compared with wire-guided excision. It is postulated that the cost-saving benefits from reduced operation times and reduced re-excision rates may provide support for the more widespread use of the technique (37).

An important benefit of the ROLL technique is that it takes advantage of the radioactive tracer that is used to detect the sentinel node. Thind et al. (38) have recently described their experience with sentinel node and occult lesion localization in patients with impalpable invasive breast cancers. In this study, the combination of ^{99m}Tc-labeled macroaggregated albumin injected into the lesion and ^{99m}Tc-labeled nanocolloid injected subdermally in the periareolar region successfully achieved

100% lesion localization rates with a 94.8% rate of clear margins and 100% sentinel node localization. Other studies have streamlined this process and demonstrated that it is possible to perform ROLL and sentinel lymph node mapping with a single injection of ^{99m}Tc-labeled nanocolloid (39–41).

A further refinement of the technique of radioisotope-guided surgery is the insertion of iodine-125 labeled titanium seed into the tumor under imaging guidance. The benefit of this procedure is that it allows seed placement up to five days prior to surgery instead of precise coordination between radiologists and surgeons for same day localization. Successful localization and retrieval of both the lesion and seed were achieved in all patients with a reduced incidence of pathologically involved margins at excision when compared with wire-guided excision (42,43).

IMAGING MODALITIES FOR LOCALIZATION
Ultrasound
Ultrasound is the preferred imaging modality for localization because it is quicker, easier for the radiologist, has real-time visualization, and is more comfortable for the patient (Fig. 24.2). It is utilized for all lesions visible under ultrasound. Also, ultrasound guidance can be used to localize a lesion that was initially biopsied under stereotactic guidance if marker clips containing gel pellets were used at the time of biopsy (44) (Fig. 24.3).

Mammography
Mammographic localization is reserved for lesions not visible on ultrasound, most commonly microcalcifications or stromal deformities. The standard mammographic positions used in aiding localization are the craniocaudal position with the patient seated upright and the lateral position with the patient sitting or lying on her side. The mammographic position is chosen so as to ensure that the distance traversed from the skin to lesion is the shortest during localization. Therefore, if the lesion is in the superior half of the breast, the patient will usually be positioned in the craniocaudal position. Localization procedures are performed with the breast under compression and are usually well tolerated by patients. However, when compared with ultrasound-guided procedures, there is a higher incidence of vasovagal episodes, especially if performed in the seated position (45).

Stereotactic guidance has the advantage of lesion localization with three-dimensional coordinates. Once the patient is positioned with the lesion visible within the stereotactic window, two stereotactic pair images are taken at +15° and −15°. The lesion to be targeted is then selected on each of the stereotactic pair images and this is double checked on the scout view to ensure accurate targeting. Dedicated computer software generates three coordinates that collectively define the position of the lesion within the breast in the x-axis (horizontal plane), y-axis (vertical plane), and z-axis (depth). These coordinates dictate the site of needle insertion on the breast surface and the depth to which the needle should be advanced. An image is then taken to ensure satisfactory position of the needle in relation to the lesion prior to deploying the wire or injecting the marker solution. Localization errors can occur if the patient moves in the time taken to acquire the paired images or if the targets chosen on the paired stereotactic films are not identical. This can be challenging with ill-defined

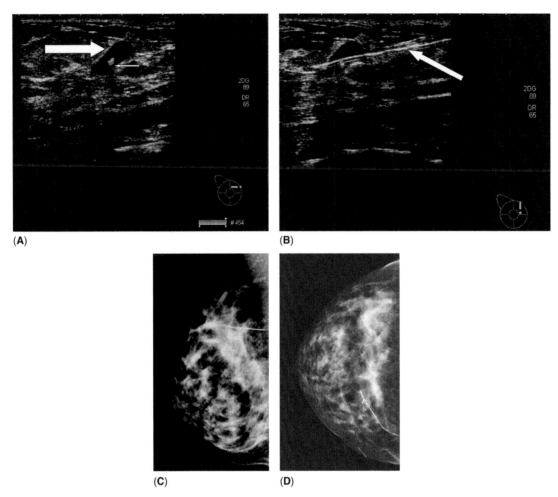

Figure 24.3 Ultrasound localization of a gel-clip marker placed following the vacuum-assisted biopsy of microcalcification 3 weeks previously. (A)Ultrasound image. Note the conspicuity of the gel plug (large arrow) and clip (small arrow). (B) The introducer needle transfixes the gel plug (arrow). (C and D) Post-procedure mammograms confirm that the wire precisely localizes the clip and residual calcifications.

lesions or with microcalcification showing minimal pleomorphism where it may be difficult to identify the same structure on both films.

Prior to the introduction of stereotactic localization for impalpable mammographic lesions, perforated plates were used (46,47). The plate was placed over the breast with a moderate degree of compression. A preliminary film localized the lesion to one of the holes in the grid. The localizer needle was inserted into the perforation overlying the lesion and the needle was advanced to a predetermined depth that had been estimated from the original image. It is important that the needle tip should pass far enough through the lesion so that its tip will still penetrate the lesion after compression is removed. A second image was then obtained in an orthogonal plane to confirm the position of the needle tip in relation to the lesion. Once the needle was in an optimal position, the wire was deployed or the marker solution was injected and the needle removed.

A variation of the perforated plate method is used successfully by some. An open plate with a grid reference on two sides is used as the compression plate, and a mammographic image obtained which includes the grid letters and numbers. A cross wire is then positioned using the grid references and casts a shadow on the skin of the breast at the site of the abnormality as seen on the mammographic image. This position is then used to guide the localization needle as described above for the perforated plate method (Fig. 24.1).

Magnetic Resonance Imaging

At present, MRI-guided intervention is available at specialist breast units and it is recommended that units offering a breast MRI service should have easy access to interventional MRI. Dedicated breast MRI coils are now available to facilitate biopsy and localization of lesions that are occult on conventional imaging. The patient lies prone with the breast moderately compressed and baseline contrast-enhanced imaging is performed to localize the lesion. The radiologist confirms the lesion to be targeted on the axial images, and the dedicated computer software calculates the lesion's coordinates in relation to a fiducial marker on the skin. These coordinates can then be transferred to a targeting device that supports a co-axial localization system. Performing intervention under MRI guidance can be labor intensive and time consuming with increased costs incurred in comparison with standard ultrasound or stereotactic guidance. Placement of an MRI-compatible marker clip following biopsy of the MRI-detected lesion is possible and provides the option of then localizing the marker clip preoperatively using conventional imaging guidance.

POST LOCALIZATION

Once the localization has been performed, the nature and accuracy of the procedure should be formally recorded and the details communicated to the surgeon. Post-localization imaging that has been performed to confirm that the correct area has been localized should be available for the surgeon during the surgical procedure (Fig. 24.2 B,C, Fig. 24.3 B,C). Following surgical excision, specimen radiography is routinely performed with the surgical specimen marked for orientation using radio-opaque clips (48). There should be an agreed policy for marking the specimen at the time of surgery, for example one clip on the anterior margin, two clips on the superior margin, and three clips on the medial margin.

The purpose of the specimen radiograph is to determine whether the targeted lesion has been successfully removed. When malignancy is confirmed preoperatively, the aim is to completely remove the lesion with a tumor-free margin. As definite information on margin status is only available after surgery, the specimen radiograph is frequently used as a surrogate to determine whether the excision has been adequate (49). In cases where a cancer is deemed close to a particular margin on the specimen radiograph (Fig. 24.2D), further tissue is removed from the surgical cavity at the same operation. Specimen radiography is therefore undertaken at the time of surgery, and the images are reviewed before the operation is completed.

CONCLUSION

The breast screening programme has generated an increasing number of mammographic abnormalities that are impalpable and require preoperative image-guided localization. Localization methods have continually improved to achieve more accurate lesion targeting and a higher rate of negative surgical margins for malignant lesions while keeping excision specimen volumes to a minimum. Preferences for the localization method and imaging guidance used vary between different institutions, and close cooperation between radiologists, surgeons, and pathologists is essential to ensure optimal results for patients.

REFERENCES

1. NHS Cancer Screening Programmes. Consolidated guidance on standards for the NHS breast screening programme. NHSBSP Publication No 60 (version 2). 2005.[Available from: www.cancerscreening.nhs.uk].
2. Frank HA, Hall FM, Steer ML. Preoperative localization of nonpalpable breast lesions demonstrated by mammography. N Engl J Med 1976; 295: 259–60.
3. Della Rovere GQ, Benson JR, Morgan M, et al. Localization of impalpable breast lesions - a surgical approach. Eur J Surg Oncol 1996; 22: 478–82.
4. Abrahamson PE, Dunlap LA, Amamoo MA, et al. Factors predicting successful needle-localized breast biopsy. Acad Radiol 2003; 10: 601–6.
5. Gallagher WJ, Cardenosa G, Rubens JR, et al. Minimal-volume excision of nonpalpable breast lesions. AJR Am J Roentgenol 1989; 153: 957–61.
6. Jackman RJ, Marzoni FA. Needle-localized breast biopsy: why do we fail? Radiology 1997; 204: 677–84.
7. Mucci B, Shaw R, Lauder J, et al. Localization of impalpable breast lesions: what are we aiming at? Breast 2009; 18: 267–9.
8. Kolpattil S, Crotch-Harvey M. Improved accuracy of wire-guided breast surgery with supplementary ultrasound. Eur J Radiol 2006; 60: 414–17.
9. Benson SR, Harrison NJ, Lengyel J, et al. Combined image guidance excision of non-palpable breast lesions. Breast 2004; 13: 110–14.
10. Bristol JB, Jones PA. Transgression of localizing wire into the pleural cavity prior to mammography. Br J Radiol 1981; 54: 139–40.
11. Davis PS, Wechsler RJ, Feig SA, et al. Migration of breast biopsy localization wire. AJR Am J Roentgenol 1988; 150: 787–8.
12. Tykka H, Castren-Persons M, Sjoblom SM, et al. Pneumothorax caused by hooked wire localisation of an impalpable breast lesion detected by mammography. Breast 1993; 2: 52–3.
13. Homer MJ. Transection of the localization hooked wire during breast biopsy. AJR Am J Roentgenol 1983; 141: 929–30.
14. Svane G. A stereotaxic technique for preoperative marking of non-palpable breast lesions. Acta Radiol Diagn (Stockh) 1983; 24: 145–51.
15. Moss HA, Barter SJ, Nayagam M, et al. The use of carbon suspension as an adjunct to wire localisation of impalpable breast lesions. Clin Radiol 2002; 57: 937–44.
16. Langlois SL, Carter ML. Carbon localisation of impalpable mammographic abnormalities. Australas Radiol 1991; 35: 237–41.
17. Mullen DJ, Eisen RN, Newman RD, et al. The use of carbon marking after stereotactic large-core-needle breast biopsy. Radiology 2001; 218: 255–60.
18. Canavese G, Catturich A, Vecchio C, et al. Pre-operative localization of non-palpable lesions in breast cancer by charcoal suspension. Eur J Surg Oncol 1995; 21: 47–9.
19. Rose A, Collins JP, Neerhut P, et al. Carbon localisation of impalpable breast lesions. Breast 2003; 12: 264–9.
20. Luini A, Zurrida S, Galimberti V, et al. Radioguided surgery of occult breast lesions. Eur J Cancer 1998; 34: 204–5.
21. Rampaul RS, Bagnall M, Burrell H, et al. Randomized clinical trial comparing radioisotope occult lesion localization and wire-guided excision for biopsy of occult breast lesions. Br J Surg 2004; 91: 1575–7.
22. Rampaul RS, MacMillan RD, Evans AJ. Intraductal injection of the breast: a potential pitfall of radioisotope occult lesion localization. Br J Radiol 2003; 76: 425–6.
23. Cremonesi M, Ferrari M, Sacco E, et al. Radiation protection in radioguided surgery of breast cancer. Nucl Med Commun 1999; 20: 919–24.
24. Rampaul RS, Dudley NJ, Thompson JZ, et al. Radioisotope for occult lesion localisation (ROLL) of the breast does not require extra radiation protection procedures. Breast 2003; 12: 150–2.
25. Zurrida S, Galimberti V, Monti S, et al. Radioguided localization of occult breast lesions. Breast 1998; 7: 11–13.
26. Sarlos D, Frey LD, Haueisen H, et al. Radioguided occult lesion localization (ROLL) for treatment and diagnosis of malignant and premalignant breast lesions combined with sentinel node biopsy: a prospective clinical trial with 100 patients. Eur J Surg Oncol 2009; 35: 403–8.
27. Lavoue V, Nos C, Clough KB, et al. Simplified technique of radioguided occult lesion localization (ROLL) plus sentinel lymph node biopsy (SNOLL) in breast carcinoma. Ann Surg Oncol 2008; 15: 2556–61.
28. Monti S, Galimberti V, Trifiro G, et al. Occult breast lesion localization plus sentinel node biopsy (SNOLL): experience with 959 patients at the European Institute of Oncology. Ann Surg Oncol 2007; 14: 2928–31.
29. Gennari R, Galimberti V, De Cicco C, et al. Use of technetium-99 m-labeled colloid albumin for preoperative and intraoperative localization of nonpalpable breast lesions. J Am Coll Surg 2000; 190: 692–8.
30. Thind CR, Desmond S, Harris O, et al. Radio-guided localization of clinically occult breast lesions (ROLL): a DGH experience. Clin Radiol 2005; 60: 681–6.
31. Nadeem R, Chagla LS, Harris O, et al. Occult breast lesions: a comparison between radioguided occult lesion localisation (ROLL) vs. wire-guided lumpectomy (WGL). Breast 2005; 14: 283–9.
32. Moreno M, Wiltgen JE, Bodanese B, et al. Radioguided breast surgery for occult lesion localization - correlation between two methods. J Exp Clin Cancer Res 2008; 27: 29.
33. Medina-Franco H, Abarca-Perez L, Garcia-Alvarez MN, et al. Radioguided occult lesion localization (ROLL) versus wire-guided lumpectomy for non-palpable breast lesions: a randomized prospective evaluation. J Surg Oncol 2008; 97: 108–11.
34. Luini A, Zurrida S, Paganelli G, et al. Comparison of radioguided excision with wire localization of occult breast lesions. Br J Surg 1999; 86: 522–5.
35. Tang J, Xie XM, Wang X, et al. Radiocolloid in combination with methylene dye localization, rather than wire localization, is a preferred procedure for excisional biopsy of nonpalpable breast lesions. Ann Surg Oncol 2011; 18: 109–13.
36. Lovrics PJ, Cornacchi SD, Vora R, et al. Systematic review of radioguided surgery for non-palpable breast cancer. Eur J Surg Oncol 2011; 37: 388–97.

37. Bland KI. Editorial on "Radioguided occult lesion localization (ROLL) versus wire-guided lumpectomy for non-palpable breast lesions: a randomized prospective evaluation" by Medina-Franco H, et al. J Surg Oncol 2008; 97: 101–2.

38. Thind CR, Tan S, Desmond S, et al. SNOLL. Sentinel node and occult lesion localization in breast cancer. Clin Radiol 2011; 66: 833–9.

39. Feggi L, Basaglia E, Corcione S, et al. An original approach in the diagnosis of early breast cancer: use of the same radiopharmaceutical for both non-palpable lesions and sentinel node localisation. Eur J Nucl Med 2001; 28: 1589–96.

40. Tanis PJ, Deurloo EE, Valdes Olmos RA, et al. Single intralesional tracer dose for radio-guided excision of clinically occult breast cancer and sentinel node. Ann Surg Oncol 2001; 8: 850–5.

41. Patel A, Pain SJ, Britton P, et al. Radioguided occult lesion localisation (ROLL) and sentinel node biopsy for impalpable invasive breast cancer. Eur J Surg Oncol 2004; 30: 918–23.

42. Gray RJ, Salud C, Nguyen K, et al. Randomized prospective evaluation of a novel technique for biopsy or lumpectomy of nonpalpable breast lesions: radioactive seed versus wire localization. Ann Surg Oncol 2001; 8: 711–15.

43. Hughes JH, Mason MC, Gray RJ, et al. A multi-site validation trial of radioactive seed localization as an alternative to wire localization. Breast J 2008; 14: 153–7.

44. McMahon MA, James JJ, Cornford EJ, et al. Does the insertion of a gel-based marker at stereotactic breast biopsy allow subsequent wire localizations to be carried out under ultrasound guidance? Clin Radiol 2011; 66: 840–4.

45. Rissanen TJ, Makarainen HP, Mattila SI, et al. Wire localized biopsy of breast lesions: a review of 425 cases found in screening or clinical mammography. Clin Radiol 1993; 47: 14–22.

46. Parekh NJ, Wolfe JN. Localization device for occult breast lesions: use in 75 patients. AJR Am J Roentgenol 1987; 148: 699–701.

47. Goldberg RP, Hall FM, Simon M. Preoperative localization of nonpalpable breast lesions using a wire marker and perforated mammographic grid. Radiology 1983; 146: 833–5.

48. NHS Cancer Screening Programmes. Quality assurance guidelines for surgeons in breast cancer screening. NHSBSP Publication No 20, fourth edition. 2009. [Available from: www.cancerscreening.nhs.uk].

49. Britton PD, Sonoda LI, Yamamoto AK, et al. Breast surgical specimen radiographs: how reliable are they? Eur J Radiol 2011; 79: 245–9.

25 The normal breast and benign breast lesions

Baljit Singh

INTRODUCTION

The breast is a modified sweat gland and the functional unit of the breast is a terminal ductal lobular unit (lobule) which drains into a complex ductal system. The ductal system coalesces into a few large ducts which open through pores in the nipple. This epithelial organ in the breast is the mammary gland which is the distinguishing feature of mammals. The breast encompasses the mammary gland and the fibrofatty matrix in which it is embedded. The breast is a rudimentary organ in males and unless otherwise specified *breast* refers to the female breast in this chapter.

EMBRYOLOGY

The breasts develop from the ectoderm and are highly specialized apocrine glands. In the seventh week of gestation a bilateral thickening of the ectoderm appears to form a *mammary ridge or milk line*, which extends from the axilla to the inguinal region (Fig. 25.1) (1). In humans most of the milk line disappears except in the thoracic region at the normal anatomic location of the nipple. In lower animals multiple bilateral mammary glands develop along the mammary ridge. In the fifth or sixth month a mass of epidermal cells from the mammary ridge grows inward and forms 16 to 20 branches in the pectoral region at the site of the adult breast (Fig. 25.2A, B, C). This epidermal growth is accompanied with mesenchymal growth which eventually matures into specialized mammary stroma and adipose tissue. In the last eight weeks of gestation the branches of epidermal cells become canalized to form the complex ductal system of the breast. The acinar glands develop by proliferation of the terminal part of the ductal system to form terminal ductal lobular units (Fig. 25.2D). The ducts initially open into a depression at the normal anatomic site of the nipple—*mammary pit*. Eventually the underlying mesoderm protrudes outward in the mammary pit to form the nipple (Fig. 25.2E). The process of invagination of ectoderm into mesenchyme explains both the absence of a true capsule surrounding the gland and how blood vessels, nerves, and lymphatics of the breast come from existing structures supplying the anterior thoracic wall. Early growth and differentiation of the breast occurs similarly in both males and females, but post-natal development occurs only in females and the breast is a vestigial structure in the adult male.

Maternal hormones stimulate the fetal breast with occasional secretion of milk (*witch's milk*). Aberrations in involution of the milk line can result in the presence of accessory nipples and breast tissue along the milk line. Occasionally the entire breast fails to form (*amastia*) or the nipple is absent (*athelia*).

PHYSIOLOGICAL STAGES OF BREAST DEVELOPMENT

Premenarchal Breast

After withdrawal of maternal hormones the breast tissue involutes. In the normal premenarchal phase the breast is inactive and composed of a ductal system without alveolar differentiation (Fig. 25.3A). In *premature thelarche* a unilateral or bilateral discoid subareolar thickening appears in premenarchal girls and microscopic examination may show papillary hyperplasia in ducts (2).

Adolescent Breast

Cyclical hormonal changes at puberty lead to breast development with proliferation of the mammary gland and fibrofatty stroma. This is physically manifest as breast mound formation. Terminal ductal lobular units (lobules) appear at the end of terminal ducts in a background of fibrofatty stroma (Fig. 25.3B) (3).

Mature Breast

The mature adult breast has 15–25 lobes and each lobe drains into a major duct which opens through a pore in the nipple. The nipple and rim of the surrounding skin (areola) have deeper pigmentation than surrounding skin and are covered by stratified squamous epithelium associated with abundant sebaceous glands. Pigmentation of the nipple becomes more pronounced during pregnancy and persists thereafter. The sebaceous glands in the areola (glands of Montgomery) open in small tubercles of Morgagni, which become more prominent during pregnancy (Fig. 25.4A). The lactiferous ducts open into pores on the nipple surface and a cluster of circular smooth muscle in the vicinity functions as a sphincter (Fig. 25.4B). Lobules and ducts are embedded in fibrofatty stroma which forms the bulk of the breast tissue. During the reproductive years breast tissue tends to have more fibrous elements and therefore appears very dense on mammography.

Lobules are composed of a variable number of acini which drain into a terminal duct (Fig. 25.5A). The lobular cells are cuboidal with indistinct cell borders and do not stain with E-cadherin (Fig. 25.5B). The ductal cells are typically columnar and show intense membranous staining with E-cadherin (Fig. 25.5C) (4). Milk is formed in lobules during lactation and extruded via the complex ductal system.

The entire lobular and ductal system is lined by two layers of cells: the inner lobular or ductal cells and the outer myoepithelial cells. The ductal and lobular layers of cells are immunoreactive for cytokeratins but other immunohistochemical stains are required to demonstrate myoepithelial cells. Calponin is a 34 kD polypeptide that interacts with actin, tropomyosin, and

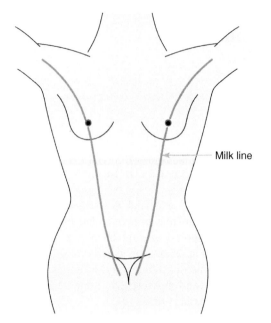

Figure 25.1 Embryology. Mammary line appears from axilla to the inguinal region.

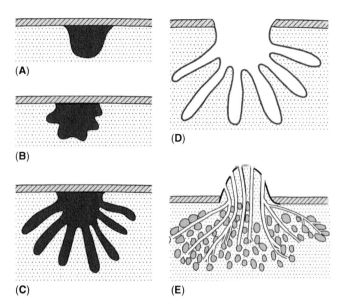

Figure 25.2 (**A–E**) Ectodermal ingrowths into the mesoderm develop into the ductal and lobular system of the mammary gland.

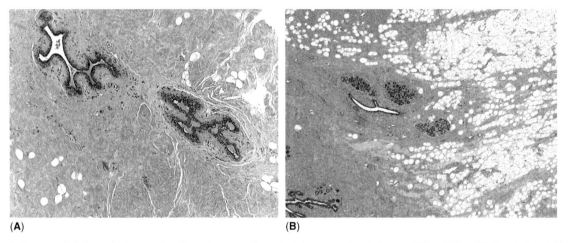

Figure 25.3 (**A**) Premenarchal phase: the breast is inactive and composed of a ductal system without alveolar differentiation. (**B**) Terminal ductal lobular units (lobule) appear at the end of terminal ducts after puberty.

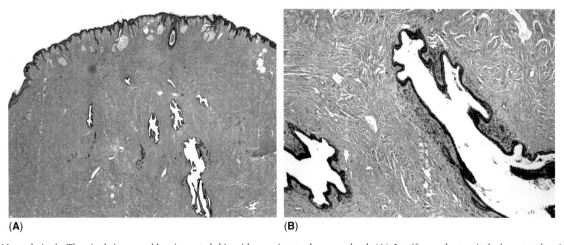

Figure 25.4 Normal nipple. The nipple is covered by pigmented skin with prominent sebaceous glands (**A**). Lactiferous ducts exit the breast at the nipple and are surrounded by clusters of smooth muscles which act as a sphincter (**B**).

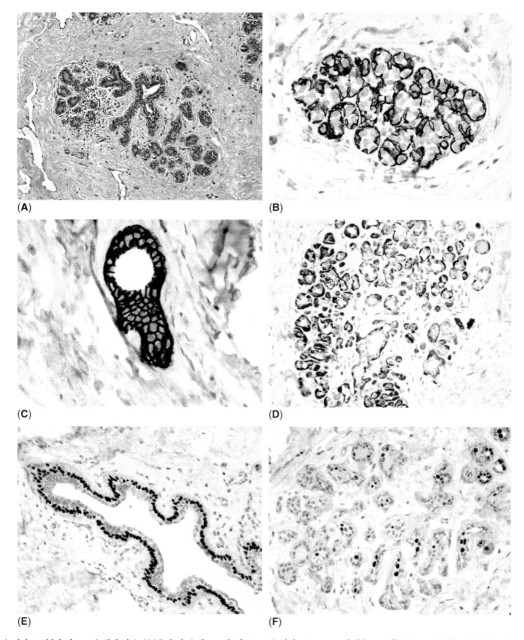

Figure 25.5 Terminal ductal lobular unit (lobule). (**A**) Lobule is formed of a terminal duct surrounded by small acinar units lined by lobular cells. Two layers of cells, inner ductal or lobular cells and outer myoepithelial cells, line all the epithelial structures in the breast. E-cadherin does not stain lobular cells (**B**) and stains ductal cells (**C**). Calponin immunohistochemical stain highlights the myoepithelial cells in a lobule (**D**). P63 highlights nuclei in myoepithelial cells in a duct (**E**) and lobule (**F**).

calmodulin and stains the cytoplasm of myoepithelial cells (Fig. 25.5D). P63 is a member of the p53 family of transcription factors and stains the nuclei of myoepithelial cells (Fig. 25.5E). Myoepithelial cells are absent in invasive carcinoma and these immunohistochemical stains are a useful adjunct for the practicing pathologist when dealing with challenging cases.

The estrogen pathway is critical in the development and physiological function of the breast, and aberrations in this pathway can lead to proliferative or neoplastic lesions. Immunohistochemical staining for estrogen receptor in the normal breast shows nuclear staining in a minority of lobular or ductal cells (Fig. 25.5F). The frequency of estrogen receptor varies during the menstrual cycle and is highest during the follicular phase of the cycle.

Cyclical hormonal changes during the menstrual cycle also impact breast anatomy. In mid-cycle the breast is least nodular on clinical examination. In the proliferative phase the acinar glands have small or no lumina with crowded lobular cells, myoepithelial cells are inconspicuous, and lobular stroma is dense. In the follicular phase increased mitotic activity is noted in the lobular cells and myoepithelial cells have clear cytoplasm and lumens can be discerned without secretions. During the luteal phase the myoepithelial cells enlarge with clear cytoplasm, the lobular cells can be columnar and some luminal secretions may be seen. In the secretory phase, secretions within the lumen are prominent and the lobular stroma is edematous. In the menstrual phase lumina tend to disappear and the stroma is less edematous and contains numerous chronic inflammatory cells.

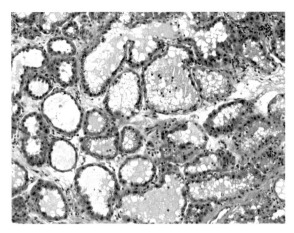

Figure 25.6 Lactational change. Lobular cells in hypertrophic lobules have vacuolated cytoplasm and proteinaceous secretion in the lumina.

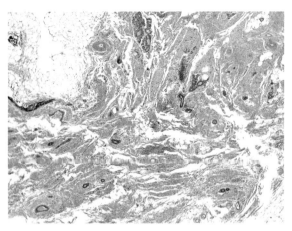

Figure 25.7 Involutional change. Small, rare atrophic lobules and attenuated ducts are seen during involution. The stroma becomes more fatty during involution (hypodense on mammography).

Pregnancy

The physiological function of the breast is to produce milk. There is a marked increase in the number of lobules during pregnancy (hyperplasia). This process may be uneven and therefore the breast may develop areas of lumpiness or more discrete lumps on clinical examination. These are called *lactational adenomas*, which is a misnomer since they are not tumors. The epidermis in the nipple and areola develops deeper pigmentation and the sebaceous glands become more prominent and form small protuberances. The marked increase in lobular formation is accompanied by attenuation of myoepithelial cells, increased vascularity, edema, and mononuclear infiltrate in the stroma. The lobular cells develop abundant vacuolated cytoplasm and secretions accumulate in the lumina (Fig. 25.6). It takes approximately three months for the breast to involute after cessation of lactation. *Pregnancy-like change* may be seen on the histological examination of breast specimens not only from women who were pregnant in the past but also in nulliparous women. Similar changes may be seen in men treated with estrogens.

Menopause

The decline in hormonal levels leads to atrophy of glandular elements, especially lobules in some women but lobular hyperplasia persists in others. In lobules undergoing *involution* the number of glands decreases with the thickening of the basement membrane and focal association with dystrophic calcification (Fig. 25.7). Myoepithelial cells continue to persist in the lobular–ductal system. This process is not uniform throughout the breast. Ducts atrophy as well and can become cystic. The stroma becomes less fibrotic and more fatty and thereby hypodense on mammography. Involution has been associated with a decreased risk of development of breast carcinoma.

APPLIED ANATOMY

The anatomy of the breast varies in different physiological stages. The nulliparous breast is hemispheric while those of multiparous women are larger and pendulous. The medial border of the breast extends to the lateral edge of the sternum and the lateral border extends up to the midaxillary line. Breast tissue extends into the lower axillary region (axillary

tail), which is an important surgical consideration. Dense connective tissue bands extend from the underlying pectoral fascia to the skin; these ligaments (Cooper's ligaments) hold the breast upward, and the loss in their tensile strength with age causes ptosis of the breast.

The breast does not have a blood supply from a single artery. Perforating branches from the internal mammary artery supply the medial and deep parts of the breast. These branches anastomose with branches from the axillary artery and the lateral thoracic artery. Branches from the thoracoacromial trunk and some intercostal vessels supply the deeper aspects of the gland. The venous drainage of the breast generally corresponds to the arterial supply. Veins beneath the areola form an anastomotic circle (circulus venosus), which together with deeper veins carries blood to the periphery of the gland where venous outflow is via the internal thoracic, lateral thoracic, and upper intercostal veins.

Lymph nodes in the axilla have been classified based on clinical, anatomical, or surgical criteria:

1. Clinical classification: medial, lateral, anterior, posterior, and apical
2. Anatomical/surgical classifications: lateral, anterior (pectoral), posterior (subscapular), central, subclavicular, and interpectoral (Rotter's)

The axillary lymph nodes are commonly defined in terms of their relationship to the pectoralis minor muscle:

1. Level I: nodes below and lateral to lateral border of muscle
2. Level II: nodes deep to muscle
3. Level III: nodes above and medial to muscle

Typically lymphatics of the breast initially drain to a group of 3–5 "sentinel" nodes located at level I. Usually there is an orderly passage of lymph from nodes at level I through level II to level III. For this reason it is unusual to find metastatic carcinoma in level III lymph nodes when those at levels I and II are uninvolved. Lymphatic channels exist which bypass the Level I axillary nodes and may account for "skip" metastases. Sentinel lymph node biopsy has become the standard of care to accurately determine the pathological status of axillary nodes (5).

INFLAMMATORY AND REACTIVE CONDITIONS
Acute Mastitis
Acute inflammation of the breast mostly occurs during lactation, especially within the first month of breastfeeding. Small cuts in the nipple region expose the underlying parenchyma containing abundant milk secretions to infection. Untreated mastitis can lead to an abscess which can rupture through the skin to form a fistula in rare cases. The most common etiologic organism is *Staphylococcus aureus* (6). This is seldom seen with appropriate antibiotic therapy and drainage of the abscess either percutaneously or by open surgery.

Fat Necrosis
In current practice fat necrosis is commonly seen after a biopsy, surgery, or radiation therapy. Traumatic fat necrosis has been observed more commonly in women with pendulous breasts who present with a painless mass. Persistent fat necrosis after surgery or biopsy can mimic a recurrent carcinoma. A zone of fat necrosis is ill defined at the outset but becomes well defined with a cystic center over time. Microscopic examination shows fat cells with foamy cytoplasm associated with chronic inflammation, granulation tissue, and fibrosis with focal cystic degeneration (Fig. 25.8). Dystrophic calcification is commonly seen with fat necrosis.

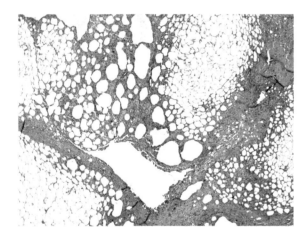

Figure 25.8 Cystic fat necrosis. Fibrofatty tissue has a cystic architecture. Fat cells have foamy cytoplasm and are associated with granulation tissue and chronic inflammation.

Mammary Duct Ectasia
Mammary duct ectasia is seen in women aged between 40 and 70 years. The presenting symptom is invariably unilateral nipple discharge which can vary in color from yellowish/cream to dark green or brown. It is rarely overtly bloodstained but may contain occult blood on cytology or dipstick testing. Duct ectasia often produces a multicolored viscous discharge associated with a burning sensation, itching, and occasional swelling. The discharge has no relation to the menstrual cycle and current medications should be documented. Younger women complain of pain and more commonly have nipple retraction than older women. The clinical and radiological presentation can mimic breast carcinoma. Microscopic examination reveals large dilated ducts with proteinaceous secretions with variable morphological features. These include association with chronic inflammation (Fig. 25.9A), foamy histiocytes, granulation tissue, granulomatous inflammation, and abscess formation. The ductal cells are typically attenuated in the dilated ducts and can be entirely absent (Fig. 25.9B). Chronic cases show dense stromal fibrosis associated with chronic inflammation. Cigarette smoking has been associated with mammary duct ectasia and therefore smoking habits should be recorded (7).

Granulomatous Mastitis
Granulomatous inflammation of the breast can masquerade as a carcinoma as it typically presents as a firm mass and unilateral nipple discharge. The lesion is typically seen in premenopausal women and an association with oral contraceptive use has been reported.

Microscopic examination reveals granulomatous inflammation which is lobulocentric (Fig. 25.10). Granulomas are well-defined clusters of epithelioid histiocytes associated with giant cells. In advanced cases the granulomas have necrotic centers and can be associated with abscess formation. Sarcoidosis or cat scratch disease should also be considered in the differential diagnosis. Carcinoma may be associated with granuloma formation and a florid granulomatous inflammation can obscure an underlying carcinoma (8). Etiological organisms cannot be demonstrated by special stains but should be performed in every case to exclude mycobacterial or fungal infection.

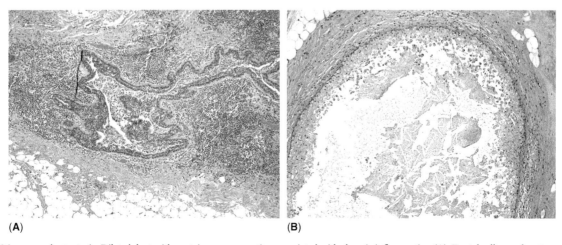

(A)   (B)

Figure 25.9 Mammary duct ectasia. Dilated duct with proteinaceous secretion associated with chronic inflammation (A). Ductal cells may be attenuated or completely absent—pseudocyst (B).

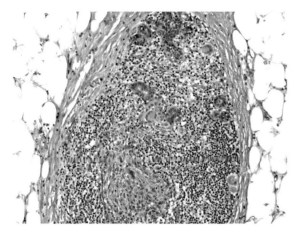

Figure 25.10 Granulomatous mastitis. Epithelioid histiocytes are arranged in clusters (granuloma) around a lobule.

Diabetic Mastopathy

Diabetic mastopathy is a self-limiting condition which presents in premenopausal women as a palpable, firm mass. It is commonly associated with type 1 insulin-dependent diabetes but has also been reported with type 2 diabetes. Microscopic examination reveals a keloid-like stroma with a perivascular chronic inflammatory infiltrate and prominent myofibroblasts (9).

Collagen Vascular diseases

Giant cell arteritis can be limited to the breast and is characterized by the presence of a chronic inflammatory infiltrate associated with giant cells in the walls of medium sized arteries. Wegener's granulomatosis rarely affects the breast and commonly patients have systemic involvement. Scleroderma, dermatomyositis, and lupus mastitis have been reported (10–12).

FIBROCYSTIC CHANGE

Fibrocystic changes are manifest clinically as a change in the texture of breast tissue which has been referred to as "*lumpy bumpy*" breasts. The term fibrocystic implies underlying fibrosis in the breast stroma and cystic change in the ductal system. A plethora of histopathological features help to categorize these age-related changes into three subtypes: *nonproliferative, proliferative type without atypia, and proliferative type with atypia*. These distinctions are important biologically as there is substantial evidence for an increased risk of breast carcinoma associated with these individual categories.

Fibrocystic Change, Nonproliferative Type

Radiological examination of "lumpy bumpy" breasts usually reveals dense tissue (fibrosis) and cystic changes. Histopathological features which distinguish nonproliferative fibrocystic change are *fibrosis*, cysts, and adenosis. Microscopic examination typically shows large areas of bland fibrosis with few stromal cells and epithelial elements (Fig. 25.11A). Fibrosis can have varying degrees of cellularity ranging from highly cellular with abundance of myofibroblasts to being almost acellular in regions of dense sclerosis.

Large *cysts* may be seen on gross examination and microscopically cysts appear as dilated ducts cut in cross section, lined by ductal cells and filled with clear fluid. Cysts are typically seen in clusters and form by dilatation of ducts but may also form by unfolding of lobules (Fig. 25.11B). Cysts contain clear proteinaceous fluid which may become milky or brown/blue with hemorrhage (so-called blue domed cysts of Bloodgood). Cysts are lined by inner ductal and outer myoepithelial cells, which become attenuated as a cyst dilates. Large cysts (macrocysts) may be clinically palpable as fluctuant masses. Fine needle aspiration of cysts done for diagnostic purposes can be curative and microscopic examination of the clear fluid typically shows a few ductal cells and foamy histiocytes. If the aspirated fluid is serosanguinous and the microscopic examination reveals a cellular specimen with atypical cells then a surgical excision is indicated for a more definitive diagnosis. Cysts rupture on occasion and can engender a painful inflammatory response. Ruptured cysts may not have an epithelial lining (pseudocyst) and contain abundant proteinaceous fluid in the lumen and are surrounded by granulation tissue associated with acute and chronic inflammation along with foreign body giant cells and hemosiderin-laden macrophages.

Apocrine metaplasia is commonly seen in cysts—the ductal cells become enlarged with pink granular cytoplasm and have prominent nuclei (Fig. 25.11C, D). The cells may have apical snouts projecting into the lumina. Nuclear pleomorphism in apocrine cells is common and the threshold for categorizing atypia in apocrine cells is higher than ductal cells. Not uncommonly papillary hyperplasia is observed in apocrine cysts.

Columnar cell change (blunt duct adenosis) is seen in the dilated smaller ducts of lobules which have become cystic and are lined by cuboidal to columnar cells in an even distribution without protruding into the lumen (Fig. 25.11E). There may be concomitant hypertrophy of myoepithelial cells. The cells may have abundant granular cytoplasm with snouts. The nuclei are not atypical, nucleoli are not discernible, and there are no mitoses. The specialized stroma in the lobules expands in the foci of columnar change. Glands with columnar cell change are typically dilated to form microcysts.

Ducts may also exhibit *mild hyperplasia* of the usual type, in which hyperplastic cells in the lumen do not cross the involved space. *Calcifications* are commonly associated with epithelial elements (such as cysts and lobules) and can be readily seen with light microscopy (Fig. 25.11F). Occasionally calcium oxalate crystals are seen in cysts which are best visualized by polarized light.

Fibrocystic change of nonproliferative type has a *relative risk* of 1.27 for development of breast carcinoma, implying that these women have a 27% increased risk in the ensuing 15 years (13). In the general population 5 out of every 100 women develop breast carcinoma with 15 years of follow-up and in women with nonproliferative fibrocystic change this figure is approximately 6 women and therefore the *absolute* increase in risk is 1 in 100 (14).

Fibrocystic Change, Proliferative Type

The term "proliferative" implies a variety of hyperplastic epithelial lesions in a background of increased fibrosis. A diagnosis of proliferative type fibrocystic change is made if any of the following features are present within the breast on microscopic examination: *sclerosing adenosis, usual ductal hyperplasia (greater than mild), papilloma, or radial scar*. The relative risk for the development of breast cancer in patients with proliferative change without atypia is 1.88 (13).

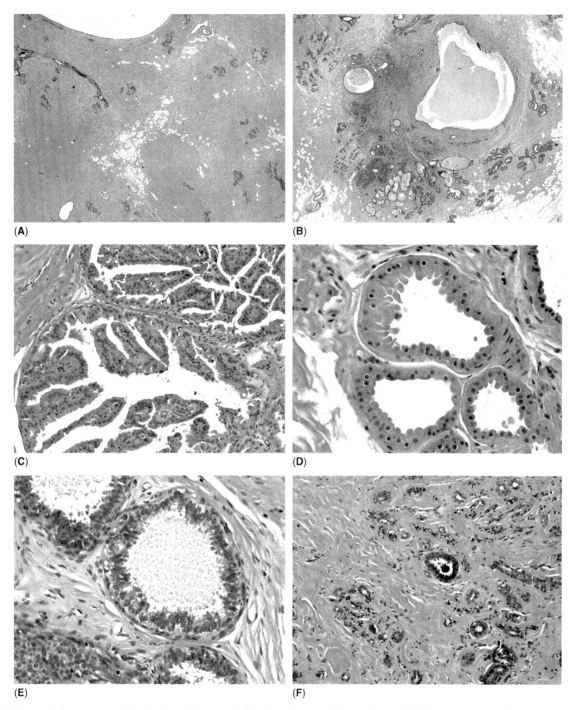

Figure 25.11 Fibrocystic change, non-proliferative type. The stroma is fibrotic and contains lobules and cysts (**A**). Microcysts are typically seen in clusters (**B**). Cysts can develop apocrine metaplasia and are lined by ductal cells with abundant granular cytoplasm (**C, D**). Clusters of enlarged acini are lined by tall columnar cells (**E**). Dystrophic calcification is commonly associated with sclerosing adenosis and small cysts (**F**).

Adenosis refers to an increase in the number of glands. *Sclerosing adenosis* is the most commonly observed epithelial change in fibrocystic change of the proliferative type. Sclerosis refers to stroma in the lobules which is densely fibrotic and adenosis implies an increase in the number of acini (Fig. 25.12A, B). The overall spherical architecture of the lobule is usually maintained in spite of stromal, lobular, and myoepithelial hyperplasia. The cells lining the lobules are small and lack cytological atypia and a lumen in small acini can typically be recognized. Foci of sclerosing adenosis can coalesce to form very complex structures which may form a clinically palpable mass and microscopically have architectural qualities similar to radial scars. These complex sclerosing lesions can be mistaken for invasive carcinoma. Immunohistochemical stains for myoepithelial cells (calponin, p63) can demonstrate the presence of both ductal and myoepithelial cells and thereby prevent this pitfall. Invasive carcinoma does not have a spherical/organoid architecture, the cells lining tubules are atypical and most importantly invasive carcinoma lacks myoepithelial cells.

Epithelial hyperplasia is typically seen in medium sized ducts. Usual ductal hyperplasia is characterized by a "streaming" architecture in which cells are aligned parallel to each other. Lumina between proliferating cells are slit like and irregular in shape and form a "sieve" like architecture. Microscopic

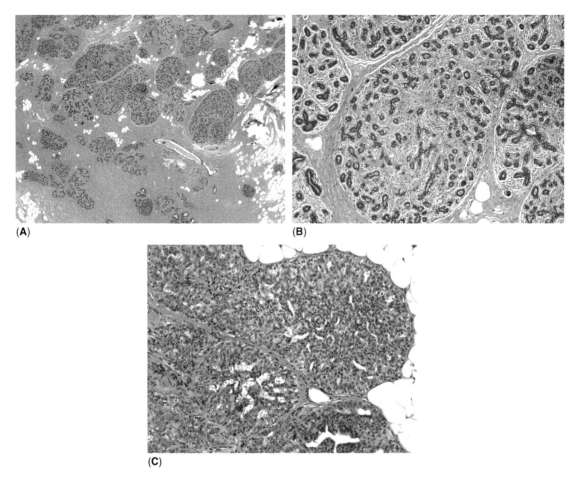

Figure 25.12 Fibrocystic change of proliferative type. The stroma is fibrotic (**A**) and contains hyperplastic lobules with sclerosing stroma—sclerosing adenosis (**B**); ducts may have usual ductal hyperplasia (**C**).

examination at high power and immunohistochemical stains (calponin, p63) show that the proliferating cells in the duct are an admixture of ductal and myoepithelial cells which overlap each other and have indistinct borders (Fig. 25.12C). The ductal cells show that no atypia are normochromic without prominent nucleoli. Epithelial hyperplasia has been categorized as mild, moderate, and florid.

*Papilloma*s are intraductal fibroepithelial neoplasms which can distend and occlude ducts. They are described in detail in the section "Intraductal Papilloma." Briefly, they have a frond-like architecture composed of fibrovascular cores lined by myoepithelial and ductal cells. Small duct papillomas are a few millimeters in largest dimension and are recognized only on microscopic examination (Fig. 25.13). Large duct papillomas are typically seen in the large nipple ducts and are described in the section, "Intraductal Papilloma."

Radial scars are a scar-like lesion with a radiating architecture (Fig. 25.14A). They are typically seen as an incidental finding on histological examination with a median size of 4.0 mm. The center of the lesion is composed of dense collagenous tissue with attenuated ducts while the periphery of the lesion has ducts with usual ductal hyperplasia and small cysts (Fig. 25.14B). Ducts within the central sclerotic zone can mimic tubular carcinoma. Moreover, the radial scar architecture can mimic invasive carcinoma on mammography and the compressed ducts in the central sclerotic zone can mimic invasive carcinoma on microscopic examination. Immunohistochemical stains are useful to demonstrate myoepithelial cells and rule out tubular carcinoma

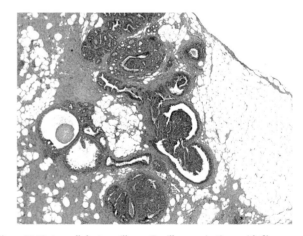

Figure 25.13 A small duct papilloma. Papillary projections with fibrovascular cores lined by ductal and myoepithelial cells are seen in small cysts.

on histological examination. The presence of a radial scar irrespective of the type of underlying fibrocystic change is associated with an increase in the subsequent development of breast cancer with a relative risk of 1.8 (15). Women with proliferative fibrocystic change with and without radial scars have a relative risk of 3.0 and 1.5 for development of breast cancer respectively as compared with women with nonproliferative fibrocystic change. Radial scars have also been associated with concurrent breast cancer and thereby a diagnosis of radial scar on core biopsy is an indication for an excisional biopsy.

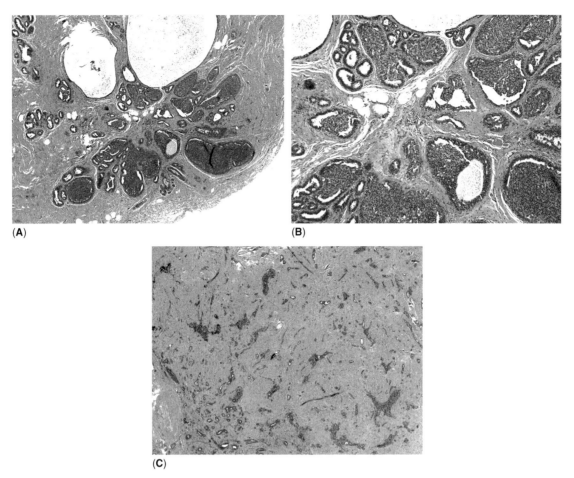

(A)

(B)

(C)

Figure 25.14 A radial scar having a dense sclerotic center (**A**) with compressed ducts and larger ducts with proliferative changes with usual ductal hyperplasia at the periphery (**B**). Sclerosing lesion has a complex architecture and is composed of coalescent sclerosing adenosis with underlying dense fibrosis (**C**).

A *complex sclerosing lesion* is a large area with complex architecture with dense sclerosis, attenuated ducts, and sclerosing adenosis which can be diagnostically challenging. Complex sclerosing lesions have a variety of morphological appearances with sclerotic stroma and compressed epithelial elements (Fig. 25.14C). Immunohistochemical stains for myoepithelial cells are very useful for the practicing pathologist to distinguish these benign lesions from invasive carcinoma which do not have myoepithelial cells compared with an abundance of this cell type in complex sclerosing lesions.

BENIGN TUMORS
Fibroadenoma
Fibroadenomas have evenly balanced stromal and epithelial components and are the most common breast tumors in premenopausal women. The relative risk for development of breast carcinoma is estimated to range from 1.6 to 2.6 in women with fibroadenomas (16). These lesions typically present as firm, well circumscribed, mobile, painless masses in the breast. They can occur in any region of the breast but have a slightly higher incidence in the upper outer quadrant of the left breast. Fibroadenomas are seldom larger than 4 cm but have been reported to grow so large as to replace the entire breast. Black adolescent girls are more prone to develop multiple fibroadenomas, which can occur synchronously and may recur after excision.

Fibroadenomas are well-circumscribed tumors on gross examination with a fleshy cut surface. They are composed of varying proportions of stromal and epithelial components in a variety of histological patterns (Fig. 25.15A). The epithelial layers lining the ducts in a fibroadenoma have an inner ductal layer and an outer myoepithelial cell layer. The two most common architectural patterns are *intracanalicular*—in which stromal overgrowth compresses ducts and *pericanalicular*—in which ducts are dilated and not compressed by the stroma. *Tubular* fibroadenomas have abundant small ducts and tubules and in the apocrine variant the ductal cells have prominent granular cytoplasm. Ductal epithelium can on occasion undergo squamous metaplasia. During pregnancy the ductal epithelium in fibroadenomas undergoes secretory change and is prone to infarction. The stromal component of fibroadenomas can vary from sclerotic to very cellular and often has a myxoid appearance. In most fibroadenomas the stromal cells do not show any atypia or mitoses. *Juvenile* fibroadenomas are characterized by stromal hypercellularity and epithelial hyperplasia. After the menopause, fibroadenomas involute like the surrounding breast tissue and become hyalinized and calcified (Fig. 25.15B). They are commonly seen in women younger than 20 years but have been observed in postmenopausal women as well. These myriad morphological changes are not indicative of a different natural history of fibroadenoma.

Complex fibroadenomas are characterized by the presence of papillary apocrine hyperplasia, cysts (Fig. 25.15C), sclerosing adenosis (Fig. 25.15D), or epithelial calcifications. They have a relative risk of 3.1 for development of subsequent

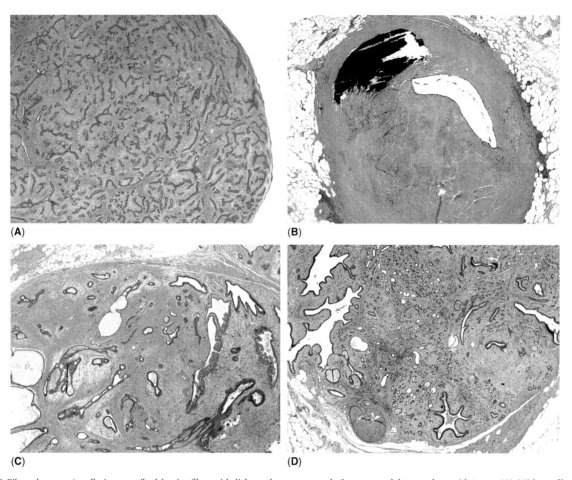

Figure 25.15 Fibroadenoma. A well-circumscribed, benign fibroepithelial neoplasm composed of compressed ducts and myxoid stroma (**A**). With age fibroadenomas become hyalinized and calcified (**B**). Complex fibroadenoma may have cysts (**C**), sclerosing adenosis (**D**), or calcifications.

breast carcinoma which is higher than the usual type fibroadenoma (16). Rarely lobular or ductal carcinoma *in situ* or invasive carcinoma in the surrounding breast may involve a fibroadenoma.

Phyllodes Tumor

A phyllodes tumor is also a fibroepithelial neoplasm with a dominant stromal component which determines the biology of this tumor. On gross examination they have a leaf-like fleshy appearance and have therefore been referred to as *cystosarcoma phyllodes*. The term is a misnomer as it implies that the tumor is always malignant (*sarcoma*). Phyllodes tumors are usually benign but can be low-grade malignant (borderline) or high-grade malignant. Benign phyllodes tumors do not metastasize but may recur; low-grade malignant tumors may metastasize (<5%) and can also recur; 25% of high-grade malignant tumors metastasize and have a propensity to recur. They manifest as unilateral masses at a median age of 45, which is approximately 20 years later than the presentation of fibroadenomas. The average size of a phyllodes tumor is 4–5 cm but they can grow to a very large size. The dominant mass may be well circumscribed but satellite nodules of tumor are not uncommonly seen in the vicinity and thereby a wide excision is necessary to remove the entire tumor (Fig. 25.16A). Histological examination shows that they characteristically have a leaf-like (intracanalicular pattern) with abundant cellular stroma with periductal hypercellularity (Fig. 25.16B). The stroma can have a variegated appearance within the same tumor with sclerotic, myxoid, and cellular areas. The morphology of the stromal cells determines the biology of phyllodes tumor. Benign phyllodes tumors are well circumscribed, with moderate stromal cellularity but stromal cells are mildly atypical with rare mitoses typically in the periductal regions (<2/high power field; hpf). Low-grade malignant tumors may be well circumscribed but can have an invasive border with hypercellular stroma with 2–5 mitoses/10 high power field (hpf) in stromal cells (Fig. 25.16C). High-grade phyllodes tumors typically have an invasive border, a fibrosarcomatous pattern with marked stromal overgrowth relative to the epithelial component of the tumor and a high rate of mitosis >5/10hpf. Malignant phyllodes tumors can have morphological features of a high-grade sarcoma with heterologous elements. The epithelial component may be proliferative and is lined by ductal and myoepithelial cells (2). A wide local excision prevents local recurrence by removing any "pseudopodia" and is the mainstay of therapy for phyllodes tumor (17).

Intraductal Papilloma

Large duct papillomas are benign neoplasms with frond-like intraductal architecture and are typically seen in the large

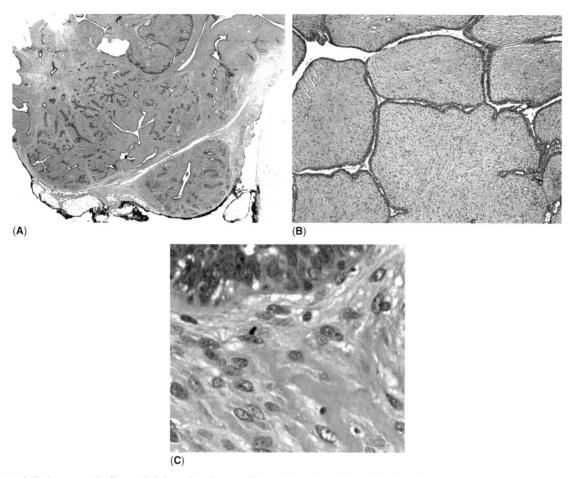

Figure 25.16 A phyllodes tumor. The fibroepithelial neoplasm has a satellite nodule at the periphery (**A**). The phyllodes tumor typically has a cleft-like architecture (**B**). Stromal overgrowth and mitotic activity (**C**) are used to determine whether a phyllodes tumor is benign, borderline, or malignant.

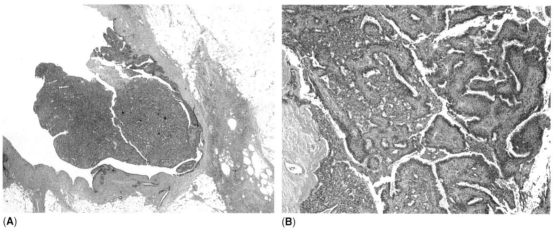

Figure 25.17 An intraductal papilloma. A mass with papillary architecture is seen protruding into a dilated duct (**A**). The papillae are formed by fibrovascular cores and are lined by myoepithelial and ductal cells (**B**).

ducts close to the nipple. They present as unilateral nipple discharge and on occasion a subareolar mass can be palpated. Multiple intraductal papillomas can also appear in the periphery of the breast. Histological examination reveals a frond-like growth into the lumen of a distended duct (Fig. 25.17A). The fronds are extensions of stroma with fibrovascular cores lined by two layers of cells: outer ductal and inner myoepithelial cells (Fig. 25.17B). The ductal cells can be cuboidal or

columnar and demonstrate moderate atypia with rare mitoses. The stromal fronds can fuse and collagenize with loss of frond-like architecture and a resultant complex architecture with compressed clusters of epithelial cells. This *sclerosing variant of intraductal papilloma* can be diagnostically challenging and immunohistochemical demonstration of myoepithelial cells definitively excludes invasive carcinoma. Rarely the intraductal portion of a papilloma is composed entirely of epithelial cells with myoepithelial cells seen only in the distended duct or not at all. This variant is called *intracystic papillary carcinoma* and behaves like intraductal carcinoma. Intraductal papillomas may be associated with either *in situ* or invasive ductal carcinoma in the surrounding breast tissue and therefore a diagnosis of intraductal papilloma on core biopsy mandates an excisional biopsy (18).

MISCELLANEOUS
Pseudoangiomatous Stromal Hyperplasia
Pseudoangiomatous stromal hyperplasia (PASH) can present as a palpable mass and is increasingly found as a well-circumscribed mass or architectural distortion on radiological screening with mammography or MRI. The lesion is seen both in men with gynecomastia and in women. The term pseudoangiomatous stromal hyperplasia is self-explanatory; the lesion is composed of stromal cells around a cleft-like space which mimics a vascular (angiomatous) proliferation (Fig. 25.18). The stromal cells stain with CD34, vimentin,

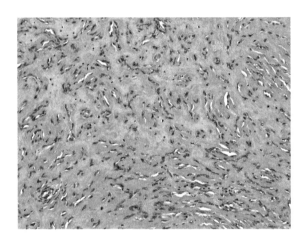

Figure 25.18 Pseudoangiomatous stromal hyperplasia. Myofibroblasts line slit-like spaces in a background of dense fibrosis. The morphological appearance mimics vascular proliferation.

desmin, and smooth muscle actin suggesting myofibroblastic differentiation in the stromal cells. No staining is seen with cytokeratin nor Factor-VIII-associated antigen. It is important that this lesion is not inadvertently categorized as angiosarcoma. In rare cases PASH can recur after excision. With increasing awareness of this lesion by radiologists and pathologists, PASH is being more commonly diagnosed as an incidental lesion in breast biopsies, but reassuringly in a series of 149 patients no case was associated with carcinoma (19). In the absence of suspicious radiological or clinical features a diagnosis of PASH on core biopsy does not necessitate an excisional biopsy.

MALE BREAST
The male breast is a rudimentary organ which is composed only of ducts and lobules that are not present normally. The most common pathological condition is unilateral or bilateral mammary enlargement—*gynecomastia*. Gynecomastia should be distinguished from *lipomastia* or *pseudogynecomastia* which is breast enlargement seen in obese men and can disappear with weight loss. A variety of etiologic factors can cause gynecomastia, including systemic diseases such as cirrhosis (impaired metabolism of estrogen), chronic renal failure, and hyperthyroidism. Several medications have been associated with gynecomastia including commonly prescribed drugs such as digitalis, tricyclic antidepressants, and the H2 antagonist cimetidine. Hormone-producing tumors such as seminomas and teratomas can also cause gynecomastia. Bilateral gynecomastia is likely to have a systemic cause while unilateral gynecomastia raises the possibility of an underlying neoplasm or idiopathic etiology. Microscopic examination of gynecomastia in the proliferative phase shows abundant ducts with epithelial hyperplasia in myxoid stroma (Fig. 25.19A). Not uncommonly the stroma shows a pseudoangiomatous stromal hyperplasia (Fig. 25.19B). When gynecomastia persists for more than 12 months the epithelial hyperplastic element regresses and the stroma becomes sclerotic.

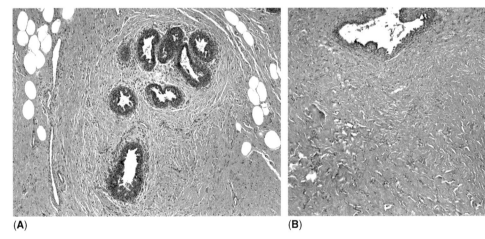

(A)   (B)

Figure 25.19 Gynecomastia. Ducts with epithelial hyperplasia are seen in myxoid stroma (A). The stroma may have a pseudoangiomatous pattern (B).

REFERENCES

1. Inderbir Singh JP. Human Embryology, 8th edn. New Delhi, India: McMillan India, 2007.
2. Rosen P. Rosen's Breast Pathology, 3rd edn. Philadelphia: Lippincott Williams & Wilkins, 2009.
3. Mills S. Histology for Pathologists, 4th edn. Philadelphia: Lippincott Williams and Wilkins, 2012.
4. Morrogh M, Andrade VP, Giri D, et al. Cadherin-catenin complex dissociation in lobular neoplasia of the breast. Breast Cancer Res Treat 2012; 132: 641–52.
5. Krag DN, Anderson SJ, Julian TB, et al. Sentinel-lymph-node resection compared with conventional axillary-lymph-node dissection in clinically node-negative patients with breast cancer: overall survival findings from the NSABP B-32 randomised phase 3 trial. Lancet Oncol 2010; 11: 927–33.
6. Eschenbach DA. Acute postpartum infections. Emerg Med Clin North Am 1985; 3: 87–115.
7. Furlong AJ, al-Nakib L, Knox WF, Parry A, Bundred NJ. Periductal inflammation and cigarette smoke. J Am Coll Surg 1994; 179: 417–20.
8. Oberman HA. Invasive carcinoma of the breast with granulomatous response. Am J Clin Pathol 1987; 88: 718–21.
9. Soler NG, Khardori R. Fibrous disease of the breast, thyroiditis, and cheiroarthropathy in type I diabetes mellitus. Lancet 1984; 1: 193–5.
10. Cernea SS, Kihara SM, Sotto MN, Vilela MA. Lupus mastitis. J Am Acad Dermatol 1993; 29: 343–6.
11. Harrison GO, Elliott RL. Scleroderma of the breast: light and electron microscopy study. Am Surg 1987; 53: 528–31.
12. Bonnetblanc JM, Bernard P, Fayol J. Dermatomyositis and malignancy. A multicenter cooperative study. Dermatologica 1990; 180: 212–16.
13. Hartmann LC, Sellers TA, Frost MH, et al. Benign breast disease and the risk of breast cancer. N Engl J Med 2005; 353: 229–37.
14. Elmore JG, Gigerenzer G. Benign breast disease—the risks of communicating risk. N Engl J Med 2005; 353: 297–9.
15. Jacobs TW, Byrne C, Colditz G, Connolly JL, Schnitt SJ. Radial scars in benign breast-biopsy specimens and the risk of breast cancer. N Engl J Med 1999; 340: 430–6.
16. Dupont WD, Page DL, Parl FF, et al. Long-term risk of breast cancer in women with fibroadenoma. N Engl J Med 1994; 331: 10–15.
17. Reinfuss M, Mitus J, Duda K, et al. The treatment and prognosis of patients with phyllodes tumor of the breast: an analysis of 170 cases. Cancer 1996; 77: 910–16.
18. Jaffer S, Nagi C, Bleiweiss IJ. Excision is indicated for intraductal papilloma of the breast diagnosed on core needle biopsy. Cancer 2009; 115: 2837–43.
19. Hargaden GC, Yeh ED, Georgian-Smith D, et al. Analysis of the mammographic and sonographic features of pseudoangiomatous stromal hyperplasia. AJR Am J Roentgenol 2008; 191: 359–63.

26 Histological risk factors, prognostic indicators, and staging

Emad A. Rakha, Sarah Pinder, and Ian O. Ellis

RISK FACTORS

Risk factors may be defined as those characteristics that impart a greater chance of developing a disease over the risk of the general population. Assessment of risk allows for improvements in the design and application of cancer-preventive strategies and intervention trials as well as improved clinical decision making. The biological risk factors for development of breast cancer are complex, multifactorial, and still remain poorly understood. Several risk factors for breast cancer are well recognized, including genetic factors, family history of breast cancer, reproductive hormone, radiation exposure, age, diet/nutrition, together with morphological factors within the breast itself. However, this chapter will concentrate on histopathological risk factors.

In the assessment of breast cancer histopathological risk indicators, premalignant lesions are by no means trivial. A multitude of proliferative hyperplastic and premalignant alterations have been identified, not uncommonly occurring synchronously with invasive carcinomas. Observational and correlative studies have identified some of these lesions as risk indicators or premalignant with potential to progress to an overtly malignant phenotype (i.e., non-obligate breast cancer precursors) (1–4). Molecular studies have demonstrated that most of these risk indicators are clonal, neoplastic proliferations which have histological, immunohistochemical, and molecular features identical to those of matched invasive breast cancers (either synchronous or metachronous). Lesions that fulfill these criteria are therefore considered breast cancer precursors. As the chance of one of these precursors progressing to invasive breast cancer rarely equates to 100%, these lesions are more accurately described as non-obligate precursors (5). Current evidence indicates that epithelial proliferative diseases, including usual-type and atypical ductal epithelial hyperplasia, lobular neoplasia, and columnar cell lesions confer an increased risk of developing breast cancer. These lesions may be discovered coincidentally in the histopathology breast screening practice and they are associated with an increased risk of breast cancer in the same breast (ipsilateral) and to a lesser degree in the contralateral breast. There is a minimally increased risk of cancer in patients with usual-type epithelial hyperplasia which is associated with a 1.5–2.0 times risk of breast cancer during the subsequent 10–15 years after diagnosis. Atypical ductal hyperplasia (ADH) is associated with a 4.6-fold increased risk, although this risk falls after 10–15 years toward that of a control population (6). However, if there is an associated family history (at least one first-degree relative), the risk associated with ADH doubles (7). Atypical lobular hyperplasia confers a four- to fivefold-increased relative risk, and

lobular carcinoma *in situ* an 8- to 10-fold increased risk (8). The presence of pure columnar cell lesions alone is associated with a mild increase in the overall breast cancer risk (risk ratio 1.47) (9,10).

These epithelial proliferative lesions may be excised coincidentally, for example in association with a lesion noted symptomatically or detected in a breast screening program, but may warrant follow-up if a sufficiently high risk is conferred. The risk incurred by the patient with these lesions and the lifetime risk for an "average" woman (which is reported as 1 in 8 for women in the United States (11)) must be interpreted with care by clinicians. The *relative risk* indicates the number of patients who develop breast cancer compared with that of the general population over a given period of time. In contrast, the *absolute risk* of developing breast cancer reflects the probability of developing breast cancer for that patient and is related to the women's age, the age-specific incidence of carcinoma, and deaths from other causes, as well as the relative risk of that individual, and is thus a more useful concept for the patient. Thus the relative risk for a 40-year-old woman with an ADH of 4.5 is reflected in an absolute risk of about 8–10% for developing invasive breast carcinoma in the following 18–20 years; however, for a 60-year-old woman with ADH, the risk is 25% within 20 years. Thus, it may be easier for a patient to understand her true individual risk of developing breast carcinoma in terms of *absolute risk*. The relative risks associated with epithelial proliferative diseases may not be long-lasting; the increased risk associated with ADH lasts only 10–15 years, therefore an indefinite follow-up at a high-risk clinic for patients with some of these lesions (and no family history) may not be justified and induce unnecessary anxiety.

Other benign conditions, such as sclerosing adenosis, radial scar, and fibroadenomas are associated with a minor increased relative risk of breast carcinoma (1.7-fold (12), 1.8-fold (13), and 2.17-fold that of the general population, respectively); however, the risk increases to 3.10-fold for "complex" fibroadenomas with foci of sclerosing adenosis or papillary apocrine change (14). These benign lesions often involve both luminal and myoepithelial cells and sometimes stromal cells, and they do not display genetic aberrations in common with those of true precursors and invasive breast cancer (15).

Prognostic Indicators

Prediction of the behavior of breast carcinoma by the use of prognostic indicators is essential; breast cancer is not a single disease entity and does not behave in a standard fashion. In particular, the range of treatment choices for patients with breast cancer has widened considerably including variation in the extent of primary breast surgery (breast conservation surgery or mastectomy), variation in the extent of axillary surgery, and differing adjuvant local and systemic therapies.

Prognostic factors are considered to have three major functions. The first purpose is to identify patients whose prognosis is so good that they require no further adjuvant treatment. The second function is to identify patients whose prognosis is so poor that an aggressive approach to treatment may be required. The third function is to identify patients who may respond or be resistant to specific therapies, thus acting as predictive agents. Therefore treatment strategies for individual patients can and should be tailored, based on the predictions of behavior for each breast tumor. Although historically the major role of the pathologist lay in providing an accurate diagnosis, it is now well recognized that much important prognostic information can be obtained from careful examination of well-fixed resected tumor and regional lymph nodes.

Pathological prognostic factors in breast cancer include time-dependent prognostic variables and biological prognostic variables. Time-dependent prognostic variables include tumor size, lymph node stage, and the extent of distant tumor spread (tumor stage/morphological features). These variables constitute all three components of the American Joint Commission on Cancer (AJCC) tumor, node, and metastasis (TNM) staging system (16). Lymph node stage and tumor size are main components of other prognostic algorithms (e.g., Adjuvant! Online (17)), guidelines (e.g., St Gallen (18)), and indices (e.g., Nottingham Prognostic Index, NPI (19)) currently used to determine the likelihood of tumor behavior and guide the use of systemic therapy for early-stage breast cancer. Biological prognostic variables are primary tumor characteristics that determine the tumor behavior and its response to therapy. Biological variables can be assessed using morphological surrogates such as tumor differentiation (e.g., tumor grade and histological type), proliferation status, growth rate, and molecular parameters such as assessment of gene/protein status individually or in consort (e.g., biomarker expression and molecular profiling at the level of DNA, RNA, or protein). There is a strong relationship between morphological and molecular features and between biological variables and tumor stage; biologically aggressive tumors are more likely to present at an advanced stage while biologically indolent tumors are likely to be slow growing and to be detected at an earlier stage. The relationship between time and tumor stage is, in fact, more obvious among tumors of similar biological characteristics. Tumor stage and not biological characteristics is the fundamental principal of breast cancer screening programs which aim for early detection of tumors regardless of their biological features. In early/operable breast cancer, knowledge about tumor stage provides important prognostic information and indicates the likelihood of recurrence or death from the disease; patients with larger primary tumors or lymph node positivity are more likely to develop recurrence or die of their disease than patients with smaller tumors or with negative lymph nodes. Despite the lack of direct predictive value, tumor stage is conventionally used to guide the use of systemic therapy by reflecting the extent of tumor burden and tumor spread and the associated prognostic information in the form of risk of tumor recurrence. On the other hand, knowledge about biological features of a given breast cancer provide information on the inherent nature and potential behavior of

that tumor and are reflected in outcome characteristics such as the time to recurrence. Typically, patients with biologically aggressive tumors either develop recurrence early after diagnosis or show long-term evidence of cure from their disease. In contrast, patients with indolent tumors are at a risk of recurrence over a more prolonged period of time (20–23). Therefore, knowledge about both tumor stage and biological variables has to be considered in combination when planning the treatment of breast cancer. Although advanced stage is usually a clear indication for systemic therapy, for early-stage disease, therapy is mainly based on biological factors.

Cancer staging can be performed using assessment with both clinical (clinical stage) and pathological (pathological stage) parameters at the time of diagnosis or after therapy or even recurrence. Patients with similar prognosis are grouped into anatomic stage/prognostic groups (stage groups). The TNM staging method incorporates an assessment of the primary tumor size (T), the regional lymph nodes (N), and distant metastases (M). Although initially proposed in 1954, several modifications have since been made. Tumor biological features are best assessed through a pathological/molecular examination of tumor tissue and stratified according to the prognostic and/or predictive value of the biological features assessed. However, assessment of biological features is not as straightforward as assessment of tumor stage. The former may suffer from inherent subjectivity and assessment may be influenced by processing and fixation of tissue, and be of limited value in small size tumors. It is not always possible to link biological features of the primary tumor to breast cancer metastasis and disease-related deaths in cases of development of intervening new primary or in-breast recurrences with different biological features.

Tumor Size

For prognostic purposes the size of tumors should be assessed by the pathologist, as clinical measurement is not sufficiently accurate; a correlation between surgical and pathological assessment of tumor size was found in only 54% of cases by the Yorkshire Breast Cancer Group (24). Benign tissue and hyperplastic changes may contribute to the apparent size of a palpable lesion. Ultrasound measurement is more useful if an estimate of clinical tumor size is required for treatment planning. In the 7th edition of the AJCC Cancer Staging Manual, microscopic measurement is considered the most accurate and preferred method to determine the size (pT) in small invasive cancers (25). Tumor size can be assessed in the fresh state and in the fixed specimen, when the margins of the tumor may be better defined. However, the Vernier scale on the microscopic stage provides the most accurate size determination of small lesions, pure *in situ* cancers, and cases with extensive *in situ* disease on tissue sections. For larger tumors, histological confirmation of size can be made on slides prepared from tumor blocks taken from four quadrants of the tumor that has been incised in a cruciate manner. As breast carcinomas often have asymmetric shape, the measurement of size is reported in terms of the largest diameter of the tumor. For prognostic value, only the size of the invasive tumor is considered. *In situ* components can be considered in the whole tumor size measurement to provide an estimate of the extent of the tumor. In cases of multifocal tumor with multiple foci separated by benign tissue, tumor size is the diameter of the largest invasive lesion (26).

A multitude of studies have confirmed the prognostic significance of breast cancer size; survival decreases with increasing tumor size (27–30). Rosen and Groshen in 1990 (31) reported a 20-year relapse-free survival rate of 88% for patients with tumors less than 10 mm in diameter, 73% for cancers measuring 11–13 mm, 65% for cancers measuring 14–16 mm, and 59% for cancers measuring 17–22 mm. Furthermore, the Nottingham/Tenovus Primary Breast Carcinoma Series (NTPBCS) has confirmed by multivariate analysis that tumor size is an important independent variable (32) forming an integral component of the NPI.

Because of the recognition of the prognostic importance of tumor size, this parameter has become an important quality assurance measure for radiologists in the United Kingdom (UK) National Health Service Breast Screening Programme (NHSBSP), with a recommendation that a target of 15 minimal invasive carcinomas per 10,000 women screened should be detected. In the ONCOPOOL series which is a retrospectively compiled database of primary operable invasive breast cancers treated in the 1990s in 10 European breast cancer units, 24% of tumors were ≤1cm and 70% were ≤2 cm (33). The terms "minimal breast cancer" and "minimal invasive breast carcinoma" have been used by different groups to represent lesions of varying sizes but there is little doubt whether lesions measuring 10 mm or less are at an earlier stage than larger tumors. Lymph node metastasis is identified in approximately 10% of tumors less than 10 mm as compared with 35% of lesions measuring greater than 15 mm in diameter (34,35). It has also been reported that in small tumors (pT1) the presence of *in situ* carcinoma is correlated with lower nodal positivity (36).

Although breast cancer size is generally considered to be a fundamental and critical determinant of lymph node positivity and clinical outcome, some molecular subtypes, in particular basal-like and BRCA1-related breast cancers, have a tendency to behave aggressively despite being of small tumor size. This observation may reflect an underlying disproportionate relationship between the number of cancer cells with metastatic potential and the size of the cancer (37).

As a prognostic marker, tumor size is used in the NPI as a continuous variable ($0.2 \times$ size in cm) in combination with lymph node stage (1–3) and histological grade (1–3) (19)). In contrast, tumor size is used as a categorical variable in the TNM system: ≤1 mm (pT1mi), >1 mm but ≤5 mm (pT1a), >5 mm but ≤10 mm (pT1b), >10 mm but ≤20 mm (pT1c), >20 mm but ≤50 mm (pT2), and >50 mm in greatest dimension (pT3). Tumors more than 50 mm carry a worse prognosis than those of lesser dimensions and are considered as locally advanced and breast conservation surgery is usually not recommended for these tumors. Small tumors (≤10 mm) have an excellent outcome which may justify local treatment as the only form of therapy when they are associated with lymph node negativity and favorable grade (grade 1 or special-type histology) (38–40).

Histological Grade and Type
Invasive breast carcinomas are morphologically subdivided according to their growth patterns and degree of differentiation, the latter reflecting how closely they resemble normal breast epithelial cells. This subdivision is achieved by assessing the histological type and grade, respectively. Both factors can be assessed by a microscopic examination of routinely stained tissue sections, although it is essential that samples be well fixed, and well-defined criteria must be used and adhered to (22). Ideally, specimens should be sent to the laboratory in the fresh state, incised immediately and placed in fixative to obtain optimum preservation of morphological details and mitotic figures.

Histological grading has become widely accepted as a powerful indicator of prognosis in addition to providing an overview of the intrinsic biological characteristics of tumors (22,41,42). Several studies have refuted earlier suggestions of lack of reproducibility if strict criteria are maintained (41). Two main methods for histological grading have evolved. One is based on nuclear features alone, and the other on both architectural and tumor cell features. The latter has been modified to give greater objectivity and has been recommended by various professional bodies internationally including the World Health Organization (WHO), AJCC, European Union (EU) and the UK Royal College of Pathologists (RCPath) (43–45). This method of histological grading assesses the three features of tubule formation, nuclear size/pleomorphism and mitotic count; each of these elements is scored 1–3 and the sum of the scores is used to categorize the tumor. If less than 10% of the carcinoma is forming luminal structures, a score 3 is given; those with 10–75% score 2, and if more than 75% of the cancer is forming tubules, a score of 1 is given. A score for tumor cell pleomorphism/size is given as 1, 2 or 3 according to whether mild pleomorphism/small cell size, moderate pleomorphism/medium size or highly pleomorphic/large nuclear size is seen. As noted above, good fixation is essential for reliable assessment of mitotic count. A score for this component is given according to the field area of the high-power lens used. Although included in the technique of Bloom and Richardson (46) for determination of histological grade, hyperchromatic (and apoptotic) nuclei should be discounted in the modified system, that is, only nuclei with definite features of metaphase, anaphase, or telophase are included. An overall sum of the three component scores of 3, 4, or 5 indicates a grade 1 cancer, a score of 6 or 7 a grade 2 tumor, and a score of 8 or 9 a carcinoma of histological grade 3. In unselected series of operable breast cancer, the distribution of histological grade is 20–25% grade 1, 35–48% grade 2, and 20–45% grade 3 tumors (41). Of note, a greater proportion of grade 1 carcinomas are found in screening programs compared with symptomatic practice.

Histological grade is a strong indicator of patient survival (Fig. 26.1). Patients with grade 1 carcinomas have a 93% 10-year survival rate, compared with a rate of less than 65% for patients with grade 3 tumors (22). In addition, histological grade provides information on prediction of response to therapy; as such, grade may also be regarded as a predictive factor in both the adjuvant (47) and advanced breast cancer settings (48). The prognostic significance of grade has become increasingly important with the shift in stage distribution due to mammographic screening, with a high proportion of tumors being T1N0M0 at diagnosis, thereby limiting the relevance of TNM staging in routine practice. In early-stage breast cancer, histological grade has prognostic value that is equivalent to that of lymph node status (19,22,49) and greater than that of

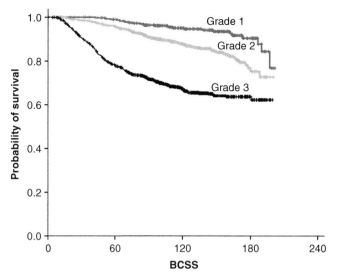

Figure 26.1 Long-term breast cancer–specific survival (BCSS) in months in the Nottingham Tenovus Primary Breast Carcinoma Series by histological grade.

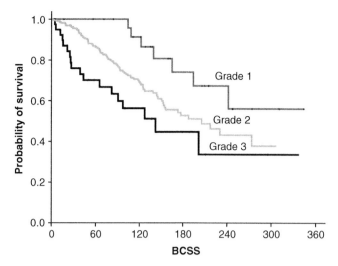

Figure 26.2 Long-term breast cancer–specific survival (BCSS in months) in the Nottingham Tenovus Primary Breast Carcinoma Series for lobular carcinoma (all subtypes) by histological grade.

tumor size (19,22,50,51). The prognostic value of grade is more important in the subgroups of breast cancer such as patients with lymph node-negative ER-positive/HER2-negative tumors or in patients with low volume lymph node metastatic disease (pN1) where the decision on use of chemotherapy cannot be determined based on risk associated with more advanced tumor stage (41,47,52). In addition to patient outcome, histological grade is associated with other clinicopathological prognostic variables such as lymph node stage, tumor size, lymphovascular invasion (22,53–55), and expression of biomarkers of prognostic and predictive value such as hormone receptor, HER2, p53, "basal" markers and P-cadherin, and prognostic gene signatures (56,57).

Breast carcinomas show a great variation in morphological appearance, and some forms of primary breast cancer, the so-called "special types," carry a significantly better prognosis than the more common "no special type" (NST)/ductal tumors (58–60). Other tumor types with varying prognoses have been recognized, and up to 15 categories of invasive tumor type are used in the Nottingham unit, excluding *in situ* and microinvasive classes (61). If a large number of mixed types are recorded, a smaller proportion of lesions will be classified as NST/ductal (approximately 55% of breast carcinomas in the authors' unit); tumors that include areas of NST with additional foci of "special-type" morphology are categorized separately. We have found that these groups of tumors behave differently, with better prognosis for ductal NST carcinomas when combined with foci of special-type carcinoma, compared with "pure" ductal NST breast carcinomas (61). An increased proportion of the good-prognosis "special types" is seen in screening compared with symptomatic practice.

The complexities of invasive breast tumor classification will not be outlined in this chapter, but for prognostication purposes several tumor types can be amalgamated into four prognostic groups according to the demonstrated 10-year survival rate from the NTPBCS (60). Those tumor types with an excellent prognosis (>90% 10-year survival rate) include tubular, invasive cribriform, mucinous, and tubulolobular carcinomas. Tumors with a good prognosis (70–90% 10-year survival rate)

include tubular mixed, alveolar lobular, and mixed ductal/NST with special type. A 10-year survival rate of 70% is seen with medullary, invasive papillary, and classical lobular carcinomas. A poor prognosis (<70% 10-year survival rate) is observed with lesions of mixed lobular, solid lobular, pleomorphic lobular, NST, mixed ductal with lobular and metaplastic types.

Tumor-type group alone provides important biological information, but is not in our opinion as valuable as histological grade for predicting any individual patient's likely prognosis. This is not only true for tumors of NST/ductal morphology in which the importance of histological grade is well recognized but is of value for all invasive breast cancers (62). For example, the majority of invasive lobular carcinomas are grade 2 morphology (scoring 3 for tubules, 2 for pleomorphism, and 1 for mitosis), but other grade subgroups (grade 1 or grade 3) may be identified and have prognostic significance (Fig. 26.2). Thus, we recommend grading all invasive breast carcinomas.

It has been suggested that histological grading was not a reproducible technique for providing prognostic information, but the same potential difficulties regarding reproducibility apply to accurate histological typing of some lesions. Although some histological tumor types, such as mucinous carcinoma, may be determined reproducibly (63), problems of typing are compounded by the larger number of type categories that must be selected from by the reporting pathologist. Issues of reproducibility may to some extent explain the variation in patient survival reported in the literature for some types of invasive breast cancer; for example, the survival of medullary carcinomas is not as favorable in the NTPBCS (59) as compared with some other studies (64). This variation in the survival of patients with medullary carcinoma is likely to be, in part, a reflection of the difficulties in establishing robust diagnostic criteria for this breast carcinoma type (65). While criteria for grading carcinomas are now strictly defined, this is less true for breast tumor typing (66).

Despite these difficulties, both histological type and grade provide important complementary prognostic information. While in multivariate analysis, grade is of much greater importance in

Table 26.1 TNM Pathological Classification for Regional Lymph Node Stage (25,73)

pNX	Regional Lymph Nodes Not Assessable
pN0	No metastasis and no additional examination performed
pN0(i–)[a]	No regional node metastasis, immunohistologically negative
pN0(i+)[a]	No regional node metastasis, immunohistologically positive, but no cluster >0.2 mm
pN0(mol–)	No regional node metastasis, negative molecular findings (RT-PCR)
pN0(mol+)	No regional node metastasis, positive molecular findings (RT-PCR)
pN1mi	Micrometastasis (>0.2 mm, but ≤2mm in the greatest dimension)
pN1	Metastasis in 1–3 ipsilateral axillary lymph nodes, and/or in internal mammary nodes with microscopic metastasis detected by SLN dissection but not clinically apparent
pN1a	Metastasis in 1–3 axillary lymph nodes (including at least one that is >2 mm, i.e., not micrometastatic)
pN1b	Metastasis in internal mammary lymph nodes with microscopic metastasis detected by SLN dissection but not clinically apparent
pN1c	Metastasis in 1–3 axillary lymph nodes *and* internal mammary lymph nodes with microscopic metastasis detected by SLN dissection but not clinically apparent
pN2	Metastasis in 4–9 ipsilateral axillary lymph nodes, or in clinically apparent ipsilateral internal mammary lymph nodes in the absence of axillary lymph node metastasis
pN2a	Metastasis in 4–9 axillary lymph nodes (including at least 1 that is >2 mm, i.e., not micrometastatic)
pN2b	Metastasis in clinically apparent internal mammary lymph nodes in the *absence* of axillary lymph node metastasis
pN3	Metastasis in ≥10 ipsilateral axillary lymph nodes or in infraclavicular lymph nodes or in clinically apparent ipsilateral internal mammary lymph nodes in the *presence* of one or more positive axillary lymph nodes; or in >3 axillary lymph nodes with a clinically negative microscopic metastasis in internal mammary lymph nodes; or in ipsilateral supraclavicular lymph nodes
pN3a	Metastasis in ≥10 axillary lymph nodes (at least one >2 mm) *or* metastasis in infraclavicular lymph nodes
pN3b	Metastasis in clinically apparent internal mammary lymph nodes in the *presence* of one or more positive axillary lymph nodes; or metastasis in >3 axillary lymph nodes and in internal mammary lymph nodes with microscopic metastasis detected by SLN dissection but not clinically apparent
pN3c	Metastasis in ipsilateral supraclavicular lymph nodes

If determined using a SLN technique alone, stage is designated "(sn)" for example, pN0 (i–)(sn).
[a]The Union for International Cancer Control, American Joint Commission on Cancer, UK, and EU (77,78) allocate single-node involvement by micrometastatic disease (deposit size 0.2–2 mm) to the node-positive Stage (TNM N1mi category) and isolated tumor cells (deposit size <0.2 mm) to the node-negative Stage, (TNM N0 category).
Abbreviations: RT-PCR, reverse transcriptase polymerase chain reaction; SLN, sentinel lymph node.

predicting survival than type, tumor typing provides additional information on behavior. For example, lobular carcinomas, particularly those of alveolar lobular type, are often estrogen receptor (ER)-positive, show different expression of markers such as E-cadherin and the catenins (67), and may also demonstrate a different pattern of metastatic disease to tumors of no special type (20).

Lymph Node Staging
Staging of breast cancer is essential in the assessment of a patient's prognosis and selection of treatment options. Reliable nodal staging of invasive breast carcinoma is imperative and a careful histological examination of lymph nodes should be carried out. Histologically confirmed regional lymph node status has repeatedly been shown to be the single most important prognostic factor in early-stage breast cancer. Numerous studies have shown that patients with involved lymph nodes have a poorer prognosis than those with no metastases in the locoregional nodes; 15–30% of node-negative patients will develop recurrence within 10 years, compared with up to 70% of patients with axillary nodal involvement (68–73). Prognosis is also related to the absolute number of positive nodes as determined by the histological examination and the level of locoregional lymph nodes involved; the greater the number of nodes involved the poorer is the overall patient survival (Table 26.1). Similarly, involvement of nodes in the "higher" levels of the

axilla, and specifically the apex, or the involvement of the internal mammary nodes carries a worse prognosis (28,73). A further refinement of lymph node staging may be provided by the size of the metastatic deposits (73–75) and the ratio of positive nodes to the total number of harvested nodes (76). In symptomatic breast cancer approximately one-third (range 30–40%) of operable breast cancer patients present with positive nodes, while 7–15% of patients present with more than three positive nodes (33). The frequency of node positivity declines to less than 20% among patients presenting through established breast mammographic screening programs.

Clinical determination of lymph node stage is notoriously inaccurate; lymph nodes may be enlarged due to reactive changes, while nodes bearing metastatic tumor may be impalpable. Although preoperative ultrasound imaging of the axilla (with guided core biopsy or fine needle aspiration cytology of suspicious lymph nodes) has now become standard practice in some centers (and should be performed for women with a clinically and sonographically node-negative invasive carcinoma of the breast), surgical axillary staging remains the gold standard to determine nodal involvement (79). Surgical staging was initially achieved by axillary lymph node dissection, but high rates of morbidity prompted alternative staging techniques (80). Moreover, the widespread use of breast cancer screening has led to more early-stage node-negative patients being detected in whom axillary dissection would now be recognized as overtreatment. As an alternative to axillary dissection, an axillary node sample, assessing a limited number of nodes (usually 3–5 nodes per case including the sentinel node) with subsequent regional axillary radiotherapy or axillary clearance for lymph node-positive disease, was adopted (81–83). Trials support this conservative approach, showing no detriment to survival or recurrence (84). Steele et al. (81) found no difference in the incidence of cases of lymph node positivity in patients with sampling or clearance and argued that, provided that at least four nodes were examined, sufficient prognostic information could be provided by sampling. The greater number of nodes obtained by clearance is associated with increased postoperative morbidity, including lymphedema and reduced shoulder mobility. Conversely, it was perceived that sampling or low axillary clearance may potentially "understage" the axilla. Therefore there was no consensus on the number of nodes that should be examined to ensure accurate staging. In our center we have adopted the axillary sampling approach from the1990's until SLN biopsy became the standard axillary staging procedure for patients with preoperatively negative nodes.

The SLN is the first node that drains the tumor and is thus potentially the site of initial metastasis (85). Current evidence demonstrates that, when performed by experienced clinicians, SLN biopsy appears to be a safe and acceptably accurate method for identifying early-stage breast cancer without involvement of the axillary lymph nodes (86). Many validation studies have shown it to be accurate and feasible for invasive breast cancer with preoperatively negative nodes (clinical, sonographical, and/or cytohistological by fine needle aspiration or core biopsy) (87–89). The status of the SLN should therefore reflect the nodal status of the axilla and provide prognostic information. The SLN concept has been validated for breast cancer and has replaced routine axillary dissection (90).

In addition, SLN biopsy has been demonstrated to be useful for more extensive ductal carcinoma *in situ*, especially those suspected of containing microinvasion or scheduled for mastectomy, as well as multifocal (86) and multicentric (91) cancers.

A weakness of some of the SLN studies is that the SLN is examined more intensively than the other nodes, which may mean that metastases in non-SLNs are missed or that small deposits in the SLN are more likely to be reported compared with conventional studies of nodal pathology in the established medical literature (88). Additional laboratory techniques, including complete embedding of the node or assessment of step sections, immunohistochemistry, and even reverse transcriptase polymerase chain reaction (RT-PCR), have been used to increase the sensitivity for detection of metastases. Complete embedding of each node and/or serial, step sectioning was employed to increase the chance of identifying metastases, as more of the node is examined (92). Immunohistochemistry increases detection (93), in part by making small metastases more visible. RT-PCR examines all the tissue submitted and it is considered as a very sensitive method that is theoretically capable of identifying a single tumor cell (94). However, most studies find that isolated tumor cells in nodes have no prognostic importance. Evidence from retrospective studies done in the pre-SLN era and two large randomized studies of SLN biopsy suggest that occult metastases identified with immunohistochemistry and not seen on H&E sections have little or no prognostic effect independent of traditional prognostic factors (95–97). From the point of view of the histopathologist, whatever the surgical extent and technique, all of the excised nodes must be examined microscopically. Whether the lymph nodes received are taken as part of an axillary sampling or as a SLN technique, blocks are taken by serial slicing of each node along the long axis in approximately 3 mm slices, thus providing the largest area of lymph node and peripheral sinus possible in one section. Ideally, each node should be examined in a separate cassette, and the majority of lymph nodes can be entirely embedded in slices in this way, although large non-SLNs may have alternate slices embedded. The workload and costs are substantially increased by examining every case of node biopsy either immunohistochemically or by serial sectioning. Guidelines in the UK for pathology specimen handling and reporting in breast cancer screening do not recommend a routine use of immunohistochemistry, step sectioning, or RT-PCR for examination of lymph nodes from patients with breast cancer (78). A few cases where features suspicious of metastatic disease are seen on H&E may be assessed immunohistochemically with anticytokeratin antibodies.

Vascular Invasion

Apart from tumor size, histological grade and lymph node stage, lymphovascular invasion (blood vessel or lymphatic space) is another independent prognostic factor for recurrence and survival on multivariate analysis (98,99). Some studies have also demonstrated that the assessment of lymphovascular invasion provides prognostic information as powerful as that provided by involvement with one or two positive lymph nodes (98,100) or by tumor size (98) in early stage–operable breast cancer. Some studies have also reported that lymphovascular invasion is a predictive factor for local recurrence after wide local excision (99) and flap recurrence in patients who have had mastectomy (101). However, other groups have not found similar correlations (102). Lymphovascular invasion is strongly associated with lymph node involvement (101,103) and provides prognostic value in node-negative patients. Therefore, it has been proposed that lymphovascular invasion could be used to identify a subgroup of lymph node-negative patients with an unfavorable prognosis who are likely to benefit from adjuvant chemotherapy (98,103,104). A wide variation in the incidence of lymphovascular invasion has been reported and may be related to the difficulties in adhering to strictly defined criteria and obtaining good fixation of specimens which must be optimal to avoid the difficulties of retraction artifacts mimicking tumor emboli.

While special techniques have been used to assess vascular invasion in breast carcinoma, these have a role to play predominantly in distinguishing artifactual shrinkage from true vascular spaces (105). Elastic stains are of little help in distinguishing ducts from vessels, and neither lymphatics nor small capillaries have elastic lamina. At present, we report vascular invasion in three categories: absent, definite, or probable. Probable vascular invasion is reported when an unequivocal endothelial lining cannot be seen but when possible tumor

Table 26.2 Proportion of Patients and Overall Survival in the Nottingham Tenovus Primary Breast Carcinoma Series by Nottingham Prognostic Index (NPI) Group: An Updated Analysis Based on Over 3700 Women with Primary Operable Breast Cancer Aged less than 71 Years

	NPI group (NPI values)				
	Excellent (<2.4)	Good (2.4≤3.4)	Moderate I (3.4–4.5)	Moderate II (4.4–5.4)	Poor (>5.4)
Number of cases	475	744	1001	891	590
Proportion of cases (%)	13	20	27	24	16
5-year survival rate (%)	97	93	85	75	42
10-year survival rate (%)	91	82	73	55	26
15-year survival rate (%)	84	74	63	46	18

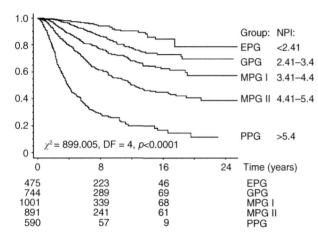

			Group:	NPI:
			EPG	<2.41
			GPG	2.41–3.4
			MPG I	3.41–4.4
			MPG II	4.41–5.4
			PPG	>5.4

$\chi^2 = 899.005$, DF = 4, $p < 0.0001$

0	8	16	24	Time (years)
475	223	46		EPG
744	289	69		GPG
1001	339	68		MPG I
891	241	61		MPG II
590	57	9		PPG

Figure 26.3 Long-term survival in the Nottingham Tenovus Primary Breast Carcinoma Series by Nottingham Prognostic Index (NPI) group: EPG, excellent; GPG, good; MPG I, moderate I; MPG II, moderate II; PPG, poor.

emboli are seen in the tissue adjacent to the invasive tumor. Although for therapeutic purposes we currently group this category with tumors showing no lymphovascular invasion, this category can benefit mostly from immunohistochemical staining with endothelial specific markers such as D2-40 (105).

In a previous study of the Nottingham breast cancer series, the features that predicted for local recurrence in patients undergoing wide local excision (without any selection criteria for surgery) in multivariate analysis included tumor size, the presence of vascular invasion, and young age (106). As a result of this analysis, our practice has been changed to advise patients with tumors larger than 3 cm clinically or radiologically against conservation surgery, especially if they are younger than 40 years of age. Postoperatively, completion mastectomy is advisable if the tumor is larger than 2 cm, histological grade 3, node positive, and shows definite lymphovascular invasion. Thus the importance of the presence of lymphovascular invasion in patient management lies in the prediction of not only survival but also recurrence and should be routinely reported in excision specimens.

Use of Prognostic Indicators
Several factors provide prognostic information in patients with primary breast cancer, and no single indicator is universally recognized to be of overall importance. The time-dependent factor of lymph node stage has been most consistently

used as a guide for stratification in most centers for patient treatment and entry into clinical trials. It should be noted however that nodal stage is of relatively poor discriminatory value; neither a group of patients with close to 100% mortality nor a group with almost normal survival can be identified by the presence or absence of lymph node metastases alone. The intrinsic biological "aggressiveness" of the tumor is also of prognostic importance and is assessed by histological grade. For each individual patient, benefit may be gained from a combination of the time-dependent and biological features of the tumor to predict prognosis.

It has long been recognized that a combination of lymph node stage and tumor differentiation is more useful than either alone in the prediction of the behavior of many epithelial malignancies. Variables that are of independent prognostic significance in multivariate analyses can be combined into a prognostic index to obtain the best prediction of survival for each individual patient. The factors of greatest prognostic importance in primary operable breast carcinoma have been found to be lymph node stage, histological grade, and tumor size. These factors have been combined with appropriate weighting from the β^2-value of multivariate analyses to form the NPI: [0.2 × tumor size (in cm)] + histological grade (scored 1–3) and lymph node stage (scored 1–3). This index was initially derived from a series of 387 patients by entry of nine separate variables in a multivariate analysis; the index has been confirmed prospectively and further confirmation of its value has come from other large and multicenter series (19,50,51,107).

The NPI is used to determine an individual patient's prognosis (Table 26.2 and Fig. 26.3) and thus, to select the appropriate treatments for those with primary operable breast cancer. Patients with an NPI <2.4 have a survival comparable to that of aged-matched controls and thus receive no systemic adjuvant treatment. Conversely, patients with a higher score receive systemic treatment based on additional data such as ER status. The NPI may also be used to compare groups of patients, and the prognosis of symptomatic and screen-detected breast carcinomas can be compared using this technique. Seventy-six percent of screen-detected carcinomas in the Nottingham unit fall within the excellent and good prognostic groups, compared with only 29% of symptomatic breast cancers. Conversely, only 4% of screening cancers are in the poor-prognosis group, compared with 17% of symptomatic tumors.

The NPI is simple to calculate and is derived from data that are relatively easy to obtain from routine histological examinations of tumor and lymph nodes. Thus it was thought that additional components should not be included to avoid making the index more cumbersome and difficult to calculate. However, with a shift in stage distribution resulting from screening, significant improvements in the identification and development of systemic and targeted therapies and increasing demand for a personalized and patient tailored therapy, there is a need for further refinement of NPI. There is a perception that the NPI cannot reveal the innate heterogeneity in clinical/survival outcomes and would benefit from greater sophistication to support more accurate personalized management of breast cancer patients. It is now recognized that the biological characteristics of breast cancer are important for clinical management and incorporation into the NPI could significantly improve the delivery of personalized medicine for breast cancer patients. Therefore, attempts have been made to incorporate other biological prognostic variables into NPI to develop a biomarker-based prognostic index, Nottingham Prognostic Index Plus (NPI+). NPI+ is based on a two tier evaluation; the initial assessment determines the biological class of the tumor and is subsequently combined with a second level analysis of traditional clinicopathological prognostic variables including lymph node status, grade, size, and lymphovascular invasion resulting in "bespoke" NPI-like formulae for each biological class (unpublished data).

ER status has been used since the mid-1970s in the clinical management of breast cancer both as an indicator of endocrine responsiveness and as a prognostic factor for early recurrence. The current gold standard to assess ER status is immunohistochemistry performed on formalin-fixed, paraffin-embedded cancer tissue (108). This diagnostic test is routinely used in the clinic, and major therapeutic decisions are dependent on the results. Existing immunohistochemical assays for ER have only modest positive predictive value (30–60%) for response to single-agent hormonal therapies. However, the negative predictive value of ER expression is high (i.e., ER negativity, which accounts for 20–25% of breast cancer, can identify the population of patients who will not benefit from endocrine therapy) (109–115). The quantitative assessment of ER immunoreactivity may be performed in several ways. In the simplest form, the percentage of tumor cells that show positive immunostaining is determined; other techniques also include an assessment of the degree of positivity (116). The modified histochemical score (H-score) is one such method, incorporating a semiquantitative assessment of both the percentage and the degree of tumor cell immunoreactivity, scored from negative (0) to strong (3) into a formula: (0 × percentage of negative cells) + (1 × percentage of weakly positive cells) + (2 × percentage of moderately stained tumor cells) + (3 × percentage strongly positive tumor cell nuclei). Thus, the H-score ranges from 0 to 300. There is good correlation between clinical response and hormone treatment, which has been demonstrated using a simplified system (Quick Score) which is based on combining intensity score with a proportion of positive cells (117). Intensity is assigned scores as 0 = none, 1 = weak, 2 = intermediate, and 3 = strong; proportion is assigned scores as 0 = none, 1 = <1%, 2 = 1–10%, 3 = 11–33%, 4 = 34–66%, 5 = >66%. The scores are added together to obtain a total score which can range from 0 to 8.

Table 26.3 Response to Tamoxifen According to ER Status Assessed with the 1D5 Antibody (Dako, Carpinteria, California, USA) on Paraffin Sections (124)

	ER-Negative (H-Score <50)	ER-Positive (H-Score >50)	Total
Response (UICC 1+2)	2	18	20
Static disease (UICC 3)	1	17	18
Progression (UICC 4)	37	15	52
Total	40	50	90

$\chi^2 = 35.7$, DF = 3, $p < 0.0001$. *Abbreviations*: ER, estrogen receptor; UICC, Union for International Cancer Control.

ER status provides a good prediction of response to hormone therapy (Table 26.3). Although most authors classify tumors with a Quick Score of 2 or less as ER negative, the American Society of Clinical Oncology guidelines indicate that patients whose breast cancers have very low levels of ER staining (>1%) should be considered as ER positive as they may still benefit from adjuvant endocrine treatment (108,117). This emphasizes the need to have sensitive reproducible techniques that can detect these very low levels. Many screen-detected breast carcinomas display good prognostic features and have an NPI <2.4, and despite showing ER positivity, patients may choose to receive no further systemic treatment. Progesterone receptor (PgR) status or other estrogen-inducible molecules should be examined in patients with breast carcinoma to assess the functioning of the ER pathway. PgR is routinely assessed immunohistochemically in most centers in the UK and elsewhere and it is recommended by the UK RCPath and NHSBSP (44). Approximately 40% of ER-positive tumors are PgR negative. Lack of PgR expression in ER-positive tumors may be a surrogate marker of aberrant growth factor signaling that could contribute to tamoxifen resistance; ER+/PR− tumors are generally less responsive than ER+/PR+ tumors (118,119). PgR status can help predict response to hormone treatment, both in patients with metastatic disease (120) and in the adjuvant setting (121–123). Determination of PgR can also be valuable for patients with low ER/high PgR values to determine whether endocrine treatment is beneficial. In addition to the prognostic value of PgR, it may help to identify cases with false-negative ER immunohistochemical staining.

Amplification of HER2 gene expression occurs in 13–20% of breast cancers, and approximately 55% of these cases are ER negative (125,126). Numerous studies have found that HER2 gene amplification/protein overexpression is a predictor of poor prognosis and response to systemic chemotherapy (127–129). Following the development of a humanized monoclonal antibody against HER2, clinical trials have demonstrated benefit from use of anti-HER2 agents in patients with HER2 positive breast cancer (130–132). Determination of HER2 amplification is a prerequisite for clinical use of anti-HER2 in patients with HER2-positive advanced disease (133) as well as in the adjuvant setting for HER2-positive early stage disease (131). The expression of ER, PgR, and HER2 may overlap, and their prognostic and predictive value can be improved by using them in combination (134). Several immunohistochemical studies have used them as surrogates to define the molecular classes initially identified by microarray gene expression profiling. For instance, ER/PgR positivity was used as a surrogate for luminal class and HER2 expression characterized the HER2-enriched groups of tumors, while the triple-negative (ER-, PgR-, HER2-) phenotype was used to define the basal-like molecular class (135,136).

OTHER MORPHOLOGICAL
AND MOLECULAR MARKERS OF PROGNOSIS

A number of other morphological factors including angiogenesis, peritumoral lymphoid infiltrate, tumor necrosis, stromal fibrosis, stromal elastosis and stromal giant cells, the former feature is of particular interest and has been suggested as useful a prognostic indicator. However, although the hypothesis that breast cancer growth and metastasis are angiogenesis dependent is logical, attractive, and supported by some studies, others have failed to confirm an association with prognosis. The neovascularization of the tumor periphery provides an increased surface area for adherence and entrance of tumor cell emboli into the circulation, but the development of new vessels may occur around foci of ductal carcinoma in situ (DCIS) (137). The growth of new vessels at the periphery of a neoplasm may thus be an early event in tumor development rather than a rate-limiting step. The assessment of angiogenesis in breast carcinomas requires the identification of so-called "hot spots" and immunohistochemical staining of these areas with subsequent counting of new vessel formation. The lack of association with prognosis in several series, including a study performed in Nottingham, may be a failure to identify these areas of highest neovascularization (72). The role of angiogenesis and angiogenetic factors in breast carcinoma may prove to be more important and interesting as therapeutic targets rather than as prognostic factors. Peritumoral lymphoid infiltrate may be another useful prognostic indicator. In a previous study of 1597 patients who received no systemic adjuvant treatment and who had a median follow-up of 9.5 years, prominent inflammation was found to be associated with high histological grades and with better survival. Grade 3 ductal NST carcinoma with prominent inflammation showed a better prognosis than grade 3 ductal NST carcinoma without prominent inflammation (59).

The significance of other morphological features is unclear; tumor necrosis has been reported predominantly in breast carcinomas of no special type. The criteria and techniques for the assessment of tumor necrosis have varied among studies, making comparison of results difficult, but the overall impression is that this is a poor prognostic feature. Both early treatment failure and reduced overall survival have been reported with tumor necrosis, but further investigation with strict reproducible criteria and evaluation of extent is required. Stromal fibrosis has also been evaluated as a potential prognostic factor. A fibrotic focus is a scar-like area consisting of a mixture of fibroblasts and collagen fibers that may occupy almost the entire center of an invasive carcinoma, replacing the necrotic central area. It may be due to intratumoral hypoxia leading to clonal heterogeneity of tumor cells. Fibrotic foci are associated with a basal subtype, an expansive growth pattern,

hypoxia, and angiogenesis, activated wound-healing signature, an adverse 76-gene signature (138) and a poorer prognosis (139,140). Perineural invasion is found in 10–25% of invasive breast cancers and tends to occur in high grade tumors with positive vascular invasion and lymph node positivity. However, this factor is not proven to be independently associated with the outcome (141).

Many invasive tumors show no or minimal associated DCIS, while a small proportion (approximately 10% of cases) are associated with abundant DCIS. The presence of extensive in situ carcinoma (EIC) has been reported to be of prognostic significance. Matsukuma et al. (142) reported that tumors with less than 20% invasive component had significantly fewer lymph node metastases and a better overall 10-year survival than tumors with a greater invasive element but other series have noted an association between a prominent in situ component and lower histological grade (143). Multivariate analyses are required to determine whether the presence of abundant DCIS is of independent significance and whether histological grade rather than EIC is the important feature.

The main risk factor for local relapse after breast-conserving surgery is residual tumor burden. Although there are data indicating that the extent of extratumoral DCIS may be a predictor of prognosis in primary operable breast carcinoma treated by breast-conserving surgery (144), the authors believe that the importance of the extent of DCIS around an invasive carcinoma lies more in determining the local recurrence risk and management after conservation treatment. Schnitt et al. (145) defined EIC as DCIS amounting to 25% or more of the overall tumor mass of an invasive carcinoma and extending beyond the confines of the infiltrating component. These authors reported that tumors with EIC had a higher local relapse rate than those without EIC (145). Assessing the completeness of DCIS excision histologically, either in a "pure" form or in association with invasive carcinoma, is notoriously difficult. This is supported by the finding that the presence of EIC predicts for residual disease in re-excision specimens - the residual disease is frequently DCIS (146). None of the 30 patients with an EIC-positive tumor developed recurrence at the site of previous excision within five years if the margins were negative or close but 50% developed local recurrence when the margins were more than focally positive (147,148). Subsequently, the same group reported that among patients treated with breast-conserving therapy and radiotherapy to the tumor bed, those with focally positive margins had a considerably lower risk of local recurrence than those with more than focally positive margins (81). These data indicate that the value of EIC in predicting outcome is very closely related to the adequacy of tumor excision. They suggest that breast carcinomas with EIC are difficult to assess histologically to ascertain whether excision is complete and that pathologists should be particularly thorough in the examination of specimen margins in these cancers. Other features have been shown to be more powerful predictors of local recurrence in multivariate analyses in some series, including patient age, nodal status, tumor size, and the presence of lymphovascular invasion (106).

Many potential molecular and genetic markers of prognosis have been described in recent years. Tumor proliferative activity represents one of the most thoroughly investigated cellular functions in breast cancer (149). Assessment of proliferation rates has been shown to provide useful information on prognosis and aggressiveness of individual cancers and can potentially be used to guide treatment protocols in clinical practice. A meta-analysis of commercially available breast cancer gene expression signatures has identified proliferation as a key biological driver in all nine prognostic signatures included in the study (150). Various techniques have been developed to quantify proliferation rates including morphological (i.e., mitotic count estimates; which represent an integral part of histological grade (151–153)) and molecular (i.e., measurement of DNA synthesis, and flow cytometry) (22,149,154,155). Other techniques include detection of antigens closely associated with proliferation using immunohistochemistry. Although most studies of different proliferation assays display concordance in outcome predictions for individual patients, there is no consensus on the best proliferation assay (156). The proliferation fraction marker Ki67 (MIB1), has been shown to provide independent prognostic value in certain subgroups of breast cancer including grade 2 tumors (157) and ER-positive/luminal class tumors (158,159) but not in ER-negative or HER2-positive molecular subgroups.

Other molecular markers, including growth factors and their receptors (e.g., epidermal growth factor receptor (EGFR) and c-erbB-3/HER3), basal cytokeratins, proteases (e.g., cathepsin D), cell adhesion markers (e.g., E-cadherin), tumor suppressor genes (e.g., *p53*), and a multitude of other factors, have not consistently shown independent prognostic significance when morphological markers such as histological grade and type, tumor size, and lymph node stage are included. Although these latter parameters appear to be rather simple and old-fashioned, histological grade and tumor type are measurements of tumor morphology reflecting a variety of complex biological changes within the tumor, including cell adhesion and structure, DNA content, and proliferation index (41). Thus, it is perhaps not surprising that individual biological markers cannot replace or surpass these well-recognized morphological prognostic factors at the present time.

SUMMARY

The place of molecular markers in the future appears to be the determination of treatment choices, with specific molecules reflecting a probable response or resistance to a particular therapy. Indeed, the value of the ER in predicting response to hormone therapy is incontrovertible, and the selection of a patient for trastuzumab therapy relies on the reproducible determination of the HER2/*neu* status of an invasive breast cancer. Other targets are on the horizon. It is possible that other non-specific biological features such as tumor angiogenesis may prove to be directly useful in anticancer treatment. It is very likely that examination of the expression of several molecular pathways will augment our understanding of the biology of breast cancer. In the last decade, the concept of molecular classification has been established after introduction of microarray gene expression profiling and the identification of multigene classifiers. Gene expression is the technical term to describe how a particular gene is active, or how many times it is expressed or transcribed, to produce the protein it encodes. This activity is measured by counting the number of mRNA molecules in a given cell type or tissue although protein and not RNA is the functional product of genes. Gene expression profiling has mainly been performed in order to (*i*) identify specific molecular classes of breast cancer (class discovery; molecular taxonomy) that have biological and clinical relevance, which are unidentifiable by conventional means (160–162); (ii) identify specific molecular profile "gene signatures" that can predict tumor behavior (163–166) and/or response to therapy (167–171) (class prediction) and (*iii*) comparison between different "predefined" classes of breast cancer (class comparison) to determine whether expression profiles are different between these classes and, if so, to identify differentially expressed genes (172–180). These multigene classifiers have the potential to complement traditional methods through provision of additional biological prognostic and predictive information in currently indeterminate risk groups.

REFERENCES

1. Dupont WD, Page DL. Risk factors for breast cancer in women with proliferati ve breast disease. N Engl J Med 1985; 312: 146–51.
2. Dupont WD, Parl FF, Hartmann WH, et al. Breast cancer risk associated with proliferative breast disease and atypical hyperplasia. Cancer 1993; 71: 1258–65.
3. Page DL, Dupont WD. Proliferative breast disease: diagnosis and implications. Science 1991; 253: 915–16.
4. Page DL, Dupont WD. Indicators of increased breast cancer risk in humans. J Cell Biochem Suppl 1992; 16G: 175–82.
5. Lopez-Garcia MA, Geyer FC, Lacroix-Triki M, et al. Breast cancer precursors revisited: molecular features and progression pathways. Histopathology 2010; 57: 171–92.
6. Page DL, Dupont WD. Anatomic markers of human premalignancy and risk of breast cancer. Cancer 1990; 66: 1326–35.
7. Page DL, Jensen RA. Evaluation and management of high risk and premalignant lesions of the breast. World J Surg 1994; 18: 32–8.
8. Page DL, Kidd TE, Dupont WD, et al. Lobular neoplasia of the breast: higher risk for subsequent invasive cancer predicted by more extensive disease. Hum Pathol 1991; 22: 1232–9.
9. Schnitt SJ. The diagnosis and management of pre-invasive breast disease: flat epithelial atypia--classification, pathologic features and clinical significance. Breast Cancer Res 2003; 5: 263–8.
10. Boulos FI, Dupont WD, Simpson JF, et al. Histologic associations and long-term cancer risk in columnar cell lesions of the breast: a retrospective cohort and a nested case-control study. Cancer 2008; 113: 2415–21.
11. Feuer EJ, Wun LM, Boring CC, et al. The lifetime risk of developing breast cancer. J Natl Cancer Inst 1993; 85: 892–7.
12. Jensen RA, Page DL, Dupont WD, et al. Invasive breast cancer risk in women with sclerosing adenosis. Cancer 1989; 64: 1977–83.
13. Jacobs TW, Byrne C, Colditz G, et al. Radial scars in benign breast-biopsy specimens and the risk of breast cancer. N Engl J Med 1999; 340: 430–6.
14. Dupont WD, Page DL, Parl FF, et al. Long-term risk of breast cancer in women with fibroadenoma. N Engl J Med 1994; 331: 10–15.
15. Washington C, Dalbegue F, Abreo F, et al. Loss of heterozygosity in fibrocystic change of the breast: genetic relationship between benign proliferative lesions and associated carcinomas. Am J Pathol 2000; 157: 323–9.
16. Edge SB, Byrd DR, Compton CC, et al. AJCC Cancer Staging Manual, 7th edn. New York: Springer, 2010.
17. Mook S, Schmidt MK, Rutgers EJ, et al. Calibration and discriminatory accuracy of prognosis calculation for breast cancer with the online Adjuvant! program: a hospital-based retrospective cohort study. Lancet Oncol 2009; 10: 1070–6.
18. Goldhirsch A, Ingle JN, Gelber RD, et al. Thresholds for therapies: highlights of the St Gallen International Expert Consensus on the primary therapy of early breast cancer 2009. Ann Oncol 2009; 20: 1319–29.
19. Galea MH, Blamey RW, Elston CE, et al. The Nottingham prognostic index in primary breast cancer. Breast Cancer Res Treat 1992; 22: 207–19.
20. Rakha EA, El-Sayed ME, Powe DG, et al. Invasive lobular carcinoma of the breast: response to hormonal therapy and outcomes. Eur J Cancer 2008; 44: 73–83.

21. Rakha EA, Elsheikh SE, Aleskandarany MA, et al. Triple-negative breast cancer: distinguishing between basal and nonbasal subtypes. Clin Cancer Res 2009; 15: 2302–10.

22. Rakha EA, El-Sayed ME, Lee AH, et al. Prognostic significance of Nottingham histologic grade in invasive breast carcinoma. J Clin Oncol 2008; 26: 3153–8.

23. Westenend PJ, Meurs CJ, Damhuis RA. Tumour size and vascular invasion predict distant metastasis in stage I breast cancer. Grade distinguishes early and late metastasis. J Clin Pathol 2005; 58: 196–201.

24. Yorkshire-Breast-Cancer-Group. Critical assessment of the clinical TNM system in breast cancer. Report from the Yorkshire Breast Cancer Group. Br Med J 1980; 281: 134–6.

25. Sinn HP, B, Helmchen Wittekind CH. TNM classification of breast cancer: changes and comments on the 7th edition. Pathologe 2010; 31: 361–6.

26. Edge SB, Byrd DR, Compton CC, eds. Breast, in AJCC Cancer Staging Manual. New York, NY: Springer, 2010: 347–76.

27. Elston CW, Gresham GA, Rao GS, et al. The cancer research campaign (kings/cambridge) trial for early breast cancer - pathological aspects. Br J Cancer 1982; 45: 655–69.

28. Fisher ER, Sass R, Fisher B. Pathologic findings from the National Surgical adjuvant Project for breast cancers (protocol No 4) X Discriminants for Tenth year treatment failure. Cancer 1984; 53: 712–23.

29. Carter CL, Allen C, Henson DE. Relation of tumour size, lymph node status, and survival in 24,270 breast cancer cases. Cancer 1989; 63: 181–7.

30. Neville AM, Bettelheim R, Gelber RD, et al. Predicting treatment responsiveness and prognosis in node-negative breast cancer. J Clin Oncol 1992; 10: 696–705.

31. Rosen PP, Groshen S. Factors influencing survival and prognosis in early breast carcinoma (T1N0M0-T1N1M0). Assessment of 644 patients with median follow-up of 18 years. Surg Clin North Am 1990; 70: 937–62.

32. Haybittle JL, Blamey RW, Elston CW, et al. A prognostic index in primary breast cancer. Br J Cancer 1982; 45: 361–6.

33. Blamey RW, et al. ONCOPOOL - A European database for 16,944 cases of breast cancer. Eur J Cancer 2009; 46: 1762.

34. Rosen PP, Groshen S, Kinne DW, et al. Factors influencing prognosis in node-negative breast carcinoma: analysis of 767 T1N0M0/T2N0M0 patients with long-term follow-up. J Clin Oncol 1993; 11: 2090–100.

35. Reger V, G, Beito Jolly PC. Factors affecting the incidence of lymph node metastases in small cancers of the breast. Am J Surg 1989; 157: 501–2.

36. Arisio R, Sapino A, Cassoni P, et al. What modifies the relation between tumour size and lymph node metastases in T1 breast carcinomas? J Clin Pathol 2000; 53: 846–50.

37. Foulkes WD, Grainge MJ, Rakha EA, et al. Tumor size is an unreliable predictor of prognosis in basal-like breast cancers and does not correlate closely with lymph node status. Breast Cancer Res Treat 2009; 117: 199–204.

38. Bergh J, Holmquist M. Who should not receive adjuvant chemotherapy? International databases. J Natl Cancer Inst Monogr 2001: 103–8.

39. Morabito A, Magnani E, Gion M, et al. Prognostic and predictive indicators in operable breast cancer. Clin Breast Cancer 2003; 3: 381–90.

40. Colpaert C, Vermeulen P, Jeuris W, et al. Early distant relapse in "node-negative" breast cancer patients is not predicted by occult axillary lymph node metastases, but by the features of the primary tumour. J Pathol 2001; 193: 442–9.

41. Rakha EA, Reis-Filho JS, Baehner F, et al. Breast cancer prognostic classification in the molecular era: the role of histological grade. Breast Cancer Res 2010; 12: 207.

42. Robbins P, Pinder S, de Klerk N, et al. Histological grading of breast carcinomas. A study of interobserver agreement. Hum Pathol 1995; 26: 873–9.

43. Pathology reporting of breast disease. A Joint Document Incorporating the Third Edition of the NHS Breast Screening Programme's Guidelines for Pathology Reporting in Breast Cancer Screening and the Second Edition of The Royal College of Pathologists' Minimum Dataset for Breast Cancer Histopathology. January 2005. NHSBSP Pub. No 58.

44. Third Edition of the NHS Breast Screening Programme's Guidelines for Pathology Reporting in Breast Cancer Screening and the Second Edition of The Royal College of Pathologists' Minimum Dataset for Breast Cancer Histopathology. PATHOLOGY REPORTING OF BREAST DISEASE. January 2005, Sheffield. NHSBSP Pub. No 58.

45. Tavassoli FA, Devilee P. World Health Organization Classification of Tumours., in Pathology and Genetics. Tumours of the Breast and Female Genital Organs. Lyon: IARC Press, 2003: 19–23.

46. Bloom HJ, Richardson WW. Histological grading and prognosis in breast cancer; a study of 1409 cases of which 359 have been followed for 15 years. Br J Cancer 1957; 11: 359–77.

47. Pinder SE, Murray S, Ellis IO, et al. The importance of the histologic grade of invasive breast carcinoma and response to chemotherapy. Cancer 1998; 83: 1529–39.

48. Robertson JFR, et al. Biological factors of prognostic significance in locally advanced breast cancer. Br Cancer Res Treat 1994; 29: 259–64.

49. Walker RA. Prognostic and Predictive Factors in Breast Cancer, 1st edn. New York: Informa Health Care, 2003: 10–17.

50. Sundquist M, Thorstenson S, Brudin L, et al. Applying the Nottingham prognostic index to a Swedish breast cancer population. South East Swedish breast cancer study group. Breast Cancer Res Treat 1999; 53: 1–8.

51. Balslev I, Axelsson CK, Zedeler K, et al. The Nottingham prognostic index applied to 9,149 patients from the studies of the Danish breast cancer cooperative group (DBCG). Breast Cancer Res Treat 1994; 32: 281–90.

52. Desmedt C, Haibe-Kains B, Wirapati P, et al. Biological processes associated with breast cancer clinical outcome depend on the molecular subtypes. Clin Cancer Res 2008; 14: 5158–65.

53. Mirza AN, Mirza NQ, Vlastos G, et al. Prognostic factors in node-negative breast cancer: a review of studies with sample size more than 200 and follow-up more than 5 years. Ann Surg 2002; 235: 10–26.

54. Rivadeneira DE, Simmons RM, Christos PJ, et al. Predictive factors associated with axillary lymph node metastases in T1a and T1b breast carcinomas: analysis in more than 900 patients. J Am Coll Surg 2000; 191: 1–6; discussion 6-8.

55. Barth A, Craig PH, Silverstein MJ. Predictors of axillary lymph node metastases in patients with T1 breast carcinoma. Cancer 1997; 79: 1918–22.

56. Putti TC, El-Rehim DM, Rakha EA, et al. Estrogen receptor-negative breast carcinomas: a review of morphology and immunophenotypical analysis. Mod Pathol 2005; 18: 26–35.

57. Fan C, Oh DS, Wessels L, et al. Concordance among gene-expression-based predictors for breast cancer. N Engl J Med 2006; 355: 560–9.

58. Rakha EA, Lee AH, Evans AJ, et al. Tubular carcinoma of the breast: further evidence to support its excellent prognosis. J Clin Oncol 2010; 28: 99–104.

59. Rakha EA, Aleskandarany M, El-Sayed ME, et al. The prognostic significance of inflammation and medullary histological type in invasive carcinoma of the breast. Eur J Cancer 2009; 45: 1780–7.

60. Pereira H, Pinder SE, Sibbering DM, et al. Pathological prognostic factors in breast cancer. IV: Should you be a typer or a grader? A comparative study of two histological prognostic features in operable breast carcinoma. Histopathology 1995; 27: 219–26.

61. Ellis IO, Galea M, Broughton N, et al. Pathological prognostic factors in breast cancer. II. Histological type. Relationship with survival in a large study with long-term follow-up. Histopathology 1992; 20: 479–89.

62. Rakha EA, El-Sayed ME, Menon S, et al. Histologic grading is an independent prognostic factor for invasive lobular carcinoma of the breast. Breast Cancer Res Treat 2008; 111: 121–7.

63. Sloane JP, Amendoeira I, Apostolikas N, et al. Consistency achieved by 23 European pathologists from 12 countries in diagnosing breast disease and reporting prognostic features of carcinomas. Virchows Arch Int J Pathol 1999; 434: 3–10.

64. Richardson WW. Medullary carcinoma of the breast; a distinctive tumour type with a relatively good prognosis following radical mastectomy. Br J Cancer 1956; 10: 415–23.

65. Jensen ML, Kiaer H, Andersen J, et al. Prognostic comparison of three classifications for medullary carcinomas of the breast. Histopathology 1997; 30: 523–32.

66. Ellis IO, Coleman D, Wells C, et al. Impact of a national external quality assessment scheme for breast pathology in the UK. J Clin Pathol 2006; 59: 138–45.

67. Gonzalez MA, Pinder SE, Wencyk PM, et al. An immunohistochemical examination of the expression of E-cadherin, alpha- and beta/gamma-catenins, and alpha2- and beta1-integrins in invasive breast cancer. J Pathol 1999; 187: 523–9.

68. Truong PT, Berthelet E, Lee J, et al. The prognostic significance of the percentage of positive/dissected axillary lymph nodes in breast cancer recurrence and survival in patients with one to three positive axillary lymph nodes. Cancer 2005; 103: 2006–14.

69. Crump M, Goss PE, Prince M, et al. Outcome of extensive evaluation before adjuvant therapy in women with breast cancer and 10 or more positive axillary lymph nodes. J Clin Oncol 1996; 14: 66–9.

70. Nemoto T, Vana J, Bedwani RN, et al. Management and survival of female breast cancer: results of a national survey by the American College of Surgeons. Cancer 1980; 45: 2917–24.

71. Smith JA 3rd, Gamez-Araujo JJ, Gallager HS, White EC, McBride CM. Carcinoma of the breast: analysis of total lymph node involvement versus level of metastasis. Cancer 1977; 39: 527–32.

72. Hilsenbeck SG, Ravdin PM, de Moor CA, et al. Time-dependence of hazard ratios for prognostic factors in primary breast cancer. Breast Cancer Res Treat 1998; 52: 227–37.

73. Singletary SE, Allred C, Ashley P, et al. Revision of the American Joint Committee on Cancer staging system for breast cancer. J Clin Oncol 2002; 20: 3628–36.

74. Reed J, Rosman M, Verbanac KM, et al. Prognostic implications of isolated tumor cells and micrometastases in sentinel nodes of patients with invasive breast cancer: 10-year analysis of patients enrolled in the prospective East Carolina University/Anne Arundel Medical Center Sentinel Node Multicenter Study. J Am Coll Surg 2009; 208: 333–40.

75. Clare SE, Sener SF, Wilkens W, et al. Prognostic significance of occult lymph node metastases in node-negative breast cancer. Ann Surg Oncol 1997; 4: 447–51.

76. Martinez-Ramos D, Escrig-Sos J, Alcalde-Sanchez M, et al. Disease-free survival and prognostic significance of metastatic lymph node ratio in T1-T2 N positive breast cancer patients. A population registry-based study in a European country. World J Surg 2009; 33: 1659–64.

77. Sobin LH, Wittekind C. In: Sobin LH, Wittekind C, eds. TNM Classification of Malignant Tumors, 6th edn. New York: Wiley, 2002.

78. Pathologists, NBSPaRCo. Pathology Reporting of Breast Disease, 3rd edn. Vol. NHSBSP Publication No 58 Sheffield: NHS Cancer Screening Programmes, 2005.

79. Sacre RA. Clinical evaluation of axillar lymph nodes compared to surgical and pathological findings. Eur J Surg Oncol 1986; 12: 169–73.

80. Chetty U, Jack W, Prescott RJ, et al. Management of the axilla in operable breast cancer treated by breast conservation: a randomized clinical trial. Edinburgh Breast Unit. Br J Surg 2000; 87: 163–9.

81. Steele RJ, Forrest AP, Gibson T, et al. The efficacy of lower axillary sampling in obtaining lymph node status in breast cancer: a controlled randomized trial. Br J Surg 1985; 72: 368–9.

82. Macmillan RD, Barbera D, Hadjiminas DJ, et al. Sentinel node biopsy for breast cancer may have little to offer four-node-samplers. results of a prospective comparison study. Eur J Cancer 2001; 37: 1076–80.

83. Macmillan RD, Rampaul RS, Lewis S, et al. Preoperative ultrasound-guided node biopsy and sentinel node augmented node sample is best practice. Eur J Cancer 2004; 40: 176–8.

84. Lamovec J, Bracko M. Metastatic pattern of infiltrating lobular carcinoma of the breast: an autopsy study. J Surg Oncol 1991; 48: 28–33.

85. Lee AH, Ellis IO, Pinder SE, et al. Pathological assessment of sentinel lymph-node biopsies in patients with breast cancer. Virchows Arch 2000; 436: 97–101.

86. Lyman GH, Giuliano AE, Somerfield MR, et al. American Society of Clinical Oncology guideline recommendations for sentinel lymph node biopsy in early-stage breast cancer. J Clin Oncol 2005; 23: 7703–20.

87. Albertini JJ, Lyman GH, Cox C, et al. Lymphatic mapping and sentinel node biopsy in the patient with breast cancer. JAMA 1996; 276: 1818–22.

88. Veronesi U, Paganelli G, Viale G, et al. Sentinel lymph node biopsy and axillary dissection in breast cancer: results in a large series. J Natl Cancer Inst 1999; 91: 368–73.

89. Tafra L, Lannin DR, Swanson MS, et al. Multicenter trial of sentinel node biopsy for breast cancer using both technetium sulfur colloid and isosulfan blue dye. Ann Surg 2001; 233: 51–9.

90. Krag DN, et al. Sentinel-lymph-node resection compared with conventional axillary-lymph-node dissection in clinically node-negative patients with breast cancer: overall survival findings from the NSABP B-32 randomised phase 3 trial. Lancet Oncol 2010; 11: 927–33.

91. Knauer M, Konstantiniuk P, Haid A, et al. Multicentric breast cancer: a new indication for sentinel node biopsy--a multi-institutional validation study. J Clin Oncol 2006; 24: 3374–80.

92. International Breast Cancer Study Group. Prognostic importance of occult axillary lymph node micrometastases from breast cancers. Lancet 1990; 335: 1565–8.

93. McGuckin MA, Cummings MC, Walsh MD, et al. Occult axillary node metastases in breast cancer: their detection and prognostic significance. Br J Cancer 1996; 73: 88–95.

94. Noguchi S, Aihara T, Nakamori S, et al. The detection of breast carcinoma micrometastases in axillary lymph nodes by means of reverse transcriptase-polymerase chain reaction. Cancer 1994; 74: 1595–600.

95. Ozao-Choy J, Giuliano AE. Prognostic significance of micrometastasis and isolated tumor cells in the sentinel lymph node. Breast Cancer Res Treat 2011; 127: 205–6.

96. Weaver DL, Ashikaga T, Krag DN, et al. Effect of occult metastases on survival in node-negative breast cancer. N Engl J Med 2011; 364: 412–21.

97. de Mascarel I, Bonichon F, Coindre JM, et al. Prognostic significance of breast cancer axillary lymph node micrometastases assessed by two special techniques: reevaluation with longer follow-up. Br J Cancer 1992; 66: 523–7.

98. Rakha EA, Martin S, Lee AHS, et al. The prognostic significance of lymphovascular invasion in invasive breast carcinoma. Cancer 2011; 118: 3670–80.

99. Pinder SE, Ellis IO, Galea M, et al. Pathological prognostic factors in breast cancer. III. Vascular invasion: relationship with recurrence and survival in a large study with long-term follow-up. Histopathology 1994; 24: 41–7.

100. Bettelheim R, Penman HG, Thornton-Jones H, et al. Prognostic significance of peritumoral vascular invasion in breast cancer. Br J Cancer 1984; 50: 771–7.

101. O'Rourke S, Galea MH, Morgan D, et al. Local recurrence after simple mastectomy. Br J Surg 1994; 81: 386–9.

102. Dawson PJ, Ferguson DJ, Karrison T. The pathological findings of breast cancer in patients surviving 25 years after radical mastectomy. Cancer 1982; 50: 2131–8.

103. Davis BW, Gelber R, Goldhirsch A, et al. Prognostic significance of peritumoral vessel invasion in clinical trials of adjuvant therapy for breast cancer with axillary lymph node metastasis. Hum Pathol 1985; 16: 1212–18.

104. Clemente CG, Boracchi P, Andreola S, et al. Peritumoral lymphatic invasion in patients with node-negative mammary duct carcinoma. Cancer 1992; 69: 1396–403.

105. Mohammed RA, et al. Objective assessment of lymphatic and blood vascular invasion in lymph node-negative breast carcinoma: findings from a large case series with long-term follow-up. J Pathol 2010; 223: 358–65.

106. Locker AP, Ellis IO, Morgan DA, et al. Factors influencing local recurrence after excision and radiotherapy for primary breast cancer. Br J Surg 1989; 76: 890–4.

107. Blamey RW, Elston CW, Ellis IO, et al. Survival of invasive breast cancer according to the Nottingham Prognostic Index in cases diagnosed in 1990-1999. Eur J Cancer 2007; 43: 1548–55.

108. Hammond ME, Hayes DF, Dowsett M, et al. American Society of Clinical Oncology/College Of American Pathologists guideline recommendations for immunohistochemical testing of estrogen and progesterone receptors in breast cancer. J Clin Oncol 2010; 28: 2784–95.

109. Nabholtz JM, Buzdar A, Pollak M, et al. Anastrozole is superior to tamoxifen as first-line therapy for advanced breast cancer in postmenopausal women: results of a North American multicenter randomized trial. Arimidex Study Group. J Clin Oncol 2000; 18: 3758–67.

110. Early Breast Cancer Trialists' Collaborative Group (EBCTCG). Effects of chemotherapy and hormonal therapy for early breast cancer on recurrence and 15-year survival: an overview of the randomised trials. Lancet 2005; 365: 1687–717.

111. Early Breast Cancer Trialists' Collaborative Group. Effects of adjuvant tamoxifen and of cytotoxic therapy on mortality in early breast cancer.

An overview of 61 randomized trials among 28,896 women. N Engl J Med 1988; 319: 1681–92.

112. Osborne CK. Steroid hormone receptors in breast cancer management. Breast Cancer Res Treat 1998; 51: 227–38.

113. Adjuvant tamoxifen in the management of operable breast cancer: the Scottish Trial. Report from the Breast Cancer Trials Committee, Scottish Cancer Trials Office (MRC), Edinburgh. Lancet 1987; 2: 171–5.

114. Early Breast Cancer Trialists' Collaborative Group. Tamoxifen for early breast cancer: an overview of the randomised trials. Lancet 1998; 351: 1451–67.

115. Fisher B, Dignam J, Bryant J, et al. Five versus more than five years of tamoxifen therapy for breast cancer patients with negative lymph nodes and estrogen receptor-positive tumors. J Natl Cancer Inst 1996; 88: 1529–42.

116. Harvey JM, Clark GM, Osborne CK, et al. Estrogen receptor status by immunohistochemistry is superior to the ligand-binding assay for predicting response to adjuvant endocrine therapy in breast cancer. J Clin Oncol 1999; 17: 1474–81.

117. Harvey JM, Clark GM, Osborne CK, et al. Estrogen receptor status by immunohistochemistry is superior to the ligand binding assay for predicting response to adjuvant endocrine therapy in breast cancer. J Clin Oncol 1999; 17: 1474–81.

118. Arpino G, Weiss H, Lee AV, et al. Estrogen receptor-positive, progesterone receptor-negative breast cancer: association with growth factor receptor expression and tamoxifen resistance. J Natl Cancer Inst 2005; 97: 1254–61.

119. Rakha EA, El-Sayed ME, Green AR, et al. Biologic and clinical characteristics of breast cancer with single hormone receptor positive phenotype. J Clin Oncol 2007; 25: 4772–8.

120. Ravdin PM, Green S, Dorr TM, et al. Prognostic significance of progesterone receptor levels in estrogen receptor-positive patients with metastatic breast cancer treated with tamoxifen: results of a prospective Southwest Oncology Group study. J Clin Oncol 1992; 10: 1284–91.

121. Bardou VJ, Arpino G, Elledge RM, et al. Progesterone receptor status significantly improves outcome prediction over estrogen receptor status alone for adjuvant endocrine therapy in two large breast cancer databases. J Clin Oncol 2003; 21: 1973–9.

122. Hilsenbeck SG, Osborne CK. Is there a role for adjuvant tamoxifen in progesterone receptor-positive breast cancer? An in silico clinical trial. Clin Cancer Res 2006; 12: 1049s–55s.

123. Dowsett M, Houghton J, Iden C, et al. Benefit from adjuvant tamoxifen therapy in primary breast cancer patients according oestrogen receptor, progesterone receptor, EGF receptor and HER2 status. Ann Oncol 2006; 17: 818–26.

124. Goulding H, Pinder S, Cannon P, et al. A new immunohistochemical antibody for the assessment of estrogen receptor status on routine formalin-fixed tissue samples. Hum Pathol 1995; 26: 291–4.

125. Slamon DJ, Clark GM, Wong SG, et al. Human breast cancer: correlation of relapse and survival with amplification of the HER-2/neu oncogene. Science 1987; 235: 177–82.

126. Dandachi N, Dietze O, Hauser-Kronberger C. Chromogenic in situ hybridization: a novel approach to a practical and sensitive method for the detection of HER2 oncogene in archival human breast carcinoma. Lab Invest 2002; 82: 1007–14.

127. Wolff AC, Hammond ME, Schwartz JN, et al. American Society of Clinical Oncology/College of American Pathologists guideline recommendations for human epidermal growth factor receptor 2 testing in breast cancer. J Clin Oncol 2007; 25: 118–45.

128. Chia S, Norris B, Speers C, et al. Human epidermal growth factor receptor 2 overexpression as a prognostic factor in a large tissue microarray series of node-negative breast cancers. J Clin Oncol 2008; 26: 5697–704.

129. Kaufmann M, von Minckwitz G, Bear HD, et al. Recommendations from an international expert panel on the use of neoadjuvant (primary) systemic treatment of operable breast cancer: new perspectives 2006. Ann Oncol 2007; 18: 1927–34.

130. Press MF, Finn RS, Cameron D, et al. HER-2 gene amplification, HER-2 and epidermal growth factor receptor mRNA and protein expression, and lapatinib efficacy in women with metastatic breast cancer. Clin Cancer Res 2008; 14: 7861–70.

131. Piccart-Gebhart MJ, Procter M, Leyland-Jones B, et al. Trastuzumab after adjuvant chemotherapy in HER2-positive breast cancer. N Engl J Med 2005; 353: 1659–72.

132. Ward S, Pilgrim H, Hind D. Trastuzumab for the treatment of primary breast cancer in HER2-positive women: a single technology appraisal. Health Technol Assess 2009; 13: 1–6.

133. Slamon DJ, Leyland-Jones B, Shak S, et al. Use of chemotherapy plus a monoclonal antibody against HER2 for metastatic breast cancer that overexpresses HER2. N Engl J Med 2001; 344: 783–92.

134. Rakha EA, Reis-Filho JS, Ellis IO. Combinatorial biomarker expression in breast cancer. Breast Cancer Res Treat 2010; 120: 293–308.

135. Carey LA, Perou CM, Livasy CA, et al. Race, breast cancer subtypes, and survival in the Carolina Breast Cancer Study. JAMA 2006; 295: 2492–502.

136. Kreike B, van Kouwenhove M, Horlings H, et al. Gene expression profiling and histopathological characterization of triple negative/basal-like breast carcinomas. Breast Cancer Res 2007; 9: R65.

137. Lee AH, Happerfield LC, Bobrow LG, et al. Angiogenesis and inflammation in ductal carcinoma in situ of the breast. J Pathol 1997; 181: 200–6.

138. Van den Eynden GG, et al. Gene expression profiles associated with the presence of a fibrotic focus and the growth pattern in lymph node-negative breast cancer. Clin Cancer Res 2008; 14: 2944–52.

139. Hasebe T, Sasaki S, Imoto S, et al. Prognostic significance of fibrotic focus in invasive ductal carcinoma of the breast: a prospective observational study. Mod Pathol 2002; 15: 502–16.

140. Marginean F, Rakha EA, Ho BC, Ellis IO, Lee AH. Histological features of medullary carcinoma and prognosis in triple-negative basal-like carcinomas of the breast. Mod Pathol 2010; 23: 1357–63.

141. Duraker N, Caynak ZC, Turkoz K. Perineural invasion has no prognostic value in patients with invasive breast carcinoma. Breast 2006; 15: 629–34.

142. Matsukuma A, Enjoji M, Toyoshima S. Ductal carcinoma of the breast. An analysis of proportions of intraductal and invasive components. Pathol Res Pract 1991; 187: 62–7.

143. Silverberg SG, Chitale AR. Assessment of the significance of the proportion of intraductal and infiltrating tumor growth in ductal carcinoma of the breast. Cancer 1973; 32: 830–7.

144. Crombie N, Rampaul RS, Pinder SE, et al. Extent of ductal carcinoma in situ within and surrounding invasive primary breast carcinoma. Br J Surg 2001; 88: 1324–9.

145. Schnitt SJ, Connolly JL, Khettry U, et al. Pathologic findings on re-excision of the primary site in breast cancer patients considered for treatment by primary radiation therapy. Cancer 1987; 59: 675–81.

146. Campbell ID, Theaker JM, Royle GT, et al. Impact of an extensive in situ component on the presence of residual disease in screen detected breast cancer. J R Soc Med 1991; 84: 652–6.

147. Schnitt SJ, Abner A, Gelman R, et al. The relationship between microscopic margins of resection and the risk of local recurrence in patients with breast cancer treated with breast-conserving surgery and radiation therapy. Cancer 1994; 74: 1746–51.

148. Pinder SE, Duggan C, Ellis IO, et al. A new pathological system for grading DCIS with improved prediction of local recurrence: results from the UKCCCR/ANZ DCIS trial. Br J Cancer 2010; 103: 94–100.

149. Daidone MG, Silvestrini R. Prognostic and predictive role of proliferation indices in adjuvant therapy of breast cancer. J Natl Cancer Inst Monogr 2001: 27–35.

150. Wirapati P, Sotiriou C, Kunkel S, et al. Meta-analysis of gene expression profiles in breast cancer: toward a unified understanding of breast cancer subtyping and prognosis signatures. Breast Cancer Res 2008; 10: R65.

151. Clayton F. Pathologic correlates of survival in 378 lymph node-negative infiltrating ductal breast carcinomas. Mitotic count is the best single predictor. Cancer 1991; 68: 1309–17.

152. Simpson JF, Gray R, Dressler LG, et al. Prognostic value of histologic grade and proliferative activity in axillary node-positive breast cancer: results from the eastern cooperative oncology group companion study, EST 4189. J Clin Oncol 2000; 18: 10.2059–69.

153. Medri L, Volpi A, Nanni O, et al. Prognostic relevance of mitotic activity in patients with node-negative breast cancer. Mod Pathol 16: 1067–75.

154. Beresford MJ, Wilson GD, Makris A. Measuring proliferation in breast cancer: practicalities and applications. Breast Cancer Res 2006; 8: 216.

155. Johnson HA, Bond VP. A method of labeling tissues with tritiated thymidine in vitro and its use in comparing rates of cell proliferation in duct epithelium, fibroadenoma, and carcinoma of human breast. Cancer 1961; 14: 639–43.

156. van Diest PJ, van der Wall E, Baak JPA. Prognostic value of proliferation in invasive breast cancer: a review. J Clin Pathol 2004; 57: 675–81.

157. Aleskandarany MA, Rakha EA, Macmillan RD, et al. MIB1/Ki-67 labelling index can classify grade 2 breast cancer into two clinically distinct subgroups. Breast Cancer Res Treat 2010; 127: 591–9.

158. Aleskandarany MA, Green AR, Benhasouna AA, et al. Prognostic value of proliferation assay in the luminal, HER2 positive and triple negative biological classes of breast cancer. Breast Cancer Res 2012; 14: R3.

159. Cuzick J, Dowsett M, Pineda S, et al. Prognostic value of a combined estrogen receptor, progesterone receptor, Ki-67, and human epidermal growth factor receptor 2 immunohistochemical score and comparison with the genomic health recurrence score in early breast cancer. J Clin Oncol 2011; 29: 4273–8.

160. Perou CM, Sørlie T, Eisen MB, et al. Molecular portraits of human breast tumours. Nature 2000; 406: 747–52.

161. Sorlie T, Perou CM, Tibshirani R, et al. Gene expression patterns of breast carcinomas distinguish tumor subclasses with clinical implications. Proc Natl Acad Sci USA 2001; 98: 10869–74.

162. Abd El-Rehim DM, Ball G, Pinder SE, et al. High-throughput protein expression analysis using tissue microarray technology of a large well-characterised series identifies biologically distinct classes of breast cancer confirming recent cDNA expression analyses. Int J Cancer 2005; 116: 340–50.

163. Foekens JA, Atkins D, Zhang Y, et al. Multicenter validation of a gene expression-based prognostic signature in lymph node-negative primary breast cancer. J Clin Oncol 2006; 24: 1665–71.

164. Van 't Veer LJ, Dai H, van de Vijver MJ, et al. Gene expression profiling predicts clinical outcome of breast cancer. Nature 2002; 415: 530–6.

165. Wang Y, Klijn JG, Zhang Y, et al. Gene-expression profiles to predict distant metastasis of lymph-node-negative primary breast cancer. Lancet 2005; 365: 671–9.

166. Ma XJ, Wang Z, Ryan PD, et al. A two-gene expression ratio predicts clinical outcome in breast cancer patients treated with tamoxifen. Cancer Cell 2004; 5: 607–16.

167. Zhang Y, Sieuwerts AM, McGreevy M, et al. The 76-gene signature defines high-risk patients that benefit from adjuvant tamoxifen therapy. Breast Cancer Res Treat 2009; 116: 303–9.

168. Jansen MP, Foekens JA, van Staveren IL, et al. Molecular classification of tamoxifen-resistant breast carcinomas by gene expression profiling. J Clin Oncol 2005; 23: 732–40.

169. Hess KR, Anderson K, Symmans WF, et al. Pharmacogenomic predictor of sensitivity to preoperative chemotherapy with paclitaxel and fluorouracil, doxorubicin, and cyclophosphamide in breast cancer. J Clin Oncol 2006; 24: 4236–44.

170. Potti A, Dressman HK, Bild A, et al. Genomic signatures to guide the use of chemotherapeutics. Nat Med 2006; 12: 1294–300.

171. Naderi A, Teschendorff AE, Barbosa-Morais NL, et al. A gene-expression signature to predict survival in breast cancer across independent data sets. Oncogene 2007; 26: 1507–16.

172. Schuetz CS, Bonin M, Clare SE, et al. Progression-specific genes identified by expression profiling of matched ductal carcinomas in situ and invasive breast tumors, combining laser capture microdissection and oligonucleotide microarray analysis. Cancer Res 2006; 66: 5278–86.

173. Ma XJ, Salunga R, Tuggle JT, et al. Gene expression profiles of human breast cancer progression. Proc Natl Acad Sci USA 2003; 100: 5974–9.

174. Porter D, Lahti-Domenici J, Keshaviah A, et al. Molecular markers in ductal carcinoma in situ of the breast. Mol Cancer Res 2003; 1: 362–75.

175. Seth A, et al. Gene expression profiling of ductal carcinomas in situ and invasive breast tumors. Anticancer Res 2003; 23: 2043–51.

176. Korkola JE, DeVries S, Fridlyand J, et al. Differentiation of lobular versus ductal breast carcinomas by expression microarray analysis. Cancer Res 2003; 63: 7167–75.

177. Zhao H, Langerød A, Ji Y, et al. Different gene expression patterns in invasive lobular and ductal carcinomas of the breast. Mol Biol Cell 2004; 15: 2523–36.

178. Turashvili G, Bouchal J, Baumforth K, et al. Novel markers for differentiation of lobular and ductal invasive breast carcinomas by laser microdissection and microarray analysis. BMC Cancer 2007; 7: 55.

179. West M, Blanchette C, Dressman H, et al. Predicting the clinical status of human breast cancer by using gene expression profiles. Proc Natl Acad Sci USA 2001; 98: 11462–7.

180. Huang E, Cheng SH, Dressman H, et al. Gene expression predictors of breast cancer outcomes. Lancet 2003; 361: 1590–6.

27 Premalignant and borderline lesions: ductal and lobular carcinoma in situ

Clive A. Wells and Evdokia Arkoumani

INTRODUCTION

A premalignant condition is one that has a potential to develop into malignancy, and can subsequently pose a threat to life (1). Premalignant lesions of the breast were investigated by Foote and Stewart (2) as early as 1945 in a comparative study that attempted to assess the risk of developing invasive carcinoma when certain types of epithelial proliferations were present in both cancerous and non-cancerous biopsies. Epithelial proliferations, sometimes associated with cytological atypia, were five times more common in breasts containing cancer than in non-cancerous breasts. This observation was not followed up until 30 years later, when, by a meticulous subgross analysis of sections, Wellings et al. (3) demonstrated that most epithelial abnormalities and carcinomas arise from the terminal duct–lobular unit (TDLU) rather than from the major ducts.

When assessing premalignant epithelial proliferations or a non-invasive carcinoma of the breast, it is clinically useful to estimate the probability of their progression to invasive carcinoma. Page (1) provided useful criteria in assessing non-invasive breast proliferations by calculating the relative risk of developing invasive carcinoma. The notion of risk factors enables the clinician to take into account the histologically assessed risk of subsequent malignancy, in addition to age, family history of breast cancer and reproductive history, and to plan suitable patient management (4). Screening mammography is effective in detecting non-palpable architectural abnormalities or calcifications. Biopsies of these lesions yield very small invasive carcinomas, carcinoma in situ, and atypical or benign epithelial proliferations. Carcinoma in situ and various epithelial proliferations are more frequently encountered nowadays than in the premammographic era. Consequently, the need to assess the risk factors for developing invasive carcinoma has never been greater in order to give patients and clinicians more information so that the most suitable treatment can be instituted. Advances in molecular pathology will also assist the clinician in making a more accurate prediction of patients at risk of developing cancer by combining genetic susceptibility and abnormal epithelial proliferations.

PATHOLOGICAL ASSESSMENT OF BIOPSIES

Frozen-section examination is not useful in the management of mammographically detected impalpable lesions, because of the risk of false-positive diagnosis in the assessment of benign lesions such as sclerosing adenosis (SA) or radial scars. Moreover, these lesions should properly be assessed as a whole, because they are usually small and sampling for frozen section

analysis may interfere with the final diagnosis. A radiograph is essential prior to processing of the specimen. This enables the radiologist and surgeon to assess the adequacy of excision of the area of microcalcification or architectural distortion noted *in vivo*. The radiograph also helps the pathologist to select the appropriate area for histological examination. The biopsy specimen, which should be orientated by the surgeon, is painted with a different colored ink to aid the histological assessment of each margin. The specimen is sliced along its long axis and the slices are re-x-rayed if no macroscopic lesion is identified. Following description of any gross abnormality, tissue blocks are taken. The whole lesion is sampled if it is small, or a minimum of four blocks including margins are taken. Microcalcification present in the specimen radiograph must be confirmed on histology. At all stages, cooperation between the radiologist, surgeon and pathologist is vital (5).

FIBROCYSTIC CHANGE AND COLUMNAR CELL LESIONS

Fibrocystic Change

Fibrocystic change is the term given to a variety of benign breast changes. The histological features include cysts, apocrine metaplasia (Fig. 27.1A), stromal fibrosis, and usual epithelial hyperplasia. Microcalcification may be present. Fibrocystic change is a very common lesion which affects more than one-third of premenopausal women. It is the most common cause of a breast lump in this age group.

Apocrine epithelium is found lining the sweat glands of the vulva and axilla. Its presence in the breast is thought either to be of similar embryological origin to the sweat glands or to arise due to metaplasia (6). The latter view is widely held because transition between the normal epithelium and apocrine epithelium can be seen in the same duct. However, apocrine metaplasia has been detected in fetal tissue, which supports the view that the epithelium is native to the breast tissue (7). Apocrine metaplasia is an integral part of fibrocystic change or gross cystic disease. The cells are large, with eosinophilic granular cytoplasm and basally located nuclei with or without apical "snouts."

There is conflicting evidence as to whether apocrine epithelium is premalignant or not. In 1932, Dawson identified apocrine epithelium in both cancerous and noncancerous breasts (6), but was unable to demonstrate carcinoma arising directly in apocrine epithelium, and concluded that this was unlikely to be a premalignant condition. These findings were disputed by Haagensen (8), who followed up patients whose biopsies had revealed apocrine metaplasia in fibrocystic disease. His patients had a fivefold risk of developing carcinoma. The significant apocrine metaplasia in Haagensen's series had mainly a papillary configuration. Although some apocrine proliferations can be florid, cytological atypia is unusual.

Using subgross analysis, Wellings et al. (9) demonstrated that apocrine metaplastic change occurred in the TDLU, the site of premalignant proliferation, and that it was a marker for an increased risk of breast cancer. This conclusion was based on the fact that apocrine metaplasia was more prevalent in cancerous than in non-cancerous breasts; hence apocrine metaplasia was a manifestation of unstable epithelium. In an earlier study, Page et al. (10) suggested that patients above the age of 45 with papillary apocrine metaplasia had twice the relative risk of developing invasive carcinoma, especially those with complex patterns. Seven years later, in a separate study, Dupont and Page (11) concluded that cysts and apocrine epithelium per se did not increase the risk of carcinoma. However, the presence of cysts in a patient with a family history of breast cancer elevated the risk slightly by 2.7 times relative to that of women without this risk factor.

Dixon et al. (12) followed up 1300 women with palpable cysts aspirated between 1981 and 1987. They reported that the overall incidence of breast cancer was three times higher than in the general population. Younger women below the age of 45 were 6 times more likely than the general population to develop cancer, compared with a relative risk of 1.7 in women aged over 55. A possible explanation for this age difference was that in younger women the breast epithelium was more susceptible to malignant change due to the proliferative activity involved in cyst formation and associated high estrogen levels. Complex apocrine papillary hyperplasia has been associated with a small increased relative risk of 2.4 of subsequent malignancy. However, 20% of cases with complex apocrine hyperplasia had associated atypical ductal hyperplasia (ADH). In the absence of ADH, the risk was not significant (13).

Following complaints from women who were paying high insurance premiums after the diagnosis of "fibrocystic disease," a consensus meeting was held in New York in 1985 by the Cancer Committee of the College of American Pathologists (14). They agreed to amend the term to fibrocystic change and concluded that cysts and apocrine metaplasia alone were not premalignant. If the general term "fibrocystic change" is to be used, the associated epithelial components must be specifically defined to allow an accurate assessment of the risk of subsequent cancer. This concept was reaffirmed at an updated consensus meeting in 1998 (15).

Molecular biological studies have demonstrated loss of heterozygosity (LOH) in apocrine epithelium. Washington et al. (16) demonstrated LOH in 10 out of 19 cases of apocrine epithelium not related to malignancy, and 7 out 14 cases of apocrine epithelium adjacent to carcinoma. In all seven cases, the carcinoma and apocrine epithelium shared LOH in one or more loci. In a separate study (17), multiple chromosomal losses and gains were present in apocrine epithelium at a similar frequency to apocrine ductal carcinoma in situ (DCIS). Earlier, Agnantis et al. (18) demonstrated immunohistochemical expression of the c-Myc and p21 Ras oncoproteins. These studies suggest that apocrine metaplasia may serve as a putative precursor of apocrine carcinoma, albeit a rare one.

Columnar Cell Lesions

Columnar cell lesions (CCLs) have been previously described by pathologists under many different terminologies (19–21). The so-called blunt duct adenosis of Foote and Stewart (2) is now regarded as a CCL. The high prevalence of CCLs has been highlighted by the use of screening mammography and needle core biopsy because many lesions tend to calcify. CCLs can exist independently of, or in association with, other benign lesions. They have been classified into three main categories: columnar cell change (CCC), columnar cell hyperplasia (CCH), and flat epithelial atypia (FEA) (22–24).

CCC is usually multifocal and may be bilateral. It affects mainly premenopausal women, but it can also be present after the menopause. As mentioned above, the vast majority of clinically detected CCC is detected mammographically, as it rarely forms a palpable lesion.

Histologically, CCC consists of variably dilated TDLUs lined by two cell layers. The cells are arranged perpendicular to the basement membrane, and apical cytoplasmic snouts are present on the luminal aspect (Fig. 27.1B). Nucleoli are inconspicuous. Luminal secretions and calcifications may or may not be present. Mitoses are rare.

In CCH, there is prominent epithelial proliferation: more than two cell layers with nuclear stratification and exaggerated apical snouts. However, true bridges are not identified. Calcification is common.

Cytological atypia can be present in both CCC and CCH and both situations are described using the term FEA (Figs. 27.1C,D) (25). Importantly, in FEA, the cytological atypia is of low grade. Schnitt (26) has emphasized that high nuclear grade is not a feature of CCLs; if high nuclear grade features are present, then the appropriate diagnosis is high-grade DCIS.

Immunohistochemical studies show that CCLs are positive for CK8/18 and CK19, indicating luminal origin and they do not express basal cytokeratins (CK5 or CK14) (27–29). There is also strong uniform expression of estrogen and progesterone receptors and in some cases androgen receptor positivity, usually a marker of apocrine change. Proliferative activity, as assessed by Ki-67 expression, is low: some studies indicate an increased expression in CCLs with atypia (5–8%) (27). HER2 and p53 are not expressed (29).

Molecular studies show LOH in the majority of cases of FEA, an indication that it may represent an early neoplastic alteration. The genetic alterations are similar to those observed in low-grade DCIS (29,30).

CCLs have been reported to coexist with lobular neoplasia and tubular carcinoma and they are considered to be related (22,31,32). Also, CCLs can coexist with ADH and DCIS, which is typically low grade, micropapillary, or cribriform without necrosis (33).

The optimum management of CCLs is uncertain and is still an issue of conflict and controversy. Based on the current data, if a CCL without atypia is detected on a core biopsy, no further excisional biopsy is required (34,35). However, if atypia is present in a core biopsy a further open biopsy or vacuum excision is recommended, since in up to 30% of the cases more significant pathology (ADH, DCIS, or invasive carcinoma) may be detected. If a CCL with atypia is identified in an excision specimen, a careful search for ADH or DCIS is warranted. This may require processing of the tissue in its entirety (36,37).

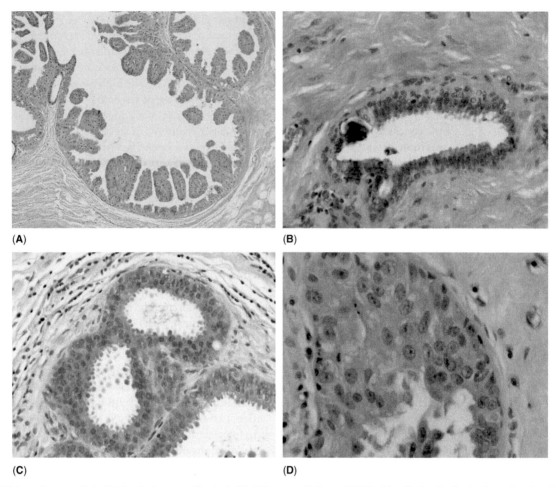

Figure 27.1 (**A**) Apocrine metaplasia (H+E stain, low magnification). (**B**) Columnar cell change (CCC) with cells showing luminal cytoplasmic tufts. Microcalcification is noted (H+E stain, medium magnification). (**C**) CCC with cytological atypia (H+E stain, medium magnification). (**D**) CCC with cytological atypia (H+E stain, high magnification).

Since current data are limited, further studies are essential to determine the clinical significance of CCLs, especially with atypia, in order to avoid under- or overtreatment.

SCLEROSING LESIONS
Sclerosing Adenosis

Jensen et al. (38) defined SA as a benign lobulocentric lesion with a disordered increase in acinar, myoepithelial, and connective tissue elements (Fig. 27.2A). The enlargement of the lobular units due to proliferation of myoepithelium and eventual destruction of the lobule with concomitant fibrosis often distorts the lobular architecture. SA is usually an incidental finding in breast specimens obtained for other reasons. On mammography, it may form an area of architectural distortion or may calcify. Less often, SA can form a palpable lump, referred to as "adenosis tumor." SA is most prevalent in perimenopausal women.

The significance of SA lies in its ability to mimic invasive cancer clinically, mammographically, macroscopically, and microscopically, especially when perineural invasion or even the formation of benign inclusions in lymph nodes is present (39). The key features are the lobulocentric pattern and the lack of desmoplastic stroma. In cases where the distinction from invasive carcinoma is difficult, immunostaining to highlight the presence of myoepithelial cells is very useful.

Jensen et al. (38) followed up patients with SA and calculated the relative risk for developing invasive breast cancer to be 2.1, regardless of the presence of atypical hyperplasia. The risk decreased to 1.7 when patients with atypical hyperplasia were excluded and increased to 6.7 when patients with atypical hyperplasia and SA were analyzed. Consequently, SA qualifies to be included as a form of proliferative breast disease without atypia, with an overall cancer risk of 1.5–2 times that of the general population. A positive family history of breast cancer in the absence of atypical hyperplasia did not significantly elevate the risk for invasive cancer. In the same study, there was a positive association of SA and atypical lobular hyperplasia (ALH), which elevated the relative risk for developing invasive cancer to 7.6. Oberman and Markey (40) and Fechner (41) independently reported an association of lobular carcinoma in situ (LCIS) and SA, although they did not consider SA a risk factor for lobular neoplasia. This association of lobular proliferations with SA should alert the pathologist to search for lobular neoplasia in the presence of sclerosing adenosis.

SA may show apocrine metaplasia of the epithelium (Fig. 27.2B): the terms used for this category are apocrine metaplasia involving SA or apocrine adenosis; the latter term has also been used for a form of adenomyoepithelioma and therefore, the former term is preferred. In this lesion, there is a risk of misdiagnosis of cancer both on cytological and on histological examination (42–44). Cytological atypia which is defined as nuclear pleomorphism, hyperchromasia, and prominent nucleoli may be present. The architectural atypia and cytological atypia in these lesions justify the use of the term atypical apocrine change within sclerosing adenosis. Seidman et al. (45) followed 37 patients with atypical apocrine change within SA for an average of 8.7 years, and four patients developed carcinoma after a mean of 5.6 years, with a relative risk of 5.5. All patients were aged over 60. Apocrine change within SA has been reported to overexpress c-ErbB-2 oncoprotein, further highlighting the malignant potential of this lesion (46,47). If atypical apocrine change within SA is detected in a core biopsy, further excision is recommended (45,48).

Radial Scar

A radial scar or complex sclerosing lesion is usually an incidental finding in breast specimens. However, if large enough they can be detected mammographically or less commonly by palpation. The significance of radial scars is that they can form stellate lesions, indistinguishable mammographically from an invasive carcinoma, especially tubular carcinoma.

The same problem may arise in histological specimens, especially in core biopsies. On microscopic examination, the radial scar is composed of a central fibroelastotic zone with small entrapped ducts, often distorted or even angular. In the periphery of the lesion, ducts, lobules, and cysts may be present (Fig. 27.2C). The entrapped glands may be confused with a tubular carcinoma, as myoepithelial cells may not be easily recognizable on hematoxylin and eosin stains. Immunohistochemistry for myoepithelial markers is used to highlight the myoepithelial cells. The most specific markers are p63 and smooth muscle myosin heavy chain. However, their positivity may be focal; occasional glands may even show a complete lack of myoepithelial cells, which may lead to a misinterpretation of the lesion.

The genesis of a radial scar is thought be due to a secondary reaction to an unknown injurious agent, possibly vascular or related to cyst rupture, which heals with central fibrosis and elastosis, resulting in the characteristic stellate configuration. Despite the benign nature of this lesion, carcinomas (in particular tubular carcinomas) have been reported to arise in association with radial scars. In an extensive study of these lesions, Linnell et al. (49) concluded that radial scars were premalignant. This view was further supported by Jacobs et al. (50) who carried out a case–control study of 1396 women with benign breast disease, 225 of whom subsequently developed cancer. Women with radial scars associated with atypical hyperplasia had a 5.8 relative risk of developing carcinoma, compared with 3.8 for those patients with ADH without a radial scar. From this study, Jacobs et al. (50) concluded that radial scars were an independent histological risk factor for developing breast cancer. However, it appears that the atypical epithelial hyperplasia was the main factor rather than the radial scar per se. Andersen and Gram (51) followed up 32 women with excised radial scars without atypical proliferation for a mean of 19.5 years, and only one developed breast cancer. In a subsequent study, Sloane and Mayers (52) reported a high association of radial scars, larger than 7 mm, with atypical hyperplasia in women aged more than 50. A similar follow-up study by Jacobs et al. (50) reported the development of cancer in 32% (32 of 99) of women with radial scars compared with 17% (223 of 1297) of the control group without radial scars. The women with radial scars who developed cancer tended to be older than 45.

In an attempt to prove the link between radial scar and tubular carcinoma, Jacobs et al. (53) performed molecular tests on the stromal elements of both lesions. In situ hybridization detected similarities in the pattern of expression of mRNA of the stromal and vascular elements in radial scars and tubular carcinomas, suggestive of similar disturbances in the stromal–epithelial interaction. Although these studies are inconclusive, most authorities will agree that local excision of a radial scar without associated atypical hyperplasia is curative, and the patients' risk of developing breast cancer is comparable to that of the general population. However, because of the difficulty in differentiating radial scars from carcinoma radiologically, all radial scars should be excised for histological examination (54). Nowadays, there is a tendency to excise radial scars without epithelial atypia with vacuum-assisted mammotomy (37,55); however, there is consensus that lesions with epithelial atypia should be surgically excised.

INTRADUCTAL PAPILLOMA

Papillomas may be central or peripheral, solitary or multiple. Solitary papillomas are usually central and multiple papillomas peripheral (56). Clinically, both can cause nipple discharge, but it is more common with solitary papillomas due to their usual location in major ducts. Multiple papillomas are more likely to be detected mammographically or may form palpable nodules which may be indistinguishable from fibrocystic change clinically. Solitary papillomas occur more often in women in their fifth and sixth decade. Multiple papillomas occur at a younger age. Their size varies from microscopic foci to areas measuring 10 cm or more.

Histologically, papillomas are an intraductal proliferation of villous-like or arborescent structures with a central fibrovascular core covered by a basal myoepithelial layer and a luminal epithelial cell layer (Fig. 27.2D). Solitary central papillomas may show apocrine metaplasia, squamous metaplasia, and infarction. Additionally, the epithelium can show proliferative changes, with either usual hyperplasia or atypical hyperplasia and even DCIS, more common in multiple papillomas. According to Page (57–59), a size of 3 mm is the cut-off point between ADH and DCIS in a papilloma; if the focus is 3 mm or less, the term atypical epithelial hyperplasia in a papilloma is recommended; if the focus is greater than 3 mm, then the term DCIS within a papilloma is used. The term "atypical papilloma" is also used, in cases where less than one-third of the papilloma is involved. Immunohistochemistry is useful to categorize these lesions. Papillomas with usual hyperplasia show a mosaic pattern of CK5 and ER in the luminal epithelium but atypical epithelial proliferations show the absence of CK5 expression and uniform strong expression of ER (60). Apocrine change, which may be atypical, is also sometimes seen (48).

The premalignant potential of papillomas has been the subject of numerous studies. In a case–control study of 368 women with intraductal papillomas, Page et al. (57) reported a relative risk of invasive carcinoma of 3.5 times that of the general population. The lesions tended to be micropapillomas (3 mm) and the risk was irrespective of family history, the presence of

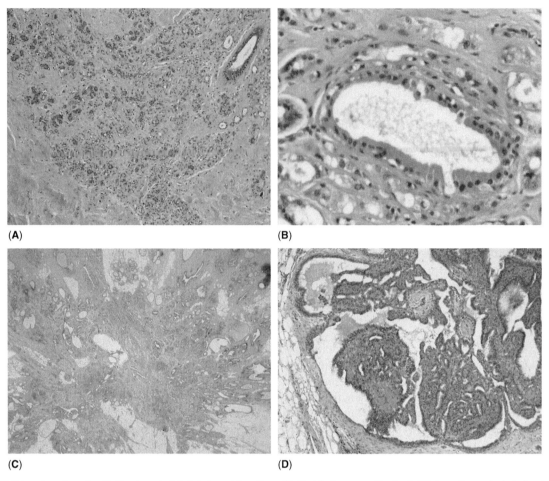

Figure 27.2 (**A**) Sclerosing adenosis with the characteristic lobulocentric pattern (H+E stain, low magnification). (**B**) Apocrine metaplasia involving sclerosing adenosis (H+E stain, high magnification). (**C**) Radial scar showing a central fibroelastotic zone with small entrapped ducts (H+E stain, low magnification). (**D**) Intraductal papilloma showing fibrovascular cores (H+E stain, low magnification).

atypical hyperplasia, or other epithelial proliferation. Papillomas larger than 3 mm had a risk 1.8 times that of the population. Page et al. (57) did not assess the significance of single versus multiple papillomas. The premalignant nature of multiple papillomas was first illustrated by Muir (61) in 1941 in his article on the evolution of carcinoma of the breast, in which relatively young women aged 50 and below, developed carcinoma in association with multiple papillomas. The carcinomas were mostly of cribriform type, either invasive or in situ. Multiple papillomas are an infrequent condition, with only 53 cases retrieved from Haagensen's files over a period of 39 years (8). The majority of the patients were aged 40 or younger, and 6 out of 53 developed breast cancer after a follow-up of 19 years. Again in this study, Haagensen emphasized the difference between central solitary papillomas and multiple peripheral papillomas.

In their study, Lewis et al. (62) calculated the relative risk for developing breast carcinoma in patients with papillomas. Solitary papillomas without atypia had a 2.04 relative risk and multiple papillomas without atypia had a relative risk of 3.01. The relative risk was higher in cases with atypia with estimates of 5.11 for solitary and 7.01 for multiple papillomas.

The management of patients with papillomas is an issue of controversy. Generally, excision is recommended in papillomas without atypia but this may be by vacuum excision. If atypia is present, surgical excision and follow-up are recommended (63).

EPITHELIAL DUCTAL HYPERPLASIA

Normal breast ducts and lobular units are lined by two cell types, consisting of an outer myoepithelial layer and an inner epithelial layer. Epithelial hyperplasia denotes an increase in the number of cells to more than two cell layers above the basement membrane (36). Like most forms of breast proliferation, hyperplasia originates from the TDLUs and varies from mild through florid to atypical proliferation, which may be virtually indistinguishable from carcinoma in situ. The relative risk for developing invasive carcinoma escalates numerically according to the degree of atypia. This was demonstrated in a large study by Dupont and Page (11) who followed up over 10,000 women who had undergone biopsy for clinically benign breast disease. The histological slides were reviewed, and the features present in biopsies of women who subsequently developed cancer were compared with those who did not. This work by Page and colleagues led to the classification of ductal epithelial proliferations into mild, moderate, or florid proliferative disease without atypia (PDWA) and ADH. These proliferations may be identified incidentally in biopsies removed for palpable abnormalities or screen-detected architectural distortion with or without calcification. ADH may also be detected as developing microcalcification in the incident round of breast cancer screening. ADH however is related to CCLs and there is no direct progression from usual hyperplasia to ADH. Although all epithelial proliferations arise from the TDLUs, the most prevalent pattern is known as "usual ductal hyperplasia" (UDH) or regular hyperplasia to distinguish it from ALH.

Usual Ductal Hyperplasia

The World Health Organization (WHO) defined UDH as a "benign ductal proliferative lesion typically characterized by slit-like secondary lumens and streaming of proliferative cells" (24). Page and Rogers (64) termed this process proliferative disease without atypia. UDH is subdivided into mild, moderate, and severe.

Mild hyperplasia is present within a duct when three layers of epithelium are seen above the basement membrane (64). The proliferation may be diffuse or focal. The latter gives rise to a corrugated luminal appearance. Tangentially cut ducts should not be labeled as hyperplasia. Mild hyperplasia is classified as a non-proliferative disease and carries the same risk of subsequent breast cancer as the general population. Its presence or absence in biopsies is not critical to patient management (4). A family history of breast cancer does not increase the risk of subsequent cancer in patients with mild hyperplasia.

Moderate hyperplasia shows increased epithelial thickness of more than three layers and it may form papillae with bridges across the ductal lumen. The papillae do not have the "rigid" appearance of micropapillary or cribriform DCIS and the cells lack the monotony of in situ carcinoma. The cytomorphology is variable, and it is important not to make a diagnosis of atypical hyperplasia or DCIS. The nuclei are bland with a delicate nuclear chromatin pattern and may be mildly hyperchromatic with small or inconspicuous nucleoli. Mitoses may be present, but are infrequent. The cytoplasm may be pale or eosinophilic, and the cells may merge into an apocrine pattern with luminal "snouts." The cells can be arranged parallel to each other, a phenomenon that Azzopardi termed "streaming" or "swirling." Malignancy should not be diagnosed in the presence of this architectural pattern.

Severe (or florid) hyperplasia shows a similar architectural and cytomorphological pattern; however, there is expansion of the ducts by an epithelial proliferation, which almost completely fills the lumen, with residual serpiginous slit-like lumina at the periphery (Figs. 27.3A,B). Rarely, central necrosis occurs in florid hyperplasia and this should not be interpreted as comedo carcinoma. The presence of apocrine change within the lesion or peripheral slit-like spaces is also a positive sign of benignity.

UDH is often seen in specimens with invasive cancer, DCIS, and other benign proliferations such as fibrocystic change, intraductal papillomas, or radial scars. It has therefore, always been assumed that UDH is the initial step in the pathogenesis of invasive cancer in a stepwise progression: UDH→ ADH→ DCIS→ invasive carcinoma. This model was challenged by Boecker et al. (65), who demonstrated that UDH and low grade DCIS were biologically different lesions with ADH and low grade DCIS having features more akin to FEA. Using double immunofluorescence, Boecker demonstrated that UDH was a CK5/14[+] progenitor cell lesion while DCIS expressed a different phenotype, more differentiated toward luminal epithelium and being CK8[+] and CK18[+]. Based on these findings, UDH is now not considered a risk factor for subsequent malignancy. The WHO (24) also supports this view that there is insufficient genetic evidence to classify UDH as a precursor lesion. The updated consensus statement on benign breast diseases assesses the risk of subsequent breast cancer of moderate or florid hyperplasia without atypia to be 1.5–2.0 times that of the general population (66).

Atypical Ductal Hyperplasia

ADH is the most controversial topic in breast pathology, and scores of papers have been dedicated to the subject. The controversy is due to the lack of definite histopathological criteria, as illustrated in the following definition of "having both architectural and cytological atypia which approximates, but falls short of that seen in carcinoma in situ" (4). This rather ambiguous definition was felt to be unacceptable by Azzopardi (67), who stated that "...the clinician should be told as unequivocally as possible whether the pathologist considers that the lesion is benign or malignant. Terms like … "'atypical hyperplasia' should be avoided as far as possible ... as such terms frighten surgeons into performing unnecessary mastectomies". Over the years, however, pathologists have come to recognize a borderline epithelial proliferation that architecturally and cytologically does not qualify for a definitive diagnosis of carcinoma in situ.

In a follow-up study of 10,542 women, 3.6% of whom had atypical epithelial proliferations, Page et al. (68) illustrated that the term "atypical hyperplasia" was appropriate for those lesions where the pattern or the cytological criteria of carcinoma in situ are partially met but not fully expressed. In that study, they outlined criteria for identifying ADH, which Page and Rogers (69) later improved. In making a diagnosis of ADH, the criteria must be based on the cytological features, histological pattern, and anatomical extent. ADH exhibits partial involvement of basement membrane-bound spaces by a cell population similar to non-comedo type low grade DCIS (cribriform) (Fig. 27.3C). These atypical cells are evenly spaced and uniform, with oval to round nuclei. The cytoplasm is pale with distinct intercellular borders (Fig. 27.3D). The non-atypical cells are columnar and further support development from CCC. They are arranged radially at the periphery of the duct, just above the basement membrane. The histological pattern is variable. This includes secondary spaces with smooth rounded "punched-out" borders of cribriform architecture with or without rigid non-tapering bars. Micropapillary structures may also be present. To qualify for ADH, the uniform cells must not completely involve two membrane-bound spaces; if they do, then DCIS is the appropriate diagnosis. ADH is usually not larger than 2–3 mm in diameter, although it may be a component in a much larger area of FEA (70). Necrosis is not a feature of ADH. High grade DCIS appears to form by a different pathway.

In spite of these criteria, there is still much inter-observer variation in the reporting of ADH, as Rosai (71) discovered when he distributed cases to five prominent breast pathologists in the United States. There was no consensus in the diagnosis of ADH versus DCIS. The root of all this disagreement lies in the fact that it may be virtually impossible to distinguish ADH from small-cell (low-grade) DCIS of cribriform type. For this reason, the consensus statement (14) asserted that only cases of severe atypia should be classified as ADH. Similarly, the United Kingdom (UK) guidelines (70) advocate that the pathologist should only make the diagnosis of ADH where a diagnosis of DCIS is seriously considered. ADH can be detected as mammographic calcification, and its presence in a needle core biopsy should prompt a biopsy by either excision or vacuum assistance, sufficient to

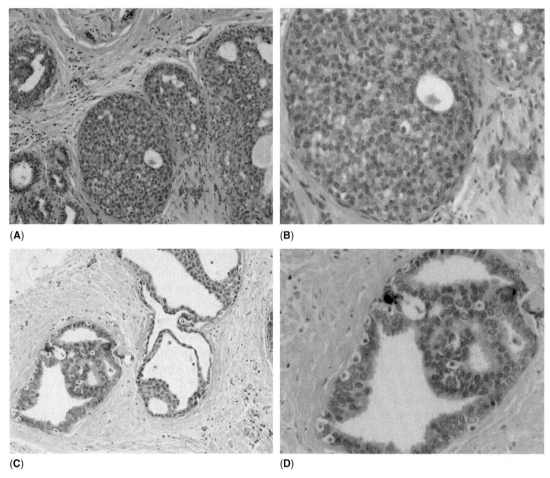

Figure 27.3 (A) Usual epithelial hyperplasia showing mild, moderate, and florid epithelial proliferation (H+E stain, low magnification). (B) Florid usual epithelial hyperplasia with solid pattern filling most of the acinus (H+E stain, high magnification). (C) Atypical ductal hyperplasia showing a cribriform pattern and microcalcification (H+E stain, low magnification). (D) Atypical ductal hyperplasia showing atypical bars and bridges, (H+E stain, high magnification).

exclude DCIS or invasive carcinoma. In this instance, the lesion should be termed "atypical intraepithelial proliferation" as its extent cannot be determined on core biopsies. ADH is a rare lesion, identified in 2% of non-screening biopsies (70), and often coexists with fibrocystic change, SA, or multiple papillomas. By contrast, the incidence of ADH is much higher in screen-detected lesions, up to 12% in some series (72).

In a 15-year follow-up study of women with ADH, Page and associates demonstrated a fourfold relative risk of developing invasive carcinoma of the breast compared with the general population. Translating this to absolute risk, approximately 10% of women with ADH will develop invasive cancer within 10–15 years of biopsy in the ipsilateral or contralateral breast. The relative risk doubles to 8–10 times if there is a family history of breast cancer (mother, sister or daughter) and the absolute risk is elevated to 20% at 15 years (73). Annual mammographic follow-up is advisable for patients with ADH.

Atypical Apocrine Hyperplasia

Atypical apocrine change in SA has been discussed earlier but there is an atypical intraductal apocrine proliferation which can be difficult to distinguish from apocrine DCIS (74). The lesion is composed of apocrine epithelium but with a complex architectural pattern and/or cytological atypia, to a degree not normally seen in papillary apocrine metaplasia. The architectural changes include Roman bridges, cribriform patterns, and

micropapillary fronds. There is nuclear enlargement with a threefold variation in nuclear size and prominent nucleoli (74). The distinction from apocrine DCIS is difficult, and the criteria to distinguish these two lesions are not clearly defined (75). The criteria used are the presence of necrosis, mitotic activity, and periductal fibrosis, features not generally seen in atypical apocrine hyperplasia. Atypical apocrine hyperplasia is insufficiently studied and its relationship to apocrine DCIS is unclear, but likely represents a precursor lesion (75,76).

LOBULAR NEOPLASIA

Haagensen et al. (77) applied the term lobular neoplasia to collectively classify proliferations currently separated into lobular carcinoma in situ (LCIS) and ALH. LCIS and ALH are cytologically identical but differ architecturally in the degree by which the cells expand the lobular units. Because of inter- and intra-observer variation, this distinction is considered by some authorities to be arbitrary; therefore, the use of "lobular neoplasia" to encompass the whole range of proliferations will improve reproducibility (78). However, this concept has not been fully embraced by pathologists (5). Rosen (79) has proposed that the term lobular neoplasia should be reserved for a spectrum of proliferations ranging from mild ALH to fully developed LCIS.

As both LCIS and ALH do not usually present with clinical or radiological abnormalities, Jacobs et al. (37) have advocated follow-up rather than local excision if these lesions are discovered as incidental findings. Both LCIS and ALH can be present in biopsies removed for a palpable lesion or a mammographic abnormality. Microcalcification is not a frequent finding but may occur. Further excision is advisable in the following situations (78,79):

- if another lesion such as ADH or DCIS is present;
- if clinical, radiological and pathological discordance is present;
- if the lesion causing the radiological abnormality has not been identified;
- if a mass lesion or an area of architectural distortion is present;
- if pleomorphic LCIS is present;
- if ALH or LCIS with mixed histological features indistinguishable from DCIS is identified;
- if central necrosis is present.

Lobular Carcinoma In Situ

LCIS was first recognized as an entity by Foote and Stewart (80) as early as 1941. LCIS is distinguished from ALH in that it shows complete distension of more than 75% of the acini in a lobular unit by a uniform population of neoplastic lobular cells (Fig. 27.4B). In classical type LCIS, the cells are arranged in a regular pattern with no intercellular spaces; intracytoplasmic mucin secretion may be present. The cells are small and round with scant cytoplasm. In the pleomorphic type of LCIS, cytological pleomorphism is present that can resemble DCIS and thus, can make the distinction difficult (Fig. 27.4D). Necrosis and calcification may rarely be observed and should not be confused with high-grade comedo DCIS. Pagetoid spread along ducts is more prevalent in LCIS than in ALH. The cells are discohesive and an alteration of E-cadherin is considered responsible for this observation. E-cadherin expression is reduced or absent in LCIS and ALH although not all cases will show this (Fig. 27.4C) (81,82). ER and PR are usually expressed and HER2/neu immunoreactivity is rare (83,84). However, pleomorphic LCIS may show HER2/neu membrane expression and loss of ER/PR expression (85,86).

Seventy percent of women with LCIS are premenopausal (87,88). The condition is present in 0.5–1.5% of screen-detected lesions (89). LCIS tends to be multifocal and bilateral: 60–85% of the patients with LCIS have multiple foci (89) and LCIS is found in the contralateral breast in 40% (90). LCIS predisposes to invasive cancer, even after a long interval. The relative risk is 4.0–12.0. In a 15-year follow-up study of 39 patients with LCIS, Page et al. (91) calculated the relative risk for developing invasive cancer to be 10–11 times that of the general population. The absolute risk of developing invasive cancer in patients with LCIS is therefore 25–30% at 15–20 years. This risk of cancer is 50–60% for the ipsilateral breast and 40–50% for the contralateral breast (92).

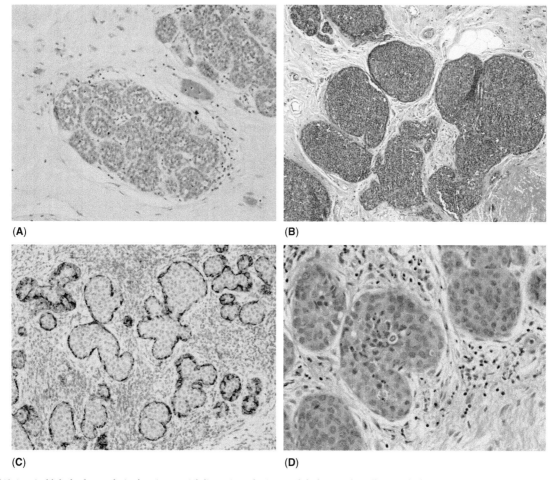

(A)   (B)

(C)   (D)

Figure 27.4 (A) Atypical lobular hyperplasia showing partial distension of acini in a lobular unit by cells typical of lobular neoplasia (H+E stain, low magnification). (B) Classical lobular carcinoma *in situ* (LCIS) showing complete distension of acini with neoplastic cells (H+E stain, medium magnification). (C) Loss of E-cadherin expression in LCIS (H+E stain, medium magnification). (D) Pleomorphic LCIS (H+E stain, high magnification).

A family history of breast cancer does not appear to have any further predictive value in identifying women who develop invasive carcinoma (91). Studies have shown that exogenous estrogen is not related to LCIS in postmenopausal women (93).

Atypical Lobular Hyperplasia

The histological criteria for ALH are met when there is partial distension of the acini in a lobular unit by a population of cells identical to those seen in LCIS with residual intercellular spaces (Fig. 27.4A) (68). The resemblance to LCIS is striking but the acini are not uniformly distended in more than 75% of the lobular units. ALH cells are usually bland and uniform, with small or inconspicuous nucleoli. Pagetoid spread of atypical cells along ducts is seen in ALH less often than in LCIS, but the latter diagnosis should not be made purely on the basis of this criterion without taking other features into consideration. As in LCIS, ALH shows reduced expression or loss of E-cadherin.

ALH is more common in perimenopausal women, with an average age of 46 (68). The relative risk for developing invasive carcinoma with ALH is 4–4.5 times that of the general population and this risk increases when associated with a family history of breast cancer (relative risk 8.5). Page et al. reported that the risk is also increased in the presence of ADH or pagetoid spread by ALH down ducts (94).

Treatment of LCIS and ALH

As mentioned, follow-up is recommended for patients with ALH and patients with LCIS. Rosen et al. proposed the use of anti-estrogens as prophylaxis (89). Fisher et al. (95) found a 56% reduction in the risk of developing invasive carcinoma. However it is not clear yet whether the rate of long-term mortality is reduced.

DUCTAL CARCINOMA IN SITU

As early as 1932, Broders (96) recognized carcinoma in situ of the breast as a neoplastic epithelial proliferation confined to the ducts and acini without migration beyond the basement membrane. Using subgross analysis, Wellings et al. (3) have demonstrated that carcinomas as well as other pre-neoplastic proliferations arise from the TDLUs and that the histological appearance of DCIS is due to the "unfolding" of lobules. According to this theory, during epithelial proliferation, the terminal ducts of a lobule enlarge and the interlobular part ceases to exist. The terminal ducts continue to dilate and incorporate themselves in a single lumen, with a resultant loss of the lobular architecture, which is termed "unfolding."

Traditionally, these structures have been called ducts and the term DCIS is used to differentiate the lesion from *lobular* carcinoma in situ. In the premammographic era, DCIS made up only 1–5% of symptomatic carcinoma (97). DCIS presented symptomatically as an ill-defined mass, nipple discharge, Paget's disease, or as an incidental finding in a clinically benign lump. However, since the introduction of breast screening mammography, DCIS has been more frequently identified as an impalpable, usually calcifying lesion, and represents 10–20% of all newly diagnosed breast cancer, depending on the breast screening unit (98). The mean age of diagnosis is between 50 and 59 years (99,100). Mammography is a sensitive diagnostic test for the detection of DCIS; 30% of the non-palpable

carcinomas detected mammographically have been proven to be DCIS (101,102). Calcifications detected by mammography are present in 70% of DCIS cases (102). Magnetic resonance imaging (MRI) is a new screening modality that may identify DCIS in the absence of calcification on mammography and may detect occult contralateral carcinoma among patients with breast cancer (103). However, MRI appears less sensitive for the detection of low-grade DCIS (103,104).

Traditionally, DCIS has been classified according to its architectural pattern into comedo and non-comedo types, disregarding cytomorphology (64). The non-comedo type has been further subclassified into cribriform, micropapillary, solid, and papillary types. Although this is a useful pathological classification in terms of pattern recognition for diagnosis, it has little therapeutic or prognostic implication. Patchefsky et al. (99) noted the heterogeneous nature of DCIS both pathologically and in biological behavior, and classified DCIS according to nuclear grade.

Investigations using biological markers, three-dimensional studies, mammographic analysis, and follow-up of patients demonstrated that the simple classification of DCIS according to architecture did not always correspond to the biological behavior. Holland et al. (105) proposed a classification of DCIS based on nuclear morphology and the presence or absence of necrosis rather than on architecture. Using these criteria, DCIS is divided into well, moderately, and poorly differentiated types. The only problem with using this terminology is that clinicians may misinterpret "differentiated" as equivalent to grade of invasive carcinomas. Similarly, the UK Coordinating Group for Breast Screening Pathology classified DCIS according to nuclear grade into high, intermediate, and low grades (106). Cytonuclear grade leads to less inter-observer variation than architectural differentiation. However, cytological and architectural features may overlap in the same breast; therefore, in situ carcinomas must be graded according to the worst area. Both the architectural and cytological features of DCIS will be discussed in relation to radiological appearance, expression of biological markers, and biological behavior.

High-Grade DCIS

High-grade DCIS with comedo necrosis is the most prevalent type of DCIS, constituting up to 85% of high-grade lesions (99). It presents clinically as an ill-defined mass or Paget's disease of the nipple. Radiologically, there is often a linear, branching, or granular pattern of microcalcification. On cut surface, breast tissue containing comedo carcinoma in situ reveals large ducts filled with yellow necrotic semisolid debris, which is easily expressed like the "comedone" of acne vulgaris. Histologically, high-grade DCIS has variable architectural differentiation or cellular polarization. The most common pattern consists of solid sheets of neoplastic cells, which line the ducts with central comedo necrosis (Fig. 27.5B). Necrosis is present in most cases, but not exclusively. Conversely, not all cases with comedo necrosis are high grade. Pure solid DCIS without necrosis is rare (Fig. 27.5A). The mammographic calcification has an amorphous histological pattern (Fig. 27.5C). The cells may lack the solid pattern, forming a pseudocribriform or micropapillary configuration. Periductal fibrosis and lymphocytic infiltration are often associated with this type of DCIS.

The cells show marked variation in nuclear size and shape (pleomorphism) and have a high nuclear-cytoplasmic ratio and condensation of chromatin. They are usually large, with pale or eosinophilic cytoplasm. The luminal layer of the epithelium is often retracted away from the necrotic debris. This feature distinguishes comedo necrosis from that occasionally seen in benign lesions such as juvenile papillomatosis, nipple adenoma, and hyperplasia of usual type (4). Mitoses are often evident, and high-grade DCIS frequently demonstrates individual cell necrosis. The pleomorphic cells often involve recognizable lobular units, in so-called "cancerization" of lobules (Fig. 27.5D).

Low-Grade DCIS

Low nuclear grade DCIS rarely presents with a palpable mass and is usually identified incidentally in a biopsy for a clinically benign lesion or by mammography. Mammographic calcification is mostly granular and is reflected histologically with a laminated crystalline pattern resembling psammoma bodies. In contrast to high-grade DCIS, low-grade DCIS tends to show architectural differentiation or cellular polarization, resulting in a cribriform or micropapillary pattern. The cribriform pattern consists of an intraductal proliferation of neoplastic cells separated by round or oval lumina (Fig. 27.6A). This must be distinguished from collagenous spherulosis and adenoid cystic carcinoma which both contain basement membrane material in the spaces seen on immunostaining with laminin or type IV collagen. The papillae of micropapillary DCIS are devoid of

fibrovascular cores and are held rigidly and perpendicular to the basement membrane. Sometimes, anastomosing arcades give rise to "Roman bridges." The cells of low-grade DCIS are small and monomorphic, with round or oval nuclei. The nuclear membrane is smooth, and the nucleolus is small or inconspicuous. Mitoses are infrequent, and individual cell necrosis is not a feature (106). Luminal necrosis is uncommon. Although this can occur in the European classification, DCIS of low nuclear grade with necrosis is classified as intermediate in the Van Nuys classification (107). Rarely, low-grade DCIS exhibits a solid proliferation mimicking LCIS (Fig. 27.6B).

Intermediate-Grade DCIS

This group of DCIS cannot be easily assigned into either the high- or low-grade categories. The architecture is variable, and cellular polarization is present with micropapillae, but is not as marked as in low-grade DCIS. Solid areas with intercellular spaces may also be present. The cytomorphology of intermediate grade lies midway between that of high- and low-grade DCIS and may show apocrine features (Figs. 27.6C,D). The cells show moderate variations in nuclear size and shape. The chromatin pattern is coarse and the nucleoli are small. Calcification may be of mixed pattern, showing both amorphous and psammomatous features in different ducts. Necrosis may or may not be present in the European classification but is uniformly present when using the Van Nuys classification (Fig. 27.6D) (107). Biological markers have justified the inclusion of this third

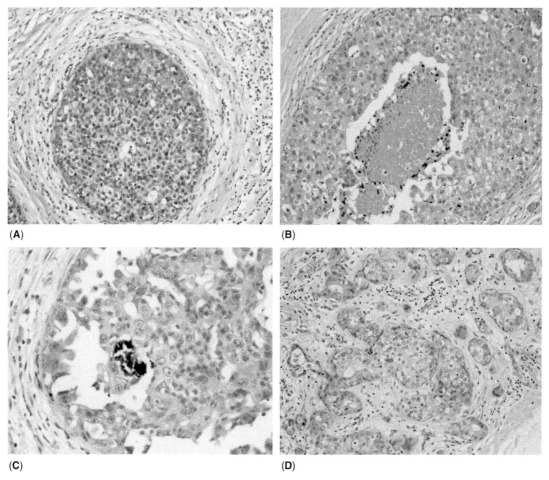

(A)　(B)　(C)　(D)

Figure 27.5 (**A**) High-grade ductal carcinoma *in situ* (DCIS), solid type, with stromal fibroblastic reaction (H+E stain, medium magnification). (**B**) High-grade DCIS with comedo necrosis (H+E stain, medium magnification). (**C**) High-grade DCIS with microcalcification (H+E stain, high magnification). (**D**) Cancerization of lobules (H+E stain, medium magnification).

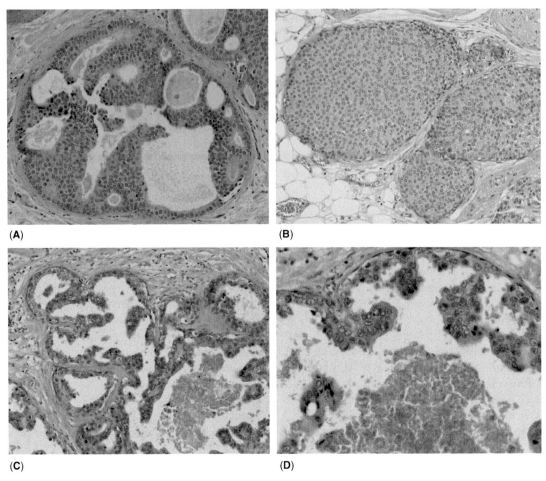

Figure 27.6 (A) Low-grade DCIS, cribriform type, (H+E stain, medium magnification). (B) Low-grade DCIS, solid type, (H+E stain, medium magnification). (C) Intermediate grade DCIS, (H+E stain, medium magnification). (D) Intermediate grade DCIS (H+E stain, high magnification).

category of DCIS (69). Clear cell and apocrine DCIS are often of intermediate nuclear grade but may be high grade also (106).

Encysted (Intracystic) Papillary Carcinoma In Situ

Intracystic papillary carcinoma is a form of DCIS that involves a grossly dilated cyst varying in size from 1 to 3 cm (64). Irrespective of the size, the important factor is that these lesions are non-invasive. Even though definite basement membrane staining may be absent in many cases, these lesions behave in an indolent fashion unless associated with more classical invasive carcinoma. Grossly, the tumor may appear solid, or a dilated duct filled with hemorrhagic debris may be evident. Histologically, the tumors may show a thick fibrous wall from which papillary excrescences arise (Fig. 27.7C). The papillae consist of a fibrovascular core covered by a layer of epithelium without intervening myoepithelial cells. The cells are small, monomorphic, and reminiscent of those seen in low-grade DCIS (Fig. 27.7D). Some lesions are so well differentiated that when Betsill et al. (108) reported papillary intraductal carcinoma, he used the term "low-grade and well-differentiated carcinoma," which would fit into the current classification of DCIS. Cribriform-type DCIS is sometimes present outside the "cystic" wall, where foci of microinvasion occasionally lurk. Carter et al. (109) followed 29 women who had had mastectomy for intracystic carcinoma, and none of them developed metastatic carcinoma after five years of follow-up. LOH on chromosome 16q in intracystic papillary carcinomas was reported to differentiate these lesions from intraductal

papillomas (110). Due to the frequent lack of peripheral myoepithelial cells, some pathologists regard these as a low grad invasive carcinoma, albeit with a prognosis similar to DCIS.

Prognostic Implication of DCIS

DCIS is a heterogeneous disease, and numerous studies have attempted to predict the behavior of this lesion. One of the first reports comes from Page et al. who followed up 28 women with non-comedo low-grade DCIS identified incidentally and treated with excision only. Overall, 28% of the women developed invasive carcinoma after a follow-up period of 15 years (111). The site of recurrence is usually close to the site of the original biopsy. The same authors, continuing the investigation with a median follow-up of 31 years, found that the percentage of subsequent carcinoma was 39.3% (112). The calculated risk factor for developing invasive cancer following a diagnosis of DCIS is 10–11 times that of the general population. Collins et al. (113) in their study that included women with unrecognized DCIS in the original biopsy, reported that 77% developed subsequent carcinoma in the ipsilateral breast; four patients were diagnosed with DCIS and six with invasive carcinoma, after a period of 2–18 years.

Several studies indicate the importance of histological features in the success of breast conservation surgery. In a retrospective study, MacDonald et al. (114) reported that the age of the patient (<40 years), high-nuclear grade, and margin of excision less than 10 mm were significantly associated with an increased risk of local recurrence. The risk was 5.39 times higher if the margin was less than 10 mm. Wong et al. (115) selected patients with a tumor size ≤2.5 cm, margin width at least 10 mm, and low or intermediate grade; 8.2% of the patients had a recurrence at a median follow-up of 40 months.

Radiotherapy is used nowadays in combination with breast conservation surgery to decrease the recurrence rate. The National Surgical Adjuvant Breast and Bowel Project (NSABP) B17 study demonstrated a 50% reduction in cases of recurrence after radiotherapy (116). The grade (intermediate or high) and architecture of DCIS (solid and cribriform) had a significant role in the outcome. Mastectomy has been the gold standard treatment for DCIS and it is still indicated for cases of widespread or multifocal disease and is associated with very low rates of recurrence (1.4%) (117).

DCIS and Microinvasion

Microinvasion is defined as the presence of an invasive focus of 1 mm or less in diameter outside the basement membrane of the duct involved by carcinoma in situ. The invasive focus can be single cells or clusters of tumor cells (Figs. 27.8A,B) (118). Detection of microinvasion can be very difficult. Features that should alarm the pathologist to search more carefully are the presence of a lymphocytic, fibroblastic, or granulomatous reaction, although microinvasion is defined as usually being outside lobular connective tissue or areas of lymphocytic infiltration. The site of a previous procedure (FNAC or needle core biopsy) can create diagnostic problems due to the displacement of epithelial cells. In the presence of brisk inflammation, visualization of the invasive focus may be difficult; in this case, if microinvasion is suspected, further levels and immunostaining for cytokeratins is the gold standard to reveal the presence of cells beyond the basement membrane. The absence of myoepithelial cells is the most convincing evidence of microinvasion, and more than one myoepithelial marker should be used.

Microinvasion is more often associated with high-grade comedo DCIS and large size. It occurs less often in other types and mammographically detected lesions (99). In the study by Walker et al. (119), microinvasion was detected in 5% of mammographically detected lesions and 13.5% of symptomatic lesions.

The main clinical significance of microinvasion is the increased risk of axillary metastases. A number of studies using sentinel lymph node mapping to assess the axillary status show metastases in less than 10% of apparently pure DCIS and up to 15% for DCIS with microinvasion (120–121).

DCIS and Expression of Biological Markers

Histological grade, lymph node status, and the application of biological markers have been used in combination to evaluate prognosis in invasive carcinomas. The commonly studied biological markers are the c-ErbB-2 and p53 proteins, and estrogen and progesterone receptors (ER and PgR). These markers have also been applied to non-invasive carcinomas in an attempt to predict their behavior.

The c-*erb*B-2 gene (also known as HER2/*neu*) encodes a transmembrane glycoprotein (c-erbB-2 oncoprotein) with

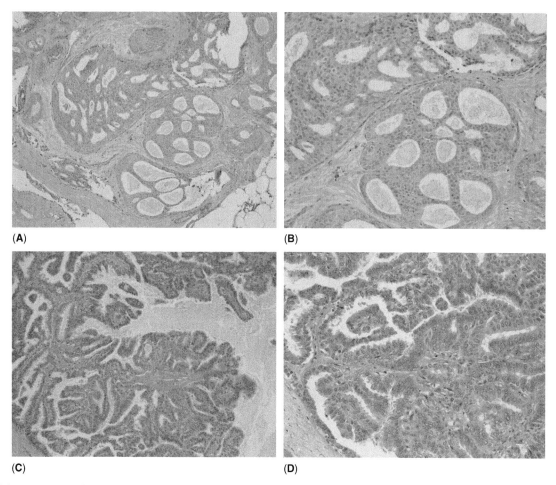

(A) (B) (C) (D)

Figure 27.7 (**A**) Apocrine DCIS showing a cribriform pattern (H+E stain, low magnification). (**B**) Apocrine DCIS (H+E stain, medium magnification). (**C**) Papillary DCIS with fibrovascular cores (H+E stain, low magnification). (**D**) Papillary DCIS with fibrovascular cores (H+E stain, medium magnification).

tyrosine kinase activity that is homologous to but distinct from the epidermal growth factor receptor (EGFR) (122). The gene is located on chromosome 17q and its amplification is associated with the overexpression of the protein product, which can be detected by immunohistochemistry as cell membrane staining (Fig. 27.8D). Overexpression of c-ErbB-2 in 20% of invasive carcinomas is associated with poor prognosis, with most of the tumors being poorly differentiated grade 3 carcinomas (123). Approximately 60–80% of high-grade DCIS strongly express the c-ErbB-2 protein (84). None of the low-grade DCIS express the c-ErbB-2 oncoprotein, but approximately 23% of intermediate-grade lesions do (124).

Poller et al. (125) demonstrated an inverse relationship between the expression of the c-ErbB-2 oncoprotein in DCIS and hormone receptor status. A similar pattern is seen in invasive carcinomas. The majority of high-grade DCIS and poorly differentiated invasive ductal carcinomas overexpress c-ErbB-2 (Fig. 27.8D) and lack ER. In this study most of the low-grade DCIS expressed ER (Fig. 27.8C) and PgR. The latter is directly modulated by estrogen, and therefore its level of expression mirrors that of ER. A separate study by Zafrani et al. (126) on mammographically detected DCIS reported a higher percentage of high-grade lesions that expressed ER as well as c-ErbB-2. The presence of both ER and PgR can be demonstrated using immunocytochemistry on wax-embedded tissue. Steroid receptors are demonstrated by nuclear staining.

The *TP53* (*p53*) tumor suppressor gene is the most commonly deleted gene in human cancers (127). It has been mapped to the short arm of chromosome 17 (17p13) (128). *TP53* encodes a nuclear phosphoprotein, p53. Mutant p53 has a longer half-life than the wild type and can be detected by immunocytochemistry (129), giving rise to positive nuclear staining, similar to hormone receptors. Sixty percent of high-grade DCIS show positive nuclear staining for p53 protein, compared with 4% of intermediate grade and none of the low-grade cases (124).

Developments in molecular genetic analysis have led to the further understanding of the biology of DCIS. It is hoped that these developments will eventually identify subgroups of lesions that are more likely to progress to invasive carcinoma. A study by Buerger et al. (130) suggests that there may be at least three different pathways for the development of DCIS, with loss of the long arm of chromosome 16 prevalent in low-grade DCIS, and gains in 17q12 and 20q13 and loss of 13q occurring in high-grade DCIS. Gains in 11q13 appear to be associated with intermediate-grade DCIS, as does loss of 11q. Loss of 16q is also a genetic alteration noted in intracystic carcinomas, which tend to be low-grade lesions.

Studies of the molecular abnormalities in DCIS suggest that although a minority of low-grade DCIS lesions with 16q loss may progress to high-grade lesions, the majority of high-grade DCIS does not show this abnormality (82,131). Those high-grade DCIS lesions showing 16q loss are ER positive, a rare

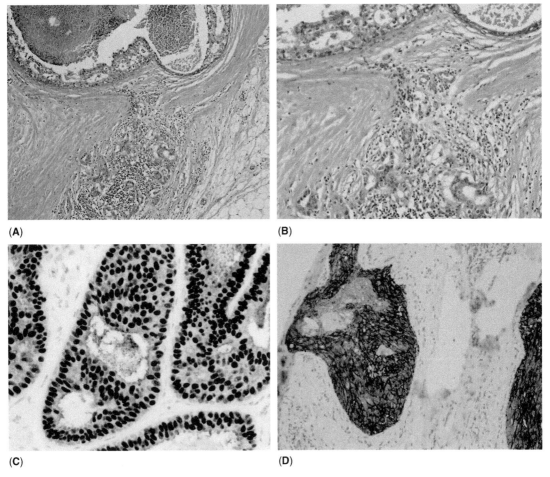

(A)   (B)

(C)   (D)

Figure 27.8 (**A**) Microinvasion from high-grade DCIS (H+E stain, low magnification). (**B**) Microinvasion (H+E stain, high magnification). (**C**) Estrogen receptor staining in low-grade DCIS (H+E stain, high magnification). (**D**) Strong membranous expression of Her-2 in high-grade DCIS (H+E stain, medium magnification).

event in high-grade lesions, but up to 50% of high-grade ER-positive DCIS does not show the characteristic 16q deletion seen in low-grade DCIS. This would suggest that there are at least two different pathways for development of high-grade DCIS (131,132). The majority of high-grade DCIS is ER negative and often overexpresses HER2. Rare "basal" type high-grade DCIS lesions are also seen (132). High-grade DCIS lesions are more heterogeneous than low-grade lesions and, while most low-grade lesions are luminal A in molecular subtype, high-grade lesions may be luminal B, HER2, basal-like, or molecular apocrine. Intermediate-grade DCIS also tends to be heterogeneous with the majority having molecular similarities to low-grade lesions and possibly representing progression of these while a smaller proportion more closely resemble high-grade lesions (133,134).

ADH has few genetic changes but those which have been documented are similar to low-grade DCIS with 1q gains and 16q losses (135). Similar changes are also seen in lobular neoplasia (ALH/LCIS) indicating that these lesions follow a low-grade pathway (131,136). Pleomorphic LCIS shows similar 1q gains and 16q losses but in addition has other genetic abnormalities; some cases show apocrine-like changes with amplification of areas of 17q and 11q while others have deletions of 8p, 13q and gains of 8q (86,137).

ACKNOWLEDGMENTS

The authors thank Dr Catherine Chinyama for her contribution to the previous edition and the Department of Pathology, Princess Alexandra Hospital for providing the slides for the illustrations.

REFERENCES

1. Page DL. Cancer risk assessment in benign breast biopsies. Hum Pathol 1986; 17: 871–4.
2. Foote FW, Stewart FW. Comparative studies of cancerous versus non-cancerous breasts. Ann Surg 1945; 121: 6–53.197–222.
3. Wellings SR, Jensen HM, Marcum RG. An atlas of the subgross pathology of human breast with special reference to possible precancerous lesions. J Natl Cancer Inst 1975; 55: 231–73.
4. Fechner RE, Mills SE, eds. Philosophy of risk assessment. Ductal carcinoma in situ. In: Breast Pathology, Benign Proliferations, Atypias and In Situ Carcinomas. Chicago: ASCP Press, 1990: 1–3.107–18.
5. Sloane JP. Pathology reporting in breast cancer screening. J Clin Pathol 1991; 44: 710–25.
6. Dawson EK. Sweat gland carcinoma of the breast. A morpho-histological study. Edin Med J 1932; 39: 409–38.
7. Viacava P, Naccarato AG, Bevilicqua G. Apocrine epithelium of the breast: Does it result from metaplasia? Virchows Arch 1997; 431: 205–9.
8. Haagensen CD. Apocrine epithelium; Solitary intraductal papilloma; Multiple intraductal papillomas; Lobular neoplasia (Lobular carcinoma in situ). In: Harris JR, Lippman ME, Morrow M, Osborne CK, eds. Diseases of the Breast. Philadelphia: WB Saunders, 1986: 82–101, 136–75, 176–91, 192–241.
9. Wellings SR, Alpers CE. Apocrine cystic metaplasia: subgross pathology and prevalence in cancer associated versus random autopsy breasts. Hum Pathol 1987; 18: 381–6.
10. Page DL, Zwaag RV, Rogers LW, et al. Relation between component parts of fibrocystic disease complex and breast cancer. J Natl Cancer Inst 1978; 61: 1055–63.
11. Dupont WD, Page DL. Risk factors for breast cancer in women with proliferative breast disease. N Engl J Med 1985; 312: 146–51.
12. Dixon JM, McDonald C, Miller WR. Risk of breast cancer in women with palpable cysts: a prospective study. Lancet 1999; 353: 1742–5.
13. Page DL, Dupont WD, Jensen RA. Papillary apocrine change of the breast: associations with atypical hyperplasia and risk of breast cancer. Cancer Epidemiol Biomarkers Prev 1996; 5: 29–32.
14. Hutter RV, et al. Consensus meeting: Is 'fibrocystic disease' of the breast precancerous? Arch Pathol Lab Med 1986; 110: 171–3.
15. Fitzgibbons PL, Henson DE, Hutter RV. Benign breast changes and risk of subsequent breast cancer: an update of the 1985 consensus statement. Cancer Committee of the College of American Pathologists. Arch Pathol Lab Med 1998; 122: 1053–5.
16. Washington C, Dalbegue F, Abreo F, et al. Loss of heterozygosity in fibrocystic change of the breast: genetic relationship between benign proliferative lesions and associated carcinoma. Am J Pathol 2000; 157: 323–9.
17. Jones C, Damiani S, Wells D, et al. Molecular cytogenetic comparison of apocrine hyperplasia and apocrine carcinoma of the breast. Am J Pathol 2001; 158: 207–14.
18. Agnantis NJ, Mahera H, Maounis N, et al. Immunohistochemical study of ras and myc oncoproteins in apocrine breast lesions with and without papillomatosis. Eur J Gynaecol Oncol 1999; 13: 309–15.
19. Bonser GM, Dossett JA, Jull JW. Neoplastic epithelial proliferation. In: Human and Experimental Breast Cancer 1961. London: Pitman Medical Publishing, 1961: 336–43.
20. Goldstein NS, O'Malley BA. Cancerization of small ectatic ducts of the breast by ductal carcinoma in situ cells with apocrine snouts. A lesion associated with tubular carcinoma. Am J Clin Pathol 1997; 107: 561–6.
21. Fraser JL, Raza S, Chorny K, et al. Columnar alterations with prominent apical snouts and secretions: a spectrum of changes frequently present in breast biopsies performed for microcalcifications. Am J Surg Pathol 1998; 22: 1521–7.
22. Rosen PP. Columnar cell hyperplasia is associated with lobular carcinoma in situ and tubular carcinoma. Am J Surg Pathol 1999; 23: 1561.
23. Rosen PP. Ductal hyperplasia. Ordinary and atypical. In: Rosen PP, ed. Breast Pathology, 2nd edn. Philadelphia, PA: Lippincott, Williams & Wilkins, 2001: 215–23.
24. Tavassoli FA, Goefler H, Rosai J, et al. Intraductal proliferative lesions. In: Tavasolli FA, Devilee P, eds. Pathology and Genetics of Tumours of the Breast and Female Genital Organs. Lyon: IARC Press, 2003: 63–7.
25. Schnitt SJ, Vincent-Salomon A. Columnar cell lesions of the breast. Adv Anat Pathol 2003; 10: 113–24.
26. Schnitt SJ. Columnar cell lesions of the breast: pathological features and clinical significance. Curr Diagn Pathol 2004; 10: 193–203.
27. Dessauvague BF, Zhao W, Heel-Miller KA, et al. Characterisation of columnar cell lesions of the breast: immunophenotypic analysis of columnar alteration of lobules with prominent apical snouts and secretion. Hum Pathol 2007; 38: 284–92.
28. Otterbach F, Bankfalvi A, Bergner S, et al. Cytokeratin 5/6 immunohistochemistry assists the differential diagnosis of atypical proliferation of the breast. Histopathology 2000; 37: 232–40.
29. Simpson PT, Gale T, Reis-Filho JS, et al. Columnar cell lesions of the breast: the missing link in breast cancer progression? A morphological and molecular analysis. Am J Surg Pathol 2005; 29: 734–46.
30. Dabbs DJ, Carter J, Fudge M, et al. Molecular alterations of columnar cell lesions of the breast. Mod Pathol 2006; 19: 344–9.
31. Sahoo S, Recant WM. Triad of columnar cell alteration, lobular carcinoma in situ and tubular carcinoma of the breast. Breast J 2005; 11: 140–2.
32. Abdel-Fatah TM, Powe DG, Hodi Z, et al. High frequency of coexistence of columnar cell lesions, lobular neoplasia and low grade ductal carcinoma in situ with invasive tubular carcinoma and invasive lobular carcinoma. Am J Surg Pathol 2007; 31: 416–26.
33. Collins LCM Achacosa NA, Nekhlyudov L, et al. Clinical and pathologic features of ductal carcinoma in situ associated with the presence of flat epithelial atypia: an analysis of 543 patients. Mod Pathol 2007; 20: 1149–55.
34. Guerra-Wallace MM, Christensen WN, White RL. A retrospective study of columnar alteration with prominent apical snouts and secretions and the association with cancer. Am J Surg 2004; 188: 395–8.
35. Schnitt SJ. The diagnosis and management of pre-invasive breast disease: flat epithelial atypia – classification, pathologic features and clinical significance. Breast Cancer Res 2003; 5: 263–8.
36. Pinder SE, Reis-Fihlo JS. Non-operative breast pathology: columnar cell lesions. J Clin Pathol 2007; 60: 1307–12.
37. Jacobs TW, Connolly JL, Schnitt SJ. Nonmalignant lesions in breast core needle biopsies: to excise or not to excise? Am J Surg Pathol 2002; 26: 1095–110.

38. Jensen RA, Page DL, Dupont WD, Rogers LW. Invasive breast cancer risk in women with sclerosing adenosis. Cancer 1989; 64: 1977–83.

39. Chen YB, Magpayo J, Rosen PP. Sclerosing adenosis in sentinel axillary lymph nodes from a patient with invasive ductal carcinoma: an unusual variant of benign glandular inclusions. Arch Pathol Lab Med 2008; 132: 1439–41.

40. Oberman HA, Markey BA. Noninvasive carcinoma of the breast presenting in adenosis. Mod Pathol 1991; 4: 31–5.

41. Fechner RE. Lobular carcinoma in situ in sclerosing adenosis. A potential confusion with invasive carcinoma. Am J Surg Pathol 1981; 5: 233–9.

42. Makunura CN, Curling OM, Yeomans P, et al. Apocrine adenosis within a radial scar: a case of false positive breast cytodiagnosis. Cytopathology 1994; 5: 123–8.

43. Simpson JF, Page DL, Dupont WD. Apocrine adenosis – a mimic of mammary carcinoma. Surg Pathol 1990; 3: 289–99.

44. Eusebi V, Casadei GP, Bussolati G, et al. Adenomyoepithelioma of the breast with a distinctive type of apocrine adenosis. Histopathology 1987; 11: 305–15.

45. Seidman JD, Ashton M, Lefkowitz M. Atypical apocrine adenosis of the breast: a clinicopathologic study of 37 patients with 8.7–year follow-up. Cancer 1996; 77: 2529–37.

46. Wells CA, McGregor IL, Makunura CN, et al. Apocrine adenosis: a precursor of aggressive cancer? J Clin Pathol 1995; 48: 737–42.

47. Selim AG, El-Ayat G. Wells CA. c-ErbB2 oncoprotein expression, gene amplification, and chromosome 17 aneusomy in apocrine adenosis of the breast. J Pathol 2000; 191: 138–42.

48. Carter DJ, Rosen PP. Atypical apocrine metaplasia in sclerosing lesions of the breast. A study of 51 patients. Mod Pathol 1991; 4: 1–5.

49. Linnell F, Ljungberg O, Anderssen I. Breast carcinoma: aspects of early stages, progression and related problems. Acta Pathol Scand 1980; 272(Suppl): 1–233.

50. Jacobs TW, Byrne C, Colditz G, et al. Radial scars in benign breast biopsy specimens and the risk of breast cancer. N Engl J Med 1999; 340: 430–6.

51. Andersen JA, Gram JB. Radial scar in the female breast. A long-term follow-up study of 32 cases. Cancer 1984; 53: 2557–60.

52. Sloane JP, Mayers MM. Carcinoma and atypical hyperplasia in radial scars and complex sclerosing lesions: importance of lesion size and patient age. Histopathology 1993; 23: 225–31.

53. Jacobs TW, Schnitt SJ, Tan X, Brown LF. Radial scars of the breast and breast carcinomas have similar alterations in expression of factors involved in vascular stroma formation. Hum Pathol 2002; 33: 29–38.

54. Rajan S, Wason AM, Carder PJ. Conservative management of screen detected radial scars: role of mammotome excision. J Clin Pathol 2011; 64: 65–8.

55. Brenner RJ, Jackman RJ, Parker SH, et al. Percutaneous core needle biopsy of radial scar of the breast: when is excision necessary? AJR Am J Roentgenol 2002; 179: 1179–84.

56. Haagensen CD, Stout AP, Phillips JS. The papillary neoplasms of the breast. I. Benign intraductal papilloma. Ann Surg 1951; 133: 18–36.

57. Page DL, Salhany KE, Jensen RA, Dupont WD. Subsequent breast carcinoma risk after biopsy with atypia in breast papilloma. Cancer 1996; 78: 258–66.

58. Mulligan AM, O'Malley FP. Papillary lesions of the breast: a review. Adv Anat Pathol 2007; 14: 108–19.

59. Raju U, Vertes D. Breast papillomas with atypical ductal hyperplasia: a clinicopathologic study. Hum Pathol 1996; 27: 1231–8.

60. Grin A, O'Malley FP, Mulligan AM. Cytokeratin 5 and estrogen receptor immunohistochemistry as a useful adjunct in identifying atypical papillary lesions of breast needle core biopsy. Am J Surg Pathol 2009; 33: 1615–23.

61. Muir R. The evolution of carcinoma of the mamma. J Pathol 1941; L11: 155–72.

62. Lewis JT, Hartmann LC, Vierkaut RA, et al. An analysis of breast cancer risk in women with single, multiple and atypical papilloma. Am J Surg Pathol 2006; 30: 665–72.

63. Collins LC, Schnitt SJ. Papillary lesions of the breast: selected diagnostic and management issues. Histopathology 2008; 52: 20–9.

64. Page DL, Rogers LW. Epithelial hyperplasia; Carcinoma in situ (CIS). In: Page DL, Anderson TJ, eds. Diagnostic Histopathology of the Breast. Edinburgh: Churchill Livingstone, 1987; 120–56: 157–92.

65. Boecker W, Moll R, Dervan P, et al. Usual ductal hyperplasia of the breast is a committed stem (progenitor) cell lesion distinct from atypical ductal hyperplasia and ductal carcinoma in situ. J Pathol 2002; 198: 458–67.

66. Fitzgibbons PL, Henson DE. Hutter RVP, for the Cancer Committee of the College of American Pathologists. Benign breast changes and the risk for subsequent breast cancer. An update of consensus statement. Arch Pathol Lab Med 1998; 122: 1053–5.

67. Azzopardi JG. Over diagnosis of malignancy. In: Azzopardi AG, ed. Problems in Breast Pathology. Philadelphia: WB Saunders, 1979: 167–91.

68. Page DL, Dupont WD, Rogers LW, Rados MS. Atypical hyperplastic lesions of the female breast: a long term follow-up study. Cancer 1985; 55: 2698–708.

69. Page DL, Rogers LW. Combined histologic and cytologic criteria for the diagnosis of mammary atypical ductal hyperplasia. Hum Pathol 1992; 23: 1095–7.

70. National Coordinating Group for Breast Screening Pathology. Pathology Reporting in Breast Cancer Screening. NHSBSP Publication 3, 2nd edn. Sheffield: NHS Breast Screening Programme, 1997.

71. Rosai J. Borderline epithelial lesions of the breast. Am J Surg Pathol 1991; 15: 209–21.

72. Owings DV, Hann L, Schnitt S. How thoroughly should needle localization breast biopsies be sampled for microscopic examination? Am J Surg Pathol 1990; 14: 578–85.

73. Page DL, Dupont WD. Indicators of increased breast cancer risk in humans. J Cell Biochem 1992; 16G (Suppl): 175–82.

74. Wells CA, El-Ayat GA. Non-operative breast pathology: apocrine lesions. J Clin Pathol 2007; 60: 1313–20.

75. O'Malley F, Bane A. The spectrum of apocrine lesions of the breast. Adv Anat Pathol 2004; 11: 1–9.

76. Page DL, Dupont WD, Jensen RA. Papillary apocrine change of the breast: associations with atypical hyperplasia and risk of breast cancer. Cancer Epidemiol Biomarkers Prev 1996; 5: 29–32.

77. Haagensen CD, Lane N, Lattes R, Bodian C. Lobular neoplasia (so-called lobular carcinoma in situ) of the breast. Cancer 1978; 42: 737–69.

78. Fulford LG, Reis-Filho JS, Lakhani SR. Lobular in situ neoplasia. Curr Diagn Pathol 2004; 10: 183–92.

79. Rosen PP. Lobular carcinoma in situ and atypical lobular hyperplasia: In: Rosen's Breast Pathology. Philadelphia: Lippincott Williams and Williams, 2009: 537–679.

80. Foote FW Jr, Stewart FW. Lobular carcinoma in situ. A rare form of mammary cancer. Am J Pathol 1941; 27: 491–5.

81. Vos CB, Cleton-Jones AM, Berx G, et al. E-cadherin in-activation in lobular carcinoma in situ of the breast: an early event in tumour genesis. Br J Cancer 1997; 76: 1131–3.

82. Reis-Filho JS, Lakhani SR. The diagnosis and management of pre-invasive breast disease: genetic alterations in pre-invasive lesions. Breast Cancer Res 2003; 5: 313–19.

83. Bur ME, Zimarowski MJ, Schnitt SL, et al. Estrogen receptor immunohistochemistry in carcinoma in situ of the breast. Cancer 1992; 69: 1174–81.

84. Raramachandra S, Machin L, Ashley S, et al. Immunohistochemical distribution of c-erbB-2 in in situ breast carcinoma- A detailed morphological analysis. J Pathol 1990; 161: 7–14.

85. Middleton LP, Palacios DM, Bryant BR, et al. Pleomorphic lobular carcinoma: morphology, immunohistochemistry and molecular analysis. Am J Surg Pathol 2002; 24: 1650–6.

86. Chen YY, Hwang ES, Roy R, et al. Genetic and phenotypic characteristics of pleomorphic lobular carcinoma in situ of the breast. Am J Surg Pathol 2009; 33: 1683–94.

87. Haagensen CD, Lane N, Lattes R. Neoplastic preoliferation of the epithelium of mammary lobules: Adenosis, lobular neoplasia and small cell carcinoma. Surg Clin North Am 1972; 52: 497–524.

88. Rosen PP, Senie R, Ashikari R, et al. Age, menstrual status and exogenous hormone usage in patients with lobular carcinoma in situ (LCIS). Surgery 1979; 85: 219–24.

89. Rosen PP, Lieberman PH, Braun DW, et al. Lobular carcinoma in situ of the breast. Detailed analysis of 99 patients with average follow-up of 24 years. Am J Surg Pathol 1978; 2: 225–51.

90. Urban JA. Biopsy of the 'normal' breast in treating breast cancer. Surg Clin North Am 1969; 49: 291–301.

91. Page DL, Kidd TE, Dupont WD, et al. Lobular neoplasia of the breast: higher risk for subsequent invasive cancer predicted by more extensive disease. Hum Pathol 1991; 22: 1232–9.

92. Page DL, Steel CM, Dixon JM. Carcinoma in situ and patients at high risk of breast cancer. BMJ 1995; 310: 39–42.

93. Newman W. Lobular carcinoma of the female breast. Report of 73 cases. Ann Surg 1966; 164: 305–14.

94. Page DL, Dupont WD, Rogers LW. Ductal involvement by cells of atypical lobular hyperplasia in the breast: a long-term follow-up study of cancer risk. Hum Pathol 1988; 19: 201–7.

95. Fisher B, Constantino JP, Wickerham DL, et al. Tamoxifen for prevention of breast cancer: report of the National Surgical Adjuvant Breast and Bowel Project P-1 Study. J Natl Cancer Inst 1998; 90: 1371–88.

96. Broders AC. Carcinoma in situ contrasted with benign penetrating epithelium. JAMA 1932; 99: 1670–4.

97. Rosner D, Bedwani RN, Vana J, et al. Non-invasive breast carcinoma Results of a national survey of the American College of Surgeons. Ann Surg 1980; 192: 139–47.

98. Lagios MD, Margolin FR, Westdahl PR, Rose MR. Mammographically detected duct carcinoma in situ. Frequency of local recurrence following tylectomy and prognostic effect of nuclear grade on local recurrence. Cancer 1989; 63: 618–24.

99. Patchefsky AS, Schwartz GF, Finkelstein SD, et al. Heterogeneity of intraductal carcinoma of the breast. Cancer 1989; 63: 731–41.

100. Silverstein MJ, Waisman JR, Gamagami P, et al. Intraductal carcinoma of the breast (208 cases): Clinical factors influencing treatment choice. Cancer 1990; 66: 102–8.

101. Ciatto S, Cataliotti L, Distante V. Nonpalpable lesions detected with mammography: review of 512 consecutive cases. Radiology 1987; 165: 99–102.

102. Stomper PC, Connolly JL, Meyer JE, et al. Clinically occult ductal carcinoma in situ detected with mammography: analysis of 100 cases with radiologic-pathologic correlation. Radiology 1989; 172: 235–41.

103. Menell JH, Morris EA, Dershaw DD, et al. Determination of the presence and extent of pure ductal carcinoma in situ by mammography and magnetic resonance imaging. Breast J 2005; 11: 382–90.

104. Pediconi F, Catalano C, Roselli A, et al. Contrast-enhanced MR mammography for evaluation of the contralateral breast in patients with diagnosed unilateral breast cancer or high risk lesions. Radiology 2007; 243: 670–80.

105. Holland R, Pertese JL, Millis RR, et al. Ductal carcinoma in situ: a proposal for a new classification. Semin Diagn Pathol 1994; 11: 167–80.

106. Pathology Reporting of Breast Disease. NHSBSP and RCPath. A Joint Document Incorporating the Third Edition of the NHS Breast Screening Programme's Guidelines for Pathology Reporting in Breast Cancer Screening and the Second Edition of The Royal College of Pathologists' Minimum Dataset for Breast Cancer Histopathology. NHSBSP Publication No. 58, 2005.

107. Silverstein MJ. The University of Southern California/Van Nuys prognostic index for ductal carcinoma in situ of the breast. Am J Surg 2003; 186: 337–43.

108. Betsill WL Jr, Rosen PP, Lieberman PH, Robbins GF. Intraduct carcinoma. Long term follow-up after treatment by biopsy alone. JAMA 1978; 239: 1863–7.

109. Carter D, Orr SL, Merino MJ. Intracystic papillary carcinoma of the breast: after mastectomy, radiotherapy or excisional biopsy alone. Cancer 1983; 52: 14–19.

110. Tsuda H, Uei Y, Fukutomi T, Hiroshoshi S. Different incidence of loss of heterozygosity on chromosome 16q between intraductal papilloma and intracystic papillary carcinoma of the breast. Jpn J Cancer Res 1994; 85: 992–6.

111. Page DL, Dupont WD, Rogers LW, et al. Inrtaductal carcinoma of the breast: Follow-up after biopsy only. Cancer 1982; 49: 751–8.

112. Page DL, Dupont WD, Rogers LW, et al. Continued local recurrence of carcinoma 15-25 years after a diagnosis of low grade ductal carcinoma in situ of the breast treated only with biopsy. Cancer 1995; 76: 1197–200.

113. Collins LC, Tamimi RM, Baer HJ, et al. Outcome of patients with ductal carcinoma in situ untreated after diagnostic biopsy: results from the Nurses' Health Study. Cancer 2005; 103: 1778–84.

114. MacDonald HR, Silverstein MJ, Mabry H, et al. Local control in ductal carcinoma in situ treated by excision alone: Incremental benefit of larger margins. Am J Surg 2005; 190: 521–5.

115. Wong JS, Kaelin CM, Troyan SL, et al. Prospective study of wide excision alone for ductal carcinoma in situ of the breast. J Clin Oncol 2006; 24: 1031–6.

116. Fisher B, Land S, Mamounas E, et al. Prevention of invasive breast cancer in women with ductal carcinoma in situ: An update of the national surgical adjuvant breast and bowel project experience. Semin Oncol 2001; 28: 400–18.

117. Boyages J, Delaney G, Taylor R. Predictors of local recurrence after treatment of ductal carcinoma in situ: a meta-analysis. Cancer 1999; 85: 616–28.

118. deMascarel I, MacGrogan G, Mathoulin-Pelissier S, et al. Breast ductal carcinoma in situ with microinvasion. A definition supported by a long-term study of 1248 serially sectioned ductal carcinomas. Cancer 2002; 94: 2134–42.

119. Walker RA, Dearing SJ, Brown LA. Comparison of pathological and biological features of symptomatic and mammographically detected ductal carcinoma in situ of the breast. Hum Pathol 1999; 30: 943–8.

120. Katz A, Gage I, Envans S, et al. Sentinel lymph node positivity of patients with ductal carcinoma in situ or microinvasive breast cancer. Am J Surg 2006; 191: 761–6.

121. Huo I, Resetkova A, Lopez A, et al. Sentinel lymph node (SLN) sampling in patients with core biopsy diagnosis of ductal carcinoma in situ (DCIS): UT M.D Anderson Cancer Center experience and future recommendations. Mod Pathol 2006; 19: 30 A.

122. Imamate T, Ikawa S, Akiyama T, et al. Similarity of protein encoded by the human c-erbB2 gene to epidermal growth factor receptor. Nature 1986; 319: 230–4.

123. Dykins R, Corbett IP, Henry JA, et al. Long term survival in breast cancer related to overexpression of c-erbB2 oncoprotein: an immunohistochemical study using monoclonal antibody NCL-CB11. J Pathol 1991; 163: 105–10.

124. Bobrow LG, Happerfield LC, Gregory WM, et al. The classification of ductal carcinoma in situ and its association with biological markers. Semin Diagn Pathol 1994; 11: 199–207.

125. Poller DN, Sneak DRJ, Roberts EC, et al. Oestrogen receptor expression in ductal carcinoma in situ of the breast: relationship to flow cytometric analysis of DNA and expression of the c-erbB2 oncoprotein. Br J Cancer 1993; 68: 156–61.

126. Zafrani B, Leroyer A, Fourquet A, et al. Mammographically-detected ductal in situ carcinoma of the breast analysed with a new classification. A study of 127 cases: correlation with oestrogen and progesterone receptors, p53 and c-erbB2 proteins and proliferation activity. Semin Diagn Pathol 1994; 11: 208–14.

127. Harris AL. Mutant p53: the commonest genetic abnormality in human cancer? J Pathol 1990; 162: 5–6.

128. Isobe M, Emmanuel BS, Giro D, et al. Localization of gene for human p53 tumour antigen to band 17p13. Nature 1986; 320: 84–96.

129. Walker RA, Daring SJ, Lane DT, Valley JM. Expression of p53 in infiltrating and in-situ breast carcinomas. J Pathol 1991; 165: 203–11.

130. Buerger H, Otterbach F, Simon R, et al. Comparative genomic hydridisation of ductal carcinoma in-situ of the breast – evidence of multiple genetic pathway. J Pathol 1999; 187: 398–402.

131. Abdel-Fatah TMA, Powe DG, Hodi Z, et al. High frequency of coexistence of columnar cell lesions, lobular neoplasia and low grade ductal carcinoma in situ with invasive tubular carcinoma and invasive lobular carcinoma. Am J Surg Pathol 2007; 13: 417–26.

132. Vincent-Salomon A, Lucchesi C, Gruel N, et al. Intergrated genomic and transcriptomic analysis of ductal carcinoma in situ of the breast. Clin Cancer Res 2008; 14: 1956–65.

133. Simpson PT, Reis-Filho JS, Gale T, et al. Molecular evolution of breast cancer. J Pathol 2005; 205: 248–54.

134. Lopez-Garcia MA, Geyer FC, Lacroix-Triki M, et al. Breast cancer presursors revisited: molecular features and progression pathways. Histopathology 2010; 57: 171–92.

135. Gong G, DeVries S, Chew KL, et al. Genetic changes in paired atypical and usual ductal hyperplasia of the breast by comparative genomic hybridization. Clin Cancer Res 2001; 7: 2410–14.

136. Etzell JE, DeVries S, Chew K, et al. Loss of chromosome 16q in lobular carcinoma in situ. Hum Pathol 2001; 32: 292–6.

137. Vargas AC, Lakhani SR, Simpson PT. Pleomorphic lobular carcinoma of the breast: molecular pathology and clinical impact. Future Oncol 2009; 5: 233–43.

28 Invasive breast carcinoma

Elena Provenzano

INTRODUCTION

Together with clinical examination and radiological investigation, histopathology is a cornerstone of triple assessment of breast lesions and the histopathologist is a key member of the multidisciplinary team. Although there have been improvements in breast cancer mortality relating to earlier detection through screening and advancements in treatment, breast cancer remains the number one cause of cancer death among women. The development of high-throughput molecular techniques such as gene expression arrays and next-generation sequencing has resulted in an exponential increase in our understanding of breast cancer and the biological pathways that drive its growth and development. It is now accepted that breast cancer is not one disease for which there is a single treatment but a group of diseases with different underlying biological mechanisms. This is reflected in the diversity of histological subtypes, many of which are associated with distinct molecular profiles and clinical behavior (1,2).

The histological reporting of breast cancer has evolved with the introduction of minimum datasets and synoptic reports, reflecting increased knowledge of the disease and the sophistication of surgical and oncological management. These developments ensure that relevant information needed by clinicians to inform the patient of their prognosis and determine the optimum clinical management is clearly and concisely presented (3,4). These essential data include information on invasive cancer size, grade, and type, the presence and extent of an *in situ* component, the presence of lymphovascular space invasion, proximity to margins, and hormone receptor and HER2 status. This chapter focuses on the different histological subtypes of breast cancer, their clinical significance, and where relevant cognate molecular characteristics. Other prognostic factors are discussed in more detail in chapter 26, and the molecular biology of breast cancer is discussed in greater depth in chapter 29.

The mode of presentation of breast cancer has changed with increasing numbers of small impalpable screen-detected lesions. Pathological workup requires a multidisciplinary team approach and relevant clinical and radiological information must accompany the surgical specimen to ensure accurate interpretation of results.

SPECIMEN HANDLING
Core Biopsies

Core biopsies (including large bore vacuum-assisted biopsies for microcalcification) have become the mainstay for preoperative diagnosis of breast lesions (Fig. 28.1). The sensitivity and specificity of core biopsy are superior to fine needle aspiration cytology; so it is the preferred diagnostic modality for screen-detected lesions (5). Additional information such as provisional tumor grade and hormone receptor and HER2 status can be obtained on core biopsy specimens allowing appropriate decisions to be made regarding neoadjuvant therapy, for which core biopsy may be the only tumor sample in the event of a complete pathological response (6).

Core biopsy specimens should be placed in formalin as soon as possible to optimize fixation. In those cases of biopsies taken for microcalcification it is helpful to identify the cores containing calcium by placing them in either a microcassette or a separate pot, in order that the pathologist knows which cores to focus attention on and performs additional levels. The pathologist should have access to the specimen X-ray, either electronically or as films; this will allow correlation between the radiological appearance (extent of the calcium) and the microscopic findings to ensure a correct diagnosis is made.

The pathologist or biomedical scientist handling the specimen should record the number of cores, their length, and appearance. An initial H&E stained slide is prepared taking care not to cut too far into the block. If no cancer is present, additional levels are often indicated to ensure the tissue has been examined thoroughly and the lesion has not been missed. This is especially true for large volume biopsies taken for microcalcification, where up to three sets of levels may need to be performed before the calcification is identified (7).

Within most national breast screening programs such as the National Health Service Breast Screening Programme (NHSBSP), there are strict guidelines for the reporting of core biopsies which together with multidisciplinary discussion ensure optimal patient management and follow-up (4). The NHSBSP recommends the use of a reporting protocol with categories B1–B5 (Table 28.1).

Diagnostic and Wide Local Excision Specimens

Accurate pathological assessment of surgical specimens requires correlation with clinical and radiological information. This is especially important in the case of microcalcification or small impalpable screen-detected masses where the lesion may not be macroscopically detectable, and in the neoadjuvant setting where there may be no residual lesion left for the pathologist to identify. Multidisciplinary cooperation is vital at every stage of the diagnostic process and continues when the specimen leaves theater and arrives on the pathologist's bench. For wide local excision (WLE) specimens correct orientation and careful handling of specimens are essential for accurate histological interpretation, especially of margins. Following wire localization, the specimen X-ray should be available to the pathologist, either electronically or as a film accompanying the specimen. This is critical for meticulous sampling of diagnostic excisions performed for microcalcification. The findings on the specimen X-ray should be included as part of the macroscopic description of the specimen (Fig. 28.2).

The surgical specimen should be weighed, measured in three dimensions, and the presence of any clips or sutures for orientation of the specimen documented. Standard orientation markings differ between individuals and institutions, although ideally a single protocol should be agreed within each unit to avoid errors. Any deviation from the standard protocol should be recorded on the request slip. Examples include a short suture superiorly and long laterally, or a short superior, double anteriorly and single long suture laterally (Fig. 28.3). An advantage of the latter method is that laterality can be confirmed by the localisation of the sutures. In cases of ductal carcinoma *in situ* (DCIS), marking of the nipple margin is also recommended as DCIS often grows along a single ductal unit toward and away from the nipple (Fig. 28.4). The external surface of the specimen is then inked according to the departmental protocol, often with different margins in different colored inks so they can be distinguished microscopically (Fig. 28.5). The margins can be assessed either as transverse sections or shave sections, depending upon unit protocols and pathologist preference (8).

For standard surgical techniques, the resection extends from the subcutis anteriorly to the pectoralis fascia on the deep aspect (Fig. 28.6). As a result, the anterior and posterior margins are

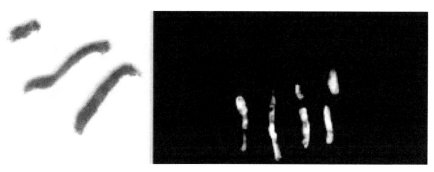

Figure 28.1 Core biopsy. Radiography is necessary for cases of microcalcification. Multiple levels may be needed for full assessment.

Table 28.1 NHS Breast Screening Programme reporting categories

B1	Normal breast tissue/or sample not representative
B2	Benign breast lesion
B3	Lesion of uncertain malignant potential. This includes atypical ductal hyperplasia, atypical lobular hyperplasia, phylloides tumour, papillary lesions, radial scar and complex sclerosing lesion
B4	Suspicious of malignancy. This includes crushed or poorly fixed cores that contain probable carcinoma but cannot provide the definitive diagnosis, neoplastic cells within blood clot outside the tissue of the core biopsy, and tiny areas of carcinoma that disappear on deeper levels for immunohistochemistry
B5	Malignant
	B5a Ductal carcinoma in situ (DCIS)
	B5b Invasive carcinoma
	B5c Carcinoma with no further assessment possible

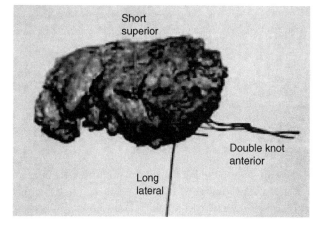

Figure 28.3 Orientation of the specimen by the surgeon with placement of three sutures: short superior, long lateral, and double knot anterior.

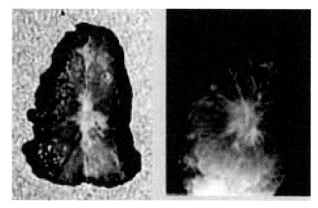

Figure 28.2 A wide local excision specimen for screen-detected cancer showing a central stellate tumor corresponding to the lesion on the accompanying X-ray.

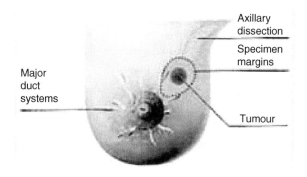

Figure 28.4 Schematic anterior view of the breast to show an excision in the upper outer quadrant. A DCIS component will grow along the duct system toward the nipple, so it is of benefit to indicate the nipple margin along with other orienting sutures to guide pathology sampling.

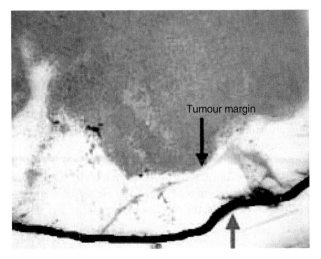

Figure 28.5 Inked excision margin enabling measurement of distance of tumor from the resection margin.

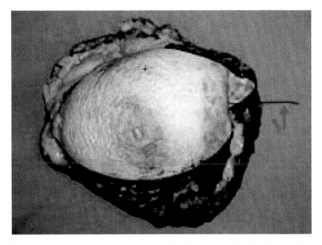

Figure 28.7 A mastectomy specimen with a long suture indicating the lateral aspect.

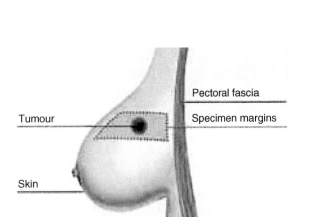

Figure 28.6 A schematic lateral view of the breast to show surgical margins in a segmental excision, which extends from the skin anteriorly to the pectoral fascia posteriorly.

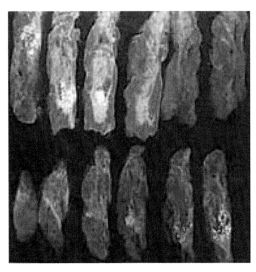

Figure 28.8 X-ray of slices of a mastectomy specimen revealing the site of microcalcifications, allowing accurate sampling of the relevant areas.

less relevant than the radial margins as no further tissue can be taken from these margins. Any deviation from this surgical practice should be recorded on the request slip.

There are three main methods for handling WLE specimens; the specimen can be sliced sagitally (medial to lateral), coronally (anterior to posterior), or in a cruciate manner. Each of these different approaches has advantages and disadvantages, and the method chosen depends on the size of the specimen, nature of the lesion, and pathologist preference (8). Requirements for the minimum dataset, particularly lesion size and margin status, must be borne in mind when handling a WLE specimen. In particular, all radial margins should be sampled even if macroscopically clear of tumor.

Resection Margin Specimens

These "cavity shavings" may be either substantial pieces of tissue taken for close margins on specimen radiology or previous surgical excision, or routine small bed biopsies taken at the time of primary surgery. The specimen is weighed and measured in three dimensions. It is important that the new outer excision margin is indicated, for example by a suture on the cavity surface, so the pathologist can orient the specimen and assess the distance of DCIS or invasive carcinoma from the new resection margin.

Mastectomy Specimens

Mastectomy specimens should be labeled and oriented according to unit protocol, for example by a suture superiorly or on the axillary tail of the specimen, and ideally with an accompanying specimen diagram indicating the site of the tumor or previous surgery as appropriate (Fig. 28.7). The specimen should be sent to the pathology department as soon as possible to allow slicing of the specimen for optimal fixation. If this is not possible, the specimen should be placed in an appropriately sized bucket with an adequate volume of formalin (at least twice the volume of the specimen). The specimen is weighed and measured in three dimensions, with a measurement of any overlying skin ellipse and description of the nipple. In nipple-sparing mastectomy, the site of the nipple must be identified by a suture to allow inking and assessment of the nipple margin.

The most popular method of handling a mastectomy specimen is to place it skin surface down, and create serial vertical slices approximately 1 cm apart. Any macroscopic lesions are clearly documented, measured in three dimensions and their location within the breast noted for purposes of correlation with imaging. In cases where there is no macroscopic lesion, such as DCIS with extensive microcalcifications, the specimen slices can be x-rayed to identify those areas to be sampled (Fig. 28.8).

Axillary Clearance

Axillary clearance specimens can be submitted as a whole with a suture marking the apex, or as individual levels. The apical lymph node may sometimes be submitted separately. The specimen is measured in three dimensions, and fat is carefully dissected off to allow identification of the lymph nodes. The yield of lymph nodes varies greatly between patients, although a minimum of at least 10 nodes should be present for accurate staging (9). All lymph nodes should be sliced at 3 mm intervals and submitted. The final pathology report should state the total number of lymph nodes retrieved and the number containing metastases. The size of the largest metastasis should be carefully recorded, indicating whether this is a micro- or a macrometastasis which impacts on TNM staging (10).

Sentinel Lymph Node Biopsy

The sentinel lymph nodes (SLNs) should be dissected from the specimen and the presence or absence of blue dye documented. SLNs are examined more thoroughly than is standard procedure for nodes in an axillary clearance specimen which minimizes the chance of false-negative results. The minimal lesion that must be identified is a macrometastasis, defined as a deposit >2 mm in size. To avoid missing any macrometastases, the recommendation is for all submitted nodes to be sliced at 2 mm intervals and embedded in their entirety (11). There is much variation in the handling of SLNs between units, with some performing additional step levels and/ or immunohistochemistry in an attempt to identify smaller deposits such as micrometastases (0.2–2 mm) or isolated tumor cells (<0.2 mm). The clinical significance of these smaller metastatic deposits remains uncertain. A subanalysis of the NSABP B-32 trial investigated the clinical significance of occult metastatic disease identified by further levels and immunohistochemistry. There was only a small difference in overall survival at 5 years (94.6% with vs. 95.8% without), suggesting that there is negligible clinical benefit from more intensive examination of originally negative SLNs (12).

Intraoperative assessment can be undertaken by frozen section or imprint cytology, with sensitivity of 76% and 62% respectively (13). Newer molecular techniques such as polymerase chain reaction (PCR) are gaining wider acceptance, with reports of high sensitivity and specificity. When alternate slices of the node are submitted for PCR and routine histological assessment, concordance rates are 93% (14). To optimize the technique, the whole node needs to be submitted for PCR. However, this leaves no material for histological assessment which may reveal other diagnoses such as lymphoma or infection. This will also preclude determination of hormone receptor and HER2 status where the nodal metastasis is the only tumor material available such as post-neoadjuvant therapy or the rare case of DCIS with nodal deposits.

HISTOLOGICAL SUBTYPES

Invasive Carcinoma of No Special Type

Definition

This is the most common type of infiltrating breast carcinoma, and accounts for up to 75% of all cancers (15). With invasive carcinoma of no special type (NST), the tumor lacks histological features associated with any of the special types of cancer described in the ensuing sections. These special type features must be present in over 50% of the lesion, and therefore invasive carcinoma (NST) is a diagnosis of exclusion. If more than 50% of the tumor has a specialized pattern, and 10–50% of the remainder is NST, the tumor is classified as mixed NST and special type or mixed NST and lobular.

NST invasive cancers are also referred to as invasive ductal carcinoma, which relates to the historical concept that these cancers arose from the ductal epithelium, in contrast to lobular cancers that arose within the lobules. It is now known that the site of origin of most breast cancers is the terminal duct lobular unit (16), which is where the mammary progenitor cells are believed to reside (17). For this reason, the NHSBSP guidelines recommend the use of the term invasive carcinoma NST rather than invasive ductal carcinoma (3).

Macroscopic Features

These cancers have no specific macroscopic features, but most commonly appear as moderately circumscribed firm gray-white masses with a stellate or rounded outline. In some cases they are indistinct, especially if the background breast tissue is very fibrous and often have a gritty cut surface, (resembling an "unripe pear"). The degree of firmness relates to the amount of fibrous stroma associated with the cancer which also confers the classical radiological appearance of a stellate lesion. Tumors with a relatively little stromal reaction may be soft and well circumscribed, thereby mimicking a benign lesion.

Microscopic Features

Invasive carcinoma NST is a heterogeneous group of cancers composed of tumor cells variably arranged in glandular structures, clusters, and trabeculae set within a fibrous stroma. Nonetheless, some high-grade lesions comprise solid sheets of cells (Fig. 28.9). In some tumors, glandular differentiation with tubule formation and the presence of lumina within cell groups may be present, the proportion of which provides one component of cancer grade (Fig. 28.10). Single-file infiltration may also be seen, but cells lack the typical cytology of lobular carcinomas, and other areas with more typical growth patterns such as nests and islands are commonly present, which provides a clue to a correct diagnosis of invasive carcinoma (NST).

Carcinomatous cells also show a great deal of variation between tumors, which is principally dependent upon the lesion grade. In low-grade cancers the cells may be small

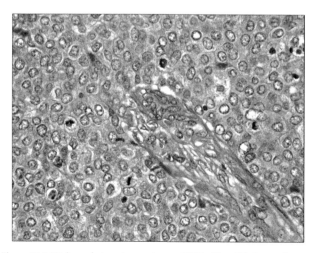

Figure 28.9 High-grade invasive carcinoma NST with solid sheets of tumor cells showing marked nuclear atypia and frequent mitoses.

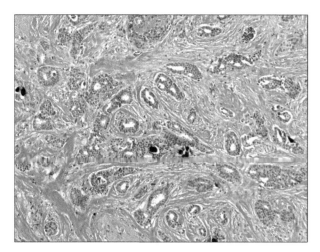

Figure 28.10 Invasive carcinoma NST with prominent tubule formation and occasional solid nests. The tumor cells show mild nuclear pleomorphism in keeping with low-grade carcinoma.

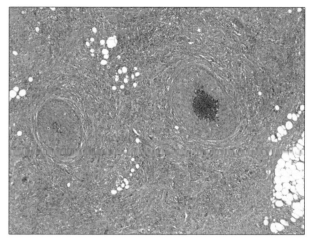

Figure 28.11 Invasive carcinoma NST with associated high-grade DCIS with central necrosis.

with a moderate amount of cytoplasm, regular round nuclei, and few mitotic figures, while high-grade tumors may comprise cells with abundant eosinophilic cytoplasm, highly pleomorphic nuclei with prominent nucleoli and frequent mitoses.

NST cancers are typically associated with a fibrous and/or elastotic stromal background, which can be either highly cellular and desmoplastic in nature or less cellular and hyalinized. The stromal component can be highly variable with some tumors having a large central zone of fibrosis with a more cellular periphery, and others having only a scant connective tissue framework. Areas of necrosis may also be present in some high-grade cancers, while other tumors may be associated with a prominent lymphoplasmacytic inflammatory infiltrate.

An associated component of DCIS may be present in up to 80% of cases (15). The grade of DCIS usually reflects that of the invasive cancer with low-grade lesions associated with low-grade DCIS and high-grade lesions having high-grade DCIS (18). The DCIS component may be confined to the invasive tumor, or extend beyond into the surrounding breast tissue (Fig. 28.11). In the latter situation the entire lesion size including DCIS must be recorded as well as the size of the invasive component. Furthermore, the distance of DCIS to excision margins must be measured (3). Microcalcification may be present within the DCIS and occasionally within the invasive component.

Immunohistochemistry
Invasive carcinomas NST typically show-positive membrane staining for E-cadherin, which can be useful in those cases where distinction from invasive lobular carcinoma (ILC) is difficult (19). However, some NST cancers are E-cadherin negative and conversely a small percentage of lobular cancers are E-cadherin positive (see the section "Invasive Lobular Carcinoma"); therefore, results must be interpreted in the context of overall histology of the tumor; cancers should not be classified on the basis of E-cadherin staining alone. E-cadherin-negative NST cancers tend to be of higher grade and are unlikely to be morphologically mistaken for lobular carcinomas (20).

Approximately 70–80% of NST cancers are estrogen receptor positive (21,22), and in population-based series around 10–20% are HER2 positive (21,23). Low-grade NST cancers tend to be of luminal subtype and are typically ER positive and HER2 negative, while high-grade cancers are more likely to be negative for ER and to be HER2 positive.

Prognosis
NST cancers constitute a heterogeneous group of tumors at both molecular and morphological levels, with variation in grade, morphology, hormone receptor, and HER2 status reflecting differences in gene expression profiles (24–26). Prognosis is influenced by factors such as grade, size, lymph node status, and the presence or absence of lymphovascular invasion, with grade and nodal involvement being the most important determinants of outcome (26,27). ER and HER2 status are major predictive factors in determining the benefit from adjuvant hormonal and chemotherapy and also have a prognostic value. Molecular studies have highlighted the degrees of heterogeneity among NST tumors at the genetic level, which has led to novel classification systems. These subclassify NST tumors into groups with distinct clinicopathological behavior and are discussed further in chapter 29 (24). The more traditional prognostic factors mentioned earlier are discussed in detail in chapter 26.

Invasive Lobular Carcinoma
Definition
This is a type of invasive carcinoma which in the classical form has a distinctive growth pattern with dyscohesive regular round cells forming single-file and targetoid arrangements around existing structures. ILC is the second most common type of invasive tumor, accounting for 5–15% of all breast cancers (15,28,29). Lobular cancers often grow around existing structures inciting minimal stromal reaction. Hence they often present clinically as ill-defined masses and radiologically may be occult or appear as an area of asymmetric stromal density. Their extent is often underestimated radiologically, and MRI is emerging as a more accurate means of determining preoperative size and detecting multifocal disease (30,31). ILC is more likely to be multifocal, and bilateral disease has been reported in 20–30% of cases (32).

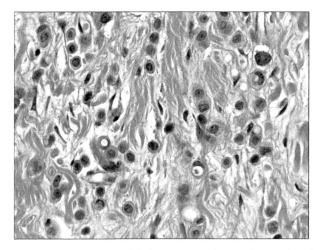

Figure 28.12 Classical invasive lobular carcinoma showing the typical single-file growth pattern. Several tumor cells have cytoplasmic mucin vacuoles.

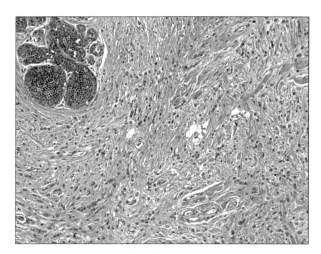

Figure 28.13 Classical invasive lobular carcinoma with associated LCIS (top left corner).

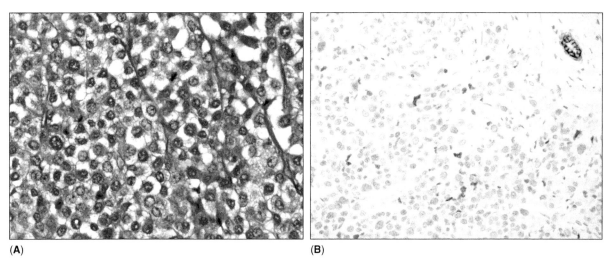

(A)   (B)

Figure 28.14 Pleomorphic invasive lobular carcinoma. The tumor cells show marked nuclear atypia with frequent mitoses (A). The cells are forming solid sheets, but have a dyscohesive pattern. The tumor cells are negative for E-cadherin (positive normal gland in the top right corner) (B).

Macroscopic Appearance

The macroscopic features of ILC are variable, with some appearing as a firm stellate white-gray lesion similar to an NST cancer, although these lobular subtypes often have an ill-defined edge. In other cases there may be no macroscopically visible lesion, with the tumor being detected as a vague area of firmness on palpation. As for radiological assessment, tumor size may turn out to be significantly greater than expected based on the macroscopic assessment.

Microscopic Appearance

Several Variants of ILC

ILC has several variants. The commonest of them is the classical variant which is composed of a proliferation of small cells with moderate amounts of esinophilic cytoplasm and regular round nuclei which may be eccentrically placed (Fig. 28.12). The cells may have intracytoplasmic lumina with central mucin, sometimes resulting in a signet-ring appearance. These cells infiltrate throughout the breast parenchyma with little stromal reaction and grow as single files or linear cords. Moreover, rather than displacing pre-existing breast elements, classical lobular tumors form concentric rings around them giving a characteristic targetoid appearance. Alternatively, the cells

may have pale foamy cytoplasm and resemble histiocytes which can be a potential trap for the unwary pathologist. Mitotic figures are rare. Up to 90% of cases are associated with LCIS (Fig. 28.13) (15,28).

The solid and alveolar variants are formed by morphologically similar cells with dyscohesive growth which forms solid sheets in the solid variant and small globular aggregates of cells in the alveolar variant. The tumor cells in these variants may show extensive nuclear atypia with more frequent mitoses.

The pleomorphic variant has a typical lobular growth pattern with dyscohesive cells growing as single files and alveolar aggregates, but these cells show severe nuclear atypia with enlarged nuclei and prominent nucleoli and often have abundant eosinophilic cytoplasm yielding an apocrine appearance (Fig. 28.14). Pleomorphic ILC is commonly associated with the pleomorphic variant of LCIS, and is a biologically more aggressive tumor (33).

The final variant of ILC is tubulo-lobular carcinoma. As its name implies this is composed of a combination of tubular structures associated with small uniform cells arranged in single files. Tubulo-lobular carcinomas have a prognosis intermediate between that of tubular carcinomas and classical lobular carcinomas, and there is some debate as to whether they should be

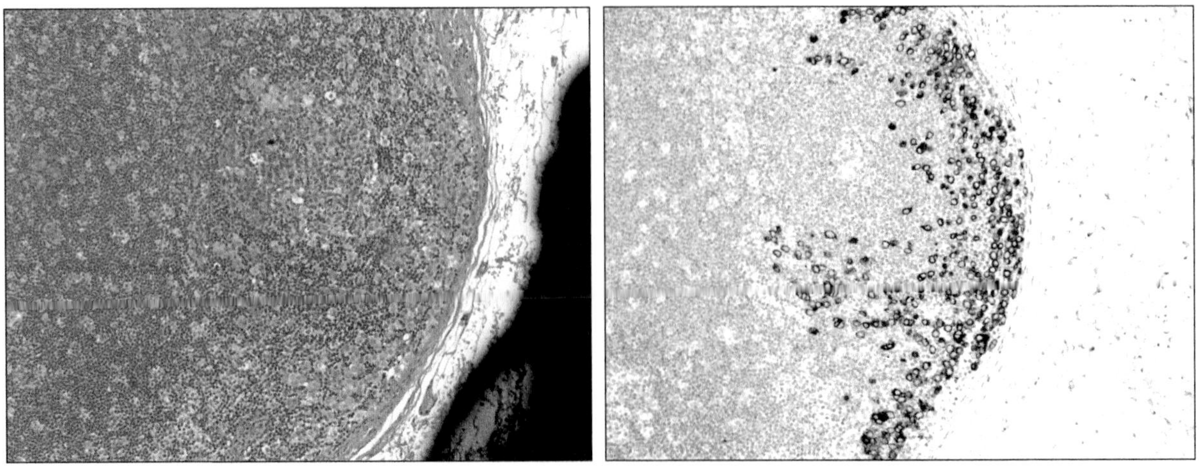

(A) (B)

Figure 28.15 Sinusoidal pattern of lymph node involvement by metastatic lobular carcinoma. The tumor cells are difficult to see on H&E staining (**A**), but show up with immunohistochemical staining for CK AE1/AE3 (**B**).

more appropriately classified with the former rather than in the lobular subgroup. On immunohistochemistry, they show positive membrane staining for E-cadherin which will support their exclusion from the lobular family of cancers (34,35).

Immunohistochemistry and Molecular Features

Invasive lobular carcinomas share many genetic changes with low-grade NST cancers, notably 16q losses and 1q gains and indeed both are believed to belong to a common low-grade neoplasia pathway (36,37). The characteristic feature of ILC is loss of function of E-cadherin, a protein involved in cell-to-cell adhesion and maintenance of cell differentiation (38). There is loss of E-cadherin expression in the majority of cases of ILC, but up to 26% of phenotypically lobular cancers may show aberrant positive staining (39–41). These lobular cancers show cytoplasmic rather than membrane localization for other members of the catenin complex such as p120. The latter is a protein which is functionally related to E-cadherin, thereby indicating disruption of cadherin–catenin complexes despite the presence of E-cadherin positivity. It is this loss of cell adhesion that gives ILC its dyscohesive appearance and typical growth pattern.

Almost all classical ILCs are of luminal type, being ER positive and HER2 negative with a low Ki-67 labeling index (32,38,42). The alveolar and solid variants are also typically ER positive (43), but pleomorphic ILC is ER negative in up to 23% of cases and HER2 positive in 14% of cases (44). The pleomorphic variant is often positive for GCDFP15, which accords with its apocrine appearance and usually has high Ki-67 labeling index (42,45). Pleomorphic ILC can belong to luminal B, HER2, or molecular apocrine genetic subtypes (2).

Prognosis

Some authors have reported a slightly better prognosis for ILC than NST cancers, while others have found similar or worse outcomes when matched for disease stage and patient age (29,32,46). The classical subtype of ILC has a more favorable prognosis than the solid or alveolar variants, with invasive pleomorphic ILC having the worst prognosis (43,45). A lower frequency of axillary metastases has been reported compared with NST cancers, although nodal involvement for ILC may be pathologically subtle with a sinusoidal pattern or isolated

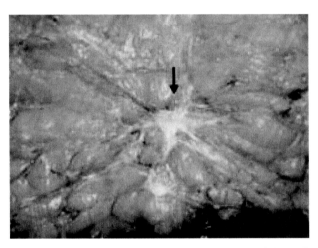

Figure 28.16 Slice of a wide local excision specimen with a central white stellate lesion, the typical macroscopic appearance of an invasive tubular carcinoma.

tumor cells (ITCs) detected by immunohistochemistry alone (Fig. 28.15). ILC has also been associated with lower response rates to neoadjuvant chemotherapy (47).

ILC tends to be associated with more unusual patterns of metastatic spread which may involve the ovaries, uterus, serosal surfaces, gastrointestinal tract, and meninges (15,32).

Tubular Cancer

Definition

Tubular carcinomas are well-differentiated tumors with an excellent prognosis. They account for up to 2% of all breast cancers, although in screen-detected series this may be as high as 9–19% (15). To fulfil the criteria for a tubular subtype, at least 90% of the tumor must be composed of angulated tubules lined by a single layer of epithelial cells set within a desmoplastic stroma which gives a spiculate appearance on mammography. Compared with NST tumors, tubular carcinomas are more likely to be smaller and screen detected (29,48).

Macroscopic Appearance

Tubular carcinomas appear as a hard spiculate gray-white mass, and the majority of lesions are less than 10 mm in size (Fig. 28.16).

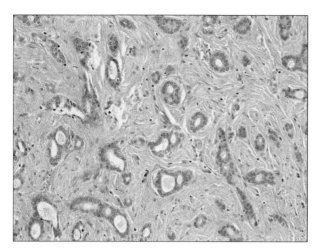

Figure 28.17 Invasive tubular carcinoma, composed of angulated tubular structures within a desmoplastic stromal background.

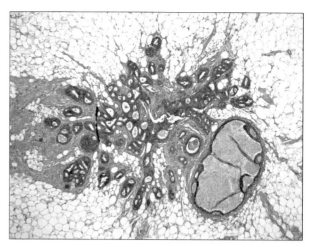

Figure 28.18 Invasive cribriform carcinoma. The tumor is formed by glands with sieve-like spaces. Myoepithelial stains were negative.

Microscopic Appearance

Tubular carcinomas are characterized by angulated or rounded tubular structures lined by a single layer of cells haphazardly distributed within a fibrous stroma (Fig. 28.17). The epithelial cells lining the tubules are small and regular with minimal nuclear atypia, and may have apical snouts. Mitoses are rare or absent. There is a cellular desmoplastic fibrous background, and the lack of a lobular arrangement is helpful in distinguishing tubular carcinomas from benign lesions such as radial scars or sclerosing adenosis.

Tubular carcinomas are commonly associated with a component of low-grade DCIS, typically with a cribriform or micropapillary pattern. Other early precursor lesions, such as atypical ductal hyperplasia (ADH) or flat epithelial atypia, may also be present. This group of lesions share common genetic changes with 16q losses and gains at 1q. These are observed in tubular cancers, lobular cancers, and low-grade NST cancers, and are considered to represent precursor lesions for the low-grade neoplasia pathway (37).

Immunohistochemistry

Tubular carcinomas belong to the luminal A subtype of cancers and are almost always strongly positive for ER and PR, negative for HER2 and have a low proliferation index (29,48). They lack a myoepithelial layer and in difficult cases can be distinguished from benign lesions such as sclerosing adenosis or radial scar by immunohistochemistry for myoepithelial markers (p63 or smooth muscle myosin heavy chain (SMMHC)) which will be negative in tubular carcinoma and positive in these benign lesions. The other differential diagnosis is microglandular adenosis which lacks a myoepithelial layer but is negative for epithelial membrane antigen which is expressed in tubular cancers.

Prognosis

When defined by strict criteria, the prognosis for pure tubular carcinomas is better than NST cancers with survival in some series reaching that of age-matched controls without cancer (46,48). Disease-free and breast cancer–specific survival is excellent, with a 5 year disease-free survival of 99% and a breast cancer–specific survival of 100% in one large series (29). Lymph node metastases are rare and when they do occur typically involve a single node only with minimal

adverse impact on outcome. Distant metastases are extremely rare (48) and the absolute benefits of sytemic adjuvant therapy are very small and perhaps considered unnecessary (48).

Invasive Cribriform Carcinoma

Definition

Invasive carcinoma composed of irregular islands of cells with a cribriform growth pattern similar to cribriform DCIS. At least 90% of the tumor should have this growth pattern, although a minor (<50%) component of tubular carcinoma is also accepted. This is an uncommon carcinoma, accounting for 1–3.5% of all breast cancers (15,29,49).

Macroscopic Appearance

There are no specific histopathological features. Cribriform carcinomas are most commonly screen-detected due to the presence a stellate mass with associated microcalcifications.

Microscopic Appearance

The tumor is composed of irregular islands of cells, often with an angulated outline, with rounded spaces forming a sieve-like or cribriform pattern (Fig. 28.18). The cells are small with mild to moderate nuclear atypia, and often have apical snouts. Mitoses are rare or absent. The islands of cells lie within a reactive fibroblastic stroma, similar to that seen in tubular carcinomas. Up to 80% of cases have an associated *in situ* component, which is most commonly low-grade cribriform DCIS (49). Luminal microcalcifications may be present in the invasive and *in situ* components.

Immunohistochemistry

Almost all cases of invasive cribriform carcinoma are strongly ER positive and HER2 negative, have a low proliferation index, and belong to the luminal A family of tumors (29). The main differential diagnosis is cribriform DCIS; invasive cribriform carcinoma lacks a myoepithelial layer on immunohistochemical staining. The other differential diagnosis is adenoid cystic carcinoma, which is ER and PR negative (see the section "Adenoid Cystic Carcinoma").

Prognosis

Pure invasive cribriform carcinoma has an excellent prognosis comparable to patients without breast cancer, with a 98%

five-year disease-free survival and overall survival (29,46). Although up to 14% of patients are reported to have axillary lymph node metastases, outcome remains favorable. Multifocality has been described in up to one-fifth of cases (49).

Mucinous Carcinoma (Colloid Carcinoma)

Definition

Mucinous carcinomas are made up of islands of tumor cells floating in pools of extracellular mucin. They account for 2–5% of all breast cancers, and are more commonly diagnosed in older patients (15,50). There is often minimal associated fibrosis and these tumors have a soft consistency with a smooth or lobulated outline resulting in an indeterminate or benign appearance on imaging.

Macroscopic Appearance

Mucinous tumors are well circumscribed with a glistening gelatinous appearance and are soft in consistency. Tumor size can range from 10 mm to 200 mm, with an average of 20–30 mm.

Microscopic Appearance

Mucinous carcinomas are composed of lakes of extracellular mucin separated by delicate fibrous septa, within which clusters and islands of tumor cells float (Fig. 28.19). The cell clusters vary in size and may involve formation of glandular lumina. The tumors are typically low grade and composed of uniform small cells with regular nuclei showing mild to moderate atypia, although high-grade cases with marked pleomorphism and mitoses can occur (50). DCIS is present surrounding the tumor in 30–75% of cases, and commonly has a solid or micropapillary pattern (15). The DCIS component may also contain extracellular mucin in the duct spaces.

Pure and mixed mucinous carcinomas are described, with the pure variant being 100% mucinous. Mixed tumors typically have an associated NST component. Pure mucinous cancers are subdivided into type A (hypocellular) and type B (cellular) variants (15,51).

Immunohistochemistry

Mucinous carcinomas belong to the luminal A subgroup and are typically ER positive and HER2 negative, although the proliferative index can be variable (29,51). They often stain positively for neuroendocrine markers, and the mucinous B subgroup form a distinct cluster with neuroendocrine breast cancers on gene expression profiling (2,52). Interestingly, pure mucinous carcinomas do not exhibit concurrent gain of 1q and 16q loss that characterizes the low-grade neoplasia family, further confirming that they are a distinct entity (51). In the same study, mixed mucinous tumors showed a similar molecular profile to pure mucinous tumors suggesting that both entities have a common clonal origin.

Prognosis

Pure mucinous carcinomas have a relatively good prognosis with five-year survival rates in excess of 90%. Hypocellular tumors have a more favorable prognosis. Some series suggest that mucinous tumors have a better outcome than NST tumors (46,50), while others report a similar outcome after a more prolonged follow-up (29). Mixed tumors have a worse prognosis, with 10-year survival rates of about 70% (15). This difference in behavior is also reflected in the incidence of axillary metastases which occur in only 3–15% of the pure variant compared with 33–46% of the mixed type (15).

Invasive Micropapillary Carcinoma

Definition

Invasive micropapillary carcinoma is composed of small clusters of tumor cells lying either within stromal spaces that resemble retraction artifact or within vascular spaces that lack an endothelial lining (Fig. 28.20). The pure form is rare and represents less than 2% of all breast cancers, but a focal micropapillary pattern may be seen in up to 6% of tumors (15). The age range is similar to that of NST cancers and the commonest presentation is as a mass lesion. There are no specific macroscopic features.

Microscopic Appearances

These carcinomas consist of hollow aggregates and morule-like clusters of cells which on sectioning resemble tubular structures lying within stromal spaces supported by a delicate fibrous framework. The tumor cells are cuboidal to columnar in shape and show moderate to severe nuclear atypia. The appearance of clusters of tumor cells within these spaces can mimic lymphovascular invasion, which is an associated feature in up to 68% of cases (53). There may be a component of micropapillary or cribriform DCIS.

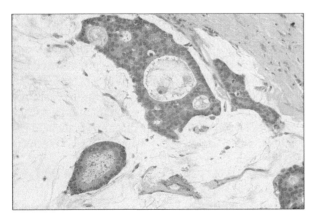

Figure 28.19 Mucinous carcinoma formed by islands of tumor cells floating within lakes of extracellular mucin.

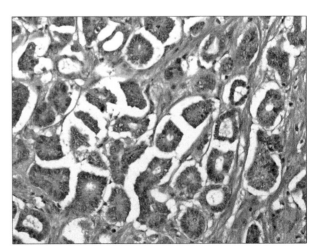

Figure 28.20 Invasive micropapillary carcinoma. The tumor is composed of morules and tubular structures lying within stromal spaces.

Immunohistochemistry

The majority of micropapillary carcinomas are ER positive (75–92%), with between 8% and 36% of cases being HER2 positive (53,54). Occasionally, HER2 can show an unusual expression pattern, with staining between cells and the central lumina rather than circumferential staining. They often have a high Ki-67 proliferative index and belong to the luminal B or HER2 molecular subtypes (54). Micropapillary cancers also have a characteristic staining pattern with epithelial membrane antigen; the positive staining of the basolateral membranes gives the tubular structures an "inside out" appearance (55). Invasive micropapillary carcinomas have a distinct genetic profile and the mixed variety (micropapillary-NST carcinomas) shows greater similarity to their pure counterparts, suggesting that they represent a discrete entity among ER-positive tumors with a more aggressive clinical behavior (2,56).

Prognosis

Invasive micropapillary carcinomas are commonly associated with lymphovascular space invasion, and three-quarters of patients have axillary node metastases at presentation (72–77%) (15). However, their prognosis is similar to NST cancers when matched for grade and stage, with one study finding a worse five-year disease-free survival (68%). Higher locoregional recurrence rates have been reported including an axillary recurrence rate of 11% in node-positive patients, but similar rates of distant metastasis-free survival (78% *vs*. 79%) and overall survival (86% *vs*. 88%) (53).

Papillary Carcinoma

Papillary lesions are characterized by fibrovascular cores lined by epithelial cells, often lying within a dilated duct or cystic space. The distinction between benign and malignant papillary lesions is dependent upon the presence of atypia within the epithelial component, and the presence or absence of a myoepithelial layer lining the fibrovascular cores and/ or externally in the surrounding cystic space (57). Benign papillomas have an intact myoepithelial layer throughout and show no cytological atypia. Papillomas can become focally or entirely involved by DCIS, in which the internal myoepithelial layer is intact but the epithelial component shows cytological and/ or architectural atypia such as the formation of cribriform spaces.

In papillary DCIS, the fibrovascular cores are often delicate and have lost their internal myoepithelial layer although the external layer lining the cyst wall is retained. The epithelium shows mild to moderate atypia and may consist of tall columnar cells.

Invasive papillary carcinomas represent 0.5–1% of invasive cancers and can be divided into three groups (58,59). Encapsulated (or intracystic) papillary carcinoma comprises a well-circumscribed lesion formed by an intricate network of delicate fibrovascular cores lined by neoplastic epithelial cells within a cystic space with a fibrous capsule (Fig. 28.21). Encapsulated papillary carcinomas show a complete or near-complete lack of myoepithelium, both internally and in the peripheral surrounding capsule, and are now regarded as an indolent form of invasive carcinoma (60–62). There may be an associated frank invasive component with infiltration of surrounding tissue, which is usually of NST. The solid variant of papillary carcinoma comprises a well-circumscribed or multinodular tumor formed by solid sheets of cells with an underlying fibrovascular stromal framework. Occasionally, the cells may have a spindle or neuroendocrine appearance. Invasive papillary carcinomas are rare, and consist of carcinoma with pure papillary morphology with an infiltrative growth pattern (Fig. 28.22).

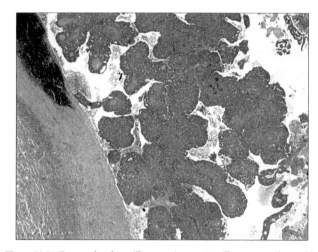

Figure 28.21 Encapsulated papillary carcinoma. Papillary tumor formed by delicate fibrovascular cores lined by neoplastic cells, lying within a cystic space lined by a fibrous capsule. This example is from a male patient, and there is an increased predominance of papillary carcinoma in men.

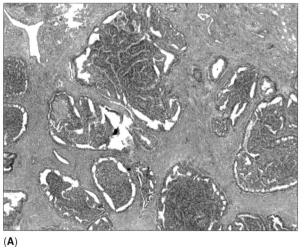

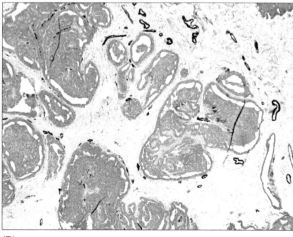

(A)   **(B)**

Figure 28.22 Invasive papillary carcinoma, made up of islands of tumor with a papillary architecture invading into fibrous breast tissue (**A**). Immunohistochemistry shows complete absence of a myoepithelial layer, with-positive staining of blood vessels (**B**).

Papillary carcinomas typically present as a mass lesion in postmenopausal patients with an average age of 70–73 years (59,61,62). Many are situated close to the nipple, where they may present with nipple discharge. Macroscopically they are often circumscribed with a friable texture, and may be associated with areas of hemorrhage. On microscopy, papillary carcinomas are typically low to intermediate grade with mild to moderate cytological atypia (61–63). About 75% of cases have an adjacent component of DCIS, often of papillary or cribriform pattern (15).

Nearly all papillary carcinomas are ER/PR positive and HER2 negative (58,62,63). They are of luminal A subtype and show similar genetic changes to low-grade NST carcinomas and have an excellent prognosis (58). The incidence of lymph node metastases is 3–6% in the absence of an associated NST component, and these are almost always micrometastases (61). Distant metastases are extremely rare and usually occur in the context of recurrent disease. The current recommendation is that in the absence of a frank invasive component, these tumors should continue to be managed in a manner similar to DCIS (57,61). In those cases with combined papillary carcinoma and associated NST (or other invasive component) the invasive carcinoma should be measured separately along with an aggregate tumor size (including the papillary carcinoma) to avoid overstaging.

Neuroendocrine Carcinoma

Focal neuroendocrine differentiation with expression of neuroendocrine markers such as S100, CD56, synaptophysin, and chromogranin is seen in up to 20% of NST cancers (64). Primary neuroendocrine carcinomas of the breast are rare, representing 2–5% of breast cancers (15). These have a similar morphological appearance to lung or gastrointestinal neuroendocrine tumors with expression of neuroendocrine markers in more than 50% of cells. They often occur in older patients and present as a discrete breast mass.

Breast neuroendocrine carcinomas have a spectrum of histological appearances similar to their lung counterparts. Better differentiated lesions resemble carcinoid tumors, and are composed of alveolar nests or solid sheets of cells separated by a delicate fibrovascular stroma. The cells may be spindle shaped with bean-shaped nuclei or large with a plasmacytoid or clear cell appearance and round nuclei with the classical salt and pepper chromatin pattern. Formation of rosettes is rare. The majority of well-differentiated neuroendocrine carcinomas are ER/PR positive and HER2 negative (15).

Poorly differentiated variants include primary small cell carcinoma of the breast and large cell undifferentiated neuroendocrine carcinoma. Small-cell carcinomas are composed of densely packed cells with minimal cytoplasm and hyperchromatic nuclei which "mold" together giving a cobblestone appearance. They are particularly mitotically active, and often contain areas of necrosis. Around 50% of cases are ER positive and these are usually HER2 negative (15). Primary small cell carcinoma of the breast is exceedingly rare, and is a diagnosis of exclusion after performing extensive imaging to look for a primary tumor elsewhere, particularly the lungs or pancreas. Large cell neuroendocrine carcinomas are high-grade tumors with a solid growth pattern formed by cells with abundant cytoplasm, vesicular or finely granular chromatin, and a high mitotic rate. Necrosis is common.

Prognosis is dependent upon the grade and stage of the tumor. Low-grade, early-stage lesions have a good prognosis with standard therapy. Although small cell carcinomas often have axillary metastases at presentation, they can respond well to chemotherapy regimens used for small cell carcinomas at other sites (65).

Apocrine Carcinoma

Apocrine carcinomas contain cytological and immunohistochemical features of apocrine cells in over 90% of tumor cells (15). Apocrine cells are large with abundant granular eosinophilic cytoplasm, and enlarged round nuclei with prominent nucleoli. The incidence of apocrine carcinoma varies between studies, as cells with apocrine differentiation can also be found in NST, papillary, micropapillary, and neuroendocrine carcinomas as well as pleomorphic lobular carcinomas. Using strict criteria approximately 4% of tumors are apocrine, and their clinical presentation and prognosis is similar to that of stage-matched NST carcinomas.

Apocrine carcinomas are usually both ER and PR negative, but can be HER2 positive. They express GCDFP and androgen receptor (15). A subset of apocrine carcinomas can be distinguished that have a distinct gene expression profile with upregulation of androgen receptor signaling pathways (66). This "molecular apocrine" signature is also seen in some pleomorphic lobular carcinomas. In contrast, NST cancers with an apocrine appearance do not tend to cluster together and belong to the luminal subtype (67).

Medullary Carcinoma

Definition

Medullary carcinoma is a controversial entity, with reported incidence ranging from 1–7% of breast cancers depending upon the stringency of criteria used (15). They are highly cellular tumors with a well-circumscribed "pushing" margin composed of sheets of poorly differentiated cells with a prominent lymphoplasmacytic inflammatory cell infiltrate (Fig. 28.23). They tend to occur in younger women and being well circumscribed and soft, they may be confused with a benign lesion both clinically and radiologically (46).

Macroscopic Appearance

Medullary carcinomas appear as a rounded, well-delineated mass with a soft texture and fleshy tan appearance. There may be associated necrosis and hemorrhage.

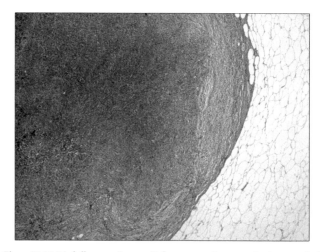

Figure 28.23 Medullary carcinoma. At low power, the tumor is circumscribed with a pushing margin and prominent lymphocytic inflammatory cell infiltrate.

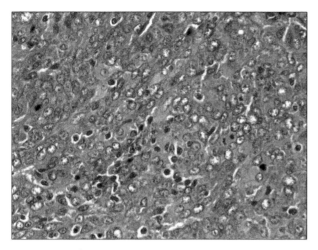

Figure 28.24 Medullary carcinoma. At high power, the tumor is composed of syncytial sheets of pleomorphic cells with a high mitotic rate.

Microscopic Appearance
There are five main criteria for diagnosis of a medullary carcinoma (68)

1. Syncytial architecture, formed by sheets of tumor cells without distinct cell boundaries, and involving over 75% of the tumor (Fig. 28.24).
2. Glandular or tubule formation is completely absent.
3. There is a diffuse stromal lymphoplasmacytic inflammatory cell infiltrate. The density of the infiltrate may vary, and in some cases is so dense it may overrun the tumor cells making them hard to see.
4. The carcinoma cells are markedly pleomorphic with abundant cytoplasm and vesicular nuclei with prominent nucleoli and a high mitotic count.
5. A circumscribed tumor with a pushing margin; the tumor is expanding as a broad front rather than infiltrating as finger-like projections.

Some definitions also include absence of an *in situ* component, which is an uncommon associated finding for these tumors. There may also be extensive tumor necrosis. Carcinomas with a syncytial growth pattern and only two or three of the other criteria have been labeled atypical medullary carcinomas, although the term NST with medullary features has been proposed as a more suitable alternative (15). Some studies have found that only classical medullary carcinomas are associated with an improved prognosis compared with grade 3 NST carcinomas, while others find a similarly improved prognosis for both medullary and medullary-like tumors (69).

Immunohistochemistry and Molecular Features
Medullary carcinomas are typically triple negative (ER, PR, and HER2) and show positive staining for basal cytokeratins CK5 and CK14 (70). They are also commonly p53 positive (69%) and have a very high Ki-67 labelling index reflecting their high mitotic count. On gene expression array analysis, they belong with the basal group of breast cancers (2).

Medullary and medullary-like carcinomas are more frequently found in BRCA1 mutation carriers, with up to 60% of tumors showing medullary features (71). Conversely, BRCA1

gene mutations have been identified in up to 11% of medullary cancers (72). In the absence of a somatic mutation there is often downregulation of BRCA1 function by other mechanisms such as gene promoter methylation. There is also a high rate of p53 mutations, with somatic p53 mutations in 40–100% of medullary carcinomas (15).

Prognosis
Despite their aggressive tumor characteristics, classical medullary carcinomas have been associated with a relatively favorable prognosis compared with grade-matched NST cancers (46,69). Less than 10% present with lymph node metastasis (15). Potential explanations for this include the presence of a florid host immune reaction, and the combination of deficient DNA repair with a high proliferation rate may confer increased sensitivity to chemotherapy (15,69). The loss of BRCA1 function may make these tumors ideal candidates for novel drugs such as PARP inhibitors that disable alternative DNA repair pathways, a concept called "synthetic lethality" (73).

Metaplastic Carcinoma
Definition
Metaplastic carcinomas are a group of tumors characterized by an admixture of adenocarcinoma with areas of spindle cell, squamous, and/ or mesenchymal differentiation (15). The metaplastic component may predominate, making distinction from a primary breast sarcoma difficult. Metaplastic carcinomas are rare and account for less than 1% of all breast cancers. Nonetheless, primary sarcomas of the breast are even rarer so a diagnosis of metaplastic carcinoma should be considered initially for all atypical spindle cell lesions of the breast.

Metaplastic carcinomas constitute a group of tumors which can be broadly subclassified as follows:

Purely epithelial: Squamous, adenosquamous, low-grade adenosquamous, spindle cell carcinoma including fibromatosis-like carcinoma.

Mixed epithelial and mesenchymal: Matrix-producing carcinoma and carcinosarcoma (where both epithelial and mesenchymal components are malignant).

Squamous and Adenosquamous Carcinoma
These are each made up of tumors showing areas of squamous differentiation, either with or without keratinization. Focal areas of squamous differentiation may be seen in up to 4% of NST tumors. When there is formation of well-developed glands admixed with nests of squamous cells, the term adenosquamous carcinoma can be used. Pure squamous cell carcinomas of the breast are exceedingly rare and must be distinguished from metastatic carcinoma from other sites particularly lung, cervix or bladder, or primary skin cancers with extension into the breast (74). They vary from well to moderately differentiated tumors with large eosinophilic cells with foci of keratinization often lining cystic spaces, to poorly differentiated cells lacking keratin with a more spindle cell appearance. There is often a fibrotic stromal background with an associated inflammatory cell infiltrate. A rare variant is the acantholytic subtype, where degenerative changes within the epithelium result in the formation of a network of anastomosing spaces that can mimic angiosarcoma.

Squamous cell carcinomas are typically negative for ER and HER2 (75–77). They stain positively for broad-spectrum

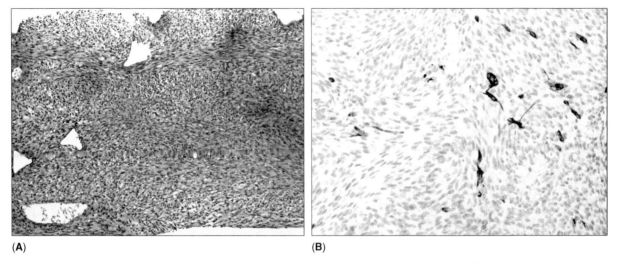

(A)   **(B)**

Figure 28.25 Tumor composed of fascicles of spindled cells with a high mitotic rate that morphologically resembles a fibrosarcoma (**A**). The cells showed focal positivity for CK14, consistent with a metaplastic carcinoma (**B**).

cytokeratins and basal cytokeratins such as CK5 and up to 86% of cases are EGFR positive (75,76). Squamous cells show nuclear positivity for p63, so this marker cannot be used to distinguish *in situ* from invasive elements (74). The acantholytic variant can be distinguished from angiosarcoma by positive staining for cytokeratins, and negative staining for endothelial markers, CD31 and CD34.

The prognosis of squamous cell carcinoma of the breast is similar to that of NST cancers when matched for age and stage of disease (74). They show limited responsiveness to chemotherapy (75).

Low-grade Adenosquamous Carcinoma
These tumors are composed of small glandular structures and solid nests of squamous cells haphazardly arranged in a cellular background stroma. The tumor has a tendency to grow within and between existing ducts and lobules, and has been described in association with sclerosing lesions such as radial scars or papillary lesions where the diagnosis can be very difficult (78,79). There is typically an associated lymphocytic infiltrate, which can be a clue to the diagnosis in this setting.

The carcinoma cells are negative for ER and HER2, but stain positively for cytokeratins including basal cytokeratins CK5 and CK14 (80). Scattered stromal spindle cells also show CK positivity, indicating that they form part of the tumor. The tumor cells can also express p63 and other myoepithelial markers such as SMMHC. In this situation the characteristic pattern of diffuse staining of cells within the group rather than a peripheral rim of staining which is typical of myoepithelial cells, is important in reaching a correct diagnosis.

Low-grade adenosquamous carcinomas have an excellent prognosis. There is a tendency for local recurrence, with lymph node metastasis being extremely rare (79).

Spindle Cell Carcinoma
As suggested by their name, spindle cell carcinomas are tumors predominantly composed of elongated spindle shaped cells that may resemble a sarcoma but show areas of epithelial differentiation and/or positive immunohistochemical staining for cytokeratins (Fig. 28.25). The diagnosis is relatively straightforward when there is an obvious NST component or associated

DCIS; however the epithelial component may be minimal and difficult to identify and cytokeratin staining can be very focal making diagnosis on core biopsy difficult (7). Extensive sampling of the excision specimen may be required to establish the correct diagnosis.

The spindle cell component can be relatively bland and uniform with variable amounts of collagen, giving a fibromatosis-like or keloidal appearance (81). There may be a highly cellular proliferation of more atypical, mitotically active spindle cells resembling a fibrosarcoma, or the spindle cells may be markedly pleomorphic giving the appearance of a poorly differentiated sarcoma. Heterologous elements, such as osseous or cartilaginous areas, may be present. The tumor may be called a carcinosarcoma if the heterologous element is malignant, such as chondrosarcoma or angiosarcoma.

The vast majority of spindle cell carcinomas are triple negative (76,81). The tumor cells show positive staining for cytokeratins, although this is often patchy and may be very focal. Pancytokeratin is positive in the majority of cases, although other cytokeratin cocktails such as Cam5.2 and AE1/AE3 can be negative in a proportion of cases (up to 80%). A panel of several cytokeratin markers including basal cytokeratins CK5 and CK14 is recommended if a spindle cell carcinoma is suspected (7,82). Spindle cell carcinomas can also show positive nuclear staining for p63 and focal positivity for other myoepithelial markers such as smooth muscle actin.

In general, metaplastic carcinomas are triple negative and belong to the basal family of breast cancers (76,83). With the exception of low-grade adenosquamous and fibromatosis-like cancers they have a worse prognosis than NST cancers even when matched for grade- and triple-negative status (46,84). They tend to be less responsive to neoadjuvant chemotherapy (47).

Adenoid Cystic Carcinoma
Adenoid cystic carcinomas of the breast share the histological features of their salivary gland counterpart. They are rare, accounting for a mere 0.1% of breast tumors (85,86). The majority of cases present as a mass, half of which occur in the subareolar region (15). Macroscopically they are well circumscribed with a microcystic change. Histologically, they are

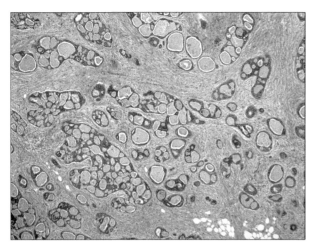

Figure 28.26 Adenoid cystic carcinoma, composed of basaloid cells forming rounded spaces containing mucin or pink basement membrane-like material.

composed of small basaloid cells with minimal cytoplasm with a solid, cribriform, or trabecular growth pattern (Fig. 28.26). The rounded spaces contain either myxoid acidic stromal mucin or cylinders of collagen representing invaginations of the stroma, or true glandular spaces containing mucin.

Adenoid cystic carcinomas are negative for ER, PR, and HER2, with most of the tumor cells having a myoepithelial phenotype with expression of basal cytokeratins, actin, p63, and c-kit (87,88). They typically have a low proliferative index (85,88). The main differential diagnosis is cribriform carcinoma, which is both ER and PR positive but does not express basal cytokeratins or c-kit. At the genetic level, adenoid cystic carcinomas are characterized by MYB overexpression, usually secondary to a translocation t(6;9) involving the MYB and NFIB genes (88). They also display low levels of genomic instability in contrast to other basal breast cancers, which may contribute to their better prognosis.

Despite being triple negative and belonging to the basal family of tumors, adenoid cystic carcinomas have an excellent prognosis with 10-year survival rates of 90–100% (88). Complete surgical resection is often curative; lymph node metastases are uncommon (0–2%) and distant metastases may rarely develop in the lungs (86).

Other rare salivary type tumors that can arise in the breast include acinic cell, oncocytic, and mucoepidermoid carcinomas (87).

Lipid-Rich Carcinoma
This is a rare variant of carcinoma in which at least 90% of tumor cells have abundant foamy cytoplasm containing lipid vesicles, comprising less than 1% of breast cancers (15). The majority are high grade with frequent lymph node metastases (70–100%) and a predictably poor prognosis with a five-year survival of only 33% (89,90). In two series examining lipid-rich cancers, all cases were ER negative and HER2 amplification was found in 71–100% of the cases (89,90). Nonetheless, there are other reports which have documented ER positivity (91).

Glycogen-Rich Carcinoma
These are rare carcinomas in which more than 90% of tumor cells have abundant clear cytoplasm containing glycogen, which can be demonstrated by positive staining for periodic acid Schiff (PAS) and negative staining for PAS diastase (15). Nonetheless, up to 60% of NST cancers contain some glycogen and therefore strict definitions must be used. The clinical and macroscopic features are similar to NST cancers. Glycogen-rich carcinomas generally have a poor prognosis with the majority of cases being high-grade and lymph node metastases present in up to 30% of cases (92). Expression of hormone receptor and HER2 is variable for this type of breast cancer.

Secretory Carcinoma
This is a rare form of carcinoma accounting for less than 0.2% of all breast cancers and often occurs in young patients, with a reported median age of 25 years (93). The typical presentation is as a discrete non-tender breast mass.

Histologically, the tumor is composed of cells with abundant pale granular cytoplasm and prominent intracytoplasmic lumina. There are variable architectural features with microcystic, solid, or tubular patterns. There is an intracellular and extracellular esinophilic milk-like secretion that is PAS positive and diastase resistant. Secretory carcinomas are usually low-grade lesions and may be associated with low-grade DCIS.

These tumors are triple negative (ER, PR, and HER2) and express basal cytokeratins (CK5 and CK14) together with EGFR and S100 (93,94). Moreover, they have a characteristic balanced gene translocation involving the ETS variant 6 (ETV6) gene on chromosome 12 and the neurotrophic tyrosine kinase receptor 3 (NTKR3) on chromosome 15. The translocation (12;15) results in a fusion gene product which is a chimeric tyrosine kinase with potent transforming activity in breast epithelial cells and fibroblasts. This has also been described in pediatric mesenchymal tumors including congenital fibrosarcoma and congenital mesoblastic nephroma.

Like adenoid cystic carcinomas, secretory carcinomas represent a subtype of basal breast cancer characterized by a gene translocation with a favorable prognosis, especially in younger patients. Local recurrence in children is rare, although delayed recurrences have been described. Axillary metastases are found in up to 15% of patients but usually involve less than four nodes (15).

Cystic Hypersecretory Carcinoma
Cystic hypersecretory carcinoma is a rare form of DCIS characterized by cystically dilated ducts containing eosinophilic secretion (similar in appearance to thyroid colloid) and lined by pleomorphic cells with a micropapillary growth pattern (Fig. 28.27) (95,96). An invasive form occurs in which cystic hypersecretory DCIS is associated with an invasive carcinoma, which is typically high-grade NST carcinoma with a solid growth pattern and triple-negative phenotype (97). The invasive tumors exhibit aggressive behavior, with over 50% of reported cases having lymph node metastases at presentation.

Microinvasive Carcinoma
Microinvasion is defined as one or more foci of invasive cancer measuring <1 mm in size (10,98). It is typically identified in the context of extensive high-grade DCIS, although rarely can be seen with low-grade DCIS (particularly papillary type) or lobular carcinoma *in situ*. Microinvasion often occurs in the setting of inflammation and a desmoplastic stromal reaction,

and immunohistochemistry to confirm the absence of a myo-epithelial cell layer around the infiltrating tumor cells may be required for a definite diagnosis. If there is any doubt about the diagnosis, the lesion should be classified as an *in situ* carcinoma.

Microinvasive carcinoma using the above definition has an excellent prognosis similar to that of pure *in situ* carcinoma, with a low incidence of axillary lymph node metastases. In cases of extensive high-grade DCIS, it is impossible to examine all the tissue, so invasive foci may be missed. The upgrade rate to invasive cancer after a core biopsy diagnosis of DCIS is up to 50% (7). In this setting, there is an argument for performing a SLN biopsy or axillary sample as part of the initial surgical management.

PAGET'S DISEASE OF THE NIPPLE

Paget's disease is reddening or an eczematous rash of the nipple due to infiltration of the epidermis by malignant cells. In 94–100% of cases there is underlying DCIS or invasive carcinoma, which is often situated centrally within the breast (99,100). More than 90% of patients with an

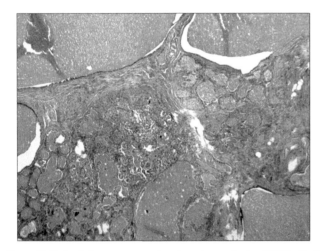

Figure 28.27 Cystic hypersecretory ductal carcinoma *in situ* (DCIS). Cystic hypersecretory change composed of dilated cystic spaces filled with colloid-like material, with a focal area of DCIS with a micropapillary architecture (central).

associated palpable mass have an invasive cancer, compared with 33% who have invasive cancer when no clinical mass is present (101). Conversely, Paget's disease is identified in 1–2% of patients with breast cancer, and in 10–30% of cases this is diagnosed on histology alone with no clinical abnormality (99).

On microscopy, there is full-thickness infiltration of the epidermis by large atypical cells with pleomorphic nuclei and abundant cytoplasm, occurring either singly and/ or in groups (Fig. 28.28). When Paget's disease is the primary presentation, the differential diagnosis is melanoma or Bowen's disease of the nipple. Pagetoid cells are positive for CK7, and negative for CK20 and melanoma markers such as HMB45 and S100. Furthermore, over 90% of these cells are HER2 positive, and the associated DCIS or invasive cancer usually shows a similar profile with HER2 positivity (102). ER expression is variable depending upon the profile of the underlying lesion; however, the majority of cases are either ER negative (86%) or of luminal B type with co-expression of ER and HER2 (12%) (102).

The prognosis of Paget's disease depends on the nature of the underlying lesion, in particular the presence and stage of any associated invasive carcinoma. In patients with DCIS only, there is almost 100% cure rate at 10 years with mastectomy (103). Breast conservation with central resection including the nipple–areola complex is an option in patients with localized disease (100,104). Careful preoperative assessment is essential, with inclusion of MRI if mammography is negative; in one series 5% of patients with no palpable mass and innocent mammography had invasive cancer and 68% had DCIS extending beyond the nipple (105).

Inflammatory Breast Cancer

Inflammatory breast cancer is a clinical diagnosis characterized by diffuse erythema and edema (*peau d'orange*) involving one-third or more of the skin of the breast (10). Both mammography and MRI show thickening of the skin and subcutaneous tissue. The histological correlate is infiltration of the dermal lymphatics by tumor cell emboli, which can be identified on punch biopsy in up to 75% of cases (106). The underlying carcinoma is often high-grade NST, which tends to be ER

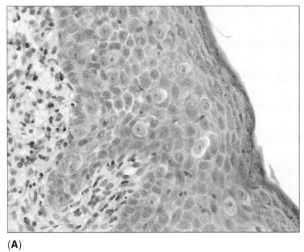

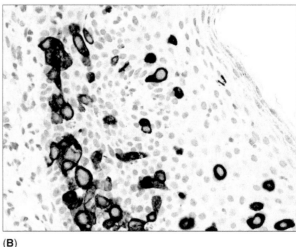

(A)   **(B)**

Figure 28.28 Paget's disease of the nipple. A section of the epidermis (A) showing infiltration by large atypical cells, confirmed by staining with Cam5.2 (B).

negative and HER2 positive and belongs to the basal or HER2-positive molecular groups (15,106).

Inflammatory cancers represent locally advanced disease, with a T component of T4d in the TNM system (10) and 60–85% of patients have axillary metastases at presentation (106). Without systemic therapy, prognosis is poor and five-year survival rates are usually less than 5% (106). Modern treatment includes neoadjuvant chemotherapy followed by mastectomy and chest wall radiotherapy. This has led to improvement in survival outcomes with five-year survival rates of 35–40%, although these exceed 80% in patients who achieve a complete pathological response. The risk of local recurrence and distant metastases is higher than for other forms of breast cancer, and in consequence immediate reconstruction is usually contraindicated.

Multicentric Breast Cancer

Multicentric cancer occurs when there is more than one focus of invasive cancer within the breast and may represent either synchronous primary tumors or intramammary spread from a single index tumor. The latter scenario is more commonly seen with invasive lobular carcinomas. The tumors may be of similar or completely different histological types. When lesions are close together it may be difficult to determine if there is only a single lesion or multiple lesions are present, particularly in the context of extensive DCIS. A distance of 5 mm or more between lesions has been arbitrarily suggested to define separate tumor foci (3,10).

The TNM stage is determined by the largest lesion present (10). The Nottingham Prognostic Index (NPI) is determined by the highest-grade tumor, as grade is given a higher weighting than size in this system (NPI score = grade + nodal score + 0.2x size). ER and HER2 status should be established for all major tumor foci, especially for synchronous primary lesions where the morphology is different. This is probably unnecessary for classical ILC with multiple satellite foci.

THERAPY-RELATED CHANGES

Neoadjuvant chemotherapy and/or endocrine therapy is increasingly being used in the management of breast cancer,

and has been shown to be as efficacious as adjuvant therapy. Established clinical indications for neoadjuvant treatment include inflammatory breast cancer and downstaging of large tumors to convert inoperable to operable disease or to allow breast conservation rather than mastectomy (107). A potential advantage of neoadjuvant therapy is it offers a unique opportunity for the evaluation of treatment response. Complete pathological response, defined as absence of invasive cancer in the breast and axillary lymph nodes, can act as a surrogate marker of survival and allow a more rapid analysis of the efficacy of new chemotherapeutic agents. Serial evaluation of biomarkers may also be of benefit in assessing response to therapy. Measurement of the Ki-67 labeling index following two weeks of neoadjuvant endocrine therapy is predictive of recurrence-free survival, with repeat testing at 12 weeks showing recovery of Ki-67 levels in some patients (108).

There can be considerable changes in the macroscopic and microscopic appearances of a tumor post neoadjuvant therapy (109). Macroscopically the lesion may become softened and ill-defined, and there may be no residual macroscopic lesion or only a vague area of fibrosis to indicate the tumor bed. In this setting, detailed clinical information regarding pre-treatment tumor location and size is vital to allow accurate pathological sampling of the lesion. Radiological placement of a marker clip to indicate the site of the tumor before commencement of treatment is very useful in the event of an excellent clinical response, and essential if breast conserving surgery is being considered (110).

Chemotherapy can alter the morphological appearances of a tumor, altering traditional histological prognostic factors. Tumor grade may change, with an increase in nuclear pleomorphism and a reduction in mitotic count. There can be a marked reduction in tumor cellularity (Fig. 28.29) and changes in the growth pattern, with typical NST cancers taking on a "lobular"-like architecture with individual cell and single-file infiltration post treatment. There may be an associated inflammatory cell infiltrate with collections of macrophages, and the stroma can show edematous or myxoid changes with central fibrosis (Fig. 28.30). A central area of fibrous scarring is commonly seen in response to neoadjuvant endocrine therapy (111).

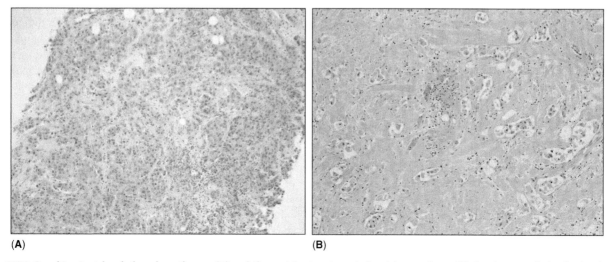

(A)   (B)

Figure 28.29 Core biopsies taken before chemotherapy (A) and the post-treatment surgical excision specimen (B) showing a marked reduction in tumor cellularity.

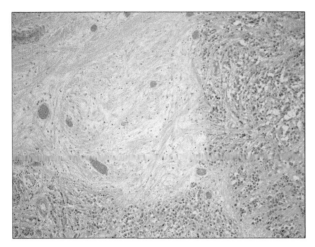

Figure 28.30 Tumor post neoadjuvant chemotherapy with a central area of reactive myxoid stroma.

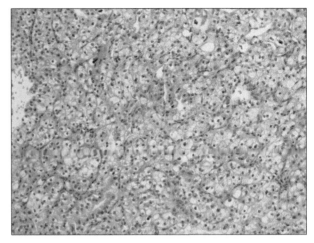

Figure 28.31 Clear cell carcinoma with a classical appearance of metastatic renal cell carcinoma.

There are also changes in the background breast tissue, with atrophy, hyalinization, and a lymphocytic infiltrate in benign lobules (112).

At present, there are no United Kingdom (UK) guidelines for the reporting of neoadjuvant chemotherapy specimens, and there are several different systems in the literature for the histological grading of chemotherapy response. Many of the systems in common use, such as the Miller–Payne system, rely on a comparison of tumor cellularity in the pretreatment core biopsy and the post-treatment resection specimen, with the grade of response determined by the percentage reduction in overall cellularity (109,113). An alternative system, the Residual Cancer Burden (RCB), has been proposed that derives a score based on tumor bed volume, average tumor cellularity, number of involved lymph nodes, and the size of the largest metastasis and relates to survival outcome (114). The score relies on absolute cellularity post treatment, without considering the change from pretreatment cellularity. Traditional tumor grading systems used in the adjuvant setting, including the NPI and the pTNM system using the prefix "y" to indicate neoadjuvant treatment, have also been shown to retain their prognostic value post chemotherapy (115,116).

Changes in breast tissue induced by irradiation can mimic malignancy and cause difficulty in interpretation of biopsies (117). The major changes include collagenization of lobules, atrophy of ductal and acinar epithelium with cytological atypia, prominence of myoepithelial cells, and the presence of atypical fibroblasts in the interlobular stroma. Elastosis and hyalinization of blood vessels may be a clue to previous radiotherapy if the relevant history has not been supplied.

Metastatic Carcinoma

Not all malignant tumors of the breast are of primary breast origin. Metastatic involvement of the breast is an uncommon presentation of a non-mammary malignancy, and there can be a delay of several years between the diagnosis of the primary tumor and development of metastases. A wide range of tumors can metastasize to the breast, including lymphoma, melanoma, and carcinoma of the lungs, ovary, kidney or stomach (118).

The presentation is usually with a rapidly growing palpable mass that is well circumscribed and superficially located. The

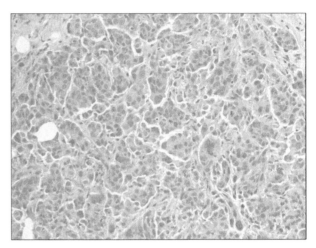

Figure 28.32 Metastatic serous papillary carcinoma with morphology similar to that of the micropapillary carcinoma of the breast.

lesions are solitary in a majority of cases (85%), and there may be accompanying axillary lymphadenopathy (119). On mammography, spiculation, and microcalcification are uncommon and support primary breast cancer diagnosis (118). On microscopy, morphological features may be present to suggest a metastatic lesion, such as pigment in melanoma or clear cell renal carcinoma (Fig. 28.31). However, about one-third of lesions do not show specific histological features and poorly differentiated carcinomas from other sites may resemble high-grade breast carcinomas (118). Other traps include metastatic signet ring cell gastric carcinoma, which can be indistinguishable from invasive lobular carcinoma, and metastatic serous papillary carcinoma of the ovary which may look like micropapillary carcinoma (Fig. 28.32). Negative staining for ER is an important clue, and should always prompt consideration of a metastasis especially in subtypes of breast cancer that are typically ER positive such as lobular carcinoma. Other potential clues are the presence of elastosis, which is rare in secondary metastases, and associated DCIS.

In cases with no history of previous cancer, immunohistochemistry can be useful in identifying the primary site. Strong, diffuse staining for ER is only seen in tumors of breast or gynecological tract origin, although tumors from other sites can show weak, focal staining (118). Breast cancers are typically

CK7 positive and CK20 negative (120). Other useful markers include GCDFP-15 which stains breast and salivary gland tumors, TTF1 for primary lung adenocarcinoma, WT1 for ovarian cancer (especially serous papillary carcinoma), and melanoma markers such as melanA or HMB45.

Recognition of metastatic malignancy is important, as extensive local surgery is often inappropriate. Breast metastases are usually a marker of extensive systemic disease, and the prognosis is dependent on the site of origin and the histological subtype.

Male Breast Cancer

Breast cancer is much rarer in men than in women and accounts for less than 1% of male cancers, although the incidence has been increasing over the last decade (121,122). It is more prevalent in older men, with an average age of 68 years, 5–10 years later than in women. Predisposing factors include an estrogen (excess) – androgen (deficiency) imbalance such as increased body mass index, testicular or liver dysfunction, exogenous estrogen administration, and Reifenstein syndrome (androgen receptor gene mutation) (121). In about 5% of cases there is a family history of breast cancer (15). Male breast cancer has been associated with BRCA2 gene mutations, with a 6% risk of developing the disease by age 70 compared with 0.1% in the general population (121). Klinefelter's syndrome, with an XXY karyotype, is associated with a 50-fold increased risk of breast cancer (121).

The most common presentation is with a subareolar mass. In one-quarter to one-half of patients there is ulceration or fixation to overlying skin, and the involvement of pectoralis muscle is more common (123). The vast majority of cancers are NST, with lobular carcinoma being extremely rare in men. There may be an associated *in situ* component, but this is usually not prominent. Papillary carcinomas are proportionally more common than in women, representing up to 12% of cases (59,124). Method of grading and staging is the same as for female patients, and the tumors are typically grade 2 or 3. Male breast cancers are commonly ER positive (90–100%) (122,124,125). The frequency of HER2 overexpression varies between studies (0–17%), although it is almost always co-expressed with ER as a luminal B subtype (122–125). Triple-negative breast cancers are rare in men, accounting for 2–4% of cases (122,125).

When matched for grade and stage, the prognosis is similar to that of female breast cancer (122). However, lymph node involvement is more common at presentation (40–55%) (121). As there is a limited amount of breast tissue in men, most patients are treated with simple mastectomy. Axillary staging with SLN biopsy has been shown to be accurate in men (123) and is widely used to select patients for axillary clearance if node positive. Adjuvant therapy with tamoxifen has been shown to be beneficial, although the effectiveness of aromatase inhibitors is doubtful as up to 20% of estrogens in men are produced in the testes via an aromatase independent pathway (123). Chemotherapy and HER2 targeted therapy should be considered if clinically indicated.

REFERENCES

1. Reis-Filho JS, Lakhani SR. Breast cancer special types: why bother? J Pathol 2008; 216: 394–8.
2. Weigelt B, Horlings HM, Kreike B, et al. Refinement of breast cancer classification by molecular characterization of histological special types. J Pathol 2008; 216: 141–50.
3. Pathology GW. GotNCCfB. Pathology Reporting of Breast Disease. Sheffield: NHS Cancer Screening Programmes, 2005.
4. Ellis I, Humphreys S, Michell M, et al. Guidelines for Non-operative Diagnostic Procedures and Reporting in Breast Cancer Screening. NHS Cancer Screening Programmes, 2001.
5. Willems SM, van Deurzen CH, van Diest PJ. Diagnosis of breast lesions: fine-needle aspiration cytology or core needle biopsy? A review. J Clin Pathol 2012; 65: 287–92.
6. Rakha EA, Ellis IO. An overview of assessment of prognostic and predictive factors in breast cancer needle core biopsy specimens. J Clin Pathol 2007; 60: 1300–6.
7. Provenzano E, Pinder SE. Pre-operative diagnosis of breast cancer in screening: problems and pitfalls. Pathology 2009; 41: 3–17.
8. Provenzano E, Pinder SE. Guidelines for the handling of benign and malignant surgical breast specimens. Curr Diagn Pathol 2007; 13: 96–105.
9. Cserni G. How to improve low lymph node recovery rates from axillary clearance specimens of breast cancer. A short-term audit. J Clin Pathol 1998; 51: 846–9.
10. AJCC. Breast. In: Edge SB, Byrd DR, Compton CC, Fritz AG, Greene FL, Trotti A, eds. Cancer Staging Handbook from the AJCC Cancer Staging Manual. Springer, 2010: 419–60.
11. Weaver DL. Pathology evaluation of sentinel lymph nodes in breast cancer: protocol recommendations and rationale. Mod Pathol 2010; 23: S26–32.
12. Weaver DL, Ashikaga T, Krag DN, et al. Effect of occult metastases on survival in node-negative breast cancer. N Engl J Med 2011; 364: 412–21.
13. Goyal A, Mansel RE. Recent advances in sentinel lymph node biopsy for breast cancer. Curr Opin Oncol 2008; 20: 621–6.
14. Douglas-Jones AG, Woods V. Molecular assessment of sentinel lymph node in breast cancer management. Histopathology 2009; 55: 107–13.
15. Ellis I, Schnitt SJ, Sastre-Garau X, et al. Invasive breast carcinoma. In: Tavassoli FA, Devilee P, eds. Pathology & Genetics Tumours of the Breast and Female Genital Tract. Lyon: IARC Press, 2003: 13–59.
16. Wellings SR, Jensen HM, Marcum RG. An atlas of subgross pathology of the human breast with special reference to possible precancerous lesions. J Natl Cancer Inst 1975; 55: 231–73.
17. Boecker W, Buerger H. Evidence of progenitor cells of glandular and myoepithelial cell lineages in the human adult female breast epithelium: a new progenitor (adult stem) cell concept. Cell Prolif 2003; 36: 73–84.
18. Gupta SK, Douglas-Jones AG, Fenn N, Morgan JM, Mansel RE. The clinical behavior of breast carcinoma is probably determined at the preinvasive stage (ductal carcinoma in situ). Cancer 1997; 80: 1740–5.
19. Moll R, Mitze M, Frixen UH, Birchmeier W. Differential loss of E-cadherin expression in infiltrating ductal and lobular breast carcinomas. Am J Pathol 1993; 143: 1731–42.
20. Rakha EA, Abd El Rehim D, Pinder SE, Lewis SA, Ellis IO. E-cadherin expression in invasive non-lobular carcinoma of the breast and its prognostic significance. Histopathology 2005; 46: 685–93.
21. Gown AM. Current issues in ER and HER2 testing by IHC in breast cancer. Mod Pathol 2008; 21: S8–S15.
22. Diaz LK, Sneige N. Estrogen receptor analysis for breast cancer: current issues and keys to increasing testing accuracy. Adv Anat Pathol 2005; 12: 10–19.
23. Walker RA, Bartlett JM, Dowsett M, et al. HER2 testing in the UK: further update to recommendations. J Clin Pathol 2008; 61: 818–24.
24. Sorlie T, Perou CM, Tibshirani R, et al. Gene expression patterns of breast carcinomas distinguish tumor subclasses with clinical implications. Proc Natl Acad Sci USA 2001; 98: 10869–74.
25. Sotiriou C, Wirapati P, Loi S, et al. Gene expression profiling in breast cancer: understanding the molecular basis of histologic grade to improve prognosis. J Natl Cancer Inst 2006; 98: 262–72.
26. Rakha EA, Reis-Filho JS, Baehner F, et al. Breast cancer prognostic classification in the molecular era: the role of histological grade. Breast Cancer Res 2010; 12: 207.
27. Carter CL, Allen C, Henson DE. Relation of tumor size, lymph node status, and survival in 24,740 breast cancer cases. Cancer 1989; 63: 181–7.
28. Dixon JM, Anderson TJ, Page DL, Lee D, Duffy SW. Infiltrating lobular carcinoma of the breast. Histopathology 1982; 6: 149–61.
29. Colleoni M, Rotmensz N, Maisonneuve P, et al. Outcome of special types of luminal breast cancer. Ann Oncol 2012; 23: 1428.

30. Mann RM, Hoogeveen YL, Blickman JG, Boetes C. MRI compared to conventional diagnostic work-up in the detection and evaluation of invasive lobular carcinoma of the breast: a review of existing literature. Breast Cancer Res Treat 2008; 107: 1–14.

31. Mann RM, Veltman J, Barentsz JO, et al. The value of MRI compared to mammography in the assessment of tumour extent in invasive lobular carcinoma of the breast. Eur J Surg Oncol 2008; 34: 135–42.

32. Arpino G, Bardou VJ, Clark GM, Elledge RM. Infiltrating lobular carcinoma of the breast: tumor characteristics and clinical outcome. Breast Cancer Res 2004; 6: R149–56.

33. Vargas AC, Lakhani SR, Simpson PT. Pleomorphic lobular carcinoma of the breast: molecular pathology and clinical impact. Future Oncol 2009; 5: 233–43.

34. Esposito NN, Chivukula M, Dabbs DJ. The ductal phenotypic expression of the E-cadherin/catenin complex in tubulolobular carcinoma of the breast: an immunohistochemical and clinicopathologic study. Mod Pathol 2007; 20: 130–8.

35. Wheeler DT, Tai LH, Bratthauer GL, Waldner DL, Tavassoli FA. Tubulolobular carcinoma of the breast: an analysis of 27 cases of a tumor with a hybrid morphology and immunoprofile. Am J Surg Pathol 2004; 28: 1587–93.

36. Lopez-Garcia MA, Geyer FC, Lacroix-Triki M, Marchio C, Reis-Filho JS. Breast cancer precursors revisited: molecular features and progression pathways. Histopathology 2010; 57: 171–92.

37. Abdel-Fatah TM, Powe DG, Hodi Z, et al. Morphologic and molecular evolutionary pathways of low nuclear grade invasive breast cancers and their putative precursor lesions: further evidence to support the concept of low nuclear grade breast neoplasia family. Am J Surg Pathol 2008; 32: 513–23.

38. Weigelt B, Geyer FC, Natrajan R, et al. The molecular underpinning of lobular histological growth pattern: a genome-wide transcriptomic analysis of invasive lobular carcinomas and grade- and molecular subtype-matched invasive ductal carcinomas of no special type. J Pathol 2010; 220: 45–57.

39. Da Silva L, Parry S, Reid L, et al. Aberrant expression of E-cadherin in lobular carcinomas of the breast. Am J Surg Pathol 2008; 32: 773–83.

40. Dabbs DJ, Kaplai M, Chivukula M, et al. The spectrum of morphomolecular abnormalities of the E-cadherin/catenin complex in pleomorphic lobular carcinoma of the breast. Appl Immunohistochem Mol Morphol 2007; 15: 260–6.

41. Rakha EA, Patel A, Powe DG, et al. Clinical and biological significance of E-cadherin protein expression in invasive lobular carcinoma of the breast. Am J Surg Pathol 2010; 34: 1472–9.

42. Jacobs M, Fan F, Tawfik O. Clinicopathologic and biomarker analysis of invasive pleomorphic lobular carcinoma as compared with invasive classic lobular carcinoma: an experience in our institution and review of the literature. Ann Diagn Pathol 2012; 16: 185–9.

43. Orvieto E, Maiorano E, Bottiglieri L, et al. Clinicopathologic characteristics of invasive lobular carcinoma of the breast: results of an analysis of 530 cases from a single institution. Cancer 2008; 113: 1511–20.

44. Simpson PT, Reis-Filho JS, Lambros MB, et al. Molecular profiling pleomorphic lobular carcinomas of the breast: evidence for a common molecular genetic pathway with classic lobular carcinomas. J Pathol 2008; 215: 231–44.

45. Middleton LP, Palacios DM, Bryant BR, et al. Pleomorphic lobular carcinoma: morphology, immunohistochemistry, and molecular analysis. Am J Surg Pathol 2000; 24: 1650–6.

46. Louwman MW, Vriezen M, van Beek MW, et al. Uncommon breast tumors in perspective: incidence, treatment and survival in the Netherlands. Int J Cancer 2007; 121: 127–35.

47. Nagao T, Kinoshita T, Hojo T, et al. The differences in the histological types of breast cancer and the response to neoadjuvant chemotherapy: the relationship between the outcome and the clinicopathological characteristics. Breast 2012; 21: 289–95.

48. Rakha EA, Lee AH, Evans AJ, et al. Tubular carcinoma of the breast: further evidence to support its excellent prognosis. J Clin Oncol 2010; 28: 99–104.

49. Page DL, Dixon JM, Anderson TJ, Lee D, Stewart HJ. Invasive cribriform carcinoma of the breast. Histopathology 1983; 7: 525–36.

50. Di Saverio S, Gutierrez J, Avisar E. A retrospective review with long term follow up of 11,400 cases of pure mucinous breast carcinoma. Breast Cancer Res Treat 2008; 111: 541–7.

51. Lacroix-Triki M, Suarez PH, MacKay A, et al. Mucinous carcinoma of the breast is genomically distinct from invasive ductal carcinomas of no special type. J Pathol 2010; 222: 282–98.

52. Weigelt B, Geyer FC, Horlings HM, et al. Mucinous and neuroendocrine breast carcinomas are transcriptionally distinct from invasive ductal carcinomas of no special type. Mod Pathol 2009; 22: 1401–14.

53. Yu JI, Choi DH, Park W, et al. Differences in prognostic factors and patterns of failure between invasive micropapillary carcinoma and invasive ductal carcinoma: matched case-control study. Breast 2010; 19: 231–7.

54. Marchio C, Iravani M, Natrajan R, et al. Genomic and immunophenotypical characterisation of pure micropapillary carcinomas of the breast. J Pathol 2008; 215: 398–410.

55. Li YS, Kaneko M, Sakamoto DG, Takeshima Y, Inai K. The reversed apical pattern of MUC1 expression is characteristics of invasive micropapillary carcinoma of the breast. Breast Cancer 2006; 13: 58–63.

56. Marchio C, Iravani M, Natrajan R, et al. Mixed micropapillary-ductal carcinomas of the breast: a genomic and immunohistochemical analysis of morphologically distinct components. J Pathol 2009; 218: 301–15.

57. Collins LC, Schnitt SJ. Papillary lesions of the breast: selected diagnostic and management issues. Histopathology 2008; 52: 20–9.

58. Duprez R, Wilkerson PM, Lacroix-Triki M, et al. Immunophenotypic and genomic characterization of papillary carcinomas of the breast. J Pathol 2011; 226: 427–41.

59. Pal SK, Lau SK, Kruper L, et al. Papillary carcinoma of the breast: an overview. Breast Cancer Res Treat 2010; 122: 637–45.

60. Collins LC, Carlo VP, Hwang H, et al. Intracystic papillary carcinoma of the breast: a reevaluation using a panel of myoepithelial cell markers. Am J Surg Pathol 2006; 30: 1002–7.

61. Rakha EA, Gandhi N, Climent F, et al. Encapsulated papillary carcinoma of the breast: an invasive tumor with excellent prognosis. Am J Surg Pathol 2011; 35: 1093–103.

62. Wynveen CA, Nehhozina T, Akram M, et al. Intracystic papillary carcinoma of the breast: An in situ or invasive tumor? Results of immunohistochemical analysis and clinical follow-up. Am J Surg Pathol 2011; 35: 1–14.

63. Nassar H, Qureshi H, Adsay NV, Visscher D. Clinicopathologic analysis of solid papillary carcinoma of the breast and associated invasive carcinomas. Am J Surg Pathol 2006; 30: 501–7.

64. Makretsov N, Gilks CB, Coldman AJ, Hayes M, Huntsman D. Tissue microarray analysis of neuroendocrine differentiation and its prognostic significance in breast cancer. Hum Pathol 2003; 34: 1001–8.

65. Rosen PP. Small cell (Oat Cell) carcinoma. In: Rosen PP, ed. Rosen's Breast Pathology. Lippincott Williams & Wilkins, 2009: 556–62.

66. Farmer P, Bonnefoi H, Becette V, et al. Identification of molecular apocrine breast tumours by microarray analysis. Oncogene 2005; 24: 4660–71.

67. Vranic S, Tawfik O, Palazzo J, et al. EGFR and HER-2/neu expression in invasive apocrine carcinoma of the breast. Mod Pathol 2010; 23: 644–53.

68. Ridolfi RL, Rosen PP, Port A, Kinne D, Mike V. Medullary carcinoma of the breast: a clinicopathologic study with 10 year follow-up. Cancer 1977; 40: 1365–85.

69. Rakha EA, Aleskandarany M, El-Sayed ME, et al. The prognostic significance of inflammation and medullary histological type in invasive carcinoma of the breast. Eur J Cancer 2009; 45: 1780–7.

70. Jacquemier J, Padovani L, Rabayrol L, et al. Typical medullary breast carcinomas have a basal/myoepithelial phenotype. J Pathol 2005; 207: 260–8.

71. Armes JE, Egan AJ, Southey MC, et al. The histologic phenotypes of breast carcinoma occurring before age 40 years in women with and without BRCA1 or BRCA2 germline mutations: a population-based study. Cancer 1998; 83: 2335–45.

72. Eisinger F, Jacquemier J, Charpin C, et al. Mutations at BRCA1: the medullary breast carcinoma revisited. Cancer Res 1998; 58: 1588–92.

73. Yap TA, Sandhu SK, Carden CP, de Bono JS. Poly(ADP-ribose) polymerase (PARP) inhibitors: exploiting a synthetic lethal strategy in the clinic. CA Cancer J Clin 2011; 61: 31–49.

74. Rosen PP. Squamous carcinoma. In: Rosen PP, ed. Rosen's Breast Pathology. Lippincott Williams & Wilkins, 2009: 506–14.

75. Hennessy BT, Krishnamurthy S, Giordano S, et al. Squamous cell carcinoma of the breast. J Clin Oncol 2005; 23: 7827–35.

76. Reis-Filho JS, Milanezi F, Steele D, et al. Metaplastic breast carcinomas are basal-like tumours. Histopathology 2006; 49: 10–21.

77. Tse GM, Tan PH, Putti TC, et al. Metaplastic carcinoma of the breast: a clinicopathological review. J Clin Pathol 2006; 59: 1079–83.

78. Denley H, Pinder SE, Tan PH, et al. Metaplastic carcinoma of the breast arising within complex sclerosing lesion: a report of five cases. Histopathology 2000; 36: 203–9.

79. Van Hoeven KH, Drudis T, Cranor ML, Erlandson RA, Rosen PP. Low-grade adenosquamous carcinoma of the breast. A clinocopathologic study of 32 cases with ultrastructural analysis. Am J Surg Pathol 1993; 17: 248–58.

80. Geyer FC, Lambros MB, Natrajan R, et al. Genomic and immunohistochemical analysis of adenosquamous carcinoma of the breast. Mod Pathol 2010; 23: 951–60.

81. Sneige N, Yaziji H, Mandavilli SR, et al. Low-grade (fibromatosis-like) spindle cell carcinoma of the breast. Am J Surg Pathol 2001; 25: 1009–16.

82. Adem C, Reynolds C, Adlakha H, Roche PC, Nascimento AG. Wide spectrum screening keratin as a marker of metaplastic spindle cell carcinoma of the breast: an immunohistochemical study of 24 patients. Histopathology 2002; 40: 556–62.

83. Weigelt B, Kreike B, Reis-Filho JS. Metaplastic breast carcinomas are basal-like breast cancers: a genomic profiling analysis. Breast Cancer Res Treat 2009; 117: 273–80.

84. Bae SY, Lee SK, Koo MY, et al. The prognoses of metaplastic breast cancer patients compared to those of triple-negative breast cancer patients. Breast Cancer Res Treat 2011; 126: 471–8.

85. Arpino G, Clark GM, Mohsin S, Bardou VJ, Elledge RM. Adenoid cystic carcinoma of the breast: molecular markers, treatment, and clinical outcome. Cancer 2002; 94: 2119–27.

86. Boujelbene N, Khabir A, Jeanneret Sozzi W, Mirimanoff RO, Khanfir K. Clinical review - Breast adenoid cystic carcinoma. Breast 2012; 21: 124–7.

87. Pia-Foschini M, Reis-Filho JS, Eusebi V, Lakhani SR. Salivary gland-like tumours of the breast: surgical and molecular pathology. J Clin Pathol 2003; 56: 497–506.

88. Wetterskog D, Lopez-Garcia MA, Lambros MB, et al. Adenoid cystic carcinomas constitute a genomically distinct subgroup of triple-negative and basal-like breast cancers. J Pathol 2011; 226: 84–96.

89. Shi P, Wang M, Zhang Q, Sun J. Lipid-rich carcinoma of the breast. A clinicopathological study of 49 cases. Tumori 2008; 94: 342–6.

90. Guan B, Wang H, Cao S, et al. Lipid-rich carcinoma of the breast clinicopathologic analysis of 17 cases. Ann Diagn Pathol 2011; 15: 225–32.

91. Reis-Filho JS, Fulford LG, Lakhani SR, Schmitt FC. Pathologic quiz case: a 62-year-old woman with a 4.5-cm nodule in the right breast. Lipid-rich breast carcinoma. Arch Pathol Lab Med 2003; 127: e396–8.

92. Rosen PP. Glycogen-rich carcinoma. In: Rosen PP, ed. Rosen's Breast Pathology. Lippincott Williams & Wilkins, 2009: 612–15.

93. Vasudev P, Onuma K. Secretory breast carcinoma: unique, triple-negative carcinoma with a favorable prognosis and characteristic molecular expression. Arch Pathol Lab Med 2011; 135: 1606–10.

94. Lae M, Freneaux P, Sastre-Garau X, et al. Secretory breast carcinomas with ETV6-NTRK3 fusion gene belong to the basal-like carcinoma spectrum. Mod Pathol 2009; 22: 291–8.

95. Guerry P, Erlandson RA, Rosen PP. Cystic hypersecretory hyperplasia and cystic hypersecretory duct carcinoma of the breast. Pathology, therapy, and follow-up of 39 patients. Cancer 1988; 61: 1611–20.

96. Shin SJ, Rosen PP. Carcinoma arising from preexisting pregnancy-like and cystic hypersecretory hyperplasia lesions of the breast: a clinicopathologic study of 9 patients. Am J Surg Pathol 2004; 28: 789–93.

97. Skalova A, Ryska A, Kajo K, et al. Cystic hypersecretory carcinoma: rare and poorly recognized variant of intraductal carcinoma of the breast. Report of five cases. Histopathology 2005; 46: 43–9.

98. Ellis IO, Lee AH, Elston CW, Pinder SE. Microinvasive carcinoma of the breast: diagnostic criteria and clinical relevance. Histopathology 1999; 35: 470–2.

99. Rosen PP. Paget's disease of the nipple. In: Rosen PP, ed. Rosen's Breast Pathology. Lippincott Williams & Wilkins, 2009: 621–36.

100. Caliskan M, Gatti G, Sosnovskikh I, et al. Paget's disease of the breast: the experience of the European Institute of Oncology and review of the literature. Breast Cancer Res Treat 2008; 112: 513–21.

101. Eusebi V, Mai KT, Taranger-Charpin A. Tumours of the nipple. In: Tavassoli FA, Devilee P, eds. Pathology & Genetics Tumours of the Breast and Female Genital Tract. Lyon: IARC Press, 2003: 104–6.

102. Sek P, Zawrocki A, Biernat W, Piekarski JH. HER2 molecular subtype is a dominant subtype of mammary Paget's cells. An immunohistochemical study. Histopathology 2010; 57: 564–71.

103. Ashikari R, Park K, Huvos AG, Urban JA. Paget's disease of the breast. Cancer 1970; 26: 680–5.

104. Dominici LS, Lester S, Liao GS, et al. Current surgical approach to Paget's disease. Am J Surg 2012; 204: 18–22.

105. Zakaria S, Pantvaidya G, Ghosh K, Degnim AC. Paget's disease of the breast: accuracy of preoperative assessment. Breast Cancer Res Treat 2007; 102: 137–42.

106. Robertson FM, Bondy M, Yang W, et al. Inflammatory breast cancer: the disease, the biology, the treatment. CA Cancer J Clin 2010; 60: 351–75.

107. Buzdar AU. Preoperative chemotherapy treatment of breast cancer–a review. Cancer 2007; 110: 2394–407.

108. Dowsett M, A'Hern R, Salter J, Zabaglo L, Smith IE. Who would have thought a single Ki67 measurement would predict long-term outcome? Breast Cancer Res 2009; 11:S15.

109. Pinder SE, Provenzano E, Earl H, Ellis IO. Laboratory handling and histology reporting of breast specimens from patients who have received neoadjuvant chemotherapy. Histopathology 2007; 50: 409–17.

110. Oh JL, Nguyen G, Whitman GJ, et al. Placement of radiopaque clips for tumor localization in patients undergoing neoadjuvant chemotherapy and breast conservation therapy. Cancer 2007; 110: 2420–7.

111. Thomas JS, Julian HS, Green RV, Cameron DA, Dixon MJ. Histopathology of breast carcinoma following neoadjuvant systemic therapy: a common association between letrozole therapy and central scarring. Histopathology 2007; 51: 219–26.

112. Aktepe F, Kapucuoglu N, Pak I. The effects of chemotherapy on breast cancer tissue in locally advanced breast cancer. Histopathology 1996; 29: 63–7.

113. Ogston KN, Miller ID, Payne S, et al. A new histological grading system to assess response of breast cancers to primary chemotherapy: prognostic significance and survival. Breast 2003; 12: 320–7.

114. Symmans WF, Peintinger F, Hatzis C, et al. Measurement of residual breast cancer burden to predict survival after neoadjuvant chemotherapy. J Clin Oncol 2007; 25: 4414–22.

115. Chollet P, Amat S, Belembaogo E, et al. Is Nottingham prognostic index useful after induction chemotherapy in operable breast cancer? Br J Cancer 2003; 89: 1185–91.

116. Carey LA, Metzger R, Dees EC, et al. American Joint Committee on Cancer tumor-node-metastasis stage after neoadjuvant chemotherapy and breast cancer outcome. J Natl Cancer Inst 2005; 97: 1137–42.

117. Girling AC, Hanby AM, Millis RR. Radiation and other pathological changes in breast tissue after conservation treatment for carcinoma. J Clin Pathol 1990; 43: 152–6.

118. Lee AH. The histological diagnosis of metastases to the breast from extramammary malignancies. J Clin Pathol 2007; 60: 1333–41.

119. Lamovec J, Wotherspoon A, Jacquemier J. Malignant lymphoma and metastatic tumours. In: Tavassoli FA, Devilee P, eds. Pathology & Genetics Tumours of the Breast and Female Genital Organs. Lyon: IARC Press, 2003: 107–9.

120. Tot T. Cytokeratins 20 and 7 as biomarkers: usefulness in discriminating primary from metastatic adenocarcinoma. Eur J Cancer 2002; 38: 758–63.

121. Reis LO, Dias FG, Castro MA, Ferreira U. Male breast cancer. Aging Male 2011; 14: 99–109.

122. Shaaban AM, Ball GR, Brannan RA, et al. A comparative biomarker study of 514 matched cases of male and female breast cancer reveals gender-specific biological differences. Breast Cancer Res Treat 2012; 133: 949–58.

123. Agrawal A, Ayantunde AA, Rampaul R, Robertson JF. Male breast cancer: a review of clinical management. Breast Cancer Res Treat 2007; 103: 11–21.

124. Ge Y, Sneige N, Eltorky MA, et al. Immunohistochemical characterization of subtypes of male breast carcinoma. Breast Cancer Res 2009; 11: R28.

125. Kornegoor R, Verschuur-Maes AH, Buerger H, et al. Molecular subtyping of male breast cancer by immunohistochemistry. Mod Pathol 2012; 25: 398–404.

29 Molecular investigation of breast cancer

Paul M. Wilkerson and J.S. Reis-Filho

INTRODUCTION

It is now widely recognized that breast cancer is a very heterogeneous disease. However, this concept is a fairly recent one; although breast cancer has been broadly classified into an estrogen receptor (ER)-positive and-negative disease (1), based on ER expression and following development of endocrine therapies in the 1970s, it was not until seminal transcriptomic studies (2–7) that the magnitude of this heterogeneity was revealed. In fact, breast cancer is now no longer viewed as a single disease, but as a collection of disparate diseases, with distinct risk factors, histopathological and molecular features, clinical behavior, and response to therapies. However, these all arise in the same microanatomical structure (i.e., the terminal duct-lobular unit) (1,8–11).

The categories of ER-positive and ER-negative breast cancers are heterogeneous at the molecular level; for example, multiple molecular subtypes of ER-negative breast cancer have been described (1,2,8–11), whose clinical significance remains to be determined. By contrast, ER-positive breast cancers form a continuum, with tumors at one end having a good prognosis and characterized by low histological grade, low proliferation rates, simple karyotypes, low levels of genomic instability, deletions of 16q, and recurrent mutations of *PIK3CA*. Tumors at the other end of the spectrum have a poor prognosis, are of high histological grade, have complex karyotypes and high levels of genetic instability, and often harbor mutations in key tumor suppressor genes (e.g., TP53) (12–17).

Despite this leap in the understanding of the molecular landscape of breast cancer, its management remains guided by a collection of histopathologically divined prognostic markers and three predictive markers [i.e., ER, progesterone receptor (PR), and HER2]. Clinical decision making guidelines or algorithms are then defined by these features (15,18–21). Although this approach has proven successful, leading to a decline in breast cancer-related mortality, the parameters only provide information for an "average" patient, and are of limited use in the implementation of personalized medicine.

The realization of personalized medicine for breast cancer will require a further paradigm shift, one that is under way. In this chapter, we will discuss the molecular techniques currently being utilized in the characterization of breast cancer. An overview of the methodology and available platforms will set the scene for a discussion of the current and future applications, and how these can help realize the transition from a largely prognostic classification system for breast cancer to a predictive model, employing biomarkers to define subpopulations of patients that are likely to respond to a given therapy.

BREAST CANCER GENOMICS
DNA Copy Number Profiling

The development of microarray technology has allowed the determination of DNA copy number in cancer to move from assessment of single loci or large chromosomal regions (22) to high-resolution genome-wide copy number profiling in a single experiment (23). Microarray-based comparative genomic hybridization (aCGH) allows for DNA copy number profiling to be performed on samples extracted from both frozen and paraffin-embedded tumor material. Essentially, in this technique, test and reference DNA are differentially labeled and then hybridized to an array of probes on a slide (e.g., bacterial artificial chromosomes, oligonucleotides, or complementary DNA probes). Slides are then scanned to produce an image of differential signal intensities. In dual-color assays, the normalized ratios of these intensities for each probe allow a genome-wide semiquantitative assessment of copy number changes at each locus in the genome (24). Single nucleotide polymorphism (SNP) arrays are made up of hundreds of thousands of oligonucleotide probes mapped to known polymorphisms and can be used to determine the relative prevalence of SNPs in a sample (e.g., the Affymetrix SNP array v6.0 contains over 900,000 SNPs as well as over 900,000 probes targeting known copy number variations), allowing the assessment of genotype and copy number silent loss of heterozygosity (i.e., SNP arrays). However, no microarray platform can detect polyploidy or balanced chromosomal translocations (24,25).

SNP arrays have been utilized in genome-wide association studies (GWAS) to identify disease-associated SNPs. Here, a disease bearing cohort is compared with a matched cohort of normal individuals and the relative prevalence of each SNP is compared between cohorts. Studies employing this approach have led to the identification of SNPs that confer an increased risk of developing breast cancer (26–33). Although the contribution of GWAS studies is unquestioned, some concerns have been voiced. The relative contribution of each SNP to the heritable risk of disease has thus far been small (34,35). Furthermore, a substantial proportion of potential disease-causing SNPs found to date map to noncoding regions (26–33). Finally, the massive number of statistical comparisons required in the analysis presents a huge potential for false-positive results (34,35).

Microarray technology is subject to a large degree of variability, due partly to differences in DNA extraction methods, probe labeling and hybridization, platform type, the number and type of sample used and the analysis/validation methods utilized (36). These issues must be taken into account when designing aCGH-based studies or when analyzing aCGH data from multiple publically available sources. A summary of the available platforms, their applications, advantages, and limitations are shown in Table 29.1.

Notwithstanding the challenges presented by the inherent variability and panoply of platforms, aCGH and its derivatives have led to a number of advances in our understanding of breast cancer, some with direct translational relevance. At the most fundamental level, studies of the pattern of copy number aberrations (CNAs) have demonstrated that ER-positive and ER-negative breast cancer are fundamentally distinct at the molecular level (37–42). Thus, while concurrent deletions of 16q and gains of 1q are a common event in ER-positive breast cancer (80% grade 1 and 50% grade 3), they are extremely rare in ER-negative breast cancer (38). Indeed, when present in ER-negative breast cancer, 16q loss is related to the deletion of chromosome 16, whereas in ER-positive disease the result of an unbalanced chromosomal translocation [i.e., der(16) t(1;16)/der(1;16)] (14,38,43,44). Although progression from ER-positive to ER-negative breast cancer is therefore unlikely to occur, given the two subtypes of breast cancer are distinct at the genetic level, progression from grade 1 to 3 breast cancer has been described (14,38). It is likely to be caused by the acquisition of genetic aberrations, including amplification at 8p11.2, 11q13-q14, 17q21, 17q23.2, and 20q13 (37–41,45).

Given the marked morphological heterogeneity of breast cancer, with the existence of 17 special histological types, it is unsurprising that this is often underpinned by distinct patterns of CNAs. By studying special histological types of breast cancer, and thus reducing the complexity of the study population a priori, distinct patterns of CNAs were identified in micropapillary, adenosquamous, mucinous, and mitochondrion-rich breast carcinomas (46–49). These studies have provided an incremental step toward a molecular taxonomy for breast cancer, which will be discussed further in the coming sections.

Copy number profiling has also provided leads on novel therapeutic strategies as well. For example, genome-wide copy number profiling of primary breast carcinomas and breast cancer cell lines identified frequent amplification at 8p12-p11.2 (10% of breast carcinomas), encompassing *FGFR1* (50–55). Preclinical functional validation of the driver nature of *FGFR1* amplification (50,52) (and its role in endocrine resistance (52)) has provided a rationale for a randomized double-blind phase IIa trial of the FGFR inhibitor AZD4547 with or without exemestane in patients with *FGFR1*-amplified breast carcinomas (ClinicalTrials.gov identifier NCT01202591). Integrative analyses of aCGH data and gene expression profiling data have also led to the identification of *FGFR2* (56) and *PPM1D* (37) as genes that are frequently amplified and overexpressed in breast cancer. Once again, functional validation has led to drug development programs and, in the case of patients with *FGFR2* amplification, phase II trials in patients with metastatic endometrial (ClinicalTrials.gov identifier NCT01244438) and gastric carcinomas (ClinicalTrials.gov identifier NCT01457846), as well as a phase I trial in advanced solid malignancies using a novel pan-FGFR inhibitor (ClinicalTrials.gov identifier NCT01004224) and a phase I trial in metastatic breast cancer using a dual VEGF and FGFR inhibitor, dovitinib (ClinicalTrials.gov identifier NCT01484041).

Integrative genomic and transcriptomic studies have demonstrated that amplicons often harbor more than one candidate driver gene. This is exemplified by the 17q12 amplicon encompassing *HER2*. Two other genes at this locus, *STARD3* and *GRB7*, have been shown to have a causal role in breast cancer development (57). The complex structure of the 8p12-p11.2 amplicon has also yielded further potential drivers and therapeutic targets. By assessing their transforming ability of MCF10A cells and using the contrasting approach of RNA interference in cell lines harboring the 8p12-p11.2 amplicon, multiple authors have identified *LSM1*, *BAG4*, *C8orf4*, *DDHD2*, *WHSC1L1*, and *PPAPDC1B* as breast cancer oncogenes within this amplicon (55,58,59). Of these candidates, *PPAPDC1B*, a transmembrane protein phosphatase, makes an attractive therapeutic target.

Of late, different phenotypes have been used as readouts in the search for amplicon drivers, including predictive markers of therapeutic resistance. One such example is *LAPTM4B* encoded at 8q22, a frequently amplified and overexpressed gene in breast cancer (60) which was found to be associated with resistance to anthracyclines, acting as a promoter of drug efflux (60,61). In fact, *LAPTM4B* was later found to also increase proliferation when overexpressed, (by promoting autophagy and stress tolerance) (62) thus, making this a potential therapeutic target not only for inhibiting tumor growth, but also modulating the response to conventional chemotherapy.

Massively Parallel DNA Sequencing

Despite the success of aCGH in cancer research, it remains a fairly blunt screening tool that provides only a rough genomic map. Regardless of the resolution, aCGH will never be able to provide information on complex modifications of regulatory or epigenetic elements, or on the presence of translocations and gene fusions that are represented by the detected copy number changes. With the rapidly falling cost of massively parallel sequencing [or next-generation sequencing (NGS)] technologies, aCGH (regardless of platform) will eventually become obsolete (63,64). Indeed, protocols and algorithms are already available both for the use of NGS for copy number assessment (65) and in the sequencing of DNA extracted from formalin-fixed paraffin-embedded (FFPE) tissues (66), making it readily applicable to clinical samples. At present, however, only targeted exome sequencing of limited sets of oncogenes has been reported for FFPE tissues (66), while whole genome coverage-based assessment of copy number has only been applied to cancer cell lines (67,68) and fresh frozen tissue (69).

First-generation (Sanger) sequencing has the inherent disadvantages of being limited to targeted sequencing of known genomic sequences, and requiring the process of electrophoresis for separation of sequences. The advent of second-generation (NGS) sequencing eliminates these limitations, allowing whole genomes to be sequenced at base pair resolution in a much more cost effective way (a whole genome can now be sequenced for approximately US$4000 at 30–40 times coverage (70)). With the falling costs and promise of a US$1000 genome in the near future (71), this technology (or a derivative) is likely to replace microarrays in characterization of cancer for diagnostic, prognostic, and predictive purposes (63,64).

Table 29.1 Currently Available Microarray Platforms

Platform	Types	Applications	Advantages	Limitations
aCGH	cDNA	Copy number gains and losses (BAC arrays optimal for single copy number gain) Amplifications and deletions	Cheap	Low sensitivity/resolution Limited types of input DNA
	BAC		Robust technology Suitable for FFPE samples Can use BACs in in situ assays for validation Established analytical pipelines	Limited commercial suppliers Challenging chip production High level copy numbers may be underestimated
	Agilent (spotted oligonuleotide) NimbleGen (photolitho-graph oligonucleotide)		High resolution Easy production High probe specificity	Requires good quality input DNA Detection of low level copy number gains and losses can be troublesome
	Affymetrix (photolithogra-phy, SNP array) Illumina (SNP bead array)	Above plus copy number neutral LOH GWAS	High resolution Easy production High probe specificity Provides allelic information	Number gains and losses can be troublesome
	MIP (spotted oligonuleotides)		Very accurate copy number analysis Suitable for FFPE samples Small amounts of input DNA required	Challenging protocol optimization Limited resolution
Gene expression arrays	cDNA microarrays	Transcriptome-wide gene expression analysis	Cheap	Early in-house platform Not commercially available
	Illumina HT12 (BeadArray)		BeadArray format allows for improved hybridization efficiency	Dynamic range narrower Considerable variability between platforms from different companies precludes comparisons
	Affymetrix HG-U133 Plus 2.0		Robust platform More bioinformatic tools freely available	Considerable variability between platforms from different companies precludes comparisons
	Agilent 244K		One and two-color assays available (can co-hybridize with normal sample) Can custom design your own arrays specific to your needs	
	NimbleGen oligonucleotide arrays 12 × 135K, 385K, or 4 × 72K		Long oligos (60mer) allows superior SNR, increased sensitivity and discrimination	
Methylation arrays	Infinium bead array - Bisul-fite DNA treatment	Genome wide DNA methylation status EWAS	Economical, automatable Good resolution (but not as good as that of massively parallel sequencing-based technologies)	Unable to distinguish methylated from hydroxy-methylated cytosine bases Many CpG sites not profiled
	HELP-chip - methylation sensitive restriction enzymes CHARM – methylation sensitive restriction enzymes		Identify hypo- or hypermethyl-ated CpG sites	Moderate resolution Limited to restriction enzyme digestion sites
	MethylCap-chip – affinity enrichment MBD-chip – affinity enrichment MeDIP-chip – affinity enrichment		Efficient assays to CGIs and repetitive sequences	Many CpG sites not profiled Less sensitive to CpG poor sites Dependent on MBD binding

Abbreviations: aCGH, microarray-based comparative genomic hybridization; cDNA, complementary DNA; BAC, bacterial artificial chromosome; CHARM, comprehensive high-throughput relative methylation; CGI, Genomic Grade Index; EWAS, epigenome-wide association studies; FFPE, formalin fixed paraffin embedded; GWAS, Genome-wide association studies; HELP, *Hpa*II tiny fragment enrichment by ligation-mediated PCR; LOH, loss of heterozygosity; MBD, methyl binding domain proteins; MeDIP, methyl DNA immunoprecipitation; MethylCap, methyl capture; MIP, molecular inversion probe; SNP, single nucleotide polymorphism; SNR, signal to noise ration.

A number of platforms are commercially available for massively parallel DNA sequencing, each with their own inherent advantages and disadvantages over each other (Table 29.2, for reviews see (72–81)). Each platform can be used for whole genome sequencing or, using exon capture kits in the library construction, for targeted or whole exome sequencing of DNA from fresh frozen tumors or cancer cell lines. Since 2008, a growing number of cancer genomes have been sequenced, together with their germ-line DNA to identify cancer-specific aberrations (see Ref. (81) for comprehensive summary). Collectively, to date, these studies have constituted a comprehensive catalogue of somatic mutations and rearrangements in cancer genomes.

This torrent of data has, first and foremost, eloquently demonstrated that cancers are far more genomically complex than first perceived and are made up of a mosaic of clonal populations (82,83). This multiclonality likely contributes to the clonal evolution of cancer genomes during the progression of the disease from primary tumor to relapse (84,85) and following interventions (such as chemotherapy and/or radiotherapy) (86). Whole genome sequencing has also revealed the high prevalence of structural rearrangements in solid cancers (82,87–89). However, the majority of fusions identified map to intergenic regions, suggesting they may be passenger events, and those that are expressed and in-frame tend to be private events (i.e., only identified in the index case). The concept of functional recurrence may rationalize this phenomenon (90), whereby different mechanisms may lead to the same phenotypic effect on a protein or pathway in different cancers (e.g., homozygous deletion in one case, inactivating mutations in another, disrupting rearrangement in a third, promoter methylation in a fourth etc., or even multiple members of a pathway being activated or inactivated in different tumors by different mechanisms).

PI3K-AKT-mTOR Pathway: Therapeutic Avenues for ER-Positive/Luminal Breast Cancers

Functioning downstream of growth factor receptor tyrosine kinases, the phosphatidylinositol 3-kinase (PI3K)-AKT-mammalian target of rapamycin (mTOR) signaling pathway (PI3K pathway) has important roles in proliferation, survival, growth, and motility (91). Although mutations in *PIK3CA* are the most frequent aberration of this pathway in breast cancers (20–40% of all invasive breast cancers (13,92–100)), several other components of the PI3K pathway are reported to be altered in breast cancer, including *AKT1* mutation, *HER2* amplification, and PTEN loss of function (101,102). *PIK3CA* mutations lead to an elevated enzymatic activity of PI3K, increased activation of the downstream signaling cascade, and induction of oncogenic transformation (103). In breast cancer, *PIK3CA* mutations have a reported prevalence of 21.3% (13.3% of catalytic domain and 8.0% of other domains) and are reported to be enriched in ER-positive breast cancers (34.5%) compared with triple-negative tumors (8.3%, (93)). Independent studies have confirmed a high frequency of *PIK3CA* mutations in ER-positive cancers (13,101,102) (http://www.sanger.ac.uk/search?db=cosmic&t= pik3ca). By contrast to other oncogenes whose mutations are associated with breast cancers of aggressive clinical behavior, and consistent with in vitro data showing that *PIK3CA* mutations increase the sensitivity of cancer cell lines to tamoxifen (104), *PIK3CA* mutations in ER-positive tamoxifen-treated patients are associated with a lower rate of node-positive disease (96) and a better outcome (13,105).

Notably, mutations in other components of PI3K pathway are less frequent in breast cancer. For example, *PTEN* and *AKT1* mutations have been identified in 2.3% and 1.4% of breast cancers, respectively (93). Unsurprisingly, *AKT1* mutations in ER-positive cancers are associated with a good outcome (93), a finding stemming from the fact that they seem to cause a similar gene expression pattern as *PIK3CA* mutations (13). Loss of PTEN expression in breast cancer (8–48% of breast cancers (106,107)) is more prevalent than *PTEN* mutation, and loss of PTEN expression is associated with ER-negative, in particular, triple-negative phenotype (108–111).

Aberrant PI3K pathway signaling represents a convergent phenotype, for which gene expression signatures have been developed (13) and classify patients as good outcome groups if PI3K pathway is activated. As expected, the survival of gene signature-mutant patients was similar to that of patients having ER-positive/HER2-negative/low-proliferation tumors (i.e., luminal A) and better than the one of ER-positive/

Table 29.2 Commercially Available Second-Generation Sequencing Technologies

Sequencing Platform	454 Ti Roche™	Illumina HiSeq™ 2000	ABI 5500	Complete Genomics
Amplification	Emulsion PCR	Bridge PCR	Emulsion PCR	PCR on DNA nanoballs
Sequence reaction	Pyrosequencing	Reverse terminator	Ligation sequencing	Combinatorial probe-anchor ligation
Read length (bp)	400	100	75	35
Run time (days)	0.4	4[a], 8[b]	3.5[a], 7[b]	12
Data yield (Gb)	0.5	150–200	90	200
Advantages	Short run times. Longer reads improve mapping in repetitive regions. Can detect large SVs	Most popular platform	Good base calling accuracy. Good multiplexing capabilities	Low error rate. Analysis and management handled by company
Disadvantages	High reagent cost. Higher error rate in repeat sequences	Short reads may miss large SVs. Low multiplexing capabilities	Short read length	Large amount of input DNA needed. Whole genome DNA sequencing only

[a]Single-end runs. [b]Paired-end runs.
Abbreviations: Gb, gigabyte of data; SVs, structural variants.

HER2-negative/high-proliferation tumors (i.e., luminal B). This is likely due to the suggestion that the worse prognosis of luminal B tumors may be underpinned by increased activity of growth factor receptors, which are upstream of PI3K (112,113). The effects of PI3K pathway activation are clearly context dependent, given the lack of correlation with outcome when this PIK3CA signature is applied to HER2-positive and ER-negative/HER2-negative subgroups of patients.

Although a gene signature has been developed to define PTEN loss of function and shown to be an independent predictor of outcome in tumors of the breast and other organs (106), it remains to be determined whether the prognostic power of this signature merely stems from the enrichment for tumors with a triple-negative phenotype in the subgroup assigned as PTEN loss of function group.

The clinical utility of gene expression signatures predicting the status of the PI3K pathway is currently debated, given the reported discordance in PI3K pathway aberrations between tumor samples of the same patient. For example, high levels of discordance in PTEN levels and PIK3CA mutations between primary tumors and metastases have been reported (114), while increased PI3K activation has been identified in recurrences of patients with ER-positive breast cancer treated with tamoxifen (115). Therefore, analysis of the primary tumor alone may not provide sufficiently accurate information to determine whether a patient will benefit from PI3K pathway inhibitors, and further studies to determine the differences in PIK3CA and PTEN status between primary tumors, circulating tumor cells, and metastases are warranted.

There is considerable heterogeneity both in the degree to which specific aberrations cause activation of the PI3K pathway and in the response to different inhibitors of the PI3K pathway. Thus, while PIK3CA mutations are only weak activators of the PI3K pathway (13,93,116), PTEN loss of function appears to result in more robust pathway activation (13,93). Some investigators have identified PIK3CA mutation as a predictive biomarker for response to PI3K pathway inhibitors (including the allosteric mTORC1 inhibitor everolimus, active-site mTORC1/mTORC2 kinase inhibitors (e.g., PP242), dual PI3K/mTOR inhibitors (BEZ235), and PI3K inhibitors (CH5132799) (117–119)) but not PTEN loss of function. Conversely, other groups have found that PIK3CA mutations are not predictive of response to rapamycin (13), or that loss of PTEN expression rather than PIK3CA mutation predicts response to the small-molecule PI3K inhibitor LY294002 (93). Further studies are required to determine the actual constellation of predictive markers of response to PI3K and mTOR inhibitors in breast cancer. It is possible that the predictive markers of response to PI3K inhibition may depend not only on the molecular features of the tumor type, but also on the type of PI3K or mTOR inhibitor used (120).

Despite these uncertainties surrounding the complex biology of the PI3K pathway, mTOR inhibitors, in particular rapamycin analogs (i.e., everolimus and temsirolimus), have been incorporated into breast cancer clinical trials (121–127) including phase III studies. Phase II studies have concluded that these drugs display antitumor activity with tolerable adverse effects (123,126,127). The phase III clinical trial BOLERO-2, which assessed progression-free survival following the addition of everolimus to exemestane in patients with metastatic ER-positive/HER2-negative breast cancer refractory to prior endocrine therapy with nonsteroidal aromatase inhibitors was halted after a positive interim analysis revealed that the regimen significantly extended progression-free survival compared with placebo plus exemestane [10.6 months compared to 4.1 months, HR 0.36 (0.27–0.47), p < 0.001] (128). It is envisaged that the tumor samples from this trial will provide an optimal dataset to determine the real predictive markers of response to this mTOR inhibitor in the ER-positive/HER2-negative subgroup of breast cancer patients.

BREAST CANCER EPIGENOMICS

The term "epigenetics" is used to encompass changes in DNA methylation, histone modification, microRNA (miRNA) expression, nucleosome positioning, and higher order chromatin and how they affect gene expression (129). Critically, these epigenetic changes do not alter the genomic sequence of a cell, and provide a further layer of transcriptional control that, until recently, has not been well studied. With the advent of new tools allowing genome-wide assessment of epigenetic changes, rapid advances have been made in our understanding of the epigenetic landscape of breast cancer (129,130). Despite this, translation of these findings to clinically effective treatments has been slow. It is hoped that the efforts of the NIH Epigenome Project (http://commonfund.nih.gov/epigenomics/overview.aspx) and The Cancer Genome Atlas (http://tcga-data.nci.nih.gov/tcga/) in breast cancer epigenomics will provide a platform for the development of more effective classification and treatment of patients with breast cancer, whereby genetic and epigenetic data will be integrated. Importantly, mutations affecting genes that control the epigenetic machinery in cancer cells have been identified by means of massively parallel sequencing, including mutations in DNA methyl transferases (e.g., DNMT3A mutations in acute myeloid leukemia (131–133)), in members of the SWI–SNF complex (e.g., ARID1A in breast cancers (134,135), granulosa cell (136), or clear cell (137) tumors of the ovary and gastric cancers (138)) and of the miRNA processing machinery (e.g., DICER1 mutations in non-epithelial ovarian cancers (139)). Hence, it remains to be determined whether the global epigenomic alterations in a cancer are underpinned by genetic aberrations.

DNA Methylation in Breast Cancer

Post-translational modification of cytosine to 5-methylcytosine in the context of CpG dinucleotides accounts for approximately 1% of all bases. In normal tissues, approximately 75% of CpG dinucleotides are methylated, 90% of which lie within repetitive elements and transposons (130,140). CpG islands are present in the 5′-regions of >60% of all genes (130), in which the majority of CpG dinucleotides are unmethylated (141). In cancer cells, however, global methylation changes have been documented (142). Half of CpG islands are associated with gene promoters of annotated genes, while the rest lie either within or between transcription units (142), some of which may still contain transcription start sites of unknown significance (143). DNA methylation at promoter regions is thought to be associated with gene transcription silencing by either (i) direct inhibition of transcription factor binding or (ii) recruitment of chromatin-modifying activities by methyl-binding domain (MBD) proteins (144,145). There are also some data suggesting DNA methylation may not directly induce transcription silencing but rather, locks the silent state (146,147); hence, whether gene promoter methylation leads to gene silencing or is a marker of silencing of that particular gene remains to be determined.

Huge strides have been made in the development of genome-wide approaches for the assessment of DNA methylation. There are essentially four approaches: (i) restriction endonuclease based analysis, (ii) bisulfate conversion of DNA, (iii) affinity and immunoprecipitation-based studies (MBD pull down or antibodies against methylcytosine, either DNA-bound or protein bound), and (iv) mass-spectrometry-based analysis (148–150). Most of these approaches have been adapted for high-throughput functionality using microarrays (Table 29.1) or massively parallel sequencing-based platforms (Table 29.2).

The clinical applications of these platforms in breast cancer are growing, including a better understanding of the limitations of the current assays [for reviews on the technical aspects of methylation profiling techniques, see references (151–153)]. Apart from defining patterns of methylation in breast cancer (150), methylation studies have proposed the existence of a CpG island methylator phenotype in breast cancer (154). How this correlates with tumor phenotypes is unclear, but it warrants further study, given that the genes targeted by this epigenomic profile are enriched for pro-metastatic pathways (129,154). Akin to the heterogeneity identified in gene expression profiling of breast cancer (see the section "Classification of ER-Positive Breast…"), methylation studies have demonstrated that different breast cancer molecular subtypes harbor distinct patterns of DNA methylation (155). Luminal B breast cancers were reported to harbor significantly more methylated CpG sites than luminal A and Basal-like cancers (155), suggesting DNA methylation has different roles in each subtype. However, when methylation profiles were compared between different molecular subtypes using different technologies, methylation profiles could not accurately predict the molecular subtype of breast cancer (156). A question that remains to be answered is related to the stability of the methylation profiles of a cancer in response to treatment, for example antiestrogenic therapies (129) and chemotherapy (157).

Histone Modification and Changes in Chromatin Structure

The post-translational modification of histone tails has long been recognized as a method of converting open chromatin that is transcriptionally active, to closed chromatin that is transcriptionally inactive (158). In breast cancer, aberrant histone modifications are frequently associated with epigenetic silencing of tumor suppressor genes and genomic instability (159), the most studied types including acetylation/deacetylation and methylation/demethylation.

Histone acetylation is a finely balanced state, regulated by the counter activities of histone acetyl transferases and histone deacetylases (HDACs). Chemical inhibition and RNA-interference mediated silencing of HDACs has been shown to modify chromatin structure and cause re-expression of aberrantly silenced genes (160–162). For example, re-expression of ER and PR has been reported in ER-negative cancer cells treated with specific HDAC inhibitors (163), which provided the rationale for a number of clinical trials exploring the efficacy of these agents in sensitizing triple-negative breast cancers to endocrine therapy (Table 29.3). HDAC inhibitors have also been shown to have synergistic activity with DNA methyltransferase inhibitors with increased ER re-expression (164) and tamoxifen responsiveness (165,166).

Reversible methylation of lysine residues on histones is a dynamic process kept in balance by the opposing actions of lysine methyltransferases and demethylases (129). Distinct patterns of methylation of lysines on the core histones (H3 and H4) are associated with either open (transcriptionally active) or closed (transcriptionally silent) chromatin (158). For example, EZH2, a conserved methyltransferase, functions as a transcription repressor (167). Overexpression of EZH2 has been reported consistently in breast cancer (168) and is associated with features of tumor aggressiveness (e.g., HER2 expression, basal subtype, and p53 mutations) (169).

Enzymes maintaining this balance of methylation therefore make attractive therapeutic targets. Preclinical data have shown that a number of agents in this class cause re-expression of target genes, induce apoptosis and inhibit proliferation and migration (170–172). Serendipitously, drugs already characterized and approved for other uses have also been shown to inhibit known methyltransferases (e.g., the HSP90 inhibitor, novobiocin and monoamine oxidase inhibitors used in the treatment of depression), potentially speeding the development of clinically useful treatments targeting these enzymes (129). However, given the wide range of effects these agents may have, it is likely that more information will be needed regarding potential off target effects before large clinical trials are conducted.

MicroRNA Expression in Breast Cancer

MicroRNAs (miRNAs) are formed in a multi-step process originating in the nucleus (involving Drosha), and culminating in final processing by Dicer and the RNA-induced silencing complex (173). MicroRNAs have ubiquitous binding patterns, using full or incomplete complementarity to the target mRNA, while the expression of target genes may be modulated by multiple miRNAs (174). Feedback networks between miRNAs result in clusters of miRNAs targeting specific pathways and exerting a coordinated and amplified effect (175).

Evidence for the role of miRNAs in breast cancer is burgeoning. Not only has aberrant expression of miRNAs been reported in breast cancer (176,177), but downregulation of miRNA machinery has also been described (178,179). Furthermore, both ER and HER2 expression has been shown to be influenced by a multitude of miRNAs (173,180). These lines of evidence together with data demonstrating an association between various miRNAs and different cancer-related processes (e.g., angiogenesis, epithelial to mesenchymal transition and metastasis) (181–183) support the proposed role for miRNAs as oncogenes or tumor suppressors. For in depth discussions of evidence pertaining to these roles, readers are directed to reviews published on the subject (173,184).

Individual miRNAs and miRNA clusters influence major biological networks (185) and appear to determine breast cancer phenotypes (186,187). For example, expression of miR-21 (one of the most extensively studied miRNAs) has been shown to be associated with shortened overall survival, advanced stage

Table 29.3 Clinical Trials Involving HDAC Inhibitors in Breast Cancer

ClinicalTrials. gov Identifier	HDAC Inhibitor	Purpose of Trial	Status	Phase
NCT00567879	Panobinostat	To identify the MTD of both intravenous and oral panobinostat plus trastuzumab in patients with metastatic HER2-positive breast cancer	Completed 8/2011	I/II
NCT00788931	Panobinostat	To identify the MTD of both intravenous and oral panobinostat when given in combination with trastuzumab and paclitaxel in patients with metastatic HER2-positive breast cancer	Completed 2/2011	I/II
NCT01194908	LBH589	To determine if re-expression of ER following treatment with LBH589 and a DNMT inhibitor (decitabine) is associated with sensitivity to tamoxifen in patients with metastatic TNBC	Recruiting	I/II
NCT00365599	Vorinostat	To explore the efficacy of vorinostat and tamoxifen combined	Completed 2/2012	II
NCT01153672	Vorinostat	To determine if vorinostat can restore sensitivity to AIs in patients with stage IV breast cancers with acquired resistance to AIs	Recruiting	II
NCT00262834	Vorinostat	To study the efficacy of neoadjuvant single agent vorinostat in patients with stage I–III breast cancer	Ongoing but recruitment ceased	II
NCT00616967	Vorinostat	To determine if vorinostat can improve the efficacy of carboplatin given in combination with paclitaxel in patients with HER-negative breast cancer	Ongoing but recruitment ceased	II
NCT01084057	Vorinostat	A dose finding and toxicity profiling study of vorinostat in combination with ixabepilone	Recruiting	I
NCT01234532	Entinostat	To determine the efficacy of combination treatment of patients with resectable TNBC with entinostat and anastrozole	Recruiting	II
NCT01434303	Entinostat	To determine the MTD and efficacy of entinostat in combination with lapatinib in patients with metastatic or recurrent HER2-positive breast cancer previously treated with trastuzumab.	Recruiting	I/II
NCT01349959	Entinostat	To determine the efficacy of entinostat in combination with azacitidine in patients with inoperable or metastatic TNBC	Recruiting	II
NCT00676663	Entinostat	To determine the efficacy of entinostat in combination with exemestane in patients with metastatic ER-positive breast cancer	Ongoing but recruitment ceased	II
NCT00828854	Entinostat	To determine the efficacy of entinostat in combination with AIs in patients with progressive ER-positive breast cancer	Completed 2/2010	II

Abbreviations: AIs, aromatase inhibitors; DNMT, DNA methyltransferases; ER, estrogen receptor; MTD, maximum tolerated dose; TNBC, triple-negative breast cancer.

(188,189), lymph node metastasis (190), high histological grade, triple-negative status (189) and loss of PTEN expression (190).

The most commonly used methods for studying miRNAs include quantitative real-time PCR(qRT-PCR, (191)), bead-based flow cytometric expression profiling (187) and miRNA microarrays (177). Owing to the small size of miRNAs and their lower risk of methylol cross-links forming between RNA and protein during tissue processing, RNA degradation is a far rarer phenomenon for miRNAs. Consequently, correlation of data generated from fresh frozen tissues and FFPE tissue is high (192).

Given the small size of miRNAs and the relative stability of their expression upon routine tissue fixation, miRNAs are attractive candidates for the development of prognostic or predictive biomarkers. Using miRNAs as prognostic markers carries a caveat related to their wide reaching effects, which may be context dependent. This is exemplified by the case of miR-21 which, despite the above cited associations, was shown to have diametrically opposite associations with outcome when patients were stratified according to ER status (189). Following encouraging preclinical data, several groups have shown that miRNA expression can be associated with therapeutic response to both endocrine therapy (193) and trastuzumab (194).

Given their stability, miRNAs expression has also been assessed in serum samples. Initial strategies using qRT-PCR have identified circulating miRNA signatures for breast cancer diagnosis (195,196), residual tumor burden assessment (195) and certain clinicopathological characteristics (196). Moving to the future, a recent study reported the use of the SOLiD sequencing platform (Applied Biosystems, sequencing by oligonucleotide ligation and detection) for more accurate genome-wide miRNA detection. This allows for more confident non-invasive diagnosis (197) and further validation of this type of approach is eagerly awaited.

Targeting miRNAs in the treatment of breast cancer is still in its infancy, but two strategies have been developed, namely (*i*) inhibiting/blocking oncomiRs and (*ii*) stimulating tumor suppressive miRNAs (129,198). The commonest agents used for oncomiRs are anti-miRNA oligonucleotides (199). Novel versions of these agents based on locked nucleic acid (LNA) technology show higher specificity and stability (200), and have produced a wealth of preclinical data demonstrating anticancer properties (194,201,202). Allowing for initial reports of severe liver toxicity following in vivo miRNA modulation (203) (which have largely been superseded by LNA-based anti-miRNAs (204)), in vivo data have reproduced preclinical results (205,206). Although early preclinical studies of miRNA replacement therapy (stimulating tumor suppressor miRNAs) have shown some positive anti-cancer effects (207), the main challenge is in improving the specificity and limiting unwanted effects of these agents (208).

Given the redundancy in miRNA targeting, it is likely that single agent antagomiRs will be superseded by strategies targeting miRNA networks. It is also hoped that a better understanding of miRNA network regulation will allow more clinically useful predictive markers to be developed from circulating miRNAs (173).

TRANSCRIPTOMICS IN BREAST CANCER
Breast Cancer Molecular Classification

Seminal microarray-based class discovery studies have demonstrated the existence of molecular subtypes within ER-positive and ER-negative breast cancers: luminal A, luminal B, HER2, basal-like, and normal breast-like (Table 29.4) (2–7). ER-negative cancers were initially subclassified into HER2, basal-like, or normal-breast like, whereas ER-positive luminal cancers could be subclassified into two or three groups (i.e., luminal A, B, and C or luminal A and B) (5,6), and different molecular subtypes were shown to have distinct clinical outcomes (2,3,5,6). Furthermore, additional molecular subtypes of ER-negative breast cancers have been identified, including molecular apocrine (8,9), interferon-rich (2), and claudin-low (3,209). It should be noted, however, that more recent microarray-based methods to identify the molecular subtypes of breast cancer show a less robust correlation between ER and HER2 status and the molecular subtypes (11,17).

Classification of ER-Positive Breast Cancer into Luminal A and Luminal B Subtypes

The use of gene expression profiling to classify breast cancer into luminal A and luminal B subtypes is driven by the expression levels of proliferation-related genes, ER and ER-related genes (2,3,18,210,211). Luminal A cancers are characterized by relatively higher levels of ER and relatively lower levels of proliferation-related genes, whereas luminal B showed the reverse pattern (1,2,15,18,211). Unsurprisingly, luminal A cancers have a significantly better outcome than luminal B cancers, likely due to the impact of proliferation on the outcome of ER-positive cancers (1,12,16).

Recent studies have questioned the validity of the subclassification of ER-positive breast cancers into luminal A and luminal B subtypes (210,212) and have suggested that ER-positive cancers form a continuum rather than segregate into distinct subtypes (16,210,211). The methodology used to develop the "intrinsic gene" molecular classification of breast cancer has some important limitations (1,213). First, a hierarchical clustering analysis has been shown to be subjective and is unsuitable for the classification of individual samples prospectively (214,215), making the subclassification of tumors into luminal A and luminal B both subjective (216) and unstable (214). Second, the development of single sample predictors (SSPs) was based on centroids for each of the molecular subtypes (i.e., the average expression profile of each molecular subtype as defined by hierarchical clustering analysis) (2,6). It is therefore not surprising that the performance of SSPs to subclassify luminal cancers is suboptimal (210,212,217). In fact, we and others have demonstrated that only basal-like breast cancers can be

Table 29.4 Breast Cancer Intrinsic Molecular Subtypes: Clinicopathological Definition and Recommendations for Treatment According to 2011 St Gallen Expert Consensus (224)

Intrinsic Subtype	Luminal A	Luminal B	Luminal B/HER2 Positive	HER2	Triple Negative/Basal-Like
Clinicopathological definition	ER and/or PR positive HER2-negative Ki67 low (<14%)	ER and/or PR positive HER2-negative Ki67 high (≥14%)	ER and/or PR positive Any Ki67 HER2 overexpressed or amplified	ER and PR-negative HER2 overexpressed or amplified	ER and PR-negative HER2-negative
Clinical management	Endocrine therapy alone	Endocrine therapy Cytotoxic drugs	Endocrine therapy Cytotoxic drugs HER2 specific therapy (trastuzumab and/or lapatinib)	Cytotoxic drugs HER2 specific therapy (trastuzumab and/or lapatinib)	Cytotoxic drugs
Notes	Ki67 cut-off has been established by comparison with PAM50 intrinsic subtyping (225). Available retrospective analysis of clinical trial data failed to show that the response to endocrine therapy differs in luminal A vs. luminal B tumors when PAM50 is applied (229,230). Cut-offs for predicting increased sensitivity to cytotoxics may differ (233)				Approximately 80% overlap between triple-negative and intrinsic basal-like breast cancers. Use of CK5/6 and/or EGFR (228) for basal-like subtyping has not been recommended. Some special histological types of breast cancer with favorable outcome, such as adenoid cystic and medullary carcinomas, fall into this category (286)

reliably identified using this approach and that the classification of breast cancers into the molecular subtypes other than basal-like is strongly dependent on the SSP used (210,212). Importantly, when the proponents of the molecular taxonomy themselves classified the same cohort of patients using two different SSPs (2,6), one by Sorlie et al. (6,218) and another by Hu et al. (2,219), the agreement was only moderate (Kappa scores = 0.527). Third, given that the levels of expression of proliferation-related genes in ER-positive disease form a continuum (12,16,220) and that subdivision of ER-positive breast cancers into the luminal A and luminal B phenotype is largely driven by the expression of proliferation-related genes (15,18,210,211), the cut-offs to define luminal A and luminal B cancer are arbitrarily set rather than emerge from a bimodal distribution of the levels of expression of these genes (12,15,16,212,220). Fourth, when breast cancers are classified using a recent version of the "intrinsic gene" classification (3,11) or based on the PAM50 assay (ARUP Laboratories, Salt Lake City, Utah, USA) (221), up to 9% of luminal A and luminal B breast cancers lacked ER expression by means of immunohistochemistry. On the other hand, up to 19% of basal-like breast cancers as defined by PAM50 were shown to express ER (3,11,221). Fifth, although PAM50 seems not to require manual microdissection of the tumors prior to RNA extraction (221), there is evidence to demonstrate that the proportion of normal cells in samples subjected to gene expression profiling interferes substantially with the results (222,223) and that samples with a large proportion of normal tissue were incorrectly assigned to less aggressive subtypes. The above observations together with those reported by Weigelt et al. (210) demonstrate that normal tissue is an important source of bias in breast genomic predictors.

The implementation of the microarray-based methods for the identification of luminal A and luminal B breast cancers into algorithms and guidelines for clinical decision making has been hampered by their limitations. At the 2011 St Gallen International Breast Cancer Conference, an expert panel recommended that therapeutic decisions should be made based on the recognition of the "intrinsic" subtypes of breast cancer (224), but that these subtypes should be defined by an immunohistochemical surrogate panel, including ER, PR, HER2, and Ki67. The distinction between luminal A and luminal B is based on the Ki67 labeling index, with a cut-off of 14% (224,225). Of note, this surrogate displayed suboptimal sensitivity (i.e., 77%; 95% CI = 64–87%) and specificity (78%; 95% CI = 68–87%) (225) when it was benchmarked using gene expression arrays as the "gold standard." Multiple immunohistochemical definitions for luminal A and luminal B breast cancers have been published, including the use of HER2 overexpression as a descriptor (226). In fact, between 8–11% and 15–24% of luminal A and luminal B breast cancers respectively, as defined by microarray-based gene expression profiling, overexpress HER2 (3,11,221).

Given that the subtypes themselves incorporate many of the risk and predictive factors used in previous consensus recommendations, use of the luminal A/luminal B nomenclature may facilitate communication between scientists, clinicians, and pathologists. The prognostic power of the molecular classification by microarrays (4–6), either PAM50 (3) or immunohistochemistry (225,227,228) is accepted; its predictive impact is yet to be fully established. PAM50-defined luminal A tumors may not display a better clinical response to endocrine therapy alone than PAM50-defined luminal B tumors (229,230). Furthermore, PAM50 stratification of breast cancers into luminal A and B subtypes was shown not to be a significant factor in multivariate models for pathological complete response and five-year recurrence-free survival after conventional neoadjuvant (231) or adjuvant (232) chemotherapy. It should be noted that the former study may not be sufficiently powered to detect a difference between these two subgroups, while in the later study, the HER2-enriched PAM50 defined subgroup was associated with an increased five-year relapse-free survival following treatment with epirubicin-containing compared with methotrexate-containing regimens. Given that the PAM50 itself may not predict response to therapy, it is questionable whether the proposed Ki67 cut-off of 14% should be employed to define the subgroup of patients with ER-positive tumors that are likely to benefit from adjuvant chemotherapy (233). Finally, the methodology for Ki67 assessment must be standardized (234) before being incorporated into clinical decision making.

The clinical and biological significance of the additional molecular subtypes thus far identified beyond luminal A and B, remains to be determined. In addition, based on the expression levels of ER-, androgen receptor- and proliferation-clusters, a further six molecular subtypes have been reported (235). A HER2 subtype was not identified; the clinically HER2-positive tumors were divided into two subgroups, namely molecular apocrine and luminal C. Likewise, class discovery studies focused on triple-negative breast cancer revealed the existence of six subtypes of triple-negative breast cancers (i.e., two basal-like, an immunomodulatory, a mesenchymal, a mesenchymal stem-like, and a luminal androgen receptor subtype) (10).

Therefore, the "intrinsic" molecular taxonomy is still a working model that is not yet ready for clinical use. The development of standardized definitions and methodologies for the identification of the molecular subtypes is important if this approach is to be employed in patient care. Although promising, validation of the robustness and clinical utility of PAM50 is still required (3,221,230).

Prognostic Gene Signatures

The challenge of preventing or reducing unnecessary treatment-related toxicity for breast cancer patients is daunting. About 70% of patients with early breast cancer currently receive adjuvant chemotherapy and are at risk of toxicity, but only 2–15% of patients derive benefit from these agents (1). Microarray-based gene signatures that are able to identify breast cancer patients with sufficiently good prognosis and may not require adjuvant chemotherapy could revolutionize breast cancer patient therapy. The commercially available breast cancer prognostic signatures are summarized in Table 29.5 and described next. For in-depth reviews, please see Kim et al. (236), Colombo et al. (237), Geyer et al. (17), and Reis-Filho & Pusztai (211).

70-Gene Signature (MammaPrint®)

MammaPrint® was developed through an empiric microarray analysis of 78 breast cancers smaller than 5 cm in diameter from lymph node-negative, systemic therapy-naive young women, who were stratified into good prognosis (i.e., no

Table 29.5 Commercially Available Prognostic and Predictive Gene Expression Signatures

Gene Signature	Assay	Platform	Tissue Type	Results	Clinical Indication	Level of Evidence[a]	FDA Approval	ASCO Recommended	Randomized Trial
MammaPrint® (Agendia)	70-gene signature	Microarray	Frozen or stabilized RNA	Good vs. poor prognosis	Prognosis in N0, <5 cm diameter, stage I/II, ER+ or ER- BC	III	Yes	No	MINDACT
MapQuant DX™ (Ipsogen)	97-gene GGI		Frozen or FFPE	GG1 (low grade) vs. GG3 (high grade)	Molecular grading in ER+, histological grade II BC		No	No	
Theros™ (Biotheranostics)	2-gene HOXB13: IL17R/ molecular grade index	qRT-PCR	FFPE	Low vs. intermediate vs. high risk	Prognosis and prediction of response to tamoxifen in ER+ BC				
EndoPredict® (Sividon Diagnostics GmbH)	11-gene EP score			Low vs. high risk	ER-positive HER2-negative patients treated with endocrine therapy alone	I			
Oncotype DX™ (Genomic Health)	21-gene RS			Low vs. intermediate vs. high risk	Prognosis and prediction of benefit from chemotherapy in ER+ N0/1-3N+ BC on tamoxifen use			Yes	TAILORx

[a]Levels of evidence as defined by Simon et al. (253).

Abbreviations: ASCO, American Society of Clinical Oncology; BC, breast cancer; ER, estrogen receptor; FDA, Food and Drug Administration; FFPE, formalin-fixed paraffin-embedded; GGI, Genomic Grade Index; N0, lymph node negative; N+, positive lymph nodes; qRT-PCR, quantitative reverse-transcriptase PCR; RS, Recurrence Score.

distant metastasis within five years) or poor prognosis groups (i.e., distant metastasis within five years) (238). The 70-gene predictor derived from this analysis identifies good-prognosis patients accurately and was partially independently validated as a predictor of outcome in a microarray analysis of a dataset comprising 295 cases (239) (which included 64 cases from the discovery cohort). This signature was subsequently converted into a Food and Drug Administration-approved prognostic test (MammaPrint®, Agendia, Amsterdam, The Netherlands), which is currently being tested in a randomized prospective phase III clinical trial called MINDACT (Microarray In Node-Negative and 1 to 3 positive lymph node Disease may Avoid ChemoTherapy). Subsequent retrospective analysis aimed to provide evidence to support the use of this gene signature in patients with lymph node-positive disease (240) and post-menopausal patients (241,242). Patients classified as of good prognosis by MammaPrint® derive minimal benefit from chemotherapy, whereas patients with poor prognosis tumors have an improved outcome following chemotherapy (243).

Genomic Grade Index

The Genomic Grade Index (GGI), a 97-gene signature, was derived following a supervised microarray comparative analysis of histological grade I and grade III breast cancers (244). Not only does the GGI classify histological grade I and grade III cancers accurately, but also sub-classifies histological grade II cancers into GGI-I and GGI-III cancers, which have significantly different outcomes. Independent groups have validated these findings using similar approaches (245). MapQuant Dx™ (Ipsogen SA, Marseille, France) is a commercial microarray-based prognostic assay based on the GGI, which has now been converted into a qRT-PCR-based test (246).

Oncotype DX™

Oncotype DX™ (Genomic Health, Redwood, California, USA) is a 21-gene signature based on qRT-PCR, developed following a reanalysis of microarray datasets and a review of the literature (247,248). FFPE material from the prospective clinical trials B-20 and B-14 was used for discovery and validation of this signature (for reviews, see (1,211,236,237)). This test involves the analysis of the expression levels of five reference genes for the standardization and relative quantification of 16 prognostic genes that are related to proliferation (i.e., Ki67, STK15, Survivin, CCNB1, and MYBL2), invasion (i.e., Stromelysin 3 and Cathepsin L2), HER2 (HER2 and GRB7), ER signaling (i.e., ER, PR, Bcl2, and SCUBE2), and other biological phenomena (i.e., GSTM1, BAG1 and CD68) (247). The output of the assay is a Recurrence Score (RS, range 0–100), which is an estimate of the 10-year distant recurrence risk. Patients are categorized into low RS (RS <18), intermediate RS (RS ≥18 and <31), and high RS (RS ≥31) (247). Oncotype DX™ RS was shown to outperform standard clinicopathological parameters for the prediction of 10-year distant recurrence risk (247,248), and has subsequently been validated as a prognostic marker in patients with ER-positive tumors with up to three positive-nodes receiving adjuvant chemotherapy (249), and in postmenopausal patients with ER-positive tumors treated with anastrozole (250). Oncotype DX™ RS has also been shown to correlate with the benefit patients derive from adjuvant chemotherapy in samples from clinical trials (248,251,252). Patients with low

RS cancers appear to derive negligible benefit from the addition of chemotherapy to tamoxifen (248). Therefore, Oncotype DX™ has also been used as a predictive marker of benefit from chemotherapy. Given that level I evidence in support of the prognostic role of Oncotype DX™ has already been accrued (253), in a complementary manner to clinicopathological features, it has received approval from the American Society of Clinical Oncology (254) and was included in the National Comprehensive Cancer Network guidelines (NCCN guidelines Breast Cancer version 1.2011 - http://www.nccn.org/) as an option to evaluate prognosis and to predict response to chemotherapy for ER-positive, node-negative breast cancer patients.

EndoPredict®

In a similar fashion, materials from the Austrian Breast and Colorectal Cancer Study Group (ABCSG)-6 (n = 378) and ABCSG-8 (n = 1,324) has been used to develop a qRT-PCR based test, EndoPredict® (Sividon Diagnostics GmbH, Cologne, Germany). This predicts the outcome of patients with ER-positive HER2-negative breast cancers (255). This test is based on eight target genes (BIRC5, UBE2C, DHCR7, RBBP8, IL6ST, AZGP1, MGP, and STC2) and three reference genes (CALM2, OAZ1, and RPL37A) and produces the EP score (a measure of the risk of distant recurrence in patients with ER-positive HER2-negative breast cancers treated with endocrine therapy alone) (255). The study design has allowed for the accrual of level I evidence for the validity of this prognostic test (253,255).

These first-generation prognostic signatures have several characteristics in common, namely:

1. Although the prognostic information provided by these signatures is independent of that provided by clinicopathological features (239,244,256), the converse is true and invariably, clinicopathological features provide prognostic information independent from that offered by the multigene predictors. As such, these signatures are at best complementary to the information offered by tumor size, lymph node status and, in some models, histological grade (15,18,210,211,237).

2. Different gene signatures identify similar (219), but not always identical (16,210,212,220,231,257) poor outcome groups of patients. In ER-positive breast cancers, although there is some degree of correlation between the poor prognosis groups identified by MammaPrint® and Oncotype DX™ and luminal B cancers (15,18,219,231), the different methods produce discordant risk prediction for individual patients (210,212,231,257). Only moderate agreement between the different methods has recently been reported [Kappa scores were 0.570 for 70-gene signature vs. 21-gene signature; 0.567 for 70-gene signature vs. PAM50 (luminal A vs. others); and 0.546 for 21-gene signature vs. PAM50 (luminal A vs. others)] (231).

3. The levels of expression of proliferation-related genes seem to drive most of the prognostic information provided by multigene predictors based on empiric approaches or histological grade (12,16,220).

In fact, reanalysis of these signatures showed that the proliferation-related genes within each signature formed a subsignature with equal if not greater prognostic power than the original, while the subsignature composed of nonproliferation-related genes was not prognostic (16,220).

4. The expression levels of proliferation-related genes in ER-positive breast cancers form a continuum (12,15,16) and thresholds to define good and poor prognosis tumors are arbitrarily set.

5. Given the high expression levels of proliferation-related genes in ER-negative breast cancer, these signatures do not have discriminatory power in ER-negative disease (Fig. 29.1) (12,16,231). In fact, fewer than 5% of ER-negative breast cancers are classified as of good prognosis using these approaches (12,16,210,211,231,239–241,243) and the rare indolent ER-negative breast cancers (e.g., adenoid cystic carcinomas) are consistently classified as of poor prognosis (258).

6. The discriminatory power of first-generation prognostic signatures wanes after five years of follow-up, and is attenuated at 10 years, including MammaPrint (259) and the 76-gene signature (260).

7. The prognostic subgroups identified by first-generation prognostic signatures have been shown to associate with benefit from chemotherapy (18,210,211,231,237,243,248,252,261). While patients with a good prognosis derive minimal if any benefit from conventional chemotherapy regimens, patients with poor prognosis tumors seem to derive significantly more benefit than those with good prognosis

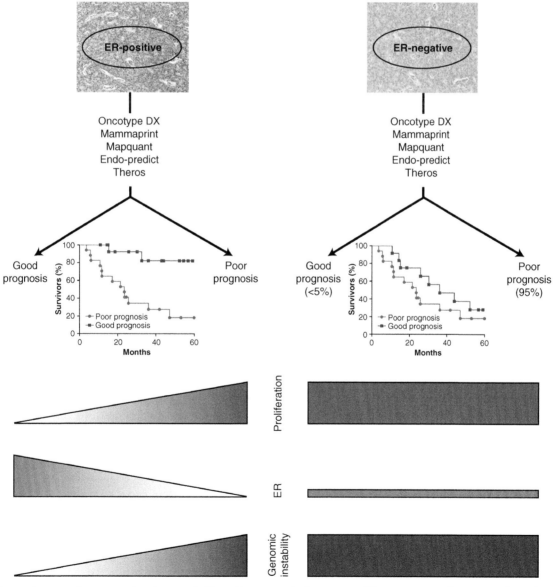

Figure 29.1 Prognostic power of gene expression signatures in ER-positive or -negative breast cancer. If breast cancers are first segregated according to expression of estrogen receptor (ER) and the various commercially available prognostic gene expression signatures, two distinct patterns emerge. For ER-positive breast cancer, good (blue line) and poor prognosis (red line) groups are defined with significant differences in outcome. However, this difference in outcome is likely to be driven by differences in the expression of proliferation-related (and to a lesser extent immune-related) genes. Likewise, ER expression is higher in the good prognosis group and genomic instability is higher in the poor prognosis group. For ER-negative disease, the two defined groups have a poor separation of survival curves, and expression of proliferation and ER-related genes is equal in both groups (high and low, respectively), with similar levels of genomic instability (high), highlighting the poor utility of these gene expression signatures in ER-negative breast cancer.

tumors. It should be noted, however, that not all poor prognosis cancers are sensitive to conventional chemotherapy regimens.

8. Oncotype DX™ and other first-generation signatures provide minimal additional prognostic information to that provided by semiquantitative immunohistochemical assessment of ER, PR, HER2, and Ki67 (262).

The importance of proliferation for the prognostication of ER-positive breast cancers has been corroborated by window-of-opportunity studies (213). Ki67 levels are measured two weeks after neo-adjuvant endocrine therapy is initiated, and changes in Ki67 before and after two weeks of endocrine therapy have been shown to predict distant recurrences better than baseline Ki67 values (213,263). It is plausible that measures of Ki67 and gene expression changes before and after therapeutic interventions may provide more robust prognostic information than that obtained from analysis of pre-therapy samples (213). The results of the trial of Perioperative Endocrine Therapy-Individualising Care (POETIC) are likely to answer this question in the near future.

It is clear that proliferation is a good predictor of outcome and, possibly, a predictive marker of response to chemotherapy in ER-positive breast cancer patients. The latest St Gallen consensus has recommended the use of Ki67 for clinical decision-making in ER-positive tumors (224). However, a number of methodological issues need to be addressed before Ki67 immunohistochemical assessment can be used as a marker for treatment decision making, including addressing the lack of standardization of Ki67 assessment in different pathology laboratories (234). A team of Breast International Group and the North American Breast Cancer Group Biomarker Working Party experts have put forward guidelines for Ki67 assessment in breast cancer, including recommendations on preanalytical and analytical assessment, and interpretation and scoring (234).

The conceptual contribution of microarray signatures has paved the way for the development of multiparameter predictors of outcome. Furthermore, the development pipeline of Oncotype DX has a bar for the standardization of the assessment of critical parameters for treatment decision making. Despite the equivalence in the prognostic information provided by Oncotype DX RS and semiquantitative assessment of ER, PR, HER2, and Ki67 (241,262), it remains to be determined if the same level of standardization and accuracy of these four immunohistochemical markers will be comparable to that of the Oncotype DX recurrence score.

Second-Generation Prognostic Signatures

Largely hypothesis-driven approaches have resulted in predictors based on the levels of immune-response genes and stroma-related genes (264–269) being developed. These predictors have been shown to have discriminatory power in highly proliferative ER-positive and triple-negative breast cancers (266,267). Interestingly, a high content of tumor-infiltrating lymphocytes, in particular CD8-positive cells (270), is significantly associated with a better survival and sensitivity to neo-adjuvant chemotherapy in triple-negative breast cancers (270,271). Although these identify a subset of triple-negative tumors with a relatively good outcome, the number of distant relapses within five years in patients classified as of good prognosis is so low that these signatures cannot be used to identify patients who could be spared chemotherapy.

Predictive Signature

As mentioned above, first-generation prognostic signatures can also be used as predictors of response to multidrug chemotherapy regimens in ER-positive breast cancers (15,18,210,211,231). Studies have demonstrated that Oncotype DX™ (248), MammaPrint® (238,243), and GGI (244,272) can be used to define which patients should receive cytotoxic medication in addition to endocrine therapy. The correlation between the expression levels of proliferation-related genes and response to multidrug chemotherapy (15,18,210,211,231,261) is the likely driving factor behind the clinical utility of these signatures in this context.

A promising approach using gene expression signatures to predict response to tamoxifen is the sensitivity to endocrine therapy (SET) index, which was developed through the transcriptomic analysis of a large series of ER-positive breast cancers (273). Gene expression profiling of 437 breast cancers led to the identification of genes whose expression is positively ($n = 109$) or negatively ($n = 59$) correlated with that of ER. Cut-offs were determined in a validation cohort of 245 patients to define three categories of sensitivity (low, intermediate, and high). Association between SET and outcome was then analyzed in three types of ER-positive cohorts receiving either adjuvant tamoxifen for five years or neo-adjuvant chemotherapy followed by endocrine therapy or no adjuvant systemic treatment. The SET index was significantly associated with the outcome of patients receiving any type of endocrine treatment but had no prognostic value in untreated patients. Unlike other multigene signatures evaluating proliferation in ER-positive tumors, the SET index seems to be predictive of benefit from endocrine therapy independently of the inherent prognosis of the tumor. A potential clinical application of the SET index is in the identification of a subset of ER-positive tumors associated with an excellent prognosis and no relapse in the tamoxifen-treated group (high SET index tumors) and in the chemoendocrine group (high and intermediate SET index) (273). This type of predictive signature may constitute one of the ways forward for the molecular stratification of ER-positive cancers.

Massively Parallel RNA Sequencing

RNA sequencing (RNA-Seq) can be used to analyze mRNA, total RNA, or miRNA/noncoding RNAs (274,275). RNA is typically fragmented and converted to cDNA before addition of adaptor molecules for sequencing. Although RNA-Seq reproduces to some extent microarray-based measurements for mRNA expression levels (276,277), it has several advantages, including (i) novel transcripts and splice variants can be identified (278), (ii) expression values are digital rather than analog, increasing the dynamic range (81), (iii) can assess allele-specific expression (279), and (iv) can refine transcript structure including read-throughs and chimeric transcripts (280,281). However, there are challenges in the identification of somatic mutations (related to adequacy/availability of frozen matched normal samples and expression levels in normal tissues) (81).

Given the current understanding that fusion genes are far more common in solid cancers than previously anticipated

(88), using RNA-Seq to identify expressed fusion genes is an attractive prospect. RNA-Seq has already been used to identify recurrent novel fusion genes in breast cancer, some of which have been functionally validated (280–283). Arguably the challenge is now to develop robust strategies for the identification of recurrent "driver" fusion events that can be targeted by available drugs, given most fusions are private events (i.e., occur in the index case only), or passenger events (i.e., by-products of the evolution of amplicons) (82,89,284,285).

CONCLUSION

The molecular investigation of breast cancer has two main goals. First, the current taxonomy for breast cancer classification, based on largely morphological features and prognostic in nature, must be revised into a molecular taxonomy that is predictive in nature. Only then can truly personalized medicine be realized. Second, by embracing new technologies, first microarrays, and now massively parallel sequencing, novel therapeutic targets can be identified and validated. The eagerly awaited results of the sequencing efforts of large consortia such as the TCGA and ICGC will provide a hugely valuable resource for the larger scientific community to tap for validation studies. Finally, the field of epigenetics is rapidly expanding, and providing insight not only into our understanding of the transcriptional control and layers of intra-tumor heterogeneity, but also with exciting leads on therapeutic agents for breast cancer patients.

ACKNOWLEDGMENTS

PMW is funded by a Wellcome Trust Clinical Fellowship grant. JSR-F is one of the recipients of the 2010 Cancer Research UK Future Leaders Prize. We also acknowledge NHS funding to the NIHR Biomedical Research Centre.

REFERENCES

1. Reis-Filho JS, Pusztai L. Gene expression profiling in breast cancer: classification, prognostication, and prediction. Lancet 2011; 378: 1812–23.
2. Hu Z, Fan C, Oh DS, et al. The molecular portraits of breast tumors are conserved across microarray platforms. BMC Genomics 2006; 7: 96.
3. Parker JS, Mullins M, Cheang MC, et al. Supervised risk predictor of breast cancer based on intrinsic subtypes. J Clin Oncol 2009; 27: 1160–7.
4. Perou CM, Sorlie T, Eisen MB, et al. Molecular portraits of human breast tumours. Nature 2000; 406: 747–52.
5. Sorlie T, Perou CM, Tibshirani R, et al. Gene expression patterns of breast carcinomas distinguish tumor subclasses with clinical implications. Proc Natl Acad Sci USA 2001; 98: 10869–74.
6. Sorlie T, Tibshirani R, Parker J, et al. Repeated observation of breast tumor subtypes in independent gene expression data sets. Proc Natl Acad Sci USA 2003; 100: 8418–23.
7. Sotiriou C, Neo SY, McShane LM, et al. Breast cancer classification and prognosis based on gene expression profiles from a population-based study. Proc Natl Acad Sci USA 2003; 100: 10393–8.
8. Doane AS, Danso M, Lal P, et al. An estrogen receptor-negative breast cancer subset characterized by a hormonally regulated transcriptional program and response to androgen. Oncogene 2006; 25: 3994–4008.
9. Farmer P, Bonnefoi H, Becette V, et al. Identification of molecular apocrine breast tumours by microarray analysis. Oncogene 2005; 24: 4660–71.
10. Lehmann BD, Bauer JA, Chen X, et al. Identification of human triple-negative breast cancer subtypes and preclinical models for selection of targeted therapies. J Clin Invest 2011; 121: 2750–67.
11. Prat A, Parker JS, Karginova O, et al. Phenotypic and molecular characterization of the claudin-low intrinsic subtype of breast cancer. Breast Cancer Res 2010; 12: R68.
12. Desmedt C, Haibe-Kains B, Wirapati P, et al. Biological processes associated with breast cancer clinical outcome depend on the molecular subtypes. Clin Cancer Res 2008; 14: 5158–65.
13. Loi S, Haibe-Kains B, Majjaj S, et al. PIK3CA mutations associated with gene signature of low mTORC1 signaling and better outcomes in estrogen receptor-positive breast cancer. Proc Natl Acad Sci USA 2010; 107: 10208–13.
14. Lopez-Garcia MA, Geyer FC, Lacroix-Triki M, Marchio C, Reis-Filho JS. Breast cancer precursors revisited: molecular features and progression pathways. Histopathology 2010; 57: 171–92.
15. Weigelt B, Baehner FL, Reis-Filho JS. The contribution of gene expression profiling to breast cancer classification, prognostication and prediction: a retrospective of the last decade. J Pathol 2010; 220: 263–80.
16. Wirapati P, Sotiriou C, Kunkel S, et al. Meta-analysis of gene expression profiles in breast cancer: toward a unified understanding of breast cancer subtyping and prognosis signatures. Breast Cancer Res 2008; 10: R65.
17. Geyer FC, Rodrigues DN, Weigelt B, Reis-Filho JS. Molecular classification of estrogen receptor-positive/luminal breast cancers. Adv Anat Pathol 2012; 19: 39–53.
18. Sotiriou C, Pusztai L. Gene-expression signatures in breast cancer. N Engl J Med 2009; 360: 790–800.
19. Weigelt B, Geyer FC, Reis-Filho JS. Histological types of breast cancer: how special are they? Mol Oncol 2010; 4: 192–208.
20. Weigelt B, Reis-Filho JS. Histological and molecular types of breast cancer: is there a unifying taxonomy? Nat Rev Clin Oncol 2009; 6: 718–30.
21. Weigel MT, Dowsett M. Current and emerging biomarkers in breast cancer: prognosis and prediction. Endocr Relat Cancer 2010; 17: R245–62.
22. Kallioniemi A, Kallioniemi OP, Sudar D, et al. Comparative genomic hybridization for molecular cytogenetic analysis of solid tumors. Science 1992; 258: 818–21.
23. Tan DS, Lambros MB, Natrajan R, Reis-Filho JS. Getting it right: designing microarray (and not 'microawry') comparative genomic hybridization studies for cancer research. Lab Invest 2007; 87: 737–54.
24. Pinkel D, Albertson DG. Array comparative genomic hybridization and its applications in cancer. Nat Genet 2005; 37(Suppl): S11–17.
25. Reis-Filho JS, Simpson PT, Gale T, Lakhani SR. The molecular genetics of breast cancer: the contribution of comparative genomic hybridization. Pathol Res Pract 2005; 201: 713–25.
26. Ahmed S, Thomas G, Ghoussaini M, et al. Newly discovered breast cancer susceptibility loci on 3p24 and 17q23.2. Nat Genet 2009; 41: 585–90.
27. Easton DF, Pooley KA, Dunning AM, et al. Genome-wide association study identifies novel breast cancer susceptibility loci. Nature 2007; 447: 1087–93.
28. Gold B, Kirchhoff T, Stefanov S, et al. Genome-wide association study provides evidence for a breast cancer risk locus at 6q22.33. Proc Natl Acad Sci USA 2008; 105: 4340–5.
29. Hunter DJ, Kraft P, Jacobs KB, et al. A genome-wide association study identifies alleles in FGFR2 associated with risk of sporadic postmenopausal breast cancer. Nat Genet 2007; 39: 870–4.
30. Stacey SN, Manolescu A, Sulem P, et al. Common variants on chromosomes 2q35 and 16q12 confer susceptibility to estrogen receptor-positive breast cancer. Nat Genet 2007; 39: 865–9.
31. Thomas G, Jacobs KB, Kraft P, et al. A multistage genome-wide association study in breast cancer identifies two new risk alleles at 1p11.2 and 14q24.1 (RAD51L1). Nat Genet 2009; 41: 579–84.
32. Zheng W, Long J, Gao YT, et al. Genome-wide association study identifies a new breast cancer susceptibility locus at 6q25.1. Nat Genet 2009; 41: 324–8.
33. Dai J, Hu Z, Jiang Y, et al. Breast cancer risk assessment with five independent genetic variants and two risk factors in chinese women. Breast Cancer Res 2012; 14: R17.
34. Gibson G. Hints of hidden heritability in GWAS. Nat Genet 2010; 42: 558–60.
35. Wang K, Li M, Hakonarson H. Analysing biological pathways in genome-wide association studies. Nat Rev Genet 2010; 11: 843–54.
36. Simon R, Radmacher MD, Dobbin K, McShane LM. Pitfalls in the use of DNA microarray data for diagnostic and prognostic classification. J Natl Cancer Inst 2003; 95: 14–18.
37. Natrajan R, Lambros MB, Rodriguez-Pinilla SM, et al. Tiling path genomic profiling of grade 3 invasive ductal breast cancers. Clin Cancer Res 2009; 15: 2711–22.
38. Natrajan R, Weigelt B, Mackay A, et al. An integrative genomic and transcriptomic analysis reveals molecular pathways and networks regulated by copy number aberrations in basal-like, HER2 and luminal cancers. Breast Cancer Res Treat 2010; 121: 575–89.

39. Andre F, Job B, Dessen P, et al. Molecular characterization of breast cancer with high-resolution oligonucleotide comparative genomic hybridization array. Clin Cancer Res 2009; 15: 441–51.

40. Chin SF, Teschendorff AE, Marioni JC, et al. High-resolution aCGH and expression profiling identifies a novel genomic subtype of ER negative breast cancer. Genome Biol 2007; 8: R215.

41. Chin K, DeVries S, Fridlyand J, et al. Genomic and transcriptional aberrations linked to breast cancer pathophysiologies. Cancer Cell 2006; 10: 529–41.

42. Jonsson G, Staaf J, Vallon-Christersson J, et al. Genomic subtypes of breast cancer identified by array-comparative genomic hybridization display distinct molecular and clinical characteristics. Breast Cancer Res 2010; 12: R42.

43. Flagiello D, Gerbault-Seureau M, Sastre-Garau X, et al. Highly recurrent der(1;16)(q10;p10) and other 16q arm alterations in lobular breast cancer. Genes Chromosomes Cancer 1998; 23: 300–6.

44. Tsuda H, Takarabe T, Fukutomi T. Hirohashi S. der(16)t(1;16)/ der(1;16) in breast cancer detected by fluorescence in situ hybridization is an indicator of better patient prognosis. Genes Chromosomes Cancer 1999; 24: 72–7.

45. Smeets SJ, Harjes U, van Wieringen WN, et al. To DNA or not to DNA? That is the question, when it comes to molecular subtyping for the clinic!. Clin Cancer Res 2011; 17: 4959–64.

46. Geyer FC, de Biase D, Lambros MB, et al. Genomic profiling of mitochondrion-rich breast carcinoma: chromosomal changes may be relevant for mitochondria accumulation and tumour biology. Breast Cancer Res Treat 2012; 132: 15–28.

47. Lacroix-Triki M, Suarez PH, MacKay A, et al. Mucinous carcinoma of the breast is genomically distinct from invasive ductal carcinomas of no special type. J Pathol 2010; 222: 282–98.

48. Marchio C, Iravani M, Natrajan R, et al. Genomic and immunophenotypical characterization of pure micropapillary carcinomas of the breast. J Pathol 2008; 215: 398–410.

49. Geyer FC, Lambros MB, Natrajan R, et al. Genomic and immunohistochemical analysis of adenosquamous carcinoma of the breast. Mod Pathol 2010; 23: 951–60.

50. Reis-Filho JS, Simpson PT, Turner NC, et al. FGFR1 emerges as a potential therapeutic target for lobular breast carcinomas. Clin Cancer Res 2006; 12: 6652–62.

51. Elbauomy Elsheikh S, Green AR, Lambros MB, et al. FGFR1 amplification in breast carcinomas: a chromogenic in situ hybridisation analysis. Breast Cancer Res 2007; 9: R23.

52. Turner N, Pearson A, Sharpe R, et al. FGFR1 amplification drives endocrine therapy resistance and is a therapeutic target in breast cancer. Cancer Res 2010; 70: 2085–94.

53. Theillet C, Adelaide J, Louason G, et al. FGFRI and PLAT genes and DNA amplification at 8p12 in breast and ovarian cancers. Genes Chromosomes Cancer 1993; 7: 219–26.

54. Gelsi-Boyer V, Orsetti B, Cervera N, et al. Comprehensive profiling of 8p11-12 amplification in breast cancer. Mol Cancer Res 2005; 3: 655–67.

55. Yang ZQ, Streicher KL, Ray ME, Abrams J, Ethier SP. Multiple interacting oncogenes on the 8p11-p12 amplicon in human breast cancer. Cancer Res 2006; 66: 11632–43.

56. Turner N, Lambros MB, Horlings HM, et al. Integrative molecular profiling of triple negative breast cancers identifies amplicon drivers and potential therapeutic targets. Oncogene 2010; 29: 2013–23.

57. Kao J, Pollack JR. RNA interference-based functional dissection of the 17q12 amplicon in breast cancer reveals contribution of coamplified genes. Genes Chromosomes Cancer 2006; 45: 761–9.

58. Bernard-Pierrot I, Gruel N, Stransky N, et al. Characterization of the recurrent 8p11-12 amplicon identifies PPAPDC1B, a phosphatase protein, as a new therapeutic target in breast cancer. Cancer Res 2008; 68: 7165–75.

59. Streicher KL, Yang ZQ, Draghici S, Ethier SP. Transforming function of the LSM1 oncogene in human breast cancers with the 8p11-12 amplicon. Oncogene 2007; 26: 2104–14.

60. Li Y, Zou L, Li Q, et al. Amplification of LAPTM4B and YWHAZ contributes to chemotherapy resistance and recurrence of breast cancer. Nat Med 2010; 16: 214–18.

61. Li L, Wei XH, Pan YP, et al. LAPTM4B: a novel cancer-associated gene motivates multidrug resistance through efflux and activating PI3K/ AKT signaling. Oncogene 2010; 29: 5785–95.

62. Li Y, Zhang Q, Tian R, et al. Lysosomal transmembrane protein LAPTM4B promotes autophagy and tolerance to metabolic stress in cancer cells. Cancer Res 2011; 71: 7481–9.

63. Shendure J. The beginning of the end for microarrays? Nat Methods 2008; 5: 585–7.

64. Ledford H. The death of microarrays? Nature 2008; 455: 847.

65. Navin N, Hicks J. Future medical applications of single-cell sequencing in cancer. Genome Med 2011; 3: 31.

66. Wagle N, Berger MF, Davis MJ, et al. High-throughput detection of actionable genomic alterations in clinical tumor samples by targeted, massively parallel sequencing. Cancer Discov 2012; 2: 82–93.

67. Chiang DY, Getz G, Jaffe DB, et al. High-resolution mapping of copy-number alterations with massively parallel sequencing. Nat Methods 2009; 6: 99–103.

68. Alkan C, Kidd JM, Marques-Bonet T, et al. Personalized copy number and segmental duplication maps using next-generation sequencing. Nat Genet 2009; 41: 1061–7.

69. Yoon S, Xuan Z, Makarov V, Ye K, Sebat J. Sensitive and accurate detection of copy number variants using read depth of coverage. Genome Res 2009; 19: 1586–92.

70. Drmanac R, Sparks AB, Callow MJ, et al. Human genome sequencing using unchained base reads on self-assembling DNA nanoarrays. Science 2010; 327: 78–81.

71. Service RF. Gene sequencing. The race for the $1000 genome. Science 2006; 311: 1544–6.

72. Pettersson E, Lundeberg J, Ahmadian A. Generations of sequencing technologies. Genomics 2009; 93: 105–11.

73. Tucker T, Marra M, Friedman JM. Massively parallel sequencing: the next big thing in genetic medicine. Am J Hum Genet 2009; 85: 142–54.

74. Voelkerding KV, Dames SA, Durtschi JD. Next-generation sequencing: from basic research to diagnostics. Clin Chem 2009; 55: 641–58.

75. ten Bosch JR, Grody WW. Keeping up with the next generation: massively parallel sequencing in clinical diagnostics. J Mol Diagn 2008; 10: 484–92.

76. Morozova O, Marra MA. Applications of next-generation sequencing technologies in functional genomics. Genomics 2008; 92: 255–64.

77. Fullwood MJ, Wei CL, Liu ET, Ruan Y. Next-generation DNA sequencing of paired-end tags (PET) for transcriptome and genome analyses. Genome Res 2009; 19: 521–32.

78. Bentley DR. Whole-genome re-sequencing. Curr Opin Genet Dev 2006; 16: 545–52.

79. Mardis ER. New strategies and emerging technologies for massively parallel sequencing: applications in medical research. Genome Med 2009; 1: 40.

80. Schadt EE, Turner S, Kasarskis A. A window into third-generation sequencing. Hum Mol Genet 2010; 19: R227–40.

81. Natrajan R, Reis-Filho JS. Next-generation sequencing applied to molecular diagnostics. Expert Rev Mol Diagn 2011; 11: 425–44.

82. Stephens PJ, McBride DJ, Lin ML, et al. Complex landscapes of somatic rearrangement in human breast cancer genomes. Nature 2009; 462: 1005–10.

83. Pleasance ED, Cheetham RK, Stephens PJ, et al. A comprehensive catalogue of somatic mutations from a human cancer genome. Nature 2010; 463: 191–6.

84. Shah SP, Morin RD, Khattra J, et al. Mutational evolution in a lobular breast tumour profiled at single nucleotide resolution. Nature 2009; 461: 809–13.

85. Ding L, Ellis MJ, Li S, et al. Genome remodelling in a basal-like breast cancer metastasis and xenograft. Nature 2010; 464: 999–1005.

86. Ding L, Ley TJ, Larson DE, et al. Clonal evolution in relapsed acute myeloid leukaemia revealed by whole-genome sequencing. Nature 2012; 481: 506–10.

87. Soda M, Choi YL, Enomoto M, et al. Identification of the transforming EML4-ALK fusion gene in non-small-cell lung cancer. Nature 2007; 448: 561–6.

88. Tomlins SA, Rhodes DR, Perner S, et al. Recurrent fusion of TMPRSS2 and ETS transcription factor genes in prostate cancer. Science 2005; 310: 644–8.

89. Campbell PJ, Stephens PJ, Pleasance ED, et al. Identification of somatically acquired rearrangements in cancer using genome-wide massively parallel paired-end sequencing. Nat Genet 2008; 40: 722–9.

90. Robinson DR, Kalyana-Sundaram S, Wu YM, et al. Functionally recurrent rearrangements of the MAST kinase and Notch gene families in breast cancer. Nat Med 2011; 17: 1646–51.

91. Vivanco I, Sawyers CL. The phosphatidylinositol 3-Kinase AKT pathway in human cancer. Nat Rev Cancer 2002; 2: 489–501.

92. Campbell IG, Russell SE, Choong DY, et al. Mutation of the PIK3CA gene in ovarian and breast cancer. Cancer Res 2004; 64: 7678–81.

93. Stemke-Hale K, Gonzalez-Angulo AM, Lluch A, et al. An integrative genomic and proteomic analysis of PIK3CA, PTEN, and AKT mutations in breast cancer. Cancer Res 2008; 68: 6084–91.

94. Samuels Y, Wang Z, Bardelli A, et al. High frequency of mutations of the PIK3CA gene in human cancers. Science 2004; 304: 554.

95. Bachman KE, Argani P, Samuels Y, et al. The PIK3CA gene is mutated with high frequency in human breast cancers. Cancer Biol Ther 2004; 3: 772–5.

96. Liedtke C, Cardone L, Tordai A, et al. PIK3CA-activating mutations and chemotherapy sensitivity in stage II-III breast cancer. Breast Cancer Res 2008; 10: R27.

97. Saal LH, Holm K, Maurer M, et al. PIK3CA mutations correlate with hormone receptors, node metastasis, and ERBB2, and are mutually exclusive with PTEN loss in human breast carcinoma. Cancer Res 2005; 65: 2554–9.

98. Perez-Tenorio G, Alkhori L, Olsson B, et al. PIK3CA mutations and PTEN loss correlate with similar prognostic factors and are not mutually exclusive in breast cancer. Clin Cancer Res 2007; 13: 3577–84.

99. Hollestelle A, Elstrodt F, Nagel JH, Kallemeijn WW, Schutte M. Phosphatidylinositol-3-OH kinase or RAS pathway mutations in human breast cancer cell lines. Mol Cancer Res 2007; 5: 195–201.

100. Ellis MJ, Lin L, Crowder R, et al. Phosphatidyl-inositol-3-kinase alpha catalytic subunit mutation and response to neoadjuvant endocrine therapy for estrogen receptor positive breast cancer. Breast Cancer Res Treat 2010; 119: 379–90.

101. Miller TW, Balko JM, Arteaga CL. Phosphatidylinositol 3-kinase and antiestrogen resistance in breast cancer. J Clin Oncol 2011; 29: 4452–61.

102. Baselga J. Targeting the phosphoinositide-3 (PI3) kinase pathway in breast cancer. Oncologist 2011; 16: 12–19.

103. Gymnopoulos M, Elsliger MA, Vogt PK. Rare cancer-specific mutations in PIK3CA show gain of function. Proc Natl Acad Sci USA 2007; 104: 5569–74.

104. Whyte DB, Holbeck SL. Correlation of PIK3Ca mutations with gene expression and drug sensitivity in NCI-60 cell lines. Biochem Biophys Res Commun 2006; 340: 469–75.

105. Kalinsky K, Jacks LM, Heguy A, et al. PIK3CA mutation associates with improved outcome in breast cancer. Clin Cancer Res 2009; 15: 5049–59.

106. Saal LH, Johansson P, Holm K, et al. Poor prognosis in carcinoma is associated with a gene expression signature of aberrant PTEN tumor suppressor pathway activity. Proc Natl Acad Sci USA 2007; 104: 7564–9.

107. Panigrahi AR, Pinder SE, Chan SY, et al. The role of PTEN and its signalling pathways, including AKT, in breast cancer; an assessment of relationships with other prognostic factors and with outcome. J Pathol 2004; 204: 93–100.

108. Perren A, Weng LP, Boag AH, et al. Immunohistochemical evidence of loss of PTEN expression in primary ductal adenocarcinomas of the breast. Am J Pathol 1999; 155: 1253–60.

109. Depowski PL, Rosenthal SI, Ross JS. Loss of expression of the PTEN gene protein product is associated with poor outcome in breast cancer. Mod Pathol 2001; 14: 672–6.

110. Marty B, Maire V, Gravier E, et al. Frequent PTEN genomic alterations and activated phosphatidylinositol 3-kinase pathway in basal-like breast cancer cells. Breast Cancer Res 2008; 10: R101.

111. Shoman N, Klassen S, McFadden A, et al. Reduced PTEN expression predicts relapse in patients with breast carcinoma treated by tamoxifen. Mod Pathol 2005; 18: 250–9.

112. Osborne CK, Shou J, Massarweh S, Schiff R. Crosstalk between estrogen receptor and growth factor receptor pathways as a cause for endocrine therapy resistance in breast cancer. Clin Cancer Res 2005; 11: 865s–70s.

113. Loi S, Sotiriou C, Haibe-Kains B, et al. Gene expression profiling identifies activated growth factor signaling in poor prognosis (Luminal-B) estrogen receptor positive breast cancer. BMC Med Genomics 2009; 2: 37.

114. Gonzalez-Angulo AM, Ferrer-Lozano J, Stemke-Hale K, et al. PI3K pathway mutations and PTEN levels in primary and metastatic breast cancer. Mol Cancer Ther 2011; 10: 1093–101.

115. Drury SC, Detre S, Leary A, et al. Changes in breast cancer biomarkers in the IGF1R/PI3K pathway in recurrent breast cancer after tamoxifen treatment. Endocr Relat Cancer 2011; 18: 565–77.

116. Vasudevan KM, Barbie DA, Davies MA, et al. AKT-independent signaling downstream of oncogenic PIK3CA mutations in human cancer. Cancer Cell 2009; 16: 21–32.

117. Weigelt B, Warne PH, Downward J. PIK3CA mutation, but not PTEN loss of function, determines the sensitivity of breast cancer cells to mTOR inhibitory drugs. Oncogene 2011; 30: 3222–33.

118. Brachmann S, Fritsch C, Maira SM, Garcia-Echeverria C. PI3K and mTOR inhibitors: a new generation of targeted anticancer agents. Curr Opin Cell Biol 2009; 21: 194–8.

119. Tanaka H, Yoshida M, Tanimura H, et al. The selective class I PI3K inhibitor CH5132799 targets human cancers harboring oncogenic PIK3CA mutations. Clin Cancer Res 2011; 17: 3272–81.

120. Shuttleworth SJ, Silva FA, Cecil AR, et al. Progress in the preclinical discovery and clinical development of class I and dual class I/IV phosphoinositide 3-kinase (PI3K) inhibitors. Curr Med Chem 2011; 18: 2686–714.

121. Andre F, Campone M, O'Regan R, et al. Phase I study of everolimus plus weekly paclitaxel and trastuzumab in patients with metastatic breast cancer pretreated with trastuzumab. J Clin Oncol 2010; 28: 5110–15.

122. Awada A, Cardoso F, Fontaine C, et al. The oral mTOR inhibitor RAD001 (everolimus) in combination with letrozole in patients with advanced breast cancer: results of a phase I study with pharmacokinetics. Eur J Cancer 2008; 44: 84–91.

123. Chan S, Scheulen ME, Johnston S, et al. Phase II study of temsirolimus (CCI-779), a novel inhibitor of mTOR, in heavily pretreated patients with locally advanced or metastatic breast cancer. J Clin Oncol 2005; 23: 5314–22.

124. Jerusalem G, Fasolo A, Dieras V, et al. Phase I trial of oral mTOR inhibitor everolimus in combination with trastuzumab and vinorelbine in pre-treated patients with HER2-overexpressing metastatic breast cancer. Breast Cancer Res Treat 2011; 125: 447–55.

125. Morrow PK, Wulf GM, Ensor J, et al. Phase I/II study of trastuzumab in combination with everolimus (RAD001) in patients with HER2-overexpressing metastatic breast cancer who progressed on trastuzumab-based therapy. J Clin Oncol 2011; 29: 3126–32.

126. Baselga J, Semiglazov V, van Dam P, et al. Phase II randomized study of neoadjuvant everolimus plus letrozole compared with placebo plus letrozole in patients with estrogen receptor-positive breast cancer. J Clin Oncol 2009; 27: 2630–7.

127. Ellard SL, Clemons M, Gelmon KA, et al. Randomized phase II study comparing two schedules of everolimus in patients with recurrent/metastatic breast cancer: NCIC clinical trials group IND.163. J Clin Oncol 2009; 27: 4536–41.

128. Baselga J, Campone M, Piccart M, et al. Everolimus in postmenopausal hormone-receptor-positive advanced breast cancer. N Engl J Med 2012; 366: 520–9.

129. Huang Y, Nayak S, Jankowitz R, Davidson NE, Oesterreich S. Epigenetics in breast cancer: what's new? Breast Cancer Res 2011; 13: 225.

130. Jovanovic J, Ronneberg JA, Tost J, Kristensen V. The epigenetics of breast cancer. Mol Oncol 2010; 4: 242–54.

131. Damm F, Kosmider O, Gelsi-Boyer V, et al. Mutations affecting mRNA splicing define distinct clinical phenotypes and correlate with patient outcome in myelodysplastic syndromes. Blood 2012; 119: 3211–18.

132. Marcucci G, Metzeler KH, Schwind S, et al. Age-related prognostic impact of different types of DNMT3A mutations in adults with primary cytogenetically normal acute myeloid leukemia. J Clin Oncol 2012; 30: 742–50.

133. Renneville A, Boissel N, Nibourel O, et al. Prognostic significance of DNA methyltransferase 3A mutations in cytogenetically normal acute myeloid leukemia: a study by the Acute Leukemia French Association. Leukemia 2012; 26: 1247–54.

134. Jones S, Li M, Parsons DW, et al. Somatic mutations in the chromatin remodeling gene ARID1A occur in several tumor types. Hum Mutat 2012; 33: 100–3.

135. Cornen S, Adelaide J, Bertucci F, et al. Mutations and deletions of ARID1A in breast tumors. Oncogene 2012; Epub ahead of print.

136. Wiegand KC, Shah SP, Al-Agha OM, et al. ARID1A mutations in endometriosis-associated ovarian carcinomas. N Engl J Med 2010; 363: 1532–43.

137. Jones S, Wang TL, Shih Ie M, et al. Frequent mutations of chromatin remodeling gene ARID1A in ovarian clear cell carcinoma. Science 2010; 330: 228–31.

138. Wang K, Kan J, Yuen ST, et al. Exome sequencing identifies frequent mutation of ARID1A in molecular subtypes of gastric cancer. Nat Genet 2011; 43: 1219–23.

139. Heravi-Moussavi A, Anglesio MS, Cheng SW, et al. Recurrent somatic DICER1 mutations in nonepithelial ovarian cancers. N Engl J Med 2012; 366: 234–42.

140. Bird A. DNA methylation patterns and epigenetic memory. Genes Dev 2002; 16: 6–21.

141. De Smet C, Loriot A, Boon T. Promoter-dependent mechanism leading to selective hypomethylation within the 5' region of gene MAGE-A1 in tumor cells. Mol Cell Biol 2004; 24: 4781–90.

142. Illingworth RS, Gruenewald-Schneider U, Webb S, et al. Orphan CpG islands identify numerous conserved promoters in the mammalian genome. PLoS Genet 2010; 6: e1001134.

143. Deaton AM, Bird A. CpG islands and the regulation of transcription. Genes Dev 2011; 25: 1010–22.

144. Klose RJ, Bird AP. Genomic DNA methylation: the mark and its mediators. Trends Biochem Sci 2006; 31: 89–97.

145. Bogdanovic O, Veenstra GJ. DNA methylation and methyl-CpG binding proteins: developmental requirements and function. Chromosoma 2009; 118: 549–65.

146. Payer B, Lee JT. X chromosome dosage compensation: how mammals keep the balance. Annu Rev Genet 2008; 42: 733–72.

147. Okamoto I, Heard E. Lessons from comparative analysis of X-chromosome inactivation in mammals. Chromosome Res 2009; 17: 659–69.

148. Ordway JM, Budiman MA, Korshunova Y, et al. Identification of novel high-frequency DNA methylation changes in breast cancer. PLoS One 2007; 2: e1314.

149. Korshunova Y, Maloney RK, Lakey N, et al. Massively parallel bisulphite pyrosequencing reveals the molecular complexity of breast cancer-associated cytosine-methylation patterns obtained from tissue and serum DNA. Genome Res 2008; 18: 19–29.

150. Ruike Y, Imanaka Y, Sato F, Shimizu K, Tsujimoto G. Genome-wide analysis of aberrant methylation in human breast cancer cells using methyl-DNA immunoprecipitation combined with high-throughput sequencing. BMC Genomics 2010; 11: 137.

151. Wong E, Wei CL. Genome-wide distribution of DNA methylation at single-nucleotide resolution. Prog Mol Biol Transl Sci 2011; 101: 459–77.

152. Martin-Subero JI, Esteller M. Profiling epigenetic alterations in disease. Adv Exp Med Biol 2011; 711: 162–77.

153. Bibikova M, Fan JB. Genome-wide DNA methylation profiling. Wiley Interdiscip Rev Syst Biol Med 2010; 2: 210–23.

154. Fang F, Turcan S, Rimner A, et al. Breast cancer methylomes establish an epigenomic foundation for metastasis. Sci Transl Med 2011; 3: 75ra25.

155. Holm K, Hegardt C, Staaf J, et al. Molecular subtypes of breast cancer are associated with characteristic DNA methylation patterns. Breast Cancer Res 2010; 12: R36.

156. Flanagan JM, Cocciardi S, Waddell N, et al. DNA methylome of familial breast cancer identifies distinct profiles defined by mutation status. Am J Hum Genet 2010; 86: 420–33.

157. Boettcher M, Kischkel F, Hoheisel JD. High-definition DNA methylation profiles from breast and ovarian carcinoma cell lines with differing doxorubicin resistance. PLoS One 2010; 5: e11002.

158. Jenuwein T, Allis CD. Translating the histone code. Science 2001; 293: 1074–80.

159. Stearns V, Zhou Q, Davidson NE. Epigenetic regulation as a new target for breast cancer therapy. Cancer Invest 2007; 25: 659–65.

160. Marson CM. Histone deacetylase inhibitors: design, structure-activity relationships and therapeutic implications for cancer. Anticancer Agents Med Chem 2009; 9: 661–92.

161. Khan O, La Thangue NB. Drug Insight: histone deacetylase inhibitor-based therapies for cutaneous T-cell lymphomas. Nat Clin Pract Oncol 2008; 5: 714–26.

162. Pruitt K, Zinn RL, Ohm JE, et al. Inhibition of SIRT1 reactivates silenced cancer genes without loss of promoter DNA hypermethylation. PLoS Genet 2006; 2: e40.

163. Keen JC, Yan L, Mack KM, et al. A novel histone deacetylase inhibitor, scriptaid, enhances expression of functional estrogen receptor alpha (ER) in ER negative human breast cancer cells in combination with 5-aza 2'-deoxycytidine. Breast Cancer Res Treat 2003; 81: 177–86.

164. Yang X, Ferguson AT, Nass SJ, et al. Transcriptional activation of estrogen receptor alpha in human breast cancer cells by histone deacetylase inhibition. Cancer Res 2000; 60: 6890–4.

165. Sharma D, Saxena NK, Davidson NE, Vertino PM. Restoration of tamoxifen sensitivity in estrogen receptor-negative breast cancer cells: tamoxifen-bound reactivated ER recruits distinctive corepressor complexes. Cancer Res 2006; 66: 6370–8.

166. Fan J, Yin WJ, Lu JS, et al. ER alpha negative breast cancer cells restore response to endocrine therapy by combination treatment with both HDAC inhibitor and DNMT inhibitor. J Cancer Res Clin Oncol 2008; 134: 883–90.

167. van der Vlag J, Otte AP. Transcriptional repression mediated by the human polycomb-group protein EED involves histone deacetylation. Nat Genet 1999; 23: 474–8.

168. Kleer CG, Cao Q, Varambally S, et al. EZH2 is a marker of aggressive breast cancer and promotes neoplastic transformation of breast epithelial cells. Proc Natl Acad Sci USA 2003; 100: 11606–11.

169. Bachmann IM, Halvorsen OJ, Collett K, et al. EZH2 expression is associated with high proliferation rate and aggressive tumor subgroups in cutaneous melanoma and cancers of the endometrium, prostate, and breast. J Clin Oncol 2006; 24: 268–73.

170. Tan J, Yang X, Zhuang L, et al. Pharmacologic disruption of Polycomb-repressive complex 2-mediated gene repression selectively induces apoptosis in cancer cells. Genes Dev 2007; 21: 1050–63.

171. Hamamoto R, Silva FP, Tsuge M, et al. Enhanced SMYD3 expression is essential for the growth of breast cancer cells. Cancer Sci 2006; 97: 113–18.

172. Luo XG, Zou JN, Wang SZ, Zhang TC, Xi T. Novobiocin decreases SMYD3 expression and inhibits the migration of MDA-MB-231 human breast cancer cells. IUBMB Life 2010; 62: 194–9.

173. Castaneda CA, Agullo-Ortuno MT, Fresno Vara JA, et al. Implication of miRNA in the diagnosis and treatment of breast cancer. Expert Rev Anticancer Ther 2011; 11: 1265–75.

174. O'Day E, Lal A. MicroRNAs and their target gene networks in breast cancer. Breast Cancer Res 2010; 12: 201.

175. Hermeking H. The miR-34 family in cancer and apoptosis. Cell Death Differ 2010; 17: 193–9.

176. Calin GA, Sevignani C, Dumitru CD, et al. Human microRNA genes are frequently located at fragile sites and genomic regions involved in cancers. Proc Natl Acad Sci USA 2004; 101: 2999–3004.

177. Saito Y, Liang G, Egger G, et al. Specific activation of microRNA-127 with downregulation of the proto-oncogene BCL6 by chromatin-modifying drugs in human cancer cells. Cancer Cell 2006; 9: 435–43.

178. Dedes KJ, Natrajan R, Lambros MB, et al. Down-regulation of the miRNA master regulators Drosha and Dicer is associated with specific subgroups of breast cancer. Eur J Cancer 2011; 47: 138–50.

179. Adams BD, Claffey KP, White BA. Argonaute-2 expression is regulated by epidermal growth factor receptor and mitogen-activated protein kinase signaling and correlates with a transformed phenotype in breast cancer cells. Endocrinology 2009; 150: 14–23.

180. Scott GK, Goga A, Bhaumik D, et al. Coordinate suppression of ERBB2 and ERBB3 by enforced expression of micro-RNA miR-125a or miR-125b. J Biol Chem 2007; 282: 1479–86.

181. Gregory PA, Bert AG, Paterson EL, et al. The miR-200 family and miR-205 regulate epithelial to mesenchymal transition by targeting ZEB1 and SIP1. Nat Cell Biol 2008; 10: 593–601.

182. Cha ST, Chen PS, Johansson G, et al. MicroRNA-519c suppresses hypoxia-inducible factor-1alpha expression and tumor angiogenesis. Cancer Res 2010; 70: 2675–85.

183. Hurst DR, Edmonds MD, Welch DR. Metastamir: the field of metastasis-regulatory microRNA is spreading. Cancer Res 2009; 69: 7495–8.

184. Andorfer CA, Necela BM, Thompson EA, Perez EA. MicroRNA signatures: clinical biomarkers for the diagnosis and treatment of breast cancer. Trends Mol Med 2011; 17: 313–19.

185. Iorio MV, Ferracin M, Liu CG, et al. MicroRNA gene expression deregulation in human breast cancer. Cancer Res 2005; 65: 7065–70.

186. Lowery AJ, Miller N, Devaney A, et al. MicroRNA signatures predict oestrogen receptor, progesterone receptor and HER2/neu receptor status in breast cancer. Breast Cancer Res 2009; 11: R27.

187. Blenkiron C, Goldstein LD, Thorne NP, et al. MicroRNA expression profiling of human breast cancer identifies new markers of tumor subtype. Genome Biol 2007; 8: R214.

188. Yan LX, Huang XF, Shao Q, et al. MicroRNA miR-21 overexpression in human breast cancer is associated with advanced clinical stage, lymph node metastasis and patient poor prognosis. RNA 2008; 14: 2348–60.

189. Qian B, Katsaros D, Lu L, et al. High miR-21 expression in breast cancer associated with poor disease-free survival in early stage disease and high TGF-beta1. Breast Cancer Res Treat 2009; 117: 131–40.

190. Huang GL, Zhang XH, Guo GL, et al. Clinical significance of miR-21 expression in breast cancer: SYBR-Green I-based real-time RT-PCR study of invasive ductal carcinoma. Oncol Rep 2009; 21: 673–9.

191. Khoshnaw SM, Green AR, Powe DG, Ellis IO. MicroRNA involvement in the pathogenesis and management of breast cancer. J Clin Pathol 2009; 62: 422–8.

192. Li J, Smyth P, Flavin R, et al. Comparison of miRNA expression patterns using total RNA extracted from matched samples of formalin-fixed paraffin-embedded (FFPE) cells and snap frozen cells. BMC Biotechnol 2007; 7: 36.

193. Rodriguez-Gonzalez FG, Sieuwerts AM, Smid M, et al. MicroRNA-30c expression level is an independent predictor of clinical benefit of endocrine therapy in advanced estrogen receptor positive breast cancer. Breast Cancer Res Treat 2011; 127: 43–51.

194. Gong C, Yao Y, Wang Y, et al. Up-regulation of miR-21 mediates resistance to trastuzumab therapy for breast cancer. J Biol Chem 2011; 286: 19127–37.

195. Heneghan HM, Miller N, Lowery AJ, et al. Circulating microRNAs as novel minimally invasive biomarkers for breast cancer. Ann Surg 2010; 251: 499–505.

196. Zhao H, Shen J, Medico L, et al. A pilot study of circulating miRNAs as potential biomarkers of early stage breast cancer. PLoS One 2010; 5: e13735.

197. Wu Q, Lu Z, Li H, et al. Next-generation sequencing of microRNAs for breast cancer detection. J Biomed Biotechnol 2011; 2011: 597145.

198. Iorio MV, Casalini P, Piovan C, Braccioli L, Tagliabue E. Breast cancer and microRNAs: therapeutic impact. Breast 2011; 20: S63–70.

199. Zhu S, Wu H, Wu F, et al. MicroRNA-21 targets tumor suppressor genes in invasion and metastasis. Cell Res 2008; 18: 350–9.

200. Frankel LB, Christoffersen NR, Jacobsen A, et al. Programmed cell death 4 (PDCD4) is an important functional target of the microRNA miR-21 in breast cancer cells. J Biol Chem 2008; 283: 1026–33.

201. Si ML, Zhu S, Wu H, et al. miR-21-mediated tumor growth. Oncogene 2007; 26: 2799–803.

202. Blower PE, Chung JH, Verducci JS, et al. MicroRNAs modulate the chemosensitivity of tumor cells. Mol Cancer Ther 2008; 7: 1–9.

203. Grimm D, Streetz KL, Jopling CL, et al. Fatality in mice due to oversaturation of cellular microRNA/short hairpin RNA pathways. Nature 2006; 441: 537–41.

204. Lanford RE, Hildebrandt-Eriksen ES, Petri A, et al. Therapeutic silencing of microRNA-122 in primates with chronic hepatitis C virus infection. Science 2010; 327: 198–201.

205. Ma L, Reinhardt F, Pan E, et al. Therapeutic silencing of miR-10b inhibits metastasis in a mouse mammary tumor model. Nat Biotechnol 2010; 28: 341–7.

206. Martello G, Rosato A, Ferrari F, et al. A MicroRNA targeting dicer for metastasis control. Cell 2010; 141: 1195–207.

207. Kota J, Chivukula RR, O'Donnell KA, et al. Therapeutic microRNA delivery suppresses tumorigenesis in a murine liver cancer model. Cell 2009; 137: 1005–17.

208. Chen Y, Zhu X, Zhang X, Liu B, Huang L. Nanoparticles modified with tumor-targeting scFv deliver siRNA and miRNA for cancer therapy. Mol Ther 2010; 18: 1650–6.

209. Herschkowitz JI, Simin K, Weigman VJ, et al. Identification of conserved gene expression features between murine mammary carcinoma models and human breast tumors. Genome Biol 2007; 8: R76.

210. Reis-Filho JS, Weigelt B, Fumagalli D, Sotiriou C. Molecular profiling: moving away from tumor philately. Sci Transl Med 2010; 2: 47ps3.

211. Reis-Filho JS, Pusztai L. Gene expression profiling in breast cancer: classification, prognostication and prediction. Lancet 2011; 378: 1812–23.

212. Haibe-Kains B, Desmedt C, Loi S, et al. A three-gene model to robustly identify breast cancer molecular subtypes. J Natl Cancer Inst 2012; 104: 311–25.

213. Weigelt B, Pusztai L, Ashworth A, Reis-Filho JS. Challenges translating breast cancer gene signatures into the clinic. Nat Rev Clin Oncol 2011; 9: 58–64.

214. Pusztai L, Mazouni C, Anderson K, Wu Y, Symmans WF. Molecular classification of breast cancer: limitations and potential. Oncologist 2006; 11: 868–77.

215. Kapp AV, Tibshirani R. Are clusters found in one dataset present in another dataset? Biostatistics 2007; 8: 9–31.

216. Mackay A, Weigelt B, Grigoriadis A, et al. Microarray-based class discovery for molecular classification of breast cancer: analysis of interobserver agreement. J Natl Cancer Inst 2011; 103: 662–73.

217. Lusa L, McShane LM, Reid JF, et al. Challenges in projecting clustering results across gene expression-profiling datasets. J Natl Cancer Inst 2007; 99: 1715–23.

218. Chang HY, Nuyten DS, Sneddon JB, et al. Robustness, scalability, and integration of a wound-response gene expression signature in predicting breast cancer survival. Proc Natl Acad Sci USA 2005; 102: 3738–43.

219. Fan C, Oh DS, Wessels L, et al. Concordance among gene-expression-based predictors for breast cancer. N Engl J Med 2006; 355: 560–9.

220. Reyal F, van Vliet MH, Armstrong NJ, et al. A comprehensive analysis of prognostic signatures reveals the high predictive capacity of the proliferation, immune response and RNA splicing modules in breast cancer. Breast Cancer Res 2008; 10: R93.

221. Nielsen TO, Parker JS, Leung S, et al. A comparison of PAM50 intrinsic subtyping with immunohistochemistry and clinical prognostic factors in tamoxifen-treated estrogen receptor-positive breast cancer. Clin Cancer Res 2010; 16: 5222–32.

222. Cleator SJ, Powles TJ, Dexter T, et al. The effect of the stromal component of breast tumours on prediction of clinical outcome using gene expression microarray analysis. Breast Cancer Res 2006; 8: R32.

223. Elloumi F, Hu Z, Li Y, et al. Systematic bias in genomic classification due to contaminating non-neoplastic tissue in breast tumor samples. BMC Med Genomics 2011; 4: 54.

224. Goldhirsch A, Wood WC, Coates AS, et al. Strategies for subtypes–dealing with the diversity of breast cancer: highlights of the St Gallen International Expert Consensus on the Primary Therapy of Early Breast Cancer 2011. Ann Oncol 2011; 22: 1736–47.

225. Cheang MC, Chia SK, Voduc D, et al. Ki67 index, HER2 status, and prognosis of patients with luminal B breast cancer. J Natl Cancer Inst 2009; 101: 736–50.

226. Carey LA, Perou CM, Livasy CA, et al. Race, breast cancer subtypes, and survival in the Carolina Breast Cancer Study. JAMA 2006; 295: 2492–502.

227. Cheang MC, Voduc D, Bajdik C, et al. Basal-like breast cancer defined by five biomarkers has superior prognostic value than triple-negative phenotype. Clin Cancer Res 2008; 14: 1368–76.

228. Nielsen TO, Hsu FD, Jensen K, et al. Immunohistochemical and clinical characterization of the basal-like subtype of invasive breast carcinoma. Clin Cancer Res 2004; 10: 5367–74.

229. Dunbier AK, Anderson H, Ghazoui Z, et al. Association between breast cancer subtypes and response to neoadjuvant anastrozole. Steroids 2011; 76: 736–40.

230. Ellis MJ, Suman VJ, Hoog J, et al. Randomized phase II neoadjuvant comparison between letrozole, anastrozole, and exemestane for postmenopausal women with estrogen receptor-rich stage 2 to 3 breast cancer: clinical and biomarker outcomes and predictive value of the baseline PAM50-based intrinsic subtype—ACOSOG Z1031. J Clin Oncol 2011; 29: 2342–9.

231. Iwamoto T, Lee JS, Bianchini G, et al. First generation prognostic gene signatures for breast cancer predict both survival and chemotherapy sensitivity and identify overlapping patient populations. Breast Cancer Res Treat 2011; 130: 155–64.

232. Cheang MC, Voduc KD, Tu D, et al. Responsiveness of intrinsic subtypes to adjuvant anthracycline substitution in the NCIC.CTG MA.5 randomized trial. Clin Cancer Res 2012; 18: 2402–12.

233. Penault-Llorca F, Andre F, Sagan C, et al. Ki67 expression and docetaxel efficacy in patients with estrogen receptor-positive breast cancer. J Clin Oncol 2009; 27: 2809–15.

234. Dowsett M, Nielsen TO, A'Hern R, et al. Assessment of Ki67 in breast cancer: recommendations from the International Ki67 in Breast Cancer working group. J Natl Cancer Inst 2011; 103: 1656–64.

235. Guedj M, Marisa L, de Reynies A, et al. A refined molecular taxonomy of breast cancer. Oncogene 2012; 31: 1196–206.

236. Kim C, Paik S. Gene-expression-based prognostic assays for breast cancer. Nat Rev Clin Oncol 2010; 7: 340–7.

237. Colombo PE, Milanezi F, Weigelt B, Reis-Filho JS. Microarrays in the 2010s: the contribution of microarray-based gene expression profiling to breast cancer classification, prognostication and prediction. Breast Cancer Res 2011; 13: 212.

238. van 't Veer LJ, Dai H, van de Vijver MJ, et al. Gene expression profiling predicts clinical outcome of breast cancer. Nature 2002; 415: 530–6.

239. van de Vijver MJ, He YD, van't Veer LJ, et al. A gene-expression signature as a predictor of survival in breast cancer. N Engl J Med 2002; 347: 1999–2009.

240. Mook S, Schmidt MK, Viale G, et al. The 70-gene prognosis-signature predicts disease outcome in breast cancer patients with 1-3 positive lymph nodes in an independent validation study. Breast Cancer Res Treat 2009; 116: 295–302.

241. Mook S, Schmidt MK, Weigelt B, et al. The 70-gene prognosis signature predicts early metastasis in breast cancer patients between 55 and 70 years of age. Ann Oncol 2010; 21: 717–22.

242. Wittner BS, Sgroi DC, Ryan PD, et al. Analysis of the MammaPrint breast cancer assay in a predominantly postmenopausal cohort. Clin Cancer Res 2008; 14: 2988–93.

243. Knauer M, Mook S, Rutgers EJ, et al. The predictive value of the 70-gene signature for adjuvant chemotherapy in early breast cancer. Breast Cancer Res Treat 2010; 120: 655–61.

244. Sotiriou C, Wirapati P, Loi S, et al. Gene expression profiling in breast cancer: understanding the molecular basis of histologic grade to improve prognosis. J Natl Cancer Inst 2006; 98: 262–72.

245. Ivshina AV, George J, Senko O, et al. Genetic reclassification of histologic grade delineates new clinical subtypes of breast cancer. Cancer Res 2006; 66: 10292–301.

246. Toussaint J, Sieuwerts AM, Haibe-Kains B, et al. Improvement of the clinical applicability of the Genomic Grade Index through a qRT-PCR test performed on frozen and formalin-fixed paraffin-embedded tissues. BMC Genomics 2009; 10: 424.

247. Paik S, Shak S, Tang G, et al. A multigene assay to predict recurrence of tamoxifen-treated, node-negative breast cancer. N Engl J Med 2004; 351: 2817–26.

248. Paik S, Tang G, Shak S, et al. Gene expression and benefit of chemotherapy in women with node-negative, estrogen receptor-positive breast cancer. J Clin Oncol 2006; 24: 3726–34.

249. Goldstein LJ, Gray R, Badve S, et al. Prognostic utility of the 21-gene assay in hormone receptor-positive operable breast cancer compared with classical clinicopathologic features. J Clin Oncol 2008; 26: 4063–71.

250. Dowsett M, Cuzick J, Wale C, et al. Prediction of risk of distant recurrence using the 21-gene recurrence score in node-negative and node-positive postmenopausal patients with breast cancer treated with anastrozole or tamoxifen: a TransATAC study. J Clin Oncol 2010; 28: 1829–34.

251. Gianni L, Zambetti M, Clark K, et al. Gene expression profiles in paraffin-embedded core biopsy tissue predict response to chemotherapy in women with locally advanced breast cancer. J Clin Oncol 2005; 23: 7265–77.

252. Albain KS, Barlow WE, Shak S, et al. Prognostic and predictive value of the 21-gene recurrence score assay in postmenopausal women with node-positive, oestrogen-receptor-positive breast cancer on chemotherapy: a retrospective analysis of a randomised trial. Lancet Oncol 2010; 11: 55–65.

253. Simon RM, Paik S, Hayes DF. Use of archived specimens in evaluation of prognostic and predictive biomarkers. J Natl Cancer Inst 2009; 101: 1446–52.

254. Harris L, Fritsche H, Mennel R, et al. American Society of Clinical Oncology 2007 update of recommendations for the use of tumor markers in breast cancer. J Clin Oncol 2007; 25: 5287–312.

255. Filipits M, Rudas M, Jakesz R, et al. A new molecular predictor of distant recurrence in ER-positive, HER2-negative breast cancer adds independent information to conventional clinical risk factors. Clin Cancer Res 2011; 17: 6012–20.

256. Wang Y, Klijn JG, Zhang Y, et al. Gene-expression profiles to predict distant metastasis of lymph-node-negative primary breast cancer. Lancet 2005; 365: 671–9.

257. Haibe-Kains B, Culhane A, Desmedt C, et al. Robustness of breast cancer molecular subtypes identification. Ann Oncol 2010; 21: iv49–59.

258. Weigelt B, Horlings HM, Kreike B, et al. Refinement of breast cancer classification by molecular characterization of histological special types. J Pathol 2008; 216: 141–50.

259. Buyse M, Loi S, van't Veer L, et al. Validation and clinical utility of a 70-gene prognostic signature for women with node-negative breast cancer. J Natl Cancer Inst 2006; 98: 1183–92.

260. Desmedt C, Piette F, Loi S, et al. Strong time dependence of the 76-gene prognostic signature for node-negative breast cancer patients in the TRANSBIG multicenter independent validation series. Clin Cancer Res 2007; 13: 3207–14.

261. Iwamoto T, Pusztai L. Predicting prognosis of breast cancer with gene signatures: are we lost in a sea of data? Genome Med 2010; 2: 81.

262. Cuzick J, Dowsett M, Pineda S, et al. Prognostic value of a combined estrogen receptor, progesterone receptor, Ki-67, and human epidermal growth factor receptor 2 immunohistochemical score and comparison with the genomic health recurrence score in early breast cancer. J Clin Oncol 2011; 29: 4273–8.

263. Dowsett M, Smith IE, Ebbs SR, et al. Prognostic value of Ki67 expression after short-term presurgical endocrine therapy for primary breast cancer. J Natl Cancer Inst 2007; 99: 167–70.

264. Bergamaschi A, Tagliabue E, Sorlie T, et al. Extracellular matrix signature identifies breast cancer subgroups with different clinical outcome. J Pathol 2008; 214: 357–67.

265. Finak G, Bertos N, Pepin F, et al. Stromal gene expression predicts clinical outcome in breast cancer. Nat Med 2008; 14: 518–27.

266. Teschendorff AE, Caldas C. A robust classifier of high predictive value to identify good prognosis patients in ER-negative breast cancer. Breast Cancer Res 2008; 10: R73.

267. Yau C, Esserman L, Moore DH, et al. A multigene predictor of metastatic outcome in early stage hormone receptor-negative and triple-negative breast cancer. Breast Cancer Res 2010; 12: R85.

268. Oh E, Choi YL, Park T, et al. A prognostic model for lymph node-negative breast cancer patients based on the integration of proliferation and immunity. Breast Cancer Res Treat 2012; 132: 499–509.

269. Bianchini G, Qi Y, Alvarez RH, et al. Molecular anatomy of breast cancer stroma and its prognostic value in estrogen receptor-positive and -negative cancers. J Clin Oncol 2010; 28: 4316–23.

270. Mahmoud SM, Paish EC, Powe DG, et al. Tumor-infiltrating CD8+ lymphocytes predict clinical outcome in breast cancer. J Clin Oncol 2011; 29: 1949–55.

271. Ono M, Tsuda H, Shimizu C, et al. Tumor-infiltrating lymphocytes are correlated with response to neoadjuvant chemotherapy in triple-negative breast cancer. Breast Cancer Res Treat 2011; 132: 793–805.

272. Liedtke C, Hatzis C, Symmans WF, et al. Genomic grade index is associated with response to chemotherapy in patients with breast cancer. J Clin Oncol 2009; 27: 3185–91.

273. Symmans WF, Hatzis C, Sotiriou C, et al. Genomic index of sensitivity to endocrine therapy for breast cancer. J Clin Oncol 2010; 28: 4111–19.

274. Wang Z, Gerstein M, Snyder M. RNA-Seq: a revolutionary tool for transcriptomics. Nat Rev Genet 2009; 10: 57–63.

275. Mortazavi A, Williams BA, McCue K, Schaeffer L, Wold B. Mapping and quantifying mammalian transcriptomes by RNA-Seq. Nat Methods 2008; 5: 621–8.

276. Morrissy AS, Morin RD, Delaney A, et al. Next-generation tag sequencing for cancer gene expression profiling. Genome Res 2009; 19: 1825–35.

277. C't Hoen PA, Ariyurek Y, Thygesen HH, et al. Deep sequencing-based expression analysis shows major advances in robustness, resolution and inter-lab portability over five microarray platforms. Nucleic Acids Res 2008; 36: e141.

278. Sultan M, Schulz MH, Richard H, et al. A global view of gene activity and alternative splicing by deep sequencing of the human transcriptome. Science 2008; 321: 956–60.

279. Wang X, Sun Q, McGrath SD, et al. Transcriptome-wide identification of novel imprinted genes in neonatal mouse brain. PLoS One 2008; 3: e3839.

280. Maher CA, Kumar-Sinha C, Cao X, et al. Transcriptome sequencing to detect gene fusions in cancer. Nature 2009; 458: 97–101.

281. Maher CA, Palanisamy N, Brenner JC, et al. Chimeric transcript discovery by paired-end transcriptome sequencing. Proc Natl Acad Sci USA 2009; 106: 12353–8.

282. Palanisamy N, Ateeq B, Kalyana-Sundaram S, et al. Rearrangements of the RAF kinase pathway in prostate cancer, gastric cancer and melanoma. Nat Med 2010; 16: 793–8.

283. Zhao Q, Caballero OL, Levy S, et al. Transcriptome-guided characterization of genomic rearrangements in a breast cancer cell line. Proc Natl Acad Sci USA 2009; 106: 1886–91.

284. Lee W, Jiang Z, Liu J, et al. The mutation spectrum revealed by paired genome sequences from a lung cancer patient. Nature 2010; 465: 473–7.

285. Berger MF, Levin JZ, Vijayendran K, et al. Integrative analysis of the melanoma transcriptome. Genome Res 2010; 20: 413–27.

286. Weigelt B, Pusztai L, Ashworth A, Reis-Filho JS. Challenges translating breast cancer gene signatures into the clinic. Nat Rev Clin Oncol 2011; 9: 58–64.

30 The role of multidisciplinary teams in breast cancer management

Cath Taylor, Amanda Shewbridge, Massimiliano Cariati, and Anand Purushotham

INTRODUCTION

The increasing complexity of treatment and management decisions for cancer patients has led to the need for relevant nursing, surgical, medical, and diagnostic experts to work closely together in order to optimize patient care. As a consequence, multidisciplinary teams (MDTs) are firmly established at the core of cancer care in many countries worldwide, defined by the United Kingdom (UK) Department of Health as *"a group of people of different health care disciplines which meets together at a given time (whether physically in one place, or by video or tele-conferencing) to discuss a given patient and who are each able to contribute independently to the diagnostic and treatment decisions about the patient."* (1).

Although central to the management of breast cancer in many health systems worldwide, a recent survey involving breast cancer specialists from 39 countries revealed wide variation in MDT practice by geographical region (2). Furthermore, although MDTs were found to be mandatory practice in many countries, only a quarter of countries reported having national or regional guidelines regarding the composition or practice of MDT working.

BREAST CANCER MDTS IN THE UK

In the UK the provision of cancer care by MDTs is mandatory. This has followed national policy recommendations starting with the Calman–Hine report in 1995 (3), and given further impetus by the publication of tumor-specific improving outcomes guidance, starting with the Breast Cancer guidance in 1996 (4). The formation of MDTs with a clearly defined core and extended membership with appropriate specialist expertise is central to the guidance, as is the need for regular (weekly) meetings to discuss and agree management recommendations for all new breast cancer cases. Subsequent cancer policy in the UK has reinforced the importance of the MDT at the core of providing optimal care to cancer patients (5,6).

In order to monitor adherence to the national guidance, the UK NHS launched a cancer peer review program in 2004 (7). The process required all MDTs to submit an annual self-assessment to a national database, which was followed by targeted validation of the data for some MDTs by an external peer-review team (made up of clinicians, patients, commissioners, and managers) who might also visit the team (see www.cquins.nhs.uk). Analysis of the findings from reviews (2009/2010) involving over 900 MDTs (including 157 breast cancer teams) showed an improvement in adherence for breast cancer teams (from a median percentage adherence of 77% in 2004–2008 to 86% in 2009–2010) (8). Despite this achievement, nearly a third of breast cancer teams had a serious concern noted, and 13% were deemed to have an immediate risk such as complex surgery taking place outside the designated center, though it was noted that most of the serious concerns for breast cancer teams related to core team membership for which the requirements were more challenging than for other tumor types. Core team membership for breast cancer teams requires two designated breast surgeons, a clinical oncologist, a medical oncologist (where the responsibility of chemotherapy is not undertaken by the clinical oncology core member), two imaging specialists, two histopathologists, two breast nurse specialists, and an MDT coordinator/secretary. The extended team members should ideally include a reconstructive/plastic surgeon, clinical geneticist/ genetics counselor, palliative care specialist, radiographer, primary care team, physiotherapist/lymphedema specialist, psychiatrist or clinical psychologist, and a social worker. It is expected that each MDT should see at least 100 new cases of breast cancer each year (1).

BENEFITS OF MDTS

In a UK national survey involving over 2000 MDT members, over 90% of respondents agreed that an effective MDT results in improved clinical decision making, more coordinated patient care, improvement to overall quality of care, more evidence-based treatment decisions, and improved treatment (9). Although MDTs had been introduced prior to conducting robust trials of their potential effectiveness, there is growing evidence that MDTs confer benefits in a number of ways.

Clinical Benefit

It is now accepted that the diagnosis, management, and survival rates of breast cancer are superior when undertaken in specialized breast teams (10–12), and similar evidence exists for other tumor types (13–15). Specifically, these benefits are seen where surgeons have workloads of more than 30 breast cancer patients per year (16), when surgeons refer to oncologists and when there is increased use of adjuvant chemotherapy or hormone therapy (17). Of greatest significance is the reduction in mortality achieved when breast specialists within a larger, teaching hospital setting manage breast cancer (18,19). It has been shown that care by specialist surgeons can confer 9% of 5-year and 8% of 10-year survival advantages to breast cancer patients (20). Appropriateness of treatments can also be measured, with fewer mastectomies and higher rates of breast-conserving surgery in specialist units (18,21,22). The use of adjuvant therapies such as chemotherapy and hormone treatments is also significantly higher in specialist units, resulting in a clear survival advantage (17,21,23,24).

Similar influences of MDT discussion on the quality of diagnostic and treatment decisions have been demonstrated in lung (25), colorectal (26), and upper GI cancers (27). This is likely to require an inclusive discussion across a range of specialists groups. In a study of breast cancer teams in the UK the proportion of breast care nurses and team workload was related to clinical performance (28). Leadership style was also found to impact on performance; teams where leadership was shared between members were most effective, but lack of clarity and conflict over leadership reduced the effectiveness. A systematic review of literature regarding MDT decision making concluded that key influences on decision making were team culture, leadership style, the quality of available information, and practical issues such as whether attendance and preparation were in job plans (29).

Education
The MDT approach to the diagnosis and management of patients offers many opportunities for education and professional development. For the standard of breast cancer care to be maintained, junior medical staff must have experience of and training within a specialist breast team. Furthermore, meetings with general practitioners to discuss common presentations in primary care and referral guidelines can assist in focusing resources appropriately and minimizing delay in the diagnosis of breast cancer. Educational opportunities could also be extended to primary caregivers and to the community through educational symposia and provision of high quality literature.

Health Professional Satisfaction
It has been shown that a well-functioning MDT can improve an individual's efficiency at work, morale, and work satisfaction. A further reported benefit is enhanced mental health of team members as a result of working within the team environment (9,30). In a national survey of over 2000 cancer MDT members, 90% felt that working in an MDT was beneficial to their mental health, and 81% felt that it increased job satisfaction (9). MDT working was confirmed as the main source of job satisfaction in a study of colorectal cancer MDT members in the UK (30). This impact may be attributed to the sharing of clinical load and diagnostic responsibility. The camaraderie associated with being part of a well-functioning team may also be beneficial.

Patient Experience
The impact of MDT working on patient experience of their care has received little attention to date though improvements to cancer patient care from national surveys undertaken in the UK have been linked to the implementation of MDTs (31). Treatment planning meetings (MDT meetings) are typically not attended by patients. Surveys of cancer health professionals' views about patient attendance in MDT meetings have shown that this is felt to be neither desirable nor practical (9), though in one survey, of breast cancer professionals and patient advocates in Australia, the patient advocates and nurses were supportive of women with breast cancer attending the meetings (32). A pilot study in Australia evaluated the impact of including women with breast cancer in MDT meetings and found it was acceptable to both staff and MDT members (33).

Further exploration of how best to ensure that patients are effectively and meaningfully involved in treatment decision making within the context of MDTs is required. The logistics of managing a large clinical caseload for discussion at every MDT should be borne in mind.

Research/Involvement in Clinical Trials
National guidelines for the management of breast cancer are directly formulated from scientific evidence obtained from clinical trials. Advances in breast cancer management are ongoing, and specialist breast cancer units that treat cohorts of patients provide the ideal setting for clinical trials. Discussion of patient eligibility for trials in MDT meetings has been associated with improved recruitment to trials (34), but confusion about which team members' are responsible for discussing trials with patients may lead to missed recruitment opportunities (35–37). Team members may also require training to ensure that this aspect of communication is effectively delivered (35). While this has not been shown to confer a survival benefit *per se*, it is vital that the MDT be committed to the development of better care for breast cancer patients and to facilitate entry into clinical trials.

OBSTACLES TO SUCCESS
It is difficult to identify disadvantages in the multidisciplinary approach to breast cancer treatment when it is properly implemented. More appropriate is the identification of obstacles to success that can be disadvantageous to both patients and team members alike.

A systematic review of decision making in MDTs concluded that factors such as time pressure, lack of information, lack of nursing input, and poor team leadership can have a negative impact on team decision making (29). Poor communication between colleagues, failure to create a flat, non-hierarchical structure within the team, clash of egos or priorities, and poor definition of the role of each team member all contribute to a dysfunctional MDT (38). It has been shown that 39% of senior oncology nurses and 33% of oncologists cite communication with colleagues as their most stressful and challenging concerns within the multidisciplinary setting (39,40). Poor communication, while stressful for team members, is also disadvantageous to the optimum care of the cancer patient. Poor teamworking in MDT meetings may lead to non-inclusive discussions resulting in information bias, with discussions being centered on the "tumor" rather than "person" (41,42). Failure of the team to consider all relevant information may lead to poor decisions, or to decisions which are not implemented as they are unacceptable to patients or clinically inappropriate (43–46). Non-implementation of MDT meeting recommendations can have both clinical and financial consequences if further discussion is required and treatment is delayed.

To our knowledge there has been no research examining what patients know, and need to know, about the MDT to be effectively involved in decisions about their care. If patients are used to being under the care of one consultant the concept of the MDT may be difficult to comprehend and may result in a perceived lack of continuity of care due to having multiple professionals involved in their care. This may result in patients losing confidence, with an accompanying feeling of depersonalization of care. This problem can be largely avoided by a clear definition of each individual member's role within the MDT, and good communication with the patient, providing reassurance that each team member is familiar with all aspects of their case. The Breast Care Nurse (BCN) role is of particular benefit and is very often the focal point for the patient and it is discussed in detail in the next section.

BREAST CARE NURSE

The recognition of the need to identify and address psychosocial concerns in women diagnosed with breast cancer led to the early development of the BCN role in the 1970s (47,48). The role has continued to evolve across the UK, Australia, North America, and Europe and plays a pivotal part in the multidisciplinary management of breast cancer. In the UK, it is expected that all patients have access to an appropriately trained BCN from the time of diagnosis to provide information and psychological support and coordinate their care throughout the treatment pathway (1). The psychosocial impact of a breast cancer can be significant (49). Holistic assessment of individual need is recognized as key to delivering patient centered care. Identified needs can be complex and multifaceted. Physical, psychological, social, spiritual, sexual, and cultural issues should be considered as part of routine assessment (50). Specialist nursing interventions include the provision of tailored information regarding decision making; emotional support; and advice about practical issues, for example finances and work and management of ongoing side effects. The BCN is usually the patient's named point of contact (key worker) (51). Studies show these nursing interactions impact on patient experience and quality of life (52,53).

Traditionally, the emphasis of the nursing role has been focused on information and support at the time of diagnosis of early breast cancer and throughout primary treatment. There has been a shift in emphasis within the past 5 years to include a greater focus on the ongoing care needs and concerns of patients beyond completion of treatment. These are known to include fatigue, physical and sexual functioning, psychosocial issues, the fear of recurrence, uncertainty, and social support needs (54). Specialist nurses play a key role in both identifying these concerns and signposting patients to appropriate services at this time. Equally important is the recognition that women with secondary breast cancer have unique needs. In the UK, it is recommended that women with secondary breast cancer have equal access to specialist nursing support (55). This has led to some services developing specific secondary breast care nursing roles (56).

COMMUNICATING SIGNIFICANT NEWS

Communication of significant news and information occurs at multiple points throughout the patient pathway. The approach to "breaking bad news" should be tailored to individual needs. The process should be via a staged approach rather than an abrupt overload of information (57). The patient needs time to digest the information and then resulting concerns should be explored. Concerns may include shock at the diagnosis and fears about mortality, uncertainty about specific treatment, and potential side effects and worries about the impact on other family members.

As the complexity of treatment of breast cancer increases, it is essential that patients are provided with relevant information about their treatment options and their efficacy to inform patient choice and decision making. Patients who feel involved in the treatment decision-making process may have fewer psychological concerns in the future (58). Written information

and details of appropriate internet sites should be offered to support face-to-face consultations. Some patients may choose to decline treatment. It is important that communication between the clinicians and the patient remains open and honest. The patient needs to be aware of the potential consequences of declining treatment and should be offered the opportunity to return to see the team for further discussions if required or if their views change (59).

THE COST OF MDTS

MDTs are a very expensive resource. There are approximately 1500 cancer MDTs in England, and based simply on the data about the time taken for radiologists and pathologists to prepare for MDT meetings (60), it has been estimated they cost £100 million a year for attendance and preparation time (31). National work is underway to determine how best to cost multidisciplinary care provision in the UK. This is important not least due to the opportunity for transferring some of the cost to the private sector, whose patients are sometimes discussed in NHS MDT meetings at no charge. Education and training of members of the team to the exacting standards required are also costly. This is counterbalanced, however, by the more efficient and effective use of resources and improved outcomes (1).

There is some indication that the provision of breast care services by an MDT within a specialist breast unit may reduce the volume and costs of litigation related to breast cancer management. In the United States, dissatisfaction with breast cancer diagnosis and treatment is the cause of one of the highest number of litigation claims (61). Good communication and provision of information to patients can go a long way toward improving satisfaction.

TECHNOLOGICAL SOLUTIONS TO MDT WORKING

Ensuring optimal team membership often requires crossing geographical boundaries and increasingly MDTs are reliant on the use of tele- or videoconferencing to facilitate collaborative decision making. Research has shown that decisions made by teams using teleconferencing are comparable in quality to those made in face-to-face meetings (62,63) and can save considerable time (64). In breast cancer there have also been major advances in the use of technology to aid decision making (see for example http://mate.cossac.org/). Based on mathematical logic, such systems are designed to be used in routine practice to improve the quality and safety of clinical decisions (65). Still under development, such technologies may further streamline MDT treatment planning meetings and enable teams to focus on the complex non-routine cases that most require their expertise.

DEFINING THE CHARACTERISTICS OF EFFECTIVE MDT WORKING

The National Cancer Action Team conducted a national survey of MDT members' perceptions of MDT working in 2009 (9). Over 2000 MDT members responded to the survey and the high level of consensus between tumor types and across professional groups led to the development of recommendations for effective teamworking in cancer MDTs. The Characteristics of an Effective MDT issued by the National Cancer Action Team (66) provides recommendations for MDT working across 17 domains of teamwork organized under five headings (Table 30.1).

Table 30.1 The Characteristics of an Effective MDT (NCAT, 2010)

Key Domain	Subdomain	Example of Recommendation
The Team	Membership	All relevant professions/disciplines—core and extended members—are represented in the team in line with the Manual of Cancer Services
	Attendance	MDT members (core and extended) have dedicated time included in their job plans to prepare for, travel to (if necessary), and attend MDT meetings; the amount of time is negotiated locally to reflect their workload and varies according to discipline and cancer type
	Leadership and chairing	There is an identified leader/chair of the MDT and a deputy to cover when necessary; the leader and the chair do not have to be the same person
	Teamworking and culture	Each MDT member has clearly defined roles and responsibilities within the team which they have signed up to and which are included in their job plans
	Personal development and training	Team members recognize the need for continued learning and individual members are supported to gain the necessary knowledge and skills for their roles and responsibilities within the MDT and for their respective professional role; support is available from the team, the organization, and nationally as appropriate and members take up relevant CPD opportunities
Infrastructure for meetings	Physical environment of meeting room	The room is environmentally appropriate in size and layout, that is, all team members have a seat and are able to see and hear each other and view all presented data (e.g., diagnostics) within and across hospital trusts
	Technology and equipment	Rooms where MDT meetings take place have: access to equipment for projecting and viewing radiology images including retrospective images; facilities for projecting and viewing specimen biopsies/resections and accessing retrospective pathology reports; connection to PACS; access to a database or proforma to enable documentation of recommendations in real time; projection facilities so members can view and validate the recommendations being recorded; facilities (when needed) to see and speak to members who are off site (e.g., videoconferencing) and share all information that will be viewed (e.g., images and reports) with them.
Meeting organization and logistics	Scheduling of MDT meetings	MDT meetings take place regularly (as set out in Manual of Cancer Services)
	Preparation prior to MDT meetings	Processes are in place to ensure that all patients diagnosed with a primary cancer have their case considered by the relevant MDT and it is clear when patient cases can be taken back to MDTs including when discussions of patients with metastatic disease/recurrence should take place
	Organization/administration during MDT meetings	It is clear who wants to discuss a particular patient and why that patient is being discussed
	Post-MDT meeting/coordination of service	Relevant items from cancer datasets are completed (if this has not been done in real time at the meeting)
Patient-centered clinical decision-making	Who to discuss?	There are local mechanisms in place to identify all patients where discussion at MDT is needed
	Patient-centered care	A patient's views/preferences/holistic needs are presented by someone who has met the patient whenever possible
	Clinical decision-making process	A locally agreed minimum dataset of information is provided at the meeting, that is, the information the MDT needs to make informed recommendations including diagnostic information (pathology and radiology); clinical information (including comorbidities, psychosocial and specialist palliative care needs); and patient history, views and preferences. It is important that any data items collected locally that are in existing national datasets or are within the NHS Data Dictionary are in line with these data definitions and codes when collected
Team governance	Organizational support	There is organizational (employer) support for MDT meetings and MDT membership demonstrated through recognition that MDTs are the accepted model by which to deliver safe and high-quality cancer care; adequate funding/resources in terms of people, time, equipment and facilities for MDT meetings to operate effectively
	Data collection, analysis, and audit of outcomes	The MDT takes part in internal and external audits of processes and outcomes and reviews audit data (e.g., to confirm that treatment recommendations match current best practice and to consider trial recruitment) taking action to change practice etc. where necessary
	Clinical governance	Significant discrepancies in pathology, radiology, or clinical findings between local and specialist MDTs should be recorded and be subject to audit

Abbreviations: CPD, continuous professional development; MDT, multidisciplinary team; NCAT, The National Cancer Action Team.

IMPROVING MDT WORKING

In the UK, now that MDTs are firmly established, attention has turned to ensuring that teams are supported to work effectively. The National Cancer Action Team, responsible for supporting the implementation of cancer policy in England, has MDT development as a key priority (66).

Addressing variability in teamworking requires valid robust assessment tools, effective teamwork and leadership interventions, and appropriate financial investment. Indeed, team members have stated a desire for valid self-assessment tools that enable them to assess the core functions of their team, and for access to team training (9). In other areas of health care, most notably surgery, team assessment tools and training interventions have been developed and there is evidence of their efficacy (67). Many skills are required for a team to work effectively, one of which is the ability to communicate well. Research has shown that communication skills can be taught and skills maintained (68,69). An evidence-based national training program is offered to all senior cancer health professionals and is a mandatory requirement for core team members who have direct clinical contact with patients (1). Extending this training to include inter- and intrateam communication skills is likely to confer additional benefit both to team members and patients. Various tools have been developed to support assessment and improvement in performance, including tools for independent observational assessment (70,71) of team performance and checklists for monitoring performance (72). The information provided to teams from using these and other such tools may provide teams with valuable feedback that may alone enhance performance (73). Crucially it is necessary for adequate investment in the necessary resources for effective MDT working, in particular ensuring that teams have the required membership, that attendance and preparation time for MDT meetings is within job plans, and that the environment and technical facilities are of the required standard for effective multidisciplinary teamworking.

CONCLUSION

The modern approach to breast cancer management involves MDT working in specialist breast units, which in turn are aligned to larger cancer centres and networks. This approach has been proven to be of benefit to patients and team members, in terms of survival, appropriateness of therapy, timely provision of services, work satisfaction, and educational and research opportunities. As the management of breast cancer continues to get even more complex with the potential introduction of molecular-based individualized treatment regimens, the role of the MDT will become even more critical. Now that the MDT's practice, purpose and outputs are clearly defined in the UK, adherence to local and national guidelines, regular audits, and interaction with user partnership groups are of paramount importance to ensure up-to-date practice and delivery of clinical excellence.

REFERENCES

1. The Department of Health. Manual for Cancer Services. London: The Department of Health, 2008.
2. Saini KS, Taylor C, Ramirez AJ, et al. Role of the multidisciplinary team in breast cancer management: results from a large international survey involving 39 countries. Ann Oncol 2012; 23: 853–9.
3. Department of Health. Policy Framework for Commissioning Cancer Services: A Report by the Expert Advisory Group on Cancer to the Chief Medical Officers of England and Wales. London: Department of Health, 1995.
4. Cancer Guidance Sub-Group of the Clinical Outcomes Group. Improving Outcomes in Breast Cancer. London: Department of Health, 1996.
5. Department of Health. Cancer Reform Strategy. London: Department of Health, 2007.
6. Department of Health. Improving Outcomes: A Strategy for Cancer. London: Department of Health, 2011.
7. The Department of Health. Manual for Cancer Services. London: Department of Health, 2004.
8. National Cancer Action Team. National Cancer Peer Review Programme Report 2009/2010: An Overview of the Findings from the 2009/2010 National Cancer Peer Review of Cancer Services in England. London: National Cancer Action Team, 2010.
9. Taylor C, Ramirez AJ. Multidisciplinary Team Members' Views About MDT Working: Results from a Survey Commissioned by the National Cancer Action team. London: National Cancer Action Team, 2009.
10. Eaker S, Dickam P, Hellstrom V, et al. Regional differences in breast cancer survival despite common guidelines. Cancer Epideimol Biomarkers Prev 2005; 14: 2914–18.
11. Houssami N, Sainsbury R. Breast cancer: multidisciplinary care and clinical outcomes. Eur J Cancer 2006; 42: 2480–91.
12. Kesson EM, Allardice GM, George WD, et al. Effects of multidisciplinary team working on breast cancer survival: retrospective, comparative, interventional cohort study of 13 722 women. BMJ 2012; 344: e2718.
13. Morris E, Haward RA, Gilthorpe MS, et al. The impact of the Calman-Hine report on the processes and outcomes of care for Yorkshire's colorectal cancer patients. Br J Cancer 2006; 95: 979–85.
14. Stephens MR, Lewis WG, Brewster AE, et al. Multidisciplinary team management is associated with improved outcomes after surgery for esophageal cancer. Dis Esophagus 2006; 19: 164–71.
15. Birchall M, Bailey D, King P; South West Cancer Intelligence Service Head and Neck Tumour Panel. Effect of process standards on survival of patients with head and neck cancer in the south and west of England. Br J Cancer 2004; 91: 1477–81.
16. Satariano ER, Swanson MG, Moll PP. Nonclinical factors associated with surgery received for treatment of early-stage breast cancer. Am J Public Health 1992; 82: 195–8.
17. Lee-Feldstein A, Anton-Culver H, Feldstein PJ. Treatment differences and other prognostic factors related to breast cancer survival. Delivery systems and medical outcomes. JAMA 1994; 271: 1163–8.
18. Selby P, Gillis C, Haward R. Benefits from specialised cancer care. Lancet 1996; 348: 313–18.
19. Hand R, Sener S, Imperato J, et al. Hospital variables associated with quality of care for breast cancer patients. JAMA 1991; 266: 3429–32.
20. Yarnold JR, Bliss JM, Brunt M, et al. Management of breast cancer. Refer women to multidisciplinary clinics. BMJ 1994; 308: 168–71.
21. Sainsbury R. Organization of breast cancer services. Cancer Treat Rev 1997; 23: S3–11.
22. Lauria MM. Continuity of cancer care. Cancer 1991; 67: 1759–66.
23. Schipper H, Dick J. Herodotus and the multidisciplinary clinic. Lancet 1995; 346: 1312–13.
24. Durant JR. How to organize a multidisciplinary clinic for the management of breast cancer. Surg Clin North Am 1990; 70: 977–83.
25. Coory M, Gkolia P, Yang I, et al. Systematic review of multidisciplinary teams in the management of lung cancer. Lung Cancer 2008; 60: 14–21.
26. Burton S, Brown G, Daniels IR, et al. MRI directed multidisciplinary team preoperative treatment strategy: the way to eliminate positive circumferential margins? Br J Cancer 2006; 94: 351–7.
27. Davies AR, Deans DA, Penman I, et al. The multidisciplinary team meeting improves staging accuracy and treatment selection for gastro-esophageal cancer. Dis Esophagus 2006; 19: 496–503.
28. Haward R, Amir Z, Borrill C, et al. Breast cancer teams: the impact of constitution, new cancer workload, and methods of operation on their effectiveness. Br J Cancer 2003; 89: 15–22.
29. Lamb BW, Brown KF, Nagpal K, et al. Quality of care management decisions by multidisciplinary teams: a systematic review. Ann Surg Oncol 2011; 18: 2116–25.

30. Taylor C, Sippitt J, Collins G, et al. A pre-post test evaluation of the impact of the PELICAN MDT-TME Development Programme on the working lives of colorectal team members. BMC Health Serv Res 2010; 10: 187.

31. Taylor C, Munro AJ, Glynne-Jones R, et al. Multidisciplinary team working in cancer: what is the evidence? BMJ 2010; 340: c951.

32. Butow P, Harrison JD, Choy ET, et al. Health professional and consumer views on involving breast cancer patients in the multidisciplinary discussion of their disease and treatment plan. Cancer 2007; 110: 1937–44.

33. Choy ET, Chiu A, Butow P, et al. A pilot study to evaluate the impact of involving breast cancer patients in the multidisciplinary discussion of their disease and treatment plan. Breast 2007; 16: 178–89.

34. McNair AGK, Choh CTP, Metcalfe C, et al. Maximising recruitment into randomised controlled trials: the role of multidisciplinary cancer teams. Eur J Cancer 2008; 44: 2623–6.

35. Jenkins V, Fallowfield LJ, Poole K. Are members of multidisciplinary teams in breast cancer aware of each other's informational roles? Qual Health Care 2001; 10: 70–5.

36. Catt S, Fallowfield L, Jenkins V, et al. The informational roles and psychological health of members of 10 oncology multidisciplinary teams in the UK. Br J Cancer 2005; 93: 1092–7.

37. Cox A, Jenkins V, Catt S, et al. Information needs and experiences: an audit of UK cancer patients. Eur J Oncol Nurs 2006; 10: 263–72.

38. Fleissig AJ, Jenkins V, Catt S, et al. Multidisciplinary teams in cancer care: are they effective in the UK? Lancet Oncol 2006; 7: 935–43.

39. Fallowfield L, Saul J, Gilligan B. Teaching senior nurses how to teach communication skills in oncology. Cancer Nurs 2001; 2424: 185–91.

40. Fallowfield L, Lipkin M, Hall A. Teaching senior oncologists communication skills: results from phase I of a comprehensive longitudinal program in the United Kingdom. J Clin Oncol 1998; 16: 1961–8.

41. Lanceley AS, Savage J, Menon U, et al. Influences on multidisciplinary team decision-making. Int J Gynecol Cancer 2008; 18: 215–22.

42. Kidger J, Murdoch J, Donovan JL, et al. Clinical decision-making in a multidisciplinary gynaecological cancer team: a qualitative study. BJOG 2009; 116: 511–17.

43. Leo F, Venissac N, Poudenx M, et al. Multidisciplinary management of lung cancer: how to test its efficacy? J Thorac Oncol 2007; 2: 69–72.

44. Stalfors J, Lundberg C, Westin T. Quality assessment of a multidisciplinary tumour meeting for patients with head and neck cancer. Acta Otolaryngol 2007; 127: 82–7.

45. Blazeby JM, Wilson L, Metcalfe C, et al. Analysis of clinical decision-making in multi-disciplinary cancer teams. Ann Oncol 2006; 17: 457–60.

46. Lamb BW, Sevdalis N, Arora S, et al. Teamwork and team decision-making at multidisciplinary cancer conferences: barriers, facilitators, and opportunities for improvement. World J Surg 2011; 35: 1970–6.

47. Maguire GP, Lee EG, Bevington DJ, et al. Psychiatric problems in the first year after mastectomy. BMJ 1978; 1: 963–5.

48. Maguire P, Brooke M, Tait A, et al. The effects of counselling on physical disability and social recovery after mastectomy. Clin Oncol 1983; 9: 319–24.

49. Burgess C, Cornelius V, Love S, et al. Depression and anxiety in women with early breast cancer: five year observational cohort study. BMJ 2005; 330: 702.

50. Richardson A, Tebbit P, Sitzia J, et al. Holistic Common Assessment of Supportive and Palliative Care Needs For Adults With Cancer: Assessment Guidance. London: National Cancer Action Team, 2007.

51. Amir Z, Scully J, Borrill C. The professional role of the breast care nurse in multidisciplinary breast care teams. Eur J Oncol Nurs 2004; 8: 306–14.

52. Redman S, Turner J, Davis C. Improving supportive care for women with breast cancer in Australia: the challenge of modifying health systems. Psychooncology 2003; 12: 521–31.

53. Halkett G, Arbon P, Scutter S, et al. The role of the breast care nurse during treatment for early breast cancer: the patient's perspective. Contemp Nurse 2006; 23: 46–57.

54. Richardson A, Addington-Hall J, Amir Z, et al. Knowledge, ignorance and priorities for research in key areas of cancer survivorship: findings from a scoping review. Br J Cancer 2011; 105(Suppl): S82–94.

55. Secondary Breast Cancer Taskforce. Guide for Commissioners. Meeting the Nursing Needs of Metastatic Breast Cancer Patients. London: Breast Cancer Care, 2008.

56. Watts K, Merser B, Conlon H, et al. A specialist breast care nurse role for women with metastatic breast cancer: enhancing supportive care. Oncol Nurs Forum 2011; 38: 627–31.

57. Fujimori M, Uchitomi Y. Preferences of cancer patients regarding communication of bad news: a systematic review of the literature. Jpn J Clin Oncol 2009; 39: 210–16.

58. Keating N, Guadagnoli E, Landrum M, et al. Treatment decision making in early-stage breast cancer: should surgeons match patients' desired level of involvement? J Clin Oncol 2002; 20: 1473–9.

59. Verhoef MJ, Rose MS, White M, et al. Declining conventional cancer treatment and using complementary and alternative medicine: a problem or a challenge? Curr Oncol 2008; 15: s101–6.

60. Kane B, Luz S, O'Briain DS, et al. Multidisciplinary team meetings and their impact on workflow in radiology and pathology departments. BMC Med 2007; 5: 15.

61. Physician Insurers Association of America. Breast Cancer Study, 3rd edn. Rockville, MD: Physician Insurers Association of America, Spring, 2002.

62. Kunkler IH, Prescott RJ, Lee RJ, et al. TELEMAN: A cluster randomised trial to assess the use of telemedicine in multi-disciplinary breast cancer decision making. Eur J Cancer 2007; 43: 2506–14.

63. Kunkler IH, Fielding RG, Macnab M, et al. Group dynamics within telemedicine-delivered and standard multidisciplinary team meetings: results from the TELEMAN randomised trial. J Telemed Telecare 2006; 12: s55–8.

64. Davison AG, Eraut CD, Haque AS, et al. Telemedicine for multidisciplinary lung cancer meetings. J Telemed Telecare 2004; 10: 140–3.

65. Fox J, Patkar V, Chronakis I, et al. From practice guidelines to clinical decision support: closing the loop. J R Soc Med 2009; 102: 464–73.

66. National Cancer Action Team. The Characteristics of an Effective MDT. London: NCAT, 2010.

67. McCulloch P, Rathbone J, Catchpole K. Interventions to improve teamwork and communications among healthcare staff. Br J Surg 2011; 98: 469–79.

68. Fallowfield LJ, Jenkins V, Farewell V, et al. Efficacy of a Cancer Research UK communications skills training model for oncologists: a randomised controlled trial. Lancet 2002; 359: 650–6.

69. Fallowfield LJ, Jenkins V, Farewell V, et al. Enduring impact of communication skills training: results of a 12-month follow up. Br J Cancer 2003; 89: 1445–9.

70. Lamb BW, Wong HW, Vincent C, et al. Teamwork and team performance in multidisciplinary cancer teams: development and evaluation of an observational assessment tool. BMJ Qual Saf 2011; 20: 849–56.

71. Taylor C, Atkins L, Richardson A, et al. Measuring the quality of MDT working: an observational approach. BMC Cancer, 2012; 12: 202 doi:10.1186/1471-2407-12-202.

72. Lamb BW, Sevdalis N, Vincent C, et al. Development and evaluation of a checklist to support decision-making in cancer multidisciplinary team meetings: MDT-QuIC. Ann Surg Oncol 2012; 19: 1759–65.

73. Jamtvedt G, Young JM, Kristoffersen DT, et al. Audit and feedback: effects on professional practice and health care outcomes. Cochrane Database Syst Rev 2006; 19: CD000259.

31 Shared decision-making for breast cancer patients

Catharine F. Clay, Alice O. Andrews, and Dale Collins Vidal

SYNOPSIS

- Healthcare decisions are complicated because they involve trade-offs between benefits and harms.
- Patients may have different values regarding the potential benefits and harms, so it is important to involve them in decision making.
- Many barriers prevent patients from participating in decision making. These arise from health system design, clinician training and practice, and patient roles and expectations.
- Tools that offer decision support, such as evidence-based decision aids, can be used to overcome some of the barriers on the part of patients. There is strong evidence that these tools can improve knowledge and engage patients in the decision-making process.
- Several models exist for implementing shared decision making (SDM) in clinical practice. The appropriate model depends on the environment, disease state, evidence about treatment options, and the clinical system in which the decision occurs.
- Successful implementation of SDM requires a system that aligns processes to foster and support this work.
- The legal standard for preference-sensitive care should move away from informed consent and toward an informed patient choice.
- The process of informing and consenting applies to all healthcare choices, and is not limited to those for which a signed form is required.

Healthcare choices are complicated and can be difficult. Such decision making often occurs when emotions are strong, outcomes are uncertain, and consequences are lifealtering. For example, a diagnosis of breast cancer initiates a series of highly emotional events over which patients may feel they have little control. Women with early-stage breast cancer face decisions at many time points, ranging from surgery and radiation therapy choices to breast reconstruction to adjuvant therapy. (1–5). The consequences of these high-stakes choices have a lasting impact on women and their families.

Having options and making choices can be empowering for patients facing serious illness, but these decisions can also be overwhelming. Each choice involves trade-offs between benefits and harms, such as the increased chance of recurrence with lumpectomy, or donor site morbidity with reconstruction. How are these decisions made? For early-stage breast cancer, research indicates that high rates of mastectomy can mean women are not informed of the breast conservation option. Conversely, high rates of breast conservation are advertised as high-quality care, when the reality may be that women are not being offered or supported in choosing mastectomy. Other studies suggest that non-clinical factors like access to radiation therapy or physician preference determine this choice. What is the "right" rate (the rate at which a fully informed women choose mastectomy or lumpectomy) of uptake of surgical options for early-stage breast cancer? We do not know, but when a choice can be based on patient preference, the patient must be an equal partner in selecting a treatment, and the goal of achieving the right rate becomes more real.

Decisions like these mentioned for breast cancer have been termed *preference-sensitive* decisions by the Dartmouth Atlas project (see sidebar). Involving patients in these decisions has been shown to result in better decision quality—a choice that is informed, consistent with the patient's value, and actionable (6) (Fig. 31.1). A high-quality decision requires that patients have adequate decision-specific knowledge and an understanding of their personal clinical circumstances and values, and make treatment choices consistent with those values (7).

A patient-centered approach to decision making is one of the six dimensions identified by the Institute of Medicine for improving quality of care and an integral part of the "Triple-Aim": improving the care experience, improving the health of populations, and reducing costs (16). The importance of such work is evident in changes to national policy since 2010. In the United Kingdom (UK), the National Health Service (NHS) has included shared decision making (SDM) as a core principle; the goal is to become a health system within which "shared decision making will become the norm: No decision about me without me" (page 3) (17). Across the Atlantic, the 2010 United States (US) Affordable Care Act includes language to promote and nurture the process of SDM between providers and patients (18).

One concern about this growing movement is that the pendulum will swing too far toward leaving patients to make medical decisions on their own. SDM does not mean ceding the medical decision over to patients completely. Moulton and King (19) discuss the historical origins in this shift from *physician beneficence*, or the duty of doctors to "promote good and act in the best interest of the patient and the health of society" (20) to a more patient-centered model. Under the principle of physician beneficence, physicians use their expertise to act as the patient's agent, meaning that they are responsible for choosing the most appropriate course of treatment even if it is contrary to or fails to take into account a patient's desires. In an effort to move away from this outdated decision-making model, Moulton and King report anecdotal evidence that doctors have reacted by using the other extreme, that of *patient autonomy*, where the patient has complete decision control

The Dartmouth Atlas (www.dartmouthatlas.org), developed by Dr John Wennberg, provides a methodology to compare rates of procedures across hospital systems and locations. In the United States, this methodology segments the country into 3436 Hospital Service Areas (HSAs) representing local markets for health care. HSAs are aggregated to 306 Hospital Referral Regions (HRRs), each of which is a market for tertiary care. All HRRs have at least one city where both cardiovascular and neurosurgeries are performed (for additional information, see http://www.dartmouthatlas.org/data/region/).

Researchers using Dartmouth Atlas data have identified striking amounts of variation across geographic regions in the United States related to the number of treatments, surgical procedures, and both hospital and doctor visits. Some of this variation remains unexplained after controlling for case mix and physician payment systems. For example, surgical procedures show up to 10-fold differences in rates (8), indicating the general consensus of the local medical community (2,8–12). Dr Wennberg refers to these differential rates as the "surgical signature" of the local area (2,12).

The first comprehensive NHS Atlas of Variation in Health Care was published in the United Kingdom in November 2010. (http://www.rightcare.nhs.uk/index.php/nhs-atlas/) This Atlas presents 34 maps of variation on topics selected by clinicians as important to their specialty. The 2011 second edition of the Atlas was greatly expanded and covers 71 indicators and 15 program budget categories. All Atlases are also available as fully interactive online maps.

Effective, Supply-Sensitive, and Preference-Sensitive Care

Dr Wennberg termed this unexplained variance an *unwarranted* variation and divided it into three types: the *underuse of effective care*, the *overuse of supply-sensitive care*, and the *misuse of preference-sensitive care* (13). Effective care refers to interventions where evidence supports their routine use; underuse of this type of care often compromises patient safety. For example, annual eye examinations for diabetics may prevent blindness, but many patients do not receive this care (retrieved October 21, 2011 from http://www.dartmouthatlas.org/keyissues/issue.aspx?con=2939). Unfortunately, effective care is often underutilized. A study by the Rand Corporation found that just 45% of adults presenting with an acute myocardial infarction received beta blockers and only 39% of adults with pneumonia received recommended care (Pneumovax, influenza vaccine, and antibiotics) (14).

Supply-sensitive care results from a lack of evidence to determine the appropriate use of services, as in the number of return visits for someone with a chronic illness. When more resources (specialists and hospital beds) are available, more care (visits and hospital stays) will occur, given a similar patient case-mix (retrieved October 21, 2011 from http://www.dartmouthatlas.org/keyissues/issue.aspx?con=2937).

Preference-sensitive care involves situations where treatment choices include multiple options with trade-offs between risks and benefits. Under these conditions, treatment choices *should* belong to patients (13) to ensure that they receive "the care patients need and no less, and the care they want, and no more[1]." For example, a Canadian study of patients with hip and knee arthritis showed that only 8–15% of patients eligible for arthroplasty definitely wanted to undergo the procedure (15). Unwarranted variation (both underuse and overuse) in preference-sensitive care is considered a "misuse" of medical resources. Often it is a situation where physician recommendation, not patient preference, drives treatment choices.

---

[1] Quotation from Dr Al Mulley, The Center for Healthcare Delivery Science at Dartmouth College.

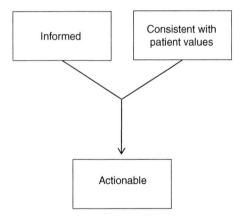

Figure 31.1 Elements of a high-quality decision.

because the decision is essentially dumped on the patient. They argue that the ethical approach requires a balance between these two extremes, and refer to this balance as *shared decision making*[2] (19), a collaborative **process** between patient and clinician that engages the patient in decision making and supports a two-way exchange of information.

---

[2] Moulton and King (2010) also note that terminology around shared decision making is confusing, and defined differently or used interchangeably with terms like decision support. Their definition refers to a process of communication that is unbiased and provides complete and balanced information about risks and benefits of treatment alternatives that engages the patient's medical goals and lifestyle preferences.

BARRIERS TO PATIENT INVOLVEMENT IN DECISION MAKING

Despite the rising consensus that patient involvement in decision making is an ethical imperative, the reality is that most preference-sensitive decisions are still dictated by providers (11,13). A Commonwealth Fund study conducted across several nations in 2004 found that nearly half of the physicians did not ask patients for their ideas about treatment and care (21). Another study found that physicians told patients about their condition over 80% of the time, but discussed the risks of procedure with patients less than a quarter of the time (22). In a 2010 editorial about the 2009 national DECISIONS study, Clarence Braddock comments that "there is a stack of evidence that clinicians do a poor job in providing patients with sufficient, balanced information and an open invitation to participate in decision making." (23).

Why does this happen? There are many barriers that interfere with patient involvement in decision making. These barriers generally can be categorized as originating from the provider, the patient, or the system and as arising from the characteristics of the individual (attitudinal) or characteristics of the situation (structural) (Table 31.1).

Attitudinal Barriers

Failure to involve patients in decision making often is attributed to provider "resistance." Given the aforementioned standard of *physician beneficence*, it is not surprising that medical training can lead physicians to rely on ingrained biases and

Table 31.1 Barriers to Involving Patients in Decision Making

	Attitudinal Barriers	Structural Barriers
Provider	• Provider preferences (based on training, experience, or personal values which may differ from those of patients) • Limitations in understanding risk data and overestimating the benefits • Lack of training in communicating risks and benefits effectively	• Limited "face" time with patients and institutional pressures for increased productivity • Limitations in the quality of evidence to support clinical decisions • Misaligned financial incentives
Patient	• Fear • Failure to explore and clarify values for potential outcomes • Difficulty understanding risk data and tendency to overestimate the benefits • Belief that "doctor knows best"	• Social supports • Role conflict (coordinating health treatments with work, family, and other obligations) • Access to treatment

beliefs about the choice that is right for their patient. Physicians also make decisions based on their prior patients' outcomes, and may prefer a particular treatment option they know has worked for most of their patients. Unfortunately, physician preferences for treatments may persist even if contrary to the clinical evidence. In today's information environment, staying current with medical literature is extremely challenging. A 1991 Pew Health Commission study estimated that if a conscientious health professional were to read two articles every day, in one year he or she would be over 800 years behind in the literature (24). The problem likely is much worse today with the explosion of information on the Internet.

Even if it were possible to read and synthesize all the scientific research, medical evidence can be wrong. John Ioannidis, an expert on the credibility of medical research, estimates that as much as 90% of published research is flawed. His model predicts that even with modest amounts of publication bias, about 80% of non-randomized trials and 25% of randomized trials would be refuted later for incorrect findings (25). Thus, figuring out an appropriate treatment choice requires that physicians understand and weigh the credibility of available evidence against their own experiences with patients.

In trying to achieve this balance, doctors may fail to recognize another factor in making treatment decisions—that patients may differently value the benefits and risks of treatment. A study by Lee and colleagues (26) found marked differences between physicians' and patients' stated top three goals of surgical treatment for breast cancer (Fig. 31.2). For example, only 7% of patients rated "keep the breast" as a top goal driving the surgery decision, whereas it was rated as such by 71% of providers. Although alignment between patients and providers was greater in discussing goals of breast reconstruction, 33% of patients said a top goal was to "avoid using a prosthesis," yet no providers rated this goal as a top priority. For chemotherapy and hormone therapy goals, providers were more likely than patients to choose "live as long as possible," while the opposite was true for "avoid lengthy treatment." While provider attitudes and communication behaviors may limit or prevent patient involvement in decision making, patients also have ingrained biases and beliefs about treatment that run contrary to evidence. Patients' fears about their illness may lead them to automatically ask for the "most aggressive" treatment without regard to whether the treatment benefits are worth the trade-off of harms for their individual situation. They may want the newest technology without regard to its

Top Three Goals and Concerns for Breast Cancer Decisions	Breast Cancer Treatment Goal	Providers	Patients
	Keep your breast	71%	7%
	Live as long as possible	96%	59%
	Look natural without clothes	80%	33%
	Avoid using prosthesis	0%	33%

Figure 31.2 The patient–provider disconnect.

effectiveness compared with older techniques, although the newer methods have a shorter track record with which to evaluate the possibility of long-term harm (27,28). In addition, patients may just fail to tell doctors their most important health concerns (29).

Patients may also lack confidence or good information upon which to base a decision or their contribution to a shared decision. They may be emotionally overwhelmed by a diagnosis or intimidated by the imbalance of power inherent in the patient–provider collaboration. They may be experiencing pressure from family or others, and they may be limited or influenced by social and financial circumstances. Patients also often assume that scientific validity supports a particular treatment, and that doctors "know best" (30). In one California poll, 65% of respondents thought that nearly all of the care they received was supported by strong evidence (30). Finally, the DECISIONS study demonstrated that patients want to do what their doctor thinks is best: 84% of women choosing breast cancer treatment rated this a "top priority" in their decision making.

COMMUNICATION BARRIERS

Even under the best circumstances, when evidence is strong and highly credible and patients are invited to provide a good description of their circumstances, communicating information about treatment risks is challenging. Both providers and patients commonly have difficulty communicating and understanding the numbers associated with the risks and benefits of treatment choices. Yet effective risk communication is essential for creating an informed patient.

Early-stage breast cancer provides a robust example. The choice of lumpectomy or mastectomy is one decision point where the evidence is strong. Randomized trials demonstrate that survival between these two groups is equivalent (31–33), but each treatment involves trade-offs. Lumpectomy is less invasive and preserves the breast, but it carries a slightly higher risk of local recurrence than mastectomy and in order to attain the lowest recurrence rate, patients must undergo radiation therapy (some mastectomy patients also require radiation). These differences are quality-of-life factors, and as such, the choice should be determined by patient preferences (34). In fact, studies have shown that an informed choice often hinges on the woman's feelings about losing a breast and her anxiety about local recurrence (35).

Without effective risk communication, it is easy to let emotion drive decision making. Emotions such as fear and risk aversion, and influences such as personal experience are important contributors to how we make decisions; these can be balanced and moderated with accurate information about all options, risks, and benefits presented in ways that patients can use. It takes time and patience to help someone understand that they do have options and that it is worth considering the benefits and costs of each option before deciding. The goal is to transform naïve, or uninformed choices to informed choices. However, improving risk communication requires more than just handing information about risk factors to patients. Edwards et al. (36) note the importance of moving beyond the traditional one-way dissemination of information from clinician to patient. They define risk communication as "the open two way exchange of information and opinion about risk, leading to better understanding and better decisions about clinical management" (page 827). The "two way" portion is critically important, yet extremely challenging to do in practice.

Research shows that few individuals understand health risks, even for common conditions such as the risk of heart attack and stroke (37). For example, a New Zealand study found no relationship between patients' perceived risk of having a future heart attack and their exposure to clinical risk factors such as age, sex, family history of myocardial infarction, diabetes, or smoking (38). The authors conclude that improving the accuracy of patients' perceptions of these risk factors could reduce anxiety and motivate behavior change. Improved accuracy requires a better approach to risk communication. However, an inherent challenge of improving risk communication is the low level of "statistical literacy," an inability to reason with or understand numbers and other mathematical concepts coupled with a low level of "health numeracy," or the degree to which individuals understand the quantitative aspects of health information (39,40). Both clinicians and patients have trouble with these numerical concepts.

In an attempt to avoid the problems inherent in communicating statistical evidence, qualitative terms often are used. For example, "the risk of infection is 'rare' or 'unlikely.'" But what does "rare" or "unlikely" mean? These terms are "elastic," in that they convey different meaning to different people under different circumstances (36). Figure 31.3 illustrates the problem with using this qualitative terminology. We asked a group of doctors and administrators the following question: "If you learn that the risk of a side effect from this medication is rare, unlikely, probable, or very likely, what do you think is the probability (percentage chance) that it will occur? For example, if 'the risk of a side effect from this medication is certain,' you might enter 100%." The figure shows the distribution and range of responses to each of these qualitative terms. Although the lines trend toward more frequent events being assigned higher probabilities, the range of responses and the overlap across categories are striking even among this very knowledgeable audience. And if you and your patient are unable to define descriptive terms in identical ways, then you have not accurately communicated the degree of benefit or risk. Thus, simplifying risk information by using qualitative language to avoid numbers actually may result in greater miscommunication.

Actual numbers can avoid the confusion resulting from these qualitative terms, but the types of numbers used to

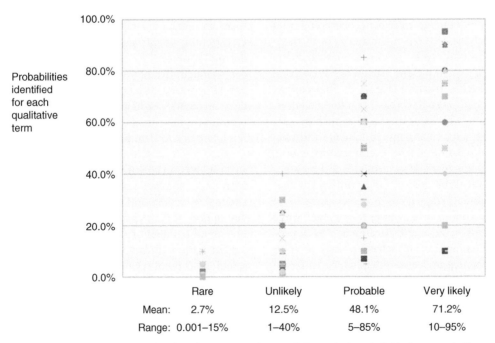

Figure 31.3 Probabilities associated with qualitative terminology. Each data point is an individual response indicating the probability associated with each term (e.g., "rarely").

present information about risk matters. Terms like "number needed to treat" may just sound like incomprehensible jargon to patients. Try to translate the numbers into terms that patients can understand. For example, steer clear of percentages; in a representative sample of US adults aged 35–70, only 25% of the population (and only 27% of individuals with post graduate degrees) could convert "1 in 1000" to 0.1%, and one in five US college graduates cannot correctly identify the larger number when asked to choose 1%, 5%, or 10% (41,42).

Absolute Vs. Relative Risk

Risk information further confuses people when it is expressed in *relative* rather than *absolute* terms. Relative risks usually make effects (both benefits and harms) sound larger than they are in absolute terms. Woloshin et al., (2009) compare these numbers to a sale at a store. A 50% discount on an item may sound very large, but whether it is worth buying depends on the base rate. For example, a 50% discount on a flat screen television is much different from a 50% discount on a tube of toothpaste in terms of the absolute dollars saved. The *base rate* matters. An advertisement for a cholesterol-lowering drug claims that "a clinical study among people with high cholesterol and heart disease found 42% fewer deaths from heart attack among those taking Zocor." When the authors of *Know Your Chances: Understanding Health Statistics* (43) rewrote the ad using absolute numbers, the sentence read as follows: "For men with heart disease and high cholesterol, Zocor reduces the 5-year chance of dying of a heart attack from 8.5 percent to 5.0 percent." The relative risk reduction of 42% is a more persuasive and also deceptive characterization of what really is a 3.5% absolute decrease in heart attack deaths (43).

Sometimes relative risks are the only available metric, such as in a case–control study where the base rate is unknown. Relative risks provide useful information when comparing treatments in a head-to-head trial. Often, however, studies report benefits as relative risks and harms as absolute risks, a bias that may lead doctors and patients to overestimate the benefits of treatment and underestimate the harms. A 2007 study found that one in three articles in the British Medical Journal, Lancet, and JAMA had mismatched framing of relative versus absolute risks for benefits and harms (44).

Better Data Presentation

Along with presenting absolute risks, another approach to better presentation of risk data is to use what is referred to as "balanced framing." A balanced frame occurs when risk is stated both as the chance of experiencing the event *and* as the chance of not experiencing the event. Patients who were told a procedure was 99% safe greatly preferred it over a procedure that had a 1% risk of complications, even though these are exactly the same data (40). In general, it is most effective to give your patients risk information in both positive and negative terms. For example, say "The risk of death from this procedure is 1 in 1000. This means that 1 out of every 1000 people who have this procedure will die, and 999 out of every 1000 people who have this procedure will survive."

Another way to improve communication of risk is to use visual displays, such as graphs and pictures. Many decision support tools show a series of faces or stick figures (often in groups of 100, as 10 rows of 10) and then shade or change the

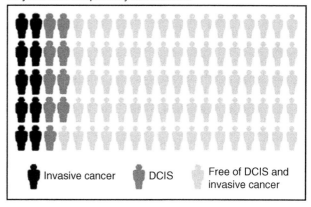

Recurrence in treated breast or other breast 10 years after lumpectomy and radiation

■ Invasive cancer   ■ DCIS   ■ Free of DCIS and invasive cancer

This chart shows what happens, on average, to 100 women in the 10 years after lumpectomy and radiation.

Figure 31.4 The absolute risk display chart.

face of the number of those figures that will experience the event described (Fig. 31.4).

Teach Back Method

A method for presenting risk information (or any medical information) that is familiar to teachers and nurses is the "teach back": building a step into the conversation to check that the person you are communicating with understands what you have told them. Employing a teach-back (or "show-me") method can help clinicians determine whether the patient's perceptions match the clinician's (45). One good way to do this that makes the step feel less like a test is to ask patients to say what they will tell a family member about the information they have just received. This exercise can help reveal areas where communication still is unclear. It also gives the patient a chance to "rehearse" what she has learned so she can communicate with others in her decision-making cohort.

STRUCTURAL BARRIERS
Time

While physician attitudes and their ability to communicate risk have a strong influence on patient involvement in decision making, even the most well-intentioned clinician who is comfortable discussing risk is stymied by numerous structural barriers that make involving patients difficult. Resource constraints in healthcare organizations mean pressure to generate more revenues. These constraints force doctors to see more patients in less time. In this environment, insufficient time is allocated to carefully carry out the two-way exchange of all the information both doctor and patient need to share in order to make a good decision. The assumption that collaborating with a well-informed patient will take more time than the standard consultation (she will have more questions, I won't be able to control the agenda as closely, I will have to listen as well as talk...) is unfounded. Both studies and anecdotal experience with using decision aids and an SDM model in breast cancer care have documented similar lengths of time and much improved use of time engaging in higher-quality conversations. In addition, we know that a woman, who leaves the consultation without having her decisional needs addressed, may actually take more time as she seeks the support and the answers she needs.

Misaligned Incentives

The second structural barrier to clinicians adopting this approach is financial; healthcare revenues today come from billing for treatments and procedures, rather than communication and collaboration, thus putting pressure on doctors to make a recommendation and move on to the next patient. At the institutional level, there may be concerns that well-informed patients will choose non-surgical treatment at a higher rate (and some evidence indicates that patients often do choose the less invasive procedure (15)). Under the current fee-for-service models, the clinician and the institution risk loss of revenues if fewer procedures are performed.

Pressure

Finally, there may be additional institutional barriers to involving patients in decision making. In breast cancer care, women are choosing between surgeries, so procedure rates will persist. However, institutional pressure may result in promoting one procedure over the other. For example, in the US, breast conservation rates have been suggested as a quality indicator, with higher rates equaling higher quality. Yet a study by Collins et al. (35) found that approximately 35% of well-informed women choose mastectomy even when breast conservation surgery is an option. Women choosing mastectomy may encounter resistance if surgeons believe breast conservation is in their best interest.

These structural barriers of time limitations, misaligned incentives, and misguided assumptions about optimal treatment choices are significant forces toward inertia; they only serve to enhance the inherent difficulties of instituting practice change. If time and money were not factors, resistance to change would still present significant challenges to integrating SDM processes into clinical care. However, if clinicians were paid to "do the right thing," if incentives were in place for both clinicians and patients, this model would find an easier path to widespread adoption.

TOWARD PATIENT INVOLVEMENT: SHARED DECISION MAKING
Shared Decision Making

Patient participation in decision making requires an approach that removes the barriers associated with physician training, uncertain evidence, difficulty with risk communication, patient fears, and structural constraints. SDM is one such approach. SDM is defined as a decision-making process that is shared by clinicians and patients, informed by the best evidence, and weighted according to the preferences and values of the patient (46). It has been argued that SDM can reduce unwarranted variations in preference-sensitive care (46,47) and that it improves overall decision quality (7). At the heart of an SDM process is the conversation between doctor and patient. A checklist of six essential steps in this conversation is as follows: (*i*) invite the patient to participate, (*ii*) present options, (*iii*) provide information on benefits and risks, (*iv*) elicit patient preferences, (*v*) facilitate deliberation and decision making, and (*vi*) assist with implementation.

DECISION AIDS

Decision aids are tools used to facilitate the SDM process. Good decision aids do more than disseminate information to educate patients; they provide both requisite knowledge and a process for engaging patients in a values clarification process (6,48). A Cochrane Collaboration meta-analysis of available randomized controlled trials of decision aids (49) defined the aims of decision aids as *providing evidence-based information*, helping patients *recognize and clarify the value-sensitive nature of the decision*, and *providing structured guidance in making a decision and communicating* with others involved in the decision (e.g., clinician, family, and friends). Decision aids are not the same as patient education materials, which lack the requirements for evidence-based, balanced presentation of all options, coaching language to help patients make use of the information, and either explicit or implicit value clarification exercises designed to help patients think about what matters to them and how much.

The Cochrane report showed that overall, patients who used decision aids felt more involved in their decisions. Decision aids also *reduced decisional conflict associated with feeling uninformed, decisional conflict related to personal values*, and *conflict related to the decision after the intervention*. Decisional conflict refers to the uncertainty surrounding decision making, such as being unclear about values and feeling uninformed or unsupported in the decision-making process (49–51). For some elective invasive surgical procedures, use of decision aids decreased the rate of surgery without affecting health outcomes or patient satisfaction.

Decision aids remove barriers to patient involvement in several ways. They are designed to include up-to-date clinical evidence, so doctors can feel comfortable that their patients are exposed to the latest scientific research. Providers may feel more comfortable sharing the decision process because they know that patients are using balanced, accurate information. When used with patient questionnaires, decision aids can reveal where patients are conflicted about their decisions and what information they still do not understand or understand incorrectly. Clinicians receiving questionnaire results can focus their limited time with patients on the issues causing conflict.

Patients benefit from decision aids beyond learning the basic facts about their treatment options. These tools are also designed to help individuals with value clarification. Patients can share the decision aids with their families, thus enlisting support that can be essential for patients going through a serious illness or major procedure.

Decision aids may also help navigate around some of the structural barriers to involving patients in decision making. For example, by prescribing a decision aid in advance of an appointment, then not having to repeat all the evidence and details about each choice option, the clinician can instead make better use of the time customizing information to make it personally relevant and answering questions.

DECISION AID STANDARDS

In order for these decision tools to truly foster SDM, they must meet standardized quality criteria. A group of interested experts, stakeholders, and practitioners convened the International Patient Decision Aid Standards (IPDAS) group to develop a checklist of criteria to assess and ensure the quality of decision aids. Table 31.2 lists the broad set of IPDAS criteria from the 2005 IPDAS collaboration background document. A more detailed checklist for evaluating patient decision aids is available at http://www.ipdasi.org/2006%20IPDAS%20Quality %20Checklist.pdf (retrieved December 31, 2011). For additional information on the IPDAS group, see http://ipdas.ohri. ca/resources.html.

Decision aids that meet IPDAS standards inform patients about treatment options and accurately specify benefits and risks in understandable terms. An inventory of decision aids, including a generic tool called the "Ottawa Personal Decision Guide©," is available on the Ottawa Hospital Research Institute (affiliated to the University of Ottawa) website at http://www.ohri.ca/DecisionAid/. It is important

to note that decision aids are designed to be adjuncts to counseling, serving as a guide in patient discussions with their clinicians and other interested parties, such as family members. They support, rather than replace, the patient-provider conversation.

SDM IN PRACTICE FOR WOMEN WITH BREAST CANCER

Decision aids, by themselves, do not constitute SDM. They must be successfully implemented into clinical practice as one tool in a process that helps patients make better decisions. Several models exist for implementing SDM into practice; which one is used depends on the optimal timing within each setting for engaging and informing patients. Decision aids can be given to patients outside the clinical visit, or completed alongside the clinician. Some are designed for specific treatments, while others are generic and may be used for any decision. They may be delivered electronically, as a hard copy video, or written on paper or discussed in an interview. New models will continue to emerge as we learn more about successful implementation strategies.

We describe in detail one comprehensive model for women with early-stage breast cancer that is used at an academic medical center in the US (52). We then present some alternative models being used in other locations.

DARTMOUTH-HITCHCOCK MEDICAL CENTER

Figure 31.5 displays a flow chart of the process a woman goes through when diagnosed with early-stage breast cancer at this institution. Her journey begins after the radiologist performs an image-guided needle biopsy. The radiologist informs the woman of the diagnosis, and a social worker who fills the role of breast care coordinator is either present during that

Table 31.2 Twelve Broad Criteria for Content and Process Requirements When Developing Patient Decision Aids

1. Systematic Development Process
2. Decision Aid Acceptability & Balance
3. Up-to-Date Evidence
4. Disclosure of Interests
5. Plain Language
6. Internet Delivery Guidelines
7. Information about Options
8. Risk Communication
9. Values Clarification
10. Structured Guidance in Deliberation & Communication
11. Balanced Display
12. Decision Process

Source: Adapted from the IPDAS background document – http://ipdas.ohri .ca/IPDAS_Background.pdf.

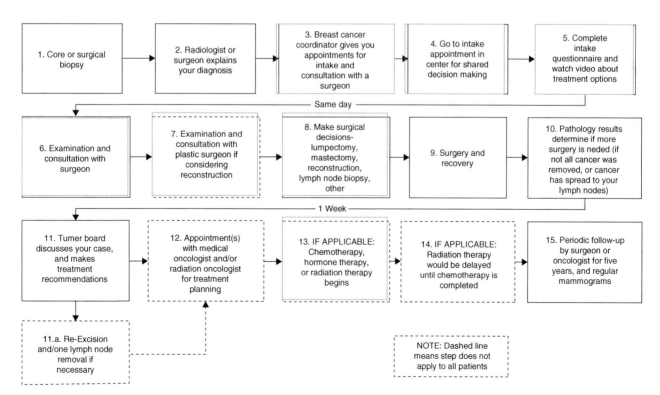

Figure 31.5 Flow chart showing the treatment process for a patient with early-stage breast cancer at one hospital. Orange boxes show where shared decision making is incorporated or decision aids are or can be used.

conversation or follows up with a call to the patient to provide support and answer questions. The breast care coordinator helps the patient understand the steps that will occur throughout the treatment process, coordinates care with the schedulers, and arranges appointments, the first of which is usually with a surgical oncologist.

After the woman receives her diagnosis, a decision aid titled "Early stage breast cancer: Choosing your surgery" (Health Dialog©, 2002–2009) is automatically mailed to her home. Decision aids about ductal carcinoma in situ, reconstruction, and adjuvant therapy may also be sent if applicable. This advance preparation is useful because it gives each patient time before meeting with a surgeon to think about the options, review the material, and integrate the information she has just learned. She can watch the DVD or read the pamphlet with family members. These decision aids are updated to include the most current evidence, and where uncertainty exists, it is explained. Patients get a more realistic view of what benefits their treatments might provide and what risks are involved, and a clear message that they are central to the decision-making process.

Viewing the decision aid before meeting with the surgeon also allows the patient to focus the surgery conversation specifically on the issues that are of most concern to her. Likewise, the surgeon does not have to explain every available option to the patient. The surgeon's role is to set the context with patient-specific diagnosis and treatment information, help each woman weigh the options, answer questions, and guide her toward the best decision for her. This process generally results in a more effective and efficient visit.

During the research phase of this project, a "Decision Quality Report" was provided to the surgeon ahead of time. Along with some general patient data, this report contained the answers to an intake questionnaire filled out by women before and after watching the decision aid; answers to questions that demonstrated a woman's knowledge and values associated with her surgical choices were summarized on the report. It also provided data on the patient's psychosocial state. If a patient appeared depressed or in need of other help or counseling, the breast care coordinator or appropriate professional could follow up.

The decision quality report helped to identify a mismatch between what the patient was choosing and what her values indicated would be the best choice for her. The decision quality report example in Figure 31.6 is based on a real patient seen by one of the authors (DCV). This woman had chosen mastectomy and was being seen to discuss reconstruction options. She placed a high value on *keeping her breast* and *avoiding reconstruction*, and a low value on *removing her breast for peace of mind*. The report also indicated that she did not correctly understand the information on recurrence and survival. It was clear that she did not have the facts needed to make an informed decision. So, rather than address treatment choices for reconstruction, the discussion focused on surgical options for early-stage breast cancer. This patient ultimately went on to choose breast conservation over mastectomy. Without the decision quality report, her reconstructive surgeon would have been unaware that the patient had basic misunderstandings about the options and the conversation would have likely focused on reconstruction options only (Table 31.3).

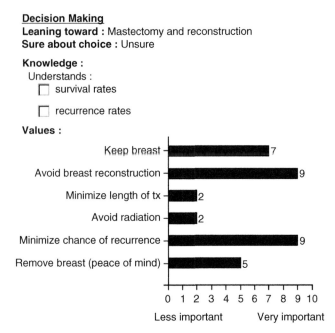

Figure 31.6 Decision quality report showing a treatment choice that is uninformed and inconsistent with the woman's personal values.

Table 31.3 Patient Case Study

Dr Collins was seeing a patient in consultation for breast reconstruction. The patient had already met with a surgical breast oncologist and she indicated that she was having a mastectomy. She was very quiet, offering little about her preferences. She confirmed that she had watched a video-based decision aid on breast reconstruction, but had not reached any conclusion about which option she would prefer.

As Dr Collins went on to probe, she noted the decision quality report on the choice for mastectomy versus breast conservation (Fig. 31.5). The surgeon noticed that she had scored highly the value questions that would typically predict a choice of breast conservation ("Keep breast" and "Avoid breast reconstruction,") and low on the option that is most associated with mastectomy ("Remove breast for peace of mind") had a low score. In addition, the patient did not understand the key knowledge questions (the boxes are not checked) about the equivalence of survival and the similar rates of recurrence associated with each option.

Dr Collins realized the patient may not have a sufficient understanding of her surgical options for breast cancer. So, rather than continuing to discuss options for reconstruction, the plastic surgeon reviewed the surgical options for early-stage breast cancer. The patient went on to choose breast conservation

---

UNIVERSITY OF CALIFORNIA AT SAN FRANCISCO

At the University of California at San Francisco, the Carol Buck Breast Care Center Decision Services unit (http://www. decisionservices.ucsf.edu/) offers a woman with breast cancer decision support in a three-step program. First, she is offered one or more of five breast cancer decision aid programs depending on the decision she is facing. Next, each woman is offered a personal coach to help brainstorm questions and concerns, as she develops a list of questions to discuss with the surgeon at the upcoming appointment. And finally, the personal coach accompanies women to appointments and makes audio recordings of the consultations (53).

NHS AND NHS WALES
NHS Direct

In the UK, several SDM efforts are under way. NHS Direct has worked to incorporate SDM tools and processes into care using their web site, http://www.nhsdirect.nhs.uk. The organization aims to be the national health line, providing expert health advice, information, and reassurance, using world-class telephone and digital services and website, and to be the NHS[1] provider of choice for telephone and digitally delivered health services.[2] One feature of the web site is a section on Decision Aids. Currently, nine decision aids are available, including one on treatment choices for newly diagnosed early-stage breast cancer. The decision aid was piloted prior to public release by breast surgeons and nurses at seven clinical sites in England. From April to November 2011, the breast cancer decision aid home page had 565 visits, and 62% of those visitors continued onto the second page of the decision aid.

MAGIC: Making Good Decisions In Collaboration

The breast care team members in Cardiff, Wales are routinely using an Option Grid (http://www.optiongrid.co.uk/) and a Decision Quality Measure (DQM; a patient questionnaire measuring knowledge, strength of values, and decision readiness). All eligible patients who have the option of mastectomy versus lumpectomy with radiotherapy receive an "Option Grid consultation," wherein the consultant or the nurse uses the Option Grid to frame a discussion around options during the diagnostic/treatment consultation. Women are asked to complete the first Decision Quality Measure (DQM1) at the end of the diagnostic consultation. In addition, they are given information about how to access BresDEX (http://www.bresdex.com/, a "Breast Cancer Decision Explorer" tool) and encouraged to make use of this interactive tool at home. The patient is seen again by the nurse during a home visit to discuss treatment options in more detail, usually within a week of the diagnostic consultation. A second, identical DQM (DQM2) is completed at the end of the home visit. The breast care team nurses use the information provided in DQM1 to tailor the home visit to each patient's individual needs, based on DQM1 responses about how much information patients have retained, what is important to them, their decision readiness, and preferred choice of treatment. The data from DQM2 are compared with data from DQM1 to assess changes in patients' knowledge, readiness to decide, and choice of treatment.

Both the diagnostic consultation and the nurse home visit are usual care; use of the Option Grid and DQM questionnaires has been adopted by clinical teams and incorporated into the existing care pathway. Results to date, although based on a small number of patients, suggest that the use of the Option Grid may have a considerable impact on patients' understanding of the key features, risks, and benefits of treatment options. Due to limitations in the scope of the project, data have not been gathered on how many patients actually access and make use of the BresDEX tool.

A summary description of decision support approaches used in 13 countries around the world, including the UK and the US, may be found in a 2011 editorial by Harter et al. and published in the German journal *Z. Evid. Fortbild. Qual. Gesundh. Wesen.* (54).

SUCCESSFUL IMPLEMENTATION REQUIRES ACCEPTING CHANGE

In our first academic medical center example, during satisfaction surveys patients gave high marks for the decision aids and were highly satisfied with the process, including delivery method and timing. Patients surveyed after using decision aids felt their understanding of options was improved. Patients commented about feeling more comfortable with their treatment decision and experiencing less decisional conflict. They also felt the process improved relationships with their providers (35).

Yet even the best decision support tools will be ineffective if they are not used. Given competing demands on their time, physicians will only adopt these methods if they believe them to improve patient care. In one study, orthopedic surgeons treating patients with knee and hip osteoarthritis gave high ratings to the use of decision aids in the treatment of their patients (55). The surgeons found the decision aids were helpful in educating patients about surgical and non-surgical options, creating more realistic expectations for outcomes and identifying patients' values and preferences in developing a treatment plan. Similar acceptance was noted among spinal surgeons. The greatest uptake has occurred in surgical decisions like breast cancer, where there are a few well-defined options at various stages of treatment.

However, successful implementation of SDM requires systems change, not just change to the specific doctor–patient interaction. True patient involvement requires a focus that moves beyond the development of tools and structures like decision aids and focuses on the engagement and interrelationships among all staff. Everyone who interacts with the patient, from the first call to the office to the end of the treatment journey must understand the value of the patient being involved. Truly patient-centered care includes consistent messaging from all staff members that demonstrates a single-minded focus on the needs of the patient, reinforcement of the value of becoming informed, making use of tools, and engaging in care decisions at every opportunity (when scheduling an appointment, during the visit, when arranging post-visit care etc.), incorporating the patient's decision-making unit (family, friends, and caregivers) by making information and opportunities for support available, and restructuring the care pathway to allow for interventions to address decisional conflict and initial and follow-up SDM conversations. In other words, successful implementation requires a high level of "relational coordination," a concept that refers to communication reinforced by high-quality relationships that allow providers to effectively coordinate work. A high level of relational coordination has been shown to positively affect quality, efficiency, and workforce satisfaction (56–59).

Successful implementation also requires support from organizational leadership. Some evidence indicates that appropriate use of decision support may reduce costs as patients explore less invasive options (53). Lower patient costs may mean lower hospital revenues if fewer procedures and tests are chosen. And currently, institutions are not reimbursed for the time or materials involved in making SDM a reality. Leadership must recognize that putting the patient at the center is the "right thing to do," and support its adoption and implementation. In fact, "identify a clinical champion who practices in the clinical setting" is the first step in the decision support implementation toolkits posted on the Dartmouth-Hitchcock Medical

Center website (see http://med.dartmouth-hitchcock.org/csdm_toolkits/step_1_leadership.html).

This sounds complicated, but all it means is that when re-engineering your care pathway to include a decision aid, a decision quality report and an SDM conversation, be sure to include all stakeholders; there is no reason to leave anyone out of the process, and there are good reasons to include everyone.

INFORMED CHOICE AS A STANDARD OF CARE

The ethical imperative to fully inform patients becomes a legal mandate when a consent form is required. The SDM steps of engaging and informing will serve to perfect informed consent by transforming it to informed choice.

O'Connor and others argue that implementation of decision aids will occur once a "tipping point" is reached and when informed patient choice becomes the standard of practice (11,47). The proposition is that the legal standard of informed consent becomes informed choice for decisions that are preference-sensitive. Informed consent in different states is divided into a patient-based standard and a physician-based standard (60). In the physician-based standard, the physician must inform the patient of risks, benefits, and alternatives that would be considered standard for a practitioner in that field. A patient-based standard involves also informing the patient of all of the above risks, benefits, and alternatives, but is based on what a *patient* would find significant (60).

A model of informed choice could center on helping the patient define the important issues, such as whether or not a treatment or procedure is worth the potential or likely undesirable outcomes, or whether that individual will experience the benefits. Implicit in defining whether or not the patient will accept the potential risks is determining the patient's values in making a decision.

Krumholz (61) suggests a way to standardize consent for elective procedures in order to facilitate an informed decision-making process. He advocates for a patient-centered approach that will provide "core information" written by experts and given to patients at least a day before treatment. The document will look quite different from the consent form we are accustomed to because it will include details about *all* available options. Krumholz notes five critical elements needed for this form: information about risks, benefits, alternatives, experience, and cost. His editorial proposes a standardized consent form, using the example of percutaneous coronary intervention. This form will help ensure that the patient is driving the decision. It will foster patient-centered communication by requiring a standardized conversation to occur between the provider and the patient. Ideally, this conversation will help to alleviate issues associated with unexpected outcomes and will improve overall patient satisfaction.

This type of consent form does have limitations. The authors note the challenge of individualizing the form; providers may be reluctant to share data on their experience or the data simply may not be available, and the evidence related to the patient's own risk might not be known. Yet true patient-centered communication requires an attempt at this type of transparency.

SUMMARY

Current practice often looks like this: paternalistic assumptions on the part of well-intentioned clinicians that they know what is best for *this* patient, informing patients of the "best" option but not all options, emphasizing the benefits and downplaying the risks to avoid unnecessarily upsetting their patients, unwittingly using words and numbers that patients do not understand, listening poorly, and failing to engage patients in decision making in the name of clinical efficiency.

What should it look like in a better, more patient-centered future? The one constant is that a conversation must occur between a clinician and a patient; it is happening now and can be improved by inserting balanced, evidence-based information, inviting each patient to share values and goals, employing techniques for accurate and understandable risk information, engaging in collaborative decision making, thus walking the talk of patient-centered care.

Health decisions, particularly preference-sensitive decisions, are complicated. We have an ethical imperative to involve patients in these choices. Individuals value the trade-offs between benefits and harms differently and these values should be incorporated into the patient–provider interaction. Taking time to include the patient and to make sure he or she understands all available options with their associated benefits and risks may sound time consuming and contrary to today's efforts to do more with less. Yet, these conversations grow in importance as treatment options become increasingly complex and the evidence for one choice over another is weak or unknown. SDM has been shown to improve the quality of care, the efficiency of the patient–provider interaction, and the degree of patient satisfaction with care. Its goal is to avoid a misuse of services and to achieve the "right rate" of treatment choices based on patients' informed choice.

REFERENCES

1. Congressional Budget Office. Geographic variation in health spending. 2008. Report by the CBO on variation in health spending.
2. Weinstein JN, Bronner KK, Morgan TS, Wennberg JE. Trends and geographic variations in major surgery for degenerative diseases of the hip, knee, and spine. Health Aff (Millwood) 2004: VAR81–9.
3. Polednak AP. Geographic variation in postmastectomy breast reconstruction rates. Plast Reconstr Surg 2000; 106: 298–301.
4. Alderman AK, McMahon L Jr, Wilkins EG. The national utilization of immediate and early delayed breast reconstruction and the effect of sociodemographic factors. Plast Reconstr Surg 2003; 111: 695–703; discussion 704–5.
5. Wanzel KR, Brown MH, Anastakis DJ, Regehr G. Reconstructive breast surgery: referring physician knowledge and learning needs. Plast Reconstr Surg 2002; 110: 1441–50. discussion 1451–4.
6. Hoffman AS, Llewellyn-Thomas H. Shared decision making. In: Kattan MW, ed. Encyclopedia of Medical Decision Making. Thousand Oaks, CA: Sage Publications, 2009: 1036–41.
7. Sepucha KR, Fowler FJ Jr, Mulley AG Jr. Policy support for patient-centered care: the need for measurable improvements in decision quality. Health Aff (Millwood) 2004: VAR54–62.
8. Birkmeyer JD, Sharp SM, Finlayson SR, Fisher ES, Wennberg JE. Variation profiles of common surgical procedures. Surgery 1998; 124: 917–23.
9. Wennberg JE. Understanding geographic variations in health care delivery. N Engl J Med 1999; 340: 52–3.
10. Wennberg JE, Fisher ES, Skinner JS, Bronner KK. Extending the P4P agenda, part 2: how medicare can reduce waste and improve the care of the chronically ill. Health Aff (Millwood) 2007; 26: 1575–85.
11. Wennberg JE, O'Connor AM, Collins ED, Weinstein JN. Extending the P4P agenda, part 1: how medicare can improve patient decision making and reduce unnecessary care. Health Aff (Millwood) 2007; 26: 1564–74.

12. Wennberg JE, Gittelsohn A, Shapiro N. Health care delivery in Maine, III: evaluating the level of hospital performance. J Maine Med Assoc 1975; 66: 298–306.

13. Wennberg JE, Roos N, Sola L, Schori A, Jaffe R. Use of claims data systems to evaluate health care outcomes. Mortality and reoperation following prostatectomy. JAMA 1987; 257: 933–6.

14. McGlynn EA, Asch SM, Adams J, et al. The quality of health care delivered to adults in the United States. N Engl J Med 2003; 348: 2635–45.

15. Hawker GA, Wright JG, Coyte PC, et al. Determining the need for hip and knee arthroplasty: the role of clinical severity and patients' preferences. Med Care 2001; 39: 206–16.

16. Berwick DM, Nolan TW, Whittington J. The triple aim: care, health, and cost. Health Aff (Millwood) 2008; 27: 759–69.

17. NHS. Equity and excellence: Liberating the NHS. July 2010; Sect. 61 (col. National Health Service).

18. Kocher R, Emanuel EJ, DeParle NA. The affordable care act and the future of clinical medicine: the opportunities and challenges. Ann Intern Med 2010; 153: 536–9.

19. Moulton B, King JS. Aligning ethics with medical decision-making: the quest for informed patient choice. J Law Med Ethics 2010; 38: 85–97.

20. Snyder L, Leffler C. Ethics manual: fifth edition. Ann Intern Med 2005; 142: 560–82.

21. Commonwealth Fund. First report and recommendations of the commonwealth fund's international working group on quality indicators: A report to health ministers of Australia, Canada, New Zealand, the United Kingdom, and the United States, 2004.

22. Braddock CH 3rd, Fihn SD, Levinson W, Jonsen AR, Pearlman RA. How doctors and patients discuss routine clinical decisions. Informed decision making in the outpatient setting. J Gen Intern Med 1997; 12: 339–45.

23. Braddock CH 3rd. The emerging importance and relevance of shared decision making to clinical practice. Med Decis Making 2010; 30: 5S–7S.

24. Pew Health Commission. Healthy America: Practitioners for 2005. San Francisco, CA: University of California San Francisco Center for the Health Professions, 1991.

25. Freedman DH. Lies, damned lies, and medical science. The Atlantic 2010.

26. Lee CN, Dominik R, Levin CA, et al. Development of instruments to measure the quality of breast cancer treatment decisions. Health Expect 2010; 13: 258–72.

27. Schwartz LM, Woloshin S. Communicating uncertainties about prescription drugs to the public: a national randomized trial. Arch Intern Med 2011; 171: 1463–8.

28. Woloshin S, Schwartz LM. Communicating data about the benefits and harms of treatment: a randomized trial. Ann Intern Med 2011; 155: 87–96.

29. Scheitel SM, Boland BJ, Wollan PC, Silverstein MD. Patient-physician agreement about medical diagnoses and cardiovascular risk factors in the ambulatory general medical examination. Mayo Clin Proc 1996; 71: 1131–7.

30. Brownlee S, Hurley V, Moulton B. Patient decision aids and shared decision making. New America Foundation [serial on the Internet]. 2011. [Available from: http://newamerica.net/publications/policy/patient_decision_aids_and_shared_decision_making]

31. Fisher B, Bauer M, Margolese R, et al. Five-year results of a randomized clinical trial comparing total mastectomy and segmental mastectomy with or without radiation in the treatment of breast cancer. N Engl J Med 1985; 312: 665–73.

32. Veronesi U, Saccozzi R, Del Vecchio M, et al. Comparing radical mastectomy with quadrantectomy, axillary dissection, and radiotherapy in patients with small cancers of the breast. N Engl J Med 1981; 305: 6–11.

33. Morris AD, Morris RD, Wilson JF, et al. Breast-conserving therapy vs mastectomy in early-stage breast cancer: a meta-analysis of 10-year survival. Cancer J Sci Am 1997; 3: 6–12.

34. Whelan T, Levine M, Willan A, et al. Effect of a decision aid on knowledge and treatment decision making for breast cancer surgery: a randomized trial. JAMA 2004; 292: 435–41.

35. Collins ED, Moore CP, Clay KF, et al. Can women with early-stage breast cancer make an informed decision for mastectomy? J Clin Oncol 2009; 27: 519–25.

36. Edwards A, Elwyn G, Mulley A. Explaining risks: turning numerical data into meaningful pictures. BMJ 2002; 324: 827–30.

37. Bachmann LM, Gutzwiller FS, Puhan MA, et al. Do citizens have minimum medical knowledge? A survey. BMC Med 2007; 5: 14.

38. Broadbent E, Petrie KJ, Ellis CJ, et al. Patients with acute myocardial infarction have an inaccurate understanding of their risk of a future cardiac event. Intern Med J 2006; 36: 643–7.

39. Gigerenzer G, Gaissmaier W, Kurz-Milcke E, Schwartz LM, Woloshin S. Helping doctors and patients make sense of health statistics. Psychol Sci Public Interest 2008; 8: 53–96.

40. Ghosh AK, Ghosh K. Translating evidence-based information into effective risk communication: current challenges and opportunities. J Lab Clin Med 2005; 145: 171–80.

41. Schwartz LM, Woloshin S, Welch HG. Can patients interpret health information? An assessment of the medical data interpretation test. Med Decis Making 2005; 25: 290–300.

42. Schwartz LM, Woloshin S, Black WC, Welch HG. The role of numeracy in understanding the benefit of screening mammography. Ann Intern Med 1997; 127: 966–72.

43. Woloshin S, Schwartz LM, Welch HG. Know Your Chances: Understanding Health Statistics. Berkeley, CA: University of California Press, 2009.

44. Sedrakyan A, Shih C. Improving depiction of benefits and harms: analyses of studies of well-known therapeutics and review of high-impact medical journals. Med Care 2007; 45: S23–8.

45. Kountz DS. Strategies for improving low health literacy. Postgrad Med 2009; 121: 171–7.

46. O'Connor AM, Llewellyn-Thomas HA, Flood AB. Modifying unwarranted variations in health care: shared decision making using patient decision aids. Health Aff (Millwood) 2004: VAR63–72.

47. O'Connor AM, Wennberg JE, Legare F, et al. Toward the 'tipping point': decision aids and informed patient choice. Health Aff (Millwood) 2007; 26: 716–25.

48. Sepucha KR, Levin CA, Uzogara EE, et al. Developing instruments to measure the quality of decisions: early results for a set of symptom-driven decisions. Patient Educ Couns 2008; 73: 504–10.

49. O'Connor AM, Bennett CL, Stacey D, et al. Decision aids for people facing health treatment or screening decisions. Cochrane Database Syst Rev 2009; 3: CD001431.

50. O'Connor AM. Validation of a decisional conflict scale. Med Decis Making 1995; 15: 25–30.

51. Legare F, Kearing S, Clay K, et al. Are you SURE?: Assessing patient decisional conflict with a 4-item screening test. Can Fam Physician 2010; 56: e308–14.

52. AHRQ. Shared Decision Making for Breast Cancer Patients Leads to High Levels of Patient Satisfaction, and Comfort with Decisions and Treatment Preferences. Rockville, MD: Agency for Healthcare Research and Quality, 2010; cited 2011 April 8, 2011.

53. Landro L. Weighty choices, in patients' hands. The Wall Street Journal [serial on the Internet]. 2009. [Available from: http://online.wsj.com/article/SB10001424052970203674704574328570637446770.html#articleTabs%3Darticle]

54. Harter M, van der Weijden T, Elwyn G. Policy and practice developments in the implementation of shared decision making: an international perspective. Z Evid Fortbild Qual Gesundhwes 2011; 105: 229–33.

55. Weinstein JN, Clay K, Morgan TS. Informed patient choice: patient-centered valuing of surgical risks and benefits. Health Aff (Millwood) 2007; 26: 726–30.

56. Gittell JH, Fairfield KM, Bierbaum B, et al. Impact of relational coordination on quality of care, postoperative pain and functioning, and length of stay: a nine-hospital study of surgical patients. Med Care 2000; 38: 807–19.

57. Gittell JH, Weinberg DB, Pfefferle SG, Bishop JA. Impact of relational coordination on job satisfaction and quality outcomes: a study of nursing homes. Hum Resour Manage J 2008; 18: 154–70.

58. Gittell JH. A relational model of how high-performance work systems work. Organ Sci 2010; 21: 490–506.

59. Havens DS, Vasey J, Gittell JH, Lin WT. Relational coordination among nurses and other providers: impact on the quality of patient care. J Nurs Manag 2010; 18: 926–37.

60. King JS, Moulton BW. Rethinking informed consent: the case for shared medical decision-making. Am J Law Med 2006; 32: 429–501.

61. Krumholz HM. Informed consent to promote patient-centered care. JAMA 2010; 303: 1190–1.

32 The evolving role of the breast care nurse in the management of patients with early breast cancer

Rebecca Llewellyn-Bennett, Jane Barker, and Zoë Ellen Winters

BACKGROUND

Breast cancer is the most common site of cancer and the second most common cause of mortality in women (1). The incidence of breast cancer has increased to a rate of 124 per 100,000 women (2008) (2). However, 80% of patients diagnosed with breast cancer are alive at 5 years (3). Breast cancer in men is rare, but still significantly affects approximately 300 men in the United Kingdom (UK) per year (4). The breast cancer screening program has diagnosed more breast cancers at an earlier stage, and ductal carcinoma in situ is the now more commonly detected since the introduction of breast cancer screening (5). The National Mastectomy and Breast Reconstruction Audit (2008–2009) highlighted the importance of surgical outcomes and patient-reported outcome measures (PROMS) to improve patient care and service provision (5). The breast care nurse (BCN) has a pivotal role in ensuring that this is provided.

THE ORIGINS OF THE BCN

Clinical nurse specialists (CNS) were introduced in the United States (US) in the 1960s (6). The UK mirrored the US in the 1980s in the development and merging roles of the CNS with creation of the stoma nurse role (7). The traditional supportive role of the BCN was developed in response to work undertaken by Maguire (1980) (8) who demonstrated the psychological and emotional needs of women following a breast cancer diagnosis. Furthermore, supportive interventions by the BCN showed a positive effect on psychological morbidity (8,9).

Initially, the role of the BCN focused on psychological support but lacked formalization and national direction until new changes were initiated for cancer services in 1995 (10). These changes promoted delivery of a uniformly high level of care to all patients with cancer across the UK. In 1996, the National Health Service (NHS) Executive (11) prepared a series of standardized guidance documents on breast cancer services to provide optimum care for those with malignant disease. The BCN was included as one of the multidisciplinary team members, and this document recommended that the BCN should work exclusively in breast care and have completed the specialist course in counseling and communication [the A11 English National Board (ENB)]. Continued psychosocial support was highlighted as a crucial requirement throughout the patient's cancer journey.

In 2001, the NHS Executive also recommended a framework of local cancer networks to assess the quality of care provided (12). Despite subsequently being updated (11), the document failed to provide national minimum standards of skills and knowledge, which were required to function competently in a specialist nurse role. This omission led to disparities in various specialist services offered along the cancer patient pathway. It was not until 2007, when the Royal College of Nursing Breast Group updated its clinical standards pertaining to working within a breast specialty, that the roles of various categories of nurses were more clearly defined (13). Currently, the framework laid out by the Royal College of Nursing provides guidance for skills, education, and experience at each level as well as defining 13 specific clinical standards, and the associated knowledge and skills to undertake each role.

The role of the BCN continues to evolve and has become progressively more diverse when compared with the original concept of someone in a traditional supportive and information-providing role.

THE CHANGING ROLE OF THE MODERN BCN

The traditional roles of the BCN were considered for many years to involve the different practices as depicted in Table 32.1. However, over the past two decades, there has been a broader evolution of the role of BCNs, and a number of factors have contributed to these changes in the traditional roles of the BCN list above.

The Reduction in Junior Doctors' Hours

The reduction in doctors' working hours, in accordance with the European Working Time Directive, led to review of tasks that appropriately qualified nurses could potentially undertake to improve the quality of patient care and service delivery (14). This approach was not mandated by national guidelines but rather allowed to develop in individual breast units, as it was believed that policies at a local level provided greater flexibility. Nursing professional bodies supported this stance. As a consequence of this, the Nurse Practitioner (NP) role developed and was gradually introduced into the healthcare setting. In parallel with these developments, BCNs began adopting additional tasks that would otherwise have been undertaken by junior doctors. These included preassessment clinics, routine surgical follow-up clinics, and drainage of seromas.

Scope of Professional Practice

The "Scope of Professional Practice" report (1992) by the Nursing and Midwifery Council proposed guidelines for clinical practitioners in order to meet the needs of patients and clients

Table 32.1 The Roles of the Breast Care Nurse

- Supporting patients at the time of breast cancer diagnosis
- Providing emotional and basic psychological support
- Providing help and guidance with decision-making
- Providing information and clarification about surgery and various treatments (and potential complications/side effects)
- Providing prosthetic fitting service
- Providing information on lymphedema
- Acting as a point of contact for patients

Table 32.2 The Extended Roles of the Breast Care Nurse

- Diagnostic clinics (history taking, clinical breast examination, breast ultrasound)
- Histopathology results conveyed in nurse-led clinics
- Nurse prescribing per standard protocols for inpatients and outpatients
- Patient advocacy role in patients' clinical decision-making
- Follow-up clinics (routine postsurgical follow-up and patients receiving primary hormone therapy clinics)
- Telephone follow-up
- Inflation of tissue expanders by BCNs
- Support to doctors when providing information to patients relating to endocrine treatment, chemotherapy, radiological interventions such as wire localization or mammotome biopsy and surgical treatments
- Autonomous requesting of appropriate radiological [mammogram, ultrasound, magnetic resonance imaging (MRI)] examination
- Liaising with other specialist teams when referring for further treatments (e.g., plastic surgeons for breast)
- Discussing clinical trials with patients

under the new concept of an "extended role" that promoted autonomous professional practice, which was responsive to the healthcare needs of patients (15).

Agenda for Change

The Secretary of State in his introduction to the "Agenda for Change" stated:

> The current pay structure inhibits staff and does not recognise that modern forms of health rely on flexible teams working across traditional skill boundaries. When these changes (pay bands) are made, nurses will no longer be confined to limitations of grade

Agenda for Change (AfC) was the biggest overhaul of NHS-wide pay and terms and conditions in more than 50 years (DoH 1999 (16)). It recreated nine pay bands that staff could be placed within which reflected the role and not the person. It also provided improved links between pay and career progression using the Knowledge and Skills Framework and enabled nurses to develop skills in relation to the post, where the previous grading structure did not. Extended roles for a State Registered Nurse prior to this were restricted to tasks such as female catheterization and administration of intravenous antibiotics.

Cancer Services Collaborative

This was founded as part of the National Cancer Plan (DoH 2000) to promote equitable care for all patients diagnosed with cancer (17). It necessitated a review of all team members' roles and facilitated delivery of high-quality services (18) in order to achieve national standards and targets that were ultimately aimed at improving rates of cancer morbidity. The collaborative recommended creation of cross-sectional or multidisciplinary teams to ensure comprehensive service delivery (19).

Teams were encouraged to map out individual patient journeys and focus on areas for improvement of care within specific time frames. Multidisciplinary teams decided who would be most appropriate to deliver specific aspects of care management (18). This resulted in a variety of independent roles being undertaken by BCNs instead of clinicians that included patient follow-up, information on diagnostic and postoperative histopathology, and endoscopy clinics.

This shift in practice raised some concerns within both the nursing and medical professions. Junior doctors felt that their own training needs were being compromised as a result of reduced learning opportunities and this was at the expense of development of nursing roles. Such opposition was greatest within general surgery (20–22), but these changes in the status quo were better received within more specialist areas (23). Nowadays, more than 15 years on, advanced skills are synonymous with the role of the BCN and are an integral part of the multidisciplinary team.

THE MULTIPLE ROLES OF THE MODERN BCN

The National Institute for Health and Clinical Excellence (NICE) recommended that all breast cancer patients should be allocated a BCN to support them throughout their journey. The BCN's task commences at the time of a patient's first diagnostic appointment at either the symptomatic or the breast screening clinic. Patients whose assessment based on symptoms and radiological and/or pathological findings indicates that support is required from specialist services are referred to a BCN.

However, this really only represents the "tip of the iceberg" in relation to the broad role of the BCN within the multidisciplinary team. Patients with early breast cancer are often followed up by the breast team for 5 years or more through formal follow-up; however, this is now for a much shorter period for selected patients in many units. This involves radiological surveillance, monitoring for recurrence, and provision of psychosocial support. Examples of specific roles undertaken by BCNs, over and above their traditional supportive roles previously described, include those illustrated in Table 32.2.

Beaver et al. (2009) reported a high level of patient satisfaction with clinical follow-up by a specialized BCN (24). This was echoed by other authors in patients with early stage I and II breast cancer (25,26).

Up to 50% of patients have clinically significant fluid or seroma collections following mastectomy with or without axillary dissection alone or combined with breast reconstruction. These may require serial aspirations at some stage postoperatively (5). Nurse-led seroma aspiration clinics provide invaluable assistance in this aspect of patient management.

Inflation of tissue expanders by BCNs is often organized alongside doctor-led clinics. This is an increasing practice in more than one-third of patients and particularly in the context of staged-delayed (two-stage) breast reconstruction where postmastectomy radiotherapy is readily anticipated (5,27).

From an economic point of view, BCNs potentially reduce costs within the NHS. As the patients' nominated key worker (a role identified within National Guidelines (28)), the BCN is the main point of contact for the patients throughout their cancer pathway. This role promotes continuity of patient care and underpins optimum coordination of a patient's overall management plan. In consequence, the BCN is often effective at identifying issues that might necessitate medical attention and enables care to be better planned, which may avert emergency admissions. BCNs also support the enhanced recovery pathway postsurgery by priming patients to manage their recovery at home and thereby minimizing the length of hospital stay (29).

Previously, concerns were raised that the ever-increasing expectations of BCNs, with acquisition of "technical" skills such as seroma aspirations, might detract from the caring role of the nurse and lead to loss of intrinsic skills that are the essence of nursing. This sentiment is prevalent in today's working environment. Macmillan et al. (30) cited a survey of CNSs showing that almost 50% of CNSs felt unable to provide the ideal quality of care they would wish for all their breast cancer patients. This impression emanated from demands of an increased workload secondary to additional duties. The National Cancer Action Team (31) reported that following expansion in breast cancer services, CNSs in this field constituted 19% of the total CNS workforce. Despite this, the expansion of the number of cancer specialist nurses has not been commensurate with the ambient pressures on this specialist service.

Fundamentally, the most important role of the BCN is and always will be patient support. Counseling skills and facilitating decision-making commence at the point of diagnosis and continue throughout the patient's cancer journey; this involves integrating all elements of the role previously described. McArdle et al. describe the crucial role of the BCN in significantly reducing psychological morbidity (32). Support for this conclusion comes from a randomized controlled trial that showed no difference in the level or quality of psychological support provided to patients who were randomized to either a CNS or a psychologist (33).

Assisting patients in decision-making is an important skill for a BCN when dealing with early breast cancer, treatment of which is becoming increasingly complex. At a time when a patient (and her family) is struggling to come to terms with a diagnosis of breast cancer, they are faced with limited time frames in which to make decisions. These decision-making branch points include various surgical options [mastectomy (with or without breast reconstruction) vs. breast conservation], neoadjuvant chemotherapy versus primary surgery, and clinical trial participation. National guidelines recommend that women should have adequate time to consider their choices (11). Overburdened clinics fail to meet the patients' needs in the decision-making process (34). A patient, once armed with a range of treatment options, will further explore these with the BCN and exploit their role of facilitating shared decision-making.

Fallowfield et al. (9) and Van Roosmalen et al. (35) demonstrated that effective communication in terms of offering patient choice, as well as patient involvement in shared decision-making, enhanced long-term psychological adjustments to breast cancer treatments. The BCN should be mindful, however,

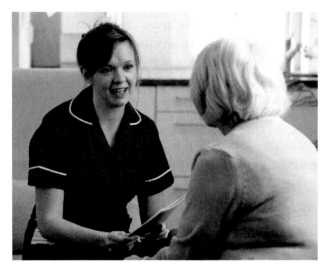

© Breast Cancer Care[1]

that decision-making is a complex issue when discussing various treatment options with a patient. Some patients wish to know what their clinicians' preferences are, if any, but value autonomy in selecting their own treatment or favor working collaboratively with their clinicians.

The BCN should be aware of current research and clinical trials that might affect the decision-making process for certain procedures. A good example is the Medical Research Council (MRC)-funded, multicenter-randomized trial called Axillary Lymphatic Mapping Against Nodal Axillary Clearance (ALMA-NAC) (36). The opportunity to introduce ALMANAC to patients was important when deciding on allocated surgical options for treating potentially involved axillary lymph nodes, axillary node clearance, or a sentinel node biopsy. The BCN uses their communication skills and knowledge of breast cancer treatment to enable a patient to make the best and most appropriate informed decision. As the patient's advocate, the BCN supports her choice of treatment, even if this may be contrary to a clinician's recommendation.

The role of a BCN necessarily demands adaptation to some extraordinary clinical scenarios, such as women who are pregnant or those younger patients who wish to have children in the future. There are additional challenges presented by elderly patients who may be mentally compromised and male breast cancer patients who require managing with appropriate sensitivity. Experience with referral to specialist services that support optimal preservation of fertility (e.g., egg preservation) is important for some women, and advice from other multidisciplinary team members should be sought. The BCN should be aware of their limitations in such circumstances.

THE FUTURE OF THE BREAST CANCER SPECIALIST NURSE
Standardizing Care

Any future role of the breast cancer specialist nurse should be standardized at a national level to ensure that equivalent levels of care are delivered to patients irrespective of location and demographics. Previous research has attempted to evaluate

---

[1] Reproduced by kind permission of the Nursing Network Breast Cancer Care (www.breastcancercare.org.uk/nursingnetwork).

this, but in the absence of internationally recognized criteria, it is impossible to make any legitimate comparisons (37,38).

The education and skills mix of BCNs has been a focal point of concern raised by both clinicians and BCNs themselves. It is acknowledged within the national cancer peer review measures (2011) that there are no national guidelines that stipulate minimum educational levels for CNSs, but there is a consensus that CNSs should undertake a period of specialist study to first degree level (28). In response, national guidelines have created the imperative for bespoke courses with education at degree and master's levels that are offered by many Universities in the UK. Presently, the UK is the only country in which the Royal College of Nursing has recognized a postgraduate higher degree such as Doctor of Philosophy (PhD) within the discipline (39).

The European Parliamentary group on breast cancer has produced European Union (EU)-agreed guidelines in 2011 on the training and role of the BCN (40). In the future, this should potentially standardize the level of training nationally and internationally (at least throughout the EU) (40) and help to highlight areas of development required by better understanding and regulation of roles.

The domains of the breast care nursing curriculum are as follows:

a) The experience of breast cancer diagnosis
b) The experience of breast cancer treatments (including side effects and their management)
c) Long-term living after breast cancer
d) Practicing in the BCN role

Service Provision

Regional service demands are constantly changing and this creates the need for flexibility and adaptation by the BCN. Initiatives such as open access clinics, mammographic surveillance only follow-up, and "pacing" decision-making are all adaptations, which have been developed throughout the UK to improve the delivery of patient care. These have been spawned by increasing numbers of patients with early breast cancer and a consequent expansion in the numbers of longer-term survivors posttreatment.

Research and Informed Decision-Making

BCNs are likely to become increasingly involved in clinical trials and part of a research group. Their role will be to help inform and guide patients' decision-making when considering trial participation as well as guiding process of care after consent according to each trial protocol. This has become a varied and unpredictable role and was not initially anticipated. In order to keep up-to-date with these national incentives, a number of workshops organized through Research Design Support Services at NHS Trusts have been established, such as mandatory training in Good Clinical Practice. This is part of the learning opportunities that are supported and funded by departments such as Research Design and Support within NHS Trusts.

Furthermore, there is a need for BCNs to be aware of current decision-making aids for breast cancer patients. An example of this is called BRESDEX (www.bresdex.com), which has been developed as a web-based online breast cancer decision-making aid that is aimed at women diagnosed with early breast cancer. PREDICT is another interactive online prognostic tool developed to aid patient–clinician consultations regarding adjuvant treatments that impact on cancer survival (38). This tool is based on a large cohort data set collated by the East Anglian Cancer Registry. It is important that BCNs are familiar with current tools and trends to deliver the optimum service to their patients. This applies especially to those tools such as BRESDEX and PREDICT, which are easily accessible by patients online (38).

Despite an explosion of resources and tools to help patient consent, some studies (41) together with the Cancer National Survey (2010) report significant variations nationally in patients' opinions about choices of treatments provided (42). The current rapidity of diagnosis and treatment might be perceived to be an obstacle that prevents some women from taking time to seek additional information from varied sources. This may be predicated on the belief that breast cancer prognosis worsens "rapidly" and therefore requires immediate interventional treatment. Patients may have become "instant decision-makers" giving a false impression of their self-confidence. Harcourt et al. (43) found the converse to be true; that the "indecisive decision-makers" were generally very anxious patients who in their attempt to derive more information became increasingly less assured of their position as a result of raising more questions than answers.

Additional factors, which can potentially compromise a patient's decision-making process, are the difficult "prioritizing" concerns versus information needs that patients wish to consider before making any decisions. Realistically, attempts to ascertain these particular factors by clinicians may not be achievable due to current constraints imposed by consultation times. This provides an opportunity for the BCN to use her advanced communication and counseling skills to elicit more complex patient concerns and thereby facilitate a patient's decision-making process.

Follow-Up of Patients

With current changes to breast cancer follow-up, the role of the BCN is pivotal for continued patient contact and they may face challenges regarding the professional execution of their role to its full potential. Traditionally, the focus of cancer services has been on breast cancer as an "acute illness" with resulting emphasis on the initial phase of treatment. Breast cancer care following primary treatment is focused on clinicalsurveillance with emphasis on symptoms and signs of recurrent disease. This clinical approach is referred to as "follow-up" care. As breast cancer incidence continues to rise annually, professionals in the field are witnessing increasing numbers of long-term cancer survivors who are challenging the resources of existing services in attempts to sustain long-term follow-up. The National Cancer Survivorship Initiative, launched in 2010 (44), encourages teams to stratify patients into the following groups for follow-up:

- Green pathway: self-management alone, with individual patient or self-referral back into system.
- Amber pathway: self-management with remote follow-up in the form of telephone clinic or remote electronic surveillance (e.g., as used for prostate cancer follow-up of patients using serial prostate-specific antigen blood tests by GP surgeries).
- Red pathway: self-management and face-to-face follow-up and support.

The BCN is fundamentally important in this phase of the patient pathway. It is necessary for the BCN at an opportune interval after treatment to spend time with the patient discussing plans for follow-up on an individual basis. The recommended options will have been discussed and agreed by the multidisciplinary team based on individual case discussion or established unit policy. The BCN plays an important role in this decision-making by highlighting sensitive and pertinent symptoms to be considered in each case. This must take account of an individual patient's level of breast awareness and potential signs and symptoms of metastatic disease. The BCN is the interface for providing readily available patient information and contact details to facilitate clinic bookings. Such opportunities for self-management in a follow-up capacity are coordinated principally by the BCN. Provision of patient counseling takes the form of courses or study days to help them prioritize and plan for the future, resume normal activities, and deal with any lingering after effects of treatments. Patients are helped with learning strategies and encouraged to gain confidence with their emotional and physical recovery. Topics include the following:

- Managing side effects of treatment (e.g., fatigue)
- Dealing with troubling thoughts/feelings
- Self-health checks
- Relaxation and mindfulness techniques
- Communication skills
- Improving physical capabilities
- Goal setting
- Finding other sources for help
- The potential benefits of diet and exercise in reduction of recurrence (45).

BCNs are responsible for organizing these sessions in conjunction with a clinical psychologist or they can arrange for patients to be referred to an appropriate center that offers this service.

Holistic Intervention

Based on recommendations by the Cancer Reform Strategy (46), BCNs are responsible for the assessments of holistic needs at timely intervals in the patient journey. Holistic needs' assessment is defined as using recognized assessment tools to identify patients who require help. This approach provides patients with an opportunity to reflect on their needs and together with their healthcare professional to consider how best to fulfill their requirements. Ultimately this helps patients to better self-manage living with the aftermath of breast cancer.

The assessment of holistic needs integrates seamlessly into a BCN-led follow-up clinic. The need to integrate all aspects of physical, social, psychological, and spiritual domains of health-related quality of life forms part of a BCN's training and professional expertise. Some BCNs prefer the flexibility of this approach by using this outside of the immediate clinical setting, within a one-to-one support session.

The BCN uses her skills in advanced communication, specialist knowledge in breast cancer, and finally their training in clinical and psychological assessment. Essential BCN training is required in using the range of specialist tools that are discussed within the *assessment of holistic needs for people with cancer* document (47). Nationally the evolution of the BCNs' role in breast cancer treatment and care is similar in clinical

teams throughout the UK. Increasing recognition of the important contribution of the BCN to the patient cancer experience has opened up new opportunities for role development leading to greater evolution of skills and specialization with recognition by the Royal College of Nursing (30). The role of the BCN is constantly adapting from one that started as a mere NP to one that is now synonymous with a CNS.

CONCLUSIONS

The BCN is an integral member of the multidisciplinary team. By using her skills and expertise, the BCN can effectively engage in information providing and communicate within specialist teams to ensure best patient care. This role potentially overlaps with that of other healthcare professionals but is evolving to meet changing demands within the breast surgical team, and further research is required to establish an evidence base for this continued development. BCNs are a costly resource although acknowledged as being an essential and integral component of a comprehensive breast cancer service. There is a need for further patient self-report to determine whether outcomes are significantly improved by the contributions of regular interaction with a BCN.

REFERENCES

1. Breast Cancer Care. Information and support for anyone affected by breast cancer. [Available from: http://www.breastcancercare.org.uk/news/media-centre/facts-statistics] [Accessed 16/08/2012].
2. Office for National Statistics. Breast Cancer. Little change in incidence. [Available from: http://www.ons.gov.uk/ons/index.html] [Accessed 16/08/2012].
3. Breast Cancer Campaign. [Available from: http://www.breastcancercampaign.org/page.aspx?pid=763] [Accessed 16/08/2012].
4. Macmillan Cancer Support. Cancer information. 2012. [Available from: http://www.macmillan.org.uk/Cancerinformation/Cancertypes/Breastmale/Aboutbreastcancerinmen/Mensbreasts.aspx] [Cited 16/08/2012].
5. The NHS Information Centre. Clinical effectiveness unit at the Royal College of Surgeons. National mastectomy and breast reconstruction audit. 2009.[Available from: http://www.ic.nhs.uk/mbr] [Accessed 30/11/2011].
6. Page NE, Arena DM. Rethinking the merger of the clinical nurse specialist and the nurse practitioner roles. J Nurs Scholarsh 1994; 26: 315–18.
7. Bousfield C. A phenomenological investigation into the role of the clinical nurse specialist. J Adv Nurs 1997; 25: 245–56.
8. Maguire P, Tait A, Brooke M, Thomas C, Sellwood R. Effect of counselling on the psychiatric morbidity associated with mastectomy. Br Med J 1980; 281: 1454–6.
9. Fallowfield LJ, Hall A, Maguire P, Baum M, Ahern RPA. Psychological effects of being offered choice of surgery for breast-cancer. Br Med J 1994; 309: 448.
10. Calman K, Hine D. A Policy Framework for Commissioning Cancer Services. England and Wales: A Report by the Expert Advisory Group on Cancer to the Chief Medical Officers, 1995.
11. National Institute for Clinical Excellence. Improving Outcomes in Breast Cancer. 2002.
12. Department of Health. Manual of Cancer Services Standards. 2001.
13. Royal College of Nursing. Clinical standards for working in a breast speciality. RCN guidance for nursing staff. 2007.[Available from: http://www.rcn.org.uk/__data/assets/pdf_file/0008/78731/003110.pdf] [Cited 16/08/2012].
14. NHS Management Executive. The New Deal. London: Junior Doctors, 1991.
15. Nursing and Midwifery Council. London: The Scope of Professional Practise, 1992.
16. Great Britain. Dept. of H. Agenda for Change: Modernising the NHS Pay System. Great Britain: Department of Health, 1999.
17. NHS Modernisation Agency. Breast Cancer service improvement guide ideal pathway. 2012.[Available from: www.ebc-indevelopment.co.uk/nhs/breast/idealpathway.html] [Accessed 28/08/2012].
18. Barker J, Turner J. The impact of the cancer services collaborative on practice. Cancer Nurs Pract 2004; 3: 21–5.

19. Jefferies H, Chan KK. Multidisciplinary team working: is it both holistic and effective? Int J Gynecol Cancer 2004; 14: 210–11.

20. West S, Weight S, Jenkins BJ, Stephenson TP. Junior doctors' hours: what do they really think? J R Soc Med 1994; 87: 331–3.

21. Higgins M. Developing and supporting expansion of the nurse's role. Nurs Stand 1997; 11: 41–4.

22. Read S, Graves K. Reduction in Junior Doctors' Hours in the Trent Region: The Nursing Contribution. 1994.

23. Snelgrove S, Hughes D. Interprofessional relations between doctors and nurses: perspectives from South Wales. J Adv Nurs 2000; 31: 661–7.

24. Beaver K, Tysver-Robinson D, Campbell M, et al. Comparing hospital and telephone follow-up after treatment for breast cancer: randomised equivalence trial. BMJ 2009; 338: a3147.

25. van Hezewijk M, Ranke GM, van Nes JG, et al. Patients' needs and preferences in routine follow-up for early breast cancer; an evaluation of the changing role of the nurse practitioner. Eur J Surg Oncol 2011; 37: 765–73.

26. Koinberg IL, Fridlund B, Engholm GB, Holmberg L. Nurse-led follow-up on demand or by a physician after breast cancer surgery: a randomised study. Eur J Oncol Nurs 2004; 8: 109–17.discussion 18-20.

27. Cordeiro PG. Breast reconstruction after surgery for breast cancer. N Engl J Med 2008; 359: 1590–601.

28. NHS National Cancer Action Team. Manual for Cancer Services. Version 2.1 London: Breast Measures, 2011.

29. National Cancer Action Team. Quality in Nursing. Excellence in Cancer Care: The Contribution of the Clinical Nurse Specialist. 2010.

30. Macmillan Cancer Support. Cancer clinical nurse specialists: an evidence review. 2011.[Available from: www.Macmillan.org.uk/servicesimpact] [Accessed 16/08/2012].

31. National Cancer Action Team. Quality in Nursing Clinical Nurse Specialists in Cancer Care; Provision, Proportion and Performance A Census of the Cancer Specialist Nurse Workforce in England 2010. 2011.

32. McArdle JM, George WD, McArdle CS, et al. Psychological support for patients undergoing breast cancer surgery: a randomised study. BMJ 1996; 312: 813–16.

33. Arving C, Sjoden PO, Bergh J, et al. Satisfaction, utilisation and perceived benefit of individual psychosocial support for breast cancer patients–a randomised study of nurse versus psychologist interventions. Patient Educ Couns 2006; 62: 235–43.

34. Fallowfield L. Participation of patients in decisions about treatment for cancer. BMJ 2001; 323: 1144.

35. van Roosmalen MS, Stalmeier PF, Verhoef LC, et al. Randomized trial of a shared decision-making intervention consisting of trade-offs and individualized treatment information for BRCA1/2 mutation carriers. J Clin Oncol 2004; 22: 3293–301.

36. Clarke D, Khonji NI, Mansel RE. Sentinel node biopsy in breast cancer: ALMANAC trial. World J Surg 2001; 25: 819–22.

37. Cruickshank S, Kennedy C, Lockhart K, Dosser I, Dallas L. Specialist breast care nurses for supportive care of women with breast cancer. Cochrane Database Syst Rev 2008: CD005634.

38. Wishart GC, Bajdik CD, Azzato EM, et al. A population-based validation of the prognostic model PREDICT for early breast cancer. Eur J Surg Oncol 2011; 37: 411–17.

39. Royal College of Nursing. Advanced Nursing Practice in Breast Cancer Care. London: 2002.

40. Eicher M, Kadmon I, Claassen S, et al. Training breast care nurses throughout Europe: the EONS postbasic curriculum for breast cancer nursing. Eur J Cancer 2012; 48: 1257–62.

41. Janz NK, Wren PA, Copeland LA, et al. Patient-physician concordance: preferences, perceptions, and factors influencing the breast cancer surgical decision. J Clin Oncol 2004; 22: 3091–8.

42. Department of Health. National Cancer Patient Experience Survey Programme. National survey report 2010.

43. Harcourt D, Rumsey N. Mastectomy patients' decision-making for or against immediate breast reconstruction. Psychooncology 2004; 13: 106–15.

44. Department of Health, Macmillan Cancer Support. NHS improvement. national cancer survivorship initiative. 2012.[Available from: http://www.ncsi.org.uk/] [Accessed 28/08/2012].

45. Fong DY, Ho JW, Hui BP, et al. Physical activity for cancer survivors: meta-analysis of randomised controlled trials. BMJ 2012; 344: e70.

46. Department of Health. Cancer report strategy. London: 2007. [Available from: www.dh.gov.uk/en/Publicationsandstatistics/.../DH_081006] [Accessed 30.08.2012].

47. National Cancer Action Team. Holistic needs assessment for people with cancer A practical guide for healthcare professionals. 2012. [Available from: http://ncat.nhs.uk/our-work/living-with-beyond-cancer/holistic-needs-assessment] [Accessed 30.08.2012].

33 Informed consent in the management and research of breast cancer

Hazel Thornton

INTRODUCTION

In the few years since writing my chapter about informed consent for the second edition of this book there has been considerable productive debate and increasing activity challenging how consent is sought and how decisions are made. The challenging practical account concerning the role of consent by Neil C. Manson and Onora O'Neill in their book *Rethinking Informed Consent in Bioethics* (1) provides a firm basis for a re-examination of the consent process. The authors lead us to reconsider what exactly is meant by "information" and to consider, for example, how good communicative practice involves sensitivity to specific audiences. We are encouraged to consider the different asymmetry of knowledge and of power that is obtained between a doctor and a patient or in the different relationship between a researcher and a patient—"who needs who." They make a case for effective informative communication rather than "disclosure." In recent years, qualitative research exploring the personal experiences of participants taking part in trials has provided good evidence to support taking that approach (2,3). Furthermore, numerous publications authored by experts in communication skills have been published, including proffering guidance for health professionals on the best way to communicate statistics, risk, and probability to citizens or patients.

Much has changed in the way that medicine is perceived and practiced in the 10 years since 2001 when I was invited by Mr Uccio Querci della Rovere to write a chapter on *informed consent in the management and research for breast cancer* for the second edition of *Early Breast Cancer from Screening to Multidisciplinary Management* (4). At that time, "Informed consent" was a new chapter to appear in the final section, *Consent and litigation*, although an accompanying chapter on medicolegal aspects had featured previously in the first edition. Ten years on, the structure and content of the third edition of this book reflects not only the scientific and technological advances that have affected the early detection and treatment of breast cancer in the intervening years, but also the changing milieu in which healthcare is offered with respect to the doctor–patient relationship; closer attention to economics; changes in culture and attitudes generally. Further changes in governance and regulation have affected standards of consent in healthcare and research, and they are a further significant factor that now needs to be considered (5). In addition to the chapters considering the multidisciplinary team and informed consent in the management of breast cancer in this new edition, space is given to the role of the breast care nurse and to shared decision-making. We have seen the development of expertise through a range of international activities concerned with shared decision-making and

risk communication, and the development of decision aids that culminated in the Salzburg Global Seminar in December 2010 with the production of the *Salzburg Statement on shared decision making* (6).

At the time of writing, there is every indication that the current preoccupation in some quarters with "improving" informed consent by persistent tightening up and tinkering with consent regulatory requirements is out of tune with current thoughts about the manner in which decisions are made and the role and definition of "information," where a more sensitively intelligent and flexible approach is being advocated. The change in title of the United Kingdom (UK) General Medical Council's (GMC) brochures offering guidance to doctors about seeking consent is significant. The 1998 brochure was entitled *Seeking patients' consent: the ethical considerations*. But the revised replacement version, published in 2008, is entitled: *Consent: patients and doctors making decisions together*. The introductory paragraphs state that "the guidance concentrates on decision-making in the context of investigations or treatments; but the principles apply more widely, including decisions on taking part in research," thus going some way to addressing the double standards (7) that had previously been the case. They also add that "the principles apply to all decisions about care: from the treatment of minor and self-limiting conditions, to major interventions with significant risks or side effects. The principles also apply to decisions about screening." How many citizens, or health professionals for that matter, realize that consent should be sought for screening; that the decision whether to be screened is theirs to make; and that it is not wrong to say "No!"? (8).

It is clear that the focus is changing from *what* is being communicated to *how* it is being communicated; from a rigid and formal approach to a more flexible approach; one that takes account of the multitude of individual and personal requirements that need to be accommodated in those consultations where consent is being sought. This applies to either research or routine clinical care, or in broaching interventions for preventive early detection to citizens, where in all cases, people need to make decisions but will need information of varying degrees of depth. The Salzburg Statement calls on patients to "recognize that they have a right to be equal participants in their care" (6). But rights also bring responsibilities and obligations which should be recognized and actively shouldered.

THE ROLE OF INFORMATION IN INFORMED CONSENT AND DECISION-MAKING

It was 20 years ago in September 1991 that "informed consent" was sought from me by my surgeon on behalf of his team to be a participant in the UK Randomised trial for the Management of Screen-detected Ductal Carcinoma of the Breast (ductal carcinoma in situ) (9). I declined. Having done so, I felt a need to explain the reasons for my refusal and to offer my explanation, not only to my surgeon but also to all the members of the trial management group for that trial. More importantly, since I was but one of many hundreds of women presented with this dilemma as a consequence of accepting the invitation to attend for population breast screening by mammography, I felt an urge and a responsibility to write about my experience so that it could be brought to the attention of the medical profession and the wider public (10).

I also wanted to draw attention to my concerns about the effects on the doctor–patient relationship brought about by the regulatory trial requirements for obtaining "informed consent" for this research. I suggested that the two-week delay imposed on a patient through being sent away for a couple of weeks to "decide" whether to participate, placed a barrier between the patient and the medical team. In my paper, I queried whether "the facts," as I had been given them—*enable genuinely "informed consent"? Or is there only, at best "partly informed consent" or, at worst, "ill-informed consent?"* I have since learned that I am not alone in having doubts about people being able to give a fully informed consent, both as citizens being approached to engage in early detection, and as patients in healthcare and research, in many different medical situations (1).

My own activity as a citizen advocating for quality in research and healthcare, and better provision of good quality information for citizens and patients, sprang from these personal frustrating attempts at decision-making which had been thwarted or misguided by a paucity of adequate accurate information. Curiously, the second of these chronologically speaking, declining participation in a trial, led to closer examination of my earlier decision to accept the invitation from the NHS Breast Screening Programme to attend for screening. Only then did I realize that my acceptance had been improperly procured since "The Facts" (11) provided then in the NHS Breast Screening Programme leaflet were insufficient (12) and biased in favor of gaining my acceptance, as is still the case today (13). Furthermore, it was worded in such a way that declining would be considered a foolish decision—if I wanted to save my life!

ACTIVE PATIENT AND PUBLIC INVOLVEMENT IN THE RESEARCH PROCESS

These experiences also led me on to believe that the responsibility for improving the situation should be a shared one, and I have advocated for active (as distinct from participatory) patient and public involvement (PPI) in the whole research process. Attempts should be made to ensure that ordinary people are educated about these things and be encouraged to see that they could, as citizens, actively contribute to improving what they find (14,15). Today, a well-informed, involved public is a crucial element in the determination of what constitutes "Good Medical Practice" (16).

A *Lancet* commentary praised the GMC's "radical reinterpretation" of what it calls "*medical professionalism in action*" for its clarity and insight (17). The GMC advises that, although the guidance is addressed to doctors, it is also intended to let the public know what they can expect from doctors. I believe that, in return, it is necessary to set out what doctors should expect from patients and the public in this partnership contract where both parties have responsibilities. There are many serious barriers and impediments to achieving this aim, including poor reporting, poor communication, imperfect understanding of research concepts, and levels of risk, together with general statistical illiteracy. Not only that, but perceptions concerning the characteristics and roles of "lay" and "professional" in this activity need further scrutiny and revision to enable people to play their full part in a productive, collaborative relationship so that we all strive together to improve research and healthcare.

CONSUMERS' ADVISORY GROUP FOR CLINICAL TRIALS

I believe that it is important that the public should be better educated about research concepts: how treatments are tested. One of the main aims of the *Consumers' Advisory Group for Clinical Trials (CAG-CT)* that I co-founded with Michael Baum in 1994 was to help the public to become educated about research (18). Another opportunity to fulfill this aim was the invitation to be a coauthor with Imogen Evans and Iain Chalmers in a book for the general public, first published by the *British Library* in 2006, entitled: *Testing treatments: better research for better healthcare*, (19), and since revised and published in a second edition (14).

SHARED DECISION-MAKING

Methods of healthcare delivery are undergoing a rapid change for a variety of reasons: economic; political; cultural, technological, and ideological. But there is hope! Here in the UK, and elsewhere, the central encounter–the consultation–is undergoing a sea-change, as shared decision-making and informed consent come increasingly under the spotlight (1,20–22). It is to be hoped that more enlightened exchanges and iterations between profession and laypeople will result in better health care generally. No longer will citizens and patients mutely accept what they read or are told: they will increasingly question, contribute, and take a more active role (15). To do this, it is essential that, not only are sources of information reliable and of good quality, but also that information is communicated effectively so that good understanding is achieved (23–25).

The pendulum has swung from one extreme to the other since the paternalistic and rather unregulated 1940s to one of shared responsibility with better understanding. Hopefully, it will find a more central, sensible, and satisfactory place with respect to consent, concordance (rather than "compliance"), regulation, governance, and practice. A united sense of purpose is needed, as well as action by those who are aware of the problems, if we are to be able to work together to improve citizens' decision-making.

I am given hope by the two important initiatives already mentioned: the recently published *Salzburg statement on shared decision-making* (26) and the review of the GMC's guidance for doctors, *Good Medical Practice* (16) which is currently out for consultation. Both call for relationships based on trust and respect, and demonstrate that it is the responsibility of both parties—patients and public, together with health professionals—to responsibly play their part in striving for a better way of working together to test and provide treatments, and to improve public health interventions, as we explain in our book (14).

Today, patients and doctors are increasingly seen as co-producers of health and equal participants in care. Doctors have an ethical responsibility to share decisions with patients. In turn, citizens must recognize their responsibility to play their part in improving what they find by working with health professionals both in respect of their own healthcare and for society in general.

Trust

I find it difficult to consider trust in that special individual relationship that occurs between patient and doctor without also considering the trust and respect that I have for the medical profession as a whole. Chambers (27) defines Medicine as "the art or science of prevention, diagnosis or cure (esp. non-surgically) of disease"; and "the practice or profession of a physician." But when I first spoke about the patient's role in research in 1994, I said that I believed that "all good art and all good science must stem from the very highest level of observation" and pleaded for the *blending* of art and science in the practice of medicine (28). Integration in medicine is increasingly called for, some of it good and necessary such as integrating qualitative with quantitative research (29). However, some not, such as integrating untested, unproven, and even useless or harmful complementary therapies into mainstream provision (30).

Trust in doctors remains high. Nearly nine in ten (88%) of adults across the UK say they trust doctors to tell the truth, making doctors the most trusted profession measured. Politicians remain the least trusted with just one in seven people (14%) saying they trust politicians in general to tell the truth. More people say they trust journalists (19%) and bankers (29%) more than politicians (31). But recent exposures in the media may rapidly alter these findings. Currently there is the Leveson inquiry into the culture, practices, and ethics of the press (32); the ongoing debate about bankers' and other executives' bonuses; the intense ongoing debate about the reorganization of the NHS which has now spent more than a year in parliament undergoing prolonged legislative scrutiny and some modification (33); the serious economic crisis in Europe and the UK. All these examples indicate a serious crisis of confidence in the integrity of those in authority. Those who regard the NHS as a gift economy feel betrayed by the current emphasis on the interests of for-profit businesses in government health policy (34). But these concerns are not new.

In the last days of 2008 in the UK, leading Bishops of the Church of England spoke out about our "morally corrupt" Labour government "beguiled by cash." The Bishop of Manchester said: "This is not just an economic issue, but a moral one. It's about what we value" (35). Cardinal Cormac Murphy-O'Connor spoke in London at his 2008 Christmas Midnight Mass, blaming the credit crunch for a breakdown in the trust felt by society (36). They, in turn, were criticized. Disestablishment threatened. Earlier that year, Rabbi Jonathan Sacks had spoken about the transformative idea of covenant in his plenary address to the Anglican Bishops at the Lambeth Conference. He said: "individuals… survive only because they are part of groups. And groups only survive on the basis of reciprocity and trust" (37). Reciprocity is an important concept to consider when thinking about building trust and improving relationships in healthcare. Cicero said "There is no duty more indispensable than that of returning a kindness …. All men distrust one forgetful of a benefit" (38). Note the word "duty."

These examples paint a grim picture of today's fractured society in which doctors work, seek to serve, and seek to retain and uphold the honor of their profession. They are not alone among professional groups bedeviled by excessive bureaucratic regulation in a culture that largely seems not to recognize the values of restraint, reticence, control, caution, or reserve—or the benefits of giving encouragement or working with community spirit. Prime Minister David Cameron's speech delivered on February 14, 2011 on the "Big Society" has been subject to many interpretations (39). Society today can seem to be an outrageously "anything goes" society in matters of speech, behavior, morals and values, spending and lifestyle, in part due to media prominence being given to individualism.

Overzealous activity by regulatory authorities does not foster feelings of well-being, confident hope, creativity, generosity of spirit, or respect for authority based on trust warmed by reciprocity. On the contrary, people are being encouraged to challenge and criticize on websites, rather than being encouraged to take more direct personal interest and action to build better relationships and better local communities (40). It has been wisely said: "if you trust someone they are much more likely to behave in a trustworthy way" (41). Niall Dickson, Chief Executive of The King's Fund, has warned of deterioration in compassion (42). People respond to the way they are treated. Mistrust thrives on suspicion; on invitations to check up and criticize; or to engage in blame games (43). How is the profession of Medicine to regain lost ground and retain respect, honor, and trust in the face of these unceasing State onslaughts? How is it to counter these threats to its professionalism? Has deference truly died? (44) And what effect will this have on the doctor–patient relationship and citizens' and patients' attempts to make informed decision in consultations?

MEDICAL PROFESSIONALISM: MOTIVATION AND MEANING

In their first editorial for 2009, *The Lancet* reminded their readers about "what being a member of the medical profession should be all about" (45). It must be taken to heart if the spirit of medicine (46) is to be revitalized and restored. As Richard Smith said in *The Guardian* in October 2006, "the battle over the soul of medicine is more profound than the battle over the NHS" (47). He also said that there is no definition of "a good doctor"; attempts at defining this are still being made. Fiona Godlee, in her BMJ editorial "Understanding the role of the doctor," (48), commenting on a consensus statement surmised that "the trust that society places in doctors may well reside to a greater extent than is currently acknowledged in their ability to go back to first principles…." What was worrying about the new Medical Schools Council Consensus Statement on the Role of the Doctor, (49), is that it concentrates on competencies but says little about the subtler matter of values that would define the conduct or attributes of character that are likely to command patients' trust and respect. Rachel Remen, in her article, Recapturing the soul of medicine (subtitled "We must remember why we started"), very nicely put her finger on what is needed when she said "Doctors need to reclaim meaning in their working lives" (50). Not only patients, but doctors too, need to work in an ambience that can foster the "continuous process of meaning creation" (51).

The 2005 Royal College of Physicians' Report *Doctors in Society*, (52), talked of a covenant relationship, requiring doctors to exercise honesty; empathy; confidentiality; humanity; and judgment in the face of uncertainty. It defined medical professionalism as "a set of values, behaviors, and relationships that underpins the trust the public has in doctors." Prof. Dame Carol Black listed aspiration to altruism; accountability; duty; service; honor; integrity; respect for others.

Trust goes hand in hand with respect. If people begin to suspect that the profession as a whole is less committed to upholding and defending the values that should underpin their calling, doubts will creep in about their will to resist any encroachments, intimidations, or violations that compromise their freedom to do what is best for their raison d'être—the patient. They must reorient themselves to have a clear view of where their primary duty lies, to the patients, and reaffirm their allegiance to professionalism.

In 2002, Richard Horton wrote in The Lancet: "Doctors can no longer remain silent about their work, leaving advocacy to a small group of medical politicians. Doctors cannot assume that they have either the trust of the public or the support of governments unless they are willing to take part in the public debate about what kind of society they want for the sick and impoverished. More doctors irrespective of their specialty, responsibility, or seniority, need to enter the public arena of dispute" (53).

To this end, Uccio Querci della Rovere, Margaret McCartney (GP and medical journalist) and myself, entered the public arena by mounting a petition and widely circulated our open letter to *The Times* in October 2007, stating "The undersigned doctors and patients believe that trust in the unique doctor–patient relationship is the bedrock of medical practice" (54) http://www.gopetition.com/online/9679.html.

COVENANT OR CONTRACT? CONDUCT OR COMPETENCE? STATE OR SOCIETY?

Trust should be built with true reciprocity. Trust should not be blindly bestowed. I chose the pen name of "Refractor" for a series of essays I wrote for *The Lancet*, with a rainbow as my logo: a symbol of hope and a covenant relationship. Do patients want a relationship with their doctor that is a covenant relationship, or one that is based on contract? What attracts a patient's trust in and respect for a doctor? Research shows that the attribute that patients value most is that the doctor listens. Most patients prefer a consultation in which they contributed but did not have sole responsibility for the decision taken; one in which they feel respected as a "player" who has made a meaningful contribution (55). Two-way respect and deference in achieving the best possible quality of an individual's informed consent in shared decision-making!

Application of business practices by the State to the practice of medicine, (with comparisons to the running of airlines, or the sale of books by Amazon) with emphasis on contracts, sharing the market goods of money and power, has inevitably

resulted in areas of competition. Does the checking of doctors' competence (prompted by the isolated and exceptional failure of the conduct of Harold Shipman) achieve the objective of producing "good doctors" and "safer patients"? (56) Wise words from Baroness O'Neill in 2002 evidently went unheeded: "The efforts to prevent the abuse of trust are gigantic, relentless, and expensive; their results are always less than perfect" (41).

What are doctors for, people might be wondering? What is government for? How has it come to pass that the doctors have allowed themselves to dance to the rhythms of imposed targets and incentives? Government has put "the patient" (whoever that might be!) on a pedestal in the center with much rhetoric about personal responsibility; being provided with choice; given "empowerment," (57) all of which put doctors on the periphery of the action fighting a defensive position in order to do that for which only they have been trained, undermining the morale of the noble profession. Is that what they want?

INFORMED CONSENT FOR SCREENING

Early detection and prevention feature increasingly prominently in today's provision of healthcare (58). Petr Skrabanek warned in 1988 of the interference by the State in the doctor's care for his patients, drawing attention to the State's power to disseminate propaganda under the general heading of "health promotion and prevention." He believed that the doctor's responsibility to his patient included protection of the patient from distortion of the concept of health, medicalization of life, and false promises of disease prevention (59). He concluded: "The ideology behind the current health promotion rhetoric is an unhealthy mix of utopian and totalitarian thinking. In processing masses of healthy people through screening mills, under a false promise of cancer prevention, the doctor ceases to be the patient's advocate and becomes an agent of State policy. His responsibility to individual patients is abrogated and substituted by the dictate of self-appointed health manipulators. The writing is on the wall." Mounting pressure from like-minded people over more than two decades has at last brought general awareness among the profession and the public that a review of the NHS Breast Screening Programme is needed (60). An independent review, led by Sir Mike Richards, is due to report this year (61).

Too often the "ought" is left out of the debate about the overall worth of breast screening, as is consideration of the need for the women themselves to be enabled to give properly informed consent. It is often forgotten that, in the enthusiasm and zeal for tackling the scourge of cancer, it does not follow that just because we CAN do something, we SHOULD do it! Considerations of distributive justice (that is, fairly and justly using available resources), for example, ought to cause us to pause and reflect before setting up a screening program, or for continuing with one when accumulating evidence indicates that it is of dubious benefit and is known to cause more harm than benefit (62,63). More important is the need to be sure that good quality evidence is thoroughly considered to ensure that, on balance, the benefit will outweigh the harm (64). "Do no harm!" should be an even more firmly-considered precept when intruding upon the lives of healthy citizens who might have wished to remain undisturbed (65). Screening is a medical intervention. Not only that, it must not be overlooked that the offer of screening is in itself an intervention. Even someone who chooses to decline screening will be left with the nagging doubt about whether they have made the "right" decision—that is human nature. Not being offered screening in the first place is very different (14).

A quarter of a century has passed since the Forrest Report was published in 1986 (66). Petr Skrabanek's prophetic comments published two years later in 1988 should make us pause and seriously reflect: we cannot say we were not clearly warned (67). He describes how those who were invited to give evidence to the working party were bound to secrecy about the matters discussed; as a result, dissent was, at least in the short term, effectively silenced. Skrabenek described the Report as "a consensus document that does not mention the arguments of the dissenting minority. Its recommendations are based on selective evidence, which ignores data that might undermine its unrealistic estimates. Published evidence is distorted. Ethical issues are avoided." The legacy and continuance of that deception are clear to see today. Skrabanek clearly described the disadvantages of screening in three concise paragraphs, which have since been confirmed and elaborated in numerous recent robust papers. Pertinently, he asks: "who will be blamed, and who will assume responsibility for screening in Britain, if, say, in 10 years' time, mortality from breast cancer shows no improvement? As Richard Feynman, the Nobel Laureate, observed after pinpointing the cause of the Challenger shuttle disaster: "Reality must take precedence over public relations, for nature cannot be fooled." "Given this history, we can see why women have never been given honest information and why reality has been suppressed in favor of promoting "public relations" in public health literature.

PREVENTION

Cancer can affect many organs of the body; each organ can be afflicted by a wide range of so-called "cancers," some intensely aggressive; others, if left alone, will never cause any problem (68). Therefore, to engage in "prevention" is not a simple matter, not only for the epidemiologists, research scientists, clinicians, policy makers, information providers, and decision makers, but also for citizens who can scarcely be expected to know about the biological variations of cancer, or about current advances in all pertinent fields. Much of what they "know" is gleaned from the press. Ben Goldacre has described this as "a broader worry." "People make real-world health-risk behaviour decisions based on information from newspapers and if that information is routinely misleading, there are real-world consequences" (69). He also said: "Numbers can kill!"

"Statistical illiteracy" and "communication of 'numbers," are topics which are of particular concern to me, (70–72), but are not given sufficient attention by health professionals when they communicate. The journey of "facts" from robust and rigorous systematic reviews compiled by expert statisticians and epidemiologists; through publications, read by clinicians, who may or may not be competent to read and understand the statistics (70); to then be communicated to patients in the clinics—requiring yet another skill—is a tortuous one indeed, requiring "translation" of the various specialist "languages" that each of these experts understands and employs. Thus, to have involvement of "consumers" in writing lay summaries of systematic reviews; in drafting information leaflets; and involvement throughout the whole research process can be

judged to be absolutely necessary if the game of "Chinese whispers" is to be avoided, and meaningful communication is to be achieved.

To Screen or Not to Screen for Breast Cancer?

There are other non-communicable diseases that affect our aging populations that are equally as unpleasant as cancer, all currently causing considerable concern worldwide. The global summit held in 2011 (58) avowed that prevention must be the cornerstone of global and national responses to non communicable diseases. Yet, like the poor, the sick are always with us, and always will be; they need care, compassion, and treatment. Where should our resources be deployed—prevention or to treating? I believe we should strive to find a sensible, middle course (73).

We must also pay careful attention to disease measurement thresholds; disease definition; and the increasing tendency toward medicalization of citizens, forewarned by Skrabanek in 1988 (59). This quotation illustrates clearly the problem of medicalization and disease risk measurement thresholds:

> "So how do we decide who has diabetes? When I was in medical school, our numerical rule was this: if you had a fasting blood sugar over 140, then you had diabetes. But in 1997, the Expert Committee on the Diagnosis and Classification of Diabetes Mellitus redefined the disorder. Now if you have a fasting blood sugar over 126, you have diabetes. So everyone who has a blood sugar between 126 and 140 used to be normal but now has diabetes. That little change turned over 1.6 million people into patients" (17).

And the following is Dr Iona Heath's (President of the UK Royal College of General Practitioners) view of disease "labeling," waste, and the Non Communicable Disease Alliance's prevention recommendations:

> "……misplaced risk factor thresholds are already causing havoc in rich countries and wasting prodigious amounts of healthcare resources. …. Yet the thresholds are being used in daily practice throughout the developed world, medicalizing health to an unprecedented degree. To allow such thresholds to be used across the developing world and in the most impoverished countries would be a tragedy on a huge scale. And the same must apply to cancer screening programmes in the context of mounting evidence of substantial harms resulting from overdiagnosis. Yet the Non-Communicable Disease Alliance has published a proposed outcomes document for the UN summit that includes establishing 'effective population-wide prevention, early detection, screening, and awareness-raising programs for NCDs targeting high risk populations."

She goes on to say:

> "Such programmes have the capacity to bankrupt publicly funded healthcare systems in rich countries let alone in poor ones and they systematically shift resources from the sick to the well and from the poor to the rich" (74).

We must beware of "turning people into patients." It must not be forgotten that screening is the business of changing people's identities, producing patients from citizens. Medical screening as an example of "institutionalization of risk" (75). It is essential that decisions about whether to offer population screening are based on the best available evidence. Screening should only be offered to the healthy people it seeks to reassure or treat if there is sound evidence that

(a) it will do more good than harm at an affordable cost;
(b) it will be delivered as part of a good-quality and well-run program (14,76).

Definitions of "Prevention"

The distinctions between prevention, secondary prevention, and early detection are not always understood. Primary prevention has been defined as that set of interventions that keeps a cancerous process from ever developing and includes health counseling and education, environmental controls and product safety as examples. Secondary prevention is that set of interventions leading to the discovery and control of cancerous or precancerous processes while localized, i.e., screening, early detection, and effective treatment (77). So, when the cause or the natural history of a particular cancer is not known, or where many factors are known to be contributory, cancer screening programs (with variable potential for "success") have been introduced with the aim of "finding it early" in the hope and belief that treating the condition before it becomes life-threatening is beneficial and not harmful. This is a flawed strategy and concept, particularly when the test for a disease is of limited efficacy (as with PSA testing and mammographic screening, for example). It leads otherwise asymptomatic people to suffer from false-positive and false-negative diagnoses, as well as the consequences of overdiagnosis and overtreatment. Not to mention resultant psychological and sociological impacts of receiving these "cancer" diagnoses for low-grade or pseudo-cancers.

The term "early" is misleading in general linguistic terms, its opposite being "late" or "too late." Early biologically or chronologically? But "early" is no guarantee of "success": "early" in the context of screening is usually equated with "small." Small is not always beautiful! Small, subclinical cancer can have already spread to establish secondaries, or may develop as interval cancers. Late, but small, cancers (thus, slow growing) with good prognosis can pose little threat to life and can be left until later. Ductal carcinoma in situ can be large and difficult to measure, impalpable, asymptomatic, diffuse, and multifocal with ill-defined, uncertain margins; it is quite often probably neither "early" nor "small," may even regress, and in many cases, is non–life threatening (78).

What Do Citizens Need to Know to Make Informed Decisions? (79–81)

They need to know

- That finding disease earlier is not necessarily a good thing (14). Earlier diagnosis does not necessarily lead to better outcomes; sometimes it makes matters worse.
- That any information they are given is honest, balanced, evidence-based, and up-to-date (82).
- That the purpose of screening is to reduce mortality in a population.

- That screened individuals can be harmed as well as helped by "finding it early"; through over-diagnosis; finding of "pseudo-disease," which would never have caused them a problem in their lifetime and that it can lead to unnecessary and costly overtreatment.
- That the repercussions of this "disease labeling" can have serious effects on their life: physical; psychological; social; employment potential; insurance problems; and inter-generational (83).
- Whether information has been provided neutrally and impartially; it is based on up-to-date reliable and robust evidence; it clearly sets out the likely benefits, harms, limitations, and consequences of being screened or tested.
- The difference between relative risk and absolute risk. Use of relative risk figures can be grossly misleading–it is important to determine individualized absolute risk.
- That they need to beware of the manipulative use of survival figures in reports. Effects on mortality should be used, not 5- or 10-year survival rates. Survival figures can convey a misleading impression of "success" of a test or program.
- That declining an invitation to be screened is a valid option (14).
- That to offer screening is itself a medical intervention with attendant harms as well as potential benefits.

Public Health Initiatives: Cancer Prevention and Cancer Screening

Encouraging behavioral change (with respect to overeating, drinking too much alcohol, smoking and failing to exercise) in order to prevent onset of various diseases, including cancers, can be difficult and costly (84). Opportunistic attempts by trained health professionals using behavioral change counseling to encourage "lifestyle changes" have at best made only a small impact.

Yet recommendations have been made by the NHS Future Forum (the body appointed to review the UK government's plans for the NHS) that doctors, nurses, and other healthcare professionals in England will be asked to question patients about their lifestyle, including smoking, diet, exercise and alcohol consumption, at every meeting, under these new plans backed by the government (85). The Forum's report states that NHS health staff should "use every contact with patients and the public to help them maintain and improve their physical and mental health and wellbeing" (86).

Barriers to Helping Citizens Make Informed Decisions

There are many barriers to helping citizens make informed decisions. High on my list would be definitions and semantics, and top of that list is that it must be remembered that people invited for screening are *citizens*, not patients. Even the BMJ published an incorrectly worded and misleading headline on the front cover of an issue entitled 'Breast screening: What leaflets don't tell patients' (February 21, 2009). Then there is the need to consider the motivation of public health departments, who may be driven by being required to achieve targets for uptake, and other personal motivations, which can bias the way they present information to citizens.

Equally important are the problems and pitfalls of risk communication in a risk averse society (24,68,87,88) Communication and exchange of information between health professionals and patients or citizens is fraught with difficulties and potential misunderstanding, both with respect to words and to "numbers" (statistics). For example:

- The terms "prevention" and "early detection" are sometimes confused; as are the terms "screening" and "diagnosis": an asymptomatic person who is "tested" is being screened, whereas a person with symptoms who is "tested" is being diagnosed. The public (and some health professionals) do not always appreciate this distinction.
- Who are we? Patients? Citizens? Consumers? People? Care needed! People approached for screening are *citizens*, not patients.
- Benefit, harm, and risk (25). The CONSORT Group defines these terms as follows: "*Benefits*: the totality of possible positive consequences of an intervention. These are the opposite of harms against which they must be compared. *Harms*: the totality of possible adverse consequences of an intervention. These are the opposite of benefits against which they must be compared. *Risk*: the probability of harm taking place. It is not possible to directly compare benefits and risks because one is an outcome while the other is the probability of an outcome" (89).
- "Research participant" is the preferred term; not research "subject"; distinction should be made between "passive research participants" and "active research participant," that is, a lay co-researcher working with health professionals.
- Indiscriminate use of the words such as advocate, patient representative, consumer, and user.
- The manipulative use of 5- and 10-year survival figures in media reporting, when mortality data should always be used.

DEMOCRATIC DELIBERATIONS

As long ago as 1941, Henry G. Sigerist stated (90):

> "The people's health is the concern of the people themselves. They must want health. They must struggle for it and plan for it. Physicians are merely experts whose advice is sought in drawing up plans and whose cooperation is needed in carrying them out. No plan, however well designed and well intentioned, will succeed if it is imposed on the people. The war against disease and for health cannot be fought by the physician alone. It is a people's war in which the entire population must be mobilized permanently."

Is there not therefore an ethical imperative to *democratically decide* how best to decide major questions about using our scarce resources for introducing public programs for early detection, and/or for undertaking public health initiatives to engage in prevention? Or to debate the continuation of a program when accumulating evidence indicates that it is doing more harm than good?

CITIZENS' DELIBERATIONS (CITIZENS' JURIES) (91,92)

I believe that we should encourage and promote the Citizens' Deliberation method: this can be used to secure public legitimacy for major questions or matters of public interest.

It is better to consider major health questions by means of Citizens' Deliberations rather than by public consultations, which tap into a poorly informed public. A Jury on Election Recounts has been described in this way by the Jefferson Center:

> The citizens jury is an intensely-involving, brain stretching, eye opening, educational experience. Every single session was a scary, emotional, wonderful experience that left me with my mind spinning, my heart pounding and a new life-changing thought process. I wish everyone could experience a process like a citizens' jury and a real live democracy in action (93).

Citizens' Juries

The idea of Citizens' Juries was developed in the last two decades of the 20th century by Professor Peter Daniel of the University of Wuppertal in Germany and Ned Crosby of the Jefferson Center in Minneapolis, Minnesota, USA. Both have organized citizens' juries on a range of subjects and for a variety of purposes.

Citizens' Deliberations can be undertaken to secure public legitimacy for major questions or matters of public interest. They provide the added advantage of simultaneously educating and informing wider sections of the public through the publicity afforded by observers who attend. At a national level, a jury deliberated on President Clinton's healthcare reforms.

What then is a Citizens' Deliberation?

- It is a small group of ordinary citizens, selected to represent a cross-section of society by using telephone surveys and criteria such as age, race, gender, and education. Jury sizes range from 12 to 24, depending on the scale of the project.
- Deliberations range from four to six days, facilitated by a trained moderator.
- Jurors are paid a modest daily stipend and this may be supplemented by compensation for loss of earnings, payments to employers, and childcare provision in some countries.
- They are informed about the issues, receive evidence, cross-examine witnesses, engage in full discussion, facilitated by the moderator who also acts as time keeper and referee.
- Jurors are sometimes allowed to amend their brief and to call on new sources of information.
- The commissioning body is expected to publicize the jury and its findings, to follow its recommendations or explain why they have not chosen to do so.

For such a system to be successful there is a need to ensure that

- The selection process delivers as representative a sample of the population as possible.
- That the initial brief does not unnecessarily limit the jury in their deliberations (framing the question).

- Information is presented in as unbiased a manner as possible.
- There is sufficient time to reach conclusions.
- The jury is not manipulated by either witnesses or moderator.
- The jury's findings are fairly reported and publicized.

It must not be overlooked that organizers of a Citizens' Deliberation have considerable powers: they brief the jury, select the witnesses, organize the presentation of information, moderate the proceedings, and report on the findings. They are accountable to the sponsors but not to the wider public. Notwithstanding this caveat, Citizens' Deliberations are a democratic way of examining important questions enabling lay people to exercise their citizenship by being involved in the decision-making process, thus sharing the responsibility for initiatives which may be undertaken arising from their conclusions (94,95).

A paper: "Making policy decisions about population screening for breast cancer: The role of citizens' deliberation" (96) reports how use of this democratic methodology produced fascinating findings with respect to citizens' decisions about attending for breast screening. It demonstrated that well-informed citizens could arrive at a different opinion from that which they held when they were unaware of all the pros and cons of a topic. The authors concluded: "A deliberative 'citizens' jury' approach is a feasible way of eliciting a well-informed, considered community view about screening or other population health initiatives."

SOME PROPOSALS AND SUGGESTIONS FOR IMPROVING "INFORMED CONSENT"

- Promote better appreciation of the inherent *uncertainties* in Medicine (2).
- Promote and encourage initiatives that emphasize the need for everybody to recognize their *responsibility to reduce uncertainties* about treatments and other interventions, including public health interventions, by participating (either actively as co-researchers, or passively as participants) in good quality research.
- Promote more *well-informed public and patient involvement* in research and generally (97). See European Science Foundation *Forward Look* Report 2011, chapter 6 and annex 6.
- Promote and encourage *better education* about the scientific principles that underlie medical research in schools (from an early age); in medical school; and in the general public.
- Promote and encourage education in *critical appraisal skills*.
- Support and promote better reporting of health matters in the media and journals.
- Encourage *better communication of "numbers"* (i.e., statistics) everywhere: in the media; in DoH communications and documents of all kinds; in press releases; in communication with patients and the public (70,98).
- Support all initiatives that encourage evidence-based shared decision-making and personal shouldering of

responsibility—both health professionals and citizens. See *Salzburg Statement* (6)

- Recognize the limitations of DoH Public Consultations. An uninformed/poorly or inadequately informed public will not be able to arrive at a well-reasoned response. (e.g., The Connecting for Health Department of Health consultation Report, November 24, 2009, on the *Secondary Uses of Patient Data*, has demonstrated how people's views can change during the course of a well-facilitated Focus Group conducted by an experienced- and skilled qualitative researcher.)
- Encourage initiatives that take steps to *reverse the increasing medicalization* of "health" which exacerbates and panders to fears, both rational and irrational (99).
- Focus on *treating* disease; seek to detect it early or prevent it *only* when evidence shows that doing so would achieve more benefit than harm in a (high risk) population, and when it will be delivered as part of a good quality and well-run program.
- Encourage use of clear, unambiguous use of language, avoiding acronyms and unnecessary medical jargon. Semantics are important.

DARE TO THINK ABOUT DOING LESS EARLY DETECTION; (14) LESS TREATMENT

Earlier diagnosis does not necessarily lead to better outcomes; sometimes it makes matters worse. More intensive treatment is not necessarily beneficial and can sometimes do more harm than good. These are important messages that should be heeded when women attempt to make decisions about screening and about treatment. Screening leads to serious harms in healthy women not only through overdiagnosis with subsequent overtreatment but also when they receive a false-positive mammogram (100). Excessive and often unnecessary treatments are used in women with pre-cancerous conditions such as screen-detected ductal carcinoma in situ. This is a serious matter, since we know that many of these women would never have suffered a problem in their lifetime if they had not attended for screening. The enthusiasm for Herceptin is another case in point. It may offer women a small chance of a longer life, but at the expense of serious side effects, or sometimes even death from the treatment itself (101,102).

DECISIONS ABOUT THE MANAGEMENT OF THE AXILLA

Deciding on how to manage the axilla is an important part of the decision that has to be made with a woman who is diagnosed with breast cancer (103). Ideally, it should be done in consultation with her doctor, taking into consideration her own personal values. Mismanagement not only prejudices the future course of the disease, but, whatever may be the outcome, also has the potential to seriously affect her quality of life and general well being. She will find many difficulties and obstacles in her way in coming to a satisfactory decision. Careful appraisal of well-founded, reliable evidence that has been placed in proper context of past evidence should be encouraged, as should a skeptical eye for media hype about "breakthroughs" and claims for superiority for the latest intervention. "New" or "more" are not always better (14).

The need for routine axillary surgery, which risks unpleasant complications affecting the arm such as lymphedema, is being increasingly challenged, since its addition to other treatments does not seem to improve survival (104). Even so, patients and their doctors should not be dictated to or deprived of choice: every decision about management of the axilla should be a shared, individualized one that takes into account the values, preferences, particular circumstances, and age of that patient, according to her needs, drawing on the latest available evidence. An individual may place more emphasis on avoiding the morbidities associated with one treatment as against another where effectiveness is similar. Or she may prefer to avoid any possible later regret she might suffer about the choice she made, by opting for the more aggressive treatment to obtain that extra 1–2% possible advantage. But choice must be allowed: persuasion or coercion should be condemned. It is unprofessional and unacceptable to say that "there really shouldn't be a choice any more" (105).

TRIAL PARTICIPATION

My recommendation to patients and the public is that they should only agree to participate in a clinical trial where patients have been involved in the research process throughout; the study protocol has been registered; the protocol refers to a systematic review of existing evidence showing that the trial is justified; and where prompt responses to reasonable questions can be obtained from the trial investigators. Finally, critically appraise all reviewed evidence-to-date that puts all robust clinical trials into context (14).

QUALITATIVE RESEARCH: BRIDGING THE GAP BETWEEN PATIENTS AND RESEARCHERS

Qualitative research work has been undertaken which, if noted and applied more generally, could lead to better ways of communicating that would take account of what might be considered by some health professionals to be "irrational uses" of patient information sheets, as opposed to the purely rational application of "fully understanding so as to be able to consent properly" (106). For example, theoretical and empirical exploration of the role of written information in "informing" participants in research has been undertaken in a qualitative study involving semistructured interviews with 29 unpaid healthy volunteers who took part in a genetic epidemiology study in Leicestershire, UK. The researchers found that people might make sense of information about research, including the content of written information, in complex and unexpected ways. The participants had high levels of confidence in the organizations conducting the research, and consequently had few concerns about their participation. Many participants saw their participation as deriving from a moral imperative, even though their understanding of the technical aspects of the study was inconsistent with what had been explained in the written information about the study. The researchers surmised that some "misunderstandings" might be a persistent and incorrigible feature of people's participation in research, raising questions about the principle of informed consent and about the role of written information (107).

Another way that social scientists can be involved is as members of research teams who formally explore sensitive aspects of illness with patients (2,3,108–110). This activity can generally improve the way in which trials are conducted.

Qualitative research with patients and members of the public can explore problems of communication that lead to misunderstandings; it can pinpoint problems of language use that confuse; it can find ways that can guide clinicians to recognize shortcoming in their communication methods and the words they use and lead to advice for improvements; it can determine how patients use information sheets; it can lead to improved patient information leaflets. In summary, this type of rigorous research work can help to achieve a better informed consent process which leads in turn to improved accrual, thus hastening the production of evidence about treatment effects and safety to the benefit of the community at large.

This type of qualitative research work is well illustrated in a clinical trial in men with localized prostate cancer. Researchers wanted to compare three very different treatments for prostate cancer—surgery, radiotherapy, or "watchful waiting." This last option, with its unfortunate description, presented difficulties both for clinicians offering the trial and for patients trying to decide whether to participate in it. Clinicians so much disliked describing the watchful waiting option that they had been leaving it to last, and describing it less than confidently because they had mistakenly thought men asked to join the trial might find it unacceptable. Social scientists had been asked to study the issue of acceptability to help determine whether a trial that included a "watchful waiting" arm was feasible (111). The researchers discovered that clinicians unknowingly used terminology that was misinterpreted by participants. For example, "trial" was sometimes interpreted as monitoring ("try and see"), and recruiters sometimes assumed that patients had refused randomization when they were really questioning monitoring. Also, the phrase intended to reflect evidence of good 10-year survival ("the majority of men with prostate cancer will be alive 10 years later") was interpreted as an (unexpected) suggestion that some might be dead in 10 years. Recruiters were thus asked to replace "trial" with "study" and to present survival in terms of "most men with prostate cancer live long lives even with the disease." It quickly became apparent that the non-radical treatment option caused difficulties for both patients and recruiters. "Conservative monitoring" was meant to emphasize regular review and lack of radical intervention. Recruiters often called it "watchful waiting," but patients interpreted this as "no treatment," as if clinicians would "watch while I die." The social scientists' results were a revelation. Their work showed that a trial offering "watchful waiting" was an acceptable third option if described as "active monitoring," if not left until last to be explained by the recruiting doctor when inviting the patient, and if the doctors were careful to describe active monitoring in terms that men could understand.

These changes to information provision and presentation of options by doctors resulted in increasingly efficient recruitment acceptable to patients and clinicians. Embedding this controversial trial within qualitative research improved recruitment. Such methods probably have wider applicability and may enable even the most difficult evaluative questions to be tackled. This research, bridging the gap between doctors and patients, had identified the particular problems that were presenting difficulties for both parties and that could easily be remedied by better attention to the finer points of recruitment processes. One result in this trial was that the rate of acceptance of men invited to join the trial (112) increased over time, from four acceptances in ten to eight* in ten. This more rapid recruitment means that the data from this trial of all three of these treatments for men with localized prostate cancer will become apparent earlier than would have been the case if the preparatory work had not been done. And, because prostate cancer is a common disease, many men stand to benefit in the future, earlier than they might have done.

WHERE ARE WE TODAY?
Thinking "outside the box" when it comes to finding ways of improving the consent process, such as suggested by Manson and O'Neill, seems not to have percolated through to the European Forum for Good Clinical Practice (EFGCP). The EFGCP organized a meeting of influential ethicists and medical researchers in Brussels in January 2012 to consider "the urgent need to do informed consent better." No mention was made in the report of any citizen involvement in the meeting, nor are we told if any social science researchers with an interest in informed consent were present. The emphasis at the meeting was focused on considering how better to enable patients to understand the implications of their study participation, their benefits, risks, and obligations. In the meeting, it was told that the organization's consent forms had tripled in length between 1995 and 2009, but, were criticized for being "20 pages of nothing." The warning was given that the process had become a box-ticking exercise focused more on offering legal protection to a trial's organizer than actually protecting patients. It seems we are a long way from achieving the effective informative communication that Manson and O'Neill advocate, (1), or of such ideas being given consideration in significant meetings.

The report also advised that the US Department of Health and Human Services is currently consulting about revising clinical trial regulations and looks likely to demand shorter, more understandable consent forms so that prospective participants "have clear and full information to use in making a decision." This has support from other organizations in the United States, who recognize that, in addition to making the process less burdensome for researchers, shorter forms could help to increase the number of patients recruited to clinical trials (113). While this is to be applauded, it is clear from this and the report of the meeting, that no thought is being given to the subtler, unsuspected ways that people use information sheets other than to "understand information" (114).

It was therefore heartening to see a call in the UK from the European Organisation for the Research and Treatment of Cancer (EORTC) for expressions of interest from members of the UK Consumer Liaison Group of the National Institute for Health Research (NIHR). This would involve being part of a small reference group, in a project seeking to improve the quality of information for UK patients taking part in the EORTC clinical research. The project is being run and supported by the EORTC, UK EORTC Liaison Office, and the NIHR Patient and Public Involvement Programme based at the NIHR Cancer Research Network Coordinating Centre. The aim of the project is to improve the quality and relevance of the Patient Information Sheets and Informed Consent given to UK patients considering taking part in EORTC clinical research activities and to ensure information is provided to the patient community about the progress of reviewed projects. EORTC stated that they believe that the experience of patients/carers, and as a member of the Consumer Liaison Group, will be invaluable in helping them to improve the information provided to patients, both for individual studies and for longer-term development of EORTC Patient Information Sheets in general (115). The UK leads the way in not only appreciating the benefits of PPI in the whole research process, but also of the necessity of providing a sound structure to enable it to happen.

CONCLUSION: "INFORMED CONCORDANCE" RATHER THAN "INFORMED CONSENT"
The complexity and inflexibility of regulatory requirements for the informed consent process resulting in overly long patient information sheets is not only an expensive, time-consuming, burdensome chore for clinicians and all others involved, but fails to achieve what is required today to properly involve citizens in coming to agreement about their participation in early detection, research, or treatment. We are a long way from putting into place the ideal of "effective informative communication" advocated by Manson and O'Neill (1) which would accord with today's model of shared decision-making and shared responsibility. Since the achievement of obtaining data from good quality research should be the desired goal of *all* citizens if we are to improve the way that disease is detected and the way that it is treated, it will seem absolutely necessary that we engage in a full and wide debate. Topics should include issues such as the purpose and method of recruiting participants; educating citizens; engaging in effective communication and using robust, systematically reviewed evidence to inform our governmental policies; our public health policies; our treatments; our personal decisions; our societal debates.

These debates should involve not only a much wider range of health professionals but also "lay" citizens. As Sigerist stated in 1942 (25), "The people's health is the concern of the people themselves." But, as I said when I spoke about patient involvement in my paper "The patient's role in research" given at *The Lancet's* "Challenge of Breast Cancer" conference in Bruges in April 1995,

> "The main impediment to implement such a proposal is the inequality of the parties. To make a useful contribution, patients will need to face unpleasant realities; learn to appreciate uncertainly; be educated to understand the dilemmas and problems of clinical research and the dilemmas of obtaining consent; understand the need for trials to evaluate new treatments and assess the value of established ones; demand quality; be aware of the diversity of opinion within the profession and be prepared to work hard to acquire understanding of all aspects of research activity, preferably when they are well, (116) so that they may effectively participate in the shared responsibility and debate."

If we are to put "Informed consent on trial" (112) we must do it properly with a full jury and a complete range of witnesses, moderated impartially, using a pre-set robust procedure

---

* Personal verbal communication 7th February 2012, Professor Michael Baum to HT

that will enable a verdict that is in accord with today's circumstances and requirements. It is unrealistic and naive to suppose that "an influential group of ethicists and medical researchers" (112) will be able to cover every aspect that needs to be exposed and considered if we are to take the necessary action to remedy the current unsatisfactory practices that go towards obtaining "informed consent." If a wide debate is engaged in, we might then be able to work hard to put the necessary requirements in place to achieve the goal of "informed concordance" both individually in consultations and also generally in public health interventions, such as screening.

We must face up to the fact that "fully informed consent" is not necessarily always desirable even were it possible to achieve.

ACKNOWLEDGMENTS

I am grateful to Prof. Mary Dixon-Woods, Professor of Medical Sociology, University of Leicester, for inviting me to present papers giving a patient's perspective in each of two workshops held in 2007 and 2009 under the auspices of the Economic Social Research Council, the first in their Science in Society program, the second in their Public Services program. The first explored the possible differences between governing medical research and medical practice; the second considered trust and the regulation of doctors. Thanks are also due to her for inviting Mr Uccio Querci della Rovere as a delegate at the first workshop.

I am also grateful to Prof. Gerald Gartlehner, Head of Department of Evidence-based Medicine and Clinical Epidemiology, Danube-University, Krems, Austria, for inviting me to present a paper at the Third European Forum for Evidence-based Prevention meeting, exploring what citizens need to know to achieve informed decision-making.

And thirdly, I am grateful to Prof. Glenn Salkeld, Associate Dean, Sydney Medical School and Head of the Sydney School of Public Health, University of Sydney, Australia, for inviting me to give a citizen's view of screening at *Screening Symposium* held in December 2011 considering the provocative and interesting question *What do the community want from screening?*

All these opportunities for involvement—and others not mentioned—widened my outlook and understanding and provided me with a wealth of fresh ideas and material to draw on for this chapter.

There are many colleagues and friends to whom I owe thanks who have been supportive and informative over the years. They know who they are, so I shall not name them individually. But without their kindness and help it would not have been possible to revise and rewrite this chapter.

> "Truth cannot be proved by power. You cannot force people to be saved.
> Coerced agreement is not consent."
> Sacks J. The Great Partnership. God, Science and the Search for Meaning. London: Hodder and Stoughton, 2011. p. 162

REFERENCES

1. Manson NC, O'Neill O. Rethinking Informed Consent in Bioethics. Cambridge: Cambridge University Press, 2007.
2. Locock L, Smith L. Personal experience of taking part in clinical trials – a qualitative study. Patient Educ Couns 2011; 84: 303–9.
3. Armstrong N, Dixon-Woods M, Rusk G, et al. Do informed consent documents for cancer trials do what they should? A study of manifest and latent functions. Sociol Health Illn 2012; in press.
4. Querci della Rovere G, Warren R, Benson JR. Early Breast Cancer, from Screening to Multidisciplinary Management, 2nd edn. London: Taylor & Francis, 2006.
5. Dixon-Woods M, Ashcroft R. Regulation and the social licence for medical research. Med Health Care Philos 2008; 11: 381–91.
6. Salzburg Global Seminar: the greatest untapped resource in healthcare? Informing and involving patients in decision about their medical care, 2010. [Available from: www.salzburgglobal.org/go/477]. BMJ 2011; 342: d1745.
7. Chalmers I, Lindley RI. Double standards on informed consent. In: Doyal L, Tobias JS, eds. Informed Consent in Medical Research. London: BMJ Books, 2001.
8. Heath I. It is not wrong to say no. BMJ 2009; 338: b2529.
9. UKCCCR (UK Co-ordinating Committee on Cancer Research). The UK randomised trial for the management of screen-detected Ductal Carcinoma in Situ (DCIS) of the breast. 1989; ISBN 1 981997 60 - 7.
10. Thornton HM. Breast cancer trials – a patient's viewpoint. Lancet 1992; 339: 44–5.
11. Health Education Authority. NHS Breast Screening. The Facts. London: Health Education Authority. 1991; ISBN 0 7521 0413 1/95 300M.
12. Jorgensen KJ, Goetzsche PC. Presentation on websites of possible benefits and harms from screening for breast cancer: a cross sectional study. BMJ 2004; 328: 148.
13. Department of Health. The Facts. 272896 9p 500k Aug 10 (HOW) (402633) Last updated 2009, and NHS Cancer Screening Programmes. NHS Breast Screening (2011) 403722 5p 500K (Jan 12) (HHC) (408649).
14. Evans I, Thornton H, Chalmers I, Glasziou P. Testing Treatments: Better Research for Better Healthcare, 2nd edn. London: Pinter and Martin 2011. [Available from: http://www.pinterandmartin.com/product/Testing_Treatments_978-1-905177-48-6].
15. Thornton H. Today's patient: passive or involved? Supplement to The Lancet 2000 1999; 354: siv48.
16. General Medical Council. Good medical practice. 2006. [Available from: http://www.gmc-uk.org/guidance/good_medical_practice/index.asp (accessed 1st February 2012)].
17. Horton R, Gilmore I. The evolving doctor. Lancet 2006; 368: 1750–1.
18. Thornton H. Patients and health professionals working together to improve clinical research: where are we going? Eur J Cancer 2006; 42: 2454–8.
19. Evans I, Thornton H, Chalmers I. Testing Treatments: Better Research for Better Healthcare. London: British Library 2006. [Available from: www.testingtreatments.org] in English and six other languages.
20. GMC review to stimulate debate for revisions of Good Medical Practice. [Available from: www.gmc-uk.org/gmp2012]
21. Emanuel EJ, Menikoff J. Reforming the regulations governing research with human subjects. N Engl J Med 2011; 365: 1145–50.
22. Stiggelbout AM, Van der Weijden T, De Wit MP, et al. Shared decision making: really putting patients at the centre of healthcare. BMJ 2012; 344: e256.
23. Fischoff B, Brewer NT, Downs JS. Communicating Risks and Benefits: An Evidence-Based User's Guide. MD, Silver Spring: FDA US Department of Health and Human Services, 2011.
24. Thornton H. Communicating to citizens the benefits, harms and risks of preventive interventions. J Epidemiol Public Health 2010; 64: 101–2.
25. Thornton H. Communicating the benefits, harms and risks of medical interventions: in journals; to patients and public. Int J Surg 2009; 7: 3–6.
26. Salzburg statement on shared decision making. Salzburg Global Seminar: the greatest untapped resource in healthcare? Informing and involving patients in decision about their medical care. 2010. [Available from: www.salzburgglobal.org/go/477] BMJ 2011.342: d1745 and Gulland A. Welcome to the century of the patient. BMJ 2011; 342: d2057.
27. Chambers. The Chambers Dictionary. New edition.
28. Thornton H. The patient's role in research. (Paper given at The Lancet "Challenge of Breast Cancer" Conference, Brugge, 1994) In: Health committee third report. Breast cancer services. Volume II. Minutes of Evidence and Appendices. London: HMSO, 1995: 112–14.
29. Dixon-Woods M, Argawal S, Young B, et al. Integrative approaches to qualitative and quantitative evidence. Report for NHS Health Development Agency 2004; ISBN 1-84279-255-5.

30. Rose LB, Garrow J. Lip service legislation. BMJ 2009; 3338: 66.

31. MORI Poll. Doctors are most trusted profession; politicians least trusted. 2011. [Available from: www.ipsos-mori.com/assets/docs/archive/polls/healthcarecommission.pdf (accessed 15th October 2012) IPSOS MORI/BMJ].

32. www.levesoninquiry.org.uk/about/terms-of-reference

33. Walshe K. The consequences of abandoning the healthcare bill. BMJ 2012; 344: e748.

34. Heath I. The NHS gift economy is in peril. BMJ 2012; 344: e590.

35. Jonathan W-J. The Sunday Telegraph, 2008.

36. BBC News, UK, Cardinal concerned over distrust 25.12.2008.

37. Sacks RJ. Plenary address to the Lambeth Conference. The Relationship between the People and God, Monday 28 July 2008. [Available from: www.lambethconference.org/daily/news.cfm/2008/7/29/ACNS4484].

38. Gouldner AW. The norm of reciprocity. A preliminery statement. Am Sociol Rev 1960; 25: 161–78.

39. Cameron D. Big society. 2011. [Available from: www.number10.gov.uk/news/pms-speech-on-big-society/].

40. Sacks J. The Home We Build Together. Recreating Society. London: Continuum Books, 2007.

41. O`Neill O. A Question of Trust. The BBC Reith Lectures. Cambridge: Cambridge University Press, 2002: 43–59.

42. Dreaper J. BBC News Correspondent. NHS 'fast losing its compassion'. 2008.

43. Heath I. The blame game. BMJ 2009; 338: 73.

44. Thornton H. The death of deference? Bmj.com rapid response to Godlee [ref. 48.]

45. Violent conflict: protecting the health of civilians. Lancet 2009; 373: 95.

46. Thornton H. The spirit of medicine blog in the International journal of surgery, 2006. [Available from: www2.le.ac.uk/departments/health-sciences/research/soc-sci/staff-pages/HazelThornton].

47. Smith R. A remedy for the soul of medicine. The Guardian, 24 October 2006.

48. Godlee F. Editorial: Understanding the role of the doctor. BMJ 2008; 337: 1425–6.

49. Medical schools council consensus statement on the role of the doctor, 2008. [Available from: www.medschools.ac.uk/AboutUs/Projects/Documents/Role of Doctor Consensus Statement.pdf (accessed 4th October 2012)].

50. Remen R. Recapturing the soul of medicine. BMJ 2001; 9: 3–4.

51. Dixon-Woods M. Writing wrongs? An analysis of published discourses about the use of patient information leaflets. Soc Sci Med 2001; 52: 1417–32.

52. Royal College of Physicians. Doctors in Society: Medical Professionalism in a Changing World. London: RCP, 2005.

53. Horton R. The doctor's role in advocacy. Lancet 2002; 359: 458.

54. Open letter: G. Querci della Rovere and Dr. Margaret McCartney, Hazel Thornton, plus 15 other signatories and 940 doctors and patients. The Times. "New check ups of doctors" 17th October 2006.

55. Thornton H, Edwards A, Elwyn G. Evolving the multiple roles of 'patients' in health-care research: reflections after involvement in a trial of shared decision-making. Health Expect. 2003; 6: 189–97.

56. Report by the Chief Medical Officer, Sir Liam Donaldson. Good Doctors, safer patients. Department of Health, 14 July 2006.

57. Thornton H. "Empowering" patient choice about participation in trials? In: Duley L, Farrell B, eds. Clinical Trials: into the New Millennium. London: BMJ Books, 2002.

58. Coombes R. World leaders sign up to tackle causes of non-communicable diseases. BMJ 2011; 343: d6034.

59. Skrabanek P. The physician's responsibility to the patient. Lancet 1988; 1: 1155–7.

60. Baum M, McCartney M, Thornton H, et al. Breast Cancer Screening Peril. Negative consequences of the breast screening programme. The Times 2009; 31. [Available from: www.dcscience.net/Times-breast-cancer screening-190209.pdf].

61. Richards M. An independent review is under way. BMJ 2011; 343: d6843.

62. Gøtzsche PC, Nielsen M. Screening for breast cancer with mammography. Cochrane Database Syst Rev 2011: CD001877, doi: 10.1002/14651858.CD001877.pub4.

63. Goetzsche PC. Mammography Screening: Truth, Lies and Controversy. Oxford: Radcliffe Publishing, 2012.

64. Jorgensen KJ, Goetzsche PC. Who evaluates public health programmes? A review of the NHS breast screening programme. J R Soc Med 2010; 103: 14–20.

65. First do no harm. Lancet Oncol 2009.10: 927 [Available from: www.thelancet.com/oncology].

66. The Forrest Report. Breast Cancer Screening. Report to the Health Ministers of England, Wales, Scotland and Northern Ireland by a working group chaired by Professor Sir Patrick Forrest. Published November 1986. ISBN 0 11 321071 X.

67. Skrabanek P. The debate over mass mammography in Britain. The case against. BMJ 1988; 297: 971–2.

68. Welch HG, Schwartz LM, Woloshin S. Over-Diagnosed: Making People Sick in the Pursuit of Health. Boston: Beacon Press, 2011: 17–18.

69. Goldacre B. How far should we trust health reporting? The Guardian. Bad Science. 17th June 2011.

70. Thornton H. Editorial: Statistical illiteracy is damaging our health. Doctors and patients need to understand numbers if meaningful dialogues are to occur. Int J Surg 2009; 7: 279–84.

71. Gigerenzer G, Gaissmaier W, Kurz-Milcke E, et al. Helping doctors and patients make sense of health statistics. Psychologic Sci Public Inter 2008; 8: 53–96.

72. Evans I, Thornton H. Editorial. Transparency in numbers. The dangers of statistical illiteracy. J R Soc Med 2009; 102: 354–6.

73. Thornton H. Is there a sensible 'middle road' for early detection of breast cancer? The Breast 2008; 17: 545.

74. Heath I. Seeming virtuous on chronic diseases. BMJ 2011; 343: d4239.

75. Giddens A. Modernity and SelfIdentity. Cambridge: Polity, 1991.

76. Raffle A, Gray M. Screening: Evidence and Practice. Oxford: Oxford University Press, 2007.

77. Spratt JS. The primary and secondary prevention of cancer. J Surg Oncol 1981; 18: 219–30.

78. Thornton H. Randomised clinical trials: the patient's point of view. In: Silverstein M, ed. Ductal Carcinoma in Situ of the Breast. Philadelphia: Williams and Wilkins, 1997. With commentary by David K. Wellisch.

79. Sense about Science. Booklet: Making Sense of Screening. London: 2009. [Available from: www.senseaboutscience.org.uk].

80. Gilbert Welch H. Should I be Tested for Cancer? Maybe Not and Here's Why. Berkeley and Los Angeles: University of California Press, 2004.

81. Thornton H. An end-user perspective of screening mammography. Mammology 2008; 3: 12–19.

82. Thornton H. The 'truth' about mammography screening? Nearing the end of a long and arduous Damascus Road. Int J Surg 2009; 7: 177–9.

83. Thornton H. Pairing accountability with responsibility – the consequences of screening 'promotion'. Med Sci Monitor 2001; 7: 531–3.

84. Pre-empt trial: Preventing disease through opportunistic, Rapid EngagEMent by Primary Care Teams using Behaviour Change Counselling (PRE-EMPT). [Available from: www.wspcr.ac.uk/pre-empt.php].

85. Mooney H. Doctors are told to "make every contact count" to promote health. BMJ 2012; 344: e319.

86. Public health in England: from nudge to nag. Lancet 2012; 379: 194.

87. Gigerenzer G. Reckoning with Risk. Learning to Live with Uncertainty. London: Penguin Books, 2002.

88. Woloshin S, Schwartz L, Welch G. Know Your Chances: Understanding Health Statistics. Berkeley: University of California Press, 2008. [Available from: www.jameslindlibrary.org].

89. Ioannidis JPA, Evans S, Goetzsche PC, et al. the CONSORT Group. Better reporting of harms in randomized trials: an extension of the CONSORT statement. Ann Intern Med 2004; 141: 781–8.

90. Sigerist HE. Medicine and Human Welfare. Yale University Press, 1941: quoted in: Silverman WA. ed. Human Experimentation. A Guided Step into the Unknown. Oxford University Press, 1985: 161.

91. Stewart J, Kendall E, Coote A. Citizens' Juries Institute for Public Policy Research. London: IPPR, 1994.

92. McIver S. Independent Evaluation of Citizens' Juries in Health Authority Settings. King's Fund Publishing, 1998.

93. Jefferson Centre. [Available from: http://www.jefferson-center.org/index.asp?Type=B_BASIC&SEC=%7B2BD10C3C-90AF-438C-B04F-88682B6393BE%7D&Design=PrintView].

94. Thornton H. To screen or not to screen? In: Peters P, Peters P. Sourcebook on Asbestos Diseases. CA: Lexis Law Publishing, a division of Reed Elsevier Inc, 1998: 177–90.

95. Thornton H. Chapter 42: Informed consent in the management and research of breast cancer. In: Querci della Rovere G, Warren R, Benson JR, eds. Early Breast Cancer, from screening to multidisciplinary management, 2nd edn. London: Taylor & Francis, 2006; Medical Books. (Third Edition in production).

96. Paul C, Nicholls R, Priest P, McGee R. Making policy decisions about population screening for breast cancer: the role of citizens' deliberations. Health Policy 2008; 85: 314–20.

97. European Science Foundation. Report Forward look: implementation of medical research in clinical practice. 2011. [Available from: www.esf.org].

98. Sense about Science and Straight Statistics. Making Sense of Statistics. London: 2010. [Available from: www.senseaboutscince.org].

99. Woloshin S, Schwartz L. Numbers needed to decide. J Natl Cancer Inst 2009; 101: 1163–5.

100. Gøtzsche PG, Jørgensen KJ, Zahl P-H, Mæhlen J. Why mammography screening has not lived up to expectations from the randomised trials. Cancer Causes Control 2012; 23: 15–21.

101. Piccart-Gebhart MJ, Procter M, Leyland-Jones B, et al. Trastuzumab after adjuvant chemotherapy in HER-2-positive breast cancer. N Engl J Med 2005; 353: 1659–72.

102. Romond EH, Perez EA, Bryant J, et al. Trastuzumab plus adjuvant chemotherapy for operable HER-2-positive breast cancer. N Engl J Med 2005; 353: 1673–84.

103. Thornton H. Patient decisions about management of the axilla. Mammology 2007; 3: 43–6.

104. Carlson GW, Woods WC. Management of axillary lymph node metastasis in breast cancer: making progress. JAMA 2011; 305: 606–7.

105. Kissin M. Two large trials favor sentinel node biopsy. [Available from: http://www.medscape.com/viewarticle/495900_print (accessed 13th December 2004)].

106. Dixon-Woods M, Tarrant C. Why do people cooperate with medical research? Soc Sci Med 2009; 68: 2215–22.

107. Dixon-Woods M, Ashcroft RE, Jackson CJ, et al. Beyond "misunderstanding": written information and decisions about taking part in a genetic epidemiology study. Soc Sci Med 2007; 65: 2212–22.

108. Hersch J, Jansen J, Irwig L, et al. How do we achieve informed choice for women considering breast cancer? Prev Med 2011; 53: 144–6.

109. Dixon-Woods M, Williams SJ, Jackson CJ, et al. Why do women consent to surgery, even when they do not want to? An interactionist and Bourdieusian analysis. Soc Sci Med 2006; 62: 2742–53.

110. Dixon-Woods M, Jackson CJ, Windridge KC, et al. Receiving a summary of the results of a trial: qualitative study of participants' views. BMJ 2006; 332: 206–10.

111. Donovan J, Mills N, Smith M, et al. the ProtecT Study Group. Quality improvement report: improving design and conduct of randomised trials by embedding them in qualitative research: ProtecT (prostate testing for cancer and treatment) study. BMJ 2002; 325: 766–70.

112. The ProtecT trial: Evaluating the effectiveness of treatment for clinically localised prostate cancer. ISRCTN201412, Current controlled trials.

113. Cressey D. Informed consent on trial. Nature 482, 16 doi: 10.1038/482016a [Available from: www.nature.com/news/informed-consent-on-trial-1.9933 (accessed 2nd February 2012)].

114. Cressey D. Informed consent on trial. Lengthy, complicated documents leave many clinical-trial participants in the dark about the risks they face. Nature 2012. [Available from: www.nature.com/news/informed-consent-on-trial-1.9933?WT.ec_id=NEWS-20 (accessed 5th February 2012)].

115. EORTC/NHS NIHR NCRN. Improving the quality of information given to UK patients considering taking part in EORTC (European Organisation for the Research and Treatment of Cancer) clinical research activities. 2012.

116. Thornton H. Commentary: a ladyplan for trial recruitment – "everyone's business!" Editorial commentary on Michael Baum's paper in same issue: new approach for recruitment into randomised controlled trials. Lancet 1993; 341: 796.

34 Ductal carcinoma *in situ* of the breast

Melvin J. Silverstein and Michael D. Lagios

INTRODUCTION

Ductal carcinoma *in situ* (DCIS) of the breast is a heterogeneous group of lesions with diverse malignant potential and a range of treatment options. It is the most rapidly growing subgroup in the breast cancer family of disease with more than 58,000 new cases diagnosed in the United States during 2011 (1). Most of the new cases (>90%) are nonpalpable and discovered mammographically.

It is now well appreciated that DCIS is a stage in the neoplastic continuum where most of the molecular changes that characterize invasive breast cancer are already present (2). All that remains on the way to invasion are quantitative changes in the expression of genes that have already been altered. Genes that may play a role in invasion control a number of functions, including angiogenesis, adhesion, cell motility, the composition of extracellular-matrix, and more. To date, genes that are uniquely associated with invasion have not been identified. DCIS is clearly the precursor lesion for most invasive breast cancers but not all DCIS lesions have the time or the genetic ability to progress to become invasive breast cancer (3–5).

Therapy for DCIS ranges from simple excision to various forms of wider excision (segmental resection, quadrant resection, oncoplastic resection using various forms of breast reduction, etc.), all of which may or may not be followed by radiation therapy. When breast preservation is not feasible, total mastectomy is performed (which is increasingly skin sparing and nipple–areola sparing) and done in conjunction with immediate reconstruction.

DCIS is a heterogeneous group of lesions rather than a single entity (6,7). Moreover, patients have a wide range of personal needs that must be considered during treatment selection and it is clear that no single approach will be appropriate for all forms of the disease and treatment must therefore be tailored to individual patients. At the current time, treatment decisions are based upon measurable parameters (tumor extent, margin width, nuclear grade, the presence or absence of comedo necrosis, age, etc.), physician experience and bias, and randomized clinical trial data. The latter suggest that all conservatively treated patients should be managed with postexcisional radiation therapy and tamoxifen.

THE CHANGING NATURE OF DCIS

There have been dramatic changes in the past 20 years that have affected the incidence of DCIS. Before mammography was common, DCIS was rare, representing less than 1% of all breast cancer (8). Today, DCIS is common, representing 20% of all newly diagnosed cases with up to 30–50% of cases of screen-detected breast cancer (1,9–13). In the past, most patients with DCIS presented with clinical symptoms, such as breast mass, bloody nipple discharge, or Paget's disease (14,15). Nowadays, most lesions are nonpalpable and often detected by imaging alone.

Until approximately 20 years ago, the treatment for most patients with DCIS was mastectomy. By contrast, almost 75% of newly diagnosed patients with DCIS are now treated with breast preservation (16). When mastectomy was common in the past, reconstruction was uncommon and when performed, was generally done as a delayed procedure. Nowadays, reconstruction for patients with DCIS treated by mastectomy is common and when performed, is generally done as an immediate procedure at the time of mastectomy. Historically, mastectomy involved excision of large amounts of skin which were discarded. It is now considered safe to perform a skin-sparing mastectomy for DCIS and in many instances, nipple–areola sparing-mastectomy.

In the past, there was little confusion about management of DCIS; all breast cancers were considered to be essentially the same and mastectomy was the only treatment. It is now recognized that all breast cancers are different and there is a range of acceptable treatments for individual lesions. For those patients who chose breast conservation surgery, there continues to be a debate as to whether radiation therapy is necessary in every case. These changes were brought about by a number of factors. Most important were increased mammographic utilization and the acceptance of breast-conservation therapy for invasive breast cancer. The widespread use of mammography changed the way DCIS was detected. In addition, it changed the nature of the disease detected by allowing us to enter the neoplastic continuum at an earlier time.

It is interesting to note the influence that mammography had on the Breast Center in Van Nuys, California in terms of the number of DCIS cases diagnosed and the way they were diagnosed (17).

From 1979 to 1981, the Van Nuys Group treated a total of only 15 patients with DCIS, five per year. Only two lesions (13%) were impalpable and detected by mammography. In other words, 13 patients (87%) presented with clinically apparent disease, detected by the old-fashioned methods of observation and palpation. Two state-of-the-art mammography units and a full-time experienced radiologist were established in 1982 and the number of new DCIS cases dramatically increased to more than 30 per year, most of them impalpable. When a third and fourth machine were added, the number of new cases increased to more than 50 per year.

The DCIS patients discussed in this chapter were accrued at Van Nuys from 1979 to 1998, at the University of Southern California (USC), Norris Comprehensive Cancer Center from 1998 to 2008, and at the Hoag Memorial Hospital Presbyterian from 2008 to September 2011. Analysis of the entire series of 1566 patients through September 2011 shows that 1386 lesions (89%) were nonpalpable (subclinical). If we look at only those diagnosed during the last five years at the USC/Norris Cancer Center, 95% were nonpalpable. At Hoag, from 2008 to 2011, 93% were nonpalpable. The second factor that changed how we think about DCIS was the acceptance of breast conservation therapy (lumpectomy, axillary node dissection, and radiation therapy) for patients with invasive breast cancer. Until 1981, the treatment for most patients with any form of breast cancer was generally mastectomy. Since that time, numerous prospective randomized trials have shown an equivalent rate of survival for selected patients with invasive breast cancer treated with breast conservation therapy (18–23). Based on these results, it made little sense to continue treating a lesser disease (DCIS) with mastectomy while treating a more aggressive invasive breast cancer with breast preservation. Current data suggest that many patients with DCIS can be successfully treated with breast preservation, with or without radiation therapy. This chapter will show how easily the available data can be used to help in the complex treatment selection process.

PATHOLOGY
Classification
Although there is no universally accepted histopathological classification, most pathologists have traditionally divided DCIS into five major architectural subtypes (papillary, micropapillary, cribriform, solid, and comedo), often comparing the first four (non-comedo) with comedo (6,13,24). Comedo DCIS is frequently associated with a high nuclear grade (6,13,24,25) aneuploidy, a higher proliferation rate (26), HER2/neu gene amplification or protein overexpression (27–31), and clinically more aggressive behavior (32–35). Non-comedo lesions tend to be just the opposite.

The division by architecture alone, comedo versus non-comedo, is an oversimplification and is impractical if the purpose of the division is to sort patients into those with a high risk of local recurrence versus those with a low risk. It is not uncommon for high nuclear grade non-comedo lesions to express markers similar to those of high-grade comedo lesions and to have a similar risk of local recurrence. Furthermore, mixtures of various architectural subtypes may coexist within a single-biopsy specimen. Within our series of patients, almost three-quarters of lesions had significant amounts of two or more architectural subtypes, thus rendering allocation to a predominant architectural subtype problematic. There is no uniform agreement among pathologists of exactly how much comedo DCIS needs to be present to classify the lesion as comedo DCIS. Although lesions exhibiting a predominant high-grade comedo DCIS pattern are generally more aggressive and more likely to recur if treated conservatively than low-grade non-comedo lesions, architectural subtyping does not reflect current biological thinking. Instead, the concept of nuclear grading has assumed greater importance and significance in classification of DCIS lesions. Nuclear grade is a better biological predictor than architecture, and has emerged as a key histopathological factor for identifying aggressive behavior (32,35–39). In 1995, the Van Nuys Group introduced a new pathological DCIS classification (40) based on the presence or

absence of high nuclear grade and comedo-type necrosis (the Van Nuys Classification).

The Van Nuys Group chose high nuclear grade as the most important factor in their classification because there was general agreement that patients with high nuclear grade lesions were more likely to have recurrence at a higher rate and in a shorter time period after breast conservation than patients with low nuclear grade lesions (32,35,38,41–43). Comedo-type necrosis was chosen because its presence also suggests a poorer prognosis (44,45) and it is easy to recognize (46).

To use the Van Nuys DCIS Classification, the pathologist, using standardized criteria as noted below, first determines whether the lesion is of a high nuclear grade (nuclear grade 3) or a non–high nuclear grade (nuclear grades 1 or 2). Then, the presence or absence of necrosis is assessed in the non-high-grade lesions. This results in three groups (Fig. 34.1). Nuclear grade is scored by previously described methods (32,38,40). Essentially, low-grade nuclei (grade 1) are defined as nuclei that are 1–1.5 red blood cells in diameter with diffuse chromatin and unapparent nucleoli. Intermediate nuclei (grade 2) are defined as those that are one to two red blood cells in diameter with coarse chromatin and infrequent nucleoli. High-grade nuclei (grade 3) are defined as nuclei that are with a diameter greater than two red blood cells, with vesicular chromatin, and one or more nucleoli. Mitotic activity is usually identifiable in high-grade DCIS, but infrequently in lower grades 1 and 2.

The Van Nuys classification does not stipulate a minimum or specific amount of high nuclear grade DCIS, nor is any minimum amount of comedo-type necrosis required for diagnosis. Occasional desquamated or individually necrotic cells are ignored and are not scored as comedo-type necrosis. The most difficult part of most classifications is nuclear grading, particularly the intermediate-grade lesions. The subtleties of the intermediate-grade lesion are not important to the Van Nuys classification; only nuclear grade 3 lesions need to be recognized. The cells must be large and pleomorphic, lack architectural differentiation and polarity, have prominent nucleoli and coarse clumped chromatin, and generally show mitoses (32,40,44). The Van Nuys classification is useful because it divides DCIS into three different biological groups with different risks of local recurrence after breast conservation therapy (Fig. 34.2). This pathological classification, when combined

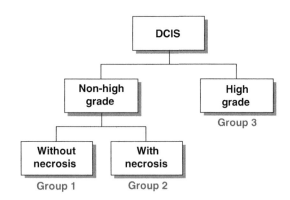

Figure 34.1 Van Nuys DCIS classification. DCIS patients are separated in high nuclear grade (grade 3) and non–high nuclear grade (grades 1 and 2). Non–high nuclear grade cases are then separated by the presence or absence of necrosis. Lesions in group 3 (high nuclear grade) may or may not show necrosis.

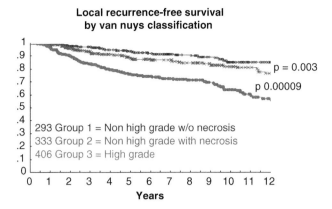

Figure 34.2 Probability of local recurrence-free survival for 1032 breast conservation patients using Van Nuys DCIS pathological classification.

with tumor size, age, and margin status, is an integral part of the USC/Van Nuys Prognostic Index (USC/VNPI), a system that will be discussed in detail.

Progression to Invasive Breast Cancer

Which DCIS lesions will become invasive and when will that happen? These are the most fundamental questions in the field of DCIS pathobiology. Currently, there is intense molecular biological interrogation regarding the progression of genetic changes in normal breast epithelium to DCIS and then to invasive breast cancer. Most of the genetic and epigenetic changes present in invasive breast cancer are already present in DCIS. To date, no genes uniquely associated with invasive cancer have been identified. As DCIS progresses to invasive breast cancer, quantitative changes in the expression of genes related to angiogenesis, adhesion, cell motility, and the composition of the extracellular-matrix may occur (2,16).

Immunohistochemical and Molecular Phenotypes in DCIS

It has been recognized for some time that there is substantial concordance between the grade of DCIS and its associated invasive carcinoma. Based on this, low-grade lesions, regardless of the classification scheme used, are generally associated with lower grade invasive carcinomas, whereas high-grade DCIS are linked with higher grade invasive carcinomas. Additionally, the frequency of specific biomarkers in DCIS varies with the grade of the lesion: estrogen and progesterone receptors are usually expressed in DCIS, but less so in high-grade DCIS, while HER-2 and elevated proliferative markers such as Ki-67 are features of high-grade DCIS. Surrogate molecular phenotypes defined by immunohistochemistry have now identified DCIS phenotypes corresponding to luminal A, luminal B, HER-2, and triple negative/basal phenotypes in invasive breast cancer. Luminal A and B DCIS phenotypes are more frequent in low intermediate-grade lesions, whereas HER-2, triple negative and basal phenotypes are more common among high-grade DCIS (47,48).

Currently, gene expression profiling for invasive carcinomas can segregate carcinomas at significantly different risks of distant relapse (10 years) and indicate the likelihood of a benefit from chemotherapy. Hannemann and colleagues were able to segregate DCIS with and without invasive carcinomas using a group of 35 genes, and stratify DCIS by another 43-gene

classifier into well-differentiated versus poorly differentiated (high grade) subtypes (49). Additionally, these authors confirmed the association of ER expression in low or intermediate DCIS and HER-2 in high-grade DCIS. Solin et al. presented a new DCIS gene signature RT-PCR assay which can separate out three risk groups based on their gene expression profiles (50). The genes were selected from the existing Oncotype DX assay, and the archived tissue from the ECOG 5194 registration trial was used for validation. The ECOG trial examined the frequency of local recurrence in DCIS patients treated by excision alone with a minimum margin of 3 mm. Low to intermediate-grade DCIS had to be 25 mm or less in the greatest extent, while high-grade DCIS could not exceed 10 mm. All patients entered into the trial had specimens examined by a serial sequential tissue protocol permitting reproducible determination of size (extent), margin widths, and exclusion of microinvasive foci. Cases which did not meet these criteria were ineligible for the study. Specimens examined by less rigorous means cannot be reliably evaluated by the assay; for example, the DCIS may exceed the size limit or exhibit margins which are suboptimal and the recurrence score (RS) reported may not be valid for the case submitted. By way of contrast, two recent nomograms, designed to predict recurrence following breast conservation therapy for DCIS, were based on archival materials that were not processed in the serial sequential method and for which data on size and margins were frequently missing. Kerlikowski and colleagues evaluated specimens which were generated from many institutions without a common protocol, and without accurately determined size or margin status (51). Rudloff and colleagues developed a nomogram which was obtained from a single institution but without a single protocol and not examined by the serial subgross technique (52). The ECOG study dichotomized DCIS into low intermediate versus high grade and only required a 3 mm margin. It will remain to be seen whether reanalysis of the pathology data will permit a greater separation of subsets of DCIS comparable to what can be achieved in the USC/VNPI.

Because most patients with DCIS have historically been treated with mastectomy, knowledge of the natural history of this disease is relatively recent. The studies of Page (53,54) and Rosen (55) provide information regarding the outcome of low-grade DCIS without treatment. In these studies, patients with non-comedo DCIS were initially misdiagnosed as benign lesions and therefore went untreated, apart from initial biopsy. The majority of these cases represented incidental foci in diagnostic excision biopsies for palpable disease. Subsequently, approximately 25–35% of these patients developed invasive breast cancer, generally within 10 years (53,54). Had the lesions been high-grade comedo DCIS, the invasive breast cancer rate likely would have been higher than 35% and the time to invasive recurrence shorter. With few exceptions, in both of these studies, the invasive breast carcinoma was of the ductal type and located at the site of the original DCIS thus implying progression of DCIS to invasive disease. However, these findings suggest that not all DCIS lesions progress to invasive breast cancer or become clinically significant (56). Page and associates updated their series in 2002 and 2005 (53,54,57). Of the 28 women with low-grade DCIS misdiagnosed as benign lesions and were treated only by biopsy between 1950 and 1968, 11 patients have recurred locally with invasive breast cancer

(39%). Eight patients developed recurrence within the first 12 years. The remaining three were diagnosed over 23–42 years. Five patients developed metastatic breast cancer (18%) and died from the disease within seven years of developing invasive breast cancer. These recurrence and mortality rates seem alarmingly high at first glance. However, they are only slightly worse than expected with long-term follow-up of patients with lobular carcinoma *in situ*, a disease that most clinicians are willing to treat with careful clinical follow-up. In addition, these patients were treated with biopsy only. No attempt was made to excise these lesions with a clear surgical margin. The natural history of low-grade DCIS can extend over a 40-year period and is markedly different from that of high-grade DCIS.

Microinvasion

The incidence of microinvasion is difficult to quantitate because there was no formal and universally accepted definition of exactly what constitutes microinvasion. The 5th edition of *The Manual for Cancer Staging* (1997) carried the first official definition of what is now classified as pT1mic and read as follows: "Microinvasion is the extension of cancer cells beyond the basement membrane into adjacent tissues with no focus more than 0.1 cm in greatest dimension. When there are multiple foci of microinvasion the size of only the largest focus is used to classify the microinvasion (do not use the sum of all individual foci). The presence of multiple foci of microinvasion should be noted, as it is with multiple larger invasive carcinomas."

The reported incidence of occult invasion (invasive disease at mastectomy in patients with a biopsy diagnosis of DCIS) varies greatly, ranging from as little as 2% to as much as 21% (58). This problem was addressed in the investigations of Lagios and colleagues (32,38).

Lagios et al. performed a meticulous serial subgross dissection correlated with specimen radiography. Occult invasion was found in 13 of 111 mastectomy specimens from patients who had initially undergone excisional biopsy of DCIS. All occult invasive cancers were associated with DCIS greater than 45 mm in extent; the incidence of occult invasion approached 50% for DCIS greater than 55 mm. In the study of Gump et al. (59), foci of occult invasion were found in 11% of patients with palpable DCIS but not in patients with clinically occult DCIS. These results suggest a correlation between the size of the DCIS lesion and the incidence of occult invasion. Clearly, as the size of the DCIS lesion increases, microinvasion and occult invasion become more likely.

If even the *smallest* amount of invasion is found, the lesion should not be classified as DCIS. It is a T1mic (if the largest invasive component is 1 mm or less) with an extensive intraductal component (EIC). If the invasive component is 1.1 mm to 5 mm, it is a T1a lesion with EIC. If there is only a single focus of invasion, these patients have a favorable prognosis. When there are many tiny foci of invasion, these patients have a poorer prognosis than expected (10). Unfortunately, the TNM staging system does not have a T category that fully reflects the malignant potential of lesions with multiple foci of invasion since they are all classified by the largest single focus of invasion. De Mascarel and colleagues have noted that microinvasive foci consisting of single cells have no impact on outcome while those comprising cohesive groups of cells are

associated with a demonstrable increase in distant recurrence and death (60).

Multicentricity and Multifocality of DCIS

Multicentricity is generally defined as DCIS in a quadrant other than the quadrant in which the original DCIS (index quadrant) was diagnosed. There must be normal breast tissue separating the two foci. However, definitions of multicentricity vary among investigators. Hence, the reported incidence of multicentricity also varies. Rates in the range of 0–78% (7,55,61,62), averaging about 30%, have been reported. Twenty-five years ago, a figure of 30% for the average rate of multicentricity was used by surgeons as the rationale for mastectomy in patients with DCIS.

Holland and colleagues evaluated 82 mastectomy specimens by taking a whole-organ section every 5 mm with each section being radiographed (63). Paraffin blocks were made from every radiographically suspicious spot. In addition, an average of 25 blocks was taken from the quadrant containing the index cancer; random samples were taken from all other quadrants, the central subareolar area, and the nipple. The microscopic extension of each lesion was verified on the radiographs. This technique permitted a three-dimensional reconstruction of each lesion. This study demonstrated that most of the DCIS lesions were larger than expected (50% were greater than 50 mm), involved more than one quadrant by continuous extension (23%), but most importantly, were unicentric (98.8%). Only one of 82 mastectomy specimens (1.2%) had "true" multicentric distribution with a separate lesion in a different quadrant. This study suggests that complete excision of a DCIS lesion is possible due to unicentricity but may be extremely difficult due to larger than expected size. In an update, Holland reported whole-organ studies in 119 patients, 118 of whom had unicentric disease (64). This information, when combined with the fact that most local recurrences are at or near the original DCIS, suggests that the problem of multicentricity *per se* is not important in the DCIS treatment decision-making process. Multifocality is defined as a separate focus of DCIS within the same ductal system. The studies of Holland et al. (63,64) and Noguchi et al. (65) suggest that a great deal of multifocality may be artifactual, resulting from looking at a three-dimensional arborizing entity in two dimensions on a glass slide. It would be analogous to saying that the branches of a tree were not connected if the branches were cut at one plane, placed separately on a slide, and viewed in cross-section (53). Multifocality may be due to small gaps of DCIS or skip areas within ducts as described by Faverly et al. (43). Multifocality is more easily recognized when a serial sequential tissue processing technique as opposed to random sampling is employed.

DETECTION AND DIAGNOSIS

The importance of quality mammography cannot be overemphasized. Currently, most patients with DCIS (more than 90%) present with a nonpalpable lesion detected by mammography. The most common mammographic finding is microcalcification, frequently clustered and generally without an associated soft-tissue abnormality. More than 80% of DCIS patients exhibit microcalcifications on preoperative mammography. The patterns of these microcalcifications may be focal, diffuse, or ductal, with variable size and shape. Patients with comedo DCIS tend to have "casting calcifications." These are linear, branching, and bizarre and are almost pathognomonic for comedo DCIS (Fig. 34.3) (66). It is important to note that many DCIS with prominent comedo necrosis fail to exhibit mammographic microcalcifications, and among others, microcalcification is seen only intermittently. Almost one-third of non-comedo lesions in this series did not have mammographic calcifications, making them more difficult to find and the patients more difficult to follow when treated with breast conserving surgery. When non-comedo lesions are calcified, they tend to have fine granular powdery calcifications or crushed stone-like calcifications (Fig. 34.4).

A major problem confronting surgeons relates to the fact that calcifications do not always delineate the entire DCIS lesion, particularly those of the non-comedo type. Even though all the calcifications are removed, in some cases, noncalcified DCIS may be left behind. Conversely, in some patients, most of the calcifications are benign and map out a lesion bigger than the true DCIS lesion. In other words, the DCIS lesion may be smaller, larger, or the same size as the calcifications that lead to its identification. Calcifications more accurately approximate

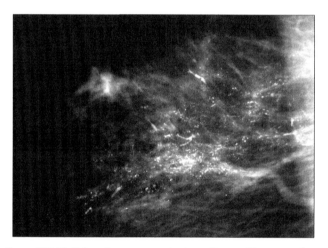

Figure 34.3 Mediolateral mammography in a 43-year-old woman shows irregular branching calcifications. Histopathology showed high-grade comedo DCIS, Van Nuys group 3.

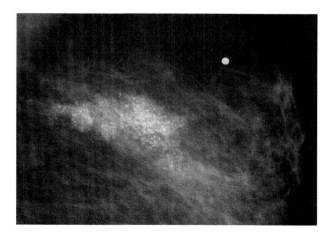

Figure 34.4 Crushed stone-type calcifications.

the size of high-grade comedo lesions than low-grade non-comedo lesions (63). Before mammography was common or of good quality, most DCIS was usually clinically apparent, diagnosed by palpation or inspection; it was gross disease. Gump and colleagues divided DCIS by method of diagnosis into gross and microscopic disease (59). Similarly, Schwartz and colleagues divided DCIS into two groups: clinical and sub-clinical (33). Both researchers thought patients presenting with a palpable mass, a nipple discharge, or Paget's disease of the nipple required more aggressive treatment. Schwartz believed that palpable DCIS should be treated as though it were an invasive lesion. He suggested that the pathologist simply had not found the area of invasion. Although it is reasonable to believe that change from nonpalpable to palpable disease is a poor prognostic sign, our group has not been able to demonstrate this for DCIS. In our series, when equivalent patients (by size and nuclear grade) with palpable and non-palpable DCIS were compared, rates of local recurrence or mortality were comparable for the two groups. If a patient's mammogram shows an abnormality, it will most likely be microcalcifications, but it could be a nonpalpable mass or an architectural distortion. At this point, additional radiological workup needs to be performed. This generally includes compression mammography and magnification views. Ultrasonography should be performed on all calcifications that require biopsy to rule out the presence of a mass that can be biopsied with ultrasound guidance. Magnetic resonance imaging (MRI) has become increasingly popular and if often used to map out the size and shape of biopsy-proven DCIS lesions or invasive breast cancers and to rule out other foci of multifocal, multi-centric or contralateral cancer.

Biopsy and Tissue Handling

If radiological workup shows an occult lesion that requires biopsy, there are multiple approaches: fine-needle aspiration biopsy (FNAB), core biopsy (with various types and sizes of needles), and directed surgical biopsy using guide wires or radioactive localization. FNAB is generally of little help for nonpalpable DCIS. With FNAB, it is possible to obtain cancer cells, but because there is minimal tissue, there is no architecture and in particular absent stroma. Thus a cytopathologist can declare that malignant cells are present but cannot determine whether or not the lesion is invasive.

Stereotactic core biopsy became available in the early 1990s, and is now widely used. Dedicated digital tables promote accurate targeting and currently large gauge vacuum-assisted needles are the tools of choice for diagnosing DCIS. Ultrasound-guided biopsy also became popular during this period but is of less value for DCIS since most lesions do not present with a mass that can be visualized on ultrasound. Nonetheless, suspicious microcalcifications should be evaluated by ultrasound since a mass will be found in 5–15% of cases (9). Open surgical biopsy should only be used if the lesion cannot be biopsied using minimally invasive techniques. This should be a rare event with current image-guided biopsy techniques and occurs in less than 5% of cases (9,67). Currently, at Hoag Memorial Hospital Presbyterian, open biopsy is performed for diagnostic purposes in only 1% of patients (more than 700 new breast cancer patients per year). Needle localization segmental resection should be a critical part of the treatment regimen, not the diagnosis (67).

Whenever a needle localization excision is performed whether for diagnosis or treatment, intraoperative specimen radiography and its correlation with the preoperative mammogram are mandatory. Margins should be inked or dyed and specimens serially sectioned with a second x-ray of the slices. The tissue sections should then be arranged and processed in sequence. Pathological reporting should include (i) a description of all architectural subtypes, (ii) a determination of nuclear grade, (iii) an assessment of the presence or absence of necrosis, (iv) the measured extent of the lesion, and (v) the margin status with measurement of all margins (especially the closest margin) (68–70). Tumor size should be determined by direct measurement or ocular micrometry from stained slides for smaller lesions. For larger lesions, a combination of direct measurement and estimation, based on the distribution of the lesion in a sequential series of slides is appropriate. The proximity of DCIS to an inked margin should be determined by direct measurement or ocular micrometry. The closest single distance between any involved duct containing DCIS and an inked margin should be reported.

If the lesion is large and the diagnosis unproven, either stereotactic or ultrasound-guided vacuum-assisted biopsy should be the first step. If the patient is motivated for breast conservation, a multiple-wire-directed oncoplastic excision can be planned. This will give the patient her best chance at two opposing goals: clear margins and good cosmesis. The best chance of successfully removing a large lesion is with a generous initial excision. Conversely, the best chance of good cosmesis is with a small initial excision. It is the surgeon's task to optimize these opposing goals. A large quadrant resection should not be performed unless there is histological proof of malignancy as this type of resection may lead to breast deformity. Should the diagnosis prove to be benign, the patient will have undergone needless and disfiguring surgery. Removal of nonpalpable lesions is best performed by an integrated team consisting of surgeon, radiologist, and pathologist. The radiologist who places the wires and interprets the specimen radiograph must be experienced, as must the surgeon who removes the lesion, and the pathologist who processes the tissue.

TREATMENT

For most patients with DCIS, there will be no single correct treatment and the patient can be offered a choice. However, these choices, although seemingly simple, are potentially complex. As the number of treatment options increase and become more complicated, frustration increases for both the patient and her physician (71,72).

Counseling the Patient with Biopsy-Proven DCIS

It is never easy to tell a patient that she has breast cancer. But is DCIS really cancer? From a biological point of view, DCIS is unequivocally cancer. But when we think of cancer, we generally think of a disease that, if untreated, runs an inexorable course toward death. That is certainly not the case with DCIS (54). We must emphasize to the patient that she has an incomplete cancerous lesion, a preinvasive lesion, which at this time is not a threat to her life. In our series of 1565 patients with DCIS, the breast cancer–specific mortality rate is 0.5% at 12 years. Numerous other DCIS series confirm an extremely low mortality rate (73–78).

Patients often ask why there is a finite mortality rate if DCIS is truly a noninvasive lesion. If DCIS recurs as an invasive lesion and the patient goes on to die from metastatic breast cancer, the source of the metastases is clear, the invasive disease. But what about the patient who undergoes mastectomy whereby only DCIS is found and sometime later develops metastatic disease, or a patient who is treated with breast preservation who never develops a local invasive recurrence but still dies of metastatic breast cancer? These latter patients probably had an invasive focus with established micrometastases at the time of their original treatment but the invasive focus was missed during routine histopathological evaluation. Routine examination of mastectomy material is inadequate for patients with DCIS and a more thorough and methodical approach utilizing specimen radiography is required. No matter how carefully and thoroughly a specimen in examined, it is still a sampling process and a small focus of invasion can be missed. One of the most frequent concerns expressed by patients once a diagnosis of cancer has been made is the fear that the cancer has spread. Patients with DCIS can be reassured that no invasion was seen microscopically and the likelihood of systemic spread is minimal.

The patient needs to be educated that the term "breast cancer" encompasses a wide range of lesions of varying degrees of aggressiveness and lethal potential. The patient with DCIS needs to be informed that she has a minimal lesion for which treatment options may include surgery, radiation therapy, an antiestrogen, or some combination of those modalities. She needs reassurance that chemotherapy is unnecessary, that her hair will not fall out and that it is highly unlikely that she will die from this lesion. Careful clinical follow-up will of course be essential.

Endpoints for Patients with DCIS

When evaluating results of treatment for patients with breast cancer, a variety of endpoints must be considered. Important endpoints include local recurrence (both invasive and DCIS), regional recurrence (namely the axilla), distant recurrence, breast cancer survival, overall survival, and quality of life. The importance of each endpoint varies depending on whether the patient has DCIS or invasive breast cancer. When treating invasive cancer, the most important endpoints are distant recurrence and breast cancer–specific survival; in other words, living or dying from breast cancer. For invasive breast cancer, a variety of systemic treatments have been shown to significantly improve survival. These include a wide range of chemotherapeutic regimens, endocrine treatments, biologic/immunological therapies, and others. Variations in the extent of local treatment were previously considered not to affect survival (23,79) but it is now recognized that this does affect local recurrence and local invasive recurrence influences survival. Meta-analyses have shown that for every four local recurrences avoided, one breast cancer death is prevented (80,81).

DCIS is similar to invasive breast cancer in respect of how local treatment determines local recurrence, but no study to date has shown a significant difference in distant disease-free or breast cancer-specific survival, regardless of any treatment (systemic or local). Moreover, no study is likely to show a difference since there are so few breast cancer deaths in patients with pure DCIS. The most important outcome measure, breast cancer-specific survival, is essentially the same whatever local or systemic treatment is given. Consequently, local recurrence has become the most commonly used endpoint when evaluating treatment for patients with DCIS.

A meta-analysis of four randomized DCIS trials involving a total of 3665 patients was published in 2007 comparing excision plus radiation therapy versus excision alone (77). Radiation therapy decreased local recurrence by 60% (statistically significant) but overall survival was insignificantly worse in the radiotherapy group with a relative risk of 1.08. These data contrast with those of the Early Breast Cancer Trialists' Collaborative Group and deserve further analysis (80,81). Half of the recurrences in the meta-analysis were DCIS and therefore would not affect survival. Of the remaining invasive recurrences, 80–90% would be cured by early detection and treatment. This should yield a trend toward a lower survival for the excision-alone group just as would be expected from the Early Breast Cancer Trialists' Collaborative Group. However, a nonsignificant trend toward a better survival in the excision-only patients was observed. The authors of the meta-analysis considered that with a longer follow-up, the higher local recurrence rate for excision alone will likely result in a lower overall survival at some point in time. Nevertheless, this has not occurred hitherto and a small detrimental effect secondary to radiation therapy must be considered a possibility. Local recurrences are psychologically demoralizing and must clearly be prevented in patients treated with DCIS. They often lead to mastectomy and when invasive, upstage the patient and constitute a threat to life. But protecting DCIS patients from local recurrence must be balanced against potential detrimental effects of treatments.

Following treatment for DCIS, almost half (40–50%) of local recurrences are invasive. Furthermore, approximately 10–20% of DCIS patients with invasive local recurrence develop distant metastases and die from breast cancer (82,83). In the long term, this could translate into a mortality rate of about 0.5 % for patients treated with mastectomy, 1–2% for breast conservation patients who receive radiation therapy (assuming no mortality from radiation therapy), and 2–3% for patients treated with excision alone. In order to preserve their breasts, many women are prepared to accept this theoretical, and as of now statistically unproven, small increase in absolute risk associated with breast conservation therapy.

Treatment Options
Mastectomy
Mastectomy is the most effective treatment available for DCIS if the main goal is simply to prevent local recurrence. Most series reveal local recurrence rates of approximately 1% with mortality rates close to zero for patients treated with mastectomy (84). In our mastectomy series of 533 patients, none of whom received radiation therapy or tamoxifen, there have been 10 local recurrences (eight invasive and two DCIS). One of the patients with an invasive local recurrence developed metastatic disease. In addition, two other patients developed metastatic breast cancer without developing a local recurrence yielding an absolute rate of distant recurrence of 0.6%. However, mastectomy is an aggressive form of treatment for patients with DCIS. It clearly provides benefit in terms of a local recurrence but only a theoretical gain in survival. Therefore, it is often difficult to justify mastectomy, particularly for otherwise healthy

women with screen-detected DCIS, during an era of increasing utilization of breast conservation for invasive breast carcinoma. Mastectomy is indicated in cases of true multicentricity (multiquadrant disease) and when a unicentric DCIS lesion is too large to excise with clear margins and an acceptable cosmetic result. Genetic positivity for one of the breast cancer–associated genes (BRCA1 and BRCA2) is not an absolute contraindication to breast preservation but many patients with genetic predisposition who develop DCIS will carefully consider bilateral mastectomy and salpingo-oophorectomy.

Breast Conservation
The most recently available Surveillance Epidemiology and End Results (SEER) data reveal that 74% of patients with DCIS are treated with breast conservation. While breast conservation is now widely accepted as the treatment of choice for DCIS, not all patients are suitable candidates. There are patients with DCIS whose local recurrence rate with breast preservation is so high (based on factors that will be discussed later in this chapter) that mastectomy is clearly the appropriate treatment. However, the majority of women diagnosed nowadays with DCIS are candidates for breast conservation. Clinical trials have shown that local excision and radiation therapy in patients with negative margins can provide excellent rates of local control (73,76–78,85–88). However, even radiation therapy may be overly aggressive since many cases of DCIS may not recur or progress to invasive carcinoma when treated by excision alone (32,54,89–93).

REASONS TO CONSIDER EXCISION ALONE
There are a number of lines of reasoning suggesting that excision alone may be an acceptable treatment for selected patients with DCIS.

1. Common Usage: Excision alone is common practice in spite of randomized data suggesting that all conservatively treated patients benefit from radiation therapy. SEER data indicate that excision alone is being used as complete treatment for DCIS in 35% of DCIS cases. American doctors and patients have embraced the concept of excision alone for DCIS.

2. Anatomic: Evaluation of mastectomy specimens using the serial subgross tissue processing technique reveals that most of the DCIS is unicentric (involves a single breast segment and is radial in its distribution (39,43,63,64,94,95). Using the same technique and evaluating patients with small extent disease (≤25 mm) more clearly established that the majority of image-detected DCIS can be adequately excised (32,38). This means that in many cases, it is possible to excise the entire lesion with a segment or quadrant resection. Since DCIS, by definition, is not invasive and has not metastasized, it can be thought of in Halstedian terms. Complete excision should cure the patient without any additional therapy. Holland and Faverly have shown that if 10 mm margins are achieved in all directions, the likelihood of residual DCIS is less than 10% (43).

3. Biologic: Some DCIS is simply not aggressive, for example small well-excised low-grade lesions bordering

on atypical ductal hyperplasia. Such lesions carry a low potential for development of invasion (about 1% per year at the most) (53,54,57,89,96,97). This is only slightly higher than for lobular carcinoma *in situ*, a lesion that is routinely treated with careful clinical follow-up.

4. Pathology Errors: The differences between atypical ductal hyperplasia and low-grade DCIS may be subtle. It is not uncommon for atypical ductal hyperplasia to be called DCIS. Such patients treated with excision and radiation therapy are indeed "cured of their DCIS."

5. Prospective Randomized Data: The prospective randomized DCIS trials show no difference in breast cancer–specific survival or overall survival, regardless of treatment after excision with or without breast irradiation (73,76–78,88). If this is true, why not strive for the least aggressive treatment?

6. Radiotherapy may do harm: Numerous studies have shown that radiation therapy for breast cancer may increase mortality from both lung cancer and cardiovascular disease (98–102). Current radiotherapy techniques, which make use of CT planning, make every attempt to spare the heart and lungs from radiation exposure but long-term date are not available. If there is no proof that breast irradiation for patients with DCIS improves survival and there is proof that radiation therapy may cause harm, it makes perfect sense to spare patients from this potentially dangerous treatment whenever possible.

7. Radiation therapy is expensive, time consuming, and is accompanied by significant side effects in a small percentage of patients (cardiac, pulmonary, etc.) (103). Radiation fibrosis continues to occur but it is less common with current techniques than it was during the 1980s. Radiation fibrosis changes the texture of the breast and skin, makes mammographic follow-up more difficult, and may result in delayed diagnosis if there is a local recurrence. This will become much less of a problem if intraoperative radiation therapy becomes an established modality for DCIS (104).

8. Some series show that there are more invasive recurrences among irradiated patients than in non-irradiated patients. In our own series, 39% of excision-only patients who recurred had invasive disease, whereas 56% of irradiated patients who recurred had invasive disease (p < 0.01). This was also found in the series of Schwartz et al. (92) and Wong et al. (105). In our series, the median time to recurrence after excision alone was 23 months compared with 58 months (p < 0.01) after excision and irradiation. This delay in diagnosis may contribute to the increased rate of invasive local recurrence among irradiated patients.

9. If radiation therapy is given for initial treatment of DCIS, it cannot be subsequently used for treatment of a small invasive recurrence. In general, in favorable patients, we prefer to withhold radiation therapy at the outset and only give it to the few that ultimately recur with invasive disease. The use of radiation therapy with its accompanying skin and vascular changes can make skin-sparing mastectomy more difficult to perform at a future date.

10. Using commonly available histopathological parameters, we can usurp the gold standard for local recurrence established by the prospective randomized trials. The "gold standard" for irradiated patients is a 16% local recurrence rate at 12 years. This was established by the National Surgical Adjuvant Breast Project (NSABP) B-17 trial (73,85–87,106). Using tools such as the USC/ VNPI, it is possible to select patients with low scores ranging from 4 to 6. These patients recur at a rate of 6% or less at 12 years without radiation therapy.

11. Finally, within the 2008 National Comprehensive Cancer Network (NCCN) Guidelines, excision without radiation therapy (excision alone) has been added as an acceptable treatment for selected DCIS patients with low risk of recurrence (107). Excision alone is now accepted and mainstream for favorable patients with DCIS.

DISTANT DISEASE AND DEATH

For a patient with DCIS, previously treated by any modality, there is a stepwise progression with development of local invasive recurrence followed by distant disease and death from breast cancer. The patient has been upstaged by development of local invasive recurrence which becomes a source of distant metastatic disease and death is now a possibility. In contrast, when a previously treated patient with DCIS develops distant disease and there has been no invasive local recurrence, a completely different sequence of events must be postulated. This sequence implies that invasive disease was present within the original lesion but was never discovered and was already metastatic at the time of the original diagnosis. The best way to avoid missing an invasive cancer is with complete sequential tissue processing at the time the original lesion is treated. Nevertheless, even the most extensive evaluation may miss a small focus of invasion. Even when a minute invasive component is found during histopathological evaluation, a woman can no longer be classified as having DCIS. She has invasive breast cancer and needs appropriate treatment for this which will involve sentinel node biopsy, radiation therapy if treated conservatively, appropriate medical oncological consultation, and aftercare.

THE PROSPECTIVE RANDOMIZED TRIALS

Prospective randomized trials have all shown a significant reduction in local recurrence for patients treated with radiation therapy compared with excision alone but no trial has reported a survival benefit, regardless of treatment (73,76,77,85–88,106,108–111). Only one trial has compared mastectomy with breast conservation for patients with DCIS and the data were incidentally accrued. NSABP performed Protocol B-06, a prospective randomized trial for patients with invasive breast cancer (61,112). There were three treatment arms: total mastectomy, excision of the tumor plus radiation therapy, and excision alone. Axillary nodes were removed regardless of treatment assignment. During central slide review, a subgroup of 78 patients was confirmed to have pure

DCIS without any evidence of invasion (61). After 83 months of follow-up, the rates of percentage of patients with local recurrences were as follows: 0% for mastectomy, 7% for excision plus radiation therapy, and 43% for excision alone (113). In spite of these large differences in rates of local recurrence for each different treatment, there were no differences among the three treatment groups in breast cancer–specific survival.

In contrast to the lack of trials comparing mastectomy with breast conservation, a number of prospective randomized trials have compared excision plus radiation therapy with excision alone for patients with DCIS: the NSABP (protocol B-17) (85), the European Organization for Research and Treatment of Cancer (EORTC), protocol 10853 (88), the United Kingdom, Australia, New Zealand DCIS trial (UK/ANZ DCIS trial) (76), and the Swedish trial (78).

The results of NSABP B-17 were updated in 1995 (109), 1998 (87), 1999 (86), 2001 (73), and 2011 (106). More than 800 patients with DCIS excised with clear surgical margins were randomized into two groups: excision alone versus excision plus radiation therapy. The main endpoint of the study was local recurrence [invasive or noninvasive (DCIS)] and the definition of a clear surgical margin was non-transection of DCIS. After 15 years of follow-up, there was a statistically significant decrease of 50% in rates of local recurrence for both DCIS and invasive breast cancer in patients treated with radiation therapy. The overall local recurrence rate for patients treated by excision alone or excision plus breast irradiation was 35% and 19.8% at 15 years respectively representing a relative benefit of 43% (106). There was no difference in distant disease-free or overall survival between these two arms. These data led the NSABP to confirm their 1993 position and to continue to recommend postoperative radiation therapy for all patients with DCIS who chose breast conservation surgery. This recommendation was based primarily on decreased rates of local recurrence for those treated with radiation therapy and secondarily on the potential survival advantage it might confer.

These early results of B-17, which favored radiation therapy for patients with DCIS, prompted the NSABP to perform protocol B-24 (86). In this trial, more than 1800 patients with DCIS were treated with excision and radiation therapy, and then randomized to receive either tamoxifen or placebo. After 15 years of follow-up, 16.6% of patients treated with placebo had recurred locally compared with 13.2% of those treated with tamoxifen (106). This difference though modest was statistically significant for invasive but not for noninvasive (DCIS) local recurrence. Data presented at the 2002 San Antonio Breast Cancer Symposium suggested that the ipsilateral benefit was seen only in estrogen receptor-positive patients (114). Again, there was no difference in distant disease-free or overall survival in either arm of the B-24 trial.

The EORTC study involved more than 1000 patients and was essentially identical to B-17 in design and margin definition. Results were published in 2000 (88,108) and updated in 2006 (110). After 10 years of follow-up, 15% of patients treated with excision plus radiation therapy had recurred locally compared with 26% of patients treated with excision alone. These results were similar to those obtained by the NSABP at the same point in their trial. As in the B-17 trial, there was no difference in distant disease-free or overall survival in either arm of the EORTC trial. In the initial report, there was a statistically

significant increase in contralateral breast cancer in patients who were randomized to receive radiation therapy. This was not maintained when the data were updated.

The UK/ANZ DCIS trial was published in 2003 (76) and updated in 2011 (111). This trial, which involved more than 1694 patients, was a two by two design in which patients could be randomized into two separate trials within a trial. The patients and their doctors chose whether to be randomized in one or both studies. After excision with clear margins (same non-transection definition as the NSABP), patients were randomized to receive radiotherapy (yes or no) and/or to tamoxifen versus placebo. This yielded four subgroups: excision alone, excision plus radiation therapy, excision plus tamoxifen, and excision plus radiation therapy plus tamoxifen. After a median follow-up of 12.7 years, those who received radiation therapy had a statistically significant decrease in ipsilateral breast tumor recurrence similar in magnitude to that observed in the NSABP and EORTC trials. However, in contrast to the B-24 study, tamoxifen significantly reduced the incidence of ipsilateral DCIS but not invasive recurrences. The incidence of new contralateral breast cancers was reduced by a magnitude similar to that of NSABP B-24. As with the NSABP and the EORTC, there were no differences in survival between any of the treatment arms in the UK DCIS trial.

The Swedish DCIS trial randomized 1067 patients into two groups: excision alone therapy versus excision plus radiation therapy. To date 1046 patients have been followed for a mean of eight years. Microscopically clear margins were not mandatory in this trial and 22% of patients had unknown or involved margins. The cumulative incidence of local recurrence at 10 years was 21.6% for excision only and 10.3% for excision plus radiation therapy. There were 15 distant metastases and breast cancer–related deaths in the excision-only arm and 18 in the excision plus radiation therapy (p = ns) (78,115).

All of these trials support the same conclusions and show that radiation therapy decreases the relative risk of local recurrence by 50% but there are no differences in survival irrespective of treatment. Two trials have shown a decrease in local recurrence and contralateral breast cancer attributable to tamoxifen.

In 2007, Viani et al. published a meta-analysis of the four prospective randomized DCIS trials comparing excision alone with excision plus radiation therapy (77). A total of 3665 patients were available for analysis and pooled data revealed a 60% reduction for both invasive and DCIS local recurrence (p < 0.00001) with the addition of radiation therapy. There was, however, no decrease in distant metastases among those who received radiation therapy nor was there any survival benefit. Patients with high-grade lesions and involved margins received proportionately greater benefit from radiation therapy.

LIMITATIONS OF THE PROSPECTIVE RANDOMIZED TRIALS

The randomized trials were designed to answer one broad question: does radiation therapy decrease local recurrence? They have accomplished that goal and have clearly shown that radiation therapy decreases rates of local recurrence overall. However, these trials cannot identify in which subgroups the benefits of adjuvant therapies are so small that patients can be safely treated with excision alone. Many of the parameters considered important in predicting local recurrence (tumor size, margin width, nuclear grade, etc.) were not prospectively collected on a routine basis during these randomized DCIS trials. Moreover, the trials did not specifically mandate marking of margins or measurement of margin width. Exact measurements of margin width occurred in only 5% of the EORTC pathology reports (108). The NSABP protocol did not require size measurements and many of their pathological data were determined by retrospective slide review. Indeed, in the initial NSABP report, more than 40% of patients had no size measurement (85). Unfortunately, if margins were not inked and tissues not completely sampled and sequentially submitted, then predictive data for recurrence can never be determined accurately by retrospective review.

The relative reduction in local recurrence rates seems to be similar for the four trials—about 50–60% for any given subgroup at any point in time. What does this relative reduction mean? If the absolute local recurrence rate is 30% at 10 years for a particular subgroup of patients treated with excision alone, radiation therapy will reduce this rate by approximately 50%. This leaves a group of patients with a 15% local recurrence rate at 10 years and radiation therapy would appear indicated for such a high local recurrence rate. But consider a more favorable subgroup, a group of patients with a 6–8% absolute recurrence rate at 10 years. These patients receive only a 3–4% absolute benefit. We must irradiate 100 women to see a 3–4% decrease in local recurrence. In these circumstances, it must be asked whether the benefits of radiotherapy outweigh the risks and costs involved.

Radiation therapy is expensive, time consuming, and accompanied by significant side effects in a small percentage of patients (cardiac, pulmonary, etc.) (103). Radiation fibrosis continues to occur but it is less common with current techniques than it was in the past. Radiation fibrosis changes the texture of the breast and skin, makes mammographic follow-up more difficult, and may result in a delayed diagnosis when there is local recurrence. The use of radiation therapy for DCIS precludes this modality as a treatment option if an invasive recurrence develops at a later date. The use of radiation therapy with its accompanying skin and vascular changes renders skin-sparing mastectomy more difficult to perform at a future date. Most importantly, when radiation therapy is given for DCIS, we must assume all of these risks and costs without any proven benefits in terms of distant disease-free or breast cancer–specific survival. Nonetheless, there will be a decrease in local recurrence. It is therefore important to carefully assess the need for radiation therapy in all conservatively treated patients with DCIS. The NSABP has conceded that not all patients with DCIS may need post-excisional radiation therapy (73). The problem is how to accurately identify those patients; those subgroups of patients with DCIS in which the probability of local recurrence after excision alone is low, may be the patients for whom the costs, risks, and side effects of radiotherapy outweigh any overall benefits.

In spite of randomized data suggesting that all conservatively treated patients benefit from radiation therapy, both doctors and patients in the United States have embraced the concept of excision alone. SEER 2003 data reveal that 74% of patients with DCIS were treated with breast conservation. Almost half of these conservatively treated patients were treated with excision alone. When all patients with DCIS are considered, 26% received mastectomy, 39% excision plus radiation therapy, and 35% were treated with excision alone. It is clear that neither American doctors nor patients are blindly following results and recommendations from prospective trials. In 2008, based on data and treatment trends, the NCCN added excision alone as an alternative treatment for patients with favorable DCIS and has upheld this recommendation in annual updates (107).

A prerequisite for calculation of the USC/VNPI is a reproducible method of determining the size or extent of DCIS in any surgical resection and evaluating margin width. Furthermore, since any focus of invasion would change the classification, great care must be taken to exclude microinvasion during examination of resected tissue. Earlier studies (13,32,38) and the Van Nuys database from its inception have employed a serial subgross sequential method of tissue examination. Briefly, this requires that an oriented, selectively inked resection is sliced into uniformly thick segments and repeat specimen radiography is employed to evaluate these segments. These are then processed in sequence in specifically identified cassettes to permit a three-dimensional reconstruction of the extent of disease and to thoroughly evaluate any margin involvement. Although this approach for DCIS is now the recommended protocol for the College of American Pathologists (68,116) this was not the case in the late 1970s and throughout most of the 1990s. There was a great reluctance to expend pathology resources and professional time on an approach that was not considered to have clinical utility, but rather constitute a cost drain.

Defining a process as DCIS alone (without invasion) and accurately calculating the size and margin width of the lesion is only possible for a resection specimen that is entirely processed. The inability of the randomized trials to replicate the USC/VNPI is a reflection of the predominant pathological technique employed, namely partial sampling. The latter approach is satisfactory for larger invasive carcinomas, but cannot determine the size or margin width for a microscopic grossly invisible lesion which often exhibits an intermittent distribution within the resection specimen and demonstrates only focal microcalcification. The randomized trials of DCIS were not empowered to define prognostic factors which are widely recognized as pertinent for DCIS. Additionally, the USC/VNPI is based on careful mammographic or other radiological correlation with pathology, an approach which was rare in the prospective trial protocols (73,76,77,85–88,106,108–111). Many retrospective attempts to evaluate the USC/VNPI and also some prospective studies (105) fail because of their inability to precisely define prognostic factors; that is, there is lack of an adequate pathological approach. In fact, current practice standards for mammographically detected and excised DCIS were not attained by any of the randomized trials.

PREDICTING LOCAL RECURRENCE IN CONSERVATIVELY TREATED PATIENTS WITH DCIS
Information is now readily available that can aid clinicians in differentiating patients who significantly benefit from radiation therapy after excision from those who do not. These same data can also indicate patients who are better served by mastectomy due to unacceptably high recurrence rates with breast conservation even with the addition of radiation therapy. Research by us (32,36,38,40,97,117,118) and others (35,44,90,91,109,119) has shown that various combinations of

nuclear grade, the presence of comedo-type necrosis, tumor size, margin width, and age are all important factors that can be used to predict the probability of local recurrence in conservatively treated patients with DCIS.

The Original VNPI and its Updated Version, the USC/VNPI

In 1995, the Van Nuys DCIS pathological classification, based on nuclear grade and the presence or absence of comedo necrosis, was developed (Fig. 34.1) (40). Nuclear grade and comedo-type necrosis reflect the biology of the lesion, but neither alone nor together are they adequate as guidelines in the treatment decision-making process. Tumor size and margin width reflect the extent of disease, the adequacy of surgical treatment, and the likelihood of residual disease, and are therefore of paramount importance. The challenge was to devise a system using these variables (each an independent factor on multivariate analysis) that would be clinically valid, therapeutically useful and user friendly. The original VNPI (37,120) was devised in 1996 by combining these factors: tumor size, margin width, and pathological classification (determined by nuclear grade and the presence or absence of comedo-type necrosis). Each of these factors had been collected prospectively in a large series of DCIS patients who were selectively treated (nonrandomized) (121). A score, ranging from 1 for lesions with the best prognosis to 3 for lesions with the worst prognosis, was given for each of the three prognostic predictors. The objective with all three predictors was to create three statistically different subgroups for each, using local recurrence as the marker of treatment failure. Cut-off points (e.g., what size or margin width constitutes low, intermediate, or high risk of local recurrence) were determined statistically, using the log rank test with an optimum p-value approach.

Size Score

A score of 1 was given for small tumors (≤15 mm), 2 for intermediate sized tumors (16–40 mm), and 3 for large tumors (≥41 mm in diameter). The determination of size required complete and sequential tissue processing along with mammographic/pathological correlation. Size was determined over a series of sections rather than being based on a single section and was the most difficult parameter to reproduce. If a 3 cm specimen is cut into 10 blocks, each block is estimated to be 3 mm thick. If a lesion measuring 5 mm in maximum diameter on a single slide appears in and out of 7 sequential blocks, it is estimated to be 21 mm (3 mm × 7) in maximum size, not 5 mm, as measured on a single slide. The maximum diameter on a single slide was the method for size estimation for most patients in the afore-mentioned prospective randomized trials.

Margin Score

A score of 1 was given for widely clear tumor-free margins of 10 mm or more. This was often achieved by re-excision when either no residual DCIS or only focal residual DCIS was found on the wall of the biopsy cavity. A score of 2 was given for intermediate margins of 1–9 mm and a score of 3 for margins less than 1 mm (involved or close margins).

Pathological Classification Score

A score of 3 was given for tumors classified as group 3 (high-grade lesions), 2 for tumors classified as group 2

(non-high-grade lesions with comedo-type necrosis), and a score of 1 for tumors classified as group 1 (non-high-grade lesion without comedo-type necrosis) (40,122). This classification system is shown diagrammatically in Figure 34.1.

The final formula for the original VNPI is as follows:

$$VNPI = pathological\ classification\ score + margin\ score + size\ score$$

The University of Southern California/Van Nuys Prognostic Index

By early 2001, a multivariate analysis at the University of Southern California revealed that age was also an independent prognostic factor and that it should be added with a weight equal to that of other factors already included in the VNPI (117,123,124). An analysis of local recurrence data from the authors' institution by age revealed that the most appropriate break points were between ages 39 and 40 and between ages 60 and 61 (Fig. 34.5). Based on these findings, a score of 3 was given to all patients 39 years old or younger, a score of 2 was given to patients aged 40–60, and a score of 1 was given to patients aged 61 years or more. The new scoring system for the USC/VNPI is shown in Table 34.1. The final formula for the USC/VNPI is derived as follows:

$$2\,USC/VNPI = pathological\ classification\ score + margin\ score + size\ score + age\ score$$

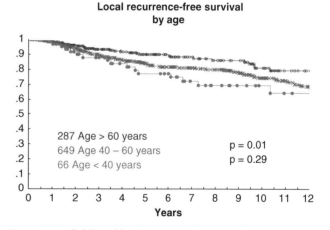

Local recurrence-free survival by age

287 Age > 60 years
649 Age 40 – 60 years
66 Age < 40 years

p = 0.01
p = 0.29

Figure 34.5 Probability of local recurrence-free survival by age group for 1032 breast conservation patients.

Table 34.1 The USC/VNPI Scoring System

	Score		
	1	2	3
Size (mm)	≤15	16–40	≥41
Margins (mm)	≥10	1–9	<1
Pathological classification	Non-high grade without necrosis	Non-high grade with necrosis	High grade with or without necrosis
Age (years)	≥61	40–60	≤39

One to three points are awarded for each of four different predictors of local breast recurrence (size, margins, pathological classification, and age). Scores for each of the predictors are totaled to yield a VNPI score ranging from a low of 4 to a high of 12.

Abbreviations: USC, University of Southern California; VNPI, Van Nuys Prognostic Index.

Scores range from 4 to 12 with this modified index. Patients least likely to recur after conservative therapy had a score of 4 or 5 (small, low grade, well-excised lesions in older women), whereas those patients most likely to recur had a score of 11 or 12 (large, poorly excised, high-grade lesions in younger women). The probability of recurrence increased as the USC/VNPI score increased.

Updated Results Using the USC/VNPI

Through September 2011, our group treated 1565 patients with pure DCIS. Patients treated with mastectomy (n = 533) were not included in the analyses that use local recurrence as the endpoint since the number of events were too few in this subgroup. However, mastectomy patients have a separate recurrence analysis by USC/VNPI (see the section "Using the USC/VNPI in Mastectomy Patients"). A total of 932 patients were treated with breast conservation (563 by excision alone and 369 by excision plus radiation therapy) and the average follow-up for all patients was 85 months (82 months for mastectomy, 109 months for excision plus radiation therapy, and 74 months for excision alone). There were 196 local failures, 92 of which were invasive (40%). The probability of local failure was reduced by 60% with radiation therapy which is almost identical to the findings in the prospective randomized trials. Local recurrence-free survival according to treatment is shown in Figure 34.6 and the probability of breast cancer specific and overall survival by treatment in Figures 34.7 and 34.8 respectively. Predictably, mastectomy had the lowest and excision alone the highest probability of local recurrence at any point in time. Two patients with palpable HER2-positive high-grade DCIS measuring ≥6 cm developed distant metastasis without developing local recurrence ever. Both patients were under 50 years of age and were treated with mastectomy and immediate reconstruction. These two patients had USC/VNPI and had scores of 11 and 12. Mastectomy specimens underwent extensive serial sectioning and were sequentially embedded but no frank invasion or microinvasion could be found. Seven patients treated with radiation therapy developed local recurrence (six in the same quadrant and one in a different quadrant) followed by development of distant metastases. Six of these patients have subsequently died from breast cancer. By contrast, three patients treated with excision alone developed local invasive recurrence followed by metastatic disease, one of whom died from breast cancer. Seventy-seven additional patients have died from other causes without evidence of recurrent breast cancer yielding a 12-year actuarial overall survival (including deaths from all causes) of 90%. Overall survival is comparable among the three treatment groups and for each of the three USC/VNPI groups (Fig. 34.9). Local recurrence-free survival for these breast conservation patients is shown by tumor size in Figure 34.10, by margin width in Figure 34.11, by pathological classification in Figure 34.2 and by age in Figure 34.5. Figure 34.12 shows grouping of patients with a low (USC/VNPI = 4, 5, or 6), intermediate (USC/VNPI = 7, 8, or 9), or high (USC/VNPI = 10, 11, or 12) risk of local recurrence and demonstrates strong statistical difference between each group.

Patients with USC/VNPI scores of 4, 5, or 6 do not show a significant local recurrence-free survival benefit from breast irradiation (Fig. 34.13) (p = NS). The 12-year local recurrence rate for patients with scores of 4, 5, or 6 treated with excision alone is 6.6%. For those patients treated with excision plus radiation, this rate is 3.0%, representing a 55% relative but only a 3.6% absolute risk reduction. Patients with USC/VNPI scores of 7, 8, or 9 benefit from irradiation (Fig. 34.14). There is a statistically significant decrease in probability of local recurrence which averages 15% throughout the curves, comparing irradiated patients to those treated by excision alone (p = 0.0003) with intermediate USC/VNPI scores. Figure 34.15 shows division of patients with USC/VNPI scores of 10, 11, or 12 into those treated by excision plus irradiation or by excision alone. Although, the difference between the two groups is highly significant (p = 0.0006), conservatively treated DCIS patients with a USC/VNPI score of 10, 11, or 12 recur at an extremely high rate even with radiation therapy.

Fine Tuning the USC/VNPI

The USC/VNPI is an algorithm based on a rigid pathology protocol which permits reproducible prospective quantification of measurable prognostic factors known to be important in predicting local recurrence in patients with DCIS. When originally published in 1996 (37) the index was based on 333 patients and treatment recommendations were grouped by scores:

Excision alone: scores 4–6
Excision plus radiation therapy: scores 7–9
Mastectomy: scores 10–12

By 2010, there were more than four and a half times as many patients and nearly twice the follow-up since the index was originally developed. Therefore, sufficient numbers of patients existed for analysis by individual score (4–12), stratified by margin width, rather than by groups of scores (125). Since current *NCCN Treatment Guidelines* have been amended to include excision alone as an acceptable alternative, but without listing any selection criteria, analysis by USC/VNPI score has become increasingly valuable (107).

The current series (1565 patients with pure DCIS), was analyzed by the following parameters:

1. Individual USC/VNPI scores (4 through 12)
2. Multiple margin widths (1, 3, 5, and 10 mm)
3. Treatment (excision plus radiation therapy *vs.* excision alone)
4. Treatment needed to achieve a local recurrence probability of less than 10%, 15%, 20%, or 25% at 12 years

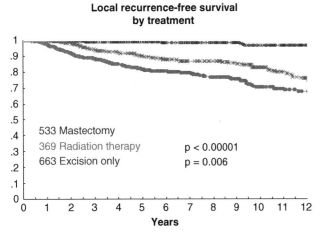

Local recurrence-free survival by treatment

533 Mastectomy
369 Radiation therapy   p < 0.00001
663 Excision only   p = 0.006

Years

Figure 34.6 Probability of local recurrence-free survival by treatment for 1565 patients with DCIS.

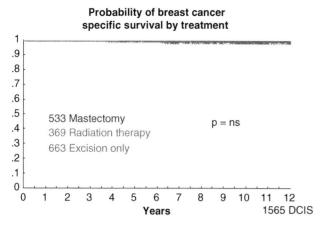

Figure 34.7 Probability of breast cancer–specific survival by treatment for 1565 patients with DCIS.

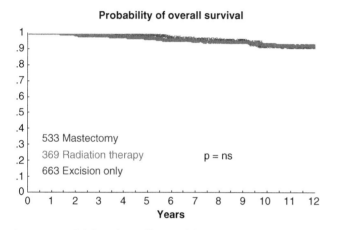

Figure 34.8 Probability of overall survival by treatment for 1565 patients with DCIS.

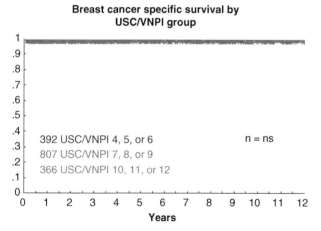

Figure 34.9 Probability of breast cancer–specific survival for 1032 breast conservation patients grouped by USC/Van Nuys Prognostic Index score (4, 5, or 6 *vs.* 7, 8, or 9 *vs.* 10, 11, or 12).

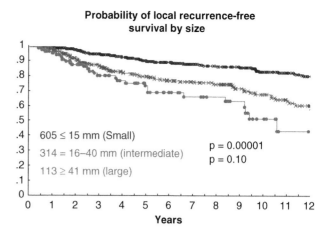

Figure 34.10 Probability of local recurrence-free survival by tumor size for 1032 breast conservation patients.

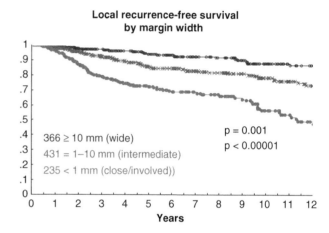

Figure 34.11 Probability of local recurrence-free survival by margin width for 1032 breast conservation patients.

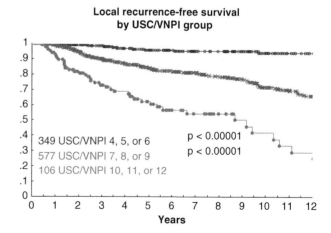

Figure 34.12 Probability of local recurrence-free survival for 1032 breast conservation patients grouped by USC/Van Nuys Prognostic Index score (4, 5, or 6 *vs.* 7, 8, or 9 *vs.* 10, 11, or 12).

Table 34.2 illustrates the treatment and margin width necessary to achieve a probability of local recurrence of 20% or less at 12 years and was derived using the Kaplan–Meier method. As the acceptable local recurrence probability is adjusted up or down, the treatment recommendations change.

To limit the chance of local recurrence to less than 25% at 12 years, these data support excision alone for patients scoring 4, 5, or 6, regardless of margin width and patients who score 7 but have a margin width ≥3 mm. Excision plus radiotherapy is appropriate for patients who score 7 and have margins <3 mm,

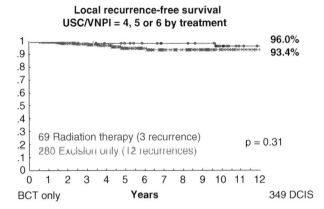

Figure 34.13 Probability of local recurrence-free survival by treatment for 349 breast conservation patients with USC/Van Nuys Prognostic Index scores of 4, 5, or 6). *Abbreviation*: BCT = breast conservation therapy.

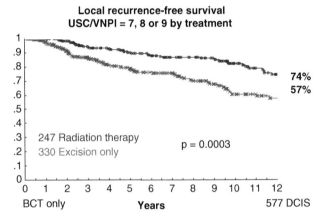

Figure 34.14 Probability of local recurrence-free survival by treatment for 577 breast conservation patients with USC/Van Nuys Prognostic Index scores of 7, 8, or 9. *Abbreviation*: BCT = breast conservation therapy.

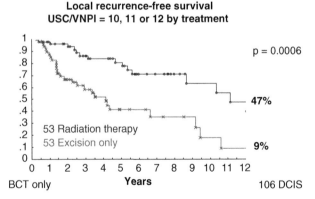

Figure 34.15 Probability of local recurrence-free survival by treatment for 106 breast conservation patients with Modified USC/Van Nuys Prognostic Index scores of 10, 11, or 12. *Abbreviation*: BCT = breast conservation therapy.

Table 34.2 Treatment and margin width necessary to achieve local recurrence of no more than 20% at 12 years

USC/VNPI Score	No. Pts 1565	Treatment Needed	12-Year Recurrence (%)
All 4, 5 or 6	392	Excision Alone	≤ 6.6
7, Margins ≥ 3 mm	176	Excision Alone	15
7, Margins < 3 mm	115	Excision + Radiation	19
8, Margins ≥ 3 mm	113	Excision + Radiation	11
8, Margins < 3 mm	174	Mastectomy	0
9, Margins ≥ 5 mm	39	Excision + Radiation	19
9, Margins < 5 mm	189	Mastectomy	0
All 10, 11 or 12	367	Mastectomy	7

Abbreviations: USC, University of Southern California; VNPI, Van Nuys Prognostic Index.

Using the USC/VNPI in Mastectomy Patients

Patients with DCIS who are treated with mastectomy seldom recur locally or develop distant metastatic disease. We explored the question of whether the USC/VNPI could predict these relatively infrequent events in mastectomy patients. There were 533 patients with pure DCIS treated with mastectomy in this series with an average follow-up of 82 months. Twelve of these patients developed recurrence: two cases of distant metastases without local recurrence, one case of distant metastasis with a preceding local recurrence, and nine local recurrences without distant metastatic disease. The majority of these recurrences were invasive (10/12) with two cases of DCIS. All 12 patients who recurred had multifocal disease, with three quarters having multicentric disease (in multiple quadrants). Using the USC/VNPI, patients scoring 4–9 are compared with those with scores of 10–12 in Table 34.3.

DCIS patients scoring 10–12 using the USC/VNPI were significantly more likely to develop recurrence after mastectomy compared with patients scoring 4–9. At particularly high risk were young patients with large high-grade tumors and close or involved mastectomy margins. These data can be used when counseling a patient who is considering post-mastectomy radiation therapy.

CURRENT TREATMENT TRENDS

In the current era of evidence-based medicine, it is reasonable to interpret prospective randomized data as support for the contention theory that all DCIS patients treated conservatively should receive post-excisional radiation therapy. However, in spite of these data, the number of patients with DCIS being treated with excision alone continues to increase. SEER data from 2003 revealed that approximately one-third of patients with DCIS in the United States are being treated with excision alone (16). As an aid to the complex treatment decision-making process, the USC/VNPI can be used as a guide to treatment options and is supported by local recurrence data. The USC/VNPI divides patients with DCIS into three groups with distinct probabilities of local recurrence after breast conserving surgery. Although there is an apparent treatment choice for each group (excision alone for patients who score 4–6, excision plus radiation therapy for patients who score 7–9, and mastectomy for those who score 10–12) the USC/VNPI is offered only as a guideline, a starting point for discussion with patients.

for patients who score 8 and have margins ≥3 mm, and for patients who score 9 and have margins ≥5 mm. Mastectomy is appropriate for patients who score 8 and have margins <3 mm, who score 9 and have margins <5 mm, and for all patients who score 10, 11, or 12, regardless of margin width. The value of the USC/VNPI has been confirmed by numerous studies and it is the only tool currently available to aid in the treatment decision-making process (126).

Table 34.3 Comparison of patient with USC/VNPI scores of 4–9 compared to those with scores of 10–12.

USC/VNPI Score	4–9	10–12	P value
N	273	260	
Average age	55	47	< 0.001
Average size	27 mm	61 mm	< 0.001
Average nuclear grade	04	73	< 0.000
Local recurrence only	1	8	02
Local recurrence then metastatic	0	1	NS
Metastatic only	0	2	NS
No. of invasive recurrence	1	9	01
Probability of recurrence at 12 years	2%	2%	< 0.001

Abbreviations: USC, University of Southern California; VNPI, Van Nuys Prognostic Index.

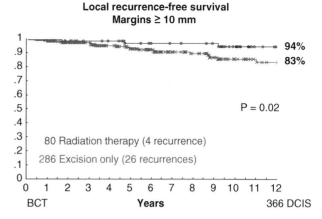

Figure 34.16 Probability of local recurrence-free survival by treatment for 366 breast conservation patients with a margin width ≥10 mm. *Abbreviation*: BCT, breast cancer therapy.

Determining size has always been the most difficult part of the USC/VNPI. Our method computes size over a series of sections (the overall extent) rather than on a single slide (unless the measurement on a single slide is larger) and correlates this with mammographic findings. For example, if an area of DCIS measuring 6 × 4 mm appears in and out of seven consecutive sections and the blocks are on average 3 mm wide, the diameter of this lesion will be recorded as a 21 mm DCIS in the USC/VNPI database (seven blocks × 3 mm average block width). However, in many other databases this will be regarded as 6 mm of DCIS, being the largest diameter on a single section.

By way of example, when the NSABP reviewed their pathological material for the B-17 study, 75–90% of their cases were measured at 10 mm or less in extent (73,127). The NSABP reported tumor size as the largest diameter on a single slide. While this is clearly the simplest and most reproducible way to measure DCIS, it is often an underestimation. Compare the NSABP sizes with our cases where only 40% (452/1032) of our conservatively treated patients had DCIS lesions measuring 10 mm or less. It is unlikely that the NSABP had twice as many smaller cases than a single group devoted to diagnosing and treating DCIS. Rather, the most likely explanation for this discrepancy lies in the way tissue was processed and the methods used for estimation of tumor size. In all likelihood, both groups treated tumors of similar size. Due to this difficulty of estimating size, we began evaluating the possibility of using margin width both as the sole predictor of local recurrence and as a surrogate for the USC/VNPI (118). The rationale for this was based on the outcome of a multivariate analysis where patients with margin width less than 1 mm were found to have a ninefold increase in the probability of local recurrence compared with patients who had a margin width of 10 mm or more. Narrow margin width was the single most powerful predictor of local failure.

In the current data set presented here, there were 366 patients with a margin width of 10 mm or more, 30 of whom (8.2%) have developed a local recurrence (4 in the radiotherapy group and 26 within the excision-only group) (Fig. 34.16). Moreover, for this group, the benefit for radiation therapy in terms of local recurrence is significant (p = 0.02). In spite of this, the actuarial local recurrence rate at 12-years for those treated with excision alone was only 17% which is almost the same as

that reported by the NSABP at 12 years for all patients treated with excision plus radiation therapy (73). There were 349 patients with USC/VNPI scores of 4, 5, or 6, of whom 15 (3%) have developed a local recurrence (3 in the radiotherapy group and 12 within the excision-only group) (Fig. 34.13). The USC/VNPI is a better predictor of local recurrence than margin width alone (half as many recurrences) and this indeed should be the case since it is based on five predictive factors, including margin width. Nevertheless, there are so few recurrences among patients with widely clear margins that for all practical purposes, margin width can be used by itself as a surrogate for the USC/VNPI.

TREATMENT OF THE AXILLA FOR PATIENTS WITH DCIS

More than 25 years ago, our group suggested that axillary lymph node dissection be abandoned for DCIS (128). In 1987, the NSABP declared that axillary node dissection for patients with DCIS be optional and done at the discretion of the surgeon. Since that time, our group has published a series of papers that continue to show that axillary node dissection is not indicated for patients with DCIS (129,130). To date, our group has performed a total of 673 node evaluations and three of which (0.4%) contained positive nodes by H&E staining. Two of these patients (both with macrometastases), were treated with adjuvant chemotherapy and were alive and well without local or distant recurrence at 8 and 10 years after their initial surgery (both patients had mastectomy and invasive cancer was likely missed during the serial sectioning of specimens). The third patient had a cluster of 40 cells discovered by immunohistochemical staining and then retrospectively they were seen on H&E. This patient was not clinically upstaged and was not treated with chemotherapy. Frykberg and colleagues in their review of the management of DCIS compiled data from nine studies with a total of 754 patients and found the incidence of axillary lymph node metastasis for patients with DCIS was only 1.7% (131).

Sentinel Node Biopsy for DCIS

Through September 2011, the senior author has performed 382 sentinel node biopsies for patients with DCIS. Nine (2.4%) were positive by IHC only, two were positive by IHC and H&E

(around 200 cells) and the rest (n = 371) were negative by both IHC and H&E. In every positive case there were only a small number of positive cells (range 4–200) and no patients were upstaged to stage II or treated with chemotherapy. All are alive and well without distant recurrence at follow-up times ranging from a few months to 15.2 years (average 3.3 years). It should be noted that not all IHC-positive cells are cancer cells; some may merely represent cytokeratin-positive debris and therefore morphology must be closely evaluated.

The authors' policy for sentinel node biopsy in patients with DCIS is as follows. Sentinel node biopsy is performed for all patients with DCIS who are undergoing a mastectomy and is performed for wide excision cases if DCIS is an upper outer quadrant high-grade lesion and the sentinel node can be easily removed through the same incision. Sentinel node biopsy is also done when DCIS is palpable or greater than 4 cm on mammography and/or MRI, or there is questionable microinvasion on core biopsy.

SUMMARY

DCIS is now a relatively common lesion and its frequency is increasing. Most of this increase is due to better and more frequent mammography available to a greater proportion of the female population. Not all cases of microscopic DCIS will progress to clinical cancer, but if a patient has DCIS which is not treated, she is more likely to develop an ipsilateral invasive breast cancer than is a woman without DCIS. The high-grade comedo subtype of DCIS is more aggressive in its histological appearance and is more likely to be associated with subsequent invasive cancer than lower grade non-comedo subtypes. High-grade comedo DCIS is more likely to have a high S-phase fraction and overexpression of HER2/neu and show increased thymidine labeling as compared with non-comedo DCIS. Comedo DCIS treated conservatively is also more likely to recur locally within the breast than non-comedo DCIS. However, separation of DCIS into two groups by architecture is an oversimplification and does not reflect the biological potential of the lesion as well as stratification by nuclear grade and comedo-type necrosis.

Most DCIS nowadays will be nonpalpable and detected by mammographic calcifications. It is not uncommon for DCIS to be larger than what is estimated by mammography, to involve more than a single quadrant and to be unicentric in its distribution. Preoperative evaluation should include mammography (preferably digital) with compression magnification and ultrasonography. MRI is becoming increasingly popular and the authors request this on every patient diagnosed with any form of breast cancer. The surgeon and the radiologist should plan the surgical excision carefully, including the need for multiple wires and the optimal approach. The first attempt at excision provides the best chance to obtain completeness with a good cosmetic result. Re-excisions often yield poor cosmetic results and these should be avoided whenever possible.

The initial breast biopsy should be an image-guided needle biopsy. After establishment of a tissue diagnosis, the patient should be counseled; if she is motivated for breast conservation, then the surgeon and radiologist should plan the procedure carefully, using multiple wires if necessary to map out the extent of the lesion.

When considering the entire population of patients with DCIS without subset analyses, prospective randomized trials have shown that post-excisional radiation therapy can reduce the relative risk of local recurrence by about 50% for conservatively treated patients. But in some low-risk DCIS patients, the costs may outweigh the potential benefits. Despite a relative reduction of 50% in the probability of local recurrence, the absolute reduction may be only a few percent. Moreover, the local recurrence rate at 15 years for the irradiated arm in the NSABP B-17 trial is 20% (106). While local recurrence is extremely important, breast cancer–specific survival is the most important endpoint for all patients with breast cancer (including patients with DCIS) and no DCIS trial has ever shown a survival benefit for radiation therapy when compared with excision alone. Moreover, radiation therapy is not without financial and physical cost. In consequence, an increasing number of selected patients with DCIS have been treated with excision alone in recent years. Furthermore, excision alone has become an acceptable form of treatment for selected patients in the 2008 NCCN Guidelines.

The USC/VNPI uses five independent predictors to estimate the probability of local recurrence after conservative treatment for DCIS. These include tumor size, margin width, nuclear grade, age, and the presence or absence of comedo necrosis. In combination, they can be used as an aid to identify subgroups of patients with extremely low probabilities of local recurrence after excision alone, for example, patients who score 4, 5, or 6 using the USC/VNPI. If size cannot be accurately determined, margin width by itself can be used as a surrogate for the USC/VNPI, although it does not provide quite as accurate risk estimates.

Oncoplastic surgery combines sound surgical oncological principles with plastic surgical techniques. Coordination of the two surgical disciplines may help to avoid poor cosmetic results after wide excision and may increase the number of women who can be treated with breast-conserving surgery by allowing larger breast excisions with more acceptable cosmetic results. Oncoplastic surgery requires cooperation and coordination of surgical oncology, radiology, and pathology. Oncoplastic resection is a therapeutic procedure not a breast biopsy and is performed on patients with a proven diagnosis of breast cancer. New oncoplastic techniques that allow for more extensive excisions can be used to achieve both acceptable cosmesis and widely clear margins, reducing the need for radiation therapy in many cases of DCIS. The decision to use excision alone as treatment for DCIS should only be made if complete and sequential tissue processing has been used and the patient has been fully informed and participated in the treatment decision-making process.

THE FUTURE

Our knowledge of DCIS genetics and molecular biology is increasing at a remarkably rapid rate. Future studies are likely to identify molecular markers that will allow us to differentiate DCIS with an aggressive potential from DCIS that is merely a microscopic finding. Once we can confidently identify DCIS that will develop the potential to invade and metastasize within a relatively short time-frame from DCIS that will not progress, the treatment selection process will be much simplified.

REFERENCES

1. Siegel R, Ward E, Brawley O, et al. Cancer statistics 2011: The impact of eliminating socioeconomic and racial disparities on premature cancer deaths. CA Cancer J Clin 2011; 61: 212–36.
2. Burstein HJ, Polyak K, Wong JS, et al. Ductal carcinoma in situ of the breast. N Engl J Med 2004; 350: 1430–41.
3. Seth A, Kitching R, Landberg G, et al. Gene expression profiling of ductal carcinomas in situ and invasive breast tumors. Anticancer Res 2003; 23: 2043–51.
4. Porter D, Lahti-Domenici J, Keshaviah A, et al. Molecular markers in ductal carcinoma in situ of the breast. Mol Cancer Res 2003; 1: 362–75.
5. Ma XJ, Salunga R, Tuggle JT, et al. Gene expression profiles of human breast cancer progression. Proc Natl Acad Sci USA 2003; 100: 5974–9.
6. Page D, Anderson T. Diagnostic Histopathology of the Breast. New York: Churchill Livingstone, 1987: 157–74.
7. Patchefsky A, Schwartz GF, Finkelstein SD, et al. Heterogeneity of intraductal carcinoma of the breast. Cancer 1989; 63: 731–41.
8. Nemoto T, Vana J, Bedwani RN, et al. Management and survival of female breast cancer: results of a national survey by The American College of Surgeons. Cancer 1980; 45: 2917–24.
9. Silverstein M, Lagios MD, Recht A, et al. Image-detected breast cancer: state of the art diagnosis and treatment. J Am Coll Surg 2005; 201: 586–97.
10. Tabar L, Smith RA, Vitak B, et al. Mammographic screening: a key factor in the control of breast cancer. Cancer J 2003; 9: 15–27.
11. Duffy SW, Tabar L, Smith RA. Screening for breast cancer with mammography. Lancet 2001; 358: 2166; author reply 2167–8.
12. Silverstein MJ, Cohlan BF, Gierson ED, et al. Duct carcinoma in situ: 227 cases without microinvasion. Eur J Cancer 1992; 28: 630–4.
13. Lagios MD. Duct carcinoma in situ: pathology and treatment. Surg Clin N Am 1990; 70: 853–71.
14. Ashikari R, Hadju S, Robbins G. Intraductal carcinoma of the breast. Cancer 1971; 28: 1182–7.
15. Silverstein MJ. Ductal carcinoma in situ of the breast. Annu Rev Med 2000; 51: 17–32.
16. Baxter N, Virnig BA, Durham SB, et al. Trends in the treatment of ductal carcinoma in situ of the breast. J Natl Cancer Inst 2004; 96: 443–8.
17. Silverstein MJ. The Van Nuys breast center - the first free-standing multidisciplinary breast center. Surg Oncol Clin N Am 2000; 9: 159–75.
18. Veronesi U, Saccozzi R, Del Vecchio M, et al. Comparing radical mastectomy with quadrantectomy, axillary dissection and radiotherapy in patients with small cancers of the breast. N Engl J Med 1981; 305: 6–10.
19. Van Dongen J, Bartelink H, Fentiman IS, et al. Randomized clinical trial to assess the value of breast-conserving therapy in stage I and II breast cancer, EORTC 10801 trial. J Natl Cancer Inst Monogr 1992: 15–18.
20. Veronesi U, Banfi A, Salvadori B, et al. Breast conservation is the treatment of choice in small breast cancer: long-term results of a randomized trial. Eur J Cancer 1990; 26: 668–70.
21. Fisher B, Redmond C, Poisson R, et al. Eight-year results of a randomized clinical trial comparing total mastectomy and lumpectomy with or without radiation therapy in the treatment of breast cancer. N Engl J Med 1989; 320: 822–8.
22. Veronesi U, Cascinelli N, Mariani L, et al. Twenty-year follow-up of a randomized study comparing breast-conserving surgery with radical mastectomy for early breast cancer. N Engl J Med 2002; 347: 1227–32.
23. Fisher B, Anderson S, Bryant J, et al. Twenty-year follow-up of a randomized trial comparing total mastectomy, lumpectomy, and lumpectomy plus irradiation for the treatment of invasive breast cancer. N Engl J Med 2002; 347: 1233–41.
24. Tavassoli F. Intraductal carcinoma. In: Tavassoli FA, ed. Pathology of the Breast. Appleton and Lange: Norwalk, Connecticut, 1992: 229–61.
25. Aasmundstad T, Haugen O. DNA Ploidy in intraductal breast carcinomas. Eur J Cancer 1992; 26: 956–9.
26. Meyer J. Cell kinetics in selection and stratification of patients for adjuvant therapy of breast carcinoma. NCI Monogr 1986: 25–8.
27. Allred D, Clark GM, Molina R, et al. Overexpression of HER-2/neu and its relationship with other prognostic factors change during the progression of in situ to invasive breast cancer. Hum Pathol 1992; 23: 974–9.
28. Barnes D, Meyer JS, Gonzalez JG, et al. Relationship between c-erbB-2 immunoreactivity and thymidine labelling index in breast carcinoma in situ. Breast Cancer Res Treat 1991; 18: 11–17.
29. Bartkova J, Barnes DM, Millis RR, et al. Immunohistochemical demonstration of c-erbB-2 protein in mammary ductal carcinoma in situ. Hum Pathol 1990; 21: 1164–7.
30. Liu E, Thor A, He M, et al. The HER2 (c-erbB-2) oncogene is frequently amplified in in situ carcinomas of the breast. Oncogene 1992; 7: 1027–32.
31. van de Vijver M, Peterse JL, Mooi WJ, et al. Neu-protein overexpression in breast cancer: association with comedo-type ductal carcinoma in situ and limited prognostic value in stage II breast cancer. N Engl J Med 1988; 319: 1239–45.
32. Lagios M, Margolin FR, Westdahl PR, et al. Mammographically detected duct carcinoma in situ. Frequency of local recurrence following tylectomy and prognostic effect of nuclear grade on local recurrence. Cancer 1989; 63: 619–24.
33. Schwartz G, Finkel GC, Garcia JC, et al. Subclinical ductal carcinoma in situ of the breast: treatment by local excision and surveillance alone. Cancer 1992; 70: 2468–74.
34. Silverstein MJ, Waisman JR, Gierson ED, et al. Radiation therapy for intraductal carcinoma: is it an equal alternative? Arch Surg 1991; 126: 424–8.
35. Solin L, Yeh IT, Kurtz J, et al. Ductal carcinoma in situ (intraductal carcinoma) of the breast treated with breast-conserving surgery and definitive irradiation. Correlation of pathologic parameters with outcome of treatment. Cancer 1993; 71: 2532–42.
36. Silverstein MJ, Poller D, Craig P, et al. Predicting local recurrence in patients with intraductal breast carcinoma (DCIS). Proc Am Soc Clin Oncol 1995; 14: 117.
37. Silverstein MJ, Lagios MD, Craig PH, et al. A prognostic index for ductal carcinoma in situ of the breast. Cancer 1996; 77: 2267–74.
38. Lagios M, Westdahl PR, Margolin FR, et al. Duct Carcinoma in situ: Relationship of extent of noninvasive disease to the frequency of occult invasion, multicentricity, lymph node metastases, and short-term treatment failures. Cancer 1982; 50: 1309–14.
39. Holland R, Peterse JL, Millis RR, et al. Ductal carcinoma in situ: a proposal for a new classification. Semin Diagn Pathol 1994; 11: 167–80.
40. Silverstein MJ, Poller DN, Waisman JR, et al. Prognostic classification of breast ductal carcinoma-in-situ. Lancet 1995; 345: 1154–7.
41. Jensen J, Handel N, Silverstein M, et al. Glandular replacement therapy (GRT) for intraductal breast carcinoma (DCIS). Proc Am Soc Clin Oncol 1995; 14: 138.
42. Jensen J, Handel N, Silverstein M. Glandular replacement therapy: an argument for a combined surgical approach in the treatment of noninvasive breast cancer. Breast J 1996; 2: 121–3.
43. Faverly D, Burgers L, Bult P, et al. Three dimensional imaging of mammary ductal carcinoma is situ: clinical implications. Semin Diagn Pathol 1994; 11: 193–8.
44. Poller D, Silverstein MJ, Galea M, et al. Ductal carcinoma in situ of the breast: a proposal for a new simplified histological classification association between cellular proliferation and c-erbB-2 protein expression. Mod Pathol 1994; 7: 257–62.
45. Bellamy C, McDonald C, Salter DM, et al. Noninvasive ductal carcinoma of the breast: the relevance of histologic categorization. Hum Pathol 1993; 24: 16–23.
46. Sloane J, Ellman R, Anderson TJ, et al. Consistency of histopathological reporting of breast lesions detected by breast screening: findings of the UK national external quality assessment (EQA) scheme. Eur J Cancer 1994: 1414–19.
47. Bryan B, Schnitt S, Collins L. Ductal carcinoma in situ with basal-like phenotype: a possible precursor to invasive basal-like breast cancer. Mod Pathol 2006; 19: 617–21.
48. Tamimi R, Baer HJ, Marotti J, et al. Comparison of molecular phenotypes of ductal carcinoma in situ and invasive breast cancer. Breast Cancer Res 2008; 10: R67.
49. Hannemann J, Velds A, Halfwerk JB, et al. Classification of ductal carcinoma in situ by gene expression profiling. Breast Cancer Res 2006; 8: R61.
50. Solin L, Gray R, Baehner FL, et al. A quantitative multigene RT-PCR assay for predicting recurrence risk after surgical excision alone without

irradiation for ductal carcinoma in situ (DCIS): A prospective validation study of the DCIS score from ECOG E5194. Breast Cancer Res Treat 2011; S4–06.

51. Kerlikowske K, Molinaro AM, Gauthier ML, et al. Biomarker expression and risk of subsequent tumors after initial ductal carcinoma in situ diagnosis. J Natl Cancer Inst 2010; 102: 627–37.

52. Rudloff U, Jacks LM, Goldberg JI, et al. Nomogram for predicting the risk of local recurrence after breast-conserving surgery for ductal carcinoma in situ. J Clin Oncol 2010; 28: 3762–9.

53. Page D, Rogers L, Schuyler P, et al. The natural history of ductal carcinoma in situ of the breast. In: Silverstein MJ, Recht A, Lagios M, eds. Ductal Carcinoma In Situ of the Breast. Philadelphia: Lippincott, Williams and Wilkins, 2002: 17–21.

54. Sanders M, Schuyler PA, Dupont WD, et al. The natural history of low-grade ductal carcinoma in situ of the breast in women treated by biopsy only revealed over 30 years of long-term follow-up. Cancer 2005; 103: 2481–4.

55. Rosen P, Senie R, Schottenfeld D, et al. Noninvasive breast carcinoma: Frequency of unsuspected invasion and implications for treatment. Ann Surg 1979; 1989: 377–82.

56. Alpers C, Wellings S. The prevalence of carcinoma in situ in normal and cancer-associated breast. Hum Pathol 1985; 16: 796–807.

57. Page D, Dupont WD, Rogers LW, et al. Intraductal carcinoma of the breast: follow-up after biopsy only. Cancer 1982; 49: 751–8.

58. Schuh M, Nemoto T, Penetrante RB, et al. Intraductal carcinoma: analysis of presentation, pathologic findings, and outcome of disease. Arch Surg 1986; 121: 1303–7.

59. Gump F, Jicha D, Ozzello L. Ductal carcinoma in situ (DCIS): a revised concept. Surgery 1987; 102: 190–5.

60. de Mascarel I, MacGrogan G, Mathoulin-Pelissier S, et al. Breast ductal carcinoma in situ with microinvasion. A definition supported by long-term study 1248 serially sectioned ductal carcinomas. Cancer 2002; 94: 2134–42.

61. Fisher E, Sass R, Fisher B, et al. Pathologic findings from the national surgical adjuvant breast project (Protocol 6) i. Intraductal carcinoma (DCIS). Cancer 1986; 57: 197–208.

62. Simpson T, Thirlby R, Dail D. Surgical treatment of ductal carcinoma in situ of the breast: 10 to 20 year follow-up. Arch Surg 1992; 127: 468–72.

63. Holland R, Hendriks JH, Vebeek AL, et al. Extent, distribution, and mammographic/histological correlations of breast ductal carcinoma in situ. Lancet 1990; 335: 519–22.

64. Holland R, Faverly D. Whole organ studies. In: Silverstein MJ, Recht A, Lagios M, eds. Ductal Carcinoma In Situ of the Breast. Philadelphia: Lippincott, Williams and Wilkins, 2002; In press.

65. Noguchi S, Aihara T, Koyama H, et al. Discrimination between multicentric and multifocal carcinomas of breast through clonal analysis. Cancer 1994; 74: 872–7.

66. Tabar L, Dean P. Basic principles of mammographic diagnosis. Diagn Imaging Clin Med 1985; 54: 146–57.

67. Silverstein M. Where's the outrage. J Am Coll Surg 2009; 208: 78–9.

68. Lester SC, Bose S, Chen YY, et al. Protocol for the examination of specimens from patients with ductal carcinoma in situ of the breast. Arch Pathol Lab Med 2009; 133: 15–25.

69. Lester SC, Connolly JL, Amin MB. College of American pathologists protocol for the reporting of ductal carcinoma in situ. Arch Pathol Lab Med 2009; 133: 13–14.

70. Consensus Conference Committee. Consensus Conference on the classification of ductal carcinoma in situ. Cancer 1997; 80: 1798–802.

71. Silverstein MJ. Intraductal breast carcinoma: two decades of progress? Am J Clin Oncol 1991; 14: 534–7.

72. Silverstein MJ. Noninvasive breast cancer: the dilemma of the 1990s. Obstet Gynecol Clin N Am 1994; 21: 639–58.

73. Fisher B, Land S, Mamounas E, et al. Prevention of invasive breast cancer in women with ductal carcinoma in situ: an update of the national surgical adjuvant breast and bowel project experience. Semin Oncol 2001; 28: 400–18.

74. Fentiman I, Fagg N, Millis RR, et al. In situ ductal carcinoma of the breast: implications of disease pattern and treatment. Eur J Surg Oncol 1986; 12: 261–6.

75. Solin L, Kurtz J, Fourquet A, et al. Fifteen year results of breast conserving surgery and definitive breast irradiation for treatment of ductal carcinoma in situ of the breast. J Clin Oncol 1996; 14: 754–63.

76. UK Coordinating Committee on Cancer Research (UKCCCR) Ductal Carcinoma in Situ (DCIS) Working Party. Radiotherapy and tamoxifen in women with completely excised ductal carcinoma in situ of the breast in the UK, Australia, and New Zealand: randomised controlled trial. Lancet 2003; 362: 95–102.

77. Viani GA, Stefano EJ, Afonso SL, et al. Breast-conserving surgery with or without radiotherapy in women with ductal carcinoma in situ: a meta-analysis of randomized trials. Radiat Oncol 2007; 2: 28–39.

78. Emdin SO, Granstrand B, Ringberg A, et al. SweDCIS: Radiotherapy after sector resection for ductal carcinoma in situ of the breast. Results of a randomised trial in a population offered mammographic screening. Acta Oncol (Madr) 2006; 45: 536–43.

79. Fisher B, Jeong JH, Anderson S, et al. Twenty-five year follow-up of a randomized trial comparing radiacal mastectomy, total mastectomy, and total mastectomy followed by irradiation. N Engl J Med 2002; 347: 567–75.

80. Clarke M, Collins R, Darby S, et al. Effects of radiotherapy and differences in the extent of surgery for early breast cancer on local recurrence and on 15-year survival. Lancet 2005; 366: 2087–106.

81. Early Breast Cancer Trialists' Collaborative Group (EBCTCG). Darby S, McGale P, Correa C, et al. Effect of radiotherapy after breast-conserving surgery on 10-year recurrence and 15-year breast cancer death: meta-analysis of individual patient data for 10,801 women in 17 randomized trials. Lancet 2011; 378: 771–84.

82. Silverstein MJ, Lagios MD, Martino S, et al. Outcome after local recurrence in patients with ductal carcinoma in situ of the breast. J Clin Oncol 1998; 16: 1367–73.

83. Romero L, Klein L, Ye W, et al. Outcome after invasive recurrence in patients with ductal carcinoma in situ of the breast. Am J Surg 2004; 188: 371–6.

84. Swain S. Ductal carcinoma in situ - incidence, presentation and guidelines to treatment. Oncology 1989; 3: 25–42.

85. Fisher B, Costantino J, Redmond C, et al. Lumpectomy compared with lumpectomy and radiation therapy for the treatment of intraductal breast cancer. N Engl J Med 1993; 328: 1581–6.

86. Fisher B, Dignam J, Wolmark N, et al. Tamoxifen in treatment of intraductal breast cancer: National Surgical Adjuvant Breast and Bowel Project B-24 randomized controlled trial. Lancet 1999; 353: 1993–2000.

87. Fisher B, Dignam J, Wolmark N, et al. Lumpectomy and radiation therapy for the treatment of intraductal breast cancer: findings from National Surgical Adjuvant Breast and Bowel Project B-17. J Clin Oncol 1998; 16: 441–52.

88. Julien J, Bijker N, Fentiman IS, et al. Radiotherapy in breast conserving treatment for ductal carcinoma in situ: first results of EORTC randomized phase III trial 10853. Lancet 2000; 355: 528–33.

89. Page D, Dupont WD, Rogers LW, et al. Continued local recurrence of carcinoma 15-25 years after a diagnosis of low grade ductal carcinoma in situ of the breast treated only by biopsy. Cancer 1995; 76: 1197–200.

90. Zafrani B, Leroyer A, Fourquet A, et al. Mammographically detected ductal in situ carcinoma of the breast analyzed with a new classification. A study of 127 cases: correlation with estrogen and progesterone receptors, p53 and c-erbB-2 proteins, and proliferative activity. Semin Diagn Pathol 1994; 11: 208–14.

91. Schwartz G. The role of excision and surveillance alone in subclinical DCIS of the breast. Oncology 1994; 8: 21–6.

92. Schwartz G. Treatment of subclinical ductal carcinoma in situ of the breast by local excision and surveillance: an updated personal experience. In: Silverstein MJ, Recht A, Lagios M, eds. Ductal Carcinoma In Situ of the Breast. Philadelphia: Lippincott, Williams and Wilkins, 2002: 308–21.

93. Silverstein M. Ductal carcinoma in situ of the breast: 11 reasons to consider treatment with excision alone. Womens Health (Lond Engl) 2008; 4: 565–77.

94. Holland R, Faverly D. Whole organ studies. In: Silverstein M, ed. Ductal Carcinoma In Situ of the Breast. Baltimore: Williams and Wilkins, 1997: 233–40.

95. Holland R, Hendriks J. Microcalcifications associated with ductal carcinoma in situ: mammographic-pathologic correlation. Semin Diagn Pathol 1994; 11: 181–92.

96. Page D, Dupont WD, Rogers LW, et al. Atypical hyperplastic lesions of the female breast. A log-term follow-up study. Cancer 1985; 55: 2698–708.

97. Lagios M. Controversies in diagnosis, biology, and treatment. Breast J 1995; 1: 68–78.
98. Early Breast Cancer Trialists' Collaborative Group (EBCTCG). Favorable and unfavorable effects on long-term survival of radiotherapy for early breast cancer: an overview of the randomized trials. Lancet 2006; 2000: 1757–70.
99. Giordano S, Kuo YF, Freeman JL, et al. Risk of cardiac death after adjuvant radiotherapy for breast cancer. J Natl Cancer Inst 2005; 97: 419–24.
100. Darby S, McGale P, Taylor CW, et al. Long-term mortality from heart disease and lung cancer after radiotherapy for early breast cancer: prospective cohort study of about 300,000 women un US SEER cancer registries. Lancet Oncol 2005; 6: 557–65.
101. Zablotska L, Neugut A. Lung carcinoma after radiation therapy in women treated with lumpectomy or mastectomy for primary breast carcinoma. Cancer 2003; 97: 1404–11.
102. Darby S, McGale P, Peto R, et al. Mortality from cardiovascular disease more than 10 years after radiotherapy for breast cancer: nationwide cohort study of 90,000 Swedish women. BMJ 2003; 326: 256–7.
103. Recht A. Randomized trial overview. In: Silverstein MJ, Recht A, Lagios M, eds. Ductal Carcinoma in Situ of the Breast. Philadelphia: Lippincott, Williams and Wilkins, 2002: 414–19.
104. Vaidya JS, Joseph DJ, Tobias JS, et al. Targeted intraoperative radiotherapy versus whole breast radiotherapy for breast cancer (TARGIT-A trial): an international, prospective, randomised, non-inferiority phase 3 trial. Lancet 2010; 376: 91–102.
105. Wong J, Kaelin CM, Troyan SL, et al. Prospective study of wide excision alone for ductal carcinoma in situ of the breast. J Clin Oncol 2006; 24: 1031–6.
106. Wapnir I, Dignam JJ, Fisher B, et al. Long-term outcomes of invasive ipsilateral breast tumor recurrences after lumpectomy in NSABP B-17 and B-24 randomized clinical trials for DCIS. J Natl Cancer Inst 2011; 103: 478–88.
107. Carlson RW, Berry DA, Burstein HJ, et al. NCCN Clincal Practice Guidelines in Oncology: Breast Cancer. 2008.[Available from: www.nccn.org]
108. Bijker N, Peterse JL, Duchateau L, et al. Risk factors for recurrence and metastasis after breast-conserving therapy for ductal carcinoma in situ: analysis of European Organization for Research and Treatment of Cancer Trial 10853. J Clin Oncol 2001; 19: 2263–71.
109. Fisher E, Costantino J, Fisher B, et al. Pathologic findings from the National Surgical Adjuvant Breast Project (NSABP) Protocol B-17. Cancer 1995; 75: 1310–19.
110. Bijker N, Meijnen P, Peterse JL, et al. Breast conserving treatment with or without radiotherapy in ductal carcinoma in situ: ten-year results of European Organization for Research and treatment of Cancer Randomized Phase III Trial 10853 - A study by the EORTC Breast Cancer Cooperative Group and EORTC Radiotherapy Group. J Clin Oncol 2006; 24: 1–8.
111. Cuzick J, Sestak I, Pinder SE, et al. Effect of tamoxifen and radiotherapy in women with locally excised ductal carcinoma in situ: long-term results from the UK/ANZ DCIS trial. Lancet Oncol 2011; 12: 21–9.
112. Fisher B, Bauer M, Margolese R, et al. Five-year results of a randomized clinical trial comparing total mastectomy and lumpectomy with or without radiation therapy in the treatment of breast cancer. N Engl J Med 1985; 312: 665–73.
113. Fisher E, Leeming R, Anderson S, et al. Conservative management of intraductal carcinoma (DCIS) of the breast. J Surg Oncol 1991; 47: 139–47.
114. Allred D, Bryant L, Land S, et al. Estrogen receptor expression as a predictive marker of effectiveness of tamoxifen in the treatment of DCIS: frindings from NSABP Protocol B-24. Breast Cancer Res Treat 2003; 76: 36.
115. Holmberg L, Garmo H, Granstrand B, et al. Absolute risk reductions for local recurrence after postoperative radiotherapy after sector rsection for ductal carcinoma in situ of the breast. J Clin Oncol 2008; 26: 1247–52.
116. Lester SC, Connolly JL, Amin MB. College of American Pathologists protocol for the reporting of ductal carcinoma in situ. Arch Pathol Lab Med 2009; 133: 13–14.
117. Silverstein MJ. The University of Southern California/Van Nuys Prognostic Index for ductal carcinoma in situ of the breast. Am J Surg 2003; 186: 337–43.
118. Silverstein MJ, Lagios MD, Groshen S, et al. The influence of margin width on local control in patients with ductal carcinoma in situ (DCIS) of the breast. N Engl J Med 1999; 340: 1455–61.
119. Ottesen G, Graversen HP, Blichert-Toft M, et al. Ductal carcinoma in situ of the female breast. Short-term results of a prospective nationwide study. Am J Surg Pathol 1992; 16: 1183–96.
120. Silverstein MJ, et al. The Van Nuys prognostic index for ductal carcinoma in situ. Breast J 1996; 2: 38–40.
121. Silverstein MJ, Lagios M, Recht A, eds. Ductal Carcinoma In Situ of the Breast, 2nd edn. Philadelphia: Lippincott, Williams and Wilkins, 2002.
122. Poller D, Silverstein MJ. The Van Nuys ductal carcinoma in situ: an update. In: Silverstein MJ, Recht A, Lagios M, eds. Ductal Carcinoma In Situ of the Breast. Philadelphia: Lippincott, Williams and Wilkins, 2002: 222–33.
123. Silverstein MJ, Buchanan C. Ductal carcinoma in situ: USC/Van Nuys prognostic index and the impact of margin status. Breast 2003; 12: 457–71.
124. Silverstein MJ. The University of Southern California/Van Nuys prognostic index. In: Silverstein MJ, Recht A, Lagios M, eds. Ductal Carcinoma In Situ of the Breast. Philadelphia: Lippincott, Williams and Wilkins, 2002: 459–73.
125. Silverstein MJ, Lagios M. Choosing treatment for patients with ductal carcinoma in situ: fine tuning the University of southern California/Van Nuys prognostic index. J Natl Cancer Inst Monogr 2010: 193–6.
126. Di Saverio S, Catena F, Santini D, et al. 259 Patients with DCIS of the breast applying USC/Van Nuys prognostic index: a retrospective review with long term follow up. Breast Cancer Res Treat 2008; 109: 405–16.
127. Fisher E, Dignam J, Tan-Chiu E, et al. Pathologic findings from the National Adjuvant Breast Project (NSABP) eight-year update of Protocol B-17: intraductal carcinoma. Cancer 1999; 86: 429–38.
128. Silverstein MJ, Rosser RJ, Gierson ED, et al. Axillary Lymph node dissection for intraductal carcinoma - is it indicated? Cancer 1987; 59: 1819–24.
129. Silverstein MJ. An argument against routine use of radiotherapy for ductal carcinoma in situ. Oncology 2003; 17: 1511–46.
130. Silverstein MJ, Barth A, Poller DN, et al. Ten-year results comparing mastectomy to excision and radiation therapy for ductal carcinoma in situ of the breast. Eur J Cancer 1995; 31A:1425–7.
131. Frykberg E, Masood S, Copeland EM, et al. Duct carcinoma in situ of the breast. Surg Gynecol Obstet 1993; 177: 425–40.

35 Principles of surgical treatment of invasive breast cancer

Starr Koslow and Rache M. Simmons

INTRODUCTION

The increased diagnosis of breast cancer at a very early stage based on the widespread use of screening mammography has led to continuous revisions to what constitutes "early breast cancer." This has been accompanied by changes in the breast TNM (tumor, lymph nodes and metastasis) staging system, now in its seventh edition, published in 2009 (1,2). Early invasive breast cancer was previously defined as carcinomas less than 1 cm, including ductal carcinoma in situ (DCIS) with microinvasion (3). Based on the aforementioned revised TNM staging system and the increased treatability of breast tumors, this definition has been revised to include any breast tumor categorized as Stage 0, I, or II.

DIAGNOSIS

While some breast tumors are detected by palpation even at an early stage, a majority of early breast cancers are detected by screening mammography. In 2009, the US Preventive Services Task Force made recommendations against routine mammography for women in their 40s. Instead, the group favored starting biennial screenings at age 50, and stated that the decision to start screening before 50 "should be an individual one and take into account patient context, including the patient's values regarding specific benefits and harms" (4). Despite their recommendations, the American Cancer Society and many other societies together with a majority of clinicians continue to advocate for annual screening mammography at the age of 40 or 10 years prior to a primary relative's diagnosis of breast cancer (5). Furthermore, studies have continued to show that mammography screening is effective in decreasing breast cancer mortality among average risk women aged 40–49 years. In a meta-analysis of eight randomized controlled trials, screening mammography was shown to reduce breast cancer mortality by 15% for women aged 39–49 years [RR 0.85, (95% CI 0.95–0.96)] (6). While mammography can potentially detect a high proportion of malignancies before they become clinically detectable, the sensitivity of mammography may be decreased in women with dense breasts, as is often the case in younger women (7). The diagnostic accuracy for mammography has been shown to be significantly increased when adding screening ultrasound for women with heterogeneously dense breast tissue, but this approach also increases the risk of false positives (8). Magnetic resonance imaging (MRI) has gained popularity in screening high-risk patients and may be more sensitive in certain cases, but it has not been shown to have any impact on overall survival (OS) (9) and can also lead to unnecessary biopsies (10). Furthermore, MRI has not been shown to be as sensitive as mammography in detecting DCIS, and it remains debatable whether breast MRI should be used routinely for a preoperative workup of patients with breast cancer (10).

Once a mass is suspected on clinical examination or breast imaging, the appropriate next step is diagnostic needle biopsy guided either by palpation or image-directed biopsy (ultrasound, stereotactic, or MRI guided) for impalpable lesions. Image-directed needle biopsy is now recommended over hand directed biopsy for palpable lesions to ensure that the needle lies within the target. A needle biopsy is less invasive than an excisional biopsy and allows adequate planning for a one-step procedure once a diagnosis has been established; therefore, it is the preferred method for biopsying the majority of breast lesions.

A core needle biopsy is preferable to fine needle aspiration cytology and has a higher innate sensitivity. A core biopsy also provides more detailed information based on histological evaluation compared with cytology alone and can distinguish between invasive and non-invasive tumors. Once a biopsy confirms a lesion to be cancerous, the next step is for the surgical oncologist to plan definitive surgery.

SURGICAL TREATMENT

Most early invasive breast cancers are amenable to breast conservation with lumpectomy. However, there are certain situations which are clear contraindications for breast conservation. For example, mastectomy will be necessary for adequate treatment when a tumor is multicentric, when there has already been radiation to the breast area in the past, or negative margins cannot be achieved by lumpectomy.

What Constitutes an Adequate Surgical Margin?

Unfortunately, there is still no consensus regarding optimal margins of excision. The National Surgical Adjuvant Breast and Bowel Project (NSABP) defines an adequate margin as "tumor not touching ink." While some studies have demonstrated decreased local recurrence rates with at least a 2 mm margin in DCIS (11), there is no agreement among surgeons as to what defines an adequate margin. In a survey of 318 surgeons who were provided with a scenario of a T1 invasive cancer, only 11% of surgeons favored margins as tumor not touching ink, while 42% preferred margins of 1–2 mm, 28% preferred margins ≥5 mm, and 19% chose a margin of >1 cm as precluding the need for re-excision before radiotherapy. Moreover, when asked about a similar scenario involving DCIS, this spectrum of opinion was replicated (12). These differences in opinion and practice were highlighted in a multi-institutional observational study by the Breast Cancer Surgical Outcomes (BRCASO) research consortium in which 2206 women with

2220 newly identified invasive breast cancers underwent breast conserving surgery (BCS). The overall re-excision rate was 22.9%, but varied widely between the 54 surgeons and 4 institutions who participated in this study. Notably, re-excision rates of positive margins (defined as tumor not touching ink) varied from 73.7% to 93.5% (p = 0.003). In this study, 14.1% of patients with positive margins did not undergo any re-excision and re-excisions performed on negative margins ranged from 1.7% to 20.9% depending on the institution (p < 0.001) (13). Positive margins have been correlated with a long-term increased risk of local recurrence (14) and a re-excision has considerable psychological and physical effects on patients, together with potential economic impact and delays in adjuvant therapy. Therefore, a clarification of standards of practice in this area is warranted.

Updates in Conservative Therapy

After decades of radical surgery for breast cancer, the NSABP initiated the B-04 clinical trial in 1971 to determine whether patients with either clinically negative or clinically positive axillary nodes who received local or regional treatments other than radical mastectomy would have outcomes similar to those achieved with radical mastectomy. The findings from this trial showed no advantage in terms of OS from radical mastectomy versus fine needle aspiration cytology and has at five years of follow-up and supported an argument for more limited operations for breast cancer (15). In 2002, Fisher et al. published 25 year follow-up data from the NSABP-04 trial which confirmed no advantage for radical mastectomy over total mastectomy with or without radiation to the axilla (16). The initial results of the B-04 trial helped pave the way for the conduct of the NSABP B-06 trial designed to evaluate even less radical surgical procedures for the treatment of early-stage breast cancer. The NSABP B-06 trial compared lumpectomy and axillary node dissection with or without breast radiation with modified radical mastectomy in patients with tumors 4 cm or less in greatest diameter. Consistent with prior reports, the latest update confirms the value of lumpectomy and breast radiation as the preferred treatment for the majority of patients with invasive operable breast cancer. After 20 years of follow-up, there continues to be no significant differences in OS, disease-free survival (DFS), or distant DFS between patients who underwent total mastectomy compared with those who underwent lumpectomy with breast radiation (17,18).

Following the National Institutes of Health Consensus Statement in 1990, BCS became more common, while mastectomy rates declined. Paradoxically, there has been a recent surge in the number of women who are otherwise suitable candidates for breast conservation, opting to undergo ipsilateral mastectomy for a diagnosed breast cancer together with contralateral prophylactic mastectomy (CPM). In November 2007, Tuttle et al. published data reporting that the use of CPM in the United States had more than doubled in the period from 1998 to 2003 (19). Rates of simultaneous occult contralateral breast cancer range from 0.5 to 6% in the literature and these alone do not support the use of CPM in average-risk women with newly diagnosed breast cancer (20). However, many women reach a decision to undergo CPM for complex emotional reasons which include avoiding the anxiety of future contralateral breast cancer or for cosmetic symmetry with the ipsilateral breast reconstruction (21).

Managing the Axilla and Micrometastatic Disease

The presence or absence of axillary lymph node metastasis in early breast cancer is the most important predictor for survival and recurrence (22). For patients with tumors less than 1 cm in size, the finding of axillary metastases will significantly alter postoperative recommendations for adjuvant systemic therapy. Sentinel node biopsy (SNB) allows accurate axillary staging of patients with invasive breast cancer and a clinically negative axilla and has less morbidity and fewer complications than traditional axillary lymph node dissection (ALND). Figure 35.1 details the technique for SNB in which the first lymph node(s) in the axillary chain are identified. SNB has been proven to be safe and effective for patients with relatively small breast cancers and clinically negative axillae. In patients with clinically node-negative disease, the sentinel node is the only involved node in 40–60% of patients undergoing SNB (23,24). NSABP B-32 was a randomized controlled trial completed at 80 centers in Canada and the United States between May 1, 1999 and February 29, 2004; the trial was designed to compare outcomes of women with invasive breast cancer who had sentinel lymph node resection plus ALND to those who had sentinel node resection alone with ALND only if the sentinel lymph nodes were positive. In 2010, Krag et al. published findings from the trial showing that OS, DFS, and regional control, were statistically equivalent between the two groups. When the sentinel lymph node is negative, SNB alone with no further axillary dissection is an appropriate, safe, and effective therapy for breast cancer patients with clinically negative lymph nodes (25,26).

In 1999, the American College of Surgeons Oncology Group (ACOSOG) sought to determine the association between survival and occult sentinel lymph node metastases detected by immunohistochemical (IHC) methods. Patients enrolled in the Z0010 trial underwent BCS, SNB, and whole breast irradiation for a clinical T1 or T2 node-negative breast cancer. Occult sentinel lymph node metastases were detected in 10.5% of patients with hematoxylin and eosin-negative sentinel nodes. The trial revealed no difference in overall or DFS in those patients with occult sentinel node metastases (95.7% vs. 95.1%, P = 0.64). The trial also addressed the question of the

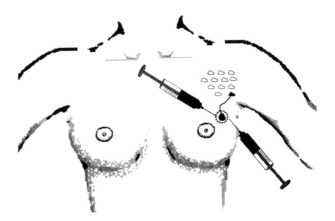

Figure 35.1 An illustration of the procedure to localize the axillary sentinel lymph node. The technique involves the injection of isosulfan or methylene blue dye with or without radioisotope to localize the sentinel lymph node.

significance of occult bone marrow metastases, which were found to be significantly associated with increased mortality. At five years, mortality rates were 5.0% (95% CI, 4.2–5.7%) for patients with IHC-negative specimens and 9.9% (95% CI, 3.9–15.5%) for those with IHC-positive specimens (P = 0. 01). However, when taking into account age and tumor size on multivariable analysis, this factor no longer remained significant. With 15 deaths among 104 women with IHC-positive bone marrow aspirate specimens, the incidence in the Z0010 trial was too low to recommend incorporating bone marrow aspirate biopsy into routine practice for patients with favorable stage disease. The ACOSOG Z0010 trial was important in being the largest prospective trial to assess IHC-detected metastases in the sentinel lymph nodes and bone marrow of women with early-stage breast cancer. As we gain a better understanding of the biology of micrometastases and as techniques to isolate tumor cells continue to improve, the detection of occult metastases in breast cancer will likely play an increasing role in the management decisions for early invasive disease (27).

Breast cancer is now diagnosed at an earlier stage than in the past, and the incidence and extent of axillary lymph node metastases has been decreasing. Our understanding of the significance of SNB findings continues to evolve. After a number of reports suggested that selected patients with sentinel node metastasis could be managed without completion ALND, ACOSOG conducted a randomized trial to formally assess this. The ACOSOG Z0011 trial, "A randomized trial of axillary node dissection in women with clinical T1 or T2 N0 M0 breast cancer who have a positive sentinel node," was a prospective trial designed to compare outcomes of patients with up to two sentinel node metastases (macro/micrometastases) who were treated with SNB alone to those treated with completion ALND without third-field axillary radiation. The primary endpoint of the trial was OS, but locoregional recurrence was also evaluated. The trial was closed prematurely in December 2004 due to lower-than-expected accrual and event rates. The trial showed no significant benefit in terms of locoregional control or DFS for completion ALND, despite the removal of axillary lymph nodes containing additional metastases. With the trial closing earlier than planned, many clinicians have been hesitant to put the treatment implications from Z0011 into practice. Moreover, there remains a need to assess the role for axillary dissection in those patients excluded from Z0011. Despite these results from the Z0011 trial and increasing evidence that many women will not have additional nodal metastases on completion ALND, the standard management of patients with clinically negative, histologically positive SNB has not changed at the time of writing. ALND remains the gold standard for treatment of axillary node positive patients in most breast units around the world though some major breast units in the United States have now abandoned completion ALND for patients with sentinel lymph node metastases who fulfill Z0011 entry criteria (24,28,29).

Cryoablation

Cryoablation represents a novel method for management of minimally invasive breast cancers with conservation surgery. The technique has already been used to treat prostate cancer and involves introduction of a cryoprobe into the center of a tumor under ultrasound guidance in order to freeze the tissue to temperatures ranging from −160 to −190°C (Fig. 35.2).

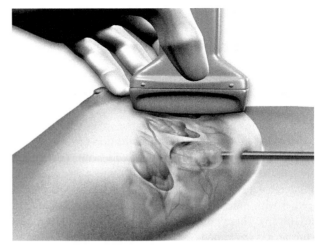

Figure 35.2 An illustration of a cryoprobe placement under ultrasound guidance. The cryoprobe creates an "ice ball" which engulfs the cancer and destroys the targeted area. *Source:* Photo courtesy of Sanarus Medical, Inc.

Several small studies have demonstrated the feasibility, safety, and efficacy of cryoablation in the treatment of benign breast tumors and breast cancer although the technique has limitations (30,31). Most of these studies have involved cryoablation followed by standard surgical resection and formed the basis for a larger multi-institutional trial sponsored by the National Cancer Institute. This may provide data supporting the use of cryoablation as an alternative to lumpectomy. The principal aim of the trial is to determine the rate of complete tumor ablation in patients with invasive ductal breast carcinoma treated with cryoablation. Patients undergo ablation using a freeze–thaw–freeze cycle and then proceed to surgical resection and SNB and/or axillary dissection within 28 days after completion of cryoablation (32). Although the prospect of such technology being used to treat breast cancer is exciting, it will likely be several years before determination of both safety and equivalence to the current standard of care.

ADJUVANT THERAPY

Adjuvant breast radiotherapy is the standard practice for patients undergoing lumpectomy. Whole-breast irradiation has been used for several decades to reduce the risk of ipsilateral breast tumor recurrence after breast-conserving surgery for early breast cancer. Even in patients where disease is only detected locoregionally, undetected deposits of both local and distant disease may remain after surgical excision. If left untreated, these could eventually develop into potentially life-threatening recurrence. Thus, adequate systemic therapies must be administered in addition to locoregional treatment. According to current guidelines, obligatory factors for decision making regarding the type of adjuvant systemic therapy include HER2 status, hormone receptor status, and menopausal status (33). Adjuvant chemotherapy, hormonal therapy, and biological therapies are recommended according to national guidelines and the status of prognostic indices.

PROGNOSIS

The prognosis of breast cancer varies widely according to stage, but early breast cancer portends an excellent prognosis overall. Treatments for breast cancer aim to increase the disease-free interval and OS. In comparison with other malignancies, the prognosis of breast cancer has improved in the last two to three decades partially as a result of mammographic screening. Axillary lymph node status has been shown to be the single most important prognostic factor for DFS and OS for patients with breast cancer (22). Since the incidence of overt systemic disease is very low for early stage breast cancer patients, most physicians do not routinely request an extent of disease workup (bone scan and CT scans of the chest, abdomen, pelvis, and brain) unless a patient has clinically suspicious metastatic disease. For women diagnosed with breast cancer in 2001 and 2002 the National Cancer Database reports a 93% five-year survival rate overall for women with Stage 0 breast cancer and figures of 88%, 81%, and 74% for Stage I, IIa, and IIb respectively (34).

Increasing understanding of the microbiology of breast tumors has led to categorization of several distinct subtypes of breast cancer that are each recognized to have their own patterns of behavior. The molecular fingerprint of a tumor is being used as a tool to determine the innate aggressiveness of a tumor and has prognostic significance. For example, triple-negative breast cancer is one tumor subtype which is characterized by being estrogen receptor negative, progesterone receptor negative, and HER2 negative. This triple-negative subtype is typically aggressive, with a relatively poor outcome even after treatment. In a cohort study designed to compare women with triple-negative disease to those with non-triple negative breast cancer, the former had an increased likelihood of distant recurrence (HR = 2.6; 95% CI 2.0–3.5; P < 0.0001) and death (HR = 3.2; 95% CI 2.3–4.5; P < 0.001) within five years of diagnosis. The pattern of recurrence was seen to peak earlier in the triple-negative group of women at approximately three years and then declined thereafter (35). In contrast, tubular and mucinous carcinomas have been shown to be associated with better prognostic features and a favorable biologic phenotype compared with infiltrating ductal carcinomas of no special type. Indeed, the survival of patients with tubular and mucinous carcinomas is similar to that of the general population (36).

The TNM staging system will continue to be revised and may even become obsolete as more is learned about the biological nature of breast cancer. The advent of high-throughput genotyping technology is leading to personalized cancer care and tailored treatments to an individual patient's biology. As more efforts are being aimed at uncovering the cause of breast cancer, prevention may replace early diagnosis and prognosis as the central tenet in breast cancer care.

SURVEILLANCE AND FOLLOW-UP

Surveillance should continue after diagnosis and treatment of early breast cancer in order to detect local recurrence or a new primary breast cancer in either the ipsilateral or contralateral breast. In accordance with the recommendations of the National Comprehensive Cancer Network (NCCN version 2.2011) mammography should be performed annually for patients undergoing BCS and physicians should perform a physical examination at intervals of four to six months to look for evidence of local recurrence and symptoms of metastatic disease (37). The ipsilateral arm should be evaluated to detect early signs of lymphedema and initiate appropriate management. The use of dedicated breast MRI may be used as an option for follow-up surveillance in those women who are at high risk of bilateral disease, such as BRCA-mutation carriers. The American Cancer Society currently makes no recommendation either for or against screening MRI in BRCA-negative women with a personal history of breast cancer.

A significant proportion of local recurrences are first detected by the patient or on clinical examination. During the follow-up period, patients should be informed about the importance of self-reporting symptoms and the limited value of routine blood tests and radiographic studies other than annual mammography. Besides a routine follow-up with history and physical examination together with yearly mammography for any retained breast tissue, optimal surveillance includes monitoring for tamoxifen-related endometrial carcinoma and bone health in women experiencing a treatment-related menopause or receiving an aromatase inhibitor (37).

Long-term follow-up studies have shown that the most common sites of recurrent disease are local soft tissue, bone, lung, liver, and brain. Guidelines do not recommend surveillance radiographs, blood counts, biochemistry, tumor markers or radionuclide scans in the asymptomatic patient. Furthermore, there is no evidence of improved survival from early detection of distant metastases (38). Conversely, patients with symptoms or physical findings suggestive of locoregional or distant relapse, or worrying abnormalities on follow-up mammography warrant a full workup and further evaluation with appropriate investigations.

REFERENCES

1. Greene FL III, Trotti A, Fritz AG, et al. eds. AJCC Cancer Staging Handbook, 7th edn. Chicago, IL: American Joint Committee on Cancer, 2010.
2. Singletary SE, Allred C, Ashley P, et al. Revision of the American joint committee on cancer staging system for breast cancer. J Clin Oncol 2002; 20: 3628–36.
3. Simmons R, Osborne M. In: Moran W, Rovere Q, eds. Surgical Treatment of Early Invasive Breast Cancer. Early Breast Cancer, 2nd edn. Taylor and Francis Publishers, 2005: 375–80.
4. US Preventive Services Task Force. Screening for breast cancer: U.S. Preventive Services Task Force recommendation statement. Ann Intern Med 2009; 151: 716–26; W-236.
5. Smith RA, Cokkinides V, Brooks D, et al. Cancer screening in the United States, 2010: a review of current American Cancer Society guidelines and issues in cancer screening. CA Cancer J Clin 2010; 60: 99–119.
6. Nelson HD, Tyne K, Naik A, et al. Screening for breast cancer: an update for the U.S. Preventive Services Task Force. Ann Intern Med 2009; 151: 727–37; W237-42.
7. Mandelson MT, Oestreicher N, Porter PL, et al. Breast density as a predictor of mammographic detection: comparison of interval- and screen-detected cancers. J Natl Cancer Inst 2000; 92: 1081–7.
8. Berg WA, Blume JD, Cormack JB, et al. Combined screening with ultrasound and mammography vs mammography alone in women at elevated risk of breast cancer. JAMA 2008; 299: 2151–63.
9. Solin LJ, Orel SG, Hwang WT, et al. Relationship of breast magnetic resonance imaging to outcome after breast-conservation treatment with radiation for women with early-stage invasive breast carcinoma or ductal carcinoma in situ. J Clin Oncol 2008; 26: 386–91.
10. Peters NH, van Esser S, van den Bosch MA, et al. Preoperative MRI and surgical management in patients with nonpalpable breast cancer: the MONET - randomised controlled trial. Eur J Cancer 2011; 47: 879–86.
11. Revesz E, Khan SA. What are safe margins of resection for invasive and in situ breast cancer? Oncology 2011; 25: 890–5.

12. Azu M, Abrahamse P, Katz SJ, et al. What is an adequate margin for breast conserving surgery? surgeon attitudes and correlates. Ann Surg Oncol 2010; 17: 558–63.

13. McCahill LE, Single RM, Aiello Bowles EJ, et al. Variability in reexcision following breast conservation surgery. JAMA 2012; 307: 467–75.

14. Singletary SE. Surgical margins in patients with early stage breast cancer treated with breast conservation therapy. Am J Surg 2002; 184: 383–93.

15. Fisher B, Montague F, Redmond C, et al. Ten year results of a randomized trial comparing radical mastectomy and total mastectomy with or without irradiation. N Engl J Med 1985; 312: 674–81.

16. Fisher B, Jeong JH, Anderson S, et al. Twenty-five-year follow-up of a randomized trial comparing radical mastectomy, total mastectomy, and total mastectomy followed by irradiation. N Engl J Med 2002; 347: 567–75.

17. Mamounas EP. NSABP breast cancer clinical trials: recent results and future directions. Clin Med Res 2003; 1: 309–26.

18. Fisher B, Anderson S, Bryant J, et al. Twenty-year follow-up of a randomized trial comparing total mastectomy, lumpectomy, and lumpectomy plus irradiation for the treatment of invasive breast cancer. N Engl J Med 2002; 347: 1233–41.

19. Tuttle TM, Habermann EB, Grund EH, et al. Increasing use of contralateral prophylactic mastectomy for breast cancer patients: a trend toward more aggressive surgical treatment. J Clin Oncol 2007; 25: 5203–9.

20. King TA, Gurevich I, Sakr R, et al. Occult malignancy in patients undergoing contralateral prophylactic mastectomy. Ann Surg 2011; 254: 2–7.

21. King TA, Sakr R, Patil S, et al. Clinical management factors contribute to the decision for contralateral prophylactic mastectomy. J Clin Oncol 2011; 29: 2158–64.

22. Fitzgibbons PL, Page DL, Weaver D, et al. Prognostic factors in breast cancer. College of American Pathologists Consensus Statement 1999. Arch Pathol Lab Med 2000; 124: 966–78.

23. Mabry H, Giuliano AE. Sentinel node mapping for breast cancer: progress to date and prospects for the future. Surg Oncol Clin N Am 2007; 16: 55–70.

24. Giuliano AE, McCall L, Beitsch P, et al. Locoregional recurrence after sentinel lymph node dissection with or without axillary dissection in patients with sentinel lymph node metastases: the American College of Surgeons Oncology Group Z0011 randomized trial. Ann Surg 2010; 252: 426–32.

25. Krag DN, Anderson SJ, Julian TB, et al. Sentinel-lymph-node resection compared with conventional axillary-lymph-node dissection in clinically node-negative patients with breast cancer: overall survival findings from the NSABP B-32 randomised phase 3 trial. Lancet Oncol 2010; 11: 927–33.

26. Benson JR. An alternative to axillary lymph node dissection. Lancet Oncol 2010; 11: 908–9.

27. Giuliano AE, Hawes D, Ballman KV, et al. Association of occult metastases in sentinel lymph nodes and bone marrow with survival among women with early-stage invasive breast cancer. JAMA 2011; 306: 385–93.

28. Giuliano AE, Hunt KK, Ballman KV, et al. Axillary dissection vs no axillary dissection in women with invasive breast cancer and sentinel node metastasis: a randomized clinical trial. JAMA 2011; 305: 569–75.

29. Morrow M, Giuliano AE. To cut is to cure: can we really apply Z11 in practice? Ann Surg Oncol 2011; 18: 2413–15.

30. Kaufman CS, Bachman B, Littrup PJ, et al. Cryoablation treatment of benign breast lesions with 12-month follow-up. Am J Surg 2004; 188: 340–8.

31. Sabel MS, Kaufman CS, Whitworth P, et al. Cryoablation of early-stage breast cancer: work-in-progress report of a multi-institutional trial. Ann Surg Oncol 2004; 11: 542–9.

32. ACOSOG Z1072: A Phase II Trial Exploring the Success of Cryoablation Therapy in the Treatment of Invasive Breast Carcinoma. NCI Clinical Trials.

33. Goldhirsch A, Ingle JN, Gelber RD, et al. Thresholds for therapies: highlights of the St Gallen International Expert Consensus on the primary therapy of early breast cancer 2009. Ann Oncol 2009; 20: 1319–29.

34. American Cancer Society. Cancer Facts and Figures 2011. Atlanta, GA: 2011.

35. Dent R, Trudeau M, Pritchard KI, et al. Triple-negative breast cancer: clinical features and patterns of recurrence. Clin Cancer Res 2007; 13: 4429–34.

36. Diab S, Clark G, Osborne C, et al. Tumor characteristics and clinical outcome of tubular and mucinous breast carcinomas. J Clin Oncol 1999; 17: 1442–8.

37. Carlson RW, Allred DC, Anderson BO, et al. The NCCN invasive breast cancer clinical practice guidelines in oncology. J Natl Compr Cancer Netw 2011; 9: 136–222.

38. Leitner SP, Swern AS, Weinberger D, et al. Predictors of recurrence for patients with small (one centimeter or less) localized breast cancer (T1a,b N0 M0). Cancer 1995; 76: 2266–74.

36 The optimum resection margin in breast conservation surgery

Lisa Newman and Jessica Bensenhaver

The application of population-based screening and surveillance mammography over the past three decades has resulted in an increased incidence of clinically occult, early-stage breast cancer. Subsequent evolution in treatment and management, supported by multiple prospective randomized trials with up to 20 years follow-up, has resulted in the use of breast conserving therapy (BCT) as the treatment standard, with established equivalent survival to mastectomy (1–8). BCT, defined as partial mastectomy with negative margins and whole-breast radiotherapy, was further sanctified in 1990 when the Consensus Conference of Breast Cancer from the National Institutes of Health recommended breast-conserving surgery followed by radiation as the preferred treatment for stages I and II breast cancer (9).

IMPACT OF MARGIN STATUS

It is well established that BCT patients hold a lifelong risk of local recurrence (LR), supported by many studies that have correlated LR and involved margins (10–13). This knowledge led to the notion that LR rates could be reduced by removing a larger volume of tissue either at the primary surgery or at the time of re-excision for margin control. However, cosmetic outcome is directly correlated with the volume of resected breast (14). With a goal of balancing LR and cosmesis, optimal margin width and margin assessment have been areas of study and debate for years.

As surgeon experience has grown, LR rates have declined steadily and are now less than 8% at 10 years of follow-up (15). Moreover, BCT treatment guidelines indicate a clear importance of adequate margin assessment noting positive margins as a frequent indication for further surgery (16). Despite decades of experience, improved technique, and known guidelines, there is no standard definition of a negative margin for breast conserving surgery. The result is a highly debated field focused at establishing a standard tumor-free resection margin, thereby maximizing local control and cosmetic outcome.

INVASIVE MAMMARY CARCINOMA
Positive Tumor Margins and LR

Over 20 years of follow-up has confirmed that positive margins result in higher rates of ipsilateral breast tumor recurrence (IBTR) (17). In 2002, a review by Singletary examined published reports addressing the clinical significance of margin width (18). Table 36.1 presents a representative sample of the available studies reviewed (11,19–51). A mean follow-up of 91 months revealed crude IBTR rates of 15.8% in cases with positive margins and 5.6% for those with free margins (as defined by tumor not touching ink) (18). Addressing the relationship between follow-up time and LR as a function of surgical margin status (using margins defined as greater than 2 mm), negative margins showed no significant change in LR rates at follow-up times ranging from 36 to 120 months ($r = -0.31$, $P = 0.35$). For positive margins, however, LR rates increased significantly with increasing follow-up times ($r = 0.75$, $P = 0.008$), thus suggesting that the adverse effects of positive margins on LR may increase over time (18).

Margin Width and LR

It is intuitive that LR could be decreased by excising a wider tissue margin around an invasive tumor; however, close margins (as defined by independent studies ranging from 1 to 3 mm) do not show consistent evidence to suggest improved local control. Table 36.1 shows no clear difference in LR rates in cases with negative surgical margins based on margin widths of 1 mm (0–7%), 2 mm (3–10%), and microscopically negative margins (2–4%) (11,18,19,32–51).

The National Surgical Adjuvant Breast and Bowel Project (NSABP) B06 trial was the prospective, randomized trial that established BCT as a suitable management option for early-stage breast cancer (7). In this trial, microscopically negative margins were defined as no tumor touching ink without specific width measurement data; no useful information can therefore be elicited from these data in regard to the effect of margin width on LR rate. Singletary's review did not suggest a relationship between margin width and rate of LR; however, it should be noted that the review included only retrospective studies and one can only anticipate uncontrolled variation between these studies in regard to factors known to influence IBTR such as systemic therapy (18).

Close Margins and LR

When addressing the impact of close margins (less than the defined negative margin width but no tumor touching ink), Singletary identified 10 studies shown in Table 36.2 that reported LR as a function of negative, positive, and close margins (11,24,34,35,40,42,43,47,52,53). The results were varied with 3 of 10 showing equivalent recurrence between close and negative margins (34,35,47), 2 of 10 showing equivalent LR between close and positive margins (40,43), one showing no difference in LR across the board (42), and the remaining four had intermediate findings (11,24,52,53). Not controlling for factors known to influence IBTR could partially explain these variable findings. Through multivariate analysis, a study from MD Anderson identified independent predictors of locoregional recurrence [young age (<50), large tumor size, positive lymph nodes, omission of chemotherapy, and/or hormonal

Table 36.1 Local Recurrence as a Function of Surgical Margin in Patients with Invasive Breast Carcinoma Treated with Breast Conservation Therapy (20)

Margin Assessment	Author (Reference)	No. of Patients	Follow-Up (Months)	Local Recurrence (%)	
				Negative Margin	Positive Margin
Positive vs. negative[a]	Cooke et al. 1995 (20)	44	50	3	13
	Pierce et al. 1997 (21)	396	60	3	10
	Heimann et al. 1996 (22)	869	60	2	11
	Burke et al. 1995 (23)	306	60	2	15
	Slotman et al. 1994 (24)	514	68	5	10
	LeBorgne et al. 1995 (25)	817	75	9	6
	Veronesi et al. 1995 (26)	289	79	9	17
	Van Dongen et al. 1992 (27)	431	96	9	20
	Fourquet et al. 1989 (28)	518	103	8	29
	Clarke et al. 1985 (29)	436	120	4	10
	DiBiase et al. 1998 (30)	453	120	13	31
	Mansfield et al. 1995 (31)	704	120	8	16
Negative >1 mm	Assersohn et al. 1999 (33)	184	57	0	3
	Recht et al. 1996 (32)	134	58	3	22
	Schnitt et al. 1994 (11)	181	60	0	21
	Gage et al. 1996 (34)	343	109	3	16[b]
	Park et al. 2000 (35)	533	127	7	19[c]
Negative >2 mm	Hallahan et al. 1989 (36)	219	36	5	9
	Solin et al. 1991 (37)	697	60	3	0
	Markiewicz et al. 1998 (38)	210	72	10	4
	Petersen et al. 1999 (39)	1021	73	8	10
	Freedman et al. 1999 (40)	480	76	7	12
	Wazer et al. 1999 (41)	509	86	4	16
	Touboul et al. 1999 (42)	528	84	6	8
	Smitt et al. 1995 (43)	303	120	2	22
	Dewar et al. 1995 (44)	663	120	6	14
	Obedien et al. 1999 (45)	984	120	2	18
	Kini et al. 1998 (46)	400	120	6	17
Negative >3 mm	Pittinger et al. 1994 (47)	183	54	3	25
Negative >5 mm	Horiguchi et al. 1999 (48)	161	47	1	11
	Schmidt-Ulrich et al. 1989 (19)	108	60	0	0
Microscopic	Spivack et al. 1994 (49)[d]	258	48	4	18
	Borger et al. 1991 (50)[e]	723	66	2	16
	Bartelinke et al. 1988 (51)[e]	585	72	2	9

Positive margins are defined as tumor cells appearing at the cut edge of the excised specimen.
[a]Negative margins not defined quantitatively.
[b]Local recurrence: 9% with focally positive margin, 28% with extensively positive margin.
[c]Local recurrence: 14% with focally positive margin, 27% with extensively positive margin.
[d]Negative margin defined as no microscopic foci of tumor cells at inked margins.
[e]Negative margins defined as greater than one microscopic field.

therapy in addition to surgical margin status] (54). Singletary found that many of these factors varied among the studies that were reviewed, with an expected influence on clinical trends. This observation further highlights the uncertainty that persists regarding the possible clinical significance of close margins, thus encouraging a conservative approach to ensuring clean margins (18).

Final Margin Recommendation for Invasive Mammary Carcinoma

From a clinical perspective, the optimal negative margin for BCT is one that results in an IBTR rate equivalent to, or better than, that seen after mastectomy (55). Successful BCT requires balancing this goal with acceptable cosmetic results. To date there is no universal definition of a negative microscopic margin. In 2010, consensus recommendations for locoregional treatment were collectively prepared and approved by an international expert panel (54). Although a large number of studies show higher rates of IBTR with positive margins, consistent evidence is lacking to support margins wider than tumor not touching ink resulting in any decrease in IBTR; moreover, a 10-year local control rate of 95% is reported when using this definition in patients receiving systemic therapy (56). The panel acknowledged that larger margins may be considered in selected cases based on clinical circumstances, but they are not routinely warranted and should be considered in the context of multiple factors known to influence local control (18,55). In the presence of inconsistent evidence, the final panel consensus endorsed the standard definition of an adequate negative margin in patients with invasive cancer as "tumor not touching ink" (57).

Table 36.2 Local Recurrence as a Function of Close, Positive, and Negative Surgical Margins in Patients with Stage I/II Invasive Ductal Carcinoma Treated with Breast Conservation Therapy (20)

Author (Reference)	Median Age	No. of Patients by Margin Assessment	Diagnosis Summary[a]	Treatment	Median Follow-Up (Months)	Local Recurrence (%)		
						Negative Margin	Close Margin	Positive Margin
Negative margin defined as >1 mm								
Recht et al. 1996 (32)	45	37 positive 28 close 69 negative	High risk	45 Gy + 16–18 Gy boost: all had chemo: 50% had chemo before XRT	45	3	11	22
Gage et al. 1996 (34)	53	131 positive 54 close 107 negative	57% T1 57% NO	45 Gy + 15 Gy boost: chemo in 31%: tamoxifen in 5%	109	3	2	16[b]
Park et al. 2000 (35)	53	188 positive 94 close 204 negative	61% T1 40% NO	Total (including boost) 60–72.5 Gy: not adjusted by margin status. Chemo in 35%, adjusted by margin status	123	7	7	19
Negative margin defined as >2 mm								
Touboul et al. 1999 (42)	53	13 positive 21 close 417 negative	79% T1 96% NO	45–50 Gy + 15 Gy boost: chemo in 22%: tamoxifen in 33%	84	6	6	8
Smitt et al. 1995 (43)	48	24 positive 17 close 157 negative	75% T1 75% NO	44–65 Gy + 2–35 Gy boost: chemo in 28%: tamoxifen in 19%	120	2	24	22
Freedman et al. 1999 (40)	55	152 positive 142 close 968 negative	66% T1 73% NO	Total 60 Gy for negative, 64 Gy for close. 66 Gy for positive. Chemo +/– tamoxifen in 28%, tamoxifen alone in 20%: adjuvant therapy adjusted by margin	76	7	14	12
Negative margin defined as >3 mm								
Pittinger et al. 1994 (47)	NS	4 positive NS 35 close 122	NS	45–60 Gy boost: chemo/ tamoxifen based on menopausal/nodal status	54	3	3	25
Negative margin defined as >1 microscopic field								
Borger et al. 1991 (50)	50	65 positive 108 close 333 negative	80% T1 71% NO	50 Gy: 25 Gy boost for positive/close,15 Gy boost for negative[c]: chemo in 21%: tamoxifen in 4%	66	2	6	16
Negative margin not defined quantitatively								
Slotman et al. 1994 (24)	52	24 positive 30 close 454 negative	77% T1 72% NO	50 Gy boost for close/ positive: chemo and tamoxifen based on menopausal/nodal status	68	3	8	10
Ryoo et al. 1989 (53)	56	23 positive 87 close 283 negative	78% T1 66% NO	46 Gy + 14–20 Gy boost: 68/77 node-positive patients received chemo	76	6	8	13

[a]High risk: all patients node positive or estrogen receptor negative or positive for lymphovascular invasion.
[b]Local recurrence 9% in focally positive, 28% in extensively positive.
[c]All patients in initial part of study received 25 Gy boost, later changed to 25 Gy for patients with positive/close margins and 15 Gy for patients with negative margins.
Abbreviations: XRT, radiotherapy; NO, node negative; NS, not specified.

DUCTAL CARCINOMA IN SITU
Special Consideration in Ductal Carcinoma In Situ
The risk of breast cancer death after any treatment of ductal carcinoma in situ (DCIS) is less than 5%, but the risk of LR varies by treatment. Half of IBTR seen after BCT for DCIS is invasive carcinoma, therefore noting the importance of minimizing LR (54). Margin width in DCIS requires more consideration than invasive carcinoma. Small lesions involving a single duct do occur; however, the lesion is frequently seen along branches of the same duct separated by areas of normal tissue. Approximately 40% of DCIS grows discontinuously, with 85% of the gaps less than 5 mm in size (57). Because skip lesions can be wider than the distance designated as a negative margin, the accuracy of a clear margin can be impacted.

Positive Tumor Margin and LR
Multiple studies have shown that a positive resection margin in DCIS increases the rate of IBTR. By defining negative margins as no tumor at the inked surface, NSABP B24 randomized patients to tamoxifen and placebo and compared women undergoing BCT with both positive and negative margins (all received whole-breast radiotherapy). When comparing IBTR in the placebo group, the IBTR rate per year was 16.05 and 30.89 per 1000 in the negative margin and positive margin groups, respectively, thus emphasizing the need for negative margins. The use of tamoxifen in both groups significantly reduced the IBTR rate; however, the failure rate was still higher in patients with positive margins (58). Singletary also reviewed the clinical significance of margin width in DCIS (20). Table 36.3 shows LR rates as a function of surgical margin in DCIS patients treated

with BCT (59–66), and like invasive carcinoma, the LR rate is significantly higher in patients with positive margins.

Margin Width and LR
The idea of benefit from more widely negative margins in DCIS is less clear. Similar to trials for invasive carcinoma, the randomized trials used the margin definition of tumor not touching ink, therefore limiting margin width information. The known multifocal nature and skip lesions associated with DCIS have led to the suggestion of improved rates of IBTR with large surgical margins. Retrospective, single-institution studies have suggested a 1-cm margin might obviate the need for RT in DCIS (60); however, prospective attempts to duplicate this have been unsuccessful (67,68). Singletary found the majority of published reports used definitions of 1–2 mm for negative margins and noted that LR as a function of margin width was not significantly higher in the DCIS studies compared with the studies of invasive carcinoma (5.3 vs. 4.6, respectively, $P = 0.59$).

A meta-analysis by Dunne et al. in 2009 reviewed both randomized and nonrandomized published works looking at patients with DCIS treated by breast conservation surgery and radiation (12). Their findings showed a higher rate of IBTR with margin definitions of 1 mm or no tumor on ink; however, a margin definition of 2 mm or greater showed no significant increase in IBTR. Although significant in suggesting an ideal width of 2 mm, it should be noted that the absolute crude rate of IBTR was still low in all groups. Table 36.4 summarizes the results from this meta-analysis of clinical studies of DCIS treated by breast conservation (12).

Table 36.3 Local Recurrence as a Function of Surgical Margin in Patients with Ductal Carcinoma In Situ Treated with Breast Conservation Therapy (20)

Margin Assessment	Author (Reference)	No. of Patients	Follow-Up (Months)	Local Recurrence (%) Negative Margin	Local Recurrence (%) Positive Margin
Positive vs. negative[a]	Fisher et al. 1995 (61)	299	60	4	10[b]
Negative >1 mm	Holland et al. 1998 (62)	129	35	2	36
	Cheng et al. 1997 (63)	232	45	4	5
	Silverstein et al. 1999 (60)	173	92	15[c]	29[d]
Negative >2 mm	Fowble et al. 1997 (64)	110	64	1	5[d]
	Vicini et al. 2001 (59)	148	86	6	13
	Weng et al. 2000 (65)	88	100	4	31
	Solin et al. 2001 (66)	418	113	9	24
Negative ≥10 mm	Silverstein et al. 1999 (60)	113	92	3	29[d]

Positive margins are defined as tumor cells appearing directly at the cut edge of the excised specimen.
[a]Negative margins not defined quantitatively.
[b]Positive or unknown margins.
[c]Negative margins 1 to <10 mm wide.
[d]Close or positive.

Table 36.4 Meta-Analysis of the Impact of Margin Width on Ipsilateral Breast Tumor Recurrence (IBTR) in Ductal Carcinoma In Situ (17)

Number of Patients	Margin	Crude IBTR (%)	Odds Ratio Vs. 0.5 mm	*p* Value
914	No tumor on ink	9.4	2.56 (1.1–7.3)	<0.05
1239	1 mm	10.4	2.89 (1.3–8.1)	<0.05
207	2 mm	5.8	1.51 (0.51–5.0)	NS
154	≥5 mm	3.9	1	

Abbreviation: NS, not significant.
Source: From Ref. (12).

Final Margin Recommendation for DCIS

The 2010 international expert panel consensus for locoregional treatment in DCIS referenced the meta-analysis by Dunne and recommended margins greater than 2 mm in patients receiving RT (12). Margins less than 2 mm are not an absolute indication for mastectomy but should be considered along with other factors known to influence IBTR, such as the amount of DCIS close to the margin, young patient age, and the findings of a post-excision mammogram (strongest predictors are age less than 40 years and positive margins of resection) (54).

OTHER FACTORS TO CONSIDER
Pathologic Evaluation of Margins

There are components of margin evaluation that must be recognized as areas of potential variation that should be taken into account when assessing margins and resection adequacy. Morrow reviewed available evidence in 2009 and noted factors to consider in margin evaluation. First, there is no benchmark regarding the number of pathologic sections that should be examined to optimize specimen evaluation. Furthermore, current techniques for margin assessment include both perpendicular sections and tangential shaved sections. In the latter, a margin is considered positive if cancer cells are present anywhere within the margin peel sections. This can, therefore, influence the likelihood of margin positivity, even though the actual distance to ink could range from 0 to 3 mm. Lastly, when assessing surgical resection adequacy, it should be understood that a negative margin does not guarantee that no residual tumor exists in the breast (55). It is recognized that when serial subgross sectioning was used to perform detailed pathology evaluation in apparently unicentric cancers, the tumor was confined to the site of clinically evident disease in only 39% of cases (69).

The Impact of Tumor Biology and Targeted Therapy in Invasive Disease

As the understanding of tumor biology continues to develop, it becomes more apparent that IBTR is due to more than just margin status. It is overly simplistic to consider margin status as the sole determinant of IBTR (55). The Early Breast Cancer Trialists' Collaborative Group (EBCTCG) overview observed that LR after mastectomy and radiation was similar to those after BCT (70). The observation that even widely negative margins achieved after mastectomy do not completely prevent local failure indicates that some LR is a manifestation of aggressive biology rather than a high residual tumor burden in

the remaining breast tissue (55). Application of Oncotype DX to subjects enrolled in NSABP B14 identified correlation of a high Oncotype Dx score with an increase in locoregional recurrence (71). This substantiates the concept that biologic factors impact on recurrence in addition to mechanical factors and further explains the known influence of systemic therapy on recurrence risk. Lastly, the impact of tumor biology as a critical component of IBTR is further supported by the effect of targeted therapy on recurrence rate. The known 50% reduction in local regional recurrence when trastuzumab and chemotherapy are used together in HER2/neu-positive cases compared with chemotherapy alone clearly shows the importance of targeted therapy (72). This is further supported by studies showing significant IBTR risk reduction in hormone-positive patients who undergo endocrine treatment (73).

Role of Mammogram in Patient Selection

Thorough preoperative clinical assessment is critical for patient selection as other factors outside of margin status can affect BCT candidacy and should be considered (74). Mammography to deselect patients with multicentric disease or with diffuse calcifications is necessary. The postsurgery mammogram is also important to exclude the presence of residual calcifications. Mammography thus has a definitive adjunctive role to treatment, decision-making, and management; however, it should be noted that the accuracy of disease present or extent, especially in younger patients and/or those with dense breasts, may be as low as 50% (75).

Positive Margin Risk Factors

Several studies have attempted to identify patient and tumor characteristics that can classify patients as high risk for positive surgical margins (18,73). Using univariate analysis, six studies found significant association with large tumor size, younger age, axillary node-positivity, presence of lymphovascular invasion, and extensive intraductal component (35,39,45,48,52,76). However, simple univariate comparisons may not give accurate assessment of risk factors, as some may be associated with each other, as opposed to having an independent association with margin status (18). When multivariate analysis was used to gain a clearer picture, two studies found large tumor size, presence of an extensive intraduct component (EIC), and lobular subtype or ductal extensions were significantly associated with positive tumor margins (76,77). Table 36.5 summarizes these findings. Considering these high-risk characteristics is

Table 36.5 Patient and Tumor Characteristics Associated with Positive Surgical Margins in Patient with Invasive Ductal Carcinoma Treated with Breast Conversation Therapy (20)

Author (Reference)	Patient No.	Analysis	Characteristics
Borger et al. 1991 (50)	904	Univariate	DCIS, LVI
Horiguchi et al. 1999 (48)	161	Univariate	None
Obedien et al. 1999 (45)	871	Univariate	A, N
Peterson et al. 1999 (39)	1021	Univariate	T, N
Park et al. 2000 (35)	533	Univariate	T, N, LVI, EIC
Tartter et al. 2000 (76)	674	Univariate	A, H, T, DCIS, EIC
		Multivariate	T
Luu et al. 1999 (77)	235	Multivariate	T, EIC, EXT

Abbreviations: A, younger age; DCIS, ductal carcinoma in situ; EIC, extensive intraductal component; EXT, lobular or ductal extension; H, positive family history; LVI, lymphovascular invasion; N, axillary node positive status; T, large tumor size.

important when developing an operative plan with the goal of maximizing the success of the primary operation through meticulous surgery and careful examination of the gross specimen and tumor cavity, therefore balancing local control with cosmesis and maximizing outcomes.

Impact of Radiotherapy and Boost

The risk of LR following partial mastectomy is effectively reduced by radiotherapy. Breast conservation therapy includes both partial mastectomy with negative margins and whole-breast radiotherapy. The large EBCTCG meta-analysis demonstrated that two of three recurrences are prevented by whole-breast radiotherapy after breast-preserving surgery (70). An additional boost of the tumor bed can further reduce the recurrence by almost a factor of two (78). Therefore, successful identification of the tumor bed, which can be aided by intraoperative clip placement, paired with a boost as part of whole-breast radiotherapy is a component of multidisciplinary treatment that should not be compromised (79).

SUMMARY RECOMMENDATIONS

The continued success of BCT has evolved from advances in surgical techniques and pathologic analyses with the application of state-of-the-art radiation and chemotherapeutic regimens (80). Based on literature review, a definition of tumor not touching ink in invasive cancer is an adequate margin; but due to the discontinuous growth pattern in DCIS, 2 mm is preferable (54). Surgical margins should always be considered in the context of the multiple factors known to influence local control and that small differences in margin width may be a reflection of differences in pathologic processing (55).

REFERENCES

1. Veronesi U, Salvadori B, Luini A, et al. Breast conservation is a safe method in patients with small cancer of the breast. Long term results of three randomized trials on 1973 patients. Eur J Cancer 1995; 31: 1574–9.
2. Fisher B, Redmond C, Poisson R, et al. Eight year results of a randomized clinical trial comparing total mastectomy and lumpectomy with or without irradiation in the treatment of breast cancer. N Engl J Med 1989; 320: 822–8.
3. Sarazin D, Le M, Arriagada R, et al. Ten year results of a randomized trial comparing a conservative treatment to mastectomy in early breast cancer. Radiother Oncol 1989; 14: 177–84.
4. Veronesi U, Salvadori B, Luini A. Conservation treatment of early breast cancer: long term results of 1,232 cases treated with quadrantectomy, axillary dissection, and radiotherapy. Ann Surg 1990; 211: 250–9.
5. Van Dongen J, Bartelink H, Fentiman I, et al. Factors influencing local relapse and survival and results of salvage treatment after breast-conserving therapy in operable breast cancer: EORTC trial 10801, breast conservation compared with mastectomy in TNM stage I and II breast cancer. Eur J Cancer 1992; 28: 801–5.
6. Lichter A, Lippman M, Danforth D, et al. Mastectomy versus breast conserving therapy in the treatment of stage I and II carcinoma of the breast: a randomized trial at the National Cancer Institute. J Clin Oncol 1992; 10: 976–83.
7. Fisher B, Anderson S, Bryant J, et al. Twenty-year follow-up of a randomized trial comparing total mastectomy, lumpectomy, and lumpectomy plus irradiation for the treatment of invasive breast cancer. N Engl J Med 2002; 347: 1233–41.
8. Veronesi U, Cascinelli N, Mariani L, et al. Twenty-year follow-up of a randomized study comparing breast-conserving surgery with radical mastectomy for early breast cancer. N Engl J Med 2002; 347: 1227–32.
9. National Institutes of Health Consensus Conference. Treatment of early-stage breast cancer. J Am Med Ass 1991; 265: 391–5.
10. Sauer R, Schauer A, Rauschecker HF, et al. Breast preservation versus mastectomy in early breast cancer – 1991 update of the GBSG 1 – protocol and prognostic factors. The German Breast Cancer Study Group. Strahlenther Onkol 1992; 168: 191–202.
11. Schnitt SJ, Abner A, Gelman R, et al. The relationship between microscopic margins of resection and the risk of local recurrence in patients with breast cancer treated with breast-conserving surgery and radiation therapy. Cancer 1994; 74: 1746–51.
12. Dunne C, Burke JP, Morrow M, Kell MR. Effect of margin status on local recurrence after breast conservation and radiation therapy for ductal carcinoma in situ. J Clin Oncol 2009; 27: 1615–20.
13. Houssami N, Macaskill P, Marinovich ML, et al. Meta-analysis of the impact of surgical margins on local recurrence in women with early-stage invasive breast cancer treated with breast-conserving therapy. Eur J Cancer 2010; 46: 3219–32.
14. Wazer DE, DePetrillo T, Schmidt-Ullrich R, et al. Factors influencing cosmetic outcome and complication risk after conservative surgery and radiotherapy for early-stage breast carcinoma. J Clin Oncol 1992; 10: 356–63.
15. Wapnir IL, Anderson SJ, Mamounas EP, et al. Prognosis after ipsilateral breast tumor recurrence and locoregional recurrences in five National Surgical Adjuvant Breast and Bowel Project node-positive adjuvant breast cancer trials. J Clin Oncol 2006; 24: 2028–37.
16. Morrow M, Harris J. ACR-ACS-CAP-SSO Practice guideline for breast conservation therapy in the management of invasive breast carcinoma. Revised 2006.
17. Kreike B, Hart AA, van de Velde T, et al. Continuing risk of ipsilateral breast relapse after breast-conserving therapy at long-term follow-up. Int J Radiat Oncol Biol Phys 2008; 71: 1014–21.
18. Singletary SE. Surgical margins in patients with early-stage breast cancer treated with breast conservation therapy. Am J Surg 2002; 184: 383–93.
19. Schmidt-Ulrich R, Wazer D, Tercilla O, et al. Tumor margin assessment as a guide to optimal conservation surgery and irradiation in early-stage breast carcinoma. Int J Radiat Oncol Biol Phys 1989; 17: 733–8.
20. Cooke AL, Perera F, Fisher G, et al. Tamoxifen with or without radiation after partial mastectomy in patients with involved nodes. Int J Radiat Oncol Biol Phys 1995; 31: 777–81.
21. Pierce LJ, Strawderman MH, Douglas KR, et al. Conservative surgery and radiotherapy for early-stage breast cancer using a lung density correction: the University of Michigan experience. Int J Radiat Oncol Biol Phys 1997; 39: 921–8.
22. Heimann R, Powers C, Halpern HJ. Breast preservation in stage I and II carcinoma of the breast. The University of Chicago experience. Cancer 1996; 78: 1722–30.
23. Burke M, Allison R, Tripcony L. Conservative therapy of breast cancer in Queensland. Int J Radiat Oncol Biol Phys 1995; 31: 195–303.
24. Slotman BJ, Meyer OWM, Njo KH, et al. Importance of timing of radiotherapy in breast conserving treatment for early stage breast cancer. Radiother Oncol 1994; 30: 206–12.
25. Leborgne F, Leborgne JH, Ortega B, et al. Breast conservation treatment of early stage breast cancer: patterns of failure. Int J Radiat Oncol Biol Phys 1995; 31: 765–75.
26. Veronesi U, Salvadori B, Luini A, et al. Breast conservation is a safe method in patients with small cancer of the breast. Long-term results of three randomized trials on 1,973 patients. Eur J Cancer 1995; 31A: 1574–9.
27. Van Dongen JA, Bartelink H, Fentiman IS, et al. Factors influencing local relapse and survival and results of salvage treatment after breast-conserving therapy in operable breast cancer: EORTC trial 10801, breast conservation compared with mastectomy in TNM stage I and II breast cancer. Eur J Cancer 1992; 28A: 801–5.
28. Fourquet A, Campana F, Zafrani B, et al. Prognostic factors of breast recurrence in the conservative management of early breast cancer: a 25-year follow-up. Int J Radiat Oncol Biol Phys 1989; 17: 719–25.
29. Clarke K, Le MG, Sarrazin D, et al. Analysis of local-regional relapses in patients with early breast cancers treated by excision and radiotherapy: experiences of the Institute Gustave-Roussy. Int J Radiat Oncol Biol Phys 1985; 11: 1137–45.

30. Dibiase SJ, Komarnicky LT, Schwartz GF, et al. The number of positive margins influences the outcome of women treated with breast preservation for early stage breast carcinoma. Cancer 1998; 82: 2212–20.

31. Mansfield CM, Komarnicky LT, Schwartz GF, et al. Ten-year results in 1070 patients with stages I and II breast cancer treated by conservative surgery and radiation therapy. Cancer 1995; 75: 2328–36.

32. Recht A, Come SE, Henderson IC, et al. The sequencing of chemotherapy and radiation therapy after conservative surgery for early stage breast cancer. N Engl J Med 1996; 334: 1356–61.

33. Assersohn L, Powles TJ, Ashley S, et al. Local relapse in primary breast cancer patients with unexcised positive surgical margins after lumpectomy, radiotherapy and chemoendocrine therapy. Ann Oncol 1999; 10: 1451–5.

34. Gage I, Schnitt SJ, Nixon AJ, et al. Pathologic margin involvement and the risk of recurrence in patients treated with breast conserving therapy. Cancer 1996; 78: 1921–8.

35. Park CC, Mitsumori M, Nixon A, et al. Outcome at 8 years after breast-conserving surgery and radiation therapy for invasive breast cancer: influence of margin status and systemic therapy on local recurrence. J Clin Oncol 2000; 18: 1668–75.

36. Hallahan DE, Michel AG, Halpern HJ, et al. Breast-conserving surgery and definitive irradiation for early-stage breast cancer. Int J Radiat Oncol Biol Phys 1989; 17: 1211–16.

37. Solin LJ, Fowble BL, Schultz DJ, Goodman RL. The significance of the pathology margins of the tumor excision on the outcome of patients treated with definitive irradiation for early stage breast cancer. Int J Radiat Oncol Biol Phys 1991; 21: 279–87.

38. Markiewicz DA, Fox KR, Schultz DJ, et al. Concurrent chemotherapy and radiation for breast conservation treatment of early-stage breast cancer. Cancer J Sci Am 1998; 4: 185–93.

39. Peterson ME, Schultz DJ, Reynolds C, Solin LJ. Outcomes in breast cancer patients relative to margin status after treatment with breast conserving surgery and radiation therapy: the University of Pennsylvania experience. Int J Radiat Oncol Biol Phys 1999; 43: 1029–35.

40. Freedman G, Fowble B, Hanlon A, et al. Patients with early stage invasive cancer with close or positive margins treated with conservative surgery and radiation have an increased risk of breast recurrence that is delayed by adjuvant systemic therapy. Int J Radiat Oncol Biol Phys 1999; 44: 1005–15.

41. Wazer DE, Jabro G, Ruthazer R, et al. Extent of margin positivity as a predictor for local recurrence after breast conserving irradiation. Radiat Oncol Investig 1999; 7: 111–17.

42. Touboul E, Buffar L, Belkacemi Y, et al. Local recurrences and distant metastases after breast-conserving surgery and radiation therapy for early breast cancer. Int J Radiat Oncol Biol Phys 1999; 43: 25–38.

43. Smitt MC, Nowels KW, Zdeblick MJ. The importance of lumpectomy surgical margin status in long term results of breast conservation. Cancer 1995; 76: 259–67.

44. Dewar JA, Arriagada R, Benhamou S, et al. Local relapse and contralateral tumor rates in patients with breast cancer treated with conservative surgery and radiotherapy (Institut Gustave Roussy 1970-1982). Cancer 1995; 76: 2260–5.

45. Obedien E, Haffty BG. Negative margin status improves local control in conservatively managed breast cancer patients. Cancer J Sci Am 1999; 6: 28–33.

46. Kini VR, White JR, Horwitz EM, et al. Long term results with breast-conserving therapy for patients with early stage breast carcinoma in a community hospital setting. Int J Radiat Oncol Biol Phys 1998; 40: 851–8.

47. Pittinger TP, Maronian NC, Poulter CA, et al. Importance of margin status in outcome of breast-conserving surgery for carcinoma. Surgery 1994; 116: 605–9.

48. Horiguchi J, Lino U, Takei J, et al. Surgical margin and breast recurrence after breast-conserving therapy. Oncol Rep 1999; 6: 135–8.

49. Spivack B, Khanna MM, Tafra L, et al. Margin status and local recurrence after breast-conserving surgery. Arch Surg 1994; 129: 952–7.

50. Borger JH. The impact of surgical and pathological findings on radiotherapy of early breast cancer. Radiother Oncol 1991; 22: 230–6.

51. Bartelink H, Borger JH, van Dongen JA, Peters JL. The impact of tumor size and histology on local control after breast-conserving therapy. Radiother Oncol 1988; 11: 297–303.

52. Kemperman H, Hart A, Peterse H, et al. Risk factors in breast conservation therapy. J Clin Oncol 1994; 12: 653–60.

53. Ryoo MC, Kagan AT, Wollin M, et al. Prognostic factors for recurrence and cosmesis in 393 patients after radiation therapy for early park mammary carcinoma. Radiology 1989; 172: 555–9.

54. Kaufmann M, Morrow M, Von Minckwitz G, et al. Locoregional treatment of primary breast cancer. Cancer 2010; 116: 1184–91.

55. Morrow M. Brest conservation and negative margins: how much is enough? Breast 2009; 18: 84–6.

56. Wapnir I, Anderson S, Mamounas E, et al. Survival after IBTR in NSABP node negative protocols B-13, B-14, B-19, B-20 and B-23 [abstract 517]. J Clin Oncol 2005; 23: 8s.

57. Faverly DR, Burgers L, Bult P, Holland R. Three dimensional imaging of mammary ductal carcinoma in situ: clinical implications. Semin Diagn Pathol 1994; 11: 193–8.

58. Fisher B, Dignam J, Wolmark N, et al. Tamoxifen in treatment of Intraductal breast cancer: National Surgical Adjuvant Breast and Bowel Project B-24 randomised controlled trial. Lancet 1999; 353: 1993–2000.

59. Vicini FA, Kestin LL, Goldstein NS, et al. Relationship between excision volume, margin status and tumor size with the development of local recurrence in patients with ductal carcinoma in situ treated with breast-conserving therapy. J Surg Oncol 2001; 76: 245–54.

60. Silverstein MJ, Lagios MD, Groshen S, et al. The influence of margin width on local control of ductal carcinoma in situ of the breast. N Engl J Med 1999; 340: 1455–61.

61. Fisher ER, Costantino J, Fisher B, et al. Pathologic findings from the National Surgical Adjuvant Breast Project (NSABP) Protocol B-17. Cancer 1995; 75: 1310–19.

62. Holland PA, Gandhi A, Knox WF, et al. The importance of complete excision in the prevention of local recurrence of ductal carcinoma in situ. Br J Cancer 1998; 77: 110–14.

63. Cheng L, Al-Kaisi NK, Gordon NG, et al. Relationship between the size and margin status of ductal carcinoma in situ of the breast and residual disease. J Natl Cancer Inst 1997; 89: 1356–60.

64. Fowble B, Hanlon MS, Fein DA, et al. Results of conservative surgery and radiation for mammographically detected ductal carcinoma in situ. Int J Radiat Oncol Biol Phys 1997; 38: 949–57.

65. Weng EY, Juillard GJF, Parker RG, et al. Outcomes and factors impacting local recurrence of ductal carcinoma in situ. Cancer 2000; 88: 1643–9.

66. Solin LJ, Fourquet A, Vicini FA, et al. Mammographically detected ductal carcinoma in situ of the breast treated with breast-conserving surgery and definitive breast irradiation: long-term outcome and prognostic significance of patient age and margin status. Int J Radiat Oncol Biol Phys 2001; 50: 991–1002.

67. Hughes L, Wang M, Page D, et al. Local excision alone without irradiation for ductal carcinoma in situ of the breast: a trial of the Eastern Cooperative Oncology Group. J Clin Oncol 2009; 27: 5319–24.

68. Wong JS, Kaelin CM, Troyan SL, et al. Prospective study of wide excision alone for ductal carcinoma in situ of the breast. J Clin Oncol 2006; 24: 1031–6.

69. Holland R, Veling SH, Mravunac M, Hendriks JH. Histologic multifocality of Tis, T1–2 breast carcinomas. Implications for clinical trials of breast-conserving surgery. Cancer 1985; 56: 979–90.

70. Clarke M, Collins R, Darby S, et al. Early Breast Cancer Trialists' Collaborative Group (EBCTCG). Effects of radiotherapy and of differences in the extent of surgery for early breast cancer on local recurrence and 15-year survival: an overview of the randomized trials. Lancet 2005; 366: 2087–106.

71. Mamounas E, Tang G, Bryant J, et al. Association between the 21-gene recurrence score assay (RS) and risk of locoregional failure in node-negative, ER-positive breast cancer: results from NSABP B-14 and NSABP B-20. Breast Cancer Res Treat 2005; S16: abstract #29.

72. Romond EH, Perez EA, Bryant J, et al. Trastuzumab plus adjuvant chemotherapy for operable HER2-positive breast cancer. N Engl J Med 2005; 353: 1673–84.

73. Nguyen PL, Taghian AG, Katz MS, et al. Breast cancer subtype approximated by estrogen receptor, progesterone receptor, and HER-2 is associated with local and distant recurrence after breast-conserving therapy. J Clin Oncol 2008; 26: 2373–8.

74. Klimberg V, Harms S, Korourian S. Assessing margin status. Surg Oncol 1999; 8: 77–84.

75. Baines CJ, Dayan R. A tangled web: factors likely to affect the efficacy of screening mammography. J Natl Cancer Inst 1999; 91: 833–8.

76. Tartter PI, Kaplan J, Bleiweiss I, et al. Lumpectomy margins, reexcision, and local recurrence of breast cancer. Am J Surg 2000; 179: 81–5.

77. Luu HH, Otis CN, Reed SP, et al. The unsatisfactory margin in breast cancer surgery. Am J Surg 1999; 178: 362–6.

78. Poortmans PM, Collette L, Horiot JC, EORTC Radiation Oncology and Breast Cancer Groups. Impact of the boost dose of 10 Gy versus 26 Gy in patients with early stage breast cancer after a microscopically incomplete lumpectomy: 10-year results of the randomised EORTC boost trial. Radiother Oncol 2009; 90: 80–5.

79. Jurgen D, Dellas K. Margins! Margins. Margins? How important is margin status in breast-preserving therapy? Breast Care 2011; 6: 359–62.

80. Hoover S, Bloom E, Patel S. Review of breast conservation therapy: then and now. ISRN Oncol 2011; 2011: 617593.

37 Skin-sparing forms of mastectomy

Gerald Gui

INTRODUCTION

Conservative surgical approaches to early breast cancer management are established (1,2). With breast cancer awareness and screening, breast conservation rates have increased further and up to 75% of screen detected cases are successfully managed by breast conservation (3). Mastectomy is still unavoidable in disease presentation that is multicentric, after failed breast conservation because of involved margins or subsequent local recurrence. Women identified to be at breast cancer risk from recognized predisposing gene mutations may seek mastectomy as part of a risk-reduction strategy. The majority of women recommended mastectomy for early stage breast cancer treatment, localized breast recurrence, and those who choose to have a mastectomy are suitable for breast reconstruction. Factors that govern decisions on the timing of breast reconstruction as either immediate or delayed procedures take into account the surgeon's recommendations, the patient's choice, and the oncological implications of neoadjuvant or adjuvant treatment. Many women are suitable for definitive immediate breast reconstruction, with the potential advantages of establishment of a breast mound at the primary surgical procedure, the esthetic placement of shorter scars, preservation of the natural breast envelope, and avoidance of the patchwork appearance of skin replacement. An important limiting factor affecting breast reconstruction decisions and outcome is the predicted or unexpected delivery of radiotherapy based on the surgical pathology.

As conservative surgery to the breast and axilla evolved, less radical approaches to the concept of a mastectomy followed. The skin-sparing mastectomy (SSM) described by Toth and Lappert in 1991 (4) was popularized to become the mainstay of immediate breast reconstruction as initial fears of oncological safety subsided (5) and patient selection criteria for the procedure were refined (6–10). SSM followed by implant alone reconstruction, autologous tissue, or a combination of both provides the basis for good long-term oncological and esthetic outcomes. The aim is to remove the entire parenchymal breast tissue while preserving the overlying skin of the breast envelope.

ONCOLOGICAL CONSIDERATIONS OF THE SKIN-SPARING CONCEPT

Early in its history, SSM was viewed by some with suspicion. A histological study by Beer et al. on skin flap thickness demonstrated inconsistency of the superficial fascial plane, noting its absence in 44% of resection specimens and identifying breast tissue up to within 0.4 mm of the skin surface (11). Ho et al. took random multiple skin samples from 30 simple mastectomy specimens and identified skin involvement away from the central breast mound in seven (23%) samples (12). Histological findings such as these, coupled with the likely operator variability in creating the mastectomy skin flaps, led to fears of potential retained occult disease or residual breast tissue in which future disease could relapse. While theoretical increases in local recurrence risk might be expected in association with SSM, mature studies with careful patient selection show equivalence of outcome compared with simple mastectomy (Table 37.1) (5–7,9,13–15). These studies consisting of retrospective patient series are subject to case selection bias with a potential tendency to perform skin-sparing approaches for less extensive, lower grade tumors in younger patients. Patients reported in retrospective series may not be adequately matched in terms of risk factors for recurrence and type of adjuvant treatment regimens when compared with historical patients undergoing conventional mastectomy. Nonetheless, overall trends in the literature, notwithstanding publication bias, support the safety of SSM as a standard procedure in current surgical practice. A meta-analysis of observational studies that compared skin-sparing versus non-skin-sparing mastectomies found no difference in locoregional recurrence rates between the two mastectomy techniques (16). The local recurrence rates with careful patient selection, of about 7% for invasive cancer with lower risks for ductal carcinoma in situ (DCIS) (4,8,17,18), lie within an acceptable range to most surgeons and their patients. Randomized data to compare skin-sparing with non-SSM are no longer feasible as the acceptance of skin-sparing mastectomy as an established technique in now entrenched. A survey of 370 Californian surgeons reports that 90% were satisfied with the oncological adequacy of SSM and 70% considered that this approach conferred superior esthetic outcome (19).

Changing patterns of early disease detection, where mastectomy is performed for the distribution of disease within the breast including DCIS or localized recurrence rather than locally advanced breast cancer, are likely to lead to lower local recurrence rates than previously reported. A proportion of patients who develop local relapse following mastectomy presents synchronously with, or later progresses to, distant disease. Whether the risk of metastatic progression is a function of the predestined overall tumor biology of the cancer or a direct result of locoregional failure will continue to be a subject of debate but improved systemic therapy options including hormonal manipulation and biological therapies are likely to offer good long-term treatment outcomes.

SSM does not delay the delivery of adjuvant systemic therapy (20). The principles that govern the multimodal treatment of breast cancer are well established and previous or planned

Table 37.1 Summary of Studies Comparing Skin-Sparing and Non-Skin-Sparing Mastectomies: All Studies Included were Retrospective Series and Provided Adequate Information on Patient Demographics, Follow-Up, and Outcome

Author	Inclusion Criteria	Patients (*n*)		Median Follow-up, Months (Range)		Local Recurrence		Distant Relapse	
		SSM	NSSM	SSM	NSSM	SSM	NSSM	SSM	NSSM
Carlson et al. 1997 (5)	Stage 0–3	327	188	5	2	9/187	8/84	NA	NA
Simmons et al. 1999 (6)	Stage 0–3	77	154	6	4	3/77	5/154	3/77	6/154
Kroll et al. 1999 (7)	T1 and T2	114	40	>60	>60	8/114	3/40	9/114	7/40
Horiguchi et al. 2001 (13)	Stage 0–3	133	910	66	81	5/133	12/910	NA	NA
Greenway et al. 2005 (9)	Stage 0–2	225	1022	49	49	16/225	55/1022	16/225	118/1022
Ueda et al. 2008 (14)	Stage 0–3	74	178	47	54	4/74	3/178	4/74	16/178
Yi M et al. 2011 (15)	Stage 0–3	799	1011	53	53	15/799	22/1011	38/799	70/1011

Abbreviations: NA, no data available; NSSM, non-skin-sparing mastectomy; SSM, skin-sparing mastectomy.

radiotherapy in particular may influence recommendations and patient choice on breast reconstruction. Large tumors may be downsized by primary chemotherapy or endocrine therapy in suitable patients to facilitate breast conservation surgery.

NIPPLE-PRESERVING MASTECTOMY

The emerging trend to preserve the nipple–areola complex (NAC) after a diagnosis of cancer was a natural extension from the notion of SSM. Maintaining the NAC retains the character of the breast and allows women to identify more readily with their breast reconstruction. In women who have had their nipple removed, subsequent nipple reconstruction provides fulfillment of completion of the breast reconstruction (21). The human eye based on previous conditioned experience and expectation is accustomed to the presence of a nipple and socially is accepted as a symbol of femininity. The majority of patients who have lost their NAC as part of the mastectomy subsequently undergo nipple reconstruction (22).

There are limitations of a reconstructed nipple, the more obvious being a loss of projection over time, the requirement to tattoo the nipple that may subsequently fade, and the lack of sensation (23,24). More subtle details that limit a perfect match to the contralateral side are differences in nipple shape, inconsistent color match, and the inability to mimic intrinsic features such as skin rugosity or the presence of Montgomery's tubercles. Although many patients are satisfied with their nipple reconstruction, perception of a surgically created nipple by individuals can be varied. There are a limited number of studies that enable a direct comparison of SSM with or without retention of the nipple and areola. Didier et al. (25) performed a questionnaire study of 159 women at least one year post nipple-sparing mastectomy and compared this group with 97 women who had undergone SSM and nipple reconstruction. These authors found that nipple preservation had a positive effect on psychological adjustment with significant enhancement of body image and patient satisfaction. The preserved nipple at SSM often retains some sensation and maintains erectile capability and thus may be perceived to be preferable to a reconstructed nipple (26–28).

Good breast form and symmetry can be obtained with nipple-sparing mastectomy techniques that can be used to give satisfactory results with implant alone, autologous only, and combined autologous and implant breast reconstruction (29,30). When radiotherapy is given to the preserved nipple,

alteration of pigmentation may occur. Petit (28) reported asymmetry of areola pigmentation following electron beam intraoperative radiotherapy (ELIOT) in 24% of cases, with radiodystrophy leading to a hyperpigmented second contour around the areola in 7.5% of cases.

ONCOLOGICAL CONSIDERATIONS OF NIPPLE-SPARING MASTECTOMY

Studies that have evaluated the presence of histologically proven cancer within the nipple removed as part of a mastectomy report prevalence figures of up to 58% (31–48). Fundamental differences of patient inclusion criteria, methods in pathological assessment, and varying definition of what constituted nipple involvement account for the wide range of findings in the literature. Studies that included patients with obvious nipple involvement at the time of mastectomy have little relevance to clinical decision making as nipple-sparing mastectomy is contraindicated. Excluding such studies still leaves an occult cancer prevalence on histological examination of the nipple of up to 31% (37,40,42,44,48). The method of sectioning the nipple at cut-up and the number of histological sections studied may further influence the reported prevalence of occult disease identified within the nipple. The findings of published studies and the varying clinicopathological methods of assessment used are summarized in Table 37.2.

Clinical factors that may help select women for nipple-sparing mastectomy need to be based on criteria that can be assessed prior to surgery. Risk factors known to predispose to positive identification of cancer within the nipple include the tumor size, the distance of the tumor from the nipple on clinical or imaging measurement, widespread multifocality, tumor type such as invasive lobular cancer, and the presence of involved lymph nodes. Mammography and ultrasound imaging may supplement clinical assessment in evaluating tumor size, multifocality, presence of extensive DCIS, and distance from the nipple but none specifically provide information that can be easily linked to occult disease in the nipple. Histological confirmation prior to surgery may enable patient selection for nipple-sparing mastectomy and Govindarajulu et al. (49) have reported the preoperative use of ultrasound-guided vacuum-assisted biopsy of the retroareolar ducts to assess for occult disease. MRI may also be a useful preoperative indicator of otherwise occult nipple involvement (50).

Table 37.2 Incidence of Occult Nipple Involvement on Pathological Assessment in Patient Series that Excluded Patients with Clinical Involvement of the Nipple

Author	Patients (*n*)	% Nipples Involved (%)	Details of Sectioning Technique	Definition of Nipple Involvement in Relation to NAC Landmark
Morimoto et al. 1985 (37)	141	31	5 mm intervals in coronal section	Full thickness of breast beneath areola
Santini et al. 1989 (40)	1240	8	Serial coronal section to 1 cm below areola	10 mm below areola skin; included LCIS
Verma et al. 1997 (42)	26	0	4 coronal sections	10 mm from nipple tip
Laronga et al. 1999 (44)	286	5.6	≥1 sagittal section if involved	3 mm from base
Rusby et al. 2008 (48)	130	26.4	3 mm coronal sections	3 mm below areola skin

Abbreviations: LCIS, lobular carcinoma in situ; NAC, nipple–areola complex.

As some of the pathology-specific criteria may only become apparent on histological examination of the surgical specimen, useful clinical decision algorithms based on readily available preoperative information may have future clinical application. Rusby et al. (48) derived a clinical algorithm based on tumor size and the distance of the tumor from the nipple on preoperative imaging in a training set consisting of 130 patients undergoing therapeutic skin-sparing mastectomies and validated their findings in a test set of patients. This model did not describe any specific cut-off criteria, but allows an individualized prediction of risk that can be used as a template for patient discussion. Loewen et al. (51) describe another model based on the distance of the primary tumor from the nipple in 116 mastectomies that predicted nipple–areola involvement when the distance was less than 4.96 cm with 82% sensitivity and 62% specificity.

SURGICAL PLANNING FOR SSM
Patient Selection
Factors that should be considered during the patient selection process are summarized in Table 37.3. Breast volume and shape are assessed with the patient upright, sitting, or standing in front of the surgeon. Useful landmarks are the midline, the breast meridian, the inframammary fold (IMF), and the lateral and upper extents of the breast. The breast meridian is marked from a point 5 cm lateral to the medial end of the clavicle and usually includes the nipple; the marking is extended to intersect the inframammary crease and is projected beyond onto the lower chest. Useful breast measurements include the sternal-notch nipple distance, inframammary crease-nipple distance, and midline-nipple distance. The attributes of the existing breast form should be taken into account, namely the transverse breast width, vertical breast height, and projection. These measurements together with the preoperative photographs form an essential part of the patient's medical record.

Reconstructive Options
The classical clinical indication for implant-based breast reconstruction after SSM is the woman with small to moderate sized breasts without significant ptosis where the skin envelope size is maintained. If the planned breast is to be larger, the ability of the submuscular implant pocket and the overlying skin to stretch should be considered. Bilateral breast reconstructions for cancer or risk reduction can also provide a scenario for achieving good symmetry. Following SSM, implant

breast reconstruction can be planned as a one-stage or two stage procedure. The stage usually refers to the need to return to the implant pocket for implant revision or exchange as it is accepted that breast reconstruction is a process to optimize the breast mound. Planned secondary procedures include other scheduled steps such as nipple reconstruction, implant port removal, scar revision, tidying up of skin folds, contour improvement, or surgery to the contralateral breast for symmetry. With implant-based reconstruction, there is also a need to consider maintenance surgery over time.

One-stage breast reconstruction may be achieved using permanent expandable implants, with an anterior fixed-volume silicone component and a posterior variable fill saline component. The volume of the saline component can be altered through a remote port placed subcutaneously on the chest wall. Round and anatomical expandable devices are available for planned one-stage procedures. Expandable implants are not tissue expanders and should be selected only when an adequate pocket can be created, with suitable soft tissue cover to match the SSM. The expandable component allows for altering implant volume and projection as an outpatient without the need for further surgery. Optimum conditions sometimes facilitate the placement of a permanent fixed-volume implant at the time of primary surgery.

Where tissue expansion is needed to create a larger implant pocket to accommodate the skin envelope, a two-stage implant reconstruction should be planned. Following tissue expansion, the definitive implant is placed at the second operation that allows an opportunity for pocket adjustment and refinement as well as contralateral surgery for symmetry. There is a wide array of implants either round or shaped, of various silicone gel cohesive types or saline fill, elastomer texture, and properties to suit individual patient needs. The second stage implant exchange has traditionally been after oncological treatment including postmastectomy radiotherapy is complete. An emerging technique that merits further evaluation is consideration of implant exchange following chemotherapy and prior to radiotherapy. In a study by Nava et al. fewer failed implant reconstructions occurred in two-stage breast reconstruction in 109 patients who had radiotherapy after implant placement (6.4% failure) compared with 50 patients who had radiotherapy while still with their tissue expanders in place (40% failures); in the control group of 98 patients who had implant surgery but no radiotherapy there were 2.3% failed implant reconstructions (52).

Table 37.3 Factors to be Considered in the Planning of Skin-Sparing Mastectomy and Immediate Breast Reconstruction

General patient features	Body mass index
	Lifestyle including work, sports and leisure activities
	Comorbid factors, for example diabetes, hypertension, smoking, obesity, etc.
	Medication history
Oncology	Cancer parameters influencing suitability for skin envelope preservation: locally advanced disease, skin and/or muscle attachment, inflammatory cancer
	Appropriateness of nipple preservation
	Previous radiotherapy exposure
	Unilateral or bilateral mastectomy
	Therapeutic or risk reduction surgery
	Adjuvant therapy requirements including likelihood of post-mastectomy radiotherapy
Breast features	Previous scars
	Skin quality and elasticity
	Size, shape, ptosis
	Skin envelope maintenance, enhancement or reduction
	Projected final nipple position
	Contralateral adjustment
Reconstruction choice	Consideration of implant and autologous options
	Characteristics of breast native skin envelope
	Previous or planned radiotherapy
	Donor site properties: quality of autologous tissue, donor site skin, existing scars, position of incisions
	Impact of donor site morbidity on lifestyle and function
Patient understanding	Surgical oncological procedure and reconstruction
	Treatment aims and recommendations
	Expectations of the reconstruction
	Adverse effects and complications

Women with small to moderate breasts generally have a lower body mass index. Depending on the available tissue, women may choose autologous tissue reconstruction with or without implants. Women with higher body mass indices are likely to have more choices for autologous breast reconstruction without implants and consideration will need to be given to available tissue for unilateral or bilateral procedures. Donor tissue can include the back based on the latissimus dorsi muscle or a perforator variant based on the thoracodorsal vessels (thoracodorsal artery perforator); the lower abdominal tissue based on the rectus muscle (transverse rectus abdominis myocutaneous, TRAM) or free flap procedures based on the inferior epigastric (freeTRAM), deep or superficial inferior epigastric vessels or their perforators (deep inferior epigastric perforator and superficial inferior epigastric artery, DIEP and SIEA respectively); the lower limb based on vessels supporting the gracilis (transverse myocutaneous gracilis) or lateral thigh (anterolateral thigh) and the gluteal flaps based on their perforator feeding vessels (superior gluteal artery perforator and inferior gluteal artery perforator). The timing of surgery for the contralateral side if offered for risk reduction purposes may be staggered depending on the reconstruction method but with TRAM, DIEP, and SIEA flap reconstructions, a synchronous procedure is necessary as the abdominal tissue needs to be transposed simultaneously. Women who rely on upper limb strength for work or sport may be directed toward an implant reconstruction or muscle-sparing autologous abdominal option as this would avoid the potential functional morbidity that may follow a latissimus dorsi flap reconstruction.

Women with large or ptotic breasts may still be suitable for implant reconstruction by utilization of a skin-sparing volume-reducing technique through a Wise pattern approach that allows reduction of the skin envelope with de-epithelialization of the inferior mastectomy skin flap. The implant is housed in a sub-musculofascial pocket formed by the pectoralis major muscle that is disconnected inferiorly from the ribcage attachments, the serratus anterior fibers along with its fascia and the de-epithelialized lower dermal adipose flap. This surgical technique is described later in this chapter. A recent publication by Nava and colleagues demonstrates oncological safety in 77 reconstructions in 65 patients with low recurrence rates of 0.5% per year and cause specific overall survival rates of 98.2% at a median follow-up of 3.6 years (53).

Women with large or advanced breast cancers and/or multiple involved axillary lymph nodes are likely to require adjuvant radiotherapy. The use of autologous tissue may be preferable in patients who have had radiotherapy in the past. Prior radiotherapy does not necessarily preclude the utilization of an implant-based reconstruction in women where skin recovery has been excellent. Clinical decisions should be made with each patient taking into account potential benefits and risks. The risks associated with prior radiotherapy in implant-based breast reconstruction are higher rates of wound infection, implant loss, poor tissue healing, and subsequent capsular contracture (54–57).

Patients undergoing a unilateral mastectomy may require a contralateral procedure for symmetrization by augmentation, mastopexy, or breast reduction. Decisions regarding the timing of contralateral surgery as a synchronous or subsequent procedure should be taken in conjunction with patients.

Temporizing Implant-Based Breast Reconstruction
A two staged approach that bridges the gap between immediate and delayed breast reconstruction employs the use of a

temporizing implant. The technique is suitable for a patient who desires an immediate breast reconstruction but is at a higher risk of requiring, or is already known to need, chest wall radiotherapy (58). Following SSM, a tissue expander is inserted and serves as an adjustable mold to preserve the skin envelope of the reconstructed breast. The amount of saline fill can be varied to meet the size of the accommodating pocket. This technique is also known as a delayed-immediate breast reconstruction.

If post-mastectomy radiotherapy is not required, the expander is exchanged for a permanent implant early, utilizing the preserved skin envelope. Implant exchange may be considered prior to systemic treatment or, more commonly, upon completion of chemotherapy to minimize avoidable delays to oncological management. If radiotherapy is necessary, the expander is usually maintained at a constant volume to facilitate radiotherapy planning and delivery. When the breast skin has recovered from the radiotherapy, a period usually of at least three to six months, a skin preserving delayed reconstruction is performed by removal of the expander and transfer of an autologous tissue flap. Sometimes, the quality of the skin may have recovered adequately despite post-mastectomy radiotherapy to consider further implant-based options. In general, the time to the second stage reconstruction may need to be longer for an implant-based procedure compared with conversion to an autologous option.

The breast envelope overlying the implant pocket can be optimized by fat transfer procedures prior to the implant exchange. The autologous injection of adipose cells with regenerative potential can improve the state of post-mastectomy tissue and at least increases the subcutaneous fatty layer before implant exchange. It remains to be seen whether this approach modifies the long-term effect of radiotherapy on implant breast reconstruction.

Acellular Dermal Matrices

The introduction of acellular dermal matrices represents a significant development in implant-based breast reconstruction (59–62). The indications for its clinical application remain to be defined (63–65) but a recent survey of plastic surgeons in the US confirms its widespread use (66). While complication rates of seroma formation and wound infection may be high in various studies (67–70), the surgical approach and patient selection may need to be focused in order to achieve the best results. Acellular dermal matrices ultimately integrate into the tissue that it is implanted into by vascularization and tissue in-growth of fibroblasts, endothelial cells, and other stromal components, hence over time provides a natural implant cover (71,72). A window of possible failure from wound infection may occur while this tissue integration is in process and complication rates may be reduced by the use of antibiotics and drains at surgery. Meticulous attention is required in the preparation of the SSM flaps. The higher rates of wound infection reported in the early experience of acellular dermal matrices may have arisen from the overambitious introduction of the technique to women with larger breasts having implant-alone reconstructions; in addition, injudicious tissue handling may have resulted in inadvertent exposure of the subdermis or interruption of the cutaneous blood supply (73).

TECHNIQUE OF SKIN-SPARING MASTECTOMY
Preoperative Marking

Full assessment of the patient with a record of the breast measurements will have been made at the time of surgical planning. Patients are marked and measured prior to surgery with the patient sitting or standing. An indelible skin marking pen, a tape measure, and breast calipers are useful tools to indicate the midline, the breast meridian, the IMF, and the lateral and upper extents of the breast. The planned skin incisions should also be indicated.

Surgical Incisions

Many surgical incisions for SSM have been described; some of the more common approaches adopted when the NAC is to be removed are shown as line drawings in Figure 37.1 with examples of postoperative photographs of patients in Figure 37.2. Common incisions to preserve the existing skin include the elliptical and short elliptical incisions (Figs. 37.1 A, B, Fig. 37.2A), often used in conjunction with a range of extensions usually laterally (Fig. 37.1C) or vertically toward the inframammary crease (Fig. 37.1D, Fig. 37.2B). A lateral envelope approach from the periphery of the breast mound is a useful incision when the skin envelope does not require significant modification (Fig. 37.1E). It is preferable to avoid extending the incision into the superior and medial sectors of the breast that compromises the reconstructed breast esthetic (Fig. 37.1F).

When the plan for immediate breast reconstruction includes the addition of a flap of autologous tissue, the surgical excision can be designed such that the intended skin paddle of the transposed myocutaneous flap accurately replaces the area of removed native breast skin (Fig. 37.2C). An optimum SSM performed through a circumareolar incision that removes the NAC can be designed such that this circular defect on which future nipple reconstructions will be based becomes the only visible disc of donor site skin (Fig. 37.1 G–I and Fig. 37.2D). Immediate nipple reconstruction may be planned in suitable patients with well-vascularized flaps, fashioning a small oval skin paddle to accommodate the circumareolar defect, leaving a perfect circle of donor site skin after nipple reconstruction to form the new areola footprint (Fig. 37.2E) that is subsequently tattooed.

The SSM may need to take into account existing scars that have arisen from a recent excision biopsy or a previous failed attempt at breast conservation that may be longstanding. A helpful classification of SSM approaches was described by Carlson (5) (illustrated in Fig. 37.1 A, J, K, L) but broadening application of skin-sparing mastectomies has seen extensive modification to adapt to current oncoplastic approaches to obtain the best results.

Instruments and Positioning

The SSM is usually performed with the patient supine with both arms out on a board to enable access to the breast and axilla. Adequate exposure should be provided when draping the patient to view the clavicles, the lateral extents of both breasts, and the lower chest. When autologous tissue is being incorporated into the breast reconstruction, exposure will need to take into account the needs of the selected donor site. The operating table used should allow intraoperative repositioning of the patient to be able to compare the shape, position, and dimensions of the reconstructed with the contralateral

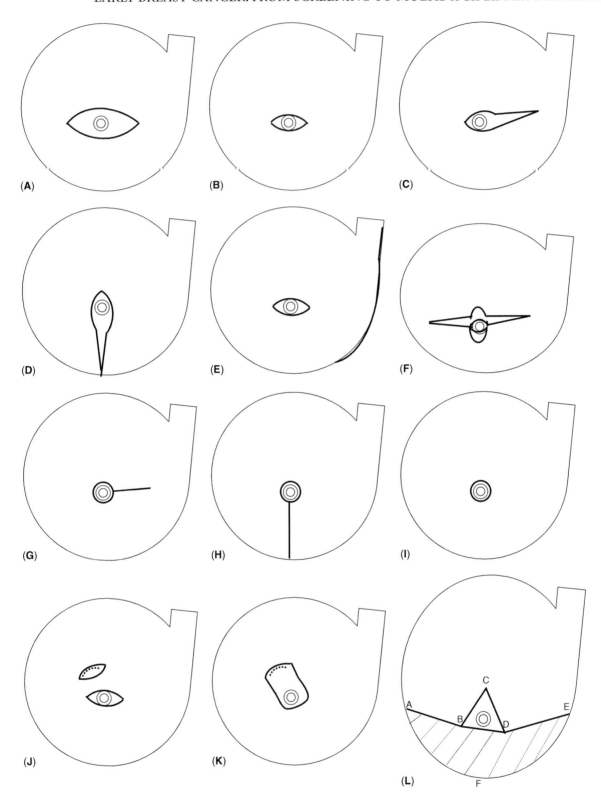

Figure 37.1 Examples of skin-sparing mastectomy incisions with excision of the nipple–areola (NAC) complex for surgical access to perform the mastectomy and breast reconstruction. (**A**) Transverse skin crease elliptical incision. (**B**) Short transverse ellipse. (**C**) Short transverse ellipse with lateral extension. (**D**) Short vertical ellipse with vertical extension. (**E**) Lateral envelope incision with short transverse ellipse to excise the NAC. (**F**) Circumareolar incision with horizontal "batswing" extensions. (**G**) Circumareolar to accept donor site skin paddle with lateral extension. (**H**) Circumareolar to accept donor site skin paddle with vertical extension. (**I**) Circumareolar incision for access without radial extension. (**J**) Short transverse ellipse with separate scar to excise previous incision. (**K**) Sector resection to incorporate pre-existing scar with NAC. (**L**) Wise pattern skin-sparing, volume-reducing mastectomy with or without de-epithelialized lower mastectomy flap (see text for description of points A–F in image (**L**)).

breast. The progressive stages of the SSM and immediate breast reconstruction can be performed with the patient supine and at varying degrees up to a complete upright sitting position.

Fiberoptic lighting or headlamps are very useful to visualize dissection through minimal access incisions. Great care must be taken to avoid trauma by traction and diathermy injury to the skin flaps. Insulated instruments are helpful when diathermy

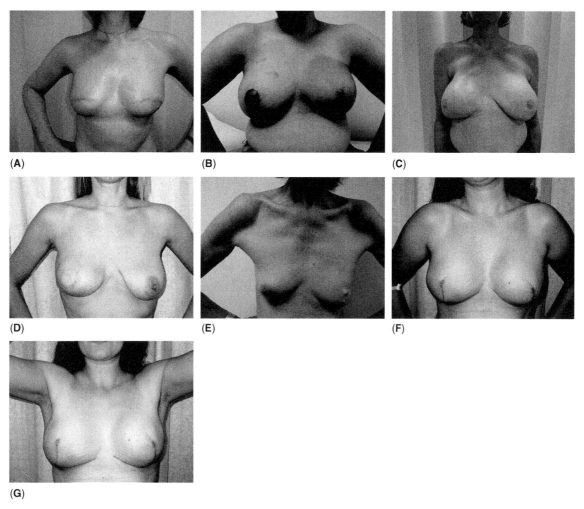

Figure 37.2 Skin-sparing mastectomy without nipple preservation. (A) Bilateral transverse skin incisions. (B) Left vertical incision with recent secondary stage nipple reconstruction and contralateral reduction mastopexy for symmetry. (C) Left implant-assisted latissimus flap through small central ellipse with nipple reconstruction and right delayed non-skin-sparing implant-assisted latissimus flap reconstruction. (D) Right implant-assisted latissimus flap through circumareola incision. (E) Left implant-assisted latissimus flap through circumareolar incision with nipple reconstruction on donor site skin prior to tattoo. (F) and (G) Wise pattern skin-sparing volume-reducing mastectomy.

dissection is used. After mastectomy, meticulous hemostasis is essential but caution should be exercised to avoid needless compromise to the network of blood vessels within the skin flaps.

Operative Surgery

At surgery, the subcutaneous plane is developed through the chosen surgical incision with the intention of removing the whole breast parenchymal tissue. Great care is taken to avoid injury to the subdermal tissue and to protect the integrity of the vascular plexus on which the skin flaps depend. Hydrodissection using local anesthetic diluted in saline may facilitate identification of tissue planes. The superior mastectomy flap is usually developed first, medial to lateral, and then the inferior subcutaneous flap is raised in a similar fashion. Preoperative marking of the upper limits of the breast is helpful to avoid over dissection into the subcutaneous non-breast tissue. When the subcutaneous plane has been fully developed, the breast can be dissected off the pectoralis major muscle from medial to lateral. Delivering the breast through the incision may facilitate the final stages of the dissection. The inframammary crease if disrupted will require to be repaired at the appropriate height and position.

Following completion of the mastectomy, attention is turned to the reconstruction. For implant-based surgery, this step involves the creation of a submuscular or submusculofascial pocket to house the implant or expander (Fig. 37.3), while in an autologous reconstruction, the focus is on transferring the donor tissue to replace the breast in the prepectoral plane and re-establishing the blood supply in a free flap or microvascular based procedure. The objectives to create the size, shape, and volume of the reconstructed breast and the intention to adjust the contralateral breast will have been preplanned.

To create a space in the submuscular plane, the fibers of pectoralis major are split 1 cm medial to the free border. The inferior surface of pectoralis major is raised off the rib cage and the dissection taken medially taking care to preserve the anterior intercostal perforators as they emerge through the intercostal spaces close to the lateral sternal edge. The medial attachment of the pectoralis major muscle should not be detached from the sternum in an immediate reconstruction. The superior dissection is taken to just beyond the marked upper pole of the projected breast mound to ensure a gentle take off of the superior reconstructed breast. For complete musculofascial implant cover, the inferior pocket is created by

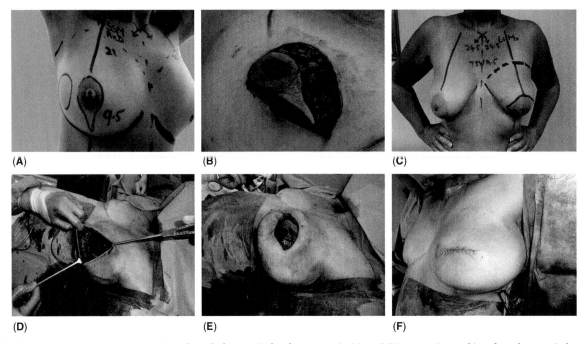

Figure 37.3 Skin-sparing mastectomy in two patients through short vertical and transverse incisions. (**A**) Preoperative markings for a short vertical scar incorporating the nipple–areola complex (NAC). (**B**) Skin incision for vertical scar approach following which the subcutaneous dissection plane is developed. (**C**) Preoperative markings for a short transverse skin incision to include the NAC. (**D**) Submuscular pocket created with adequate mobilization of pectoralis major and serratus anterior; a drain is placed in each of the subcutaneous and submuscular pockets. (**E**) Demonstration of complete musculofascial cover of the implant. (**F**) Reconstructed breast mound upon completion of surgery with a well-defined breast form and inframammary crease.

disconnecting the attachment of pectoralis major to the rib-cage from within the pocket. This takes the dissection on to a plane in continuity with the anterior rectus sheath, allowing the lower pole of the breast reconstruction to rise on the inferior implant surface. This inferior dissection should be limited by the marking of the existing or new inframammary crease. Sparing the contents of the IMF facilitates this dissection and avoids buttonholing of the thin fascia that can exist below the fibers of the pectoralis attachment. In implant breast reconstruction, if the lower fibers of pectoralis are not adequately dissected, the implant will ride high on the chest wall.

Partial musculofacial cover of the implant pocket is a recognized technique and involves a simpler surgical dissection. Advocates argue that placing the expander or implant in the subpectoral space alone allows for quicker operative time, less painful surgery, less discomfort after surgery including during subsequent tissue expansion, and better definition of the IMF. The pectoralis major muscle is dissected free at its lateral border. The muscle is elevated and detached inferiorly at its insertion. Medially the dissection is carried to the parasternal region, but the muscle should not be detached from the sternum. The free inferior border of pectoralis major muscle should be tacked down usually to the lower mastectomy skin flap as the muscle would otherwise retract providing for poor implant cover. This approach creates a breast that may be more easily placed on the chest wall and is unrestricted by the lower attachment of the pectoralis major to the rib cage. By avoiding disruption of the serratus anterior and rectus fascia, there is less muscle morbidity and postoperative pain. The technique can provide predictable and cosmetically pleasing outcomes but usually needs to be performed as a two-stage procedure. The pocket can be refined at the secondary procedure and the tissue expander exchanged for a fixed-volume implant (74). As implant cover

inferiorly may be thin, lower pole rippling can be more evident. Fat transfer techniques can be utilized as a secondary procedure to improve subcutaneous cover over the implant.

Incorporation of an Acellular Dermal Matrix
If an acellular dermal matrix sheet is to be used in the reconstruction, the dissection and creation of the submuscular pocket are simplified. The pectoralis major is freed at its lateral edge and detached from the ribs at the inferior border, maintaining the attachment at the lower sternum. The selected acellular dermal matrix sheet is cut to shape and sutured to interposition the area between the lower free pectoralis major muscle border and the inframammary crease to provide lower pole implant cover (Fig. 37.4). The acellular dermal matrix thus acts as an extension of the pectoralis major muscle, providing for an adequate sized pocket to house the implant in immediate breast reconstruction. The size of the matrix sheet, its pliability and elasticity are variable depending on product type. In the short term, the matrix acts as a barrier, adding a layer of protection under the SSM flaps.

Careful assessment of the patient and accurate breast markings to re-create the inframammary crease at the correct level is essential. The combined arc length of the IMF and lateral fold is measured to determine the length of the matrix needed. A fixed-volume implant can often be used to create a planned one-stage breast reconstruction. Expandable implants can also be used but it is unlikely that the acellular matrix itself lends itself well to postoperative shape alteration by expansion as any stretch is taken up by the muscular component of the pocket that provides implant cover.

The use of acellular dermal matrices has extended the role of one-stage implant reconstruction. Conventionally, the latissimus dorsi flap has been used to provide implant cover in this

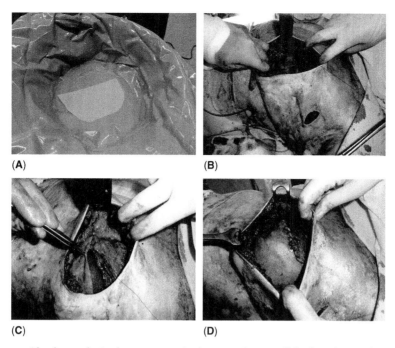

(A)   (B)

(C)   (D)

Figure 37.4 Skin-sparing mastectomy with submuscular implant reconstruction incorporating an acellular dermal matrix (ADM). (**A**) ADM sheet cut to size. (**B**) The inferior suture line securing the ADM to the inframammary crease is complete; the first suture anchoring the ADM to the medial inferior border of freed pectoralis major from its rib attachment is in place. (**C**) Commencement of the superior suture line with the implant sitting comfortably within its fully created pocket with no indentation. (**D**) ADM sewn into position, acting as an extension of the pectoralis major muscle free of bunches and wrinkles, providing a total cover for a permanent implant.

overlapping group of patients but with increasing acellular dermal matrix use, it is likely that the indications for implant-assisted latissimus flaps will decline.

SKIN-SPARING VOLUME-REDUCING MASTECTOMY

In women with larger and ptotic breasts, the use of a Wise pattern approach provides excellent access to perform a mastectomy (Fig. 37.1L). The lower mastectomy-skin flap is de-epithelialized and used to provide lower pole implant cover as an autogenous dermal sling. This approach usually results in a smaller breast mound that corrects for ptosis and is the prime example of a skin-sparing volume-reducing technique. The implant reconstruction can usually be performed with a fixed-volume device or an expandable implant as a one-stage procedure. As the implant pocket is usually pliable, gentle expansion with an expandable implant enables the subsequent creation of a larger breast than the skin envelope initially permits at the end of surgery, should this be required. Planning a two-stage procedure has some advantages of returning to optimize the pocket but may not be an essential second step as good control of the pocket can be achieved with this technique. A two-stage technique can also be used to expand the skin envelope to create a significantly larger breast with implant exchange at the second planned operation. The procedure is well suited to bilateral cases. In unilateral cases, the contralateral breast will usually require a reduction mammoplasty for symmetry. The ability to use the de-epithelialized lower flap often negates the requirement for an acellular dermal matrix in this type of operation.

Preoperative Markings for Wise Pattern Skin-Sparing Volume-Reducing Mastectomy

With the patient upright, the position of the new nipple is marked in the breast meridian, at a typical distance of 19–23 cm from the sternal notch. The markings are as for a breast reduction or mastopexy approach as the geometry of this surgery is based on similar principles. As for a reduction mammoplasty, the length of the two segments that form the vertical limb are typically 5–10 cm allowing a planned nipple to inframammary crease distance to be adjusted in relation to the height of the breast (taking into account the areola diameter) according to the esthetic requirement of each case. The angle between the limbs varies from 45 to 90 degrees depending on the amount of skin required to be conserved and the matching up of the skin reduction to the length of the inframammary crease. The larger the angle between the two limbs, the greater the extent of skin reduction. The vertical limb should align with the projected breast meridian and intersect the inframammary crease at this point, the final scar resembling an inverted T.

With expandable implants and the lower dermal flap for cover, ultraconservative skin preservation may be used by minimal skin resection between the vertical limbs. Care must be taken to avoid too acute an angle between the vertical limbs and the upper border of the dermal flap (the angle formed by CBA and CDE in Fig. 37.1L) to maintain the vascularity of the skin.

Surgical Technique of Wise Pattern Skin-Sparing Volume-Reducing Mastectomy

The lower mastectomy skin flap that forms the dermal sling is the area between the line joining the lower ends of the vertical limbs to the medial and lateral extents at which they meet the IMF; the lower border is formed by the sector circumference of the inframammary crease (shaded area in Fig. 37.1L). This area is de-epithelialized to form the dermal sling that supports the lower implant. The triangle between the vertical limbs and inferior mastectomy flap that bears the nipple is to be excised

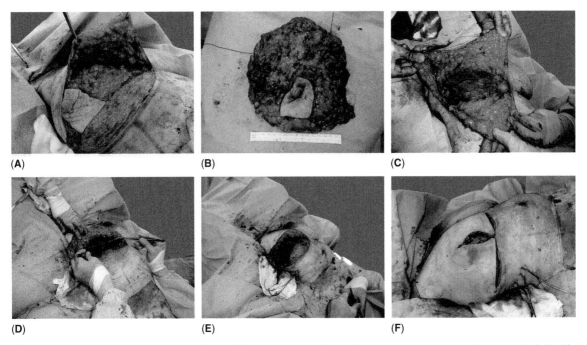

Figure 37.5 Skin-sparing volume-reducing mastectomy utilizing a Wise pattern approach providing a lower implant cover with a de-epithelialized lower mastectomy flap. (**A**) The upper flaps are raised, medial followed by lateral. (**B**) Mastectomy specimen orientated for histology. (**C**) View of subcutaneous pocket prior to raising the pectoralis major muscle to create the submuscular pocket. (**D**) Demonstration of the disconnected inferior attachment of the pectoralis major muscle from the chest wall to create the submuscular pocket. (**E**) Pectoralis major sutured to the de-epithelialized mastectomy skin flap prior to closing the lateral aspect of the pocket with the mobilized anterior fibres of serratus anterior. (**F**) Approximation of the horizontal and vertical limbs to complete the reconstruction.

with the mastectomy (area formed by B-C-D in Fig. 37.1L). The skin incision is made along the lines between the vertical and horizontal limbs (line A-B-C-D-E in Fig. 37.1L) and the subcutaneous plane developed as described for a standard SSM. At the end of the operation, the skin flaps at the base of the vertical limbs B and D meet at point F in the inframammary crease in the meridian of the new breast mound.

Operative photographs of this surgical technique of SSM through a Wise pattern approach are shown in Figure 37.5. As the upper medial and lateral flaps are raised in the subcutaneous plane, wide access to complete the mastectomy is obtained. It is also usually possible to perform the axillary surgery through the Wise pattern incision without the need for a separate incision. When the upper border of the breast is reached, the breast can be dissected off the pectoralis major and the chest wall in a craniocaudal direction. The inferior mastectomy flap is dissected in the subcutaneous plane down to the inframammary crease, the only difference in thickness to a standard mastectomy flap being the de-epithelialized external skin surface. It is essential that the vascularity of the de-epithelialized dermal flap is maintained through the subdermal vasculature entering from the inframammary crease as ischemic necrosis causing gangrene and sepsis can occur. The subcutaneous dissection meets the deep subglandular dissection in the IMF and the breast is removed and orientated for pathological assessment.

Following this, for an implant reconstruction, the submuscular pocket is created by splitting the pectoralis major muscle 1 cm medial to the lateral free border. The inferior attachment of the pectoralis muscle is dissected off the chest wall, paying attention not to damage the perforating anterior intercostal vessels at the medial extent. The lateral pocket is created by

raising the lateral fibers of the pectoralis major and some fibers of the serratus anterior with the intervening fascia between the two muscles. The implant or expander is placed in the submuscular plane and the lower de-epithelialized dermal flap is sutured to the inferior border of the pectoralis muscle and the corresponding lateral pocket to provide a total implant cover. Using an expander or expandable implant allows the inflation process to continue in outpatients facilitating closure without tension on the skin flaps, in particular at the junction between the vertical and horizontal limbs where the skin blood supply may be vulnerable. Partial implant cover by raising the pectoralis major muscle alone at the lateral free border and disconnecting the inferior attachment from the lower rib cage is also a variation of this technique.

In autologous tissue reconstruction, the donor tissue is positioned over the pectoralis muscle without the need to create a submuscular plane. The dissection to access the recipient vessels in a free flap transfer is performed as required.

SURGICAL TECHNIQUE
OF NIPPLE-SPARING MASTECTOMY

Nipple-sparing mastectomy can be performed through a range of surgical incisions (Fig. 37.6). In patients with small breasts, the SSM may be performed through a periareolar incision alone (Fig. 37.6A and Fig. 37.7A). Access may be improved using lateral or vertical incisions of varying lengths (Fig. 37.6B, C, D, Fig. 37.7B, C). If the nipple needs to be repositioned, this can be achieved by incorporating a crescentic skin excision if the movement is to be in the line of the meridian, or on a de-epithelialized ring, ellipse, or segment (Fig. 37.6G, H, I, L, N) to its new position to accommodate the planned meridian. The blood supply of the nipple must be carefully maintained

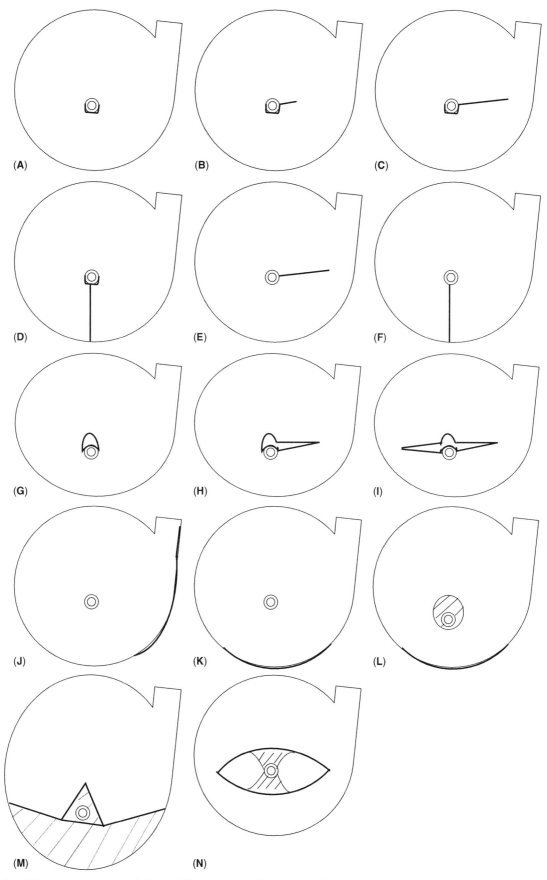

Figure 37.6 Examples of skin-sparing mastectomy incisions with preservation of the nipple–areola complex (NAC). (**A**) Inferior periareolar incision. (**B**) Inferior periareolar with short lateral extension. (**C**) Inferior periareolar with long lateral extension. (**D**) Inferior periareolar with vertical extension. (**E**) Lateral incision alone. (**F**) Vertical incision alone. (**G**) Circumareolar crescentic incision to adjust skin envelope and nipple position. (**H**) Circumareolar crescentic incision with lateral skin resection to adjust skin envelope and nipple position. (**I**) Circumareolar crescentic incision with "batswing" lateral and medial extensions to adjust skin envelope and nipple position. (**J**) Lateral perimeter envelope incision. (**K**) Inframammary crease incision. (**L**) Inframammary crease incision with sector de-epithelialization to reduce skin envelope and adjust nipple position. (**M**) Wise pattern skin-sparing, volume-reducing mastectomy with de-epithelialized lower mastectomy flap, preserving NAC on superior-medial dermal pedicle. (**N**) Elliptical incision to reduce skin envelope with nipple preservation on superior and inferior de-epithelialized dermal bridges.

on an adequate dermal bridge. The larger the increase in size or alteration in breast form from the original breast envelope the more unpredictable the final nipple position on the reconstructed breast mound can be and great care needs to be taken in surgical planning. The new nipple position must be aligned at the appropriate height in the existing or new breast meridian to match the contralateral side. Delayed nipple repositioning can be planned if the blood supply to the nipple is considered compromised.

Lateral breast perimeter or envelope incisions provide excellent access to the breast and with nipple preservation, avoids incisions on the breast mound itself (Fig. 37.6J). The acceptance of nipple preservation in some patient subgroups has also renewed interest in the inframammary crease approach (Fig. 37.6K, L, Fig. 37.7D, E). Both the lateral and inframammary crease incisions are best used to reconstruct a breast of similar size without the need to alter the existing nipple position. The use of acellular dermal matrix sheets interpositioned between the lower freed border of pectoralis major and the surgically created inframammary crease facilitates good cover of the skin envelope over the lower pole of the implant. The skin-sparing volume-reducing technique described above can be adapted for nipple preservation supported on a dermal bridge of the upper skin flap, either from both limbs of the upper half of the inverted V incision or as a rotation based on the superomedial or superolateral wing of the inverted V (Fig. 37.6M, Fig. 37.8) (75).

Careful attention to safeguarding the anterior intercostal perforators and the integrity of the subdermal vascular plexus is integral to the preservation of the nipple blood supply. As the vascularity of the retained nipple is dependent on that of the skin (76), the orientation of the surgical incisions in relation to the nipple may influence the rates of nipple ischemia. Radially orientated incisions, particularly lateral extensions may be associated with a lower risk of ischemia (77,78). The vertical extension has the esthetic advantage of being incorporated into the surgical incision of any future secondary procedure more readily and for the scar to resemble that of a mastopexy.

The nipple core may be excised by sharp dissection or using point diathermy. Intraoperative frozen section of the nipple base or nipple core to confirm a clear nipple margin of resection can be helpful. The false-negative rate of intraoperative nipple frozen section is reported to be 1–13% (79–81). Potential disadvantages of intraoperative frozen section include the distortion of tissue morphology from freezing artifact, the loss of tissue during preparation, and inadvertent false negative reporting. Final clinical decisions still need to be based on the formal paraffin-fixed analysis of the nipple core and retroareolar tissue.

The role of focal radiotherapy to treat the retained nipple in therapeutic mastectomy is uncertain. Petit et al. (28) employed the ELIOT radiotherapy to allow preservation of a retroareolar pad of tissue without compromising oncological outcome. Histologically proven cancer extension into the nipple at the time of surgery is best treated by primary nipple resection. Preservation of the areola with excision of the nipple may be one option (45). Delayed identification of nipple involvement when the results of standard histological assessment are known may pose a dilemma on further management. The option of targeted radiotherapy may have a role and may be an alternative to the more common recommendation of secondary nipple excision.

RECURRENCE RISK FOLLOWING NIPPLE-SPARING MASTECTOMY

Studies of oncological outcome after nipple-sparing mastectomy with adequate follow-up are limited by differences in patient selection and variation in adjuvant treatment regimens between studies to enable direct comparison. Earlier studies from the 1980s and 1990s appear to have a higher incidence of subsequent cancer occurrence within the nipple of 5–12% (38,82) while the trend in later studies shows a lower subsequent cancer incidence of under 5% within the nipple (80,83–86), possibly reflecting a more refined case selection for nipple preservation. Thus, with careful patient assessment, the overall incidence of future nipple cancer recurrence is small and contemporary studies comparing nipple-sparing mastectomies to skin-sparing mastectomy without nipple preservation show equivalent outcomes with both techniques (87,88).

Petit et al. 2009 (81) reported their experience in 63 patients with positive definitive histology of the nipple margin; seven patients underwent subsequent excision of the nipple and the remainder received intraoperative ELIOT radiotherapy. No nipple relapse was seen after 19 months of follow-up with an overall survival rate of 99.6% at 5 years. Benediktsson et al. reported 216 patients treated by subcutaneous mastectomies with an overall survival rate of 76.4% after a 13-year median follow-up in a study that included women with tumors larger than 3 cm or with multifocal disease that were deemed unsuitable for breast conservation (89). Horiguchi (13) reported 5- and 10-year overall survival in a study of 131 patients after subcutaneous mastectomy of 98.4% and 94.4% respectively.

The place of nipple-sparing mastectomy is likely to gain in popularity as mastectomies become more conservative. Its role in risk-reducing mastectomy is established (90–92). While concerns that a new primary could arise in both the skin and the retained nipple-areola, the incidence rate is low and few subsequent cancers, if any, arise in the nipple.

MANAGING SKIN AND NIPPLE NECROSIS
Ischemic Necrosis of the Skin Envelope
Native skin flap necrosis is reported to occur in about 10% of cases in SSM (5) and is associated with a history of smoking, vascular disease, obesity, hypertension, and diabetes; similar risk factors are associated with nipple ischemia. The complication is best prevented by careful preparation of the mastectomy skin flaps, avoiding iatrogenic diathermy injury, unnecessary exposure of the undersurface of the dermis, and interruption of the subdermal vascular plexus. Overexpansion should be avoided and implants may be deflated should the skin envelope appear threatened in the early postoperative phase.

Small areas of superficial skin necrosis can be left to granulate from below, the surface eschar acting as its own dressing. Skin loss can be managed by dressings that absorb exudates and de-sloughing agents or surgical debridement to encourage granulation. The implant is usually protected by the underlying muscle layer but partially covered implants are at a higher risk of extrusion. Larger areas of ischemic necrosis and

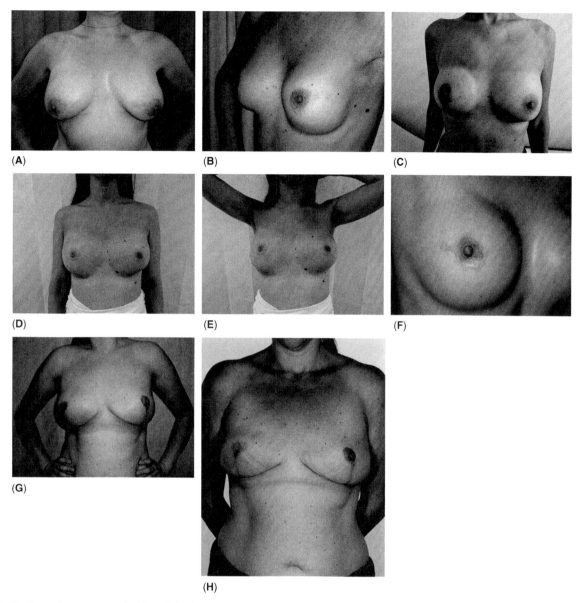

Figure 37.7 Nipple-sparing mastectomy incisions. (**A**) Bilateral inferior periareolar incisions in a woman with sizable areolas for access and immediate reconstruction using submuscular implants and acellular dermal matrices. (**B**) Inferior periareolar incision with lateral extension and submuscular implant showing a well-healed scar. (**C**) Right inferior periareolar incision with vertical extension. (**D**) Initial bilateral expanders placed through inferior periareolar incisions with subsequent exchange for fixed-volume implants through bilateral inframammary crease incisions. (**E**) Patient in image (**D**) with arms elevated. (**F**) Partial inferior areola ischemia managed conservatively with slight loss of pigmentation and Montgomery's tubercles in affected segment upon recovery. (**G**) Near total loss of nipple–areola complex managed conservatively with subsequent recovery. (**H**) Shows the patient in image (**G**) 4 months post surgery with flat nipple and some loss of areola pigmentation, on which future nipple reconstruction may be based.

full-thickness skin loss are best treated by early surgical resection. Expanders and expendable implants can be deflated if necessary or exchanged for a smaller device to hold the skin envelope while the skin loss is managed. Thorough irrigation of the implant cavity and antibiotics are needed to protect the implant. Even if implant salvage is initially successful, with significant skin necrosis, the subsequent risk of capsule formation is high.

Ischemic Necrosis of the Nipple

The incidence of nipple ischemia following nipple-sparing mastectomy is reported to be up to 10% (27,28,80,84,85,93–95). A practical guide for patients is that the risk of nipple necrosis is

1–10%, a higher risk within that range of partial necrosis and a lower risk of total nipple–areola loss. Most episodes of partial necrosis can be managed by supportive nursing care and dressings. Partial nipple loss may still recover to provide a reasonable nipple match (Fig. 37.7F, G, H). Greater degrees of nipple ischemia result in dry gangrene, which is best managed by early surgical excision and primary closure. Secondary complications following nipple necrosis include the risk of implant loss through infection and a higher rate of middle- to long-term capsule formation. Delayed nipple reconstruction can be performed when the breast mound is finally optimized.

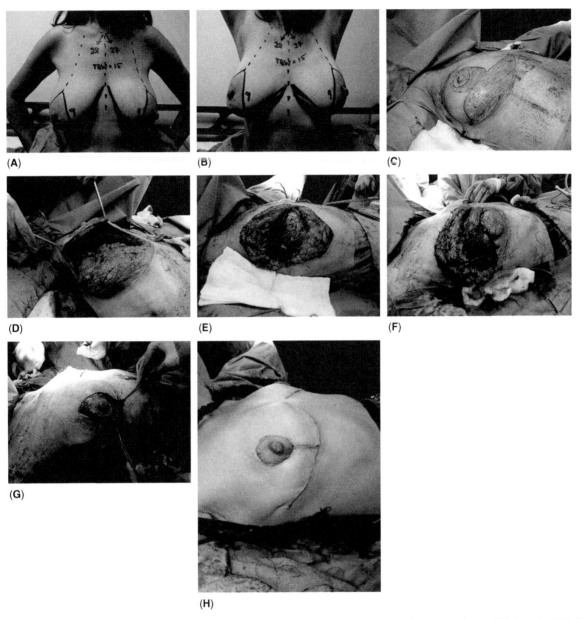

Figure 37.8 Nipple-sparing mastectomy using a skin-sparing volume-reducing technique preserving the nipple on a superior-medial dermal pedicle. (**A**) Preoperative markings. (**B**) The same patient in image (**A**) with arms up. (**C**) De-epithelialization of the zone between the vertical limbs and the future inferior dermal flap. (**D**) Completion of the superior subcutaneous dissection. (**E**) Breast removed and the de-epithelialized inferior mastectomy skin flap folded back to show the disconnected pectoralis major muscle from its inferior rib cage attachments. (**F**) Submusculofascial implant cover provided by suturing the freed lower border of the pectoralis muscle medially and the disconnected anterior fibers of serratus anterior laterally to the inferior de-epithelialized lower mastectomy flap. (**G**) Nipple preserved on superior-medial dermal bridge. (**H**) Nipple rotated on its dermal pedicle to final position on the reconstructed breast mound.

REFERENCES

1. Veronesi U, Cascinelli N, Marubini E, et al. Twenty-year follow-up of a randomized study comparing breast-conserving surgery with radical mastectomy for early breast cancer. N Engl J Med 2002; 17: 1227–32.
2. Fisher B, Anderson S, Bryant J, et al. Twenty-year follow-up of a randomized trial comparing total mastectomy, lumpectomy, and lumpectomy plus irradiation for the treatment of invasive breast cancer. N Engl J Med 2002; 347: 1233–41.
3. NHS Breast Screening Program and Association of Breast Surgery. An audit of screen detected breast cancers for the year of screening April 2009-March 2010. [Available from: http://www.cancerscreening.nhs.uk/breastscreen/publicationsbaso2009-2010.pdf]
4. Toth BA, Lappert P. Modified skin incisions for mastectomy: the need for plastic surgical input in preoperative planning. Plast Reconstr Surg 1991; 87: 1048–53.
5. Carlson GW, Bostwick J III, Wood WC, et al. Skin-sparing mastectomy. Oncologic and reconstructive considerations. Ann Surg 1997; 225: 570–5.
6. Simmons RM, Fish SK, Osborne MP, et al. Local and distant recurrence rates in skin-sparing mastectomies compared with non-skin sparing mastectomies. Ann Surg Oncol 1999; 6: 676–81.
7. Kroll SS, Khoo A, Singletary SE, et al. Local recurrence risk after skin-sparing mastectomies compared with non-skin sparing mastectomies. Ann Surg Oncol 1999; 6: 676–81.
8. Medina-Franco H, Vasconez LO, Fix RJ, et al. Factors associated with local recurrence after skin-sparing mastectomy and immediate breast reconstruction for invasive breast cancer. Ann Surg 2002; 235: 814–19.
9. Greenway RM, Schlossberg L, Dooley WC. Fifteen-year series of skin-sparing mastectomy for stage 0 to 2 breast cancer. Am J Surg 2005; 190: 918–22.
10. Spiegel AJ, Butler CE. Recurrence following treatment of ductal carcinoma in situ with skin-sparing mastectomy and immediate breast reconstruction. Plast Reconstr Surg 2003; 111: 706–11.
11. Beer GM, Varga Z, Budi S, et al. Incidence of the superficial fascia and its relevance in skin-sparing mastectomy. Cancer 2002; 94: 1619–25.

12. Ho CM, Mak CK, Lau Y, et al. Skin involvement in invasive breast carcinoma: safety of skin-sparing mastectomy. Ann Surg Oncol 2003; 10: 102–7.

13. Horiguchi J, Iino JH, Takei H, et al. A comparative study of subcutaneous mastectomy with radical mastectomy. Anticancer Res 2001; 21: 2963–7.

14. Ueda S, Tamaki Y, Kano K, et al. Cosmetic outcome and patient satisfaction after skin-sparing mastectomy for breast cancer with immediate reconstruction of the breast. Surgery 2008; 143: 414–25.

15. Yi M, Kronowitz SJ, Meric-Bernstam F, et al. Local, regional, and systemic recurrence rates in patients undergoing skin-sparing mastectomy compared with conventional mastectomy. Cancer 2011; 117: 916–24.

16. Lanitis S, Tekkis PP, Sgourakis G, et al. Comparison of skin-sparing mastectomy versus non-skin-sparing mastectomy for breast cancer. Ann Surg 2010; 251: 632–9.

17. Meretoja TJ, Rasia S, von Smoitten KA, et al. Late results of skin-sparing mastectomy followed by immediate breast reconstruction. Br J Surg 2007; 94: 1220–5.

18. Vaughan A, Dietz JR, Aft R, et al. Patterns of local recurrence after skin-sparing mastectomy and immediate breast reconstruction. Am J Surg 2007; 194: 438–43.

19. Shen J, Ellenhorn J, Qian D, et al. Skin-sparing mastectomy: a survey based approach to defining standard of care. Am Surg 2008; 74: 902–5.

20. Allweis TM, Boisvert ME, Otero SE, et al. Immediate reconstruction after mastectomy for breast cancer does not prolong the time to starting adjuvant chemotherapy. Am J Surg 2002; 183: 218–21.

21. Wellisch DK, Schain WS, Noone RB, et al. The psychological contribution of nipple addition in breast reconstruction. Plast Reconstr Surg 1987; 80: 699–704.

22. Nahabedian MY, Tsangaris TN. Breast reconstruction following subcutaneous mastectomy for cancer: a critical appraisal of the nipple-areola complex. Plast Reconstr Surg 2006; 117: 1083–90.

23. Jabor MA, Shayani P, Collins DR Jr, et al. Nipple-areola reconstruction: satisfaction and clinical determinants. Plast Reconstr Surg 2002; 110: 457–63.

24. Shestak KC, Gabriel A, Landecker A, et al. Assessment of long-term nipple projection: a comparison of three techniques. Plast Reconstr Surg 2002; 110: 780–6.

25. Didier F, Radice D, Gandini S, et al. Does nipple preservation in mastectomy improve satisfaction with cosmetic results, psychological adjustment, body image and sexuality? Breast Cancer Res Treat 2009; 118: 623–33.

26. Benediktsson KP, Perbeck L, Geigant E, et al. Touch sensibility in the breast after subcutaneous mastectomy and immediate reconstruction with a prosthesis. Br J Plast Surg 1997; 50: 443–9.

27. Denewer A, Farouk O. Can nipple-sparing mastectomy and immediate breast reconstruction with modified extended latissimus dorsi muscular flap improve the cosmetic and functional outcome among patients with breast carcinoma? World J Surg 2007; 31: 1169–77.

28. Petit JY, Veronesi U, Orecchia R, et al. Nipple-sparing mastectomy in association with intra operative radiotherapy (ELIOT): a new type of mastectomy for breast cancer treatment. Breast Cancer Res Treat 2006; 96: 47–51.

29. Mori H, Umeda T, Osanai T, et al. Esthetic evaluation of immediate breast reconstruction after nipple-sparing or skin-sparing mastectomy. Breast Cancer 2005; 12: 299–303.

30. Mosahebi A, Ramakrishnan V, Gittos M, et al. Aesthetic outcome of different techniques of reconstruction following nipple-areola-preserving envelope mastectomy with immediate reconstruction. Plast Reconstr Surg 2007; 119: 796–803.

31. Smith J, Payne WS, Carney JA. Involvement of the nipple and areola in carcinoma of the breast. Surg Gynecol Obstet 1976; 143: 546–8.

32. Parry RG, Cochran TC Jr, Wolfort FG. When is there nipple involvement in carcinoma of the breast? Plast Reconstr Surg 1977; 59: 535–7.

33. Andersen JA, Gram JB, Pallesen RM. Involvement of the nipple and areola in breast cancer. Value of clinical findings. Scand J Plast Reconstr Surg 1981; 15: 39–42.

34. Lagios MD, Gates EA, Westdahl PR, et al. A guide to the frequency of nipple involvement in breast cancer. a study of 149 consecutive mastectomies using a serial subgross and correlated radiographic technique. Am J Surg 1979; 138: 135–42.

35. Wertheim U, Ozzello L. Neoplastic involvement of nipple and skin flap in carcinoma of the breast. Am J Surg Pathol 1980; 4: 543–9.

36. Quinn RH, Barlow JF. Involvement of the nipple and areola by carcinoma of the breast. Arch Surg 1981; 116: 1139–40.

37. Morimoto T, Komaki K, Inui K, et al. Involvement of nipple and areola in early breast cancer. Cancer 1985; 55: 2459–63.

38. Kissin MW, Kark AE. Nipple preservation during mastectomy. Br J Surg 1987; 74: 58–61.

39. Menon RS, van Geel AN. Cancer of the breast with nipple involvement. Br J Cancer 1989; 59: 81–4.

40. Santini D, Taffurelli M, Gelli MC, et al. Neoplastic involvement of nipple-areolar complex in invasive breast cancer. Am J Surg 1989; 158: 399–403.

41. Suehiro S, Inai K, Tokuoka S, et al. Involvement of the nipple in early carcinoma of the breast. Surg Gynecol Obstet 1989; 168: 244–8.

42. Verma GR, Kumar A, Joshi K. Nipple involvement in peripheral breast carcinoma: a prospective study. Indian J Cancer 1997; 34: 1–5.

43. Vyas JJ, Chinoy RF, Vaidya JS. Prediction of nipple and areola involvement in breast cancer. Eur J Surg Oncol 1998; 24: 15–16.

44. Laronga C, Kemp B, Johnston D, et al. The incidence of occult nipple-areola complex involvement in breast cancer patients receiving a skin-sparing mastectomy. Ann Surg Oncol 1999; 6: 609–13.

45. Simmons RM, Brennan M, Christos P, et al. Analysis of nipple/areolar involvement with mastectomy: can the areola be preserved? Ann Surg Oncol 2002; 9: 165–8.

46. Afifi RY, El-Hindawy A. Analysis of nipple-areolar complex involvement with mastectomy: can the nipple be preserved in egyptian patients receiving skin-sparing mastectomy? Breast J 2004; 10: 543–5.

47. Vlajcic Z, Zic R, Stanec S, et al. Nipple-areola complex preservation: predictive factors of neoplastic nipple-areola complex invasion. Ann Plast Surg 2005; 55: 240–4.

48. Rusby JE, Brachtel EF, Othus M, et al. Development and validation of a model predictive of occult nipple involvement in women undergoing mastectomy. Br J Surg 2008; 95: 1356–61.

49. Govindarajulu S, Narreddy S, Shere MH, et al. Preoperative mammotome biopsy of ducts beneath the nipple areola complex. Eur J Surg Oncol 2006; 32: 410–12.

50. Friedman EP, Hall-Craggs MA, Mumtaz H, et al. Breast MR and the appearance of the normal and abnormal nipple. Clin Radiol 1997; 52: 854–61.

51. Loewen MJ, Jennings JA, Sherman SR, et al. Mammographic distance as a predictor of nipple-areola complex involvement in breast cancer. Am J Surg 2008; 195: 391–4.

52. Nava MB, Pennati AE, Lozza L, et al. Outcome of different timings of radiotherapy on implant based breast reconstructions. Plast Reconstr Surg 2011; 128: 353–9.

53. Nava MB, Ottolenghi J, Pennati A, et al. Skin/nipple preserving mastectomies and implant-based breast reconstruction in patients with large and ptotic breast: oncological and reconstructive results. Breast 2012; 21: 267–71.

54. Clough KB, Thomas SS, Fitoussi AD, et al. Reconstruction after conservative treatment for breast cancer: cosmetic sequelae classification revisited. Plast Reconstr Surg 2004; 114: 1743–53.

55. Cordeiro PG, Pusic AL, Disa JJ, et al. Radiation after immediate tissue expander/implant breast reconstruction: outcomes, complications, aesthetic results, and satisfaction among 156 patients. Plast Reconstr Surg 2004; 113: 877–81.

56. Tallet AV, Salem N, Moutardier V, et al. Radiotherapy and immediate two-stage breast reconstruction with a tissue expander and implant: complications and esthetic results. Int J Radiat Oncol Biol Phys 2003; 57: 136–42.

57. Behranwala KA, Dua RS, Ross GM, et al. The influence of radiotherapy on capsule formation and aesthetic outcome after immediate breast reconstruction using biodimensional anatomical expander implants. J Plast Reconstr Aesthet Surg 2006; 59: 1043–51.

58. Kronowitz SJ. Delayed-immediate breast reconstruction: technical and timing considerations. Plast Reconstr Surg 2010; 125: 463–74.

59. Topol BM, Dalton EF, Ponn T, et al. Immediate single-stage breast reconstruction using implantsand human acellular dermal matrix with adjustment of the lower pole of the breast to reduce unwanted lift. Ann Plast Surg 2008; 61: 494–9.

60. Becker S, Saint-Cyr M, Wong C. Alloderm versus DermaMatrix in immediate expander-basedbreast reconstruction: a preliminary comparison of complication profiles and material compliance. Plast Reconstr Surg 2009; 123: 1–6.

61. Salzberg CA, Ashikari AY, Koch RM, et al. An 8 year experience of direct-to-implant immediate breast reconstryction using acellular dermal matrix (Alloderm). Plast Reconstr Surg 2011; 127: 514–24.

62. Cassileth L, Kohanzadeh S, Amersi F. One-stage immediate breast reconstruction with implants: a new option for immediate reconstruction. Ann Plast Surg 2012; 69: 134–8.

63. Collis GN, Terkonda SP, Waldorf JC, et al. Acellular dermal matrix slings in tissue expander breast reconstruction: are there substantial benefits? Ann Plast Surg 2012; 68: 425–8.

64. Joanna Nguyen T, Carey JN, Wong AK. Use of human acellular dermal matrix in implant based breast reconstruction: evaluating the evidence. J Plast Reconstr Aesthet Surg 2011; 64: 1553–61.

65. de Blacam C, Momoh AO, Colakoglu S, et al. Cost analysis of implant-based breast reconstruction with acellilar dermal matrix. Ann Plast Surg 2011; Epub ahead of print.

66. Gurunluoglu R, Gurunluoglu A, Williams SA, et al. Current trends in breast reconstruction: survey of American Society of Plastic Surgeons 2010. Ann Plast Surg 2011; Epub ahead of print.

67. Lanier ST, Wang ED, Chen JJ, et al. The effect of acellular dermal matrix use on complication rates in tissue expander/ implant breast reconstruction. Ann Plast Surg 2010; 64: 674–8.

68. Chun YS, Verma K, Rosen H, et al. Implant based breast reconstruction using acellular dermal matrix and the risk of postoperative complications. Plast Reconstr Surg 2010; 125: 429–36.

69. Liu AS, Kao HK, Reish RG, et al. Post-operative complications in prosrthesis-based breast reconstruction using acellular dermal matrix. Plast Reconstr Surg 2011; 127: 1755–62.

70. Rawlani V, Buck DW II, Johnson SA, et al. Tissue expander breast reconstruction using prehydrated human acellular dermis. Ann Plast Surg 2011; 66: 593–7.

71. Menon NG, Rodriguez ED, Byrnes CK, et al. Revascularization of human acellular dermis ib full-thickness abdominal wall reconstruction in the rabbit model. Ann Plast Surg 2003; 50: 523–7.

72. Buinewicz B, Rosen B. Acellular cadaveric dermis (Alloderm): a new alternative for abdominal hernia repair. Ann Plast Surg 2004; 52: 188–94.

73. Newman MI, Swartz KA, Samson MC, et al. The true incidence of near-term post-operative complications in prosthetic breast reconstruction utilizing human acellular dermal matrices: a meta-analysis. Aesthetic Plast Surg 2011; 35: 100–6.

74. Spear SL, Pelletiere CV. Immediate breast reconstruction in two stages using integrated, integrated-valve tissue expanders and breast implants. Plast Reconstr Surg 2004; 113: 2098–103.

75. Rusby JE, Gui GP. Nipple sparing mastectomy in women with large or ptotic breasts. J Plast Reconstr Aesthet Surg 2010; 63: 754–5.

76. Nakajima H, Imanishi N, Aiso S. Arterial anatomy of the nipple-areola complex. Plast Reconstr Surg 1995; 96: 843–5.

77. Wijayanayagam A, Kumar AS, Foster RD, et al. Optimizing the total skin-sparing mastectomy. Arch Surg 2008; 143: 38–45.

78. Regolo L, Ballardini B, Gallarotti E, et al. Nipple sparing mastectomy: an innovative skin incision for an alternative approach. Breast 2008; 17: 8–11.

79. Vlajcic Z, Zic R, Stanec S, et al. Nipple-areola complex preservation: predictive factors of neoplastic nipple-areola complex invasion. Ann Plast Surg 2005; 55: 240–4.

80. Crowe JP, Patrick RJ, Yetman RJ, et al. Nipple-sparing mastectomy update: one hundred forty-nine procedures and clinical outcomes. Arch Surg 2008; 143: 1106–10.

81. Petit JY, Veronesi U, Rey P, et al. Nipple-sparing mastectomy: risk of nipple-areolar recurrences in a series of 579 cases. Breast Cancer Res Treat 2009; 114: 97–101.

82. Bishop CC, Singh S, Nash AG. Mastectomy and breast reconstruction preserving the nipple. Ann R Coll Surg Engl 1990; 72: 87–9.

83. Gerber B, Krause A, Reimer T, et al. Skin-sparing mastectomy with conservation of the nipple-areola complex and autologous reconstruction is an oncologically safe procedure. Ann Surg 2003; 238: 120–7.

84. Caruso F, Ferrara M, Castiglione G, et al. Nipple sparing subcutaneous mastectomy: sixty-six months follow-up. Eur J Surg Oncol 2006; 32: 937–40.

85. Sacchini V, Pinotti JA, Barros AC, et al. Nipple-sparing mastectomy for breast cancer and risk reduction: oncologic or technical problem? J Am Coll Surg 2006; 203: 704–14.

86. Paepke S, Schmid R, Fleckner S, et al. Subcutaneous mastectomy with conservation of the nipple-areola skin: broadening the indications. Ann Surg 2009; 250: 288–92.

87. Gerber B, Krause A, Dietrich M, et al. The oncological safety of skin sparing mastectomy with conservation of the nipple-areola complex and autologous reconstruction: an extended follow-up study. Ann Surg 2009; 249: 461–8.

88. Boneti C, Yuen J, Santiago C, et al. Oncologic safety of nipple skin-sparing or total skin-sparing mastectomies with immediate reconstruction. J Am Coll Surg 2011; 212: 686–93.

89. Benediktsson KP, Perbeck L. Survival in breast cancer after nipple-sparing subcutaneous mastectomy and immediate reconstruction with implants: a prospective trial with 13 years median follow-up in 216 patients. Eur J Surg Oncol 2008; 34: 143–8.

90. Ashikari RH, Ashikari AY, Kelemen PR, et al. Subcutaneous mastectomy and immediate reconstruction for prevention of breast cancer for high-risk patients. Breast Cancer 2008; 15: 185–91.

91. Yiacoumettis AM. Two staged breast reconstruction following prophylactic bilateral subcutaneous mastectomy. Br J Plast Surg 2005; 58: 299–305.

92. Hartmann LC, Schaid DJ, Woods JE, et al. Efficacy of bilateral prophylactic mastectomy in women with a family history of breast cancer. N Engl J Med 1999; 340: 77–84.

93. Margulies AG, Hochberg J, Kepple J, et al. Total skin-sparing mastectomy without preservation of the nipple-areola complex. Am J Surg 2005; 190: 907–12.

94. Psaila A, Pozzi M, Barone Adesi L, et al. Nipple sparing mastectomy with immediate breast reconstruction: a short term analysis of our experience. J Exp Clin Cancer Res 2006; 25: 309–12.

95. Stolier AJ, Sullivan SK, Dellacroce FJ. Technical considerations in nipple-sparing mastectomy: 82 consecutive cases without necrosis. Ann Surg Oncol 2008; 15: 1341–7.

38 Locoregional recurrence of breast cancer

John R. Benson and Katy Teo

INTRODUCTION

The term recurrence refers to the reappearance of breast cancer at the local, regional, or systemic level. The propensity for relapse depends upon both innate tumor characteristics and stage at presentation as well as types of treatment administered, be this surgery, radiotherapy, or chemohormonal therapy. Determination of factors predictive of relapse has been hampered by failure to distinguish between local and regional recurrence in the published literature and to separate cases of isolated locoregional disease from those with distant metastases. Local recurrence in the context of breast cancer can refer to either (*i*) recurrence of tumor in the soft tissues of the chest wall after mastectomy or (*ii*) recurrence of disease in the same breast following breast conservation surgery (BCS): ipsilateral breast tumor recurrence (IBTR).

Regional recurrence is defined as reappearance of disease within the ipsilateral axillary nodes, which may or may not involve the overlying skin. It should be noted that the current American Joint Committee on Cancer staging system classifies supraclavicular nodal involvement as regional and not systemic recurrence (pN3M0 IIIC).

The psychological impact of local recurrence can be devastating and more traumatic than disclosure of the primary breast cancer diagnosis. It can sometimes undermine the patient's confidence in her initial treatment, particularly when a minimal approach has been adopted. Breast conservation treatment has become established over the past 30 years as the preferred standard of surgical management for women with early stage breast cancer. Longer term follow-up data are now available from several prospective randomized controlled trials demonstrating survival equivalence for breast conservation therapy (BCT) compared with modified radical mastectomy.

There is longstanding controversy over the significance of IBTR following conservation surgery and whether rates of local recurrence affect overall survival. Of particular concern is the relationship to distant relapse and whether local recurrence within the conserved breast acts as a source of distant metastases or is a marker of risk for development of distant disease and de facto poor prognosis. Several studies have confirmed that local recurrence confers an increased risk of distant relapse of approximately three to fourfold (1–4). Nonetheless, for individual trials this does not translate into survival differences suggesting that no causal relationship exists between IBTR and distant disease. These findings have promoted the view that recent falls in breast cancer mortality are largely attributable to a combination of screening and application of systemic therapies with minimal contribution from any improvements in locoregional treatments.

An overview by the Early Breast Cancer Trialists' Collaborative Group (EBCTCG) revealed that moderate differences in rates of local recurrence at five years can impact upon breast cancer mortality after a more prolonged follow-up of 15 years (1). This suggests that local recurrence has a determinant role with patients developing disseminated disease as a direct consequence of failure to remove residual, but viable cancer cells at the time of primary treatment. By implication, inadequate locoregional treatment may compromise survival and it is "important to distinguish local recurrences linked to increased risk of distant spread from those due to inadequate treatment" (2).

The variable natural history and enigmatic behavior of breast cancer at a clinical level has been recognized for many years. The development of molecular technologies with genetic profiling of individual tumors has emphasized the heterogeneous nature of breast cancer and the therapeutic challenges this presents (3,4). A patient's clinical fate and overall survival are ultimately determined by the presence of distant metastases and their levels of dormancy. Competing sources of distant metastases are pertinent to some patients. If no distant micrometastases exist at presentation or have been obliterated with systemic therapy, then local treatments are relatively more important as prevention of local recurrence avoids a potential source of distant metastases. In order to gain a survival benefit from local control, there must be no significant competing risk from uncontrolled distant disease arising from either the activation of dormant micrometastatic foci present at the time of diagnosis or a greater propensity to form distant metastases due to innate biological properties of the tumor.

BIOLOGICAL PARADIGMS IN BREAST CANCER

Two dominant biological paradigms have provided a conceptual rationale for management strategies in breast cancer over the past century. These two paradigms espouse opposing views on the significance of local recurrence and the influence of local treatments on mortality from the disease. With a longer term follow-up of clinical trials and application of meta-analysis methodology, an intermediate paradigm appears to be more relevant. This encompasses elements of both the "centrifugal theory" (*Halstedian paradigm*) and biological predeterminism (*Fisherian paradigm*), which may better inform contemporary management of the disease.

Halstedian Paradigm

According to the Halstedian paradigm, breast cancer is a localized disease at inception which commences as a single focus and spreads in a centrifugal manner encroaching upon ever more distant structures with progressive and sequential spread

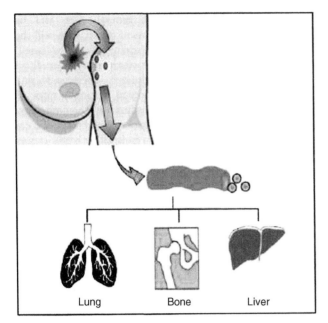

Figure 38.1 Halstedian paradigm: sequential spread of breast cancer from single focus within the breast. Lymph node involvement is necessary for hematogenous dissemination.

along fascial planes and lymphatics (5). Metastatic spread to distant organs by hematogenous dissemination is preceded by infiltration of lymph nodes which provide a circumferential line of defense and initially serve as barriers but subsequently permit access of tumor cells into the circulation when their filtration capacity is exhausted (Fig. 38.1). Local recurrence is considered to be a cause of distant metastases and the chance of cure related to the extent of primary locoregional treatment. At the extreme, mastectomy will minimize local recurrence, but acceptable rates of local control can be achieved with "adequate" wide excision and radiotherapy. Where local recurrence is a determinant of distant disease, treatment at relapse may prevent distant metastases and the timing of diagnosis and initiation of treatment is critical. Though systemic treatment has been shown to be effective in prolonging overall survival of breast cancer patients, other modalities of treatment such as surgery and radiotherapy have until recently no proven benefit on long-term survival. Nonetheless, although more extensive surgery does not improve survival for the majority of patients, there may be a subgroup with truly localized disease. For these patients, local therapy involving surgical excision (plus radiotherapy) might be curative and thus influence the natural course of the disease. Analysis of long-term survival of patients treated for stage I disease prior to the widespread use of adjuvant systemic therapy suggests that breast cancer is a locoregional process in up to 75–80% of node negative cases who may be considered statistically "cured" (6,7). In a series of patients from Memorial Sloan–Kettering Cancer Center, with node negative and node positive tumors less than or equal to 2 cm (T_1N_0 and T_1N_1), a comparison of observed to expected survival at a median follow-up of 18 years revealed that 89% of patients with node negative tumors less than or equal to 1 cm were estimated to be cured, with survival curves becoming parallel or congruent during the second decade of follow-up (0.89; 95% CI 0.80–0.98) (7). For tumors between 1 and 2 cm the figure was slightly lower at 77% (0.77; 95% CI

0.70–0.85). Though the time taken to attain parallelism was 13 years for tumors <1 cm and 18 years for tumors between 1 and 2 cm there was no statistically significant difference between the observed and expected curves after 10 years. Any divergence of the curves beyond 20 years is unlikely to detract from the conclusion that a substantial proportion of patients will not die of breast cancer and are likely to have achieved a "personal cure" and to succumb from non–breast cancer-related causes (Fig. 38.2).

Patients with early stage breast cancer currently have 10-year survival rates in excess of 80% (8). Despite improved outcomes being largely attributable to adjuvant chemohormonal therapies, about 50–60% of breast cancer patients will survive for this period with locoregional treatments only. This implies that disease is confined to the breast and lymph nodes and is adequately managed with local treatments or that some tumors possess low innate biological aggressiveness with stringent dormancy. William Halsted commented that "*the efficiency of a breast cancer operation is measured truer in terms of local recurrence than of ultimate cure....*" (5). Treatments which allowed en bloc resection of a tumor together with adjacent locoregional tissues offered the best chance of "cure" and minimized its local recurrence. In an attempt to increase cure rates, Urban proposed an extended radical mastectomy involving partial removal of the chest wall and internal mammary nodes. Though this reduced rates of parasternal recurrence for inner quadrant tumors, there was no difference in overall survival (9,10). This has been confirmed with a 30-year follow-up of the Milan randomized trial of radical mastectomy versus extended radical mastectomy (737 patients). Interestingly, a paper by Gaffney et al. suggests a possible survival advantage from internal mammary node dissection for patients with inner quadrant tumors (11).

These results support the Halstedian paradigm as does the reduction in mortality from breast cancer screening which aims to detect cancers during the preclinical phase when they remain localized without micrometastatic dissemination (12). Between one-third to one-half of documented mortality reductions for breast cancer are attributed to screening (13), but an analysis from Norway suggests that only 10% of the decrease in breast cancer–specific mortality results from screening *per se* with the remainder due to improvements in systemic treatments and formalization of multidisciplinary care (14).

Fisherian Paradigm
This presupposes that breast cancer is a predominantly systemic disease at the outset and challenges the concept of a progressive centrifugal spread according to anatomical, mechanical, and temporal criteria. Thus cancer cells can enter the bloodstream at an early stage of tumor development via the leaky vessels of the neovasculature and lymphaticovenous communications. Initially, circulating cells may be destroyed by the immune system and fail to establish viable foci of micrometastases (Fig. 38.3). A corollary of Fisher's conclusions is that current forms of treatment have modest effects on reduction of mortality from breast cancer. Though a primary tumor can be excised surgically or may regress completely with chemotherapy and/or radiotherapy, it is the presence of micrometastases at the time of presentation which will determine a patient's clinical fate. Local recurrence is viewed as an indicator of poor prognosis and

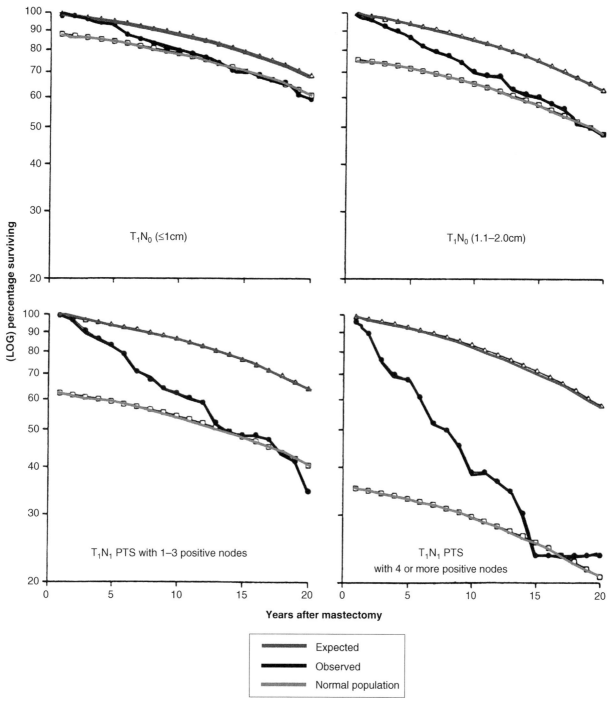

Figure 38.2 Observed and expected survival curves for T_1N_0 and T_1N_1 patients with tumors either 1 cm (Group A) or 1.1–2.0 cm (Group B).

reflects a host–tumor relationship which favors the development of distant disease or activation of processes leading to "kick start" of micrometastases (15). The biological potential of residual tumor cells within the breast is resonant with this more aggressive phenotype. Distant disease and mortality are governed by innate pathobiological features of the disease and not the extent of locoregional treatments. An intermediate or a spectrum paradigm is less restrictive than either paradigm in pure form and acknowledges that some breast cancers behave in a more Halstedian manner while others are more likely to disseminate early on in accordance with biological predeterminism. The latter was based on the results of clinical trials demonstrating equivalence of survival between mastectomy

(radical/modified radical) and BCS. However, it is the significance attributed to local recurrence that is perhaps of greater interest and has until now been underestimated. An update of the largest breast conservation trial (NSABP B-06) with a 20-year follow-up confirms that postoperative irradiation improves local recurrence-free survival and in particular rates of early local recurrence (16). Of note, distant disease-free and overall survival are similar in the three arms of the trial, namely wide local excision (WLE), WLE with radiotherapy, and modified radical mastectomy. In the NSAPB B-06 trial 39.2% of patients undergoing WLE only (negative surgical margins) had developed local recurrence at 20 years' follow-up compared with only 14.3% of those receiving radiotherapy post lumpectomy. Despite a great variation in the incidence of IBTR, this did not translate into survival differences and it was concluded that no causal relationship existed between IBTR and distant disease (Fig. 38.4). Differences in distant-disease-free survival were examined between patients with and without IBTR using a Cox regression model based on the fixed covariates of age, nodal status, tumor size and grade together with the time varying covariate of IBTR. IBTR was found to be the strongest predictor for distant disease and was considered to be a marker for increased risk but not a cause of distant metastases

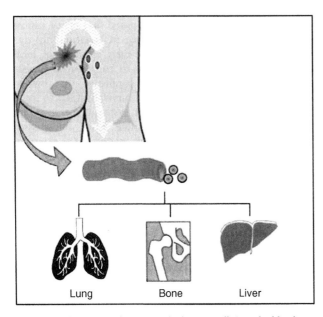

Figure 38.3 Fisherian paradigm: spread of tumor cells into the bloodstream occurs early in tumorigenesis and precedes lymph node infiltration.

(3.41-fold increased risk, 95% CI 2.70–4.30) (17). Early local recurrence was associated with a shorter distant disease free interval and IBTR was better correlated with distant disease than tumor size which has been reported to be highly predictive for development of distant metastases. IBTR is an independent predictor of distant disease and a marker of risk, but not an instigator of distant metastases. Though locoregional treatment in the form of surgery or radiotherapy may prevent or reduce chance of expression of the marker, such therapy does not alter the intrinsic risk of developing distant disease. The prognostic significance of IBTR has also been addressed by other workers. Haffty and colleagues examined the prognostic significance of IBTR among a group of almost 1000 patients with invasive breast cancer treated with BCS and radiotherapy (18). Overall rates of distant metastases were higher in patients with IBTR (50%) compared with those without local breast relapse (17%; $p < 0.01$). In particular, early IBTR was a significant predictor for distant metastases. However, the authors were unable to conclude whether IBTR was a marker of risk or a determinant of distant disease. Similar conclusions were reached by a Japanese group who evaluated outcomes in 1901 patients who underwent BCS (with or without irradiation) for invasive tumors measuring ≤3 cm (19). They used a Cox proportional hazards model to estimate the risk of distant metastases following IBTR. Though IBTR strongly correlated with subsequent development of distant metastases (hazard rate 3.93, $p < 0.0001$), it was unclear whether IBTR was an indicator or a cause of distant disease relapse. Survival data have been presented from the Nottingham group on 970 patients with and without local recurrence treated between 1990 and 1999 with BCT (20). The relative risk of recurrence from avoidance of IBTR was 0.69, that is, IBTR per se contributed to approximately one-third of the overall recurrence risk (Fig. 38.5). A Cox analysis involving the covariates of tumor size, grade, lymph node status, and

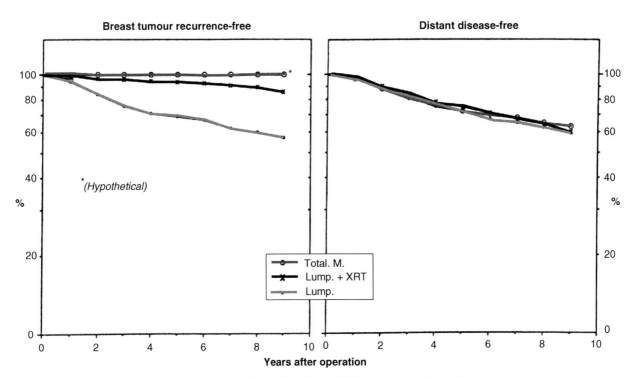

Figure 38.4 Relationship of IBTR to distant-disease-free survival (DDFS) within the NSABP B-06 trial. Variations in local recurrence within the conserved breast due to local treatment differences do not translate into differences in DDFS.

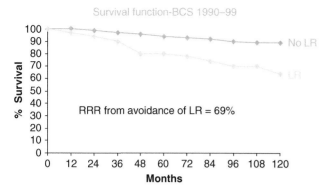

Figure 38.5 Ipsilateral breast cancer recurrence contributes approximately one-third to the overall recurrence risk within the Nottingham data set.

lymphovascular invasion revealed that IBTR was the single most important risk factor and an independent prognostic factor for survival (ß = 1.41; SE 0.15 p < 0.001). However, this analysis did not indicate whether IBTR was causal or just associated with survival. Whether IBTR is causal or merely associated with survival, treatments that reduce local recurrence definitely impact on survival and therefore efforts to minimize recurrent disease in the conserved breast are justified.

A longer term follow-up (25 years) of the NSABP B-04 trial also reveals equivalent overall survival for clinically node-negative patients undergoing radical mastectomy compared with total mastectomy and radiotherapy or total mastectomy alone (none of whom received adjuvant systemic therapies) (21). Results of these trials individually support the contention that local treatments for breast cancer have minimal impact on overall survival outcomes and local recurrence is a marker of risk for development of distant disease which reflects intrinsic biology of the tumor. Residual cancer cells are a determinant of local failure but not of clinically relevant distant disease (20).

LOCAL RECURRENCE AFTER BREAST CONSERVING SURGERY
Extent of Local Surgery
The overview by the EBCTCG confirmed that long term mortality was also influenced by reduction in locoregional disease attributable to more extensive surgery as well as addition of radiotherapy. With improvements in surgical margins of clearance, the absolute benefits from radiotherapy in terms of local control will be less in the future. BCS is now an established surgical modality and is the preferred standard of care for management of women with early stage breast cancer. Introduction of conservative forms of breast surgery has coincided with instigation of widespread mammographic screening over the past 25 years. With a smaller average tumor size at presentation, the majority of patients are eligible for BCS though rates of mastectomy are variable at both institutional and geographical levels (22). Within the United Kingdom, rates of mastectomy vary from 9% to 57% with an average of 24% (23). These variations in patterns of surgical management are likely to reflect differences in philosophy and training among surgeons together with an element of fear and concern about recurrence. Selection of patients for BCS is of crucial importance with an inverse relationship between the oncologic demands for surgical radicalism on the one hand and cosmesis on the other.

There is a balance between the risk of local recurrence and cosmetic results. Most patients deemed eligible for BCS will have a favorable tumor to breast size ratio and be suitable for conventional forms of WLE in which the tumor is excised with an approximate 2 cm margin of surrounding breast tissue without any formal breast remodeling. It is no longer acceptable to merely attain gross macroscopic clearance of the tumor at operation; all radial margins should be clear of tumor at the microscopic level. The NSABP and others have reported higher rates of local recurrence with microscopically positive margins, with rates increasing significantly with duration of follow-up compared with negative margin tumors [regression coefficients of 0.75 (p = 0.008) and −0.31 (p = 0.35) respectively] (24–28). However, some studies have found no correlation between local recurrence and positive resection margins (29,30), although relapse rates may have been influenced by modification of radiotherapy regimens with a proportionate increased booster dose to "compensate" for positive margins.

Ipsilateral Breast Tumor Recurrence
Two factors emerge as principal determinants of true local recurrence within the ipsilateral breast (*i*) "margin status" and (*ii*) the presence or absence of an "extensive intraductal component" (EIC) (24,31). Other factors have been implicated in determining the risk of local relapse, but correlations are in general much weaker than for margin status and EIC. Among these, lymphatic invasion, young age (35 years), and absence of chemohormonal therapy have been shown to be primary predictors for increased risk of local recurrence (32–34). Consistent associations have been found for a larger tumor size (>2 cm) and a higher histological grade but not for tumor subtype or nodal status. These findings are consistent with the notion that local recurrence develops from regrowth of residual cancer cells in peritumoral tissue. Increased rates of local recurrence associated with positive margins and EIC suggest that incomplete removal of tumor may contribute to local recurrence. A web-based tool has been developed as a predictive nomogram for IBTR after BCS. This uses relative risk ratios for seven clinicopathological variables and a modification of the original nomogram has been devised using two independent population-based data sets. The nomogram predicts an overall risk of IBTR of 4.0% at 10 years with an observed estimate of 2.8%. The nomogram is accurate for most patients at low (<3%) to moderate (3–5%) risk of recurrence but overestimates risk in a minority of higher risk patients (35). The risk of local recurrence, both within the breast after BCS and the chest wall following mastectomy, can be predicted from gene microarray data which have classified breast tumors into distinct biological subtypes (luminal A, luminal B, normal, basal, and HER2). The basal subtype appears to be associated with a higher risk of local recurrence after BCS and mastectomy compared with luminal subtypes and may have stronger and more consistent associations than some of the conventional histopathological factors (grade, subtype, and nodal status) (36). Voduc and colleagues analyzed local and regional relapse associated with each molecular subtype among a group of almost 3000 patients with early stage breast cancer (37). A semiquantitative analysis was undertaken using a validated six-marker immunohistochemical panel involving expression of estrogen receptor (ER), progesterone receptor (PR), HER2, EGFR, and CK 5/6. After a

mean period of follow-up of 12 years there were 325 local and 227 regional recurrences reported. For those patients undergoing BCS the local recurrence risk at 10 years was 8% for luminal A tumors compared with 21% for HER2-enriched and 14% for basal tumors. Similarly, the rates of regional relapse were significantly higher for the nonluminal subtypes (Table 38.1 and Fig. 38.6A and B). Interestingly, rates of both local and regional relapse after mastectomy were higher for luminal B, HER2-enriched, and basal subtypes. Nonetheless, rates of chest wall

recurrence for the mastectomy patients in this study were relatively high which might have been a reflection of more node positive cases and a lower proportion of mastectomy patients receiving chemotherapy compared with BCS patients. It has been suggested that BCS should be avoided in HER2-enriched tumors, but is probably safe provided a booster dose is given to the tumor bed. The 21-gene recurrence score has been derived from a set of node negative, ER-positive tamoxifen-treated patients in the NSAPB B-14 and B-20 trials. The recurrence score correlated with the risk of relapse for both BCS and mastectomy patients, though there was a more consistent relationship for the latter. The risk of locoregional relapse overall was 4.3%, 7.2%, and 15.8% for low (≤ 18), intermediate (18–30), and high (≥ 31) recurrence scores (Fig. 38.7) (38).

Surgical Margins

There has been lack of uniformity in definition of a positive resection margin and this in turn has compounded issues relating to microscopically negative margins and degrees of surgical clearance: how wide must a negative margin be to result in acceptable rates of local recurrence (<1–1.5% per annum) (31)? Some authors have defined a further category of "close margins" and found correlations between margin status and local recurrence based on strict and consistent criteria (30). Several studies have examined the impact of close margins (≤2 mm) on rates of local recurrence. Although these are relatively small studies with some variability in other factors, such as age, EIC, and systemic therapies, they all reveal a statistically significant increase in rates of local recurrence for "close" compared with negative margins (39–42). Freedman

Table 38.1 Score Risk of Locoregional Relapse (10 years)

Score	Risk (%)
Low (≤18)	4
Intermediate (18–30)	7.2
High (≥31)	15.5

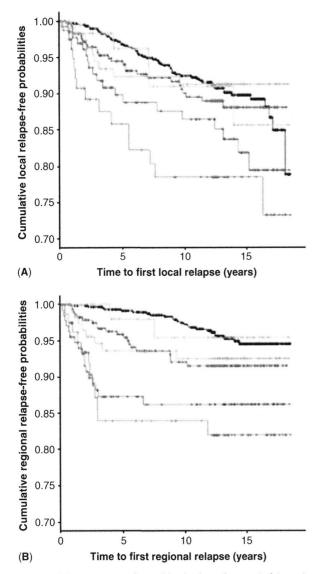

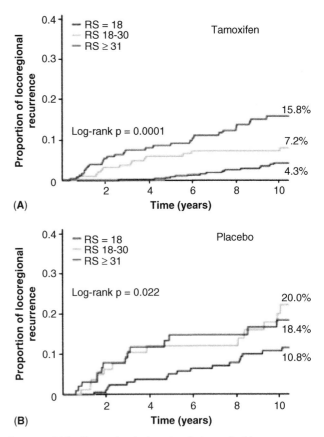

Figure 38.6 (**A**) Univariate analysis of local relapse-free survival in patients treated with breast conserving therapy reveals significant differences among breast cancer intrinsic subtypes. (**B**) Univariate analysis of regional relapse-free survival among patients treated with breast conserving therapy reveals statistically significant differences among breast cancer intrinsic subtypes. (violet line = luminal A; light blue = luminal human epidermal growth factor receptor (HER2); dark blue = luminal B; gold = 5-marker negative phenotype; red = basal; beige = HER2 enriched). *Source*: Figure courtesy of the Journal of Clinical Oncology.

Figure 38.7 Risk of locoregional relapse in relation to the 21-gene recurrence score assay.

and colleagues reported 10-year actuarial local recurrence rates of 14% when surgical margins were ≤2 mm and 7% when margins exceeded 2 mm (median follow-up 76 months) (42). Similar figures were found by Park and colleagues at a median follow-up of 82 months (17% vs. 9% respectively) (43). Many surgeons consider a margin clearance of 2–3 mm to be appropriate, though up to 45% of American radiation oncologists consider a margin as negative provided there are no tumor cells at the inked edge (44). A survey of 200 breast surgeons from the United Kingdom found wide variation in opinions on adequacy of margins, with 65% aiming for a margin of ≥2 mm and one-quarter accepting a clearance of just over 1 mm (45). Further surgery may be necessary to obtain the requisite radial margin clearance, be this 1 mm, 2 mm, or 5 mm (46). Most studies confirm that tumor size, lobular phenotype, lymphovascular invasion, and nodal involvement are associated with close margins (43,46–49). About 30% of breast units in continental Europe and a mere 10% in the United States strive for a radial margin clearance of 5 mm. However, a wider margin mandate can lead to re-excision rates of almost 50% without necessarily resulting in lower recurrence rates compared with a less stringent margin policy (46). The authors' group has reported a five-year actuarial rate of 1.1% for IBTR following BCS for invasive breast cancer when a 5 mm margin was enforced (50). This compares favorably with average contemporary rates of 3.5–10% at 10 years (51). There is less chance of finding further tumor when re-excision is performed to achieve a wider margin rather than a negative margin *per se*. Thus Pittinger and colleagues found residual disease in 44% of cases with involved margins, 24% of cases with free margins of ≤3 mm, and no further tumor in wider excision/mastectomy specimens when the free margin exceeded 3 mm (52). An analysis of data from the authors unit has shown that residual disease is found in 60% of patients with involved margins, 40% of those with negative margins up to 2 mm, and only 6% for patients with a margin of 2–5 mm [OR: 2–5 mm margin vs. involved margin = 0.05 (p = 0.004)] (53). Others have similarly reported a low probability of finding residual disease upon further resection when the margin of clearance is at least 2 mm (2.3%) compared with one-third of cases when the clearance is between 0.1 mm and 0.9 mm (46). Singletary has provided a useful analysis which shows median rates of IBTR of 3%, 6%, and 2% when margins of clearance were 1 mm, 2 mm, or just clear respectively (54). Thus patients with no tumor cells within one microscopic field of the cut edge had the lowest rates of recurrence ranging from 2% to 4%. When studies of local recurrence are grouped according to how a negative margin is defined, there is a consistent and statistically significant difference between positive and negative margins (Fig. 38.8). Thus although rates of recurrence are determined by negative margin status, no direct relationship exists between margin width and rates of local recurrence. When the first re-excision fails to achieve surgical clearance, mastectomy is often indicated and becomes necessary if margins remain positive after a "reasonable" number of surgical attempts (55). Larger tumor size and a lobular phenotype are more likely to be associated with close/positive margins and patients should be warned of being at a higher risk for re-excision or mastectomy. It remains unclear whether a mandate

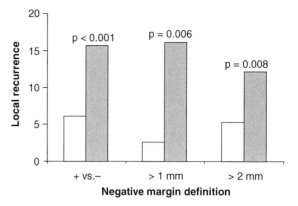

Figure 38.8 Relationship of local recurrence to margin status (defined as "positive" and "negative").

of 2–3 mm pertains equally to ductal carcinoma in situ (DCIS) as for invasive malignancy. Some have advocated the need for a wider margin of clearance for DCIS (of up to 10 mm) (56). Nonetheless, a meta-analysis suggests that a 2 mm margin of clearance is adequate when radiotherapy is administered to the whole breast postoperatively (57) and this accords with the current National Institute of Clinical Excellence guidance (58).

Oncoplastic Surgery
The newer techniques of oncoplastic surgery are advancing the limits of surgical resection which may be associated with an increased chance of tumor-free margins though not necessarily lower rates of IBTR (Fig. 38.9). Furthermore, positive margins under these circumstances usually reflect extensive disease for which mastectomy (rather than re-excision) is indicated. Down and colleagues undertook a retrospective analysis to compare margin width and re-excision rates for conventional WLE (121 patients) versus an oncoplastic resection (37 patients) (59). The latter included techniques such as therapeutic mammoplasty, subaxillary fat pad rotation mammoplasty, thoracoepigastric flap, and central flaps (e.g., Grisotti flap). The oncoplastic group had significantly larger tumors than the WLE group (23.9 mm vs. 17.6 mm; p = 0.002) and higher mean specimen weights (231.1 g vs. 58.1 g; p = 0.0001). Furthermore, the width of margin clearance was greater in the oncoplastic group compared with the WLE group (14.3 mm vs. 6.1 mm; p = 0.0001). Finally, this study found that rates of surgical re-excision were significantly lower for the oncoplastic group with less potential delay in commencing adjuvant therapies (5.4% vs. 28.9%; p = 0.002). These authors employed a 5 mm mandate for radial margin clearance which perhaps accounted for a relatively high rate of re-excision in the WLE group. It has been suggested that the chance of local relapse could be reduced by more aggressive approaches to BCS (60) but there are currently no data on the longer-term follow-up of these oncoplastic procedures. Moreover, there is no information from clinical trials on the safety of BCS for invasive tumors in excess of 4 cm (61). Though margin status and the presence or absence of an extensive in situ component are the principal determinants of local recurrence, consistent associations have been found for tumors >2 cm in size (62). For node positive patients, tumor size exceeding 5 cm was the only risk factor for local recurrence on multivariate analysis (63). Therefore it is likely that the risk of relapse would remain high for

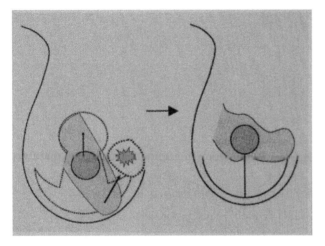

Figure 38.9 Glandular transposition can permit filling of defects secondary to wide excision of tumors and potentially avoid the need for mastectomy and whole breast reconstruction.

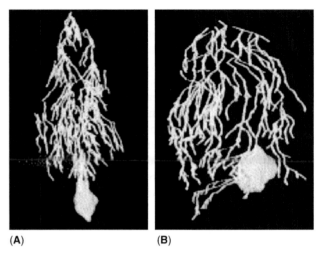

(A)   **(B)**

Figure 38.10 Computer generated 3-D image of a central type (A) and peripheral type (B) of intraductal extension of an invasive carcinoma. *Source*: Courtesy of Wiley-Liss, Inc., a subsidiary of John Wiley and Sons, Inc).

larger tumors despite adequate surgical clearance. Nonetheless, it may be possible to excise large areas of non–high grade DCIS (>4 cm) with clear margins and partially reconstruct the breast with autologous tissue replacement. The size categories for the Van Nuys Prognostic Index are <15 mm, 16–40 mm, and >40 mm and it is possible to have a VNPI score involving DCIS in excess of 40 mm which can be safely managed with BCS and breast radiotherapy (as opposed to mastectomy). Age less than 35 years and family history of breast cancer are additional factors which must be considered when selecting patients for either oncoplastic surgery with a high percentage breast volume excision or skin-sparing mastectomy (SSM) with whole-breast reconstruction (higher risk of local recurrence or de novo cancer risk). Though it may not be feasible in routine clinical practice to formally estimate the percentage excision from radiological measurements of tumor and breast size, consideration of MRI assessment of the breast is advisable. This can confirm unifocality or exclude multifocal disease involving different quadrants. Where imaging is equivocal and tumor parameters are borderline for BCS, it may be preferable to undertake a two-stage procedure; initial "wide" local excision of tumor permits full histopathological evaluation with assessment of margins. A definitive oncoplastic procedure can subsequently be carried out either two to three weeks later or following radiotherapy to the breast. A one-stage procedure is optimal and avoids any technical difficulties relating to the sequelae of previous surgery and radiotherapy (scarring and fibrosis). There are less likely to be problems with skin viability when completion mastectomy is undertaken after a simple excision of tumor compared with a more complex oncoplastic procedure with parenchymal undermining and transposition (64).

Influence of Breast Duct Anatomy and Wound Healing Response on Local Recurrence

Mannino and colleagues have proposed a hypothesis to reconcile some of the inconsistencies between rates of IBTR and the extent of locoregional resection (65). Increasing tumor-free resection margins have not yielded the expected gains in local control within the conserved breast, especially for women under

the age of 35 years. Changes secondary to breast involution and related changes in duct anatomy with age were considered in conjunction with intraductal spread and independence of the duct systems. These authors propose that higher rates of relapse in younger women are related to a degree of intraductal tumor extension which is precluded in older women due to physiological involution of the duct system. Furthermore, it was tantalizingly suggested that wider resections might be counterproductive and can exert stimulatory effects locally via cytokines and promote growth of residual cancer cells. Radiotherapy can modify the tumor bed microenvironment and counterbalance a "negative" effect of surgery-induced wounding on tumor progression (Figure 38.10).

Clinical Presentation of Ipsilateral Breast Tumor Recurrence

Most cases of local recurrence following breast conservation treatment present as a mass lesion within the breast which is either palpable or detected mammographically on routine annual surveillance (Fig. 38.11). The majority of symptomatic recurrences are found by patients themselves between routine follow-up visits. Any recurrence occurring within a different quadrant from the original tumor (several centimeters from the scar/boosted volume) is considered a new primary tumor. A new primary is more likely when there is a prolonged period between initial presentation and recurrence (more than eight years) and local recurrence within two years has a greater chance of being associated with distant disease. It is unusual for IBTR to involve the skin and in this respect differs from chest wall recurrence after mastectomy.

Local Treatments at Presentation Vs. Relapse

Where local recurrence is a determinant of distant disease, treatment at relapse may prevent distant dissemination and the timing of diagnosis and initiation of treatment will be critical. However, where IBTR develops against a background of pre-existing micrometastatic disease and distant relapse risk, it represents a marker for distant disease which would have developed whatever was the extent of primary locoregional treatment. For the former group, it is important to administer

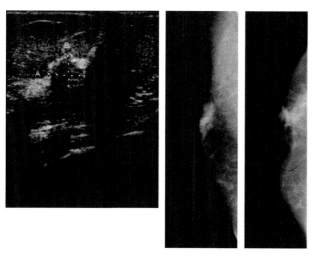

Figure 38.11 Local recurrence of a right breast cancer treated previously with breast conserving surgery. An asymmetric density is present on the right side corresponding to a palpable tumor mass.

maximal locoregional therapy at the time of initial diagnosis with curative intent. For the latter group, minimal early locoregional treatment would suffice, as any local recurrence developing secondary to "inadequate" locoregional treatment would not impact on survival, but be an indicator of a relationship between tumor and host which favored distant relapse. It would be an indication for maximal treatment at the time of local recurrence, including systemic therapy.

LOCAL RECURRENCE AFTER MASTECTOMY
Skin-Sparing Techniques and Immediate Breast Reconstruction

In contrast to local recurrence following BCT, local failure after mastectomy is more closely correlated with the conventional histological parameters of tumor size, histological grade, and nodal status. Chest wall recurrence is also increased when lymphovascular invasion is prominent. Historical values for the reported rates of loco-regional relapse following either radical or modified radical mastectomy are highly variable, ranging from 3% to 48%. An extensive review by Clemons in 2001 concluded that the overall incidence of local chest wall recurrence was 13% at 10 years (interquartile range 9–26%). Furthermore, approximately one-third of patients with local recurrence after mastectomy will have antecedent or concomitant (synchronous) distant metastases (66).

Breast Reconstruction

A pertinent issue which often concerns patients is locoregional recurrence and its detection following breast reconstructive surgery. Several studies have now confirmed that reconstruction does not influence the chances of detection of local recurrence with disease-free and overall survival being comparable between breast reconstruction patients and those with similar stage disease without reconstruction. This applies to both immediate and delayed reconstruction with equivalence of survival irrespective of the timing of reconstruction (67). Most cases of chest wall recurrence are manifest as either cutaneous nodules or subcutaneous lumps. It is uncommon for local recurrence in this situation to be confined to a deeply sited deposit within the chest wall musculature. Rates of local recurrence in breast reconstruction patients at five years were reported to be comparable to those for non-reconstructed patients (68). Though these rates were relatively high (20.1%), more than 90% of recurrences occurred within the first 5 years. Moreover, the interval from mastectomy to first local recurrence was not increased by reconstruction (68). In the case of implant reconstruction with subpectoral placement of an expander prosthesis, the site of local recurrence is essentially lifted forward, that is the skin, subcutaneous tissue, and pectoralis major muscle. However, with TRAM flap reconstruction, there is a theoretical risk that the flap may conceal local recurrence which is more deeply situated on the musculature of the chest wall. A longer follow-up is required for a more recent series of TRAM flap reconstruction to determine whether any subgroup of patients developing local recurrence are disadvantaged by the transfer of a myocutaneous flap to a zone where potential local relapses can occur.

Skin-Sparing Mastectomy

Earlier concerns that mastectomy in the context of immediate breast reconstruction may be oncologically compromised have not been substantiated. In particular, SSM techniques with preservation of much of the breast skin envelope are not associated with increased rates of local recurrence in the short term (69) or with longer follow up beyond 5 years (70). The perception that ablative techniques which spared much of the breast skin would represent an incomplete mastectomy has not been justified and biopsies taken from the zone of the skin which would otherwise have been resected in a conventional mastectomy have not shown evidence of any residual breast duct epithelium (71).

Several series have now been published confirming that SSM techniques are not associated with higher rates of chest wall recurrence with a follow-up ranging from 42 to 72 months (72–80). Most of these studies involve patients with stage I or IIa disease who have relatively small tumors with no skin tethering or direct skin infiltration (72). There is a risk with SSM that the anterior margin will not be clear surgically which increases the chance of native breast flap recurrence. Several authors have emphasized the importance of resecting the skin and subcutaneous tissue overlying the tumor in higher risk patients. One of the earliest studies evaluating rates of local (and distant) recurrence following SSM was published by Simmons and colleagues in 1999 (72) with a median follow-up of 15.5 months and subsequently updated in 2002 (81). This is one of several series, which compares patients undergoing SSM with a conventional, non-skin-sparing mastectomy (NSSM). Among a total of 236 patients, 101 had an SSM and were followed up for a mean period of 45 months. A comparison group of 136 patients underwent NSSM for whom the follow-up was slightly longer (59 months). There was no statistically significant difference in rates of local recurrence between the SSM (3.0%) and NSSM (2.9%) groups (p > 0.05). Most patients in this series had stage 0, I, or II disease with a median tumor diameter of 1.8 cm (0.1–7.5 cm) which may partially account for these low rates of local recurrence. Of note, younger women and those with smaller tumors were more likely to undergo SSM.

Most studies to date testify to the oncological adequacy of SSM and confirm that rates of local recurrence are comparable to conventional non–skin-sparing forms of mastectomy. These rates of local recurrence range from 1.7% to 6.7% and tumor size is a main predictor and risk factor for local recurrence. Nowadays tumors exceeding 5 cm in size are often managed with induction chemotherapy to downstage disease prior to definitive surgery. Furthermore, sentinel lymph node (SLN) biopsy is increasingly being undertaken in advance of mastectomy and immediate breast reconstruction and negative nodal status is reassuring. Nonetheless, a positive SLN biopsy or confirmed nodal metastases on ultrasound-guided core biopsy of ipsilateral axillary nodes is not a contraindication to SSM and immediate breast reconstruction. The majority of patients will receive some form of systemic therapy, be this chemotherapy, hormonal therapy or a biological therapy such as Herceptin or an antiangiogenic agent (bevacizumab). These systemic treatments alone or in combination collectively reduce the chance of local recurrence by approximately one-third. A potential weakness of many studies comparing SSM with NSSM is variability in adjuvant treatments including systemic therapies and radiotherapy to the chest wall/supraclavicular fossa (82). Furthermore, many of these studies examining local, regional, and systemic recurrence following SSM have been small case series with limited follow-up and heterogeneous groups of patients in terms of stage and adjuvant therapies. Yi and colleagues reported outcomes of SSM from a single institution over a period from 2000 to 2005 (83). A total of 1810 patients with stage 0–III disease underwent either SSM (799 patients) or conventional mastectomy (1011 patients). At a median follow-up of 53 months, overall recurrence rates were similar for the two groups (7.6% and 5.3% respectively; p = 0.04). The proportion of these patients with isolated locoregional disease was about 9% for both groups and combined locoregional and systemic recurrence between 20 and 25%. More than two-thirds of patients in both groups had systemic recurrence only and there were no significant differences in disease-free survival rates after adjustment for clinical stage. These authors reported relatively low local recurrence rates of 0.8% and 1.5% for SSM and conventional mastectomy respectively when analysis was confined to invasive disease with local relapse rates progressively increasing from stage I (0.32%) to stage III disease (3.31%).

Though all patients undergoing breast conserving surgery receive some form of breast irradiation, radiotherapy is applied more selectively to the chest wall following mastectomy. All trials have consistently shown that post-mastectomy radiotherapy (PMRT) reduces the proportional risk of local failure by two-thirds to three-quarters. Moreover, 2 randomized studies of PMRT have shown a survival benefit of approximately 10% in a subgroup of premenopausal node positive patients (84,85). Results of the EBCTCG overview that was previously referred to showed an overall survival benefit at 15 years from local radiation treatment to either the breast following BCT or the chest wall after mastectomy.

The Cambridge Breast Unit has derived a PMRT index to use as a clinical tool for selection of patients for chest wall radiotherapy. This ranks patients by a scoring system that is related to known risk factors for locoregional failure (Table 38.2). Patients receive PMRT if the score is ≥3 (actuarial local recurrence rates at 5 years 9%, 4%, and 4% for high, intermediate, and low risk groups) (86).

Clinical Presentation of Chest Wall Recurrence

More than three-quarters of chest wall recurrences following mastectomy involve the scar or skin flaps. There are four patterns of recurrence; localized spot lesions appear as reddened nodules which are raised from the skin.

Table 38.2 Post-Mastectomy Radiotherapy Index

Score	3	2	1
Number of Positive Nodes or lymphovascular invasion (LVI)	> 4 positive nodes	1–3 positive nodes	lympho-vascular invasion
Tumor Size	>5 cm/T4	3–5 cm	2–2.9 cm
Excision Margins	Pectoral muscle involvement or deep margin <1 mm	–	–
Tumor Grade	–	–	Grade 3

1. Single spot
2. Multiple spots
3. Widespread disease (including cancer *en cuirasse*)
4. Ulcerating/fungating lesion

Several authors have specifically commented that detection of local recurrence is not hampered by immediate breast reconstruction in the context of SSM (79,82). Patients often require reassurance on this issue and it should be emphasized that local recurrence rarely occurs deep to any autologous flap or implant. In the study of Newman and colleagues from MD Anderson Cancer Center, 96% of patients (22/23) with local recurrence presented with a skin flap mass, confirming that most cases of local recurrence following SSM are clinically detected in the skin and subcutaneous tissues of the chest wall and are not masked by the volume and bulk of the reconstructed breast whether this be an implant and/or autologous tissue (75).

AXILLARY RECURRENCE

Rates of regional recurrence following axillary lymph node dissection vary from 0.8% to 2.5% with a median time interval to regional recurrence after nodal dissection of 19 months. The chance of axillary recurrence is related to the absolute number of lymph nodes removed (Table 38.3).

Reported rates of axillary recurrence following negative SLN biopsy are very low (<0.5%) (Table 38.4) (87–90). Among a selected group of patients who have declined further axillary surgery after a positive SLN biopsy, rates of axillary recurrence are higher but still remain relatively low (2%) (89). It may appear counterintuitive that rates of recurrence should be lower for SLN biopsy than axillary lymph node dissection, but the former is a targeted procedure and is more likely to remove the biologically relevant node(s). Dauphine and colleagues reported only one case of axillary recurrence among 139 patients (0.7%) who underwent a negative SLN biopsy at a median follow-up of 52 months (90). Low rates of axillary recurrence are consistently reported in the literature and compare favorably with axillary lymph node dissection (91). Furthermore, the median time interval to regional recurrence after nodal dissection (19 months) is a shorter period than the median follow up period for most studies of axillary recurrence after a negative SLN biopsy to date. Finite rates of false negativity associated with the SLN biopsy technique do not appear to translate into higher rates of axillary relapse. However, any residual disease within the axillary nodes will be low volume and a longer follow-up is required

Table 38.3 Relationship between the Risk of Axillary Recurrence the Number of Nodes Removed

Number of Nodes Removed	Chance of Axillary Recurrence at 5 Years (%)
0	19
<3	10
<5	5
>5	3

Table 38.4 Rates of Axillary Recurrence Following Negative Sentinel Lymph Node Biopsy

Author	Number of Patients	Median Follow-Up (Months)	Axillary Recurrence No (%)
Giuliano 2000	67	39	0
Veronesi 2001	285	14	0
Roumen 2001	100	24	1 (1)
Reitsamer 2002	116	22	0
Chung 2002	206	26	3 (1.4)
Veronesi 2003	167	46	0
Blanchard 2003	685	29	1 (0.1)
Winchester 2004	614	28	1 (0.16)
Janssen 2004	401	26	2 (0.5)
Dauphine 2010	139	52	1 (0.7)

Source: From Ref. (89).

to substantiate these early observations. It should be noted that in the mastectomy-only arm of the NSABP-B04 trial, rates of axillary recurrence were sixfold higher (18%) than the axillary dissection group (3%). Moreover, three-quarters of these cases occurred within two years of follow-up. It is essential that rates of axillary relapse following SLN biopsy for node negative disease do not exceed those for axillary lymph node dissection, which is the "gold standard" for axillary management. A short communication revealed an actual recurrence rate of 5% at a median follow-up of 6.5 years with a prediction that up to 10% of patients may ultimately develop isolated axillary recurrence after a negative SLN biopsy (92).

Chemohormonal therapy will reduce axillary recurrence by approximately one-third and thus long term rates of recurrence are unlikely to exceed 1%.

CAN LOCAL TREATMENT INFLUENCE MORTALITY?

There is limited but increasingly cogent evidence that not all cases of breast cancer are systemic at the outset and that a subgroup of patients with early breast cancer exists for whom micrometastatic spread has not occurred before clinical (or mammographic) detection. As mentioned above, two randomized studies of PMRT have shown a survival benefit (approximately 10%) in a subgroup of premenopausal node positive patients receiving chemotherapy suggesting that persistence of local or regional disease can lead to distant metastases and impaired survival (84,85). In the smaller Canadian study, 318 node positive women were randomized to mastectomy and chemotherapy, with or without irradiation. At 15-year follow-up, the overall survival rates were 54% and 46% for these two groups respectively. In the larger Danish trial, 1708 node positive or stage III breast cancer patients were

similarly randomized and overall survival rates at 10 years were 54% for the irradiated group compared with 48% for the non-irradiated group (p < 0.001). The results of these trials have generated some controversy due to the low number of nodes harvested at axillary dissection and potential understaging of patients due to suboptimal management of the axilla. Some have cautiously interpreted results of the Danish and British Columbia trials due to poor nodal retrieval rates and concerns that some patients received inadequate axillary surgery and in consequence had residual locoregional disease or "oligometastases" (93).

Local Recurrence After Breast Conservation Surgery and Survival

Vinh-Hung and colleagues performed a pooled meta-analysis of 14 randomized trials comparing radiotherapy versus no radiotherapy after breast BCS among almost 10,000 patients (94). The outcomes were IBTR and death from any cause; this study attempted to resolve some of the published discrepancies on the risks associated with omission of radiotherapy (95–97). A pooled random-effects model was employed with formal assessment of heterogeneity using the Cochran Q test. WLE alone without radiotherapy was found to increase the relative risk (RR) of IBTR by 3.00 (95% CI 2.65–3.40) which translated into a marginal increase in breast cancer–related deaths (RR 1.086; 95% CI 1.003–1.175). This corresponded to a small excess of mortality (8.6%) when radiotherapy was withheld following WLE. The more definitive meta-analysis by the EBCTCG suggests an overall survival benefit at 15 years from local radiation treatment to either the breast following BCT or the chest wall after mastectomy (1). Data were available on 9000 women in 14 randomized comparisons of breast conservation with or without radiotherapy. There was no significant heterogeneity between trials and some patients received systemic therapy. Adjuvant radiotherapy reduced the rate of isolated local recurrence by two-thirds with a recurrence rate ratio of 0.32. Rates of local recurrence were reduced at 15 years from 28.3% to 10.4% in node negative patients and from 39.9% to 10.9% in node positive patients for whom there was a greater absolute difference in local recurrence. Much of the effect of radiotherapy on local recurrence was evident in the first five years. The corresponding absolute breast cancer mortality reductions were 3% and 7.8% at 15 years for node negative and node positive patients respectively. The overall proportional reduction in breast cancer mortality was 17% with a breast cancer death rate ratio of 0.83 (SE 0.04 95% CI 0.75–0.91; 2p = 0.002). There is as yet no statistically significant difference in deaths from all causes. Of note, patient age and tumor grade (but not size) were significant predictors of five-year local recurrence risk. Younger women benefited more from radiotherapy in terms of local relapse with local recurrence gains at five years of 5.5% and 18% for women ≥50 years and <50 years age respectively. The overall gain in mortality at 15 years was 5% but node negative older women (50–59 years, 60–69 years, and 70+ years) with well-differentiated tumors did not derive any survival benefit from radiotherapy after BCT.

Local Recurrence after Mastectomy and Survival

PMRT prevents two-thirds of local recurrences on the chest wall with much of the effect within the first five years. There is an absolute mortality reduction of 6.2% at 20 years (63.6% vs.

57.4%; 2p = 0.0007). For node negative patients (one-third of whom had systemic treatment) the absolute gains for local recurrence at five years were relatively small (3.4%) with a negligible increase in survival at 20 years (2.1%; 2p > 0.1). Indeed, there was evidence for increased mortality in a subgroup of older women receiving PMRT for node negative disease. There was a mortality loss of 2.2% with one woman in 50 being "killed" by radiotherapy due to adverse cardiac effects of radiation (correlation between cardiac mortality and mean cardiac dose).

These results therefore confirm an overall survival benefit at 15 years from local radiation treatment to either the breast following BCS or the chest wall after mastectomy. For those treatment comparisons where the difference in local recurrence rates at 5 years was less than 10%, survival was unaffected (Fig. 38.12). Among the 25,000 women where differences in local relapse were substantial (>10%), there were moderate reductions in breast cancer–specific and overall mortality (Fig.38.13). The absolute reduction in local recurrence at five years was 19% and the absolute reduction in breast cancer mortality at 15 years was 5%. This represents one life saved for every four locoregional recurrences prevented by radiotherapy at 5 years. It is unclear precisely what the proportional

contribution of local versus regional reductions was as nodal recurrence rates were very low. Though clinical trials should provide conclusive evidence on whether surgery affects local or distant relapse, there are now relatively fewer relapse events. If rates of local recurrence can be minimized in the first five years, this will eventually impact on overall survival (*Halstedian paradigm*). The exact relationship between local recurrence and mortality rather constitutes a "moving target" (93); nonetheless, the 4:1 ratio derived from the EBCTCG meta-analysis is a useful "rule of thumb" and emphasizes that prevention of local recurrence can save lives. Interestingly, a reanalysis of the Danish Breast Cancer Group 82b and 82c trials involving 1000 high-risk patients has found that the magnitude of survival benefit from reduction of local recurrence varies between patient subgroups based on relative risk of locoregional relapse and competing risks for uncontrolled distant metastatic disease (98). Kaplan–Meier plots were used to define three prognostic categories for local recurrence risk: (*i*) good, (*ii*) intermediate, and (*iii*) poor. The "good" group had at least four favorable pathological criteria: ≤3 positive nodes, tumor size < 2 cm, grade 1, and ER or PR positive or HER2 negative. By contrast, the "poor" group had at least two of the

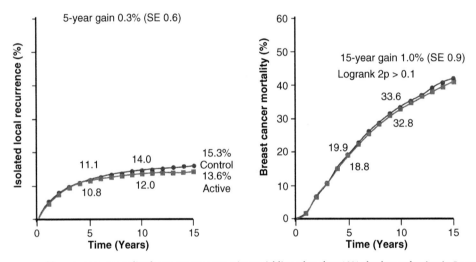

Figure 38.12 Local recurrence and breast cancer mortality for treatment comparisons yielding a less than 10% absolute reduction in 5-year local recurrence risk.

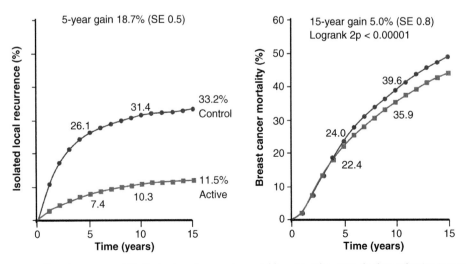

Figure 38.13 Local recurrence and breast cancer mortality for treatment comparisons yielding more than 10% absolute reduction in 5-year local recurrence risk.

following: >3 nodes positive, tumor size >5 cm or grade 3, while the intermediate group was in between. The smallest absolute reduction in local recurrence risk after PMRT occurred in the good prognostic group [11%; (33% vs. 22%)]. By contrast, the greatest absolute reduction in local recurrence risk was seen in the poor prognostic group [36%; (50% vs. 14%)]. These reductions are consistent with the EBCTCG overview (1). However, spectrum analysis revealed that there was variability in how these reductions of local recurrence translated into any survival benefit. Continuously improved breast cancer–specific and overall survival following PMRT was observed in the good and intermediate prognostic subgroups but no survival gains were evident in the poor prognostic group. Thus the corresponding reductions in 15-year mortality for the good and poor prognostic groups were 11% (61% vs. 50%) and 0% (81% vs. 81%) respectively (Fig. 38.14) (98). The authors surmise that patients in the poor prognostic group are more likely to have established distant micrometastases at initial presentation which are unresponsive to systemic therapy and fail to be eradicated. Micrometastatic foci eventually develop into overt metastatic disease from which the patient succumbs: they are the driver of mortality and represent a competing risk for distant metastatic disease over and above that which is derived from locoregional recurrence. PMRT can only impact on overall survival when it prevents local recurrence from acting as a source for distant micrometastases. However, these findings conflict with the recent results from the EBCTCG overview in which the largest mortality reduction was reported for patients at the highest risk of local recurrence. Though high risk groups were defined from probability of recurrence risk in both these studies, subgroups in the Danish Breast Cancer 82b and 82c studies were constructed from prognostic markers as opposed to outcome parameters. The high-risk category in the Danish analysis was likely to contain a greater proportion of intrinsically more aggressive tumors with increased tendency to form distant micrometastases leading to earlier death. Further improvements in systemic therapies (taxanes, Herceptin, and other biological agents) may reduce the proportion of patients with unresponsive distant micrometastases and permit emergence

of a survival benefit from PMRT in the higher-risk subgroups. The SUPREMO trial will help clarify the role of PMRT in patients with one to three positive nodes who may have a smaller proportion with unresponsive distant micrometastases and hence less chance of competing uncontrolled distant metastatic disease (99).

Therefore the 4:1 ratio is an overall average based on all prognostic categories. The estimated ratios for the "good," "intermediate," and "poor" groups are 1:1, 2:1 and 0 respectively. The proportional benefit from each local recurrence avoided is greater in the "good" prognostic group members who have a lower likelihood of coexistent distant micrometastases which represent a competing cause of mortality. Within this prognostic category, an absolute reduction of 11% in local recurrence translates into a mortality gain of 11% at 15 years. This reflects a more favorable ratio approaching one death prevented for each local recurrence avoided (98).

There is some evidence that local recurrence might be a cause of distant metastases from analysis of hazard rates for distant metastases in patients who have undergone BCS with and without local control (100). Those patients with local control demonstrate a peak in the hazard rate at about two years after which there is a continuous decline in the rate of distant metastases. By contrast, for those patients with local failure, a second hazard peak was seen at or beyond five years which was absent in those patients without local recurrence (Fig. 38.15A). It should be noted that the hazard rate for metastases is always higher in patients with local failure compared with those with local control. The first peak which is seen in patients with or without local control represents micrometastases present at the

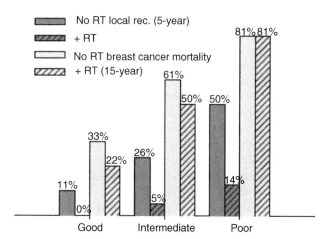

Figure 38.14 Survival benefit from reduction in local recurrence depends on the relative risk of local relapse (good, intermediate and poor groups). No survival gain is evident in the poor prognostic group due to competing risks for uncontrolled distant metastatic disease.

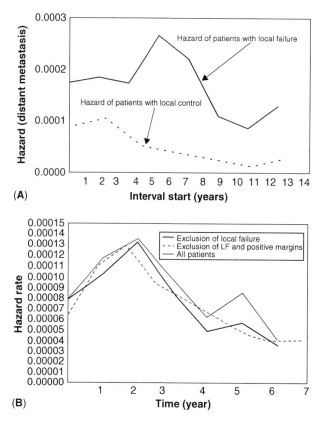

Figure 38.15 (**A**) Hazard rate for distant metastases for patients with and without local control. (**B**) Effect on late mortality peak from exclusion of patients with local failure or local failure together with positive margins.

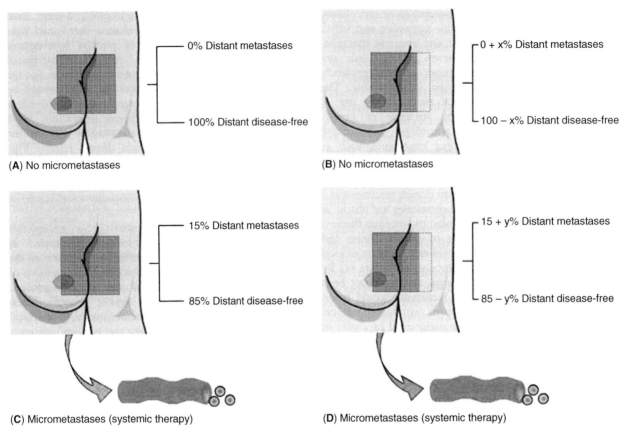

Figure 38.16 (**A**) Adequate locoregional treatment is potentially curative in the absence of micrometastases. (**B**) When locoregional control is inadequate, residual tumor cells will cause local recurrence and possibly distant disease in a proportion (x) of patients. Despite the absence of micrometastases, Survival is reduced because of poor locoregional management. (**C**) In the presence of micrometastases about 15% of patients will relapse at distant sites despite therapies with local recurrence being an indicator of poor prognosis. (**D**) Even with micrometastases, inadequate locoregional treatment will reduce the efficacy of systemic therapy, leading to a reduction (y) in the number of patients remaining free of distant disease.

time of diagnosis. When patients with local failure are excluded from the analysis, the late mortality peak is reduced in amplitude and actually disappears when patients with local failure and positive margins are excluded (Fig. 38.15B) (101). It therefore appears that local failure has a causative relationship to this late mortality peak and this second peak is evidence that local failure can be a source of new distant metastases and subsequent mortality; when this occurs, patients are more likely to have suffered early locoregional or contralateral recurrence.

LOCAL RECURRENCE AS A DETERMINANT OR AN INDICATOR OF DISTANT METASTASES

Locoregional treatments such as surgery or radiotherapy are potentially curative in the absence of micrometastases when disease is confined to the breast and lymph nodes. Under these circumstances, when local management is incomplete, cancer cells persist within locoregional tissues and can develop into distant metastases at a later date (Fig. 38.16A and B). Therefore, where micrometastases are absent at presentation or have been obliterated by systemic therapy, local recurrence is a determinant of distant disease and assumes a different significance from Fisher's postulate of local recurrence being a marker for distant disease. By contrast, where micrometastases exist and have not been ablated with systemic therapy, local recurrence would be an indicator of poor prognosis, with foci of residual tumor and distant occult disease maintained in a state of dynamic equilibrium until some event triggers recurrence (Fig. 38.16C) (2).

However, studies have revealed partial independence among prognostic factors in determining the potential for local and distant relapse. In their study of IBTR in more than 2000 patients undergoing BCS with quadrantic resection, Veronesi and colleagues found that tumor size and nodal status are correlated with distant but not local disease recurrence while young age and peritumoral invasion predict for both local and to a lesser extent distant disease relapse (102). Local recurrence conferred an overall increased risk of distant relapse of 4.62-fold (95% CI 3.34–6.39). There was actually evidence of an inverse relationship between nodal status and local recurrence which may be due to confounding effects of concomitant chemotherapy. Furthermore, EIC predicts for local recurrence only, which under these circumstances represents inadequate local treatment and is not a marker for inherently increased risk of distant metastases. Where there are both invasive and DCIS components to local recurrence after BCT, it is the invasive element which confers the increased risk of distant failure. In situ disease does not contribute to distant metastases, and when local recurrence is exclusively DCIS, the systemic risk is determined by features of the original primary tumor (20).

Of interest, the benefits of chemotherapy may be compromised when locoregional control is inadequate due to the reduced efficacy of chemotherapy in the presence of a greater tumor cell burden in locoregional tissues (Fig. 38.16D). Any persistent locoregional disease could become a source of distant metastases (oligometastases) (103). Within the trials of breast conservation, most of the cases of local recurrence occur against a background of micrometastatic disease and therefore represent a marker of distant relapse. Those patients without micrometastases at presentation and who undergo adequate locoregional treatment have the same outcome irrespective of the type of surgery. However, where there is an inadequate or incomplete locoregional therapy, survival differences may emerge because local recurrence is a determinant of distant disease and may render systemic therapy less effective. It is perhaps not surprising that no survival difference is detectable in BCT trials because the majority of patients have received adequate primary locoregional treatment (with or without mastectomy at the time of relapse) and local recurrence is not a cause of distant disease. Those cases where local recurrence is a determinant of distant failure are probably too few and follow-up too short to have any statistical impact. Molecular profiling may allow distinction between these two basic groups and avoid under- and overtreatment with both locoregional and systemic therapies (104,105).

Though randomized clinical trials have previously failed to identify any group of patients for whom local recurrence produces a decrement in survival, these may not have possessed the power to detect any effect of attenuated locoregional treatment on overall survival. The number of events is relatively small and some cases of distant recurrence may not yet have occurred at the time of analysis. The EBCTCG overview implies that survival and local recurrence are related, but not in a simple one to one manner (as discussed earlier). Interestingly, in the EBCTCG overview, those patients in whom the difference in local relapse rates was <10% had presumably received adequate locoregional treatment from surgery alone with little further reduction from more surgery or radiotherapy (1). These latest clinical results accord with the intuitive assumption that viable cancer cells remaining in the peritumoral tissue of the breast following conservation surgery will ultimately proliferate and metastasize to distant sites.

MANAGEMENT OF LOCAL RECURRENCE

There is variation in time to relapse, site of recurrence, and previous therapies for locally recurrent breast cancer and it is therefore impossible to formulate a single management strategy that is applicable to all patients. Furthermore, treatment recommendations have been reported to differ considerably among oncologists in the context of limited evidence from prospective randomized clinical trials (106). Each patient should be assessed individually with a precise and tailored treatment plan.

Patients presenting with locally recurrent breast cancer should always undergo re-staging with the following investigations which are recommended by the European Society of Medical Oncology (ESMO) Clinical Practice Guidelines (107):

- Routine blood tests (full blood count, liver function tests, bone profile, and calcium)
- Bone scan (for symptomatic bone metastases)
- CT scan chest, abdomen, and pelvis with bone windows (asymptomatic metastases)

Clinically suspected locoregional recurrence should be confirmed by imaging where appropriate and patients should be fully staged irrespective of symptoms suggestive of distant disease. However, a formal bone scan is only indicated in symptomatic patients. A full clinical history should be undertaken to ascertain relevant comorbidities and performance status which will influence the choice of therapies. Cardiac assessment is important in HER2 positive patients and may involve echocardiography or a MUGA scan to measure left ventricular function.

Until recently, the management of locally recurrent disease has been guided by biological characteristics of the primary tumor. However, there is now greater appreciation that receptor expression can change with tumor progression or secondary to previous therapies. Histopathological studies have shown various degrees of immunohistochemical discordance for ER, PR, and c-erbB2 expression between local or distant sites of recurrence and the primary tumor (108–111). Moreover, Thompson and colleagues found that switch in receptor status at the time of recurrence led to an alteration in treatment plan in 17.5% of cases (109). Of note, change in PgR status was especially evident and loss of PgR correlated with a poorer prognosis (108,111). These studies emphasize the importance of routine re-evaluation of ER, PgR, and c-erbB2 in locally advanced and metastatic breast cancer both for prognostic and therapeutic purposes.

The various treatment options for recurrent disease mirror those for the treatment of primary breast cancer and include surgery, radiotherapy, and systemic therapies (chemotherapy and hormonal therapy). The choice of treatment must reflect the previous therapies that have been followed by failure of local disease control. A crucial determinant of management strategy is the presence or absence of concomitant systemic disease.

ISOLATED LOCOREGIONAL DISEASE
Ipsilateral Breast Tumor Recurrence
BCT without radiotherapy is associated with a local recurrence rate in excess of 30% overall. However, for smaller tumors in older women which are of favourable grade or special type, acceptable rates of local recurrence with surgery only may be feasible. In principle, under these circumstances local recurrence could be treated with further wide excision followed by radiotherapy, provided that satisfactory cosmesis could be maintained. When both surgical resection and radiotherapy have already been employed as treatment for the primary tumor, recurrence in the breast should be treated by mastectomy. This yields a 10-year disease-free survival rate of 50–60% and the rates of complications for salvage mastectomy are comparable to those for primary mastectomy despite surgery within an irradiated field (112–115). In those cases where the axilla has not previously been treated, a formal axillary dissection should be carried out at the time of salvage mastectomy. In a study by Kurtz and colleagues involving 118 patients, approximately a half of them were treated with salvage mastectomy and the other half with further BCT. Rates of subsequent local recurrence were higher in patients treated with an additional conservation procedure. These authors advocate the selective use of further BCS which should be restricted to local recurrences that are isolated mobile lesions of 2 cm diameter or smaller occurring in an originally node-negative patient. However, larger recurrences can be successfully managed with initial induction chemotherapy either to render them operable or to permit further BCS (112).

Of late, it has been emphasized by several leading experts that more treatment options should be available for local recurrence after BCT (115–117). In most countries, including the United States, completion mastectomy is the only surgical treatment commonly practiced for IBTR. Further BCS should perhaps be considered after MRI imaging of the breast and it may be feasible to consider reirradiation with brachytherapy where a booster dose has not been employed at the time of primary treatment. A small study from a single institution reported use of reirradiation for 12 locoregional recurrences among eight patients. The mean dose of reirradiation was 46.7Gy usually administered in a twice daily regimen (mean initial dose 57.1Gy). Local control was achieved in most cases (11 of 12 recurrences) at a median follow-up time of 30 months. Half of these patients developed late skin and soft tissue toxicity which included fibrosis and telangiectasia, and a single case of rib fracture was reported (117).

A modified technique for SSM with immediate breast reconstruction is appropriate in selected patients with recurrent tumor foci measuring less than 3 cm in diameter and without skin or chest wall infiltration, nodal involvement, or distant metastases. In a study of 60 patients undergoing SSM with immediate reconstruction for locally recurrent disease, Linford and colleagues reported rates of local control in excess of 90% at 66 months' follow-up (118). Larger foci of recurrence can be managed initially with induction chemotherapy to render them operable (mastectomy) or amenable to further breast conservation in certain highly selected cases with the above caveats applying (119).

With widespread adoption of SLN biopsy for primary surgical management of patients with clinically and sonographically negative nodes, increasing numbers of patients are now presenting with IBTR (or chest wall recurrence after mastectomy) who have previously undergone a negative SLN biopsy without a formal axillary dissection. Reports suggest that when a repeat SLN biopsy is undertaken in these circumstances and no further axillary surgery is undertaken for negative SLN biopsy result, then axillary recurrence rates are very low (120–122). Kothari and colleagues have undertaken a useful review of this topic and reported on six nonrandomized, retrospective studies involving 327 patients. The overall rate of successful SLN identification at reoperation was 69% (227/327 patients). A limited subgroup analysis of those patients with fewer than nine nodes removed, rates of SLN identification reached 83% (165/199) and 86% of these patients were node negative. No cases of axillary recurrence were documented for this selected subgroup of patients with a negative SLN biopsy at reoperation at a follow-up ranging from 26 to 46 months (122). Several of these studies commented on higher rates of aberrant lymphatic drainage of recurrent breast tumors to extra-axillary nodal locations but the clinical significance of these extra-axillary nodes remains uncertain. Nonetheless, there may be a role for lymphoscintigraphy in cases of repeat SLN biopsy (120,122).

Chest Wall Recurrence

Chest wall recurrence following mastectomy can be classified according to the extent of recurrent disease and its management is likewise dependent on the extent of recurrent disease (Table 38.5). It should be noted that the presence of an implant

Table 38.5 Treatment of Chest Wall Recurrence Following Mastectomy

Type of Recurrence	Treatment
Single spot	Wide excision + radiotherapy (if not used previously)
Multiple spots	Radiotherapy (not previously used) or wide excision (± flap)
Widespread disease	Radiotherapy (not previously used) and/or chemotherapy
Ulcerating/ fungating tumor	Excision of necrotic tissue for palliation/ control of bleeding sites; topical charcoal for odor control/antibiotics

does not interfere with the treatment of local recurrence by surgical excision; a portion of the pectoralis major muscle can be removed without breaching the capsule around the implant (68). In other circumstances, chest wall recurrence may mandate a more extensive resection of native mastectomy skin flaps and importation of a myocutaneous flap for chest wall coverage. Irradiation of the chest wall with external beam radiotherapy is usually recommended when patients have not previously received PMRT, but reirradiation of the chest wall is possible. This should be cautiously applied to minimize complications such as rib fractures and chronic chest wall pain (116,117). Bethke concluded that reirradiation of the chest wall up to a dosage of 60Gy was feasible for local recurrence following either mastectomy (chest wall radiotherapy) or breast conserving surgery (whole breast radiotherapy) when hypothermia was practiced. Reirradiation was associated with acceptable late morbidity and improved prognosis for this group of patients in whom the median preradiation exposure was 54Gy (115).

Axillary Recurrence

Isolated axillary recurrences when operable should be treated by a formal level II/III axillary lymph node dissection when this has not been undertaken as part of the primary treatment, that is, SLN biopsy or axillary sampling with or without radiotherapy. Recurrences following axillary clearance can sometimes be treated with local excision but this can be challenging when tumor is adherent to vital structures such as the axillary vein. CT imaging can be useful in determining the operability of an axillary mass, especially when this lies relatively high in the axilla. It may be possible to confidently discern a plane of dissection between the mass and the major axial vessels or the latter may be encased in tumor (thus precluding surgery as a treatment option). Radiotherapy to the axilla and supraclavicular fossa can be considered as an alternative option and is necessary for cases of inoperable axillary recurrence. This can be employed in conjunction with chemoendocrine therapies to maximize response and obtain local control of the disease.

Systemic Treatment for Isolated Locoregional Disease

In the absence of distant metastases, it remains unclear who should receive systemic treatment at the time of IBTR. A proportion of patients with local recurrence apparently in the absence of systemic disease will have micrometastases and are at a high risk of subsequent overt metastatic disease at distant sites. The chance of distant metastases is significantly greater when the interval between recurrence and primary treatment is less than two years. Local treatment alone is potentially curative in the absence of distant metastases and recurrent tumor nodules must be excised with clear margins. It is suggested that systemic treatment should be considered for the following:

1. Patients whose original disease was node positive
2. Evidence of lymphovascular invasion at the time of IBTR
3. High nuclear grade
4. Short time interval to local recurrence (IBTR)

There is evidence that systemic treatments administered at the outset influence not only distant disease-free and overall survival, but also reduce the risk of locoregional recurrence as the first site of relapse (EBCTCG) (123). The magnitude of proportional risk reduction is about 30% and the principle applies to all forms of systemic therapy including chemotherapy, hormonal therapy, and biological agents such as Herceptin. These locoregional effects of systemic treatments will tend to reduce the impact of surgery and radiotherapy on mortality; the chance of any persistent or recurrent disease in the breast and regional nodes acting as a source for distant disease will be minimized and patients are more likely to succumb from competing risks of pre-existent distant metastases. Techniques of gene profiling can potentially characterize the biology of individual tumors and provide a molecular "portrait" which can guide treatment strategies. Recurrence scores predicting the risk of both local and distant relapse can be incorporated into clinical decision-making processes once rigorous clinicopathological correlation has been achieved (38,104).

The efficacy of chemotherapy after IBTR is unknown; the BIG 1-02 trial is an international collaboration which will randomize patients to chemotherapy (investigators choice) or observation (124). Patients with a recurrence of HER2 positive disease in the breast should receive Herceptin. HER2 status should be reassessed at the time of IBTR as 10–12% can change from being HER2 negative to positive upon recurrence. There is currently no evidence that treatment with chemotherapy at the time of IBTR will prolong survival and many patients treated with taxanes at the time of IBTR will eventually develop distant metastases.

ER and progesterone receptor status should be measured at the time of IBTR and if positive, endocrine therapy should be either changed or introduced. Tamoxifen can prevent further local recurrence but does not improve overall survival in this situation.

LOCOREGIONAL RELAPSE IN THE PRESENCE OF SYSTEMIC DISEASE

Where local recurrence occurs in the setting of metastatic disease, local and systemic therapies are of palliative nature only, but can provide useful relief of symptoms. The development of local recurrence simultaneously with distant metastases accounts for approximately 10% of all patients with local failure after BCS. Furthermore, the dual manifestation of local and distant disease is the strongest argument for IBTR being a marker rather than determinant of distant disease.

CONCLUSION

There is now convincing evidence that prevention of local recurrence following either BCS or mastectomy can save lives in the longer term and is a worthwhile aim. Management of breast cancer patients must now be guided by an "intermediate" or a spectrum paradigm which encompasses elements of both Halsted and Fisher but has inherent flexibility and can accommodate contradiction. It is difficult for clinicians to ascertain precisely how a tumor will behave within this conceptual "coalition" but genetic profiling may offer insight into innate risks of relapse and allow more tailored treatments which avoid under- and overtreatment. Such techniques may ultimately select those patients for whom more aggressive locoregional treatment at the outset may confer a survival advantage. This is likely to include younger patients for whom the risk of local recurrence in the conserved breast is almost twice as high compared with older women. Avoidance of death from breast cancer gains more additional years of life expectancy for younger women. With the stage shift witnessed in recent years, fewer women will in theory have micrometastases at presentation and local recurrence assumes a greater significance and consequence as a source and determinant of distant metastases. It is important that this group of women receive adequate locoregional treatment to both breast and axilla, especially if systemic therapy is minimal. Low volume residual disease within the breast, chest wall, and axillary tissues may not be manifest as distant disease and translate into any detriment in survival for many years and clinicians should be wary about "reductionist" approaches to locoregional treatments based on trials with limited years of patient follow-up (78).

REFERENCES

1. Early Breast Cancer Trialists Collaborative Group (EBCTCG). Effects of radiotherapy and of differences in the extent of surgery for early breast cancer on local recurrence and 15 year survival: an overview of the randomized trials. Lancet 2005; 366: 2087–106.
2. Veronesi U, Marubini E, Del Vecchio M, et al. Local recurrences and distant metastases after conservative breast cancer treatments: partly independent events. J Natl Cancer Inst 1995; 87: 19–27.
3. Perou CM, Sorlie T, Eisen MB, et al. Molecular portraits of human breast tumours. Nature 2000; 406: 747–52.
4. Curtis C, Shah S, Chin S-H, et al. The genomic and transcriptomic architecture of 2000 breast tumours reveals novel groups. Nature 2012; 486: 346–52.
5. Halsted WS. The results of radical operations for the cure of cancer of the breast performed at the Johns Hopkins Hospital from June 1889 to January 1894. Ann Surg 1898; 20: 497–55.
6. Hellman S. Natural history of small breast cancers. J Clin Oncol 1994; 12: 2229–34.
7. Rosen PP, Groshen S, Saigo PE, et al. A long term follow up study of survival in stage I (T1M0) and stage II (T1N1) breast carcinoma. J Clin Oncol 1989; 7: 355–66.
8. info.cancerresearchuk.or/cancerstats
9. Urban JA. Radical mastectomy in continuity with en bloc resection of the internal mammary lymph node chain. Cancer 1952; 5: 992–1008.
10. Veronesi U, Marubini E, Mariani L, et al. The dissection of internal mammary nodes does not improve the survival of breast cancer patients. 30 year results of a randomized trial. Eur J Cancer 1999; 35: 1320–5.
11. Gaffney T, Tsodikov A, Wiggins CL, et al. Diminished survival in patients with inner quadrant versus outer quadrant breast cancers. J Clin Oncol 2003; 21: 467–72.
12. Gotzsche PC, Nielsen M. Screening for breast cancer with mammography. Cochrane Database Syst Rev 2006; 3: CD001877.

13. Berry DA, Cronin KA, Plevritis SK, et al. Effect of screening and adjuvant therapy on mortality from breast cancer. N Engl J Med 2005; 353: 1784–92.

14. Kalager M, Zelen M. LangmarkF, et al. Effect of screening mammography on breast cancer mortality in Norway. N Engl J Med 2010; 363: 1203–10.

15. Baum M, Benson JR. Current and future roles of adjuvant endocrine therapy in management of early carcinoma of the breast. In: Senn H-J, Goldhirsch RD, Gelber RD, Thurlimaan B, eds. Recent Results in Cancer Research 140 -Adjuvant Therapy of Breast Cancer V. Berlin, Heidelberg, New York: Springer - Verlag, 1996: 215–26.

16. Fisher B, Anderson S, Bryant J, et al. Twenty-year follow up of a randomized trial comparing total mastectomy, lumpectomy and lumpectomy plus irradiation for the treatment of invasive breast cancer. N Engl J Med 2002; 347: 1233–12.

17. Fisher B, Anderson S, Fisher ER, et al. Significance of ipsilateral breast tumour recurrence after lumpectomy. Lancet 1991; 338: 327–31.

18. Haffty BG, Reiss M, Beinfield M, et al. Ipsilateral breast tumour recurrence as a predictor of distant disease: implications for systemic therapy at the time of local relapse. J Clin Oncol 1996; 14: 52–7.

19. Komoike Y, Akiyama F, Iino Y, et al. Ipsilateral breast tumour recurrence (IBTR) after breast conserving treatment for early breast cancer: risk factors and impact on distant metastases. Cancer 2006; 106: 35–41.

20. Benson JR, Querci della Rovere G. Ipsilateral breast cancer recurrence. Breast 2008; 17: 12.e1–12.e13.

21. Fisher B, Joeng J-H, Anderson S, et al. Twenty-five year follow up of a randomized trial comparing radical mastectomy, total mastectomy and total mastectomy followed by irradiation. N Engl J Med 2002; 347: 567–75.

22. Locker G, Sainsbury R, Cuzick J. Breast surgery in the ATAC trial: women in the United States are more likely to have mastectomy. Breast Cancer Res Treat 2002; 76: S35.

23. NHS Breast Screening Programme and Association of Breast Surgery. Audit of screen detected breast cancers 2010–2011.

24. Schnitt SJ, Abner A, Gelman R, et al. The relationship between microscopic margins of resection and the risk of local recurrence in patients with breast cancer treated with breast-conserving surgery and radiation therapy. Cancer 1994; 74: 1746–51.

25. Ryoo MC, Kagan AT, Wollin M, et al. Prognostic factors for recurrence and cosmesis in 393 patients after radiation therapy for early mammary carcinoma. Radiology 1989; 172: 555–9.

26. Kurtz JM, Jacquemir J, Amalric R, et al. Risk factors for breast recurrence in premenopausal and postmenopausal patients with ductal cancers treated by conservation therapy. Cancer 1990; 65: 1867–78.

27. Boger J, Kemperman H, Hart A, et al. Risk factors in breast conservation therapy. J Clin Oncol 1994; 12: 653–60.

28. Di Biase S, Komarnicky LT, Schwartz GF, et al. The number of positive margins influences the outcome of women treated with breast preservation for early stage breast carcinoma. Cancer 1988; 82: 2212–20.

29. Schmidt-Ulrich R, Wazer D, Tercilla O, et al. Tumour margin assessment as a guide to optimal conservation surgery and irradiation in early-stage breast carcinoma. Int J Radiat Oncol Biol Phys 1989; 17: 733–8.

30. Solin LJ, Fowble BL, Schultz DJ, Goodman RL. The significance of the pathology margins of the tumor excision on the outcome of patients treated with definitive irradiation for early stage breast cancer. Int J Radiat Oncol Biol Phys 1991; 21: 279–87.

31. Schnitt SJ. Risk factors for local recurrence in patients with invasive breast cancer and negative surgical margins of excision. Am J Clin Pathol 2003; 120: 485–8.

32. Mirza NQ, Vlastos G, Meric F, et al. Predictors of loco-regional recurrence amongst patients with early-stage breast cancer treated with breast-conserving therapy. Ann Surg Oncol 2002; 9: 256–65.

33. Wallgren A, Bonetti M, Gelber RD, et al. Risk factors for locoregional recurrence among breast cancer patients: results from International Breast Cancer Study Group Trials I through VII. J Clin Oncol 2003; 21: 1205–13.

34. Park CC, Mitsumori M, Nixon A, et al. Outcome at 8 years after breast conserving surgery and radiation therapy for invasive breast cancer: influence of margin status and systemic therapy on local recurrence. J Clin Oncol 2000; 18: 1668–75.

35. Sanghani M, Truong PT, Taad RA, et al. Validation of a web-based predictive nomogram for ipsilateral breast tumour recurrence after breast conservation treatment. J Clin Oncol 2010; 28: 718–22.

36. Nguyen PL, Taghian AG, Katz MS, et al. Breast cancer subtype approximated by estrogen receptor, progesterone receptor and HER2 is associated with local and distant recurrence after breast conserving therapy. J Clin Oncol 2008; 26: 2373–8.

37. Voduc KD, Cheang MCU, Tyldesley S, et al. Breast cancer subtypes and the risk of local and regional relapse. J Clin Oncol 2010; 28: 1684–91.

38. Mamounas EP, Tang G, Fisher B, et al. Association between the 21-gene recurrence score assay and risk of locoregional recurrence in node negative, estrogen receptor positive breast cancer: Results from NSABP B-14 and NSABP B-20. J Clin Oncol 2010; 28: 1677–83.

39. Smitt MC, Nowels K, Carlson RW, et al. Predictors of re-excision findings and recurrence after breast conservation. Int J Radiat Oncol Biol Phys 2003; 57: 979–85.

40. Petersen ME, Schultz DJ, Reynolds C, et al. Outcomes in breast cancer patients relative to margin status after treatment with breast-conserving surgery and radiation therapy: The University of Pennsylvania experience. Int J Radiat Oncol Biol Phys 1999; 43: 1029–35.

41. Wazer DE, Schmidt-Ulrich RK, Ruthazer R, et al. Factors determining outcome for breast-conserving irradiation with margin-directed dose escalation to the tumor bed. Int J Radiat Oncol Biol Phys 1998; 40: 851–8.

42. Freedman G, Fowble B, Hanlon A, et al. Patients with early stage invasive cancer with close or positive margins treated with conservative sugery and radiation have an increased risk of breast recurrence that is delayed by adjuvant systemic therapy. Int J Radiat Oncol Biol Phys 1999; 44: 1005–15.

43. Park CC, Mitsumori M, Nixon A, et al. Outcome at 8 years after breast-conserving surgery and radiation therapy for invasive breast cancer: influence of margin status and systemic therapy on local recurrence. J Clin Oncol 2000: 1668–167.

44. Taghian A, Mohiuddin M, Jagsi R, et al. Current perceptions regarding surgical margin status after breast conserving therapy: results of a survey. Ann Surg 2005; 241: 629–39.

45. Young OE, Valassiadou K, Dixon M. A review of current practices in breast conservation surgery in the UK. Surg Oncol 2007; 89: 118–23.

46. Ward ST, Jones BG, Jewkes AJ. A two millimeter free margin from invasive tumour minimizes residual disease in breast conserving surgery. Int J Clin Pract 2010; 64: 1675–80.

47. Moore MM, Borossa G, Imbrie JZ, et al. Association of infiltrating lobular carcinoma with positive surgical margins after breast conservation therapy. Ann Surg 2000; 231: 877–82.

48. Dillon MF, Hill AD, Fleming FJ, et al. Identifying patients at risk of compromising margins following breast conservation for lobular carcinoma. Am J Surg 2006; 191: 201–5.

49. Dillon MF, Hill ADK, Quinn CM, et al. A pathological assessment of adequate margin status in breast conserving surgery. Ann Surg Oncol 2006; 13: 333–9.

50. Liau S-S, Cariati M, Noble D, et al. Local recurrence following breast conservation surgery with 5mm target margin and 40-Gray breast radiotherapy for invasive breast cancer. Eur J Cancer 2008; 6: 204.

51. Morrow M, Schmidt R, Hassett C. Patient selection for breast conservation therapy with magnification mammography. Surgery 1995; 118: 621–6.

52. Pittinger TP, Maronian NC, Poulter CA, et al. Importance of margin status in outcome of breast conserving surgery for carcinoma. Surgery 1994; 116: 605–9.

53. Forouhi P, Brahmbhatt DH, Benson JR. Breast conservation: factors predictive of residual disease following reoperation for narrow surgical margins. Cancer Res 2009; 69: 355.

54. Singletary SE. Surgical margins in patients with early-stage breast cancer treated with breast conservation therapy. Am J Surg 2002; 184: 383–93.

55. Morrow M, Harris JR. Practice guidelines for breast conserving therapy in the management of invasive breast cancer. J Am Coll Surg 2007; 205: 362–76.

56. Silverstein M, Lagios M, Groshen S, et al. The influence of margin width on local control of ductal carcinoma of the breast. N Engl J Med 1999; 340: 1455–61.

57. Dunne C, Burke JP, Morrow M, et al. Effect of margin status on local recurrence after breast conservation and radiation therapy for ductal carcinoma in situ. J Clin Oncol 2009; 27: 1615–20.

58. NICE Clinical Guideline 80; early and locally advanced breast cancer: diagnosis and treatment. 2009.

59. Down SK, Burger A, Jha PK, Hussien MI. Oncological advantages of oncoplastic breast conserving surgery in early breast cancer. Scheduled for publication in Breast J 2013; 19; early view available from Sep.

60. Veronesi U, Volterrani F, Luini A, et al. Quadrantectomy versus lumpectomy for small size breast cancer. Eur J Cancer 1990; 26: 671–3.

61. Asgeirsson K, McCulley S, Pinder S, MacMillan R. Size of invasive breast cancer and risk of local recurrence after breast conserving therapy. Eur J Cancer 2003; 39: 2462–9.

62. Van Dongen JA, Bartelink H, Fentimen I, et al. Factors influencing local relapse and survival and results of salvage treatment after breast conserving treatment in operable breast cancer. EORTC 10801. Eu J Cancer 1992; 28A: 808–15.

63. Fisher BJ, Perera FE, Cooke AL, et al. Long term follow up of axillary node positive breast cancer patients receiving adjuvant systemic therapy alone: patterns of recurrence. Int J Radiat Oncol Biol Phys 1997; 38: 541–50.

64. Clough KB, Lewis JS, Couturaud B, et al. Oncoplastic techniques allow extensive resection for breast conserving therapy of breast carcinomas. Ann Surg 2003; 237: 26–34.

65. Mannino M, Yarnold J. Effect of breast-duct anatomy and wound-healing responses on local tumour recurrence after primary surgery for early breast cancer. Lancet Oncol 2009; 10: 425–9.

66. Clemons M, Danson S, Hamilton T, et al. Locoregionally recurrent breast cancer: incidence, risk factors and survival. Cancer Treat Rev 2001; 27: 67–82.

67. Johnson CH, van Heerden JA, Donohue JH, et al. Oncological aspects of immediate breast reconstruction following mastectomy for malignancy. Arch Surg 1989; 124: 819–24.

68. Noone RB, Farzier TG, Noone GC, et al. Recurrence of breast carcinoma following immediate breast reconstruction: a 13 year review. Plast Reconstr Surg 1994; 93: 96–106.

69. Kroll SS, Shusterman MA, Tradjalli HE, et al. Risk of recurrence after treatment of early breast cancer with skin-sparing mastectomy. Ann Surg Oncol 1997; 4: 193.

70. Doddi S, Singhal T, Kasem A, Desai A. A single institution experience with skin-sparing mastectomy and immediate breast reconstruction. Ann R Coll Surg Engl 2011; 93: 382–4.

71. Slavin SA, Schnitt SJ, Duda RB, et al. Skin-sparing mastectomy and immediate reconstruction: oncologic risk and aesthetic results in patients with early-stage breast cancer. Plast Reconstr Surg 1997; 102: 49–62.

72. Simmons RM, Fish SK, Gayle L, et al. Local and distant recurrence rates in skin-sparing mastectomies compared with non-skin-sparing mastectomies. Ann Surg Oncol 1999; 6: 676–81.

73. Carlson GW. Local recurrence after skin-sparing mastectomy: a manifestation of tumour biology or surgical conservatism? Ann Surg Oncol 1998; 5: 571–2.

74. Carlson GW, Styblo TM, Lyles RH, et al. Local recurrence after skin-sparing mastectomy: tumour biology or surgical conservatism. Ann Surg Oncol 2003; 10: 108–12.

75. Newman LA, Kuerer HM, Hunt KK, et al. Presentation, treatment and outcome of local recurrence after skin-sparing mastectomy and immediate breast reconstruction. Ann Surg Oncol 1998; 5: 620–6.

76. Greenway R, Scholssberg L, Dooley WC. Fifteen-year series of skin-sparing mastectomy for stage 0 to 2 breast cancer. Am J Surg 2005; 190: 933–8.

77. Medina-Franco H, Vasconez LO, Fix FJ, et al. Factors associated with local recurrence after skin-sparing mastectomy and immediate breast reconstruction. Ann Surg 2002; 235: 814–19.

78. Foster RD, Esserman LJ, Anthony JP, et al. Skin-sparing mastectomy and immediate breast reconstruction: a prospective cohort study for the treatment of advanced stages of breast carcinoma. Ann Surg Oncol 2002; 9: 462–6.

79. Patani N, Mokbel K. Oncological and aesthetic considerations of skin-sparing mastectomy. Breast Cancer Res Treat 2008; 111: 391–403.

80. Drucker-Zertuche M, Robles-Vidal C. A 7 year experience with immediate breast reconstruction after skin-sparing mastectomy for cancer. Eur J Surg Oncol 2007; 33: 140–6.

81. Simmons RM, Burrell W, Brennan M, et al. Society of Surgical Oncology. Denver CO: 2002: abstract no. 14 SCNA.

82. Downes KJ, Glatt BS, Kanchwala SK, et al. Skin-sparing mastectomy and immediate reconstruction is an acceptable treatment option for patients with high-risk breast carcinoma. Cancer 2005; 103: 903–13.

83. Yi M, Kronowitz S, Meric-Bernstam F, et al. Local, regional and systemic recurrence rates in patients undergoing skin-sparing mastectomy compared with conventional mastectomy. Cancer 2011; 117: 916–24.

84. Overgaard M, Hansen PS, Overgaard J, et al. Post-operative radiotherapy in high risk pre-menopausal women with breast cancer who receive adjuvant chemotherapy. N Engl J Med 1997; 337: 949–55.

85. Ragaz J, Jackson SM, Le N, et al. Adjuvant radiotherapy and chemotherapy in node positive pre-menopausal women with breast cancer. N Engl J Med 1997; 337: 956–62.

86. Wilson CB, Haba Y, Wishart GC. The identification of patients for post-mastectomy radiotherapy using the Cambridge index: audit of a prospective series (abstract 4093). Breast Cancer Res Treat 2007; 106: S198.

87. Chung MA, Steinhoff MM, Cady B. Clinical axillary recurrence in breast cancer patients after a negative sentinel node biopsy. Am J Surg 2002; 184: 310–14.

88. Blanchard DK, Donohue JH, Reynolds C. Relapse and morbidity in patients undergoing sentinel lymph node biopsy alone or with axillary dissection for breast cancer. Arch Surg 2003; 138: 482–8.

89. Naik AM, Fey J, Gemignani M, et al. The risk of axillary relapse after sentinel lymph node biopsy for breast cancer is comparable with that of axillary lymph node dissection. Ann Surg 2004; 240: 462–71.

90. Dauphine C, Nemtsev D, Rosing D, Vargas HI. Axillary recurrence after sentinel lymph node biopsy for breast cancer. Am Surg 2010; 76: 1127–9.

91. Van der Ploeg IM, Nieweg OE, van Rijk MC, et al. Axillary recurrence after a tumour-negative sentinel node biopsy in breast cancer patients: A systematic review and meta-analysis of the literature. Eur J Surg Oncol 2008; 34: 1277–84.

92. Kujit GP, Roumen RMH. Second thoughts on sentinel lymph node biopsy in node negative breast cancer. Br J Surg 2008; 95: 310–11.

93. Benson JR, Querci della Rovere G. The biological significance of ipsilateral local recurrence of breast cancer: determinant or indicator of poor prognosis. Lancet Oncol 2002; 3: 45–9.

94. Vinn-Hung V, Verschraegen C. Breast conserving surgery with or without radiotherapy: pooled analysis for risks of ipsilateral breast tumour recurrence and mortality. J Natl Cancer Inst 2004; 96: 115–12.

95. Whelan TJ, Lada BM, Laukkanen E, et al. Breast irradiation in women with early stage invasive breast cancer following breast conservation surgery. Provincial Breast Disease Site Group. Cancer Prev Control 1997; 1: 228–40.

96. Early Breast Cancer Trialists Collaborative Group. Favourable and unfavourable effects on long term survival for early breast cancer: an overview of the randomized trials. Lancet 2000; 355: 1757–70.

97. Vinh-Hung V, Burzykowski T, Van de Steene J, et al. Post-surgery radiation in early breast cancer: survival analysis of registry data. Radiother Oncol 2002; 64: 281–90.

98. Kyndi M, Sorensen FB, Knudsen H, et al. Estrogen receptor, progesterone receptor, HER2 and response to postmastectomy radiotherapy in high risk breast cancer: the Danish Breast Cancer Cooperative Group. J Clin Oncol 2008; 26: 1419–26.

99. www.supremo-trial.com

100. Demechelli R, Valagussa P, Bonadonna G. Double peaked time distribution of mortality of breast cancer patients undergoing mastectomy. Breast Cancer Res Treat 2002; 75: 127–34.

101. Fortin A, Larochelle M, Laverdiere J, et al. Local failure is responsible for the decrease in survival for patients with breast cancer treated with conservative surgery and post-operative radiotherapy. J Clin Oncol 1999; 101: 104–9.

102. Veronesi U, Marubini E, Del Vecchio D et al. Local recurrences and distant metastases after conservative breast cancer treatments: partly independent events. J Natl Cancer Inst 1995; 87: 19–27.

103. Hellman S. Stopping metastases at their source. N Engl J Med 1997; 337: 996–7.

104. Paik S, Shak S, Tang G, et al. A multigene assay to predict recurrence of tamoxifen treated, node negative breast cancer. N Engl J Med 2004; 351: 2817–26.

105. Reis-Filho JS, Pusztai L. Gene expression profiling in breast cancer: classification, prognostication and prediction. Lancet 2011; 378: 1812–23.

106. Clemons M, Hamilton T, Mansi J, et al. Management of recurrent locoregional breast cancer: oncologist survey. Breast 2003; 12: 328–37.

107. Cardoso F, Fallowfield L, Costa A, et al. Locally recurrent or metastatic breast cancer: ESMO clinical practice guidelines for diagnosis, treatment and follow up. Ann Oncol 2011; 22: 25–30.

108. Bogina G, Bortesi L, Marconi M, et al. Comparison of hormonal receptor and HER2 status between breast primary tumours and relapsing tumours: clinical implications of progesterone receptor loss. Virchows Arch 2011; 450: 1–10.

109. Thompson AM, Jordan LB, Quinlan P, et al. Prospective comparison of switches in biomarker status between primary and recurrent breast

cancer: the Breast Recurrence in Tissues Study (BRITS). Breast Cancer Res 2010; 12: R02.

110. Idirisinghe PKA, Thike AA, Cheok PY, et al. Hormone receptor and c-erbB2 status in distant metastatic and locally recurrent breast cancer: pathologic correlations and clinical significance. Am J Clin Pathol 2010; 133: 416–29.

111. Nishimura R, Osako T, Okumura Y, et al. Changes in the ER, PgR, HER2, p53 and Ki-67 biological markers between primary and recurrent breast cancer: discordance rates and prognosis. World J Surg Oncol 2011; 9: 131.

112. Kurtz JM, Amalric R, Brandone H, et al. Results of salvage surgery for mammary recurrence following breast conserving surgery. Ann Surg 1988; 207: 347–51.

113. Osborne MP, Simmons RM. Salvage surgery for recurrence after breast conservation surgery. World J Surg 1994; 18: 93–7.

114. Osteen RT. Risk factors and management of local recurrence following breast conservation surgery. World J Surg 1994; 18: 76–80.

115. Bethke KP. Breast conservation: predictors and treatment of local recurrence. Semin Surg Oncol 1996; 12: 332–8.

116. Muller AC, Eckert F, Heinrich V, et al. Re-surgery and chest wall re-irradiation for recurrent breast cancer: a second curative approach. BMC Cancer 2011; 11: 197.

117. Harkenrider MM, Wilson MR, Dragun AE. Reirradiation as a component of the multidisciplinary management of locally recurrent breast cancer. Clin Breast Cancer 2011; 11: 171–6.

118. Linford AJ, Metetoja TJ, von Smitten KA, et al. Skin-sparing mastectomy and immediate breast reconstruction in the management of locally recurrent breast cancer. Ann Surg Oncol 2010; 17: 1669–74.

119. Stebbing JJ, Gaya A. The evidence-base use of induction chemotherapy in breast cancer. Breast Cancer 2001; 8: 23–37.

120. Boughey JC, Ross MI, Babiera GV, et al. Sentinel lymph node surgery in locally recurrent breast cancer. Clin Breast Cancer 2006; 73: 248–53.

121. Taback B, Nguyen P, Hansen N, et al. Sentinel lymph node biopsy for local recurrence of breast cancer after breast conserving therapy. Ann Surg Oncol 2006; 13: 1099–104.

122. Kothari MS, Rusby JE, Agusti AA, et al. Sentinel lymph node biopsy after previous axillary surgery: a review. Eur J Surg Oncol 2011; 38: 8–15.

123. Early Breast Cancer Trialists Collaborative Group (EBCTCG). Effects of chemotherapy and hormonal therapy for early breast cancer on recurrence and 15 year survival: an overview of the randomised trials. Lancet 2005; 365: 1687–1771.

124. Wapnir IL, Aebi S, Gelber S, et al. Progress on BIG 1-02/IBCSG 27-02/NSABP B-37, a prospective randomised trial evaluating chemotherapy after local therapy for isolated locoregional recurrences of breast cancer. Ann SurgOncol 2008; 15: 3227–3231.

39 Management of the axilla I

John R. Benson and Mattia Intra

INTRODUCTION

Surgical techniques for locoregional management of breast cancer have become progressively more conservative with respect to both parenchymal and nodal resections. Despite the widespread introduction of breast conservation surgery (BCS), a formal axillary lymph node dissection (ALND) was, until recently, the standard procedure of choice for management of the axilla in the majority of patients irrespective of primary tumor characteristics. Breast screening programs and heightened public awareness of the disease have led to a stage shift with smaller average tumor size at presentation and a lower proportion of patients with nodal involvement. Almost two-thirds of patients are eligible for some form of BCS, and skin-sparing techniques are increasingly being employed in the context of immediate breast reconstruction following mastectomy. Approximately half of patients had nodal disease in the past (1), and removal of tumor foci within axillary nodes obviated locoregional relapse, and crucial information for guiding selection of patients for adjuvant systemic therapies was provided by ALND. Furthermore, axillary nodal status remains the single most important prognostic factor in breast cancer and has yet to be superceded by newer molecular indices (1,2). However, breast cancer is a heterogeneous disease in terms of pathobiology and natural history, which renders any blanket approach to the management of the axilla inappropriate. A selective policy based on thresholds of probability for nodal involvement may be justified, which incorporates alternative options, including sampling, sentinel lymph node (SLN) biopsy, and observation alone. Node positivity rates are determined principally by tumor size although are influenced by other factors such as grade and type of tumor together with the presence or absence of lymphovascular invasion (1,3). It is not the absolute incidence of nodal micrometastases or macrometastases which is important per se, but rather the proportion of these that develop into clinically relevant disease—manifest either as regional relapse or as distant disease from acting as a source for tertiary spread (4). Management decisions on adjuvant chemotherapy are increasingly based on primary tumor characteristics (including molecular forecasting (5)) rather than nodal status, which often reinforces but does not change any systemic treatment plan. Indications for postmastectomy radiotherapy (PMRT) are less dependent on stratification of patients into one to three or four or more positive nodes (6). These developments coupled with the failure of ALND to confer any clear survival benefit (7,8) have prompted exploration of less intrusive staging methods for determining which patients have nodal metastases and thus require ALND. These include sampling and SLN biopsy, which may be associated with less morbidity and lower costs (9–11). Axillary ultrasound in combination with percutaneous node biopsy for tissue acquisition is yielding useful preoperative staging information on regional nodes (12). SLN biopsy has been embraced around the world as a standard of care for breast cancer patients and ideally incorporates dual localization techniques using both blue dye and radioisotopic localization. Although SLN biopsy is now the dominant method for staging the axilla in clinically node-negative patients, technical aspects mandate standardization and confirmation is awaited that longer-term survival is not impaired as a consequence of either withholding systemic therapies of failing to remove non-sentinel nodes in the context of false negativity.

In the current era of the "sentinel rush" (13)", there has been a tendency to apply some form of axillary staging to all patients with early disease. Any form of axillary surgery—be it for staging or therapeutic purposes—might safely be omitted in some patients, without significant clinical detriment in terms of locoregional control and overall survival (14). Conversely, other groups of patients have a relatively high chance of nodal metastases and could be offered ALND at the outset.

PATHOBIOLOGICAL ASPECTS OF THE LYMPHATIC SYSTEM

Biological Models of Tumor Dissemination

The lymphatics of the breast form an extensive and complex network of periductal and perilobular vessels, which drain principally to the axillary nodes (Fig. 39.1). Moreover, the intraparenchymal lymphatics are linked to vessels within the dermis, which accounts for preferential drainage of cutaneous malignancy and tracer agents to axillary nodes. Although the internal mammary nodes are a route for lymphatic drainage from medial and central zones of the breast (15), the majority of breast cancers metastasize to the axillary nodes irrespective of the index quadrant. Fewer than 10% of node-positive tumors involve the internal mammary nodes exclusively, and clinical manifestations of such metastases are rare. The biological significance of internal mammary node involvement is uncertain (16), and significant morbidity can ensue from surgical extirpation of these nodes with no overall survival advantage from more aggressive resections (17).

Solid epithelial tumors commonly invade local structures and spread in a progressive and sequential manner to regional lymph nodes. The lymphatic vessels provide anatomical continuity to this process by acting as a link between primary tumor and regional nodes. Metastatic dissemination of breast cancer occurs predominantly via the lymphatic system in accordance

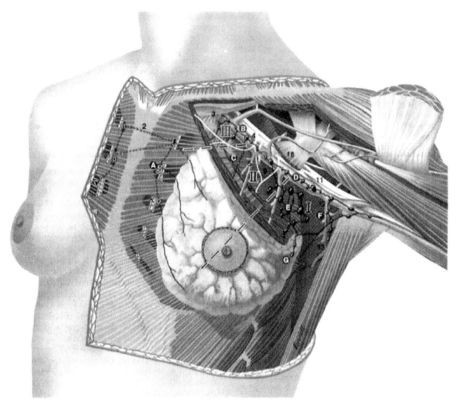

Figure 39.1 Lymphatic drainage of the breast showing lymph node groups and levels. 1. Internal mammary artery and vein; 2. substernal cross-drainage to contra-lateral internal mammary lymphatic chain; 3. subclavius muscle and Halsted ligament; 4. lateral pectoral nerve (from the lateral cord); 5. pectoral branch from thoracoacromial vein; 6. pectoralis minor muscle; 7. pectoralis major muscle; 8. lateral thoracic vein; 9. medial pectoral nerve (from the medial cord); 10. pectoralis minor muscle; 11. median nerve; 12. subscapular vein; 13. thoracodorsal vein; A. internal mammary lymph nodes; B. apical lymph nodes; C. interpectoral (Rotter) lymph nodes; D. axillary vein lymph nodes; E. central lymph nodes; F. scapular lymph nodes; G. external mammary lymph nodes; level I lymph nodes: lateral to lateral border of pectoralis minor muscle; level II lymph nodes: behind pectoralis minor muscle; level III lymph nodes: medial to medial border of pectoralis minor muscle.

with the Halstedian paradigm. Nonetheless, 30% of node-negative patients will eventually relapse with distant disease, and it is acknowledged that a significant proportion of breast cancers are systemic at the time of diagnosis due to tumor cells entering the bloodstream at an early stage of the neoplastic continuum. Furthermore, such hematogenous dissemination is not conditional upon lymph node involvement, and access to the circulation can occur through both lymphaticovenous communications in regional nodes (18) and "leaky" endothelium of the tumor neovasculature.

The SLN Hypothesis

The principle of the SLN hypothesis was first proposed by Cabanas in 1977 in the context of inguinal lymphatic drainage from penile cancer (19). This concept was applied to melanoma by Morton et al. at the beginning of the 1990s (20) and subsequently pioneered in breast cancer patients by Guiliano et al. (21). This technique is a diagnostic test for assessing the histological status of nodes in the axillary basin. According to the SLN hypothesis, there is a single node that receives drainage from the primary breast tumor and acts as "first port of call." The SLN hypothesis is Halstedian and presupposes a sequential and orderly spread of cancer cells from the primary tumor to the first draining, or sentinel node, whence passage to higher echelon nodes occurs. If the SLN does not contain metastases, the remaining non-sentinel nodes are likewise presumed to be tumor free. Conversely, if tumor deposits are found in the SLN,

it is implicit that there is a finite probability of non-sentinel lymph node (NSLN) involvement, and completion axillary dissection is undertaken. The concept of the SLN hypothesis in its pure form has proved to be slightly imperfect and does not accord with our understanding of lymphatic drainage patterns of the breast derived from anatomical studies or the pathophysiology of disordered lymphatic flow (Fig. 39.2). Lymphatic drainage is based on an intricate system of channels that arborize extensively in multiple directions (22). These lymphatics converge toward a group of three to five lymph nodes at level I of the axilla (below and lateral to the pectoralis minor muscle). From these nodes, there is a predictable passage of lymph toward level II and, in turn, level III nodes with a low incidence of "skip" metastases (23). However, the "plasticity" of the lymphatic system potentially allows skip metastases to occur in which nodes at levels II and III become involved in the absence of disease affecting level I nodes. In a study of the distribution of nodal metastases, Veronesi and colleagues reported skip metastases in only 4% of cases (24). In this study, level I nodes alone were found to be involved in 58%, levels I and II nodes in 22%, and all three levels in 16% of patients. Despite the occurrence of skip lesions, there is generally an orderly passage of lymph from nodes at level I through levels II and III. When nodes at levels I and II are tumor free, the chance of skip metastases at level III is only 2–3%. For this reason, a standard ALND involves clearance of nodes at levels I and II (partial ALND) only without routine removal of level III nodes. When at least

Sentinel node hypothesis

(A) Pure form

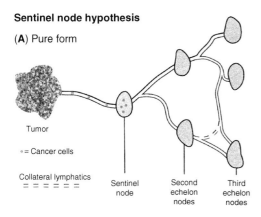

(B) 'Imperfect' form

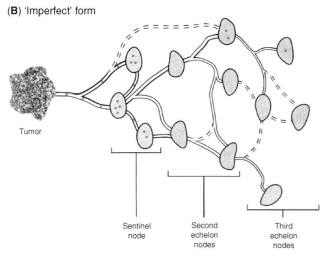

Figure 39.2 Patterns of lymphatic drainage from a primary tumor. According to the SLN hypothesis, in its pure form, cancer cells pass from primary tumor focus to first draining node or SLN, from where sequential passage to second and third echelon nodes occurs (**A**). In reality, cancer cells drain initially to a group of three to five nodes (**B**), which should all be classed as SLNs if they are blue, hot, blue and hot, or palpably suspicious. Plasticity of lymphatic system allows cancer cells to travel via collaterals to non-sentinel nodes. This accounts for the finite false-negative rate of SLNB. *Abbreviations*: SLN, sentinel lymph node; SLNB, sentinel lymph node biopsy.

10 nodes have been removed during a partial ALND, the axilla should be correctly staged in 96% of patients with primary breast cancer. When fewer than 10 negative nodes are resected, there is less confidence that the axillary basin is truly negative, and involved nodes may have been left behind in a nontargeted dissection. Conversely, when overtly malignant nodes are present at levels I and II, it is customary to undertake a complete ALND that includes level III nodes.

This branching network of lymphatic vessels permits a degree of adaptability, and detailed anatomical studies undertaken in the 1950s revealed no evidence of a first or "sentinel" lymph node at the gates of the axilla. Usually, more than a single node is identified as being "sentinel" or the true SLN is not apparent, leading to the removal of several nodes that, in effect, constitutes a targeted sampling. The average number of nodes retrieved at SLN biopsy is between two and three, and false-negative rates are lower when multiple nodes are harvested (25). Indeed, when palpably suspicious nodes are removed at operation and included as sentinel, many studies report an average of almost four nodes (26). Nonetheless, in addition to a low incidence of "skip" metastases (2%), the

negative predictive value of the technique is high with a figure of about 97% reported in most studies (27). A crucial parameter is the false-negative rate, which is the proportion of patients incorrectly diagnosed as node negative. The false-negative rate is usually quoted as approximately 5%, which is only slightly higher than the rate for conventional axillary dissection and is considered acceptable. However, in the latter case, nodal tissue is excised, and the effects of false negativity and potential under-staging are less consequential. By contrast, with SLN biopsy, inappropriate management decisions may ensue, and undetected tumor deposits in NSLNs may become as source of distant metastases, with impairment of locoregional and overall survival. Many studies quote false-negative rates above 5%, and rates as high as 17% have been cited. Calculation of the rate may yield a misleadingly low figure in some studies (the denominator should be the number of patients with positive nodes and not the total number of patients) (28,29).

Sophisticated methods of axillary imaging with computed tomography (CT), magnetic resonance imaging (MRI), and positron emission tomography (PET) cannot provide resolution at the microscopic tumor level, although ultrasound-guided percutaneous core biopsy (CB) or fine needle aspiration cytology (FNAC) permits tissue acquisition and is a promising complementary technique (30).

SLN BIOPSY

The advent of SLN biopsy has generated much enthusiasm as a method for pathological evaluation of nodal tissue and identification of those patients (who by implication do not require axillary clearance) without metastatic involvement of axillary lymph nodes. This can potentially avoid unnecessary surgical dissection and concomitant morbidity among an increasing proportion of node-negative patients (stage shift). A plethora of publications of variable quality have emerged on the topic of SLN biopsy in breast cancer over the past decade. The majority of published data on SLN biopsy come from validation studies in which clinically node-negative patients have undergone SLN biopsy followed by immediate completion ALND. These studies have provided important information on the success rate and accuracy of SLN biopsy, but have not yielded any comparative data for SLN biopsy alone without concomitant ALND. Furthermore, these single and multi-institutional validation studies have invariably involved relatively small numbers of patients.

Clinical Data
Nonrandomized Controlled Studies
The technique of SLN biopsy is now widely practiced in many centers around the world and has become a standard of care. The main issue with SLN biopsy is how best to identify the group of sentinel nodes, and initial studies assessed in peer-reviewed pilot studies employed blue dye alone (Patent Blue V, isosulfan blue, and methylene blue). These dyes initially identified the SLN in only 65.5% of cases, and a learning curve for the technique was evident as further experience was accrued (21). Krag and colleagues introduced radioactive tracers (technetium-99m colloid) as an alternative method with detection of "blue" and "hot" nodes (31). This combined approach allowed successful identification of the SLN in more than 95% of cases and is associated with the shortest learning

curve (21,31–33). Morrow et al performed a randomized study comparing the use of blue dye alone with blue dye and isotope and found these two methods to be of similar performance (34). A review by the American Society of Clinical Oncology Technology Assessment panel re-affirmed that dual localization techniques with a combination of blue dye and isotope maximize identification rates (>90%) and are associated with high negative predictive values (>95%) and a short learning curve (35). The overall false-negative rate for the SLN biopsy technique was 8.4% with a range of 0–29%. This analysis involved more than 10,000 patients who underwent SLN biopsy followed by completion ALND for validation. Patients were distributed between 69 single and multi-institutional studies, and sensitivity rates varied from 71% to 100%. False-negative rates are minimized by intraoperative digital examination and removal of nodes that are suspicious but neither hot nor blue. Although there is international consensus that a combination of dye and isotope is optimal for localization of SLN(s), much variation exists in details of methodology, and there is an urgent need for standardization of techniques to maximize sensitivity and specificity (36).

Prospective Randomized Controlled Studies
Krag and colleagues reported technical and clinical outcomes from the NSABP B-32 trial, which is the largest of five randomized controlled trials, comparing SLN biopsy to conventional ALND in clinically node-negative breast cancer patients (37,38). Three of these were of similar design to the NSABP B-32 trial and compared SLN biopsy + ALND versus SLN biopsy alone, that is, A + B versus A (39,40,11). The ALMANAC trial compared A versus B, and those patients randomized to ALND (or four-node sampling) did not receive initial SLN biopsy (Table 39.1) (41). The primary end points of NSABP B-32 and other trials were survival, regional control, and morbidity. Mature data on the accuracy and technical aspects of SLN biopsy within the context of NSABP B-32 trial are consistent with other studies and confirm that SLN biopsy is a safe and accurate method for staging the axilla with an acceptable false-negative rate (9.8%) and high negative predictive value. These results reinforced the need to remove palpably suspicious nodes and also to ensure that more than a single node is removed to minimize false-negative rates. Although these were secondary end points, they represented important results from a large trial of more than 5000 women

recruited from 80 centers and operated upon by more than 200 surgeons (37).

The primary outcomes of overall survival, disease-free survival, and regional control from the NSABP B-32 trial were published in late 2010 (38). Despite being a large multicenter trial, with a relatively high ratio of surgeons to number of cases (1–20), both surgeons and pathologists followed specific protocols, and performance audits were done periodically as part of quality control (42). Nonetheless, a potential criticism of this otherwise well-designed and robust trial is the number of participating centers and surgeons performing the SLN biopsy cases; there is no indication of case load distribution between different centers, and it is noteworthy that within the ALMA-NAC trial, almost one-third of cases were undertaken by a single surgeon! Based on the figures supplied for the NSABP B-32 trial, the average number of cases performed annually during the accrual period was only five. There was much emphasis on training and proctoring of surgeons/pathologists in the initial phase of this trial with a detailed audit process. The use of intraoperative assessment with touch imprint cytology (TIMC) was (and remains) controversial, but this does not detract from the principal objectives of the NSABP B-32 study. Omission of routine immunohistochemistry (IHC) was important in terms of categorization of patients as SLN negative; routine use of IHC could potentially upstage some cases and remove a subgroup of patients from the SLN biopsy-negative group who might otherwise produce a decrement in overall survival (42).

Longer-term data on locoregional control and overall survival in SLN biopsy-negative patients had been eagerly awaited prior to publication of primary outcomes from the NSABP B-32 study (38). Up until then, other SLN biopsy trials had addressed neither disease-free nor overall survival and focussed on morbidity and rates of locoregional control. It is of crucial importance to ascertain whether the finite proportion of patients with residual axillary disease (falsely negative SLN without completion ALND) have any detrimental effect on overall survival, which is clinically relevant. The NSABP B-32 trial was designed to detect a modest 2% survival difference at five years, thereby acknowledging that any reduction in morbidity must not occur at the expense of impaired survival. With a mean follow-up of 96 months, the authors reported no significant differences in the primary end points of overall survival, disease-free survival, and regional control. Data on overall

Table 39.1 Randomized Trials of SLNB

Trial	Study Population	Study Groups
ALMANAC (UK) (41)	Any invasive tumor, clinical N0; (n = 1260)	ALND or ANS vs. SLNB (if positive SLN, proceeded to ALND or RT to axilla; if negative SLN, observed)
NSABP B-32 (USA) (37,38)	Clinical T1–T3, N0; (n = 4000)	SLNB + ALND vs. SLNB (if positive SLN, proceeded to ALND; if negative SLN, observed)
SNAC (Australia/New Zealand) (71)	≤30 mm invasive tumor, clinical N0; (n = 1060)	SLNB + ALND vs. SLNB (if positive SLN, proceeded to ALND; if negative SLN, observed)
European Institute of Oncology (Milan, Italy) (39)	T1, N0; (n = 516)	SLNB + ALND vs. SLNB (if positive SLN, proceeded to ALND; if negative SLN, observed)
Cambridge (UK) (11)	N0; (n = 253)	SLNB + ALND vs. SLNB (if positive SLN, proceeded to ALND; if negative, observed)

Abbreviations: ALMANAC, axillary lymphatic mapping against nodal axillary clearance; ALND, axillary lymph node dissection; ANS, axillary node sampling; RT, radiotherapy; SLNB, sentinel lymph node biopsy; SNAC, sentinel node versus axillary clearance.

survival have been carefully analyzed with tests for interaction of treatment with stratification variables; groups 1 and 2 were well matched for patient characteristics and adjuvant treatments. Interestingly, there was a trend for improved survival in the axillary dissection group with an unadjusted hazard ratio of 1.2 (p = 0.12) and an adjusted ratio of 1.19 (p = 0.13). The authors offer possible explanations for this observed trend based on random events favoring group 1 and the presence of 75 patients in this group with a positive NSLN. These would be analyzed as node negative and receive appropriate systemic adjuvant therapy, whereas the unknown non-sentinel node-positive patients in group 2 would be treated as SLN biopsy negative. Although the number of events documented for nodal recurrences was small within each group (and consistent with other studies), there were almost twice as many regional recurrences in the SLN biopsy only arm (14 vs. 8)—these might arguably be clinically if not statistically significant but do not appear to translate into any impaired overall survival.

It is notable that more than 80% of patients had tumors ≤2 cm (T1) in size indicating a moderately favorable prognostic group (the proportion of SLN biopsy-positive patients in groups 1 and 2 were 29.5% and 28.3%, respectively). The conclusions of this trial in terms of the appropriateness, safety, and effectiveness of SLN biopsy are justified for this particular population but may not necessarily apply to patients with larger T2 (2–5 cm) or multifocal tumors who commonly undergo SLN biopsy.

The NSABP B-32 trial constituted the largest randomized trial of SLN biopsy, and results for the primary end points of locoregional recurrence and overall survival justify contemporary practices for axillary staging and provide support for a reduction in extent of surgery for the majority of breast cancer patients.

Technique of SLN Biopsy
Standard Methodology
There is international consensus that a combination of blue dye and isotope is optimal in terms of identification rates and learning curves for the SLN biopsy technique in the hands of beginners (27,31,32,35). Nonetheless, since around 2010, many breast units in the United Kingdom (UK) have ceased routinely using blue dye for SLN biopsy and employ radioisotope only. This change in practice has been prompted by persistent residual staining of the breast and reports of adverse reactions to blue dye (43). Other surgeons omit injection of blue dye on table when there is a strong localized signal from the gamma probe placed percutaneously in the axilla. Other aspects of methodology such as site of injection and lymphoscintigraphy remain more contentious. The dye–isotope can be injected as intratumoral, peritumoral, subcutaneous, intradermal, or subareolar (Fig. 39.3). However, routine use of lymphoscintigraphy does not yield additional useful staging information, and ablative therapy is not routinely directed at extra-axillary nodal sites at the present time. Although intratumoral injection of dye–isotope is no longer used, peritumoral, subcutaneous, intradermal, and subareolar sites are practiced. There is evidence that the skin envelope shares a common pattern of lymphatic drainage with the parenchyma of the breast, and these converge upon the same SLN(s) (44). There is a trend toward subareolar injection that gives less "shine through" but requires more prolonged massage, which may encourage migration of tumor cells to the

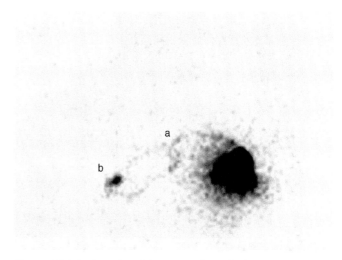

Figure 39.3 Injection of radioisotope in the right breast (intradermal/subareolar): the lymphatic vessels (a) and only one lymph node (b) at the right axilla.

SLN (so called traumets) (45). These could become a potential source of micrometastases. Conversely, benign epithelial cells may be similarly displaced and interpreted as a false-positive result on IHC (46). Periareolar injections give poorer visualization of the internal mammary chain, and when lymphoscintigraphy is used, it is preferable to inject deeper within the breast parenchyma (closer to the parenchymal fascia) (47). Reduced volumes of blue dye may be appropriate in smaller breasted women and avoid prolonged staining of the tissues postoperatively.

Blue Dye-Assisted Node Sampling
Some centers do not have access to radioisotope facilities, and others cannot afford to use this technique. Blue dye-assisted node sampling (BDANS) could be a more pragmatic and cheaper approach for some centers around the world. Standard four-node axillary sampling has evolved into a blue dye-assisted variant, which permits a more targeted sampling and better standardization of technique (Fig. 39.4) (48,49). Interestingly, the preexistence of a minimalist staging procedure in the UK has led some to question the additional benefits of SLN biopsy using dual localization procedures (dye and isotope), which have cost implications. A survey undertaken in 1999 revealed that 47% of British surgeons used axillary sampling (either blind or dye guided) and this figure increased to 64% in 2001 (50). In the absence of nuclear medicine facilities, the standard four-node sample has been adapted as a BDANS. This is a practical option for identification of three to four relevant nodes and avoids the use of isotope, which may present financial and logistical problems for some breast units. Some surgeons have opted to use BDANS despite availability of radioisotope, and with increasing experience of conventional SLN biopsy, removal of three to four nodes seems optimal afterall! Bleiweiss refers to a "sentinel node plus" technique in which surgeons remove a similar number of nodes as for a BDANS (51). The original definition of the SLN was strict: the first node draining the tumor. Not only is there usually more than one SLN in the axillary basin, but lymphoscintigraphy may reveal nodes in the internal mammary chain or supraclavicular zones. The existence of multiple candidate

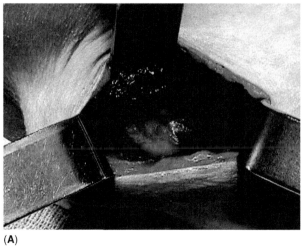
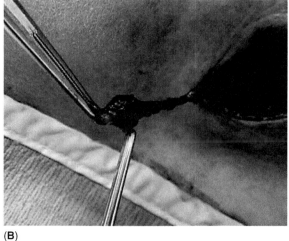

(A)   (B)

Figure 39.4 Blue dye-assisted node sampling: (**A**) blue lymphatic in the right axilla and (**B**) SLN. *Abbreviation*: SLN, sentinel lymph node.

SLNs is a potential flaw in the pathophysiology of the SLN hypothesis; the number of nodes detected is to some extent a time-dependent phenomenon. Dye or isotope will be retained for an indeterminate period in the "sentinel" lymph node(s) before proceeding to higher echelon nodes. Methodological issues such as the time interval between injection and node harvesting together with colloid particle size are critical determinants of sensitivity and specificity. Hypothetically, if there were a range of different colored dyes (blue, yellow, green, etc.), there would be a cognate SLN for each color.

Number of Sentinel Nodes
The average number of axillary SLNs is two or three, but McCarter et al. reported that three nodes were required to identify 99% of positive patients (52). Removal of three or four SLNs from the axilla really represents a sophisticated form of sampling. Nodes that are judged palpable at operation (clinically node negative preoperatively) are always removed irrespective of whether they are blue or hot. Where several nodes are blue the presence of a blue afferent lymphatic does not necessarily indicate sentinel status. Some surgeons now choose to remove all blue-stained nodes and sometimes adjacent nodal tissue as a kind of "limited orientated axillary dissection." These techniques that potentially remove more than two to three nodes may be relevant to recent trends for omission of completion axillary dissection in selected SLN biopsy-positive patients (53). Those patients with a higher metastatic ratio (one out of four) are less likely to harbor NSLN metastases than patients with a single positive SLN or one out of two nodes positive. Thus the proportion of retrieved nodes that contain metastases may be a critical factor in determining NSLN involvement and ultimately the risk of regional recurrence when any further axillary surgery is omitted (21). Thus there are degrees of sampling and some advocate a limited orientated axillary dissection, which is a kind of super-sampling and may avoid the need for further surgery in cases of isolated sentinel node positivity (54). It is often difficult to decide at operation when to stop sampling further nodes; there is general consensus that SLN biopsy should aim to remove all nodes that are blue, hot, blue and hot, or palpably suspicious. Some surgeons consider any radioactive node to be "hot" and aim to remove all such nodes. Use of count ratios can limit the

Table 39.2 Location of the SLN in Relation of Surgical Levels in the Axilla

Level I	83.0%
Level II	15.6%
Level III	0.5%
Internal mammary	0.5%
Supraclavicular	0.1%

number of nodes excised when activity levels are more diffuse and relatively high among three or more nodes. A hot node can be defined in terms of either the SLN:background count (3:1) or the ex vivo count (10:1) (55). In the NSABP B-32 trial, all nodes were removed containing at least 10% of the activity of the hottest node (37).

Location of the Sentinel Node
The SLN is usually found in the lower part of the axilla among level I nodes. Identification and removal are relatively straightforward and morbidity low. Occasionally, the SLN is located at level II (56) and rarely at level III, when removal can incur significant insult (Table 39.2). A delayed axillary dissection is technically challenging, and it might be argued that when the SLN is encountered at higher levels, a formal dissection should be undertaken at the same time. Extra-axillary sites may be found to harbor the SLN when radioactive tracers are used.

Internal Mammary Nodes
The internal mammary nodes receive up to one-quarter of lymphatic flow as an accessory drainage pathway, and the internal mammary chain can be identified on routine lymphoscintigraphy for SLN biopsy in about 15% of cases (Fig. 39.5) (57). Substantial surgical morbidity can result from removal of internal mammary nodes with no demonstration of any gains in overall survival (58). Moreover, it is uncommon for the internal mammary nodes to be involved in the absence of metastases in the axillary nodes (9%), which undermines its value as additional staging information. The biological significance of internal mammary chain disease remains uncertain, and the use of adjuvant therapies is often prompted by concomitant axillary nodal disease. Thus the necessity for internal mammary node biopsy is controversial; it is acknowledged

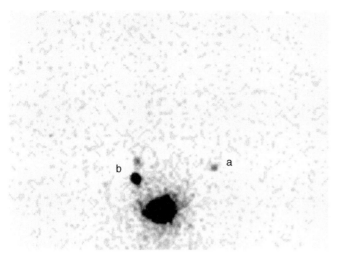

Figure 39.5 Deep injection of the radioisotope in the inner quadrant of the left breast: lymph nodes drain both to the axilla (a) and to the internal mammary chain (b).

that microscopic involvement of the internal mammary nodes may be significant for medially placed tumors with positive axillary nodes. It should be noted that trials of PMRT that have shown an improvement of about 10% in overall survival included irradiation of the internal mammary chain (59,60). Nonetheless, clinical manifestation of internal mammary node recurrence is rare. The indications for irradiation of the internal mammary nodes are unclear at the present time, but CT-based simulation with new planning techniques may minimize the volume of the heart and lungs exposed to radiation and hence related morbidities such as pericarditis and coronary artery disease.

LYMPHEDEMA
Axillary Lymph Node Dissection
More radical resection of axillary nodes is associated with greater upper limb morbidity including lymphedema, shoulder stiffness, pain, and paresthesia (61). The benefits of ALND in terms of regional disease control, staging information, and prognostication must be balanced against these potential sequelae, of which lymphedema is the most serious concern. The overall incidence of lymphedema is cited between 10% and 30% (62–64). Rates are generally lower for a level II ALND (10–15%) compared with a level III ALND (25%). The combination of a complete ALND with irradiation of the axilla can lead to rates of lymphedema as high as 40%. There is rarely any justification for combined axillary dissection and irradiation nowadays. Furthermore, surgeons often loosely refer to level II/III ALND in the literature, and this confounds interpretation of data on rates of lymphedema formation. A complete ALND to level III removes up to 30 lymph nodes, while a partial ALND confined to levels I and II only removes between 10 and 15 nodes on average. A standard axillary dissection refers to clearance of nodes at levels I and II only (in the absence of grossly abnormal nodes at these levels), and it is unusual for level III nodes to contain metastases when nodes at levels I and II are tumor free (24). It has been suggested that removal of an additional three to four nodes maximum at level III is unlikely to significantly impact on documented rates of lymphedema. The ipsilateral

supraclavicular nodes can subsequently be irradiated when extensive nodal involvement is confirmed histologically at levels II and III. Lymphedema remains a common complication, which can lead to major physical and psychological morbidity (65) and in the longer term to the rare complication of lymphangiosarcoma (Stewart–Treves syndrome) (66). Although it is often the nondominant upper limb that is affected (most breast cancers occur on the left side), lymphedema causes symptoms of heaviness and discomfort with associated functional impairment and an unsightly appearance. The accumulation of protein-rich fluid within the extracellular compartment renders the limb prone to recurrent superficial infection, which contributes to more chronic inflammatory changes with fibrosis. Disruption and blockage of the lymphatics raises hydrostatic pressure within other parts of the lymphatic system and promotes further tissue edema by hampering absorption of excess fluid back into the lymphatic vessels. The precise etiology of lymphedema remains unclear, but it is related to the extent of extirpation of axillary nodes. The latter disrupts lymphatic drainage pathways and thus compromised function is more likely when surgical dissection is more extensive.

SLN Biopsy
There is an a priori assumption that a major rationale and justification for SLN biopsy is a reduction in upper limb morbidity, particularly lymphedema. There is a paucity of published material comparing rates of lymphedema in patients undergoing SLN biopsy versus ALND (11,41). Interestingly, some of the differences in morbidity (in favor of SLN biopsy) seen in the ALMANAC trial at three and six months were attenuated at 12 months (although the rate of lymphedema in the SLN biopsy arm was less at 12 months, this was not statistically significant). Documented rates of lymphedema for routine SLN biopsy can be as high as 5–8%, and the chance of lymphedema is independent of node harvest (67,68).

PATHOLOGICAL ASSESSMENT
The SLN has been subjected to much more intensive pathological scrutiny than nodal tissue from a conventional ALND, in which the node is only bisected and a single section from each half examined. The SLN is typically serially sectioned at intervals of 150–200 μm, which, for example, would yield six "slabs" of tissue for a node with a maximum longitudinal diameter of 12 mm. Sections are routinely stained with hematoxylin-eosin (H&E), and IHC is reserved for equivocal cases on H&E, where metastases may be present. Multiple step sections greatly increase the chance of finding tumor cells (diameter 15 μm) (69). In order to validate the SLN hypothesis, it has been essential to exhaustively examine the node to confidently declare it free of tumor. Less intensive protocols would increase false-negative rates and undermine the premise upon which the SLN hypothesis is based. Using both H&E and immunohistochemical methods, the probability of NSLN involvement when the SLN is free of tumor relates to several factors including tumor size and the nature of deposits in the SLN— whether macrometastases (>2 mm), micrometastases (≤2 mm, >0.2 mm), or isolated tumor cells (ITCs; ≤0.2 mm). Some pathologists have suggested that *any* intraparenchymal deposit

measuring ≤0.2 mm constitutes a micrometastasis and consider these intraparenchymal foci to be more biologically important than subcapsular deposits. A meta-analysis by Cserni revealed that when the SLN contains micrometastases only, the probability of NSLN involvement is approximately 15% when the analysis is confined to "high-quality" studies (70). The NSLN metastases have usually been detected by H&E and are macrometastases or larger micrometastases. By contrast, when ITCs only are detected (usually by immunohistochemical methods) the incidence of NSLN positivity is only 9%. Of particular concern is the finding of macrometastases in NSLN when only micrometastases are present in the SLN. This could indicate a "false-negative" result but might suggest that the latter has lower biological priority and that patterns of lymphatic flow exist, which preferentially direct tumor cells to these NSLNs (71). A meta-analysis by Kim and colleagues found that almost half of cases of positive SLN biopsy had NSLN involvement, leading the authors to recommend completion ALND for all cases of a positive SLN based on H&E evaluation (irrespective of tumor load) (72). Others have reported NSLN involvement in 25–30% of patients with micrometastases in the SLN and 10% of those with ITCs (≤0.2 mm). However, the clinical relevance of ITCs is uncertain, and few would recommend completion ALND for ITCs alone. American guidelines currently advise completion ALND for all cases of micrometastases irrespective of whether detectable by H&E or IHC only, but these are under review (35). A nomogram can be used to calculate the probability of NSLN involvement based on a number of variables (73). It would be useful to identify a subgroup of SLN-positive patients, with an acceptably low probability of NSLN involvement, for whom further axillary surgery is unnecessary. Three studies have indirectly addressed this issue of NSLN involvement and stratify risk based on metastatic load in the SLN. Outcomes for the American College of Surgeons Surgical Oncology Group (ACOSOG)-Z0011 trial have been published, and results for the International Breast Cancer Study Group (IBCSG) 23-01 trial were presented at the 31st San Antonio Breast Cancer Symposium in December 2011 (74,75). These results and their implications for clinical practice are discussed in more detail in the next chapter, but both of these trials have shown no difference in either locoregional recurrence or overall survival for selected groups of SLN biopsy-positive patients randomized to either completion ALND or observation only. It should be emphasized that omission of completion axillary dissection is not predicated on a low probability of NSLN involvement per se, but rather a minimal residual tumor load in the NSLNs that can be treated adequately with adjuvant therapies such as breast radiotherapy and systemic treatments. Studies addressing the issue of completion axillary surgery in SLN-positive patients are summarized in Table 39.3 (74–76).

The absolute incidence of node positivity is higher when the SLN biopsy technique is used compared with conventional examination of ALND dissection specimens. Much of this upstaging is attributable to the detection of micrometastases (often by immunohistochemical methods), and the clinical significance of these and ITCs was controversial even before the advent of SLN biopsy and a fragile consensus exists (77–79). The term "staging" implies a discontinuous concept, yet in reality there is a continuum in extent of nodal involvement that reflects the propensity to form distant metastases.

Table 39.3 Trials Investigating Management of Sentinel Node-Positive Patients

Trial	Sentinel Node Status	Randomization
ACOSOG-Z0011 (74)	Macrometastases/micrometastases	ALND vs. no further surgery
IBCSG 23-01 (75)	Micrometastases	ALND vs. no further surgery
AMAROS (76)	Macrometastases/micrometastases	ALND vs. axillary radiotherapy

Abbreviation: ALND, axillary lymph node dissection.

The definition of micrometastasis is arbitrary, and there is no sudden transition from low to high risk and whatever the degree of pathological involvement of the "sentinel node(s)," this tumor load is likely to be clinically relevant in only a small proportion of patients with smaller tumors. If the NSLNs were examined as intensely as the SLN, it is likely that some would be deemed positive. This enhanced scrutiny of the SLN has two consequences. First, it tends to favor a good correlation between sentinel and non-sentinel nodes—when the latter are positive, there is less chance that the SLN will be reported as falsely negative because there is greater likelihood of finding metastatic foci (especially micrometastases <2 mm). Second, it leads to upstaging of disease in approximately 10% of patients and increases rates of isolated SLN positivity to levels above the expected node positive rate for standard ALND (for any particular tumor size). Most validation studies have not examined NSLNs as intensively as the SLN, and it is possible that occult disease is present in some patients who are otherwise SLN biopsy negative and who may not receive chemotherapy as a component of systemic therapy. However, in a multicenter validation study, Weaver and colleagues examined the distribution of occult and non-occult metastases in SLNs and NSLNs among 431 patients by taking additional sections at a depth of 100 and 200 μm into paraffin blocks (80). Sections were stained with both routine H&E and IHC. Metastases were found in only 4.2% of NSLNs, and the odds ratio for metastases in NSLN was more than 10-fold higher for SLN positive than for SLN-negative patients ($p < 0.001$; 95% CI 6.7–28.1). These results validated the SLN hypothesis, although provided no indication of the clinical significance of occult metastatic disease in the SLN.

Circulating tumor cells must undergo both arrest and proliferation to form viable metastatic foci (81). Recent results from the Z0011 and 23-01 studies suggest that systemic therapies may effectively abort this process and contribute to regional disease control with improved disease-free and overall survival (74,75).

INTRAOPERATIVE NODE ASSESSMENT

Several different approaches are currently practiced for intraoperative assessment of SLNs in breast cancer patients with no single method perceived as having any overall advantage in terms of performance, patient care, logistics, and cost. These include frozen section (FS) (82–85), TIMC (83,85,86), and the newer molecular biological assays based on reverse-transcription technologies (87,88).

Rationale

The main purpose for intraoperative nodal assessment is avoidance of a completion ALND undertaken as a delayed, secondary procedure. Axillary reoperation can be technically challenging due to adhesions and fibrosis, but there is no objective evidence for increased morbidity when ALND follows SLN biopsy and median hospital stay is similar for delayed and primary ALND (89). When completion ALND is performed as an *isolated* procedure, there are potential benefits from intraoperative assessment in terms of cost savings, patient convenience, and avoidance of further general anesthesia. When completion ALND rather than radiotherapy is recommended for patients with a positive SLN (tumor deposits >0.2 mm in size), this is often combined with a breast surgical procedure—hence abrogating some advantages relating to cost and inconvenience (90). Clinical decision making for breast cancer patients increasingly incorporates neoadjuvant systemic schedules and immediate breast reconstruction. SLN biopsy can be undertaken either in advance or after neoadjuvant chemotherapy and prior to mastectomy and immediate breast reconstruction (91,92). Whenever node positive, completion ALND is undertaken at the time of definitive surgery without necessity for any separate surgical episode to complete axillary surgery. There would be little advantage from intraoperative node examination with advance SLN biopsy, and completion ALND at this juncture would be inappropriate. For those patients who require a re-excision or completion mastectomy for positive margins following wide excision, further axillary surgery can be done at the same time. The benefits of any intraoperative nodal assessment would be diminished for these patients for whom primary tumor characteristics mandate further surgery. There also exist subgroups of older patients and those with comorbidities for whom a single-stage axillary operation is recommended at the outset. Similarly, selected women might safely avoid completion ALND with minimal chance of regional relapse or impact on longer-term survival. In the "post-Z0011" era, any decision for selective omission of completion ALND should be based on full histopathological parameters relating to both axillary nodes and primary tumor; ironically, some patients may be committed to completion ALND when intraoperative node assessment is available and confirms positivity. Preliminary results from the AMAROS trial suggest that axillary radiotherapy could substitute for completion ALND in some patients with low-volume nodal disease for whom intraoperative assessment would not apply.

Axillary Ultrasound

Sonographic examination with CB of any suspicious axillary nodes is being incorporated into routine clinical assessment of early breast cancer patients and can potentially deselect a subgroup of patients for SLN biopsy based on either a positive nodal CB result or suspicious nodes with or without a negative CB. Published reports suggest that up to 40–50% of node positive patients can be identified by percutaneous biopsy of axillary nodes and as many as 90% of those with four or more positive nodes (93). Nonetheless, this procedure has limited sensitivity (25%) for the detection of micrometastases, which constitute between 20% and 40% of tumor deposits when only a single SLN is positive (94).

Recall Rates for Isolated ALND

Modern approaches to axillary management can potentially contribute to a reduction in absolute numbers of patients who need a completion ALND performed as an isolated, delayed procedure requiring surgical scheduling and readmission to hospital. The recall rate for isolated completion ALND within the authors' unit is about 10% (9.2%) for those patients initially considered suitable for SLN biopsy (95). Intraoperative nodal assessment is not practiced, but all patients undergo preoperative axillary ultrasound and SLN biopsy prior to both immediate breast reconstruction and neoadjuvant chemotherapy.

Molecular Assays

In the light of the preceding comments, it is appropriate to ask whether intraoperative nodal assessment can be justified for all SLN patients or at least those having SLN biopsy as a component of primary surgery. This question acquires greater prescience in view of inconsistency and variable sensitivity of both FS and TIMC, which have not yet been surpassed by molecular assays based on quantitative reverse transcription-polymerase chain reaction (RT-PCR). Conventional examination of the SLN using paraffin-embedded H&E sections remains the reference standard for histopathological evaluation and has a minimum sensitivity for detection of micrometastases or macrometastases of 83.4% (96). It is estimated that routine processing of the SLN misses 10–15% of clinically relevant metastases (96,97). Both FS and TIMC employ rapid H&E staining methods but, like formalin-fixed tissue sections, examine less than 5% of the node and have other limitations. Interpretation is subjective, and for TIMC (which only examines clusters of cells), the distinction between micrometastases and macrometastases may be unclear. The reported patient-based sensitivities for both FS and TIMC are highly variable at 36–96% and specificity of 95–100% (83–86). FS examination has a false-negative rate of about 25% and although TIMC is reported to be more accurate when immunohistochemical staining is used, a "blinded" trial of a single-section approach using facing halves of a bivalved SLN revealed equivalence of accuracy (98). A meta-analysis reported a sensitivity of 75% (95% CI 65–84) and 63% (95% CI 57–69) for FS and TIMC, respectively, with TIMC having significantly lower pooled sensitivity for micrometastases (22%) compared with macrometastases (81%) (99).

Immediate pathological evaluation of the sentinel node is not routinely available in many centers due to resource constraints (100). Molecular based technologies for intraoperative nodal assessment objectively measure expression of genes normally expressed in breast tissue but not in lymph nodes. The most commonly used gene codes for the cytoskeleton protein CK19, which is expressed in most breast cancer cells (101). Operating parameters are set such that quantitative RT-PCR detects macrometastases and micrometastases and not ITCs. The use of multiple gene markers reduces the potential problem of amplification of pseudogenes within genomic DNA segments, but recent innovations such as reverse transcription-loop-mediated isothermal amplification (RT-LAMP) provide high specificity for target mRNA with minimal genomic amplification (102). Validation studies suggest these molecular technologies are almost as accurate as conventional histological evaluation but examination of different nodal slabs ultimately prevents complete concordance (100). Overall concordance levels between RT-PCR scores and permanent H&E sections are 93.7% for the GeneSearch breast lymph node assay (Veridex) and 98.2% for the one-step nucleic acid assay (OSNA), which typically analyze 50% of fresh nodal tissue (103). The remaining available molecular assay (OSNA) takes approximately 30 minutes to process one node (five minutes per additional node) with a mean time saving of 18 minutes compared with TIMC or FS (104). Although breast resection (wide local excision/mastectomy) is undertaken during this period, in reality intraoperative assessment incurs additional operating time of up to 30 minutes per case with cumulative delays and cost implications. SLN biopsy-positive patients will subsequently require node clearance, which consumes further operating time.

Cost–Benefit Analysis

It seems unlikely, therefore, that any of the current methods for intraoperative lymph node assessment can increase the efficiency of breast cancer surgery and may not necessarily lead to net cost savings when the absolute number of cases of isolated completion ALND is modest. With a recall rate of <10%, the cost of performing intraoperative node assessment in all SLN biopsy cases is unlikely to offset the costs of any delayed axillary surgery. A recent analysis reported net cost savings of 10–15% when intraoperative assessment was omitted in T1a and T1b and only macroscopic inspection done for T1c breast cancers. No distinction was made between isolated and combined completion ALND, which might otherwise have favored omission in larger tumors too (105). Addition of TIMC is reported to half the recall rate for ALND in patients with negative preoperative axillary ultrasound examination (106). The recall rate with TIMC was 9%, which is comparable to the authors' figure *without* intraoperative nodal assessment. A prospective study found about 10% of patients were spared further axillary surgery when TIMC was employed (107). If half of these patients need concomitant breast surgery, the impact of TIMC on absolute numbers of isolated ALND is relatively modest (<5%).

Intraoperative node examination may be more difficult to justify for all patients in the context of contemporary practice, which either deselects patients for SLN biopsy or dictates that completion ALND is performed alongside definitive or additional breast surgery. Formal cost analysis is warranted to compare intraoperative node assessment for all cases of SLN biopsy in relation to the small number of cases of isolated completion ALND. Recall rates for completion ALND might be further reduced, but the overall cost–benefit of routine intraoperative nodal assessment remains questionable, and allocation of node evaluation cases to separate operating lists is impractical (90,105). Development of noncommercial open access molecular assays (home recipes) as alternatives may significantly influence cost–benefit analyses of intraoperative assessment.

**TIMING OF SLN BIOPSY
AND NEOADJUVANT THERAPY**

Patient selection and timing of SLN biopsy in the context of primary chemotherapy continue to evolve. Before the advent of SLN biopsy, all neoadjuvant chemotherapy patients underwent ALND at the time of definitive surgery following induction chemotherapy. In consequence, pretreatment nodal status was unknown for any individual patient, some of whom were converted from being node positive to node negative. For the majority of patients, this lack of staging information upfront had no influence on surgical treatment and minimal impact on adjuvant therapy decisions. The purpose of SLN biopsy was to permit some primary surgical patients to potentially avoid ALND, but neoadjuvant patients remained obligated to undergo ALND despite being eligible for BCS after downstaging of their breast tumor.

A dichotomy of practice emerged among clinicians in attempts to define how SLN should be optimally incorporated into the neoadjuvant setting; SLN biopsy either was carried out in conjunction with a completion ALND *after* chemotherapy as part of prospective clinical trials to assess the safety and accuracy of this technique or was done *before* initiation of chemotherapy as a separate surgical procedure.

SLN Biopsy Prior to Neoadjuvant Chemotherapy

This will minimize the risk of a false-negative result and may allow more accurate initial staging of patients (108–111). Much surgical experience has now accrued with SLN biopsy pretreatment (as for primary surgical treatment), and high rates of identification (98–100%) and node positivity (29–67%) are reported. Completion ALND can safely be avoided at the time of definitive surgery with low regional recurrence rates ranging from 0% to 3.6%, with rates generally <0.5% at more prolonged follow-up of 37–48 months (112). Upfront SLN biopsy provides important information on prognostication and can guide treatment decisions for adjuvant radiotherapy, systemic therapy, and axillary surgery. It should be noted that a complete nodal remission after neoadjuvant chemotherapy is a predictor of disease-free survival (B-18) (113). However, in general, there is no quantification of regional metastatic load with upfront approach, and the total number of positive nodes at the commencement of treatment remains unknown—although there may be a minimum number of positive nodes from SLN biopsy in excess of two or even three. Knowledge of pretreatment nodal status potentially influences the decision to give chemotherapy if the primary tumor is relatively small together with type of chemotherapy (e.g., taxanes and trastuzumab for node-positive tumors). Furthermore, decisions for chest wall and supraclavicular radiotherapy postoperatively are more reliable when there is accurate information about initial staging of disease. Interestingly, patients with larger estrogen receptor-positive tumors, which are confirmed to be node negative on SLN biopsy but have a low oncotype-DX score, could be treated with neoadjuvant hormonal therapy rather than a combination of chemohormonal therapy (114). A common criticism of upfront SLN biopsy is that patients require two separate operations, but patients who are SLN positive or SLN negative with clinically positive/sonographically suspicious nodes at the outset still require a completion ALND. Moreover, SLN biopsy is undertaken in advance of mastectomy and immediate breast reconstruction postchemotherapy in order to avoid any delayed ALND when facilities for intraoperative node assessment are not available.

Concerns have been expressed about possible delays in commencement of definitive treatment with prechemotherapy SLN biopsy, which relates to delays consequent to scheduling issues and wound complications such as seromas and infection. An audit was undertaken in the author's unit of 24 patients undergoing SLN biopsy prechemotherapy (115). The mean time from tissue diagnosis to SLN biopsy was 7.3 days (range 5–22 days), and the mean time from SLN biopsy to start of chemotherapy was 9.2 days (range 2–23 days). Finally, the mean time from tissue diagnosis to chemotherapy was 16.5 days (range 13–25 days), which was significantly longer than average time period of 8.3 days for a group of patients not undergoing SLN biopsy (t-test; p = 0.00002). However, this delay of more than 2 weeks was not considered detrimental to outcome in the context of clinically and sonographically node-negative disease.

SLN Biopsy after Neoadjuvant Chemotherapy

Some advocate SLN biopsy *after* primary chemotherapy (113,116) in order to take advantage of nodal downstaging and avoidance of axillary dissection in up to 40% of patients, particularly those with triple negative or HER2-positive disease. Where facilities for intraoperative node assessment are available, this permits a "single" operation with associated advantages of patient convenience and cost. Between 30% and 70% of patients will be committed to ALND with upfront SLN biopsy. It should be noted that axillary ultrasound was infrequently performed in many of the earlier studies leading to higher rates of node positivity at the time of SLN biopsy. Rates of complete pathological nodal response vary from 20% to 36% (and may be higher for micrometastases alone) in patients with needle biopsy confirmed positive nodes prechemotherapy (117,118). It has been suggested that knowledge of *nodal response* to chemotherapy is more relevant for prognostication/PMRT decisions than initial *nodal status* per se. There is some evidence that primary chemotherapy may modify lymphatic drainage patterns and lead to differential downstaging between sentinel and non-sentinel nodes (113). Cancer cells reach the SLN first and subsequently pass to the NSLN (*front to back*). However, chemotherapy may yield an earlier response in NSLN than SLN, which might render SLN biopsy less accurate postchemotherapy (*back to front*) (114). Reports from the past few years have shown false-negative rates of 8–11% with a pooled estimate of 12% for SLN biopsy following chemotherapy in clinically node-negative patients (119,120). These figures are similar to false-negative rates for primary surgery (NSABP B-32 = 9.7%) but may not be strictly comparable; for example, only a subset of patients in the neoadjuvant studies had SLN biopsy postchemotherapy and there may have been some bias related to patient selection and surgeon experience. Furthermore, much variation in technique for SLN biopsy (blue dye alone, isotope alone, combination) was employed in these studies. There are mixed reports on false-negative rates for cytologically/CB-proven positive nodes prechemotherapy with only three published studies relating specifically to this group of patients (Table 39.4).

A meta-analysis of all trials since 2004 has shown wide variability in false-negative rates ranging from 5% to 25% with a mean of 9% (124). Limited data are available on omission of completion ALND in node-positive patients with a subsequent

Table 39.4 Rates of False Negativity for SLN Biopsy when Performed After Preoperative Chemotherapy for Patients with Documented Nodal Metastases at Presentation

Author	No. of Patients	False-Negative Rate (%)
Shen et al (121)	69	25
Lee et al (122)	238	5.6
Newman et al (123)	54	10.7

negative SLN biopsy after neoadjuvant chemotherapy; it is unclear from studies whether rates relate to patients with either positive or negative initial nodal status. Moreover, there is confounding due to up to 30% of patients having ALND. Hunt and colleagues reported axillary recurrence rates of 1.2% at a median follow-up of 55 months (125). Further information is required on rates of regional recurrence—these are likely to be higher when there is residual non-sentinel nodal disease after a false-negative SLN biopsy postchemotherapy (126).

SLN biopsy can be performed either before or after neoadjuvant chemotherapy, and there are advantages and limitations with both approaches. A National Cancer Institute (NCI) conference recommended SLN biopsy *before* or *after* for clinically node-negative disease (127). Nonetheless, it remains uncertain whether a "negative" SLN biopsy after primary chemotherapy can avoid the need for ALND. Ideally, there should be an "all-or-none" response of nodes to chemotherapy—either all nodes respond or none do so. Micrometastases and ITCs may have different biological significance if they represent downstaged macrometastases. Implications from the ACOSOG-Z0011 trial cannot be readily extrapolated to the neoadjuvant setting as patients with a positive SLN biopsy after chemotherapy will not undergo further chemotherapy (although they may receive breast irradiation). It is reasonable to consider SLN biopsy postchemotherapy in clinically (and sonographically) node-negative patients for whom pretreatment nodal status would not impact on choice of chemotherapy or radiotherapy.

SLN BIOPSY IN SPECIAL CIRCUMSTANCES
Pregnancy

The development of breast cancer during pregnancy presents unique emotional and management problems. Although termination may be advocated in the first trimester, surgical treatments can be safely undertaken in any trimester of pregnancy (128,129). Adjuvant therapies including radiotherapy and chemohormonal therapies are usually deferred until after delivery although chemotherapy (but *not* tamoxifen) can be safely administered in the second trimester when organogenesis is complete and teratogenic effects are minimal (130). Radiotherapy is absolutely contraindicated in the gravid state, but interestingly the dose of radiation from exposure to technetium radiocolloid in SLN biopsy is only 20 MBq. This is well below the safe upper limit for pregnant women, and therefore SLN biopsy using isotopic localization only could be employed; note that blue dye will stain placental and fetal tissue and must be avoided. If there are concerns about the use of radioisotope, axillary staging could be carried out as a delayed procedure (if ALND at the outset is deemed inappropriate). For further information on breast cancer and pregnancy, please refer to chapter 48.

Male Breast Cancer

Cadaver studies have confirmed that the pattern of lymphatic distribution and drainage is similar in males and females (131); the cutaneous plexus of lymphatics is linked to lymphatics within the breast parenchyma via specialized subareolar and circumareolar plexuses that drain directly to axillary nodes (22). Based on this common anatomy and physiology, SLN biopsy should be feasible in clinically node-negative male patients, and there is no a priori reason to suppose that the technique is less accurate in men (35). A limited number of publications have emerged in the literature supporting this contention, demonstrating high rates of detection and low rates of false negativity and axillary recurrence (132–137). However, the numbers of patients in these studies are necessarily very low, and calculations of relevant performance indicators must be interpreted with caution. Cimmino et al. reported on 18 male patients treated for breast cancer, of whom six underwent SLN biopsy (133). Most of these had a confirmatory ALND (4/6) and half had a positive SLN biopsy (mean tumor size 1.6 cm). The authors concluded that SLN biopsy was suitable for male breast cancer patients with clinically node-negative tumors measuring ≤2 cm (T1). It was unclear whether the technique could be applied to larger tumors where the chance of nodal involvement and false-negative rates were higher. Gentilini et al. reported an identification rate of 100% among a group of 32 male patients who underwent SLN biopsy for mainly T1 tumors (75%) (136). The mean number of SLNs removed at operation was 1.5 (range 1–3). Twenty six of these 32 patients were SLN negative and were spared ALND. Among the six SLN biopsy-positive patients, only two had involvement of NSLNs with no axillary recurrences in SLN-negative patients at 30 months follow-up. Other studies have confirmed high rates of identification of the SLN in clinically node-negative male patients using dual localization techniques with or without lymphoscintigraphy. Boughey et al. emphasized that male patients present with larger tumors on average than females and are more likely to be SLN positive (37.0% vs. 22.3%; p = 0.1) and to harbor additional disease in NSLN (62.5% vs. 20.7%; p = 0.01) (135). These conclusions were echoed in a recent series of 78 male breast cancer patients from Memorial Sloan-Kettering Cancer Center. The SLN was successfully identified in 76 patients (97%), and 37 of these had a positive SLN (node positivity rate 49%). Both patients with a failed SLN biopsy proceeded to ALND and were found to have nodal metastases. Furthermore, in three patients with a negative SLN (8%), a positive NSLN was found by digital palpation at operation.

The overall benefits of SLN biopsy for men may be less than for their female counterparts who undergo regular breast screening and present with earlier stage disease or "minimal" breast cancer (29). Nonetheless, the procedure is feasible and appears safe and justified in a selected group of younger, clinically node-negative patients with tumors ≤2 cm.

Ductal Carcinoma In Situ

There is consensus that patients with ductal carcinoma *in situ* (DCIS) which is extensive (on imaging) and requiring mastectomy (+/− reconstruction) or those presenting as a palpable mass should undergo SLN biopsy. An incidental invasive component will be found in up to 20% of those cases of DCIS mandating mastectomy (138). Detailed studies on the incidence of nodal metastases in the pre-sentinel era failed to reproducibly identify a group of patients with invasive cancer whose risk of axillary disease was <10%, with the exception of those with pure tubular tumors ≤1 cm in size. Many reports of node positivity in DCIS relate to ITCs or micrometastases only and are probably clinically irrelevant. The risk of nodal involvement, which is acceptable if left undetected, is a subjective judgment; patients with a very low risk of nodal disease might be spared the minimal but finite morbidity of SLN biopsy with concomitant cost savings. However, there is consensus that patients with a typical screen-detected focal area of DCIS, which represents up to 80% of cases in a screening program, should not undergo SLN biopsy or any other form of surgical staging of the axilla. SLN biopsy is preferable in cases of DCIS with microinvasion diagnosed on CB as a significant proportion of those patients with microinvasion on core needle biopsy will have further invasive foci on definitive histology (particularly when the target of biopsy is not microcalcifications). These foci of overt invasion (>1 mm) mandate some form of axillary staging, and up to 10% of patients with microinvasion on initial CB will be SLN biopsy positive (139). Moreover, between 10% and 15% of lesions diagnosed as DCIS using large bore vacuum devices will demonstrate invasion on complete excision. Nonetheless, despite reports of node positivity rates approaching 15% in high-risk DCIS and DCIS with microinvasion (140), it should be re-iterated that many cases involve ITCs or micrometastases only, which are of questionable biological significance (141).

Multifocal and Multicentric Tumors

These were initially found to be associated with high false-negative rates and were considered a contraindication to SLN biopsy (142). This was consonant with the erroneous assumption that tumors located in different quadrants of the breast drain through mutually exclusive lymphatic pathways, and therefore SLN biopsy would lead to inaccurate axillary lymph node staging (142). Some publications refute this viewpoint, and SLN biopsy is no longer precluded by the presence of multiple tumor foci either within the same (multifocality) or different (multicentricity) quadrants of the ipsilateral breast (142–144). Information from lymphoscintigraphy supports the notion that the various quadrants of the breast share common lymphatic drainage channels, which converge upon the subareolar region (145).

Elderly Patients

SLN biopsy should be employed in most elderly patients with clinically node-negative breast cancer but might be avoided in some older patients who have a low probability of nodal involvement. Perhaps a more pertinent issue is whether completion ALND should be undertaken for a positive SLN in older patients. Even before publication of the ACOSOG-Z0011 trial, completion ALND was selectively omitted in certain older patients, particularly those with only micrometastases in the SLN, as these may not be biologically important. A publication from the Memorial Sloan-Kettering Cancer Center reported that rates of axillary relapse in patients with a positive

SLN who, for various reasons, had no further axillary surgery were very low (2% at three years) (146). Some elderly patients will decline completion ALND when fully informed of risks and benefits of this procedure; these group of patients are very unlikely to have residual disease, which would develop into any troublesome regional recurrence or compromise longer-term survival in any clinically meaningful way.

NEWER TECHNIQUES FOR SLN IDENTIFICATION
Fluorescence Mapping
There are potential drawbacks associated with the use of radio-isotopes as a tracer agent for localization of the SLN. These include cumulative radiation exposure for healthcare workers and problems with surgical waste disposal, which place restrictions on access to isotopes secondary to mandatory licensing. The radioisotope is usually injected a few hours preoperatively in the nuclear medicine department, and this requires a coordinated effort between different disciplines. Moreover, these particular radioisotopes are formed as a bi-product of the nuclear industry and supply might become unpredictable with more widespread usage in the future. This may lead to an increase in the differential cost between radiocolloid and blue dye. Localization techniques using a combination of blue dye and another nonradioactive tracer, which has comparable accuracy to blue dye and isotope, therefore warrant investigation. The indocyanine green (ICG) fluorescent navigation system is a promising new method for identification of SLNs, which is claimed to be more reliable and easier to use than conventional isotope methods in smaller district hospitals. Less training may be required, although dissection of the fluorescent lymphatics can be awkward at times with the need to dim theater lights. There is potential for ICG fluorescence to replace radioisotope, and comparison of blue dye and isotope with blue dye and ICG fluorescence is justified. The injection of radioisotope while the patient is awake is uncomfortable and may involve the inconvenience of a separate visit to the hospital the day before surgery in some units (or possibly an overnight stay). Fluorescence navigation not only permits co-injection with blue dye after induction of anesthesia but also avoids radioisotope and lymphoscintigraphy (Fig. 39.6).

Japanese workers have investigated use of ICG fluorescence mapping for lymphatic drainage pathways in gastric cancer

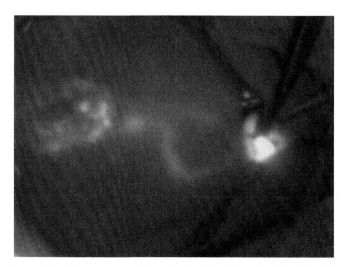

Figure 39.6 Fluorescent mapping with ICG dye for sentinel lymph node localization. *Abbreviations*: ICG, indocyanine green

(147,148). Within subcutaneous tissues, ICG binds to albumin that drains to the lymphatic vessels and, in turn, to lymph nodes. The principle of fluorescence imaging has subsequently been applied to SLN mapping in breast cancer. An early validation study used ICG alone in place of blue dye for SLN biopsy. The SLN was identified in almost 80% of cases using ICG as the sole tracer agent. All patients underwent a completion ALND, and calculated concordance rates for final nodal status were high (96.1%) (149). A further study by Kitai and colleagues explored the use of ICG alone and attempted to utilize both its green color and fluorescence to detect SLNs among a group of 31 patients. Identification rates in excess of 90% were reported, but these were reliant mainly on the fluorescent properties of ICG, which permitted immediate visualization of lymphatic channels within seconds of injection and real-time observation of passage of dye through the lymphatic system. Although more than three-quarters of lymphatics were visibly green, only half of the SLNs were green, but all were fluorescent (150).

Subsequent practice has favored a combination of ICG with either blue dye or radioisotope, which allows both conventional and fluorescent visualization of the lymphatic vessels and nodes. These have all shown high levels of nodal recognition by fluorescence with few nodes (<5%) being classified as blue and/or hot but not fluorescent (151).

Several groups from Japan have reported highly successful identification of SLNs using both ICG and blue dye. Among a group of 411 patients, 408 (99%) had fluorescent-positive SLNs. Detection rates for blue dye alone within this multicenter study ranged from 83% to 93%. The sentinel node positivity rate was 9.5%, and all nodes with tumor deposits >0.2 mm were fluorescent (151).

An interesting prospective study directly compared the performance of ICG and radioisotope in node-negative patients with tumors <3 cm (152). Identification rates were 98.7% and 96.9% for ICG and radioisotope, respectively, when combined individually with blue dye. Node positivity rates and false-negative rates were equivalent for the two techniques, but ICG was notably cheaper. Murawa and colleagues investigated the relative performance of ICG and Tc-labeled sulfur radiocolloid in a small group of 20 patients, all of whom underwent ALND following SLN biopsy. The SLN was identified in all 20 patients with ICG and in 17 patients with radiocolloid. Moreover, the false-negative rate was threefold higher for radiocolloid compared with ICG (23% vs. 8%) (153).

All these studies investigating fluorescence imaging for SLN biopsy have consistently shown near 100% identification rates and confirmed that combination with either blue dye or isotope is the optimal technique. A conjugated form of ICG adsorbed onto human serum albumin (ICG:HSA) has been explored in an attempt to limit the number of fluorescent nodes. Mieog and colleagues reported the use of ICG:HSA as a third tracer in 24 breast cancer patients undergoing conventional localization with blue dye and isotope. All SLNs were fluorescent, and the average nodal count was 1.45 (154). A further study involving 49 consecutive breast cancer patients has compared ICG alone (after first 28 patients) with ICG:HSA (next 21 patients). There was no statistically significant difference between the number of SLNs detected with these two tracers, suggesting that conjugation of ICG to a carrier molecule may be unnecessary (155).

Blue SLNs 1 and 2   **ICG fluorescence in SLNs 1 and 2 but not fat**

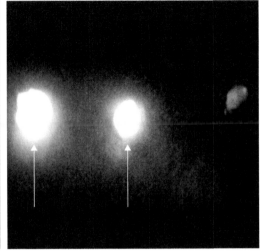

Figure 39.7 Fluorescent sentinel lymph nodes seen ex vivo; the piece of tissue to the right of the field is fat only.

One of the authors (J.R.B.) has now completed recruitment of 100 patients into a feasibility study, which was undertaken to validate and confirm the sensitivity and safety of ICG as a tracer agent for SLN identification in early breast cancer patients. The primary objective of this study was to determine the sensitivity of ICG when combined with blue dye and isotope. Patients received triple injection of blue dye, radiocolloid, and ICG at the time of SLN biopsy in order to avoid any potential increase in false-negative rates. Nodal staining characteristics were recorded numerically, and the sensitivity of ICG fluorescence was calculated as the percentage of SLNs detected by blue and/or radioisotope that were also fluorescent with ICG. A definitive analysis of the entire cohort of 100 patients has confirmed that fluorescence imaging using ICG provides high sensitivity for detection of the sentinel nodes (100%), and combined nodal sensitivity is higher for blue dye and ICG (95.0%) compared with the standard combination of blue dye and radioisotope (73.1%). The procedural node positivity rate was 17.3%, and all nodes containing macrometastases/micrometastases were blue, hot, and fluorescent and represented the first nodes removed. Moreover, ICG appears to be a safe agent with no adverse reactions, and fluorescence imaging provides an additional dimension to the procedure of SLN biopsy (Fig. 39.7) (156).

Microbubbles

This is a novel method that aims to improve the preoperative diagnosis of axillary lymph node metastases using enhanced ultrasound technology with a special contrast agent (microbubbles). This can potentially identify the SLN preoperatively, which can then be removed percutaneously without the need for an open surgical operation. The contrast agent employed is sulfur hexafluoride, which is injected intradermally. Following massage of the breast, the contrast can be traced to the axilla using ultrasound and the first draining (i.e., sentinel) node identified. This can then be comprehensively biopsied with the intention of removing the entire node. All material is sent for histological analysis, and those patients with confirmed metastases can proceed directly to axillary dissection. At the present time, the negative predictive value of this technique is insufficiently accurate to omit SLN biopsy in the absence of any tumor in a percutaneously biopsied node; nonetheless, this remains a possibility in the future. For the time being, microbubbles do offer the chance of improving the preoperative diagnosis rate for lymph node metastases. A preliminary report by Jones and colleagues, involving 70 consecutive patients, indicated that the SLN could be accurately identified with microbubbles in 87% of cases (61), and a guidewire successfully placed to locate the node that was subsequently removed at the time of conventional SLN biopsy (157). This methodology is being further evaluated in the unit of one of the authors (J.R.B.) to specifically ascertain whether the identified SLN node can be removed percutaneously.

TRAINING

There is a learning curve associated with the SLN biopsy technique. Surgeons must be appropriately trained, and validation undertaken with a predefined number of consecutive cases (between 20 and 30 cases). In principle, a minimum rate of SLN identification and correspondingly low false-negative rate (5–10%) should be confirmed before an individual surgeon or institution can use this method for staging the axilla in routine practice. There will be a constant stream of new trainees for instruction in the SLN biopsy technique; at the inception of SLN biopsy, it was decreed that validation be carried out on selected patients who will undergo mandatory completion axillary dissection. However, this is both unethical and impractical with medicolegal implications. Instead, surgical trainees must now be proctored when undertaking SLN biopsy cases by recognized trainers in accredited breast units. From initially having a "head start" from experience with blind sampling techniques, British surgeons rapidly moved toward a "NEW START" with introduction of the world's largest structured, multiprofessional, and validated SLN biopsy training program (158). The latter is based on a combined technique for localization using a combination of blue dye (Patent Blue V) and isotope (^{99m}Tc-albumin colloid) in order to ensure consistency and reproducibility. The program was spearheaded by the Royal College of Surgeons of England and was rapidly rolled out across the UK with designated training centers and a system of proctoring for all breast surgeons. The program facilitated the rapid transfer of relevant knowledge and technical skills to ensure that surgeons could deliver safe and competent SLN biopsy throughout breast units in the UK. A particular feature of NEW START was the formalized training of multiprofessional teams with emphasis on both theory and practical aspects of SLN biopsy. Almost 90% of patients (5849/6685) underwent immediate axillary staging after SLN biopsy (mentorship model). Surgeons had to perform 30 cases (first five supervised by an accredited NEW START trainer) and achieve an identification rate of >90% and a false-negative rate of <10%. More than 200 SLN biopsy naïve surgeons entered the program and although localization rates and false-negative rates improved with surgeon caseload, there was no significant learning curve and false-negative rates fell to <10% after 20 cases. Therefore, a training program for SLN biopsy can yield satisfactory performance standards and guarantee patient safety during the period of training.

CONCLUSION

The advent of SLN biopsy as a surgical innovation has revolutionized the management of the axilla over the past 15 years. Nonetheless, it is probably true to state that SLN biopsy has generated much controversy and debate with emergence of more questions than answers. These relate to several aspects including methodology, interpretation, and clinical significance of nodal metastases and the timing of the procedure in relation to neoadjuvant therapy and reconstruction. Despite recent seminal publications, there remain lingering concerns about longer-term outcome in terms of locoregional control and overall survival for both node-negative patients and node-positive patients for whom completion axillary dissection is omitted. Axillary surgery encompasses both staging and therapeutic procedures, and it is important to select patients appropriately to avoid under- and over-treatment of patients, respectively. SLN biopsy is associated with much reduced surgical morbidity and is now the dominant and preferred method for staging the axilla. False-negative rates must be kept to a minimum by routine use of dual localization techniques and intraoperative digital examination with removal of all nodes, which are not only hot/blue but also palpably suspicious. Radionucleotide facilities are not universally available, and SLN biopsy can be adapted into a more pragmatic technique of BDANS with harvesting of about four axillary lymph nodes. However, reports of allergic reactions to blue dye and persistent staining of the breast have led some surgeons to abandon blue dye and perform SLN biopsy with only radioisotope. Other tracer agents are being investigated at the present time but are not yet in common practice and must be evaluated alongside existing standard methods for SLN localization. In the future, it may be possible to identify the SLN preoperatively and perform percutaneous sampling and even removal of the SLN and hence obviate the need for any form of surgical staging.

Individualized recommendations based on the risk of relapse, which includes formal analysis of the risks, benefits, and cost of treatment, are the ideal approach to management of the axilla. This strategy should incorporate a spectrum of options including ALND, targeted sampling, and observation alone.

REFERENCES

1. Carter CL, Allen C, Henderson DE. Relation of tumour size, lymph node status and survival in 24,740 breast cancer cases. Cancer 1989; 73: 505–8.
2. Rosen PP, Groshen S, Saigo PE, et al. Pathologic prognostic factors in stage I (T1N0M0) and stage II (T1N1M0) breast carcinoma: a study of 644 patients with median follow up of 18 years. J Clin Oncol 1989; 7: 1239–125.
3. Cady B, Stone MD, Schuler J, et al. The new era in breast cancer: invasion, size and nodal involvement dramatically decreasing as a result of mammographic screening. Arch Surg 1996; 131: 301–8.
4. Querci della Rovere G, Bonomi R, Ashley S, Benson JR. Axillary staging in women with small invasive breast tumours. Eur J Surg Oncol 2006; 32: 733–7.
5. Caldos C, Aparicio SA. The molecular outlook. Nature 2002; 415: 484–5.
6. Recht A, Edge SB, Solin LJ, et al. Post-mastectomy radiotherapy: clinical practice guidelines of the American Society of Clinical Oncology. J Clin Oncol 2001; 19: 1539–69.
7. Fisher B, Montague F, Redmond C, et al. Ten-year results of a randomized trial comparing radical mastectomy and total mastectomy with or without radiation. N Engl J Med 1985; 312: 674–81.
8. Baum M, Coyle PJ. Simple mastectomy for early breast cancer and the behaviour of the untreated nodes. Bull Cancer 1977; 64: 603–10.
9. Rampaul RS, Mullinger K, MacMillan RD, et al. Incidence of clinically significant lymphoedema as a complication following surgery for primary operable breast cancer. Eur J Cancer 2003; 39: 2165–7.
10. Purushotham AD, MacMillan RD, Wishart G. Advances in axillary surgery for breast cancer–time for a tailored approach. Eur J Surg Oncol 2005; 31: 929–31.
11. Purushotham AD, Upponi S, Klevesath MB, et al. Morbidity following sentinel lymph node biopsy in primary breast cancer–a randomized controlled trial. J Clin Oncol 2005; 23: 4312–21.
12. Britton PD, Goud A, Godward S, et al. Use of ultrasound-guided axillary node core biopsy in staging of early breast cancer. Eur Radiol 2009; 19: 561–9.
13. Querci della Rovere G, Benson JR. The case for axillary dissection. Adv Breast Cancer 2004; 1:3–8.
14. Querci della Rovere G, Bonomi R, Ashley S, Benson JR. The incidence of axillary nodal metastases in older women with small non-high grade tumours. Breast Cancer Res Treat 2005; 94: S41.
15. Borgstein PJ, Meijer S, Pijpers RJ, et al. Functional lymphatic anatomy for sentinel node biopsy in breast cancer: echoes from the past and the periareolar blue dye method. Ann Surg 2000; 232: 81–9.
16. Mansel RE, Goyal A, Newcombe RG. Internal mammary node drainage and its role in sentinel node biopsy: the initial ALMANAC experience. Clin Breast Cancer 2004; 5: 279–84.
17. Veronesi U, Cascinella N, Greco M, et al. Prognosis of breast cancer patients after mastectomy and dissection of internal mammary nodes. Ann Surg 1985; 202: 702–7.
18. McMinn RMH. Last's Anatomy (Regional and Applied), 18th edn. Edinburgh: Churchill Livingstone, 1990.
19. Cabanas RM. An approach for the treatment of penile carcinoma. Cancer 1997; 39: 456–66.
20. Morton DL, Wen DR, Wong JH, et al. Technical aspects of intraoperative lymphatic mapping for early stage melanoma. Arch Surg 1992; 127: 392–9.
21. Guiliano AE, Kirgan DM, Guenther JM, Morton DL. Lymphatic mapping and sentinel lymphadenectomy for breast cancer. Ann Surg 1994; 220: 391–401.
22. Romrell LJ, Bland KI. Anatomy of the breast, axilla, chest wall and related metastatic sites. In: Bland KI, Copeland EM, eds. The Breast, 3rd edn. Chapter 2, Vol I Philadelphia: Saunders, 2004.
23. Veronesi U, Luini A, Galimberti V, et al. Extent of metastatic axillary involvement in 1446 cases of breast cancer. Eur J Surg Oncol 1990; 16: 127–33.
24. Veronesi U, Rilke R, Luini A, et al. Distribution of axillary node metastases by level of invasion. Cancer 1987; 59: 682–7.
25. Goyal A, Newcombe RG, Mansel RE. Clinical relevance of multiple sentinel nodes in patients with breast cancer. Br J Surg 2005; 92: 438–42.
26. Rescigno J, Taylor LA, Aziz MS, et al. Predicting negative axillary lymph node dissection in patients with positive sentinel lymph node biopsy: can a subset of patients be spared axillary dissection? Breast Cancer Res Treat 2005; 94: S35.

27. Veronesi U, Paganelli G, Galimberti V, et al. Sentinel node biopsy to avoid axillary dissection in breast cancer with clinically negative nodes. Lancet 1997; 349: 1864–7.

28. Mcmasters KM, Giuliano AE, Ross MI, et al. Sentinel lymph node biopsy for breast cancer: not yet standard of care. N Engl J Med 1998; 349: 1864–7.

29. Sachdev U, Murphy K, Derzie A, et al. Predictions of non-sentinel lymph node metastases in breast cancer patients. Am J Surg 2002; 183: 213–17.

30. Damera A, Evans AJ, Cornford EJ, et al. Diagnosis of axillary node metastases by ultrasound guided core biopsy in primary operable breast cancer. Br J Cancer 2001; 89: 1310–13.

31. Krag D, Weaver D, Ashikaga T, et al. The sentinel node in breast cancer. A multicentre validation study. N Engl J Med 1998; 339: 941–6.

32. Albertini JJ, Lyman GH, Cox C, et al. Lymphatic mapping and sentinel node biopsy in the patient with breast cancer. JAMA 1996; 276: 1818–22.

33. Cody HS. Management of the axilla in early stage breast cancer: will sentinel node biopsy end the debate? J Surg Oncol 1999; 71: 137–9.

34. Morrow M, Rademaker AW, Bethke KP, et al. Learning sentinel node biopsy: Results of a prospective randomized trial of two techniques. Surgery 1999; 126: 714–22.

35. Lyman GH, Guiliano AE, Somerfield MR, et al. The American society of clinical oncology guideline recommendations for sentinel lymph node biopsy in early stage breast cancer. J Clin Oncol 2005; 23: 7703–20.

36. Benson JR, Querci della Rovere G. Management of the axilla in women with breast cancer. Lancet Oncol 2007; 8: 331–48.

37. Krag DN, Anderson SJ, Julian TB, et al. Technical outcomes of sentinel-lymph node resection and conventional axillary lymph node dissection in patients with clinically node negative breast cancer: results from the NSABP B-32 randomised phase III trial. Lancet Oncol 2007; 8: 881–8.

38. Krag D, Anderson SJ, Julian TB, et al. Sentinel lymph node resection compared with conventional axillary lymph node dissection in clinically node negative patients with breast cancer: overall survival findings from the NSABP B-32 randomised phase 3 trial. Lancet Oncol 2010; 11: 927–33.

39. Veronesi U, Paganelli G, Viale G, et al. A randomized comparison of sentinel node biopsy with routine axillary dissection in breast cancer. N Engl J Med 2003; 349: 546–53.

40. Gill PG. Sentinel lymph node biopsy versus axillary clearance in operable breast cancer. The RACS SNAC trial, A Multicenter randomised trial of the Royal Australian College of Surgeons (RACS) Section of Breast Surgery, in collaboration with the National Health and Medical Research Council Clinical Trials Center. Ann Surg Oncol 2004; 11: 216S–21S.

41. Mansel RE, Goyal A, Fallowfield L, et al. Sentinel node biopsy versus standard axillary treatment: results of the randomized multicentre UK ALMANAC trial. J Natl Cancer Inst 2006; 98: 599–609.

42. Benson JR. An alternative to axillary lymph node dissection. Lancet Oncol 2010; 11: 908–9.

43. Manson AL, Juneja R, Self R, et al. Anaphylaxis to Patent Blue V: a case series. Asia Pac Allergy 2012; 2: 86–9.

44. Nathanson SD, Wachna DL, Gilman D, et al. Pathways of lymphatic drainage from the breast. Ann Surg Oncol 2001; 8: 837–42.

45. Rosser RJ. Safety of sentinel lymph node dissection and significance of cytokeratin micrometastases. J Clin Oncol 2001; 19: 1882–3.

46. Bleiweiss IJ, Legmann MD, Nagi CS, Jaffer S. Sentinel lymph nodes can be falsely positive due to iatrogenic displacement and transport of benign epithelial cells. J Clin Oncol 2006; 24: 2013–18.

47. Tanis PJ, Neiweg OE, Valdes Olmos RA, et al. Anatomy and physiology of lymphatic drainage of the breast from the perspective of sentinel node biopsy. J Am Coll Surg 2001; 192: 399–409.

48. Chetty U. Axillary node sampling to evaluate the axilla. World J Surg 2001; 25: 773–9.

49. Steel RJ, Forrest APM, Chetty U. The efficacy of lower axillary sampling in obtaining lymph node status in breast cancer: a controlled randomized trial. Br J Surg 1985; 72: 368–9.

50. Gaston MS, Dixon JM. A survey of surgical management of the axilla in UK breast cancer patients. Eur J Cancer 2004; 40: 1738–42.

51. Bleiweiss I. Sentinel lymph nodes in breast cancer after 10 years: rethinking basic principles. Lancet Oncol 2006; 7: 686–92.

52. McCarter MD, Yeung H, Fey J, et al. The breast cancer patients with multiple sentinel nodes: when to stop? J Am Coll Surg 2001; 192: 692–7.

53. Benson JR, Wishart GC. Axillary dissection for sentinel node positive patients with early stage breast cancer. Br J Surg 2011; 98: 1499–500.

54. Salmon RJ, Marcolet A, Vieira M, et al. Sentinel node biopsy or limited orientated axillary dissection. Eur J Surg Oncol 2005; 31: 949–53.

55. Kuehn T, Bembenek A, Decker T, et al. A concept for the clinical implementation of sentinel lymph node biopsy in patients with breast carcinoma with special regard to quality assurance. Cancer 2004; 103: 451–61.

56. Roumen RMH, Valkenburg JGM, Geuskens LM. Lymphoscintigraphy and feasibility of sentinel lymph node biopsy in 83 patients with primary breast cancer. Eur J Surg Oncol 1997; 23: 495–502.

57. Borgstein PJ, Meijer S, Pijpers RJ, van Diest PJ. Functional lymphatic anatomy for sentinel node biopsy in breast cancer: echoes from the past and the periareolar blue dye method. Ann Surg 2000; 232: 81–9.

58. Veronesi U, Cascinella N, Greco M, et al. Prognosis of breast cancer patients after mastectomy and dissection of internal mammary nodes. Ann Surg 1985; 202: 702–7.

59. Overgaard M, Hansen PS, Overgaard J, et al. Post-operative radiotherapy in high risk pre-menopausal women with breast cancer who receive adjuvant chemotherapy. N Engl J Med 1997; 337: 949–55.

60. Ragaz J, Jackson SM, Le N, et al. Adjuvant radiotherapy and chemotherapy in node positive pre-menopausal women with breast cancer. N Engl J Med 1997; 337: 956–62.

61. Kissin MW, Querci della Rovere G, Easton D, et al. Risk of lymphoedema following the treatment of breast cancer. Br J Surg 1986; 73: 580–4.

62. Jacobsson S. Studies of the blood circulation in lymphoedematous limbs. Scand J Plast Reconstr Surg 1967; 3: 1–81.

63. Schuneman J, Willich N. Lympheodema of the arm after primary treatment of breast cancer. Anticancer Res 1998; 18: 2235–6.

64. Mortimer PS, Bates DO, Brassington HD, et al. The prevalence of arm oedema following treatment for breast cancer. Q J Med 1996; 89: 377–80.

65. Pain SJ, Purushotham AD. Lymphoedema following surgery for breast cancer. Br J Surg 2000; 87: 1128–41.

66. Stewart FW, Treves N. Lymphangiosarcoma in post-mastectomy oedema. Cancer 1948; 1: 64–8.

67. Sener SF, Winchester DJ, Martz CH, et al. Lymphoedema after sentinel lymphadenectomy for breast cancer. Cancer 2001; 92: 748–52.

68. Newman L. 30th San Antonio Breast Cancer Symposium; Texas, United States of America, December 2010.

69. Viale G, Bosari S, Mazzarol G, et al. Intra-operative examination of axillary sentinel lymph nodes in breast carcinoma patients. Cancer 1999; 85: 2433–9.

70. Cserni G, Gregori D, Merletti F, et al. Non-sentinel node metastases associated with micrometastatic sentinel nodes in breast cancer: meta-analysis of 25 studies. Br J Surg 2004; 91: 1245–52.

71. Cserni G. Evaluation of sentinel nodes in breast cancer. Histopathology 2005; 46: 697–702.

72. Kim T, Agboola O, Giuliano A, et al. Lymphatic mapping and sentinel lymph node sampling in early stage breast cancer: A meta-analysis. Cancer 2006; 106: 4–16.

73. Van Zee KJ, Manasseh DM, Bevilacqua JL, et al. A nomogram for predicting the likelihood of additional nodal metastases in breast cancer patients with a positive sentinel node biopsy. Ann Surg Oncol 2002; 10: 1140–51.

74. Giuliano AE, Hunt K, Ballman K, et al. Axillary dissection vs no axillary dissection in women with invasive breast cancer and sentinel node metastases: a randomized clinical trial. JAMA 2011; 305: 569.

75. Galimberti V, Cole BF, Zurrida S, et al. Update of International Breast Cancer Study Group Trial 23-01 to compare axillary dissection versus no axillary dissection in patients with clinically node negative breast cancer and micrometastases in the sentinel node. Cancer Res 2011; 71: 102s.

76. Straver ME, Meijnen P, van Tienhoven G, et al. Sentinel node identification rate and nodal involvement in the EORTC 10981-22033 AMAROS trial. Ann Surg Oncol 2010; 17: 1854–61.

77. De Mascarel I, Bonichon F, Coindre JM, et al. Prognostic significance of breast cancer axillary lymph node micrometastases assessed by two special techniques. Reevaluation with longer follow up. Br J Cancer 1992; 66: 523–7.

78. Millis RR, Springall R, Lee AH, et al. Occult axillary lymph node metastases are of no prognostic significance in breast cancer. Cancer 2002; 86: 396–401.

79. Weaver DL, Ashikaga T, Krag D, et al. Effect of occult metastases on survival in node negative breast cancer. N Engl J Med 2011; 364: 412–21.

80. Weaver DL, Krag DN, Ashikaga T, et al. Pathologic analysis of sentinel and nonsentinel lymph nodes in breast carcinoma. Cancer 2000; 88: 1099–107.

81. den Bakker MA, van Weeszenberg A, de Kanter AY, et al. Non-sentinel lymph node involvement in patients with breast cancer and sentinel node micrometastases; too early to abandon axillary clearance. J Clin Pathol 2002; 55: 932–5.

82. Dixon JM, Mammam U, Thomas J. Accuracy of intraoperative frozen-section analysis of axillary nodes. Edinburgh Breast Unit team. Br J Surg 1999; 86: 392–5.

83. Brogi E, Torres-Matundan E, Tan LK, Cody HS. The results of frozen section, touch preparation and cytological smear are comparable for intraoperative examination of sentinel lymph nodes: a study in 133 breast cancer patients. Ann Surg Oncol 2005; 12: 173–8.

84. Dowlatshahi K, Fan M, Anderson JM, Bloom KJ. Occult metastases in sentinel nodes of 200 patients with operable breast cancer. Ann Surg Oncol 2001; 8: 675–81.

85. Van Diest PJ, Torrenga H, Borgstein PJ, et al. Reliability of intra-operative frozen section and imprint cytological investigation of sentinel lymph nodes in breast cancer. Histopathology 1999; 35: 14–18.

86. Lambah PA, McIntyre MA, Chetty U, Dixon JM. Imprint cytology of axillary lymph nodes as an intraoperative diagnostic tool. Eur J Surg Oncol 2003; 29: 224–8.

87. Blumencranz P, Whitworth PW, Deck K, et al. Sentinel node staging for breast cancer: intraoperative molecular pathology overcomes histological sampling errors. Am J Surg 2007; 194: 426–32.

88. Viale G, Dell'Orto P, Biasi MO, et al. Comparative evaluation of an extensive histopathologic examination and a real-time reverse-transverse transcription polymerase chain reaction assay for mammoglobin and cytokeratin 19 on axillary sentinel lymph nodes of breast carcinoma patients. Ann Surg 2008; 247: 136–42.

89. Goyal A, Newcombe RG, Chhabra A, Mansel RE. Morbidity in breast cancer patients with sentinel node metastases undergoing delayed axillary lymph node dissection compared with immediate ALND. Ann Surg Oncol 2008; 15: 262–7.

90. Benson JR, Wishart GC. Is intra-operative nodal assessment essential in a modern breast practice? Eur J Surg Oncol 2010; 36: 1162–4.

91. Schrenk P, Hochreiner G, Fridrik M, et al. Sentinel node biopsy performed before preoperative chemotherapy for axillary node staging in breast cancer. Breast J 2003; 9: 282–7.

92. Benson JR, Wishart GC, Forouhi P, Provenzano E. Sentinel lymph node biopsy prior to mastectomy and immediate breast reconstruction. Eur J Surg Oncol 2009; 35: 1233.

93. MacMillan RD, Blamey RW. The case for axillary sampling. Adv Breast Cancer 2004; 1: 9–10.

94. Benson JR, Wishart GC, Forouhi P, et al. The incidence of nodal involvement following completion axillary lymph node dissection for sentinel node positive disease. Eur J Surg Oncol 2006; 32: 104.

95. Benson JR, Wishart GC, Forouhi P, Provenzano E. How often does a positive lymph node biopsy prompt an isolated delayed axillary lymph node dissection? Cancer Res 2010; 70: 135S.

96. Yared MA, Middleton LP, Smith TL, et al. Recommendations for sentinel lymph node processing in breast cancer. Am J Surg Pathol 2002; 26: 377–82.

97. Cserni G. What is a positive sentinel lymph node in breast cancer patients? A practical approach. Breast 2007; 16: 152–60.

98. Vanderveen KA, Ramsamooj R, Bold RJ. A prospective, blinded trial of touch prep analysis versus frozen section for intraoperative evaluation of sentinel lymph nodes in breast cancer. Ann Surg Oncol 2008; 15: 2006–11.

99. Tew K, Irwig L, Matthews A, et al. Meta-analysis of sentinel node imprint cytology in breast cancer. Br J Surg 2005; 92: 1068–80.

100. Mansel RE, Goyal A, Douglas-Jones A, et al. Detection of breast cancer metastasis in sentinel lymph nodes using intra-operative real time GeneSearch BLN Assay in the operating room: results of the Cardiff study. Breast Cancer Res Treat 2009; 115: 595–600.

101. Chu PG, Weiss LM. Keratin expression in human tissues and neoplasms. Histopathology 2002; 40: 403–39.

102. Notomi T, Okayama H, Masubuchi H, et al. Loop-mediated isothermal amplication of DNA. Nucleic Acids Res 2000; 28: E63.

103. Tsujimoto M, Nakabayashi K, Yoshidome K, et al. One-step nucleic acid amplification for intra-operative detection of lymph node metastases in breast cancer patients. Clin Cancer Res 2007; 13: 4807–16.

104. Bernet L, Martinez-Benaclocha M, Cano-Munoz R, et al. One-step nucleic acid amplification (OSNA) for sentinel node intra-operative diagnosis: advantages from the classical procedures. 7th European Breast Cancer Conference, Barcelona, 2010; abstract 337.

105. Canavese G, Bruzzi P, Catturich A, et al. Intra-operative evaluation of the sentinel lymph node for T1-N0 breast cancer patients: Always or never? A risk/benefit and cost/benefit analysis. Eur J Surg Oncol 2010; 36: 737–44.

106. Shrestha DB, Nayagam M, Pittam M, et al. Effect of combined preoperative axillary ultrasound and intraoperative imprint cytology of the sentinel lymph node biopsy on the recall rate for axillary lymph node dissection. Miami Breast Cancer Conference, 2010; abstract 133.

107. Hamidian Jahromi A, Narayanan S, MacNeill F, et al. Testing the feasibility of intra-operative sentinel lymph node touch imprint cytology. Ann R Coll Surg Engl 2009; 91: 336–9.

108. Schrenk P, Hochreiner G, Fridrik M, et al. Sentinel node biopsy performed before preoperative chemotherapy for axillary node staging in breast cancer. Breast J 2003; 9: 282–7.

109. Schrenk P, Tausch C, Wolfl S, et al. Sentinel node mapping performed before preoperative chemotherapy may avoid axillary dissection in breast cancer patients with negative or micrometastatic sentinel nodes. Am J Surg 2008; 196: 176–83.

110. Menard J-P, Extra J-M, Jacquemier J, et al. Sentinel lymphadenectomy for the staging of clinical axillary node negative breast cancer before neoadjuvant chemotherapy. Eur J Surg Oncol 2009; 35: 916–20.

111. Straver ME, Rutgers EJT, Russel NS, et al. Towards rational axillary treatment in relation to neoadjuvant therapy in breast cancer. Eur J Cancer 2009; 45: 2284–92.

112. Bergkvist L, de Boniface J, Jonsson PE, et al. Axillary recurrence after negative sentinel lymph node biopsy in breast cancer: 3 year follow up of the Swedish Multicentre Cohort Study. Ann Surg 2008; 247: 150–6.

113. Mamounas E, Brown A, Anderson S, et al. Sentinel node biopsy after neoadjuvant chemotherapy: results of the National Surgical Adjuvant Breast and Bowel Project B-27. J Clin Oncol 2005; 23: 2694–702.

114. Sabel M. Sentinel lymph node biopsy before or after neoadjuvant chemotherapy: pros and cons. Surg Oncol Clin N Am 2010; 19: 519–38.

115. Benson JR, Wishart GC, Ambler G, Provenzano E. Sentinel lymph node biopsy before primary chemotherapy in breast cancer patients. Eur J Cancer 2010; 8: 29.

116. Gianni L, Baselga J, Eiermann W, et al. First report of the European Cooperative Trial in operable breast cancer (ECTO): effects of primary systemic therapy (PST) in local-regional disease. Proc Am Soc Clin Oncol 2002; 21: 34a (abstr 132).

117. Hennessy BT, Hortobagyi GN, Rouzier R, et al. Outcome after pathologic complete eradication of cytologically proven breast cancer axillary node metastases following primary chemotherapy. J Clin Oncol 2005; 23: 9304.

118. Beatty JD, Precht LM, Lowe K, et al. Axillary conserving surgery is facilitated by neoadjuvant chemotherapy of breast cancer. Am J Surg 2009; 197: 637–42.

119. Xing Y, Foy M, Cox DD, et al. Meta-analysis of sentinel lymph node biopsy after pre-operative chemotherapy in patients with breast cancer. Br J Surg 2006; 93: 539–46.

120. Van Deurzen CH, Vriens BE, Tjan-Heijnen VC, et al. Accuracy of sentinel lymph node biopsy after neoadjuvant chemotherapy. Eur J Cancer 2009; 45: 3124–30.

121. Shen J, Gilcrease MZ, Babiera GV, et al. Feasibility and accuracy of sentinel lymph node biopsy after preoperative chemotherapy in breast

cancer patients with documented axillary metastases. Cancer 2007; 169: 1255–63.

122. Lee S, Kimey EY, Kang SH, et al. Sentinel lymph node identification rate, but not accuracy is significantly decreased after pre-operative chemotherapy in axillary node positive breast cancer patients. Breast Cancer Res Treat 2007; 102: 283–8.

123. Newman EA, Sabel MS, Nees AV, et al. Sentinel lymph node biopsy performed after neoadjuvant chemotherapy is accurate in patients with documented node positive breast cancer at presentation. Ann Surg Oncol 2007; 14: 2946–52.

124. Mamounas EP, Bellon JR. Loco-regional therapy considerations in patients receiving preoperative chemotherapy. In: Harris JR, Lippman ME, Morrow M, et al. eds. Diseases of the Breast, 4th edn. Philadelphia: Lippincott Williams & Wilkins, 2010: 730–44.

125. Hunt KK, Yi M, Mittendorf EA, et al. Sentinel lymph node surgery after neoadjuvant chemotherapy is accurate and reduces the need for axillary dissection in breast cancer patients. Ann Surg 2009; 250: 558–66.

126. Sabel MS. Locoregional therapy of breast cancer: maximising control, minimising morbidity. Expert Rev Anticancer Ther 2007; 6: 1261–79.

127. Bucholtz TA, Lehman CD, Harris JR, et al. Statement of Science concerning loco-regional treatments after pre-operative chemotherapy for breast cancer: a National Institute Conference. J Clin Oncol 2008; 26: 791–7.

128. Theriault RL. Breast cancer during pregnancy. In: Singletary SE, Robb GL, eds. Advanced therapy of Breast Disease. chapter 18 Ontario: BC Decker Inc, 2000: 167–73.

129. Berry DL, Theriault RL, Holmes FA, et al. Management of breast cancer during pregnancy using a standardized protocol. J Clin Oncol 1999; 17: 855–61.

130. Doll DC, Ringenberg QS, Yarbro JW. Antineoplastic agents and pregnancy. Semin Oncol 1989; 16: 337–46.

131. Suami H, Pan WR, Mann GB, Taylor GI. The lymphatic anatomy of the breast and its implications for sentinel lymph node biopsy: a human cadaver study. Ann Surg Oncol 2008; 15: 863–71.

132. Hill AD, Borgen PI, Cody HS III. Sentinel node biopsy in male breast cancer. Eur J Surg Oncol 1999; 25: 442–3.

133. Cimmino VM, Degnim AC, Sabel MS, et al. Efficacy of sentinel lymph node biopsy in male breast cancer. J Surg Oncol 2004; 86: 74–7.

134. Rusby JE, Smith BL, Dominguez FJ, Golshan M. Sentinel lymph node biopsy in men with breast cancer: a report of 31 consecutive procedures and review of the literature. Clin Breast Cancer 2006; 7: 406–10.

135. Boughey JC, Bedrosian I, Meric-Bernstam F, et al. Comparative analysis of sentinel lymph node operation in male and female breast cancer patients. J Am Coll Surg 2006; 203: 475–80.

136. Gentilini O, Chagas E, Zurrida S, et al. Sentinel lymph node biopsy in male patients with early breast cancer. Oncologist 2007; 12: 512–15.

137. Flynn LW, Park J, Patil SM, et al. Sentinel lymph node biopsy is successful and accurate in male breast carcinoma. J Am Coll Surg 2008; 206: 616–21.

138. Meyer JE, Smith DN, Lester SC, et al. Large-core needle biopsy of nonpalpable breast lesions. JAMA 1999; 281: 1683–41.

139. Intra M, Zurrida S, Maffini F, et al. Sentinel lymph node metastasis in microinvasive breast cancer. Ann Surg Oncol 2003; 10: 1160–5.

140. Zavotsky J, Hansen N, Brennan MB, et al. Lymph node metastasis from ductal carcinoma in situ with micro-invasion. Cancer 1999; 85: 2439–43.

141. Klauber-DeMore N, Tan LK, Liberman L, et al. Sentinel lymph node biopsy: is it indicated in patients with high-risk ductal carcinoma in situ and ductal carcinoma in situ with microinvasion? Ann Surg Oncol 2000; 7: 636–42.

142. Goyal A, Newcombe RG, Mansell RE, et al. ALMANAC Trialist Group. Sentinel lymph node biopsy in patients with multifocal breast cancer. Eur J Surg Oncol 2004; 30: 475–9.

143. Gentilini O, Trifiro G, Soleldo J, et al. Sentinel lymph node biopsy in patients with multicentric breast cancer. The experience of the European Institute of Oncology. Eur J Surg Oncol 2006; 32: 507–10.

144. Toumisis E, Zee KJV, Fey JV, et al. The accuracy of sentinel lymph node biopsy in multicentric and multifocal invasive breast cancers. J Am Coll Surg 2003; 197: 529–34.

145. Holwitt DM, Gillanders WE, Aft RL, et al. Sentinel lymph node biopsy in patients with multicentric/multifocal breast cancer: low false-negative rate and lack of axillary recurrence. Am J Surg 2008; 196: 562–5.

146. Naik AM, Fey J, Gemignani M, et al. The risk of axillary relapse after sentinel lymph node biopsy for breast cancer is comparable with that of axillary lymph node dissection: a follow up study of 4008 procedures. Ann Surg 2004; 240: 462–8.

147. Nimura H, Narimiya N, Mitsumori N, et al. Laparoscopic sentinel node navigation achieved by infra-red ray electronic endoscopy system in patients with gastric cancer. Br J Surg 2004; 91: 575–9.

148. Tajima Y, Yamazaki K, Masuda Y, et al. Sentinel node mapping guided by indocyanine green fluorescence imaging in gastric cancer. Ann Surg 2009; 249: 58–62.

149. Motomura K, Inaji H, Komoike Y, et al. Sentinel node biopsy guided by indocyanine Green dye in breast cancer patients. Jap J Clin Oncol 1999; 29: 604–7.

150. Kitai T, Inomoto T, Miwa M, Shikayama T. Fluorescence navigation with indocyanine green for detecting sentinel lymph nodes in breast cancer. Breast Cancer 2005; 12: 2111–215.

151. Sugie T, Kassim KA, Takeuchi M, et al. A novel method for sentinel lymph node biopsy by indocyanine green fluorescence technique in breast cancer. Cancers 2010; 2: 713–20.

152. Tagaya N, Tsumuraya M, Nakagawa A, et al. Indocyanine green (ICG) fluorescence imaging versus radioactive colloid for sentinel lymph node identification in patients with breast cancer. J Clin Oncol 2010; 28:674.

153. Murawa D, Hirche C, Dresel S, et al. Sentinel lymph node biopsy in breast cancer guided by indocyanine green fluorescence. Br J Surg 2009; 96: 1289–94.

154. Mieog JSD, Troyan SL, Hutteman M, et al. Toward optimization of imaging system and lymphatic tracer for near-infrared fluorescence sentinel lymph node mapping in breast cancer. Ann Surg Oncol 2011; 18: 2483–91.

155. Polom K, Murawa D, Nowaczyk P, et al. Breast cancer sentinel lymph node mapping using near-infrared guided indocyanine green and indocyanine green-human serum albumin in comparison with gamma emitting radioactive colloid tracer. Eur J Surg Oncol 2011; 38: 137–42.

156. Wishart GC, Jones LC, Loh S-W, Benson JR. Fluorescence mapping with indocyanine green (ICG) for sentinel lymph node detection in early breast cancer.–results of the ICG-10 study. Eur J Surg Oncol 2012; 38:465.

157. Jones P, Jones S, Mills P, et al. Identification of sentinel lymph nodes preoperatively using microbubble enhanced ultrasound in patients with breast cancer. Proc Am Soc Clin Oncol 2009; abstract 44.

158. Goyal A, MacNeill F, Newcombe RG, et al. Results of the UK NEW START sentinel lymph node biopsy training programme: A model for future surgical training. Proc Am Assoc Surg Oncol 2009; abstract 25.

40 Management of the axilla II

Laura S. Dominici and Mehra Golshan

INTRODUCTION

Over the last several decades, the surgical management of breast cancer has been evolving toward less invasive therapy due to emphasis on a multidisciplinary approach and results of randomized prospective studies. Many women with early-stage disease undergo less invasive surgery with breast conservation rather than mastectomy. Results of seven large randomized prospective studies (with the two largest having more than a 20-year follow-up) show equivalence in terms of survival between these two surgical techniques (1,2). In the past, women with locally advanced disease were relegated to mastectomy but with an increasing use of neoadjuvant therapy, selected women who present with locally advanced breast cancers may become candidates for breast conservation. The safety of breast conserving therapy in this setting has been evaluated in many randomized trials that have demonstrated equivalence in survival and local recurrence as well as an increase in rates of breast conserving therapy (3–6).

During the same period, systemic therapies have become tailored to an individual patient's tumor biology. Advances include endocrine therapy with aromatase inhibitors, novel chemotherapeutic agents, and targeted therapies. Radiation therapies which traditionally focused on whole-breast irradiation are now being examined in partial and accelerated forms. In conjunction with advances in local therapy to the breast and systemic therapies, the status of axillary lymph nodes and method of evaluation remains an important part of staging a patient's breast cancer in addition to improving local control and providing information for adjuvant treatment recommendations (7).

Surgical management of the axilla has likewise moved toward a less invasive approach. A woman with a clinically negative axilla now undergoes sentinel lymph node biopsy (SNB) rather than axillary lymph node dissection (ALND) in many parts of the world (8,9). Sentinel node status is used to make decisions for adjuvant therapy and will direct any decision on further axillary surgery. For related groups of patients SNB can provide comparable control to ALND. For women who have a positive sentinel node with micrometastatic disease or greater, the standard of care has been to perform an ALND although this has been challenged (7). With the publication from the American College of Surgeon's Oncology Group, controversy has arisen on whether or not all patients with a positive sentinel lymph node need to undergo completion axillary dissection for either prognostic and/or therapeutic purposes.

AXILLARY LYMPH NODE DISSECTION

ALND remains the standard of care for patients with a clinically positive axilla and was performed on all patients with breast cancer prior to introduction of SNB. In the era of the Halsted radical mastectomy all three levels of the axilla were resected, while over the past 40 years this has transitioned to resections of levels I and II. The purpose of ALND is to provide prognostic information, improve local control, and potentially improve survival. The National Surgical Adjuvant Breast and Bowel Project (NSABP) B-04 trial did not reveal significant differences in survival among patients who were clinically node negative and were randomized to radical mastectomy, total mastectomy with postoperative radiation therapy, or total mastectomy with ALND only (10). However, this study was not powered to detect small survival differences. In contrast, some studies have projected a small survival benefit (11,12). Following ALND, rates of local recurrence are extremely low, ranging from 0% to 2.1% with a follow-up of 40–180 months (13). Nonetheless, ALND is associated with significant morbidity in terms of lymphedema, pain, paresthesiae, and reduction of arm mobility. In consequence, less invasive approaches to the management of the axilla have been explored. Studies addressing trends in practice have already revealed a significant decrease in the number of patients with a positive SNB who do not undergo completion ALND. An American Society of Clinical Oncology survey, found that only 22% of members always recommend ALND for micrometastatic disease and many radiation oncologists increasingly consider axillary radiation as an alternative to further surgery. Studies done using the SEER database also confirm a significant number of patients are no longer proceeding to completion ALND after a positive sentinel node and that the proportion of patients in this category is increasing (14–16).

IMPLEMENTATION OF SENTINEL NODE BIOPSY

Following pivotal research done by Morton and colleagues at the John Wayne Cancer Institute with use of SNB in melanoma, this technique was applied to breast cancer (17). Initial validation studies using either blue dye or technetium (17,18) involving SNB followed by completion ALND revealed that SNB was a safe and accurate procedure with acceptable false-negative rates. Subsequently, several retrospective studies have sought to confirm these findings (19). The sentinel node procedure is feasible to perform in both academic and community settings (20), and multiple mapping methods have been used (21). The average false-negative rate for SNB is 8.4% with a majority of studies having values below 10% (7). A group from the Memorial Sloan-Kettering Cancer Center (MSKCC) found the risk of axillary relapse after negative SNB to be comparable to that of ALND in their dataset (9) and several other publications have now confirmed this finding (22). The Cancer Institute in Milan examined this in a randomized fashion, and found no differences in local recurrence between patients who had SNB compared with ALND (23). The NSABP B-32 presented data showing no significant differences in overall survival, disease-free survival, and regional control in patients undergoing SNB alone versus SNB followed by ALND in node-negative patients. This was the largest prospective randomized trial to examine this question and had a median follow-up of more than over 90 months (24).

MORBIDITY OF AXILLARY SURGERY

The procedure of SNB is associated with significantly less morbidity than that of ALND (Table 40.1). A prospective multicenter trial revealed decreased mobility, increased pain, increased seroma formation, and more frequent numbness in patients undergoing ALND versus SNB. There were also significant differences in rates of lymphedema at a follow-up of 29–31 months with rates of 3.5%, 15.7%, and 19.1% for patients having SLNB, ALND without radiotherapy, and ALND with radiotherapy (25). The American College of Surgeons Oncology Group (ACOSOG) Z0011 trial randomized patients with a positive SNB (micro/macro metastases) to completion ALND versus no further surgery. Patients were assessed both subjectively and objectively for postoperative morbidity, including lymphedema. There was no significant difference in arm circumference at one year, but a significantly high number of patients complained of subjective swelling in the ALND group. One quarter of patients having SLNB only complained of postoperative symptoms, while 70% of those in the ALND group had postoperative complaints (26). The authors' own group reviewed the morbidity of SNB and found a significant decrease in morbidity of the procedure when compared with ALND (27). Notwithstanding these comments, SNB does have side effects including lymphedema in up to 5% of cases, but can significantly reduce morbidity associated with a more extensive removal of axillary nodes.

SENTINEL NODE POSITIVITY
AND PREDICTION MODELS

In general, patients with sentinel nodes containing micro or macrometastases are recommended to undergo completion ALND. Studies suggest that in 40–60% of cases, the sentinel node is the only positive node (28). Therefore, ALND could potentially be avoided if it could be determined with a high degree of accuracy that the sentinel nodes were the only involved nodes. This is of relevance in terms of local recurrence and risk of distant failure from leaving positive nodes within the axilla. Several predictive models have been devised to calculate the likelihood of residual axillary disease.

Van Zee and colleagues at Memorial Sloan-Kettering Cancer Center (MSKCC) created a nomogram for prediction of non–sentinel lymph node metastases. This included tumor and nodal characteristics but did not consider the size of metastases and used detection by immunohistochemistry (IHC) as a surrogate for size. This analysis was initially performed retrospectively and then validated prospectively, with the receiver operating characteristic being 0.76 and 0.77 respectively (29). This model was subsequently validated on a database of 200 consecutive patients from MD Anderson Cancer Center. The nomogram was found to be reliable for those with either a relatively low probability of nodal metastases and could be useful for counseling purposes in these patients. Unfortunately, the sensitivity and specificity for prediction of a 10% or 15% probability of additional node positivity was low (30).

A validation study for this nomogram was also undertaken at the Institut Curie, involving 588 consecutive patients with a positive SNB. Though this model worked well for patients with macrometastatic deposits, it was not valid for those with micrometastases (defined as foci ≤2 mm). These micrometastases were detected by IHC in 44% of the patient population in this French study, compared with only 5–9% of patients studied at MSKCC (31). It was suggested that an alternative model might be necessary for patients with only micrometastases in the sentinel node (32). There have been other attempts to validate this nomogram, some of which have revealed limitations in the nomogram pertaining to the particular dataset used (33–38).

The Stanford model was developed by Kohrt and colleagues and emphasized the interrelation among factors such as primary tumor size, lymphovascular invasion, and the size of metastases. Data from this alternative model suggested that it was more strongly correlated with the presence of non–sentinel node metastases than the MSKCC model. Nonetheless, reliability of both models was further reduced when applied to a different patient population (39). The Cambridge and Tenon models take account of the size of sentinel node metastasis (40), while Cho et al. at Seoul National University designed a scoring system which incorporates preoperative evaluation of the axilla by ultrasound (41). The University of Louisville created an integer-based model for prediction (42). Other scoring systems have been developed by the University of Texas MD Anderson Cancer Center (43), with a nomogram taking into account nodal ratio of involvement and size of metastasis as a continuous variable (44).

It is recognized that nomograms may be limited predictors of additional disease in the context of micrometastases only in the sentinel node. Meretoja and colleagues published results of an analysis based on a series of 484 patients with isolated tumor cells (ITCs) or micrometastatic disease; these data were used to create a nomogram to predict a greater than 10% chance of additional axillary disease. The area under the curve was 0.791 in the validation series but the model has not yet been independently validated (45).

Table 40.1 Comparison of Morbidity Following Sentinel Lymph Node Biopsy with and Without Completion Axillary Dissection (26)

Outcome	Sentinel Lymph Node Biopsy (%)	Completion Axillary Lymph Node Dissection (%)
Lymphedema	3.5	19.1
Impaired shoulder range of motion	3.5	11.3
Shoulder/arm pain	8.1	21.1
Shoulder/arm numbness	10.9	37.7

For all comparisons, p < 0.0001.

Other studies have commented on the sensitivity and specificity of the most commonly used predictive models. These models have all been determined retrospectively, and their performance is highly dependent upon the database evaluated. When a particular model is chosen, its limitations must be explained to the patient and validation with the clinical local data set is preferable (46,47) Moreover, in the event that axillary node dissection is no longer performed for some patients with positive sentinel nodes, then the use of nomograms becomes less relevant.

EXISTING DATA REGARDING OMISSION OF AXILLARY DISSECTION

For women who are node negative (pN0) overall survival is comparable irrespective of whether they undergo SNB or extensive ALND (48). With a more detailed pathological analysis of sentinel nodes controversy has arisen as to what should be considered a positive sentinel node. At present, those patients with ITCs (only positive on IHC), do not usually undergo completion ALND. Most studies suggest that these patients have a similar outcome to patients who are node negative (49,50), though some reports suggest that these ITCs may be clinically relevant (51) and may reflect significant residual nodal disease in the axilla (52). ACOSOG released the results of the Z0010 trial which revealed that sentinel node metastases detected only by IHC do not appear to have any significant effect on overall survival (53). This would suggest that these women with ITCs should be treated as node negative. There are now questions regarding the treatment of the axilla with a single positive sentinel node or low volume axillary disease.

There have been both retrospective and prospective studies examining omission of ALND in patients with low-volume lymph node metastases. Most patients in these studies were considered to be at a relatively low risk for additional disease in the axilla based on older age, smaller tumors of lower grade,

and estrogen receptor–positive disease. Most of these studies are nonrandomized and include many patients who did not undergo ALND due to their disease not being identified intraoperatively. Furthermore, many of these patients did receive adjuvant breast radiation in the context of breast conserving therapy. Trials included both patients undergoing mastectomy as well as breast conservation, but these groups were not analyzed separately. Table 40.2 details outcomes of the studies examining patients who did not undergo ALND after a positive SNB.

The largest prospective randomized trial, ACOSOG Z0011, reported results for women with clinically node-negative disease, undergoing breast conserving therapy followed by whole breast irradiation with a positive SNB. There were no differences in locoregional recurrence, disease-free survival, or overall survival for women with one or two positive sentinel nodes (macro-/micrometastases), who were randomized to ALND completion or no further axillary surgery. These patients had clinical T1 or T2 tumors and the majority (>80%) had hormone receptor–positive tumors. All underwent breast conservation and received whole-breast radiation (54). With a median follow-up of 6.3 years, local and regional recurrences were similar between the SNB-only arm and the ALND arm. Criticism of this trial includes early closure with accrual of less than one-half of the original target (1900) and lack of power to determine a survival benefit. The radiation oncologists were not blinded to surgical therapy, and there was no standardization of radiation fields. Efforts are currently ongoing to ascertain precise details of radiation fields used for treatment among the 115 centers participating in the trial. Among patients who underwent completion ALND, the proportion of additional positive lymph nodes (27%) was much lower than previously reported in the literature, suggesting that a longer follow-up is necessary to determine whether equivalence of outcomes for the two treatment groups persists.

Table 40.2 Axillary Recurrence After Positive Sentinel Lymph Node Biopsy and no ALND

Author	Date	Number	Follow-up (months)	Size of Axillary Metastasis (mm)	Axillary Recurrence Number (%)
Galper (55)	2000	418	96	NR	6 (1.4)
Ganaraj (60)	2003	17	30[a]	<2 mm	0
Guenther (61)	2003	16	32[b]	<2 mm	0
Fant (62)	2003	27	30[a]	<2 mm	0
Fournier (63)	2004	6	12[a]	≤2 mm	0
Fan (64)	2005	27	29[b]	≤2 mm	1
Schrenk (65)	2005	16	48[b]	>0.2 mm ≤2 mm	0
Carlo (66)	2005	21	60[b]	<2 mm	0
Chagpar (49)	2005	12	40[b]	>0.2 mm ≤2 mm	0
Takei (67)	2007	127	34[b]	NR	0
Hwang (68)	2007	90	30[b]	>0.2 mm ≤2 mm	0
Zakaria (69)	2008	85	30[b]	any	0
Langer (25)	2009	27	77[b]	>0.2 mm ≤2 mm	0
Golshan (70)	2009	131	59[b]	any	0
Giuliano (54)	2010	446	74[b]	any	(1.3)
Pernas (71)	2010	45	60[b]	>0.2 mm ≤2 mm	0

[a]Mean.
[b]Median.
Abbreviations: ALND, axillary lymph node dissection; NR, Not reported.

ALTERNATIVE AXILLARY THERAPY

While controversy exists as to whether ALND is primarily diagnostic or a therapeutic procedure, there are other non-surgical options for obtaining local control within the axilla. Radiation has been suggested as an alternative to completion ALND in patients with low volume axillary disease. As mentioned previously, the NSABP B-04 trial found that radiation therapy is equivalent to ALND in terms of regional control for women with a clinically negative axilla. Retrospective data from the Joint Center of Radiation Therapy also support these conclusions and show that only 1.4% of women developed regional nodal failure after undergoing axillary radiation without ALND or after removal of five or fewer nodes (55). Two prospective single-arm trials have shown a low rate of axillary failure in patients for whom axillary radiation was substituted for ALND in patients with a positive SNB (56,57).

A large prospective phase III trial in Europe called After Mapping of the Axilla: Radiotherapy or Surgery (AMAROS) is currently in progress. This study will evaluate patients undergoing both mastectomy and breast conservation. Only patients undergoing breast conservation were included in ACOSOG Z0011 and all received whole breast radiation with tangents that would have treated a portion of the axilla. However, it should be emphasized that these patients were not treated with formal axillary radiation fields. Further investigation is underway to determine the details of the actual radiation fields utilized in that study and whether there are potential differences between the outcome from formal axillary radiation and that of the tangential breast field radiation, which captures the lower axilla. Elucidation of these details has implications for treatment of these and other patients. Results of the ACOSOG Z0011 study are only applicable to women who have undergone breast conservation, and further investigation is needed to determine management of the positive sentinel node in mastectomy patients.

Systemic therapies effectively treat disease in the axillary nodes. In National Surgical Adjuvant Breast and Bowel Project (NSABP) B-18 trial, significantly more women were node negative (58%) after receiving preoperative doxorubicin and cyclophosphamide than those undergoing surgery first (42%). For those with confirmed nodal disease on fine needle aspiration cytology (FNAC) pretreatment, 32% converted to node-negative disease after preoperative therapy (58). In biopsy-proven node positive HER2-positive disease, 74% of patients receiving trastuzumab-based preoperative chemotherapy were found to be node negative at the time of definitive surgery (59). As targeted systemic therapies continue to become more effective, treatment of axillary metastases will likely continue to improve. A recently completed study, ACOSOG Z1071, evaluated the role for completion axillary dissection in patients with positive axillary nodes prior to preoperative systemic therapy. The data from this study are still being compiled, but will lead to future trials in this patient population. If sterilization of the axilla by neoadjuvant therapy can accurately be predicted from SNB post-chemotherapy, completion axillary dissection may be avoidable for this subgroup of patients who present with node positive disease.

FUTURE DIRECTIONS

The indications for ALND continue to evolve and will be influenced by continued trends for less invasive surgical approaches in breast cancer coupled with improvements in targeted systemic therapy and radiation techniques. The standard of care for patients with a positive sentinel lymph node remains ALND, although this has been challenged by provocative results from the ACOSOG Z0011 trial. There is likely a group of women with sentinel-node positive disease for whom an ALND can be safely omitted, but further follow-up and investigation with randomized trials is needed to safely determine appropriate subsets of patients. Nomograms can be used to guide the decision-making process while understanding their limitations. Whenever a nomogram is used, validation with the local clinical dataset is critical for applicability. Nomograms cannot provide definitive answers as to which patients should undergo completion ALND, but can only indicate the likelihood of additional disease in the non-sentinel nodes. At present, the decision to omit ALND is made on a case-by-case basis with careful consideration given to individual patient characteristics. Multidisciplinary discussions between the surgeon, radiation/medical oncologists and the patient can help in development of a tailored treatment plan. In the future, individual tumor biology (based on molecular profiling) may more accurately predict risk of regional recurrence thus permitting appropriate and safe omission of completion ALND in selected patients.

REFERENCES

1. Veronesi U, Casinelli N, Mariani L, et al. Twenty-year follow-up of a randomized study comparing breast-conserving surgery with radical mastectomy for early breast cancer. N Engl J Med 2002; 347: 1227–32.
2. Fisher B, Anderson S, Bryant J, et al. Twenty-year follow-up of a randomized trial comparing total mastectomy, lumpectomy and lumpectomy plus irradiation for the treatment of invasive breast cancer. N Engl J Med 2002; 347: 1233–41.
3. Rastogi P, Anderson SJ, Bear HD, et al. Preoperative chemotherapy: updates of national surgical adjuvant breast and bowel project protocols: B-18 and B-27. J Clin Oncol 2008; 26: 778–85.
4. Van der Hage JA, van de Velde CJH, Julien JP, et al. Preoperative chemotherapy in primary operative breast cancer: results from the European organization for research and treatment of cancer trial 10902. J Clin Oncol 2001; 19: 4224–37.
5. Smith IE, Walsh G, Jones A, et al. High complete remission rates with primary neoadjuvant infusional chemotherapy for large early breast cancer. J Clin Oncol 1995; 13: 424–9.
6. Scholl SM, Asselain B, Palangie T, et al. Neoadjuvant chemotherapy in operable breast cancer. Eur J Cancer 1991; 27: 1668–71.
7. Lyman GH, Giuliano AE, Somerfield MR, et al. American Society of clinical oncology guideline recommendations for sentinel lymph node biopsy in early-stage breast cancer. J Clin Oncol 2005; 23: 7703–20.
8. Giuliano AE, Kirgan DM, Guenther JM, et al. Lymphatic mapping and sentinel lymphadenectomy for breast cancer. Ann Surg 1994; 220: 391–401.
9. Krag D, Weaver D, Ashikaga T, et al. The sentinel node in breast cancer—a multi-center validation study. N Engl J Med 1998; 229: 941–6.
10. Fisher B, Jeong JH, Anderson S, et al. Twenty-five year follow-up of a randomized trial comparing radical mastectomy, total mastectomy and total mastectomy followed by irradiation. N Engl J Med 2002; 347: 567–75.
11. Orr RK. The impact of prophylactic axillary node dissection on survival: a Bayesian Model Analysis. Ann Surg 1999; 6: 109–16.
12. Early Breast Cancer Trialists Collaborative Group (EBCTCG). Effects of radiotherapy and of differences in the extent of surgery for early breast cancer on local control and 15-year survival: an overview of the randomized trials. Lancet 2005; 366: 2087–106.
13. Naik AM, Fey J, Gemignani M, et al. The risk of axillary relapse after sentinel lymph node biopsy for breast cancer is comparable with that of axillary lymph node dissection. Ann Surg 2004; 240: 462–71.
14. Rescigno J, Zampbell JC, Axelrod D. Patterns of axillary surgical care for breast cancer in the era of sentinel lymph node biopsy. Ann Surg Oncol 2009; 16: 687–96.

15. Wasif N, Maggard MA, Ko CY, et al. Underuse of axillary dissection for the management of sentinel node micrometastases in breast cancer. Arch Surg 2010; 145: 161–6.

16. Yi M, Giordano SH, Meric-Bernstam F, et al. Trends in and outcomes from sentinel lymph node biopsy (SLNB) alone vs. SLNB with axillary lymph node dissection for node-positive breast cancer patients: experience from the SEER database. Ann Surg Oncol 2010; 17: S343–51.

17. Morton DL, Wen DR, Wong JH, et al. Technical details of Intraoperative lymphatic mapping for early stage melanoma. Arch Surg 1992; 127: 392–9.

18. Krag DN, Weaver DL, Alex JC, et al. Surgical resection and radiolocalization of the sentinel lymph node in breast cancer using a gamma probe. Surg Oncol 1993; 2: 335–9.

19. Veronesi U, Paganelli G, Galimberti V, et al. Sentinel-node biopsy to avoid axillary dissection in breast cancer with clinically negative lymph-nodes. Lancet 1997; 349: 1864–7.

20. Lucci A Jr, Kelemen PR, Miller C, et al. National practice patterns of sentinel lymph node dissection for breast carcinoma. J Am Coll Surg 2001; 192: 453–8.

21. Miltenberg DM, Miller C, Karamlou TB, et al. Meta-analysis of sentinel lymph node biopsy in breast cancer. J Surg Res 1999; 84: 138–42.

22. Veronesi U, Paganelli G, Viale G, et al. A randomized comparison of sentinel-node biopsy with routine axillary dissection in breast cancer. N Engl J Med 2003; 349: 546–53.

23. Jeruss JS, Winchester DJ, Sener SF, et al. Axillary recurrence after sentinel node biopsy. Ann Surg Oncol 2005; 12: 34–40.

24. Krag DN, Anderson SJ, Julian TB, et al. Primary outcome results of NSABP B-32, a randomized phase III clinical trial to compare sentinel node resection (SNR) to conventional axillary dissection (AD) in clinically node-negative breast cancer patients. J Clin Oncol 2010; 28: 18S.

25. Langer I, Guller U, Berclaz G, et al. Morbidity of sentinel lymph node biopsy (SLN) alone versus SLN and completion axillary lymph node dissection after breast cancer surgery: a prospective Swiss multicenter study on 659 patients. Ann Surg 2007; 245: 452–61.

26. Lucci A, McCall LM, Beitsch PD, et al. Surgical complications associated with sentinel lymph node dissection (SLND) plus axillary lymph node dissection compared with SLND alone in the American College of Surgeons Oncology Group Trial Z0011. J Clin Oncol 2007; 25: 3657–63.

27. Bafford A, Gadd M, Gu X, et al. Diminishing morbidity with the increased use of sentinel node biopsy in breast carcinoma. Am J Surg 2010; 200: 374–7.

28. Kim T, Giuliano AE, Lyman GH. Lymphatic mapping and sentinel node lymph node biopsy in early stage breast carcinoma: a meta-analysis. Cancer 2006; 106: 4–16.

29. Van Zee KJ, Manasseh DM, Bevilacqua JL, et al. A nomogram for predicting the likelihood of additional nodal metastases in breast cancer patients with a positive sentinel node biopsy. Ann Surg Oncol 2003; 10: 1140–51.

30. Lambert LA, Ayers GD, Hwang RF, et al. Validation of a breast cancer nomogram for predicting nonsentinel lymph node metastases after a positive sentinel node biopsy. Ann Surg Oncol 2006; 13: 310–20.

31. Alran S, DeRycke Y, Fourchotte V, et al. Validation and limitations of use of a breast cancer nomogram predicting the likelihood of non-sentinel node involvement after positive sentinel node biopsy. Ann Surg Oncol 2007; 14: 2195–201.

32. Erb KM, Julian TB. Completion of axillary dissection for a positive sentinel node: necessary or not? Curr Oncol Rep 2009; 11: 15–20.

33. Smidt ML, Kuster DM, van der Wilt GJ, et al. Can the Memorial Sloan-Kettering Cancer Center nomogram predict the likelihood of nonsentinel lymph node metastases in breast cancer patients in the Netherlands? Ann Surg Oncol 2005; 12: 1066–72.

34. Pal A, Provenzano E, Duffy SW, et al. A model for predicting non-sentinel lymph node metastatic disease when the sentinel lymph node is positive. Br J Surg 2008; 95: 302–9.

35. Soni NK, Carmalt HL, Gillett DJ, et al. Evaluation of a breast cancer nomogram for prediction of non-sentinel lymph node positivity. Eur J Surg Oncol 2005; 31: 958–64.

36. Ponzone R, Maggiorotto F, Mariani L, et al. Comparison of two models for the prediction of nonsentinel node metastases in breast cancer. Am J Surg 2007; 193: 686–92.

37. Cripe MH, Beran LC, Liang WC, et al. The likelihood of additional nodal disease following a positive sentinel lymph node biopsy in breast cancer patients: validation of a nomogram. Am J Surg 2006; 192: 484–7.

38. Klar M, Jochmann A, Foeldi M, et al. The MSKCC nomogram for predicting the likelihood of non-sentinel node involvement in a German breast cancer population. Breast Cancer Res Treat 2008; 112: 523–31.

39. Kohrt HE, Olshen RA, Bermas HR, et al. New models and online calculator for predicting non-sentinel lymph node status in sentinel lymph node positive breast cancer patients. BMC Cancer 2008; 8: 66.

40. Barranger E, Coutant C, Flahault A, et al. An axilla scoring system to predict non-sentinel lymph node status in breast cancer patients with sentinel lymph node involvement. Breast Cancer Res Treat 2005; 91: 113–19.

41. Cho J, Han W, Lee JW, et al. A scoring system to predict nonsentinel lymph node status in breast cancer patients with metastatic sentinel lymph nodes: a comparison with other scoring systems. Ann Surg Oncol 2008; 15: 2278–86.

42. Chagpar AB, Scoggins CR, Martin RC, et al. Prediction of sentinel lymph node-only disease in women with invasive breast cancer. Am J Surg 2006; 192: 882–7.

43. Hwang RF, Krishnamurthy S, Hunt KK, et al. Clinicopathologic factors predicting involvement of nonsentinel axillary nodes in women with breast cancer. Ann Surg Oncol 2003; 10: 248–54.

44. Mittendorf EA, Hunt KK, Boughey JC, et al. Size matters: incorporation of sentinel lymph node (SLN) metastasis size into a nomogram predicting non-SLN involvement in SLN-positive breast cancer patients (abstract PD 106-108). Cancer Res 2010; 70(Suppl): 117s.

45. Meretoja TJ, Strien L, Heikklla PS, et al. A simple nomogram to evaluate the risk of nonsentinel node metastases in breast cancer patients with minimal sentinel node involvement. Ann Surg Oncol 2012; 19: 567–76.

46. Gur AS, Unal B, Johnson R, et al. Predictive probability of four different breast cancer nomograms for nonsentinel axillary lymph node metastasis in positive sentinel node biopsy. J Am Coll Surg 2009; 208: 229–35.

47. Gur AS, Unal B, Ozmen V, et al. Validation of breast cancer nomograms for predicting the nonsentinel lymph node metastases after a positive sentinel lymph node biopsy in a multi-center study. Eur J Surg Oncol 2010; 36: 30–5.

48. Moon HG, Han W, Noh DY. Comparable survival between pN0 breast cancer patients undergoing sentinel node biopsy and extensive axillary dissection: a report from the Korean Breast Cancer Society. J Clin Oncol 2010; 28: 1692–9.

49. Chagpar A, Middleton LP, Sahin AA, et al. Clinical outcome of patients with lymph node-negative breast carcinoma who have sentinel lymph node metastasis detected by immunohistochemistry. Cancer 2005; 103: 1581–6.

50. Hansen NM, Grube BJ, Te W, et al. Clinical significance of axillary micrometastasis in breast cancer; how small is too small? Proc Am Soc Clin Oncol 2001; 20: A91.

51. Colleoni M, Rotmensz N, Peruzzotti G, et al. Size of breast cancer metastases in axillary lymph nodes: clinical relevance of minimal lymph node involvement. J Clin Oncol 2005; 23: 1379–89.

52. Cserni G, Gregori D, Merletti F, et al. Meta-analysis of non-sentinel node metastases associated with micrometastatic sentinel node in breast cancer. Br J Surg 2004; 91: 1245–52.

53. Cote R, Giuliano AE, Hawes D, et al. ACOSOG Z0010: a multicenter prognostic study of sentinel node (SN) and bone marrow (BM) micrometastases in women with clinical T1/T2 N0 M0 breast cancer. J Clin Oncol 2010; 28: 18S.

54. Giuliano AE, McCall LM, Beitsch PD, et al. ACOSOG Z0011: a randomized trial of axillary node dissection in women with clinical T1-2 N0 M0 breast cancer who have a positive sentinel node. J Clin Oncol 2010; 28: 18S.

55. Galper S, Recht A, Silver B, et al. Is radiation alone adequate treatment to the axilla for patients with limited axillary surgery? Implications for treatment after a positive sentinel node biopsy. Int J Radiat Oncol Biol Phys 2000; 48: 125–32.

56. Gadd M, Harris J, Taghian A, et al. Prospective study of axillary radiation without axillary dissection for breast cancer patients with a positive sentinel node (abstract 25). Presented at The Annual San Antonio Breast Cancer Symposium. San Antonio, TX, USA, 8–11 December 2005.

57. Yegiyants S, Romero LM, Haigh PI, et al. Completion axillary lymph node dissection not required for regional control in patients with breast cancer who have micrometastases in a sentinel node. Arch Surg 2010; 145: 564–9.

58. Newman EA, Sabel MS, Nees AV, et al. Sentinel lymph node biopsy performed after neoadjuvant chemotherapy is accurate in patients with documented node-positive breast cancer at presentation. Ann Surg Oncol 2007; 14: 2946–52.

59. Dominici LS, Gonzalez VM, Buzdar AU, et al. Cytologically proven axillary lymph node metastases are eradicated in patients receiving preoperative chemotherapy with concurrent trastuzumab for HER-2 positive breast cancer. Cancer 2010; 116: 2884–9.

60. Ganaraj A, Kuhn JA, Jones RC, et al. Predictors for nonsentinel node involvement in breast cancer patients with micrometastases in the sentinel lymph node. Proc (Bayl Univ Med Cent) 2003; 16: 3–6.

61. Guenther JM, Hansen NM, DiFronzo LA, et al. Axillary dissection is not required for all patients with breast cancer and positive sentinel nodes. Arch Surg 2003; 138: 52–6.

62. Fant JS, Grant MD, Knox SM, et al. Preliminary outcome analysis in patients with breast cancer and a positive sentinel lymph node who declined axillary dissection. Ann Surg Oncol 2003; 10: 126–30.

63. Fournier K, Schiller A, Perry RR, et al. Micrometastasis in the sentinel lymph node of breast cancer does not mandate completion axillary dissection. Ann Surg 2004; 239: 859–63.

64. Fan YG, Tan YY, Wu CT, et al. The effect of sentinel node tumor burden on non-sentinel node status and recurrence rates in breast cancer. Ann Surg Oncol 2005; 12: 705–11.

65. Schrenk P, Konstantiniuk P, Wolfi S, et al. Prediction of non-sentinel lymph node status in breast cancer with a micrometastatic sentinel node. Br J Surg 2005; 92: 707–13.

66. Carlo JT, Grant MD, Knox SM, et al. Survival analysis following sentinel lymph node biopsy: a validation trial demonstrating its accuracy in staging early breast cancer. Proc (Bayl Univ Med Cent) 2005; 18: 103–7.

67. Takei H, Suemasu K, Kurosumi M, et al. Recurrence after sentinel lymph node biopsy with or without axillary lymph node dissection in patients with breast cancer. Breast Cancer 2007; 14: 16–24.

68. Hwang RF, Gonzalez-Angulo AM, Yi M, et al. Low locoregional failure rates in selected breast cancer patients with tumor-positive sentinel lymph nodes who do not undergo completion axillary dissection. Cancer 2007; 110: 723–30.

69. Zakaria S, Pantvaidya G, Reynolds CA, et al. Sentinel node positive breast cancer patients who do not undergo axillary dissections: are they different? Surgery 2008; 143: 641–7.

70. Golshan M, Bellon J, Smith B, et al. Can axillary node dissection be omitted in a subset of patients with low local and regional failure rates? (abstract 219). American Society of Clinical Oncology Breast Cancer Symposium. San Francisco, CA, USA, 8–10 October 2009.

71. Pernas S, Gil M, Benitez A, et al. Avoiding axillary treatment in sentinel lymph node micrometastases of breast cancer: a prospective analysis of axillary or distant recurrence. Ann Surg Oncol 2010; 17: 772–7.

41 Radiation therapy following breast conserving surgery or mastectomy

Ian Kunkler

INTRODUCTION

Breast conserving therapy consisting of a wide local excision and postoperative whole-breast radiotherapy (WBRT) has now been established as the standard of care for the majority of women presenting with early invasive breast cancer for over three decades. It was Sir Geoffrey Keynes, who first proposed the procedure of wide local excision and implantation of the breast with radium needles as an alternative to the Halsted mastectomy (1). However, Keynes's observations were insufficient to challenge Halstedian dogma and it took over a half century for the safety of breast conservation to be accepted. No detriment in overall survival was demonstrated in randomized trials comparing breast conservation with mastectomy (2–5). These were followed by a series of randomized trials demonstrating a 4–5-fold reduction in local recurrence from the addition of postoperative whole-breast irradiation to breast conserving surgery (BCS) (6–9). Of late, a more conservative form of radiotherapy (RT) (partial breast irradiation, PBI) has been investigated as an alternative to whole-breast irradiation. In addition, "low-risk" subsets of patients with invasive breast cancer have been sought from whom postoperative RT might be omitted completely. Important developments have been the introduction of shortened dose fractionation schedules, three-dimensional CT-based treatment (3D-CT) planning, and intensity modulated radiotherapy (IMRT). 3D-CT planning has played an important role in reducing cardiac toxicity by minimizing the volume of the heart that is irradiated. The role of postmastectomy irradiation has expanded for node-positive disease, although its role in intermediate-risk breast cancer remains controversial.

ADVANCES IN RADIOTHERAPY TECHNIQUE

There have been significant advances in radiation oncology planning and delivery which have improved the quality of radiation therapy for breast cancer, both by improving dose homogeneity within the breast and/or regional nodal areas and reducing dosage to critical normal tissues, particularly the lungs, heart, and brachial plexus. Breathing adapted gating techniques (e.g., switching on the X-ray beam in deep inspiration when the heart has moved away from posterior edge of the tangential field) reduces cardiac irradiation (10). These developments have the potential to improve locoregional control and/or diminish acute and late radiation-induced morbidity.

The 3D-CT planning allows dosimetric evaluation of the breast not just in a single plane but at all levels. Achieving a homogeneous dose distribution in the breast is challenging because its contour changes in both craniocaudal and sagittal planes. To compensate for the changing contour of the breast, wedge-shaped beam attenuators are positioned in the radiation field, thus attenuating the beam from a minimum along the chest wall to a maximum in the subareolar region. They compensate for the diminishing tissue volume from the chest wall to the apex of the breast by differentially reducing the intensity of the beam from the chest wall to the nipple–areola complex. Wedges compensate for dose heterogeneity in two dimensions (2D), normally optimized in the central plane of the breast. While 2D planning can achieve excellent dose homogeneity along the central axis of the breast, dose homogeneity is poorer in the upper and lower regions resulting in marked "hot spots" in areas of the breast away from the central axis (11). Tangential beam plans can be optimized to ensure that significant volumes of the breast do not exceed 105% of the prescribed dose. IMRT in which the X-ray beam is dynamically collimated to modified its influence, allows the dose to be "painted" to the breast/chest wall and peripheral lymphatics while minimizing the passage of unwanted dose to critical adjacent structures. IMRT attenuates the radiation beam differentially in multiple planes, improving homogeneity throughout the breast. The "field-in-field" technique [also called "field in field forward planned intensity-modulated radiotherapy (FiF-IMRT)] enables areas of suboptimal dose homogeneity to be improved, reducing "hot spots" such as the inframammary fold and the thin area of the breast close to the nipple–areola complex (11,12). In a comparison of dosimetry in 201 breast cancer patients treated with FiF-IMRT and 131 patients treated with a standard wedged 3D technique for postoperative treatment of whole-breast (according to breast size and supraclavicular node irradiation) homogeneity of dose distribution significantly improved with forward IMRT, irrespective of breast size or supraclavicular nodal irradiation (13). Scattered dose to the contralateral breast is also reduced with FiF-IMRT techniques (14). In a randomized trial comparing acute breast toxicity after conventional 3D CT planning with IMRT in 358 patients with early breast cancer treated by BCS and whole-breast irradiation, moist desquamation and breast pain were significantly less with IMRT and associated with improved quality of life and better dose homogeneity compared with standard RT (15). Longer term follow-up will be needed to see if late radiation changes such as breast fibrosis are also reduced by IMRT. This seems likely since a United Kingdom (UK) randomized trial comparing 2D wedges to 3D IMRT showed at five years a significant improvement in the breast appearance (16). Another advantage of the improved dose homogeneity of IMRT is that it may diminish the risk of breast fibrosis and impaired cosmesis from large fraction sizes used in accelerated whole-breast irradiation (11). It is known that "hot spots" in 2D plans are enhanced with the larger doses per fraction. IMRT techniques can also deliver radiation to the whole breast, while simultaneously "boosting" the tumor bed (so-called concomitant or simultaneous integrated boost). This can shorten the overall treatment duration (compared to a sequential boost). A small Canadian study has shown the feasibility and acceptable toxicity levels of giving simultaneous integrated boost of 10 Gy to supplement a whole-breast dose of 42.5 Gy in 16 fractions (17). IMRT might also allow chemotherapy to be given concurrently with postoperative RT after BCS where there have been concerns that concurrent treatment, while improving local control in some patients, may enhance acute and late radiotoxicity (18).

Traditionally patients have been irradiated in the supine position. However, the prone position has a number of advantages (19). Firstly, dose homogeneity is improved since dose buildup in the inframammary fold is avoided. Secondly, dose to the lung and heart is minimized and thirdly, respiratory motion is reduced and there is no need for complex gating mechanisms. In a consecutive series of 97 patients (minimum follow-up six months) receiving hypofractionated treatment in the prone position (40 with 3-dimentional conformal radiotherapy (3D-CRT) and 57 with IMRT) grade 2 dermatitis occurred in 13% of the 3D-CRT group and 2% in the IMRT group (19). In addition, with both 3D-CRT based planning and IMRT the prone position can improve nodal coverage (20). However, experience is required to achieve a stable setup in the prone position. A small randomized trial at the Royal Marsden Hospital identified a higher rate of set-up error with prone compared to conventional supine treatment position (21).

POSTOPERATIVE RADIOTHERAPY
AFTER BCS FOR INVASIVE CANCER

The combination of BCS and postoperative RT has been established as the standard of care for over 70% of women with early breast cancer and is underpinned by a large body of level 1 evidence with long-term follow-up (22). Improvements in local control over the last decade are probably multifactorial in origin. They include better appreciation of tumor extent on imaging, mammographic screening, attention to surgical margins, and better systemic therapy. As a result, five-year breast failure rates have fallen from around 5% to 2–3% at present (23).

OXFORD OVERVIEW

Perhaps the most influential source of information on the effects of adjuvant breast irradiation is the Early Breast Cancer Trialists' Collaborative Group meta-analysis and overview. The important benefit of this approach is that the very large numbers of patients analyzed allow the detection of treatment effects that may not be detected within individual trials. The most recent update (22) reports on 10-year recurrence rates on over 10,000 women in 17 randomized trials. In contrast to previous overviews, where the focus was on locoregional recurrence as first recurrence, the primary endpoint in the 2011 overview was on any first recurrence whether locoregional or distant. RT reduced the 10-year risk of any recurrence by 15.7% (35–19.3%; (95% CI 13.7–17.7, 2p = <0.00001) and 15-year mortality from 25.2% to 21.4% [an absolute reduction of 3.8% (95% CI 1.6–6.0, 2p = 0.00005)]. In 7287 women with a pathologically node-negative

axilla (pN0), the equivalent risk reductions were from 31% to 15.6%, absolute reduction in recurrence of 15.4% (95% CI 13.2–17.6, 2p = <0.00001), and an absolute reduction in mortality of 3.3% from 20.5% to 17.2%. There were far fewer women with pathologically involved axillary nodes (pN1) (1050) in whom the 10-year risk reduction was higher at 21.2% (95% CI 14.5–27.9, 2p = <0.00001) from 63.7% to 42.5% with an 8.5% reduction in 15-year breast cancer mortality (95% CI 1.8–15.2, 2p = 0.01) from 51.3% to 42.8%. The 10-year risks of any recurrence varied with age, tumor size, grade, ER status, use of tamoxifen, and extent of surgery as shown in Figure 41.1. While the proportional reduction in any recurrence is the same for younger and older women, the absolute reduction in risk is substantially lower for women over the age of 70, although the older group is much less represented. This is largely due to historical exclusion of patients over the age of 70 in many trials. The most marked reduction in recurrence after RT was achieved in ER-positive patients not receiving tamoxifen. The differences in risk of breast cancer mortality according to reduction in first recurrence for different risk groups according to pathological nodal status are shown in Figure 41.2. Patients with pN0 disease were ascribed a 10-year absolute reduction in risk of recurrence (large, intermediate, and lower) based on their characteristics and features of the trial in which they participated.

While the primary analysis was on first recurrence, the majority (75%) were locoregional. Locoregional recurrences were higher in the no-RT groups (25%) compared with 8% in the irradiated arms. The maximal effect on locoregional recurrence from RT was in the first year. Nonetheless, the impact even up to years 5–9 was substantial.

The observation in the Oxford overview of RT that for every 4 recurrences prevented, one breast cancer death was avoided (24), was confirmed in the latest overview (22) confined to breast conservation. The overview shows that there is a causal relationship between locoregional control and survival. Eradication of persistent local disease by RT is a key factor in preventing death from metastatic breast cancer. However this is a complex relationship. As has been pointed out (25), for locoregional RT to impact on survival, there must be persistent disease after BCS not eradicated by systemic therapy. RT must be effective in sterilizing local disease and finally patients must not have micrometastatic disease to distant sites. The risk of residual disease is influenced by other factors including tumor size, axillary nodal status, grade, ER status, and age. The "4 to 1" ratio might also vary with stage and type of surgery. Overall, despite unquantifiable differences in individual sensitivity to radiation, RT is highly effective in sterilizing much of the local residual tumor burden. The overall impact of RT on any recurrence was an impressive proportional reduction of 50%. This is higher than that achieved by chemotherapy or hormonal therapy (25). The benefit conferred by RT varies with breast cancer subtype, with a relatively greater benefit in ER-positive disease (about 60% reduction in recurrence) than in ER-negative disease (35%) which argues for investigation of more intensive radiation schedules for the latter group (25).

BREAST BOOST AFTER BCS

There is level I evidence that a boost of irradiation to the site of excision after BCS improves local control irrespective of age. In the EORTC boost trial over 5000 T1/2N0/NIM0

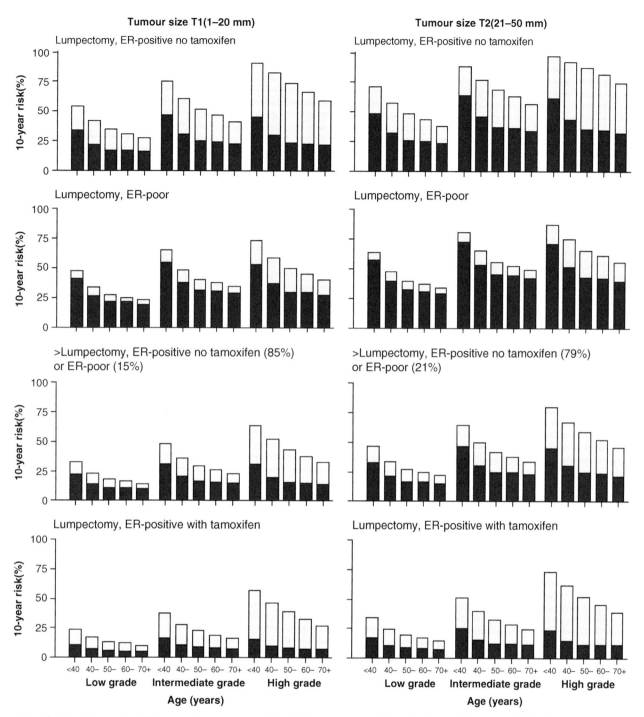

Figure 41.1 Absolute 10-year risks (%) of any (locoregional or distant) first recurrence with and without radiotherapy (RT) following breast-conserving surgery (BCS) in pathologically node-negative women by patient and trial characteristics, as estimated by regression modeling of data for 7287 women. Further details are in webappendix pp 27–30. Results for 5-year risks are in webappendix pp 31–34. Bars show 10-year risks in women allocated to BCS only, dark sections show 10-year risks in women allocated to BCS plus RT, light sections show absolute reduction with RT. *Abbreviation*: ER, estrogen receptor. *Source*: Courtesy of the Lancet.

patients were randomized after BCS with clear margins and whole-breast irradiation (50 Gy) to a boost of 16 Gy in eight fractions or no boost. At five years the benefit of the boost for local control was only statistically significant in women <50 years (26). However, at 10 years a statistically significant benefit was seen in older as well as younger women (27), although the reduction in ipsilateral breast tumor recurrence (IBTR) (7.3% vs. 3.8%) was only 3.5% for women >60 years.

IS THERE A SUBGROUP OF OLDER PATIENTS FROM WHOM POSTOPERATIVE RADIOTHERAPY CAN BE OMITTED?

It would be beneficial, particularly to older patients, if one could identify selection criteria for the omission of postoperative RT without compromising local control. Older patients, in particular, find the practicalities of attending for several weeks of RT burdensome.

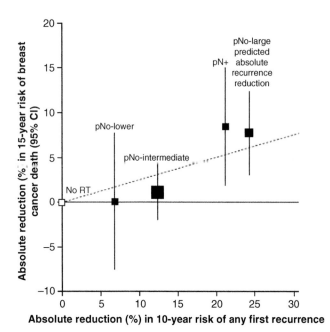

Figure 41.2 Absolute reduction in 15-year risk of breast cancer death with radiotherapy (RT) after breast-conserving surgery versus absolute reduction in 10-year risk of any (locoregional or distant) recurrence. Women with pN0 disease are subdivided by the predicted absolute reduction in 10-year risk of any recurrence suggested by regression modeling (pN0-large ≥20%, pN0 intermediate 10–19%, pN0-lower <10%; further details are in webappendix pp 35–39). Vertical lines are 95% CIs. Sizes of dark boxes are proportional to amount of information. Dashed line: one death from breast cancer avoided for every four recurrences avoided. *Abbreviations*: pN0, pathologically node-negative; pN+, pathologically node-positive. *Source*: Courtesy of the Lancet.

Whether postoperative RT can be safely omitted for any subset of patients remains controversial. To date no such subgroup has been identified. WBRT reduces the risk of IBTR in all subgroups of patients. However the absolute benefit of RT in low-risk, small (<2 cm), axillary node negative, low grade, hormone receptor-positive tumors is very modest.

The principal source of level I evidence in older patients evaluating the omission of postoperative RT in "low-risk" women after BCS is the United States (US) Cancer and Leukemia Group B (CALGB) trial (28,29). More than 600 women 70 years of age or older with T1N0M0 hormone receptor-positive breast tumors were randomized after BCS and tamoxifen to whole-breast irradiation or no RT. At five years there was a modest 3% reduction in IBTR (4% vs. 1%) from adjuvant irradiation (28). There was more breast radiotoxicity in the irradiated arm (breast edema, skin fibrosis, and pain). The small reduction in local recurrence led to the questioning of the value of RT (30). Two limitations of the trial were the absence of an axillary surgical staging procedure and statistical underpowering. Another concern if WBRT is omitted is the cumulative risk of local recurrence with time (1% per year at least up to 10 years) (31). This is substantiated by the 10-year analysis of the CALGB trial showing that the difference in local recurrence has widened to 7% (2% in the RT group and 9% in the no-RT group) (29).

In the Italian 55–75 trial (32), 749 women with T1-T2 (<2.5 cm) N0/1, M0 breast cancer were randomized to WBRT (50 Gy in 2 Gy fractions) or no RT after quadrantectomy and systemic therapy. Axillary node status was assessed on sentinel lymph node (SLN) biopsy. SLN biopsy–positive patients went on to an axillary clearance. The cumulative incidence of IBTR

was 2.5% in the surgery alone arm and 0.7% in the surgery plus RT arm (median follow-up 53 months). The smaller difference in IBTR (1.8%) in the Italian 55–75 trial compared with the CALGB trial probably reflects the greater extent of surgery. In excess of 1300 patients with node-negative breast cancers measuring less than 3 cm were randomized after BCS and adjuvant endocrine therapy to whole-breast irradiation (40–50 Gy) or no WBRT in the ongoing PRIME 2 trial (33). Age was found to be an independent risk factor in a Canadian trial (7), with a higher locoregional recurrence rate (LRR) for patients under 50 years. The authors could not identify a low-risk group with an LRR of less than 10%. In the Milan III trial, women over 55 years had a lower risk of recurrence (3.8%) compared with 8.8% for the whole population. In the Scottish conservation trial (8), a trend toward lower local recurrence with age was observed, in particular between 60 and 70 years. No difference in local recurrence was seen in the NSABP B-06 trial for women less than or over 50 years (34). However the upper age limit for eligibility was not stated. International consensus remains that postoperative RT after BCS should be the standard of care for all fit patients irrespective of age (35). However, with the evidence that local recurrence rates are falling after breast conserving therapy (23), the absolute benefits of RT in low-risk older patients are likely to diminish even further. In addition it may be that particular molecular subtypes (e.g., luminal A in the ELIOT study of intraoperative RT) (36) may identify patients at sufficiently low risk to justify the omission of RT.

ALTERED FRACTIONATION
Conventionally adjuvant RT after BCS and mastectomy has been delivered in 1.8–2.0 Gy fractions to total doses of 45–50 Gy over five weeks. In the UK, shorter 15-day schedules have long been used in the north of England where RT centers served widely dispersed populations. There would therefore be substantial advantages to patients in terms of convenience and quality of life if treatment schedules could be shortened (hypofractionated) without compromising local control or increasing toxicity.

The biological hypothesis of hypofractionation is based on differences in sensitivity of normal and cancer cells to dose per fraction. The linear quadratic model provides an explanation for these differences. The alpha to beta ratio is inversely related to fractionation sensitivity and distinguishes between acutely responding normal tissues such as skin and late responding tissues such as the spinal cord. It is thought that breast cancer is probably similar to some acutely responding tissues with an alpha to beta ratio of 4–5 (37). However the linear quadratic model does not take account of effects of dose per fraction on tumor repopulation, oxygenation, or redistribution in the cell cycle (38).

There is now a substantial body of level 1 evidence underpinning the value of hypofractionated RT. There have been four large randomized trials from United Kingdom, Canada, and France (START A, START B, Royal Marsden Hospital/Gloucester Oncology Centre) which have compared conventional fractionation with hypofractionation (39–43). The START A trial recruited 2236 patients treated with BCS and mastectomy and randomized to two hypofractionated schedules: 39 Gy in 13 fractions of 3 Gy or 42.6 Gy in 13 fractions of 3.2 Gy compared with a standard of 25 fraction of 2 Gy over five weeks. START B compared 15 fractions of 2.87 Gy over three weeks to the same standard as in START A. The ipsilateral local control rates for the intervention arms of START A were 94.8% and 96.5% respectively and 96.4% for the standard arm at a median follow-up of five years. The equivalent rates for START B for the intervention and standard arms were 97.8% and 96.7% respectively. There were no statistically significant differences between the intervention arms and control in either trial. In the Royal Marsden Hospital/Gloucester Oncology Centre trial three regimens (2 test arms) (42.9 Gy in 13 fractions and 39 Gy in 13 fractions, and 50 Gy in 25 fractions) were compared. The local recurrence rate at 10 years was less than 15% in both groups. However there was a trend to higher local recurrence in the hypofractionated arm of 39 Gy. In the Canadian trial (42) eligible patients were restricted to low-risk clinical node-negative patients in a non-inferiority design; 1234 patients were randomized to 43.5 Gy in 16 fractions or to a standard arm of 50 Gy in 25 fractions. At a median follow-up of 12.5 years local control was 93.8% for the hypofractionated schedule and 91% in the standard arm.

Toxicity of Hypofractionated Radiotherapy

The toxicity data from the START and Canadian trial are reassuring with very similar cosmesis for standard and hypofractionated arms. In the Canadian trial, 69.8% of patients treated with hypofractionation had good or excellent cosmesis at 10 years compared with 71.3% in the standard arm with no case of severe breast fibrosis. In addition, the START and Canadian trials showed no increase in late radiation-induced cardiac morbidity. The START trial showed no increase in ischemic heart disease at five years, but it should be noted that late cardiac events are likely to occur over a much longer timescale at 10 years or longer after RT. The Canadian trial has 12 years of follow-up. Cardiac related deaths were 1.5% in the standard arm and 1.95% in the hypofractionated arm. This provides more confidence in the absence of late cardiac effects of hypofractionation. However, longer term follow-up will be needed to confirm this. It should also be noted that most of the Canadian centers participating in the trial will have used 3D treatment planning which is known to reduce cardiac irradiation. It therefore cannot be assumed that hypofractionation is safe from the perspective of cardiac toxicity if centers do not have access to modern 3D planning. Other complications such as rib fracture and pneumonitis were not increased with hypofractionated RT. There is also evidence from a long-term follow-up of older patients treated with hypofractionated RT that late toxicity is acceptable (44).

Selecting Patients Suitable for Hypofractionated Breast Irradiation

With the rising tide of obesity, large breast size is an increasing challenge for the radiation oncologist. For these patients there is likely to be greater dose inhomogeneity which is increased by hypofractionation through a combination of higher total dose to parts of the breast and higher dose per fraction to some areas (38). Of note, patients with large breasts (breast separation more than 25 cm along the central axis) were ineligible for the Canadian trial. The START trial radiotherapy quality assurance restricted the dose variation to within 5% on the central axis. Despite including some patients with a separation of more than 25 cm, no adverse effect on cosmesis in relation to breast size was demonstrated.

While the equivalence in local control of hypofractionated RT compared with standard fractionation is well accepted from the START and Canadian trials, there is less consensus on the generalizability of their findings to clinical practice. The American Society for Radiation Oncology (ASTRO) consensus guidelines on hypofractionation after BCS (45) argue that the Canadian trial data are relevant to older (>50 years) patients with lower-risk node negative and predominantly ER-positive tumors. It is not clear what the role of the boost is after hypofractionated RT in this population since they did not receive a boost in the trial. The ASTRO consensus argues that the trial data are not applicable to patients receiving chemotherapy or peripheral irradiation since these were excluded from the Canadian trial and had limited representation in the START trials. The criteria adopted by ASTRO are shown in Table 41.1. In contrast the guidance of the National Institute of Clinical Excellence (46) in the UK has recommended 40 Gy in 15 fractions as the standard dose fractionation for post conservation and post-mastectomy radiotherapy (PMRT) based on the START trial results, supporting the broad generalizability of level 1 evidence to adjuvant breast irradiation.

PARTIAL BREAST IRRADIATION

The topic of PBI remains controversial. With this approach RT is given either to the site of excision of the primary tumor alone or in higher dose to this region. The potential benefits of PBI are in reducing the volume of the breast irradiated and thus reducing radiation-induced toxicity as well as shortened treatment time and reduced treatment costs. PBI may be particularly attractive to older patients where avoidance of several weeks of tiring external beam RT might be avoided. Nonetheless, it is particularly important that the safety of this approach is underpinned by the results of randomized trials given the recent evidence from the Oxford overview of trials of RT after BCS (in which the whole breast was irradiated) showing that a 19% reduction in local recurrence at five years translates into a 5% reduction in 15-year breast cancer mortality (22). This sets a high standard of treatment efficacy for partial breast irradiation to match. There remain uncertainties over patient selection, treatment, and clinical outcomes for PBI (47).

Table 41.1 ASTRO Criteria for Hypofractionated Whole-Breast Irradiation after Breast Conserving Surgery: Evidence for the Equivalence with Conventional Whole-Breast Irradiation for Patients Who Meet All of these Criteria

1. Patient is 50 years or older at diagnosis
2. Pathologic stage is T1-2 N0 and patient has been treated with breast-conserving surgery
3. Patient has not been treated with systemic chemotherapy
4. Within the breast along the central axis, the minimum dose is no less than 93% and maximum dose is no greater than 107% of the prescription dose (±7%) (as calculated with 2D treatment planning without heterogeneity corrections)

Source: Courtesy of the International Journal of Radiation Oncology, Biology and Physics.

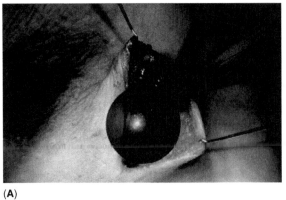 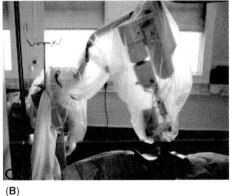

(A)   **(B)**

Figure 41.3 Targeted intraoperative radiotherapy technique with the Intrabeam system. (A) The applicator being placed in the tumor bed. (B) The X-ray source is delivered to the tumor bed by use of a surgical support stand. The sterile applicator is joined with a sterile drape that is used to cover the stand during treatment delivery. *Source:* Courtesy of the Lancet.

The rationale for PBI is that breast recurrences mainly occur at or close to the site of excision (9,34). A variety of techniques are being investigated in clinical trials including intraoperative kilovoltage (Fig. 41.3) Targeted intraoperative radiotherapy (TARGIT) (48), ELectron IntraOperative Therapy (ELIOT) (49), intraoperative or postoperative brachytherapy, (50), and external beam Intensity Modulated and Partial Organ Radio-Therapy (IMPORT LOW) (51). A review of the rationale and indications for these techniques is recommended reading (52).

To date the only level 1 evidence on PBI is the TARGIT A trial (48). Eligibility included age 45 years or older, T2-T3, N0-N1. However, the majority of patients recruited were mainly low-risk postmenopausal patients, probably reflecting clinicians' concerns about entering higher-risk patients. They were randomized to either intraoperative radiotherapy using Intrabeam (Zeiss) (Fig. 41.3) with 50 kV X rays (a dose of 20 Gy in a single fraction delivered to the surface of the applicator) or to whole-breast RT. It was assumed that a dose of 20 Gy at the surface was equivalent to a fractionated dose of 70 Gy with a dose of 5 Gy at 1 cm from the applicator being equivalent to a fractionated dose of 18 Gy (47). The concern is that the fall off in dose is quite marked with distance from the applicator and the dose may be insufficient to sterilize residual disease not immediately adjacent to the applicator. The IBTR was very low in both arms of the trial but the follow-up was relatively short (median follow-up 24 months). The Kaplan–Meier estimate of IBTR at four years was 1.20% (95% CI 0.53–2.71) in TARGIT A and 0.95% (0.39–2.31) in the external beam RT group. A confounding factor however is that the investigators could supplement intraoperative radiotherapy with external beam if they thought that there were additional risk factors for recurrence identified on pathology of the excised specimen (53). One of the principal limitations of this technique is that treatment is given before the margins of excision can be assessed pathologically.

Intraoperative electrons (3–12 MeV) (ELIOT) using a mobile linear accelerator delivering a single dose of 21 Gy to the 90% isodose are being investigated by the European Institute of Oncology in Milan, shielding the chest wall with lead if required (49). Results of "off trial" use of ELIOT have been reported in 1822 patients (36). The actuarial local recurrence rate was 4.84% (annual rate 1.21%). Two-thirds of the recurrences were in the same quadrant and a third in another quadrant. However the median follow-up was short at 36 months.

Postoperative brachytherapy after a wide local excision with low dose rate interstitial implantation over four to five days or high dose rate typically twice daily for five days gives good local control (54,55).

Consensus on Partial Breast Irradiation

Largely in response to the adoption of PBI outside of clinical trials, predominantly in the US and some parts of Europe, consensus guidelines for the use of PBI have been published by ASTRO and GEC-ESTRO (45,50). While the ASTRO and GEC-ESTRO guidelines may be a pragmatic approach to off study use of PBI, their limitation is that they are not based on level 1 evidence. This may further encourage the use of accelerated PBI (APBI) outside an investigational setting, when a sufficient body of level 1 evidence to support it is lacking. Indeed at the St Gallen breast cancer consensus meeting, a US/European consensus panel (56) and the DEGRO guidelines (57) concluded that PBI should still be considered experimental, although the St Gallen consensus did acknowledge that it might be routinely acceptable for patients over the age of 60 with favorable features (58). The National Comprehensive Cancer Network (NCCN) 2011 guidelines (59) permit breast RT to be omitted in patients meeting most of the eligibility of the ASTRO "suitable" group. The lack of consensus between guidelines almost certainly reflects the paucity of level I evidence. As results of ongoing or completed trials are published, a more unified consensus will hopefully emerge. In the meantime, patients should be informed, as the ASTRO guidelines recommend (45), that whole-breast irradiation has a much longer track record of safety and efficacy. Until further information on level 1 evidence is available, PBI should, in the author's view, remain investigational.

POSTMASTECTOMY IRRADIATION

The evolution of post-mastectomy radiotherapy (PMRT) has seen a remarkable transformation since the first overview of RT trials in 1987 (60) involving 7941 women from randomised controlled trials (RCTs). This showed that the 25-year survival rate was 42% in the postmastectomy group (simple/radical) compared with 51% after surgery alone. The excess of deaths occurred beyond 10 years, mainly due to cardiac causes in the irradiated group. In the 1994 update of that analysis it was shown that the excess mortality in irradiated patients was due to cardiac damage and that was probably balanced by a reduction in breast cancer mortality (61). No direct effect between vascular causes of death and RT could be shown since data on the laterality of the primary tumor was not included in the analysis. Previous meta-analyses and randomized trials of locoregional RT had shown that the risk of locoregional failure was diminished by two-thirds with PMRT directed to the chest wall and peripheral lymphatics including the axillary, supraclavicular, and internal mammary nodes (61–63). However the impact on overall and breast cancer–specific survival was unclear. Two further meta-analyses (62,63) showed improvement in locoregional control from PMRT but with no overall survival benefit. The 10-year-risk of locoregional failure was reduced from 27.2% to 8.8% (2p = < 0.00001) and at 20 years from 30.1% to 10.4% (2p = < 0.00001). Overall survival at 10 and 20 years was not significantly different (54.5% in control and 56.6% for RT; 35.9% for control and 37.1% for RT respectively) (2p = 0.06). There was, however, a statistically significant fall in breast cancer deaths in the RT group, counterbalanced by an increase in non-breast cancer deaths, particularly from vascular causes (death rate ratio 1.30, p = 0.0007). However, interpretation of how these overviews should apply to clinical practice was difficult since there was a mixture of patients treated by different types of surgery (simple/modified radical mastectomy, BCS), with or without differing types of systemic therapy, radiation dose fractionation schedules, and treatment volumes and techniques. In the older trials many patients were treated with orthovoltage techniques where the dose to the heart was higher. None of the trials were subject to RT quality assurance.

In 1997, two landmark trials from the Danish (64) and Canadian groups (65) showed not only a reduction in locoregional failure but for the first time a 9–10% survival advantage from the addition of adjuvant postmastectomy locoregional irradiation to systemic therapy in high-risk premenopausal patients and subsequently in high-risk postmenopausal patients treated with tamoxifen (66). In the Danish 82b trial, the 10-year overall survival was 54% in the irradiated group and 45% in the CMF (cyclophosphamide, methotrexate, and fluorouracil) alone arm (p = < 0.001). PMRT reduced locoregional failure (9% vs. 32%, p = < 0.001) and improved disease-free survival (36% vs. 24%, p = <0.001). In the smaller British Columbia trial of 318 premenopausal node positive patients receiving CMF with or without PMRT were compared. PMRT reduced locoregional failure by 56% (RR 0.44, 95% CI 0.26–0.77, p = 0.003), breast cancer mortality by 29% (RR 0.71, 95% CI 0.51–0.99) and improved 10-year disease-free survival (48% vs. 34%, p = 0.003). Moreover, 15-year overall mortality was reduced by 26% (RR 0.74, 95% CI, 0.53–1.02). An update of the trial showed a 30% reduction in overall mortality at 20 years (RR 0.70, p = 0.02) (67). Surgery consisted of mastectomy and level III clearance in both trials. RT was given to the chest wall, axilla, and internal mammary chain (IMC) at a dose of 48–50 Gy in 22–25 fractions over 5–5.5 weeks. In the Danish trials electron beam was used to treat the medial part of the chest wall and IMC and matched to the megavoltage photon fields treating the lateral part of the

chest wall and the axilla. The Danish and British Columbia trials provide the most compelling level 1 evidence for benefit of PMRT on disease-free and overall survival. As a result of these key practice changing publications PMRT has been established as the standard of care for women with high-risk breast cancer (i.e., at least 20% risk of locoregional failure at 10 years) (68). This includes those with four or more positive axillary nodes and patients with tumors 5 cm or greater or tumors invading the skin, muscle, or chest wall (69–73). There is evidence that the use of regional nodal irradiation (RNI) has increased since 1997 (74).

A meta-analysis confined to patients who had received systemic therapy from 18 trials predominantly in node-positive pre- and postmenopausal patients showed that locoregional RT reduced the risks of any recurrence (OR 0.69, 95% CI 0.58–0.83, p = 0.00004) locoregional failure (OR 0.25, 95% CI 1.9–0.34, p < 0.000001), and mortality (OR 0.83, 95% CI 0.74–0.94, p = 0.004) (75).

ROLE OF POSTMASTECTOMY RADIOTHERAPY FOR INTERMEDIATE-RISK BREAST CANCER

The role of PMRT in the intermediate-risk group (i.e., women with a 10–19% 10-year risk of locoregional recurrence) who have one to three involved axillary nodes or are axillary node negative with other risk factors such as grade 3 histology and/ or lymphovascular invasion remains controversial (76,77). These categories are currently being investigated in the MRC/ EORTC BIG 2-04 SUPREMO trial (78). One of the key issues in the controversy is the generalizability of the Danish and British Columbia trials to clinical practice. The locoregional failure rates in the Danish 82b and 82c trials and the British Columbia trials were higher than in many contemporary non-randomized American series. The higher loco-regional recurrences may be partly explained by inadequate axillary surgery with a median of only seven nodes removed from the axilla in the Danish trials and eleven in the British Columbia trial. Indeed 40% of all locoregional recurrences were in the axilla. In addition, the duration of CMF chemotherapy changed over the course of the Danish trial. One of the other criticisms was the intensity of chemotherapy (68). CMF was initially given for 12 months but this was subsequently reduced to six months. In the Danish 82c trial only one year of adjuvant tamoxifen was given compared with the current standard of five years. It has been estimated that the risk of local relapse in intermediate-risk patients is in the range of 5–15% (79) and that further reductions in risk by PMRT might be too low to justify irradiation, especially if some of the heart is irradiated. The Oxford overview of randomized RT trials did not provide any definitive data since results were not reported by nodal subgroup. Selection of patients at the highest risk of locoregional relapse is, therefore, based on subgroup analyses of individual trials and multivariate analyses of prospective cohort studies (73). In an analysis of 2016 patients recruited in three East Cooperative Oncology Group (ECOG) trials, treated with a variety of systemic therapies including anthracycline containing regimes, CMF, CMF + prednisone, and tamoxifen, the risk of locoregional failure with or without distant failure was 12.9% at 10 years in the one to three node-positive group and 28.7% in women with four or more positive nodes (79). It is likely that the proportional reduction in locoregional failure by two-thirds will be similar in the one to three node-positive group as the four or more node-positive group but the absolute size of the reduction will be less in the one to three node-positive group (73). The heterogeneity of RT treatment in the Early Breast Cancer Collaborative Group trials was addressed by reclassifying the trials according to (*i*) predefined biologically equivalent dose, (*ii*) insufficient or excessive dose of irradiation and (*iii*) an inappropriate target volume (80). Optimum dosage was defined as 40–60 Gy in 2 Gy fractions. Insufficient dosage was defined as <40 Gy and excessive dosage as >60 Gy, and insufficient target coverage less than the chest wall and peripheral lymphatics. In category 1 trials with adequate dosage and target coverage, the odds of death were less than category 2 trials (inadequate or excessive dosage; 3% lower) and category 3 trials (inadequate coverage; 26% lower). Unfortunately, quality assurance protocols were not applied to the trials in the Oxford overview. Nonetheless, Gebski's findings underpin the importance of RT quality assurance and its influence on treatment outcome. By contrast, quality assurance procedures for RT are in place for the MRC/EORTC SUPREMO trial to standardize dosage, dose prescription, and limits of lung and cardiac irradiation (78). Others have argued that the criterion used by Gebski and colleagues with the inclusion of axillary nodes was inappropriate given the low risk of axillary recurrence after an adequate clearance and that axillary fields increase the risk of radiation-induced brachial plexopathy, lung toxicity, lymphedema, and shoulder dysfunction (77). In addition, these authors contend that the risk of locoregional failure is lower than in the Oxford overview (63) due to better attention to surgical technique in the axilla and the adoption of more effective anthracycline-based regimens. Finally they suggest that nodal ratios may be the parameter for assessing degrees of axillary nodal involvement for risk of local recurrence (81).

Largely in response to criticisms of the adequacy of axillary clearance in the original DBCG 82b and c trials, (64,66), an unplanned subgroup analysis was reported of a subset of 1152 node-positive patients with eight or more nodes removed from the axilla (82). The 15-year overall survival was increased by 9% in those patients with one to three positive nodes. While the benefit in local control was lower in the one to three node positive group than the 4 or more node-positive group, the survival benefit was similar in both groups. Some argue that the separation of the one to three node-positive group from the four or more node-positive group is an artificial distinction and that locoregional risk of relapse rises linearly with the number of involved axillary nodes (76). These authors and others (83) make the case that comprehensive PMRT is appropriate for all node-positive patients (76). Others argue that more definitive evidence is needed from randomized trials (73,77). This difference is reflected in consensus statements. The UK National Institute for Clinical Excellence guidelines recommend that patients with one to three-positive nodes are entered in the MRC SUPREMO trial (46), while the NCCN clinical practice guidelines strongly recommend consideration of chest wall and supraclavicular irradiation in women with one to three involved nodes (59). However there were differences of opinion among NCCN panel members with some in favor of making PMRT as standard for the one to three node-positive group with others

opposing any mandatory recommendation (59). In part the NCCN guidelines probably reflect less equipoise among American clinicians on this question where a previous trial (SWOG 9928) addressing the role of PMRT in the one to three node-positive patients closed prematurely due to inadequate accrual.

POSTMASTECTOMY RADIOTHERAPY AND BIOLOGICAL SUBTYPE

It is likely that biological subtype also plays a role in identifying which patients are most likely to benefit from PMRT, adding greater complexity to the question of which patients are likely to benefit on an individual basis. In a subgroup analysis of 1000 patients in the DBCG 82b and c trials (84) assessed for estrogen receptor (ER), progesterone receptor (PR), and HER2 status, a significantly improved overall survival after PMRT was seen only among patients characterized by good prognostic markers such as hormone receptor–positive and HER2-negative patients (including the ER- and PR-positive subtypes). No significant overall survival improvement after PMRT was found among patients with an *a priori* poor prognosis, the hormone receptor–negative and HER2-positive patients, and in particular the Rec-negative/HER2-positive subtype. Improved overall survival after PMRT was observed only among patients in good prognosis, hormone receptor–positive, and HER2-negative patients (including the two Rec-positive subtypes). PMRT did not improve overall survival among poor prognosis, hormone receptor-negative, and HER2-positive patients, especially the ER/PR-negative/HER2-positive subtype.

A further intriguing finding from a separate subgroup analysis of 1000 patients from the DBCG82b and c trials (85) is that the greatest improvement in overall survival from a reduction in local recurrence was seen in the good prognosis group. A possible explanation for these findings and those on biological subtype is that patients with more aggressive biological subtypes and poor prognosis tumors are more likely to have developed micrometastatic disease and therefore their overall survival is unlikely to be impacted on by locoregional RT. More data are needed to confirm this observation from biological substudies which are an integral component of contemporary prospective RCTs such as SUPREMO (78).

NODAL IRRADIATION

The role of elective regional nodal irradiation (RNI) remains controversial and this has been heightened by the adoption of sentinel lymph node biopsy (SNB) as an alternative to axillary node dissection for increasing numbers of patients with early breast cancer. This poses a new therapeutic dilemma for the clinical/radiation oncologist as to whether to irradiate the axilla in patients with macro or micrometastases in the sentinel node in those circumstances when axillary dissection is not carried out.

There are two principal points of view on the impact of RNI. The first is the Halstedian hypothesis that locoregional treatment prevents dissemination. The second is that regional nodal involvement is simply a marker of disseminated disease and therefore RNI is unlikely to affect survival. From the discussion earlier on PMRT, there is evidence that locoregional RT does improve survival but whether it is the chest wall or peripheral nodes are the key determinant in the survival benefit is unclear. Most recurrences seem to occur on the chest wall rather than in the axilla (if the latter is adequately treated). The chest wall recurrence rate in patients from four ECOG trials involving PMRT showed that at 10 years, 12% of recurrences were on the chest wall and only 4% in the axilla (79). This implies that the axilla may be a less critical target for an overall survival benefit from RT. RNI might impact on survival if systemic therapy eradicated distant metastases but not regional disease (86).

The American College of Surgeons Oncology Group (ACOSOG) (87) addressed the question as to whether axillary clearance could be omitted after BCS, even with a positive sentinel node biopsy. A total of 891 patients with a clinically negative axilla but one to two positive sentinel nodes were randomized to axillary clearance or no additional axillary surgery. The five-year failure rate in the axilla was higher in the SNB-only arm (0.9% vs. 0.5%) but the difference was not significantly different. There have been a number of criticisms of the trial. Firstly, it was underpowered since it did not reach its intended accrual of 1900 patients and secondly, there was no quality assurance of the RT aspects of the trial to ensure that the upper limits of the tangential breast fields were similar in both arms of the trial (i.e., the radiation oncologist was not tempted to place the upper border of these fields more cranial to treat more of the axilla in patients randomized to SNB alone). These weaknesses in trial design limit the generalizability of the findings to contemporary practice. Various explanations have been offered for the low rate of axillary recurrence in the SNB-alone arm of the ACOSOG trial. These include the use of hormonal therapy, control of low volume axillary disease by immune surveillance mechanisms (analogous to patients with bone marrow micrometastases who do not develop clinically overt metastases), or inadvertent inclusion of the lower axillary nodes in the tangential fields (88). As these authors have emphasized (88), the results of the ACOSOG trial should not be generalized to patients treated by partial breast irradiation, intraoperative RT, patients treated in the prone position or other techniques in which the axilla is not irradiated or mastectomy without radiation.

Other non-randomized studies report a low axillary recurrence rate after a positive SLN biopsy without axillary dissection at six years of follow-up (2% in the Memorial Sloan-Kettering series). However in a recent Dutch study (89) of 857 patients with node-negative disease, 795 patients with isolated tumor cells and 1028 patients with micrometastases in the SLN in which axillary treatment was omitted, the five-year regional recurrence rates were 2.3%, 2.0%, and 5.6% respectively. Risk factors for axillary recurrence were doubling of tumor size and grade 3 and negative hormone receptor status. Given the uncertainties inherent in the interpretation of the ACOSOG trial, patients with macrometastases in axillary nodes should be treated by axillary dissection or in less fit or older patients by axillary irradiation until more definitive level 1 evidence emerges to inform practice. For axillary micrometastases, a pragmatic approach taking into account different risk factors for axillary recurrence is suggested by Haffty et al. (88) (Table 41.2).

Table 41.2 Suggested Approach for Radiation Field Design in Patients with Positive Sentinel Node Biopsy without Axillary Lymph Node Dissection

Clinical and Pathological Parameters	No. of Positive Sentinel Nodes	Total no. of Sentinel Nodes Sampled	Probability of Additional Nodes[a] (%)	Probability of Additional Nodes[b] (%)	Probability of Four or More Nodes Involved[c] (%)	Field Design
IDC, 1.0 cm, LVI negative, ER positive	1 (IHC only)	3	3	8	<1	Tangents only
IDC, 1.8 cm, G3, LVI negative, ER-positive, unifocal	1 (macro)	2	27	24	2	High tangents
IDC, 2.0 cm, ER negative, LVI-positive	2 (macro)	2	63	55	30	High tangents/ consider full nodal irradiation
ILC, 4.0 cm, ER-positive, multifocal, LVI negative	2 (macro)	2	77	64	40	High tangents/ consider full nodal irradiation
IDC, 3.0 cm, ER negative, LVI-positive, multifocal	3 (macro with ENE)	3	78	95	80	Full nodal irradiation

[a]On the basis of the Memorial-Sloan Kettering Cancer Center nomogram.
[b]On the basis of the MD Anderson Center nomogram.
[c]Katz et al.
Abbreviations: ENE, extranodal extension; ER, estrogen receptor; G, grade; IDC, infiltrating ductal carcinoma; IHC, immunohistochemistry; ILC, infiltrating lobular carcinoma; LVI, lymphovascular invasion; Macro, macroscopic.
Source: From Ref. (88).

INTERNAL MAMMARY NODE IRRADIATION

The role of internal mammary node (IMN) irradiation remains controversial. Clinical internal mammary nodal recurrence is rare (around 1%) but this may partly reflect underdiagnosis and there may be increased recognition of radiological but not clinical signs of IMN disease with wider use of CT-based breast RT planning. The largest randomized trial assessing the role of internal mammary node and periclavicular irradiation is the EORTC 22922 trial of 4004 patients (90). The final analysis of this trial has been deferred to 2014 due to lack of events. A smaller French RCT of 1334 patients with a follow-up of eight years showed no difference in overall survival (91). Given the low event rate in the EORTC trial it seems unlikely that IMN irradiation will confer a clinically significant benefit in survival and at present it is not recommended as part of standard practice.

RADIATION-INDUCED TOXICITY

The benefits of adjuvant locoregional RT have to be balanced against radiation-induced toxicity. Perhaps the most important of these is cardiac toxicity. However this is highly dependent upon the technique. Older RT trials using obsolescent orthovoltage techniques and higher doses per fraction largely account for a 2% reduction in breast cancer mortality in the Oxford overview of RT trials being counterbalanced by a similar level of increased non–breast cancer mortality, mainly vascular in origin (63). Modern megavoltage RT techniques, in particular the use of 3D-CT based treatment planning, allow a comprehensive assessment of the relationship of the heart to the irradiated volume and allow beam modification to minimize cardiac dosage. It should be noted that the follow-up of these modern studies are relatively short and the wider use of cardiotoxic anthracycline-containing regimens and trastuzumab may increase long-term risks of cardiotoxicity. Most radiation-related cardiac events tend to occur 10 or more years after irradiation so a very long-term follow-up is needed to monitor these risks. Studies with short follow-ups suggest that the combination of trastuzumab with left-sided RT is safe if CT planning is used with the rider that the internal mammary nodes were not generally treated in this study (92).

Adjuvant irradiation of the breast normally includes some of the lung. The risk of clinically apparent pneumonitis is low at around 1% (93). The risk of rib fracture (94) and brachial plexopathy (95) are generally around 2% in older series and are likely to be even lower with modern RT techniques. The risks of lymphedema after axillary RT alone are about 2% after an axillary node sample (96) and but rises to 30–40% if combined with axillary dissection (97).

Most patients treated by adjuvant breast irradiation after BCS experience good to excellent cosmesis. Increasing breast size correlates with worse cosmesis as does the use of a breast boost after whole-breast irradiation (98).

REFERENCES

1. Keynes G. Conservative treatment of cancer of the breast. Br Med J 1937; 2: 643–66.
2. Fisher B, Redmond C, Poisson R, et al. Eight-year results of a randomized clinical trial comparing total mastectomy and lumpectomy with or without irradiation in the treatment of breast cancer. N Engl J Med 1989; 320: 822–8.
3. Sarrazin D, Lê MG, Arriagada R, et al. Ten-year results of a randomized trial comparing a conservative treatment to mastectomy in early breast cancer. Radiother Oncol 1989; 14: 177–84.
4. van Dongen JA, Bartelink H, Fentiman IS, et al. Factors influencing local relapse and survival and results of salvage treatment after breast-conserving therapy in operable breast cancer: EORTC trial 10801, breast conservation compared with mastectomy in TNM stage I and II breast cancer. Eur J Cancer 1992; 28A: 801–5.
5. Lichter AS, Lippman ME, Danforth DN Jr, et al. Mastectomy versus breast-conserving therapy in the treatment of stage I and II carcinoma of the breast: a randomized trial at the National Cancer Institute. J Clin Oncol 1992; 10: 976–83.
6. Liljegren G, Holmberg L, Adami HO, et al. Sector resection with or without postoperative radiotherapy for stage I breast cancer: five-year results of a randomized trial. Uppsala-Orebro Breast Cancer Study Group. J Natl Cancer Inst 1994; 86: 717–22.
7. Clark RM, McCulloch PB, Levine MN, et al. Randomized clinical trial to assess the effectiveness of breast irradiation following lumpectomy and axillary dissection for node-negative breast cancer. J Natl Cancer Inst 1992; 84: 683–9.
8. Forrest AP, Stewart HJ, Everington D, et al. Scottish Cancer Trials Breast Group. Randomised controlled trial of conservation therapy for breast cancer: 6-year analysis of the Scottish trial. Lancet 1996; 348: 708–13.
9. Veronesi U, Cascinelli N, Mariani L, et al. Twenty-year follow-up of a randomized study comparing breast-conserving surgery with radical mastectomy for early breast cancer. N Engl J Med 2002; 347: 1227–32.
10. Korreman SS, Pedersen AN, Nøttrup TJ, et al. Breathing adapted radiotherapy for breast cancer: comparison of free breathing gating with the breath-hold technique. Radiother Oncol 2005; 76: 311–18.
11. Haffty BG, Buchholz TA, McCormick B, et al. Should intensity-modulated radiation therapy be the standard of care in the conservatively managed breast cancer patient? J Clin Oncol 2008; 26: 2072–4.
12. Hoover S, Bloom E, Patel S. Review of breast conservation therapy: then and now. ISRN Oncol 2011; 2011: 617593.
13. Morganti AG, Cilla S, de Gaetano A, et al. Forward planned intensity modulated radiotherapy (IMRT) for whole breast postoperative radiotherapy. Is it useful? When? J Appl Clin Med Phys 2011; 12: 3451.
14. Borghero YO, Salehpour M, McNeese MD, et al. Multileaf field-in-field forward-planned intensity-modulated dose compensation for whole-breast irradiation is associated with reduced contralateral breast dose: a phantom model comparison. Radiother Oncol 2007; 82: 324–8.
15. Pignol JP, Olivotto I, Rakovitch E, et al. A multicenter randomized trial of breast intensity-modulated radiation therapy to reduce acute radiation dermatitis. J Clin Oncol 2008; 26: 2085–92.
16. Donovan E, Bleakley N, Denholm E, et al. Randomised trial of standard 2D radiotherapy (RT) versus intensity modulated radiotherapy (IMRT) in patients prescribed breast radiotherapy. Radiother Oncol 2007; 82: 254–64.
17. Teh AY, Walsh L, Purdie TG, et al. Concomitant intensity modulated boost during whole breast hypofractionated radiotherapy–a feasibility and toxicity study. Radiother Oncol 2012; 102: 89–95.
18. Toledano A, Garaud P, Serin D, et al. Concurrent administration of adjuvant chemotherapy and radiotherapy after breast-conservative surgery enhances late toxicities. Cancer Radiother 2006; 10: 158–67.
19. Hardee ME, Raza S, Becker SJ, et al. Prone hypofractionated whole-breast radiotherapy without a boost to the tumor bed: comparable toxicity of IMRT versus a 3D conformal technique. Int J Radiat Oncol Biol Phys 2012; 82: e415–23.
20. Sethi RA, No HS, Jozsef G, et al. Comparison of three-dimensional versus intensity-modulated radiotherapy techniques to treat breast and axillary level III and supraclavicular nodes in a prone versus supine position. Radiother Oncol 2012; 102: 74–81.
21. Kirby AM, Evans PM, Helyer SJ, et al. A randomised trial of supine versus prone breast radiotherapy (SuPr study): comparing set-up errors and respiratory motion. Radiother Oncol 2011; 100: 221–6.
22. Early Breast Cancer Trialists' Collaborative Group. Effect of radiotherapy after breast-conserving surgery on 10-year recurrence and 15-year breast cancer death: meta-analysis of individual patient data for 10,801 women in 17 randomised trials. Lancet 2011; 378: 1707–16.
23. Mannino M, Yarnold JR. Local relapse rates are falling after breast conserving surgery and systemic therapy for early breast cancer: can radiotherapy ever be safely withheld? Radiother Oncol 2009; 90: 14–22.

24. Clarke M, Collins R, Darby S, et al. Early Breast Cancer Trialists' Collaborative Group (EBCTCG). Effects of radiotherapy and of differences in the extent of surgery for early breast cancer on local recurrence and 15-year survival: an overview of the randomised trials. Lancet 2005; 366: 2087–106.

25. Buchholz TA. Radiotherapy and survival in breast cancer. Lancet 2011; 378: 1680–2.

26. Bartelink H, Horiot JC, Poortmans P, et al. Recurrence rates after treatment of breast cancer with standard radiotherapy with or without additional radiation. N Engl J Med 2001; 345: 1378–87.

27. Bartelink H, Horiot JC, Poortmans PM, et al. Impact of a higher radiation dose on local control and survival in breast-conserving therapy of early breast cancer: 10-year results of the randomized boost versus no boost EORTC 22881-10882 trial. J Clin Oncol 2007; 25: 3259–65.

28. Hughes KS, Schnaper LA, Berry D, et al. Lumpectomy plus tamoxifen with or without irradiation in women 70 years of age or older with early breast cancer. N Engl J Med 2004; 351: 971–7.

29. Hughes KS, Schnaper LA, Cirrincione C, et al. Lumpectomy plus tamoxifen with or without irradiation in women age 70 or older with early breast cancer. J Clin Oncol 2010; 28: 507.

30. Smith IE, Ross GM. Breast radiotherapy after lumpectomy - no longer always necessary. N Engl J Med 2004; 351: 1021–3.

31. Montgomery DA, Krupa K, Jack WJ, et al. Changing pattern of the detection of locoregional relapse in breast cancer: the Edinburgh experience. Br J Cancer 2007; 96: 1802–7.

32. Tinterri C, Gatzemeier W, Zanini V, et al. Conservative surgery with and without radiotherapy in elderly patients with early-stage breast cancer: a prospective randomised multicentre trial. Breast 2009; 18: 373–7.

33. Kunkler I. PRIME II breast cancer trial. Clin Oncol 2004; 16: 447–8.

34. Fisher B, Anderson S, Redmond CK, et al. Reanalysis and results after 12 years of follow-up in a randomized clinical trial comparing total mastectomy with lumpectomy with or without irradiation in the treatment of breast cancer. N Engl J Med 1995; 333: 1456–61.

35. Wildiers H, Kunkler I, Biganzoli L, et al. Management of breast cancer in elderly individuals: recommendations of the International Society of Geriatric Oncology. Lancet Oncol 2007; 8: 1101–15.

36. Veronesi U, Orecchia R, Luini A, et al. Intraoperative radiotherapy during breast conserving surgery: a study on 1,822 cases treated with electrons. Breast Cancer Res Treat 2010; 124: 141–51.

37. Khan A, Haffty BG. Hypofractionation in adjuvant breast radiotherapy. Breast 2010; 19: 168–71.

38. Schoenfield JD, Harris JR. Abbreviated course of radiotherapy (RT) for breast cancer. Breast 2011; S3: S116–27.

39. START Trialists' Group. Bentzen SM, Agrawal RK, Aird EG, et al. The UK Standardisation of Breast Radiotherapy (START) Trial A of radiotherapy hypofractionation for treatment of early breast cancer: a randomised trial. Lancet Oncol 2008; 9: 331–41.

40. START Trialists' Group. Bentzen SM, Agrawal RK, Aird EG, et al. The UK Standardisation of Breast Radiotherapy (START) Trial B of radiotherapy hypofractionation for treatment of early breast cancer: a randomised trial. Lancet 2008; 371: 1098–107.

41. Whelan T, MacKenzie R, Julian J, et al. Randomized trial of breast irradiation schedules after lumpectomy for women with lymph node-negative breast cancer. J Natl Cancer Inst 2002; 94: 1143–50.

42. Whelan TJ, Pignol JP, Levine MN, et al. Long-term results of hypofractionated radiation therapy for breast cancer. N Engl J Med 2010; 362: 513–20.

43. Owen JR, Ashton A, Bliss JM, et al. Effect of radiotherapy fraction size on tumour control in patients with early-stage breast cancer after local tumour excision: long-term results of a randomised trial. Lancet Oncol 2006; 7: 467–71.

44. Kirova YM, Campana F, Savignoni A, et al. Institut Curie Breast Cancer Study Group. Breast-conserving treatment in the elderly: long-term results of adjuvant hypofractionated and normofractionated radiotherapy. Int J Radiat Oncol Biol Phys 2009; 75: 76–81.

45. Smith BD, Arthur DW, Buchholz TA, et al. Accelerated partial breast irradiation consensus statement from the American Society for Radiation Oncology (ASTRO). J Am Coll Surg 2009; 290: 269–77.

46. NICE. Early and Locally Advanced Breast Cancer: Diagnosis and Treatment. London: National Institute for Clinical Excellence, 2009.

47. Orecchia R, Leonardo MC. Intraoperative radiation therapy: is it a standard now? Breast 2011; 20: S111–15.

48. Vaidya JS, Joseph DJ, Tobias JS. Targeted intraoperative radiotherapy versus whole breast radiotherapy for breast cancer (TARGIT-A trial): an international, prospective, randomised, non-inferiority phase 3 trial. Lancet 2010; 376: 91–102.

49. Orecchia R, Veronesi U. Intraoperative electrons. Semin Radiat Oncol 2005; 15: 76–83.

50. Polgár C, Van Limbergen E, Pötter R, et al. GEC-ESTRO Breast Cancer Working Group. Patient selection for accelerated partial-breast irradiation (APBI) after breast-conserving surgery: recommendations of the Groupe Européen de Curiethérapie-European Society for Therapeutic Radiology and Oncology (GEC-ESTRO) breast cancer working group based on clinical evidence (2009). Radiother Oncol 2010; 94: 264–73.

51. Coles C, Yarnold J; IMPORT Trials Management Group. The IMPORT trials are launched (September 2006). Clin Oncol 2006; 18: 587–90.

52. Stewart AJ, Khan AJ, Devlin PM. Partial breast irradiation: a review of techniques and indications. Br J Radiol 2010; 83: 369–78.

53. Cameron D, Kunkler I, Dixon M, et al. Intraoperative radiotherapy for early breast cancer. Lancet 2010; 376: 1142.

54. Vicini FA, Baglan KL, Kestin LL, et al. Accelerated treatment of breast cancer. J Clin Oncol 2001; 19: 1993–2001.

55. Polgár C, Sulyok Z, Fodor J, et al. Sole brachytherapy of the tumor bed after conservative surgery for T1 breast cancer: five-year results of a phase I/11 study and initial findings of a randomized phase III trial. J Surg Oncol 2002; 80: 121–8.

56. Kaufmann M, Morrow M, von Minckwitz G, et al. Locoregional treatment of primary breast cancer: consensus recommendations from an International Expert Panel. Cancer 2010; 116: 1184–91.

57. Sautter-Bihl ML, Budach W, Dunst J, et al. DEGRO practical guidelines for radiotherapy of breast cancer I: breast-conserving therapy. Strahlenther Onkol 2007; 183: 661–6.

58. Goldhirsch A, Ingle JN, Gelber RD, et al. Thresholds for therapies: highlights of the St Gallen International Expert Consensus on the primary therapy of early breast cancer 2009. Ann Oncol 2009; 20: 1319–29.

59. Carlson RW, Allred C, Anderson BO, et al. Invasive breast cancer. J Natl Compr Canc Netw 2011; 9: 136–22.

60. Cuzick J, Stewart H, Peto R, et al. Overview of randomized trials comparing radical mastectomy without radiotherapy against simple mastectomy with radiotherapy in breast cancer. Cancer Treat Rep 1987; 71: 7–14.

61. Cuzick J, Stewart H, Rutqvist L, et al. Cause-specific mortality in long-term survivors of breast cancer who participated in trials of radiotherapy. J Clin Oncol 1994; 12: 447–53.

62. Early Breast Cancer Trialists' Collaborative Group. Effects of radiotherapy and surgery in early breast cancer. An overview of the randomized trials. N Engl J Med 1995; 333: 1444–55.

63. Early Breast Cancer Trialists' Collaborative Group. Favourable and unfavourable effects on long-term survival of radiotherapy for early breast cancer: an overview of the randomised trials. Lancet 2000; 355: 1757–70.

64. Overgaard M, Hansen PS, Overgaard J, et al. Postoperative radiotherapy in high-risk premenopausal women with breast cancer who receive adjuvant chemotherapy. Danish Breast Cancer Cooperative Group 82b Trial. N Engl J Med 1997; 337: 949–55.

65. Ragaz J, Jackson SM, Le N, et al. Adjuvant radiotherapy and chemotherapy in node-positive premenopausal women with breast cancer. N Engl J Med 1997; 337: 956–62.

66. Overgaard M, Jensen MB, Overgaard J, et al. Postoperative radiotherapy in high-risk postmenopausal breast-cancer patients given adjuvant tamoxifen: Danish Breast Cancer Cooperative Group DBCG 82c randomised trial. Lancet 1999; 353: 1641–8.

67. Ragaz J, Olivotto IA, Spinelli JJ, et al. Locoregional radiation therapy in patients with high-risk breast cancer receiving adjuvant chemotherapy: 20-year results of the British Columbia randomized trial. J Natl Cancer Inst 2005; 97: 116–26.

68. Goldhirsch A, Coates AS, Colleoni M, et al. Radiotherapy and chemotherapy in high-risk breast cancer. N Engl J Med 1998; 338: 330–1.

69. Recht A, Bartelink H, Fourquet A, et al. Postmastectomy radiotherapy: questions for the twenty-first century. J Clin Oncol 1998; 16: 2886–9.

70. Harris JR, Halpin-Murphy P, McNeese M, et al. Consensus Statement on postmastectomy radiation therapy. Int J Radiat Oncol Biol Phys 1999; 44: 989–90.

71. Scottish Intercollegiate Guidelines Network. Breast Cancer in Women: A National Guideline. SIGN Publication no 29. Edinburgh: SIGN, 1998.

72. Recht A, Edge SB, Solin LJ, et al. Postmastectomy radiotherapy: clinical practice guidelines of the American Society of Clinical Oncology. J Clin Oncol 2001; 19: 1539–69.

73. Truong PT, Olivotto IA, Whelan TJ, et al. Clinical practice guidelines for the care and treatment of breast cancer: 16. Locoregional post-mastectomy radiotherapy. CMAJ 2004; 170: 1263–73.

74. Chua B, Olivotto IA, Weir L, et al. Increased use of adjuvant regional radiotherapy for node-positive breast cancer in British Columbia. Breast J 2004; 10: 38–44.

75. Whelan TJ, Julian J, Wright J, et al. Does locoregional radiation therapy improve survival in breast cancer? A meta-analysis. J Clin Oncol 2000; 18: 1220–9.

76. Marks LB, Zeng J, Prosnitz LR. One to three versus four or more positive nodes and postmastectomy radiotherapy: time to end the debate. J Clin Oncol 2008; 26: 2075–7.

77. Russell NS, Kunkler IH, van Tienhoven G, et al. Postmastectomy radiotherapy: will the selective use of postmastectomy radiotherapy study end the debate? J Clin Oncol 2009; 27: 996–7.

78. Kunkler IH, Canney P, van Tienhoven G, et al. MRC/EORTC (BIG 2-04) SUPREMO Trial Management Group. Elucidating the role of chest wall irradiation in 'intermediate-risk' breast cancer: the MRC/EORTC SUPREMO trial. Clin Oncol 2008; 20: 31–4.

79. Recht A, Gray R, Davidson NE, et al. Locoregional failure 10 years after mastectomy and adjuvant chemotherapy with or without tamoxifen without irradiation: experience of the Eastern Cooperative Oncology Group. J Clin Oncol 1999; 17: 1689–700.

80. Gebski V, Lagleva M, Keech A, et al. Survival effects of postmastectomy adjuvant radiation therapy using biologically equivalent doses: a clinical perspective. J Natl Cancer Inst 2006; 98: 26–38.

81. Woodward WA, Vinh-Hung V, Ueno NT, et al. Prognostic value of nodal ratios in node-positive breast cancer. J Clin Oncol 2006; 24: 2910–16.

82. Overgaard M, Nielsen HM, Overgaard J. Is the benefit of postmastectomy irradiation limited to patients with four or more positive nodes, as recommended in international consensus reports? A subgroup analysis of the DBCG 82 b&c randomized trials. Radiother Oncol 2007; 82: 247–53.

83. Poortmans P. Evidence based radiation oncology: breast cancer. Radiother Oncol 2007; 84: 84–101.

84. Kyndi M, Sørensen FB, Knudsen H, et al. Danish Breast Cancer Cooperative Group. Estrogen receptor, progesterone receptor, HER-2, and response to postmastectomy radiotherapy in high-risk breast cancer: the Danish Breast Cancer Cooperative Group. J Clin Oncol 2008; 26: 1419–26.

85. Kyndi M, Overgaard M, Nielsen HM, et al. High local recurrence risk is not associated with large survival reduction after postmastectomy radiotherapy in high-risk breast cancer: a subgroup analysis of DBCG 82 b&c. Radiother Oncol 2009; 90: 74–9.

86. Xie L, Higginson DS, Marks LB. Elective regional nodal irradiation in patients with early-stage breast cancer. Semin Radiat Oncol 2011; 21: 66–78.

87. Giuliano AE, Hunt KK, Ballman KV, et al. Axillary dissection vs no axillary dissection in women with invasive breast cancer and sentinel node metastasis: a randomized clinical trial. JAMA 2011; 305: 569–75.

88. Haffty BG, Hunt KK, Harris JR, et al. Positive sentinel nodes without axillary dissection: implications for the radiation oncologist. J Clin Oncol 2011; 29: 4479–81.

89. Pepels MJ, de Boer M, Bult P, et al. Regional recurrence in breast cancer patients with sentinel node micrometastases and isolated tumor cells. Ann Surg 2012; 255: 116–21.

90. Matzinger O, Heimsoth I, Poortmans P, et al. EORTC Radiation Oncology & Breast Cancer Groups. Toxicity at three years with and without irradiation of the internal mammary and medial supraclavicular lymph node chain in stage I to III breast cancer (EORTC trial 22922/10925). Acta Oncol 2010; 49: 24–34.

91. Romestaing P, Belot A, Hennequin C, et al. Ten-year results of a randomised trial of internal mammary chain irradiation after mastectomy. Int J Rad Oncol Biol Phys 2009; 75: SI.

92. Halyard MY, Pisansky TM, Dueck AC, et al. Radiotherapy and adjuvant trastuzumab in operable breast cancer: tolerability and adverse event data from the NCCTG Phase III Trial N9831. J Clin Oncol 2009; 27: 2638–44.

93. Lind PA, Marks LB, Hardenbergh PH, et al. Technical factors associated with radiation pneumonitis after local +/- regional radiation therapy for breast cancer. Int J Radiat Oncol Biol Phys 2002; 52: 137–43.

94. Pierce SM, Recht A, Lingos TI, et al. Long-term radiation complications following conservative surgery (CS) and radiation therapy (RT) in patients with early stage breast cancer. Int J Radiat Biol Phys 1992; 23: 915–23.

95. Powell S, Cooke J, Parsons C. Radiation-induced brachial plexus injury: follow-up of two different fractionation schedules. Radiother Oncol 1990; 18: 213–20.

96. Chetty U, Jack W, Prescott RJ, et al. Management of the axilla in operable breast cancer treated by breast conservation: a randomized clinical trial. Edinburgh Breast Unit. Br J Surg 2000; 87: 163–9.

97. Larson D, Weinstein M, Goldberg I, et al. Edema of the arm as a function of the extent of axillary surgery in patients with stage I-II carcinoma of the breast treated with primary radiotherapy. Int J Radiat Oncol Biol Phys 1986; 12: 1575–82.

98. Fowble B, Freedman G. Cancer of the breast. In: Wang CC, ed. Clinical Radiation Oncology: Indications, Techniques and Results, 2nd edn. Wiley-Liss, 2000: 258.

42 Partial breast irradiation

Charlotte Coles, Mukesh Mukesh, and Martin Keisch

INTRODUCTION

Standard breast radiotherapy consists of radiation to the whole breast and this has been discussed in detail in chapter 41. A group of techniques have been developed in recent years, collectively referred to as partial breast irradiation (PBI), which decrease both the volume of breast tissue irradiated and the duration of treatment. PBI is an alternative strategy whereby only the tumor bed and surrounding tissue are irradiated following breast conserving surgery. More than three-quarters of true in-breast recurrences occur at the site of lumpectomy and therefore, irradiation of the whole breast may be unnecessary. This approach focuses on the tumor bed and a zone of surrounding tissue to a variable depth with the aim of minimizing radiation dose to sensitive normal structures such as the heart, lungs, and breast tissue distant from the tumor bed. The advent of computed tomography (CT) based treatment planning in the late 1980s minimized exposure of normal tissues and helped radiotherapists cope with the challenges resulting from the peculiar shape of the breast and contiguity of important surrounding structures. It is hypothesized that PBI will decrease the late radiation-induced normal tissue side effects, while maintaining the low rates of local recurrence observed with whole-breast irradiation (WBI). Consequently, patients at a low risk of local recurrence are usually selected for this approach. This chapter will critically review the rationale for PBI, discuss the results of reported randomized controlled trials (RCTs), and describe the various radiation techniques required to deliver PBI following breast conservation surgery.

RATIONALE FOR PARTIAL BREAST IRRADIATION

The rationale for PBI is based on pathological studies demonstrating the distribution of tumor foci from the index cancer, clinical studies showing spatial patterns of relapse and the postulated (modest) effects of radiotherapy on other quadrant ipsilateral recurrence. In addition, it is suggested that reducing the breast volume irradiated will result in lower normal tissue toxicity and will also facilitate accelerated partial breast irradiation (APBI). Shortened overall treatment times with APBI have attractions for both patients and healthcare providers. Each of these aspects will be discussed in detail.

Observations from Clinicopathological Studies

It is frequently reported that the majority of breast cancer relapses occur within the vicinity of the original tumor bed. In reality, there are conflicting data regarding the spatial pattern of ipsilateral breast tumor relapse, which does not always correspond closely to pathological findings. This observation is reviewed in detail by Mannino and Yarnold and is summarized here (1). Five prospective RCTs of breast conservation surgery with or without whole-breast radiotherapy, have reported a 76–90% "same site" spatial pattern of relapse (2–6). In contrast, the European Organization for Research and Treatment of Cancer (EORTC) boost versus no-boost trial reported a 42% rate of relapse outside the original tumor area following a median follow-up of more than 10 years (7). This discrepancy in the spatial pattern of recurrence within RCTs could possibly be explained by differences in the definition of "same site" relapse. For example, the EORTC reported these relapses as within the tumor bed or scar, whereas other studies used different definitions such as the index quadrant or some arbitrary distance from the tumor bed/scar.

Pathological studies have also been used to analyze the pattern of breast relapse. One such study examined 264 mastectomy samples from women with tumors ≤4 cm (8). This pathological study illustrated that the density of tumor foci decreased with distance from the reference tumor: tumor foci could be identified in 41% (14% invasive, 27% non-invasive) and 11% (7% invasive, 4% non-invasive) of cases at distances more than 2 cm and 4 cm from the edge of the main tumor respectively. The high incidence of multifocality and distance from the index lesion may relate to the era of these studies by Holland et al. in which mammographic techniques were less sensitive and a higher proportion of tumors were palpable (9). A similar subsequent study analyzed 30 mastectomy specimens from patients who would have been eligible for breast conserving surgery, using a combination of pathology and imaging to detect multicentric tumor foci. This showed that 47% and 20% of cases had tumour foci more than 2 cm and 4 cm respectively from the edge of the index tumor (9). These observations suggest that multicentric tumor deposits are relatively common, but may not necessarily translate into clinical relapses following breast conserving therapy. Another elegant subgross and stereomicroscopic pathologic study by Ohtake et al. examined quadrantectomy specimens and found that the average value for maximum extension of ductal carcinoma in situ (DCIS) from the primary tumor was 11.9 mm for all patients and 9 mm for patients over 50 years of age (10). Imamura et al. processed 253 mastectomy specimens and determined that the maximal extension of DCIS from invasive cancers was less than 9 mm for all patients over 40 years of age (11).

Other studies have focused on analyzing re-excision margins following breast surgery. In a pathologic review of 441 breast conservation cases undergoing re-excision, the maximal distance of residual disease from the initial excision margin was available for measurement in 333 cases. This study showed that in 90% of patients with negative initial margins, residual disease was limited to within 10 mm of the original excision margin (12). The apparent discrepancy between this study and the two other pathological studies could be explained by assuming that tumor foci were present beyond the limits of the re-excision margin, and/or tissue damage due to diathermy/pathology processing may have resulted in loss of breast tissue immediately around the surgical excision borders.

Effect of Radiotherapy on Other Quadrant Ipsilateral Recurrence

One of the arguments used to justify APBI is that the ipsilateral breast tumor recurrence (IBTR) rate in quadrants distant from the original tumor is similar to the rates of contralateral breast cancer (CLBC). This was based on the results from the Milan I trial, which tested quadrantectomy and whole-breast radiotherapy against mastectomy (2). It showed similar rates of other-quadrant IBTR and CLBC: 0.42 and 0.66 per 100 women-years respectively. A possible interpretation of these data is that whole-breast radiotherapy is ineffective in preventing other IBTR in non-index quadrants, which are likely to be new primaries arising with the same frequency as CLBC.

In contrast, there are at least seven RCTs of breast conservation therapy suggesting that CLBC rates may be greater than other quadrant IBTR (4,5,13–18). The Early Breast Cancer Trialists Collaborative Group reported a 1.18 rate ratio for CLBC in irradiated patients, which takes into account the possibility of radiotherapy causing an increased rate of CLBC (19). A more recent analysis of both IBTR after breast conserving surgery and whole-breast radiotherapy and of CLBC in a United Kingdom (UK) radiotherapy fractionation trial, suggests that whole-breast radiotherapy does appear to reduce the risk of other-quadrant IBTR, including new primaries (20).

The Volume Effect of Breast Irradiation

To date, there is a paucity of data relating to the normal tissue consequences of PBI. Over a decade ago, Emami commented in a seminal paper that "there is a critical need for more accurate information about the tolerance of normal tissue to radiation." This is not only related to time–dose parameters, but specifically to the *partial volumes* of normal tissue receiving variable dose levels (21). Since the publication by Emami and colleagues, the dose volume effect of radiation on normal tissues has been updated in the Quantitative Analyses of Normal Tissue Effects in the Clinic (QUANTEC) report (22). Despite there being very good evidence for a radiation dose volume effect in many organs including lung and rectum, there appears to be little published data on the dose–volume effects of radiation on breast tissue including the QUANTEC report.

Level I evidence is available from the EORTC "boost versus no boost" trial, which randomized 5318 patients with early breast cancer between an additional dose of radiation to the tumor bed (16 Gy boost) and no boost treatment after WBI (7). On a univariate analysis it was reported that the boost volume was associated with an increased risk of moderate or severe breast fibrosis 10 years following radiotherapy (23). Vrieling et al. from the same group had previously reported worse cosmetic outcomes in patients with a boost volume >200 cm³ compared with ≤200 cm³ (odds ratio 0.47; 95% CI 0.29–0.76; p = 0.002) after three years of follow-up (24). However, these

conclusions were based on a univariate analysis; boost volume was not a significant variable affecting fibrosis and cosmesis on multivariate analysis.

Borger et al. (level IV evidence) reported on dose and volume effects on breast fibrosis after using a brachytherapy boost (25). A total of 404 patients were treated with external ream radiotherapy (50 Gy in 2 Gy daily fractions to the whole breast) followed by a low dose rate iridium implant boost. At a median follow-up of 70 months, a fourfold higher risk of fibrosis was observed for each 100 cm³ increase in irradiated boost volume. Those dose–volume relationships make the concept of PBI attractive as normal tissue toxicity is likely to decrease with smaller volumes of breast tissue irradiated.

Accelerated Partial Breast Irradiation

Accelerated radiotherapy is defined as more than the standard once daily treatments (fractions) delivered five times a week. This can be achieved by treating over the weekend or more commonly with PBI, twice daily. In addition, the dose per fraction often exceeds the standard dose of 2 Gy and is called hypo-fractionated radiotherapy. Hypofractionated radiotherapy can result in a higher incidence of normal tissue side effects unless care is taken to adequately reduce the total dose and/or reduce the volume irradiated (26). The postulated lower risk of normal tissue side effects with a smaller PBI volume makes the concept of APBI (hypofractionated) attractive.

The potential advantages of APBI can be divided into issues relating to health economics, patient satisfaction, and radiobiological factors. Firstly, a substantial reduction in the number of radiotherapy fractions will be an advantage for many institutions where resources are limited; breast irradiation constitutes a significant proportion of the total radiotherapy workload (approximately 30% in the UK). Secondly, a shorter overall treatment time is appealing to patients particularly those residing in remote areas, where patients may opt for mastectomy rather than having to travel long distances over a period of weeks for radiotherapy (27). Lastly, there is compelling evidence from five RCTs of hypofractionated whole-breast radiotherapy in breast cancer patients (n > 7000) suggesting no significant differences in local tumor control and normal tissue toxicity (with a trend for reduced toxicity) compared with conventional WBI schedules (28–32). This implies that breast tumors are at least as sensitive to dose per fraction as late reacting tissues and therefore hypofractionation may be advantageous in terms of breast cancer radiobiology (33).

Despite some areas of conflicting data, there does appear to be a sound rationale for PBI in selected subgroups of patients. It is clear that local recurrence rates for all breast cancer patients following breast conserving surgery is falling. This can be attributed to a combination of better multidisciplinary team working, improved imaging, increased attention to surgical margins, and more effective adjuvant therapies (systemic drugs and local radiotherapy) (34). In consequence, any increase in the relative risk of local relapse with PBI compared with whole-breast radiotherapy is likely to translate into only a modest absolute increase in risk of local recurrence.

SUMMARY OF RANDOMIZED TRIALS OF PBI

RCTs to date involving PBI are outlined in Table 42.1. An early UK trial conducted in the 1980s randomized 708 breast conservation patients to limited field (LF) radiotherapy to

Table 42.1 Phase II–III Randomized Controlled Trials Comparing Whole-Breast Radiotherapy *Vs.*PBI

Trial/Institute	Control Arm (WBI)	Test Arm (PBI): Treatment Modality	Median Follow-up (months)	Target Accrual	Reported
Christie group trial (35)	WBI 40 Gy in 15 fractions with matched field for regional nodes	PBI: 40–42.5 Gy in 8 fractions using electrons	65	708	Yes
Yorkshire Breast Cancer Group trial (36)	WBI 40 Gy in 15 fractions with 15 Gy boost	PBI using direct cobalt, cesium, or electrons beam or a small mega-voltage tangential pair to a dose of 55 Gy in 20 fractions	96	174 (premature closure)	Yes
Hungarian National Institute of Oncology (37)	WBI using cobalt or photons beam to a dose of 50 Gy in 25 fractions over 5 wks	HDR Ir-192 (85 pts) to a dose of 36.4 Gy in 7 fractions over 4 days or electrons (40 pts) to a dose of 50 Gy in 25 fractions prescribed to the 80% isodose	66	258	Yes
TARGIT (39)	WBI 40–56 Gy with optional boost of 10–16 Gy	PBI: 20 Gy single fraction using Intraoperative 50 kV photons	24	2232	Yes
ELIOT (66)	WBI 50 Gy in 25 fractions with 10 Gy boost	PBI: Intraoperative electrons 21 Gy in single fraction	NA	1200 (activated 2000)	No
IMPORT LOW (58,67)	WBI 40 Gy in 15 fractions, no boost	Arm 1: 36 Gy in 15 fractions to the low-risk volume of the breast and 40 Gy in 15 fractions to the index quadrant. Arm 2 (PBI): 40 Gy in 15 fractions over 3 wks to the index quadrant only	NA	2000 (closed 2010)	No
GEC-ESTRO (68)	WBI 50–50.4 Gy in 25–28 fractions with 10 Gy optional boost	PBI: 32 Gy in 8 fractions or 30.3 Gy in 7 fractions HDR or 50 Gy PDR	NA	1170 (activated 2004)	No
NSABP-39 (41)	WBI 50–50.4 Gy in 25–28 fractions with 10–16 Gy optional boost	PBI: 34 Gy in 10 fractions over 5 days using single/multisource brachytherapy or 38.5 Gy in 10 fractions over 5 days using 3D-CRT	NA	4300 (activated 2005)	No
RAPID (69)	WBI 42.5 Gy in 16 fractions with optional 10 Gy boost	PBI: 38.5 Gy in 10 fractions bd twice daily over 5–8 days using 3D-CRT	NA	2128 (activated 2006)	No
IRMA (70)	WBI 45 Gy in 18 fractions or 50 Gy in 25 fractions or 50.4 Gy in 28 fractions with optional 10–16 Gy boost	PBI: 38.5 Gy in 10 fractions bd over 5 days using 3D-CRT	NA	3302 (activated 2007)	No
Danish Breast Cancer Cooperative Group (59)	WBI 40 Gy in 15 fractions	PBI: 40 Gy in 15 fraction using 3D-CRT	NA	628 (activated 2009)	No
SHARE (71)	WBI 50 Gy in 25 fractions + 16 Gy boost or WBI 40–42.5 Gy in 15–16 fractions without boost	PBI: 40 Gy in 10 fractions bd over 5 to 7 days using 3D-CRT	NA	2796 (activated 2010)	No

Abbreviations: b.d., twice daily; 3D-CRT, 3-dimensional conformal radiotherapy; HDR, high dose rate; LDR, low dose rate; NA, not applicable; PBI, partial breast irradiation; PDR, pulsed dose rate; WBI, whole-breast irradiation.

the tumor bed or to wide field (WF) radiotherapy to the whole breast and regional nodes (35). The LF technique consisted of 40–42.5 Gy in 8 fractions over 10 days using 8–14 MeV electrons. By contrast, WF consisted of 40 Gy in 15 fractions over 21 days using photons. Marked fibrosis was seen in 14% of LF patients compared with 5% of WF patients.

The overall survival was 72.7% and 71.2% for the LF and WF groups respectively. The actuarial breast recurrence rate (first event) was 15% (LF) versus 11% (WF) for infiltrating ductal carcinoma, whereas for infiltrating lobular carcinoma, the recurrence rate was 34% (LF) versus 8% (WF). A high actual recurrence rate of 21% (LF) and 14% (WF) was also found for patients with an extensive intraductal component (EIC).

Even when lobular carcinoma and EIC were excluded from the analysis, there remained a higher recurrence rate in the LF group. This may have been due to geographical tumor miss in the LF treatment arm, as radiotherapy planning was based on clinical assessment rather than using specific imaging techniques. This illustrates an important issue with PBI: the need to accurately localize and treat the tumor bed and surrounding tissue. In addition, risk factors such as node positivity (nodal status was unknown in all) and positive margins (present in more than half of patients) may have contributed to the higher recurrence rate in the LF group.

Another early UK trial by the Yorkshire Breast Cancer Group randomized 174 patients between WBI (40 Gy in 15 fractions over 21 days) followed by tumor bed boost (15 Gy in five fractions) and PBI using a variety of techniques, including a direct cobalt or cesium beam, electrons or a small mega-voltage tangential pair to a dose of 55 Gy in 20 fractions over 28 days (36). The trial closed prematurely due to poor accrual with higher locoregional recurrence rates in the PBI group compared with the WBI group (24% versus 9%). It has been suggested that higher locoregional recurrence in the PBI arm was secondary to difficulty in accurate definition of the tumor bed. Treatment related morbidity with PBI and WBI was not reported.

Both of these trials pioneered the concept of PBI at a time when patient selection and techniques for tumor bed localization were at an early stage of development. Subsequent randomized trials have used more stringent protocols relating to both of these factors and some have recently reported outcomes. These include the Hungarian National Institute of Oncology PBI trial (37), the GEC ESTRO Working Group trial (38), and the TARGIT trial (39).

The Hungarian PBI trial randomized 258 patients with T1 N0-1 (grade I/II) breast cancer to WBI or PBI following breast-conserving surgery (37). WBI was delivered with a cobalt source or photon beam to a dose of 50 Gy in 2 Gy-daily fractions while PBI was administered using a high dose rate Iridium-192 brachytherapy (85 pts) to a dose of 36.4 Gy in 5.2 Gy per fraction over four days. Alternatively some patients received electrons (40 pts) to a dose of 50 Gy in 2 Gy daily fractions prescribed to the 80% isodose. At a median follow-up of 66 months (range 18–101 months), local recurrence rates were not significantly different in the two arms of the trial. The cosmetic results using Harvard criteria (40) were favorable in the PBI arm. The rate of excellent to good cosmesis was 77.6% for the PBI group and 62.9% for the WBI group (p = 0.009). Longer term results of other trials listed in Table 42.1 are still awaited. The largest ongoing trial to date is the National surgical adjuvant breast and bowel project (NSABP)/Radiation Therapy Oncology Group (RTOG) RCT which is scheduled to complete accrual of 4300 patients in 2012 (41). Nonetheless, this trial was closed to low risk patients after recruitment of approximately 2500 patients and an interim analysis revealing a high probability of the study being underpowered if low risk patients continued to be included.

USE OF PBI OUTSIDE CLINICAL TRIALS

Despite ongoing trials evaluating the efficacy of PBI versus whole-breast radiotherapy, there has been a notable increase in use of PBI outside of clinical trials (42–45). This has prompted the emergence of guidelines to try and ensure that "appropriate" patients are selected for PBI. Examples of such guidelines from the American Society of Radiation Oncology (ASTRO) and the Groupe Européen de Curiethérapie-European Society for Therapeutic Radiology and Oncology (GEC-ESTRO) are shown in Tables 42.2 and 42.3 (46,47). Additional, more flexible guidelines are in existence in other organizations such as the American Brachytherapy Society, the American Society of Breast Surgeons, and the American College of Radiation Oncology (Table 42.4). Attempts have been made to validate the criteria on which these guidelines are based. To date there has been no evidence from any single institution data that any selection

Table 42.2 Comparison of ASTRO and GEC-ESTRO Guidelines for Patient Selection for Partial Breast Irradiation Outside Clinical Trials

	ASTRO	GEC-ESTRO
Age	≥ 60 yrs	≥ 50 yrs
Tumor size	≤ 2 cm	≤ 3 cm
T stage	T1	T1-T2
Margins	≥ 2 mm	≥ 2 mm
Tumor	Unicentric, unifocal	Unicentric, unifocal
Histology	Invasive ductal or favorable subtype, not invasive lobular	Invasive ductal or favorable subtype, not invasive lobular
Pure DCIS	No	No
Grade	Any	Any
Lymphovascular space invasion	No	No
Extensive intraductal component	No	No
LCIS	Allowed	Allowed
ER	Positive	Any
N stage (SLNB or ALND)	pN0	pN0
Neoadjuvant chemotherapy	No	No
BRCA mutation	No	–

Abbreviations: ALND, axillary lymph node dissection; ASTRO, American Society of Radiation Oncology; DCIS, ductal carcinoma *in situ*; ER, estrogen receptor; GEC-ESTRO, Groupe Européen de Curiethérapie-European Society for Therapeutic Radiology and Oncology; LCIS, lobular carcinoma *in situ*; SLNB, sentinel lymph node biopsy.

Table 42.3 Patients are Good Candidates for Accelerated Partial Breast Irradiation Only in Context of Clinical Trials Based on ASTRO and GEC-ESTRO Guidelines

	ASTRO	GEC-ESTRO
Age	50–59 yrs	>40–50 yrs
Tumor size	2.1–3 cm	≤ 3 cm
T stage	T0-T2	T1-T2
Margins	Close but < 2 mm	Negative but <2 mm
Tumor	Clinically unifocal (microscopic multifocality allowed if total lesion between 2.1 and 3 cm)	Multifocal (limited to 2 cm of the index lesion)
Histology (invasive lobular)	Allowed	Allowed
Pure DCIS	≤ 3 cm	Allowed
Grade	Any	Any
Lymphovascular space invasion	Limited/focal	No
Extensive intraductal component	≤ 3 cm	No
LCIS	Allowed	Allowed
ER	Negative	Any
N stage	pN0	pN1mi, pN1a (ALND)
Neoadjuvant chemotherapy	No	No
BRCA mutation	No	–

Abbreviations: ALND, axillary lymph node dissection; ASTRO, American Society of Radiation Oncology; DCIS, ductal carcinoma *in situ*; ER, estrogen receptor; GEC-ESTRO, Groupe Européen de Curiethérapie-European Society for Therapeutic Radiology and Oncology; LCIS, lobular carcinoma *in situ*.

Table 42.4 ASBrS, ABS, and NSABP/RTOG Appropriateness Criteria for APBI

ASBrS (72)	ABS (73)	NSABP/ RTOG (41)
Age ≥45 (IDC), ≥50 (DCIS)	Age ≥45	Age >18
Histology: IDC, DCIS	Unifocal IDC	DCIS or any histology
Size ≤3 cm	≤ 3 cm	≤ 3 cm
Negative microscopic margins	No tumor on ink	No tumor on ink
LN negative	LN negative	Up to 3 LNs +[a]

Abbreviations: ABS, American Board of Surgery; ASBrS, American Society of Breast Surgeons; DCIS, ductal carcinoma in situ; IDC, invasive ductal carcinoma; LN, lymph node; NSABP, National Surgical Adjuvant Breast and Bowel Project; RTOG, Radiation Therapy Oncology Group.

criteria can be applied which will determine the candidacy for APBI and ensure uniformly low recurrence rates at 5–10 years in these non-controlled studies (Table 42.5).

The off-trial use of PBI is partially attributable to the Federal Drug Agency (FDA) approval of the balloon brachytherapy device in 2002 and subsequent Medicare reimbursement. Several groups have now reported on the efficacy of this technique with conflicting data on the correlation between balloon volume and overall cosmesis/fibrosis (48–52). The American Society of Breast Surgeons (ASBrS) MammoSite Breast Brachytherapy Registry trial is the largest series published to date and with more than five years of follow-up only 50 local failures have occurred among 1440 patients (3.61% actuarial rate of local recurrence) (53). Furthermore, a matched pair analysis versus SEER database patients receiving WBI also shows no difference in any endpoint (54). However, concerns have been raised regarding appropriate patient selection and the premature adoption of this treatment for early stage breast cancer before the long-term efficacy of PBI has been fully demonstrated. Hattangadi et al. examined the SEER database and identified 3556 patients treated with accelerated PBI with brachytherapy from 2000 to 2007. Only 32% of these patients would have been classified as suitable for PBI based on the ASTRO consensus statement (44). Smith et al. (45) examined the Medicare claim of 130,000 patients with early breast cancer treated with lumpectomy followed by adjuvant radiotherapy

for the period 2000–2007. The use of APBI with brachytherapy increased from 1% in 2000 to 13% in 2007 and the incidence of mastectomy at five years of follow-up was 3.8% in brachytherapy patients compared with only 2% after WBI (p < 0.001). It must be noted that the study by Smith and colleagues was based solely on billing claims data and not clinical information; therefore the reasons for additional surgery is unknown. Concerns relate not only to in-breast recurrence but also the possibility of higher axillary failure rates due to the lack of radiation treatment to the low axilla. Many physicians feel that tangential breast fields help treat and control the axilla (55,56). Nonetheless, data from William Beaumont Hospital showed an actuarial axillary failure rate of only 0.19% at five years among 534 patients treated with various APBI techniques including interstitial implant, balloon brachytherapy, and 3D-CRT (53).

In summary, PBI should be used cautiously outside a clinical trial until longer term follow-up data from the majority of ongoing studies become available. Patterns of local recurrence for lower grade cancers appears to be different from higher grade lesions in poor risk patients; relapses can occur more than 10 years following treatment for lower grade tumors (57). ASTRO guidelines state that patients who fulfill the criteria for recommending PBI should still be counseled before proceeding with PBI and be informed that it has not been proven to be safer than or even as effective as whole-breast radiotherapy (47).

Table 42.5 IBTR Rate by ASTRO Consensus Panel Group

Study	N	Median F/u	Suitable	Cautionary	Unsuitable	Notes
Shah, et al. (62)	199	10.7 yrs	4.4% (n = 95, 12-yr)	7.4% (n = 63, 12-yr)	2.4% (n = 41, 12-yr)	No difference in IBTR between groups (p = 0.61)
Vicini, et al. (74)	199	9.3 yrs	2.6% (n = 95, 10-yr)	7.8% (n = 63, 10-yr)	2.5% (n = 41, 10-yr)	No increased IBTR between groups (p = 0.86). Young age associated with increased IBTR.
Leonardi, et al. (75)	1797	Not reported	1.5% (n = 294, 5-yr)	4.4% (n = 691, 5-yr)	8.8% (n = 812, 5-yr)	ELIOT non-randomized trial. Alternate definition of ER negative (<1%) used. Difference between groups noted (p<0.001)
Shah, et al. (76)	39	7.1 yrs	–	–	2.2% (n = 39, 5-yr)	Lymph node positive patients only
McHaffie, et al. (77)	136	5.0 yrs	1.6%	4.8%	6.6%	No statistical increase in IBTR rates.
Shaitelman, et al. (78)	1,025	4.5 yrs	2.6% (n = 419, 5-yr)	5.4% (n = 430, 5-yr)	5.3% (n = 176, 5-yr)	No difference in IBTR between groups (p = 0.19)
Jeruss, et al. (79)	194	4.5 yrs	–	3.4% (5-yr)	–	Pure-DCIS patients only
Wilkinson, et al. (80)	202	4.1 yrs	1.4% (n = 182, 5-yr)	0% (n = 20, 5-yr)	–	Receptor positive *vs.* triple negative
Zaulis, et al. (81)	183	3.8 yrs	–	–	–	IBTR by ASTRO CP group not reported. DFS/OS not different between groups
Park, et al. (82)	53	3.6 yrs	–	0% (n = 53, 5-yr)	–	Pure-DCIS patients only

Abbreviations: ASTRO, American Society of Radiation Oncology; DCIS, ductal carcinoma *in situ*; DFS, disease-free survival; ER, estrogen receptor; IBTR, ipsilateral breast tumor recurrence; OS, overall survival.

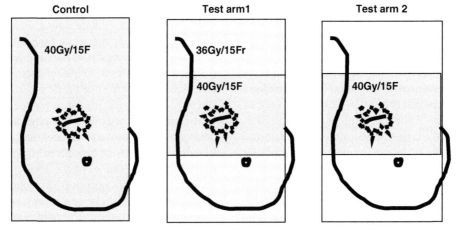

Figure 42.1 An IMPORT LOW trial schema.

RADIATION TECHNIQUES FOR PBI
External Beam Techniques
UK "IMPORT LOW" Technique

The UK Intensity Modulated Partial Organ Radiotherapy trial (58) for women at low risk of recurrence (IMPORT LOW) is outlined schematically in Figure 42.1. This RCT closed to recruitment in 2010 with more than 2000 patients entered. The control arm schedule was the UK standard of 40 Gy in 15 fractions (2.67 Gy each) over 3 weeks. Test arm 2 consisted of partial breast radiotherapy to the index quadrant using shortened tangential fields. Test arm 1 included whole-breast radiotherapy with a modest dose reduction to 36 Gy. This 10% decrease in dose intensity is expected to reduce late adverse effects significantly with a disproportionately small effect on local tumor control.

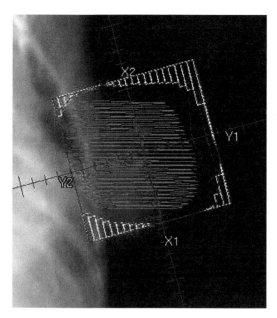

Figure 42.2 IMPORT LOW trial field arrangement.

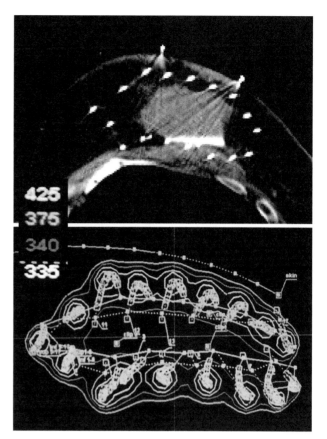

Figure 42.3 CT image and corresponding isodose curves of an interstitial multicatheter implant. *Source:* Courtesy D. Arthur.

The partial breast test arm used simple shortened tangential fields, so that the treated partial breast volumes were on average larger than those treated with APBI over five days. Three-dimensional compensation was most commonly achieved using simple forward planned intensity modulated fields and adequate uniformity obtained with three or four segments per beam. A typical field arrangement for the partial breast trial arm is shown in Figure 42.2.

IMPORT LOW was designed to evaluate the volume effect of partial breast radiotherapy; identical total dose and fractionation was used for the control and partial breast test arms, with breast volume being the only variable. This IMPORT LOW and the Danish Breast Cancer Cooperative Group trial (59) are the only randomized trials adopting this approach with all other trials incorporating variable dose-fractionation schedules.

3D Conformal Radiation Technique

Three-dimensional conformal radiotherapy is a form of APBI which employs conventional external beam technology to treat smaller volumes than WBI. Despite being a non-invasive form of APBI, there are technical problems with achieving high levels of conformity. Multiple non-coplanar beams with CT-designed blocking are typical. The equipment is widely available, but the technique can be challenging due to limitations in the ability to minimize the treatment volume leading to much less conformality than with brachytherapy techniques. Patient motion, respiratory motion, and set-up error all must be considered. In a phase III trial 58 patients were treated to 38.5 Gy in 10 fractions over five days. At a median follow-up of 4.5 years the study showed excellent tolerance and an IBTR rate of 6% (60). The technique employed in trials to date requires that the heart and lung dose be maintained below those associated with WBI. Other approaches being evaluated include prone techniques and intensity modulated radiation therapy. The latter delivers more conformed dose distributions and improves homogeneity (61). A handful of small patient studies have been published with encouraging results. The RTOG performed a phase I–II pilot trial that led to the inclusion of the technique in the NSABP/RTOG 0413 trial which is assessing three techniques for ABPI (3D conformal, interstitial brachytherapy, and MammoSite). This trial aims to evaluate these in comparison with WBI using the primary endpoints of local recurrence, disease-free, and overall survival together with quality of life as a secondary endpoint (41).

Brachytherapy Techniques

Modern Image-Guided Multicatheter Interstitial Implants

Modern APBI began in the early 1990s, employing careful computer calculated brachytherapy techniques for placement of multiplanar interstitial catheter implants after lumpectomy to treat the tumor bed plus a margin of tissue to a depth of 1–2 cm (Fig. 42.3). Treatment was delivered to a total dose of 34 Gy delivered twice daily in five treatment days and therefore permitted brachytherapy to be completed within one week rather than five or six weeks as was standard at the time in the United States. Initially rigid template guided techniques predominated, but freehand techniques have become increasingly popular. Various forms of image guidance are employed including CT, ultrasound, and stereotactic mammography. Care in Planning Target Volume (PTV) coverage allows for narrower margins and likely improves toxicity ratios. In the William Beaumont series of patients, careful use of these techniques in appropriately selected patients has shown excellent results with follow-up to 12 years. A matched pair analysis with WBI patients shows similar results for all endpoints (62). The RTOG published a phase I–II trial performed at multiple institutions which likewise demonstrated excellent outcomes in terms of recurrence and cosmesis (63).

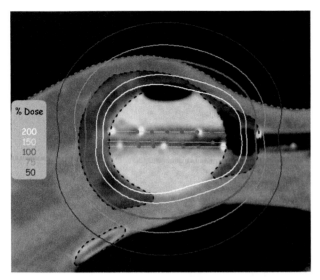

Figure 42.4 Typical dose distribution around a multilumen balloon brachytherapy applicator. *Source:* Courtesy Hologic Inc.

Intracavitary Balloon-Based Brachytherapy

MammoSite® (Hologic, Inc., Bedford, Massachusetts, USA) is an inflatable double lumen balloon catheter which is placed in the surgical cavity and acts as a breast brachytherapy applicator. The introduction of MammoSite has overcome some of the perceived complexities and technical barriers to the multicatheter approach, including a steep learning curve, and challenging quality assurance. The device fills the surgical cavity and delivers a dose of radiation that is highest at the surface of the balloon but falls off rapidly as the surrounding breast tissue is irradiated to a depth of 1 cm. The device delivers a total dosage of 34 Gy in 10 fractions (a high dose rate remote afterloader with Iridium 142). Since the approval of MammoSite by the FDA, the device has become a frequently employed method for PBI in the United States with over 4000 physicians in more than 1000 centers now trained in its use. In excess of 70,000 patients are estimated to have been treated using the original MammoSite device or other similar product such as the Contura balloon™ (SenoRx, Inc., Irvine, CA) or SAVI™ (Cianna Medical, Aliso Viejo, CA). The device was initially a single treatment lumen applicator but subsequently multiple treatment lumens have become available allowing more flexibility in dosimetry prescription. The previously mentioned ASBrS Registry trial represents the largest collection of patients treated to date with excellent results at six years of follow-up with respect to local control (54), cosmetic outcome (64), and toxicity (65).

Figure 42.4 shows a typical multilumen balloon implant and the resulting dose distribution.

SUMMARY

A growing interest in PBI is evidenced by the multitude of techniques under investigation around the world. Although randomized controlled data are currently limited, the outlook for these techniques seems optimistic. Additional research is needed to clarify subsets of patients best served by these techniques.

REFERENCES

1. Mannino M, Yarnold J. Accelerated partial breast irradiation trials: diversity in rationale and design. Radiother Oncol 2009; 91: 16–22.
2. Veronesi U, Cascinelli N, Mariani L, et al. Twenty-year follow-up of a randomized study comparing breast-conserving surgery with radical mastectomy for early breast cancer. N Engl J Med 2002; 347: 1227–32.
3. Fisher ER, Sass R, Fisher B, et al. Pathologic findings from the National Surgical Adjuvant Breast Project (protocol 6). II. Relation of local breast recurrence to multicentricity. Cancer 1986; 57: 1717–24.
4. Liljegren G, Holmberg L, Bergh J, et al. 10-Year results after sector resection with or without postoperative radiotherapy for stage I breast cancer: a randomized trial. J Clin Oncol 1999; 17: 2326–33.
5. Clark RM, Whelan T, Levine M, et al. Randomized clinical trial of breast irradiation following lumpectomy and axillary dissection for node-negative breast cancer: an update. Ontario Clinical Oncology Group. J Natl Cancer Inst 1996; 88: 1659–64.
6. Malmstrom P, Holmberg L, Anderson H, et al. Breast conservation surgery, with and without radiotherapy, in women with lymph node-negative breast cancer: a randomised clinical trial in a population with access to public mammography screening. Eur J Cancer 2003; 39: 1690–7.
7. Bartelink H, Horiot JC, Poortmans PM, et al. Impact of a higher radiation dose on local control and survival in breast-conserving therapy of early breast cancer: 10-year results of the randomized boost versus no boost EORTC 22881-10882 trial. J Clin Oncol 2007; 25: 3259–65.
8. Holland R, Veling SH, Mravunac M, Hendriks JH. Histologic multifocality of Tis, T1-2 breast carcinomas. Implications for clinical trials of breast-conserving surgery. Cancer 1985; 56: 979–90.
9. Vaidya JS, Vyas JJ, Chinoy RF, et al. Multicentricity of breast cancer: whole-organ analysis and clinical implications. Br J Cancer 1996; 74: 820–4.
10. Ohtake T, Abe R, Kimijima I, et al. Intraductal extension of primary invasive breast carcinoma treated by breast-conservative surgery. Computer graphic three-dimensional reconstruction of the mammary duct-lobular systems. Cancer 1995; 76: 32–45.
11. Imamura H, Haga S, Shimizu T, et al. Relationship between the morphological and biological characteristics of intraductal components accompanying invasive ductal breast carcinoma and patient age. Breast Cancer Res Treat 2000; 62: 177–84.
12. Vicini FA, Kestin LL, Goldstein NS. Defining the clinical target volume for patients with early-stage breast cancer treated with lumpectomy and accelerated partial breast irradiation: a pathologic analysis. Int J Radiat Oncol Biol Phys 2004; 60: 722–30.
13. Veronesi U, Marubini E, Mariani L, et al. Radiotherapy after breast-conserving surgery in small breast carcinoma: long-term results of a randomized trial. Ann Oncol 2001; 12: 997–1003.
14. Fisher B, Anderson S, Bryant J, et al. Twenty-year follow-up of a randomized trial comparing total mastectomy, lumpectomy, and lumpectomy plus irradiation for the treatment of invasive breast cancer. N Engl J Med 2002; 347: 1233–41.
15. Forrest AP, Stewart HJ, Everington D, et al. Randomised controlled trial of conservation therapy for breast cancer: 6-year analysis of the Scottish trial. Scottish Cancer Trials Breast Group. Lancet 1996; 348: 708–13.
16. Fisher B, Bryant J, Dignam JJ, et al. Tamoxifen, radiation therapy, or both for prevention of ipsilateral breast tumor recurrence after lumpectomy in women with invasive breast cancers of one centimeter or less. J Clin Oncol 2002; 20: 4141–9.
17. Winzer KJ, Sauer R, Sauerbrei W, et al. Radiation therapy after breast-conserving surgery; first results of a randomised clinical trial in patients with low risk of recurrence. Eur J Cancer 2004; 40: 998–1005.
18. Potter R, Gnant M, Kwasny W, et al. Lumpectomy plus tamoxifen or anastrozole with or without whole breast irradiation in women with favorable early breast cancer. Int J Radiat Oncol Biol Phys 2007; 68: 334–40.
19. Clarke M, Collins R, Darby S, et al. Effects of radiotherapy and of differences in the extent of surgery for early breast cancer on local recurrence and 15-year survival: an overview of the randomised trials. Lancet 2005; 366: 2087–106.
20. Gujral DM, Sumo G, Owen JR, et al. Ipsilateral breast tumor relapse: local recurrence versus new primary tumor and the effect of whole-breast radiotherapy on the rate of new primaries. Int J Radiat Oncol Biol Phys 2011; 79: 19–25.
21. Emami B, Lyman J, Brown A, et al. Tolerance of normal tissue to therapeutic irradiation. Int J Radiat Oncol Biol Phys 1991; 21: 109–22.
22. Bentzen SM, Constine LS, Deasy JO, et al. Quantitative Analyses of Normal Tissue Effects in the Clinic (QUANTEC): an introduction to the scientific issues. Int J Radiat Oncol Biol Phys 2010; 76: S3–9.

23. Collette S, Collette L, Budiharto T, et al. Predictors of the risk of fibrosis at 10 years after breast conserving therapy for early breast cancer: a study based on the EORTC Trial 22881-10882 'boost versus no boost'. Eur J Cancer 2008; 44: 2587–99.

24. Vrieling C, Collette L, Fourquet A, et al. The influence of patient, tumor and treatment factors on the cosmetic results after breast-conserving therapy in the EORTC 'boost vs. no boost' trial. EORTC Radiotherapy and Breast Cancer Cooperative Groups. Radiother Oncol 2000; 55: 219–32.

25. Borger JH, Kemperman H, Smitt HS, et al. Dose and volume effects on fibrosis after breast conservation therapy. Int J Radiat Oncol Biol Phys 1994; 30: 1073–81.

26. Yarnold J, Bentzen SM, Coles C, Haviland J. Hypofractionated whole-breast radiotherapy for women with early breast cancer: myths and realities. Int J Radiat Oncol Biol Phys 2011; 79: 9.

27. Vicini FA, Remouchamps V, Wallace M, et al. Ongoing clinical experience utilizing 3D conformal external beam radiotherapy to deliver partial-breast irradiation in patients with early-stage breast cancer treated with breast-conserving therapy. Int J Radiat Oncol Biol Phys 2003; 57: 1247–53.

28. Bentzen SM, Agrawal RK, Aird EG, et al. The UK Standardisation of Breast Radiotherapy (START) Trial A of radiotherapy hypofractionation for treatment of early breast cancer: a randomised trial. Lancet Oncol 2008; 9: 331–41.

29. Bentzen SM, Agrawal RK, Aird EG, et al. The UK Standardisation of Breast Radiotherapy (START) Trial B of radiotherapy hypofractionation for treatment of early breast cancer: a randomised trial. Lancet 2008; 371: 1098–107.

30. Whelan TJ, Pignol JP, Levine MN, et al. Long-term results of hypofractionated radiation therapy for breast cancer. N Engl J Med 2010; 362: 513–20.

31. Agrawal RK, Alhasso A, Barrett-Lee PJ, et al. First results of the randomised UK FAST Trial of radiotherapy hypofractionation for treatment of early breast cancer (CRUKE/04/015). Radiother Oncol 2011; 100: 93–100.

32. Owen JR, Ashton A, Bliss JM, et al. Effect of radiotherapy fraction size on tumour control in patients with early-stage breast cancer after local tumour excision: long-term results of a randomised trial. Lancet Oncol 2006; 7: 467–71.

33. Yarnold J, Ashton A, Bliss J, et al. Fractionation sensitivity and dose response of late adverse effects in the breast after radiotherapy for early breast cancer: long-term results of a randomised trial. Radiother Oncol 2005; 75: 9–17.

34. Mannino M, Yarnold JR. Local relapse rates are falling after breast conserving surgery and systemic therapy for early breast cancer: can radiotherapy ever be safely withheld? Radiother Oncol 2009; 90: 14–22.

35. Ribeiro GG, Magee B, Swindell R, Harris M, Banerjee SS. The Christie Hospital breast conservation trial: an update at 8 years from inception. Clin Oncol (R Coll Radiol) 1993; 5: 278–83.

36. Dodwell DJ, Dyker K, Brown J, et al. A randomised study of whole-breast vs tumour-bed irradiation after local excision and axillary dissection for early breast cancer. Clin Oncol (R Coll Radiol) 2005; 17: 618–22.

37. Polgar C, Fodor J, Major T, et al. Breast-conserving treatment with partial or whole breast irradiation for low-risk invasive breast carcinoma–5-year results of a randomized trial. Int J Radiat Oncol Biol Phys 2007; 69: 694–702.

38. Strnad V, Ott OJ, Hildebrandt G, et al. First clinical results of the GEC-ESTRO Breast WG Phase III multicentric APBI trial (OC 88). Radiat Oncol 2012; 103:S35–6.

39. Vaidya JS, Joseph DJ, Tobias JS, et al. Targeted intraoperative radiotherapy versus whole breast radiotherapy for breast cancer (TARGIT-A trial): an international, prospective, randomised, non-inferiority phase 3 trial. Lancet 2010; 376: 91–102.

40. Harris JR, Levene MB, Svensson G, Hellman S. Analysis of cosmetic results following primary radiation therapy for stages I and II carcinoma of the breast. Int J Radiat Oncol Biol Phys 1979; 5: 257–61.

41. Wolmark N, Curran W; On behalf of NSABP and RTOG of the American College of Radiology (ACR). NSABP Protocol B-39. RTOG Protocol 0413. A randomized phase III study of conventional whole breast irradiation versus partial breast irradiation for women with stage 0, I, or II breast cancer. National surgical adjuvant breast and bowel project (NSABP). Trial protocol March 13, 2007. p. 1–132. [Available from: http://clinicaltrials.gov/ct2/show/NCT00103181]

42. Smith GL, Xu Y, Buchholz TA, et al. Brachytherapy for accelerated partial-breast irradiation: a rapidly emerging technology in breast cancer care. J Clin Oncol 2011; 29: 157–65.

43. Abbott AM, Habermann EB, Tuttle TM. Trends in the use of implantable accelerated partial breast irradiation therapy for early stage breast cancer in the United States. Cancer 2011; 117: 3305–10.

44. Hattangadi JA, Taback N, Neville BA, Harris JR, Punglia RS. Accelerated partial breast irradiation using brachytherapy for breast cancer: patterns in utilization and guideline concordance. J Natl Cancer Inst 2012; 104: 29–41.

45. Smith GL, Xu Y, Buchholz TA, et al. Association between treatment with brachytherapy vs whole-breast irradiation and subsequent mastectomy, complications, and survival among older women with invasive breast cancer. JAMA 2012; 307: 1827–37.

46. Polgar C, Van Limbergen E, Potter R, et al. Patient selection for accelerated partial-breast irradiation (APBI) after breast-conserving surgery: recommendations of the Groupe Europeen de Curietherapie-European Society for Therapeutic Radiology and Oncology (GEC-ESTRO) breast cancer working group based on clinical evidence (2009). Radiother Oncol 2010; 94: 264–73.

47. Smith BD, Arthur DW, Buchholz TA, et al. Accelerated partial breast irradiation consensus statement from the American Society for Radiation Oncology (ASTRO). J Am Coll Surg 2009; 209: 269–77.

48. Vicini F, Beitsch P, Quiet C, et al. Five-year analysis of treatment efficacy and cosmesis by the American Society of Breast Surgeons MammoSite Breast Brachytherapy Registry Trial in patients treated with accelerated partial breast irradiation. Int J Radiat Oncol Biol Phys 2011; 79: 808–17.

49. Johansson B, Karlsson L, Liljegren G, Hardell L, Persliden J. Pulsed dose rate brachytherapy as the sole adjuvant radiotherapy after breast-conserving surgery of T1-T2 breast cancer: first long time results from a clinical study. Radiother Oncol 2009; 90: 30–5.

50. Cuttino LW, Keisch M, Jenrette JM, et al. Multi-institutional experience using the MammoSite radiation therapy system in the treatment of early-stage breast cancer: 2-year results. Int J Radiat Oncol Biol Phys 2008; 71: 107–14.

51. Chao KK, Vicini FA, Wallace M, et al. Analysis of treatment efficacy, cosmesis, and toxicity using the MammoSite breast brachytherapy catheter to deliver accelerated partial-breast irradiation: the william beaumont hospital experience. Int J Radiat Oncol Biol Phys 2007; 69: 32–40.

52. Dragun AE, Harper JL, Jenrette JM, Sinha D, Cole DJ. Predictors of cosmetic outcome following MammoSite breast brachytherapy: a single-institution experience of 100 patients with two years of follow-up. Int J Radiat Oncol Biol Phys 2007; 68: 354–8.

53. Shah C, Vicini F, Keisch M, et al. Outcome after ipsilateral breast tumor recurrence in patients who receive accelerated partial breast irradiation. Cancer 2012; 118: 4126–31.

54. Shah C, Ben Wilkinson J, Lyden M, et al. Comparison of survival and regional failure between accelerated partial breast irradiation and whole breast irradiation. Brachytherapy 2012; 11: 311–15.

55. Russo JK, Armeson KE, Rhome R, Spanos M, Harper JL. Dose to level I and II axillary lymph nodes and lung by tangential field radiation in patients undergoing postmastectomy radiation with tissue expander reconstruction. Radiat Oncol 2011; 6: 179.

56. Rabinovitch R, Ballonoff A, Newman F, Finlayson C. Evaluation of breast sentinel lymph node coverage by standard radiation therapy fields. Int J Radiat Oncol Biol Phys 2008; 70: 1468–71.

57. Rakha EA, El-Sayed ME, Lee AH, et al. Prognostic significance of Nottingham histologic grade in invasive breast carcinoma. J Clin Oncol 2008; 26: 3153–8.

58. Coles C, Yarnold J. The IMPORT trials are launched (September 2006). Clin Oncol (R Coll Radiol) 2006; 18: 587–90.

59. Danish Breast Cancer Co-operative Group. Partial breast versus whole breast irradiation in elderly women operated on for early breast cancer. [Available from: http://clinicaltrials.gov/ct2/show/NCT00892814]

60. Vicini F, Winter K, Wong J, et al. Initial efficacy results of RTOG 0319: three-dimensional conformal radiation therapy (3D-CRT) confined to the region of the lumpectomy cavity for stage I/II breast carcinoma. Int J Radiat Oncol Biol Phys 2010; 77: 1120–7.

61. Formenti SC, Truong MT, Goldberg JD, et al. Prone accelerated partial breast irradiation after breast-conserving surgery: preliminary clinical

results and dose-volume histogram analysis. Int J Radiat Oncol Biol Phys 2004; 60: 493–504.

62. Shah C, Antonucci JV, Wilkinson JB, et al. Twelve-year clinical outcomes and patterns of failure with accelerated partial breast irradiation versus whole-breast irradiation: results of a matched-pair analysis. Radiother Oncol 2011; 100: 210–14.

63. Arthur DW, Winter K, Kuske RR, et al. A Phase II trial of brachytherapy alone after lumpectomy for select breast cancer: tumor control and survival outcomes of RTOG 95-17. Int J Radiat Oncol Biol Phys 2008; 72: 467–73.

64. Vicini FA, Keisch M, Shah C, et al. Factors associated with optimal long-term cosmetic results in patients treated with accelerated partial breast irradiation using balloon-based brachytherapy. Int J Radiat Oncol Biol Phys 2012; 83: 512–18.

65. Khan AJ, Arthur D, Vicini F, et al. Six-year analysis of treatment-related toxicities in patients treated with accelerated partial breast irradiation on the American Society of Breast Surgeons MammoSite Breast Brachytherapy registry trial. Ann Surg Oncol 2012; 19: 1477–83.

66. Orecchia R, Ciocca M, Lazzari R, et al. Intraoperative radiation therapy with electrons (ELIOT) in early-stage breast cancer. Breast 2003; 12: 483–90.

67. Yarnold J, Coles C; On behalf of the IMPORT LOW Trial Management Group. Intensity- Modulated and Partial Organ Radiotherapy. Randomised trial testing intensity-modulated and partial organ radiotherapy following breast conservative surgery for early breast cancer. Trial protocol, version 6; 2009, Institute of Cancer Research, Sutton, UK. p 1-74. [Available from: http://clinicaltrials.gov/ct2/show/NCT00814567]

68. Strnad V, Polgar C; On behalf of the European Brachytherapy Breast Cancer GEC-ESTRO Working Group. GEC-ESTRO APBI Trial: Interstitial brachytherapy alone versus external beam radiation therapy after breast conserving surgery for low risk invasive carcinoma and low risk duct carcinoma in-situ (DCIS) of the female breast. 2006.[Available from: http://www.apbi.uni-erlangen.de/outline/outline.html]

69. Ontario Clinical Oncology Group (OCOG), Canadian Institutes of Health Research (CIHR), Canadian Breast Cancer Research Alliance. RAPID: Randomized Trial of Accelerated Partial Breast Irradiation. 2008. [Available from: http://clinicaltrials.gov/ct2/show/NCT00282035]

70. [Available from: http://groups.eortc.be/radio/res/irma/synopsis_trial_irma1.pdf]

71. Belkacemi Y, Lartigau E; On behalf of Federation Nationale des Centres de Lutte Contre le Cancer. Standard or Hypofractionated Radiotherapy Versus Accelerated Partial Breast Irradiation (APBI) for Breast Cancer (SHARE). 2010.[Available from: http://clinicaltrials.gov/ct2/show/NCT01247233]

72. American Society of Breast Surgeons, Consensus statement for Accelerated Partial Breast Irradiation. [Available from: www.breastsurgeons.org]

73. Arthur DW, Vicini FA, Kuske RR, Wazer DE, Nag S. Accelerated partial breast irradiation: an updated report from the American Brachytherapy Society. Brachytherapy 2003; 2: 124–30.

74. Vicini F, Arthur D, Wazer D, et al. Limitations of the American Society of Therapeutic Radiology and Oncology Consensus panel guidelines on the use of accelerated partial breast irradiation. Int J Radiat Oncol Biol Phys 2011; 79: 977–84.

75. Leonardi MC, Maisonneuve P, Mastropasqua MG, et al. How do the ASTRO consensus statement guidelines for the application of accelerated partial breast irradiation fit intraoperative radiotherapy? A retrospective analysis of patients treated at the European Institute of Oncology. Int J Radiat Oncol Biol Phys 2012; 83: 806–13.

76. Shah C, Wilkinson JB, Shaitelman S, et al. Impact of lymph node status on clinical outcomes after accelerated partial breast irradiation. Int J Radiat Oncol Biol Phys 2012; 82: e409–14.

77. McHaffie DR, Patel RR, Adkison JB, et al. Outcomes after accelerated partial breast irradiation in patients with ASTRO consensus statement cautionary features. Int J Radiat Oncol Biol Phys 2011; 81: 46–51.

78. Shaitelman SF, Vicini FA, Beitsch P, et al. Five-year outcome of patients classified using the American Society for Radiation Oncology consensus statement guidelines for the application of accelerated partial breast irradiation: an analysis of patients treated on the American Society of Breast Surgeons MammoSite Registry Trial. Cancer 2010; 116: 4677–85.

79. Jeruss JS, Kuerer HM, Beitsch PD, Vicini FA, Keisch M. Update on DCIS outcomes from the American Society of Breast Surgeons accelerated partial breast irradiation registry trial. Ann Surg Oncol 2011; 18: 65–71.

80. Wilkinson JB, Reid RE, Shaitelman SF, et al. Outcomes of breast cancer patients with triple negative receptor status treated with accelerated partial breast irradiation. Int J Radiat Oncol Biol Phys 2011; 81: e159–64.

81. Zauls AJ, Watkins JM, Wahlquist AE, et al. Outcomes in women treated with MammoSite brachytherapy or whole breast irradiation stratified by ASTRO Accelerated Partial Breast Irradiation Consensus Statement Groups. Int J Radiat Oncol Biol Phys 2012; 82: 21–9.

82. Park SS, Grills IS, Chen PY, et al. Accelerated partial breast irradiation for pure ductal carcinoma in situ. Int J Radiat Oncol Biol Phys 2011; 81: 403–8.

43 Targeted intraoperative radiotherapy for breast cancer: not all cancers in the breast will grow

Jayant S. Vaidya, John R. Benson, and Jeffrey S. Tobias

INTRODUCTION

Radiotherapy is considered mandatory for most patients undergoing breast conservation therapy which involves resection of the primary tumor with clear margins, axillary surgery (sentinel lymph node biopsy or axillary lymph node dissection), and radiotherapy to the remaining breast tissue. Radiation treatment is normally given as external beam radiotherapy with tangential fields in 15 to 30 daily fractions over a three- to six- weeks period. The total dosage to the breast is usually 40–50 Gy, usually with a boost to the tumor bed of 10–15 Gy. The most common side effects are skin reactions with occasional nausea and vomiting; pneumonitis resulting from irradiation of the lung occurs in fewer than 2% of patients. Older regimens inadvertently included the heart and the anterior descending coronary artery, leading to an excess cardiac mortality which was most conspicuous in those with left-sided breast cancers. Newer regimens including intensity-modulated radiotherapy have been devised to reduce the cardiac dose and consequent morbidity. However, the heart and the lungs still receive a substantial dose of radiation and one cannot yet be certain that there is no cardiac toxicity with newer external beam radiotherapy techniques.

The most recent meta-analysis by the Oxford group (published in 2011), examined the outcomes among more than 10,000 women in 17 randomized trials of breast conservation therapy and yielded the following conclusions:

- Radiotherapy provides highly effective local control, preventing local recurrence in more than 80% of those treated.
- Cardiac side effects can be significant, but the trend is to reduce complications to as few as possible with modern treatment approaches.

It is worth reiterating the fundamental observation that for every four recurrences prevented at five years, one life is saved at 15 years. Nonetheless, an analysis suggests that this ratio of 4:1 varies with the stage of the primary tumor and that for background local recurrence rates of less than 10%, radiotherapy has little or no effect on overall survival (Fig. 43.1). A large study from Canada together with the Standardisation of Radiotherapy (START) trial in the UK has shown that the breast is more sensitive to fraction size than previously appreciated (2). The START Trial B found that a three-week regimen was associated with equivalent results to a conventional five- to six-week regimen in terms of local recurrence rates at five-year follow-up. This has prompted the trial of "faster radiotherapy

for breast cancer patients," which is investigating whether one week of therapy can be as effective as conventional longer courses but without side effects. When taken to the extreme, the ultimate hypofractionation regimen is to give radiotherapy in a single dose intraoperatively and targeted to the tumor bed.

Intraoperative radiotherapy (IORT) is a technique that permits the administration of a high dose of radiation as a single fraction at the time of surgery. It can be employed either alone or in combination with conventional external beam therapy as an irradiation boost. The technique allows precise application of radiation dosage to the target area with minimal exposure of surrounding tissues, which are retracted and shielded during delivery of the radiation. IORT facilitates an integrated approach to the multidisciplinary treatment of cancer (3) and emphasizes the interaction between surgery and radiotherapy in the following principal aspects:

- It reduces the chance of residual disease at the site of surgery by eliminating microscopic tumor foci.
- Although the physical dose is low, the radiobiologically effective dose of targeted intraoperative radiotherapy has been modelled to be similar to external beam radiotherapy.
- It optimizes combined surgical and radiotherapy treatment with early irradiation, reducing the risk of tumor recurrence secondary to growth of residual disease at the site of surgery.
- It has been shown to effectively change the tumor microenvironment. When the wound fluid, collected in the first 24 hours after lumpectomy, is placed on breast cancer cell lines, it is found to stimulate proliferation, motility, and invasiveness. This stimulation is abrogated if the patient had received targeted intraoperative radiotherapy (TARGIT) treatment (4).
- As it is done during surgery, the radiation can be aimed and focused to the target tissues with minimal error (or geographical miss).
- It is given immediately, so any delay (or temporal miss) (5) in giving radiation is eliminated.

IORT therefore potentially intensifies the tumor-kill effect of surgery and radiotherapy and minimizes the chance of local failure. For patients with disease confined to locoregional tissues, this may increase the chance of definitive cure. Its use does not preclude the administration of chemotherapy or other systemic adjuvant therapies. Furthermore, as the total dose given with the TARGIT technique is low, whole-breast radiotherapy (WBRT)

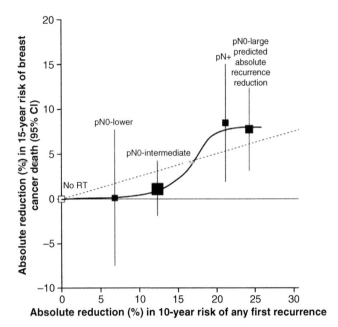

Figure 43.1 The sigmoid black line that has been superimposed on the existing Figure 5 from the latest Oxford overview (1) may be a more likely representation of the relationship between reduction in local recurrence and reduction in mortality than the dashed red line.

can be added if adverse prognostic factors are found postoperatively; a pragmatic approach in which one can expect 15–20% of patients to receive WBRT treatment.

Initial experience with IORT dates back to the 1920s, but poor technical facilities restricted its use to the palliative treatment of locally unresectable tumors. With the development of orthovoltage equipment in the 1940s, the potential role of intraoperative radiotherapy in conjunction with external beam radiation became better defined. During the 1960s, generation of electron beams from linear accelerators replaced low-energy radiation (6) with the advantages of more homogeneous dose distribution, sparing of underlying tissue due to lower exit dose, and a reduction in total duration of treatment.

An important advancement with IORT occurred in the mid-1990s with the development of miniaturized mobile linear accelerator prototypes (7). These devices can be readily positioned in proximity to the operating table and possess an arm that can be manipulated into the required position for irradiation. These accelerators have a variable spectrum of electron energy and have the particular advantage of being accommodated in any operating theater without major structural modifications. Mobile shields can be positioned appropriately in relation to the operating field to provide maximum radioprotection. This avoids any transfer of the patient, and surgical time is prolonged by approximately 20–30 minutes only. One such device includes sources of low-energy X-rays (approximately 50 kV) and can used in any operating room (8). It can be also secured to a stereotactic support for precise placement within any body cavity.

TECHNIQUES FOR INTRAOPERATIVE RADIOTHERAPY
Targeted Intraoperative Radiotherapy (TARGIT)
TARGIT technique uses a miniaturized x-ray source (9) that is attached to an articulated arm that can be positioned

according to stereotactic coordinates or as required by the surgeon and radiation oncologist accurately targeting the appropriate tissues. This distribution around the source is approximately spheroidal, thus ensuring that the dose distribution is isotropic when the source is placed at the center of a spheroidal applicator. The 50KeV X-rays have a steep dose gradient, with rapid attenuation of dose with increasing distance from the source and the dose rate is 2 Gy/min for a spheroidal applicator 2 cm in diameter. The principal advantages of this system are limited penetration at depth (20 Gy near the surface and 6 Gy at 1 cm in water), a relatively long period for delivery of a therapeutic dose (20–30 min), that will allow normal cells but not tumor cells to repair their DNA and protection of normal tissues from the side effects of radiation. Solid spherical applicators of various diameters (1.5 cm–5.0 cm with 0.5 cm increments) are available to provide peritumoral irradiation following a wide local excision (WLE). An ionization camera with flat parallel electrodes used in a water puppet allows evaluation of basal and applicator-specific dosimetry. These measurements can be integrated with data from radiochromic films or thermoluminescent detectors analyzed through a microdensitometer.

TARGIT technique has been developed over the last 14 years for use after WLE of early-stage breast cancer and has been tested in randomized trials. The TARGIT technique employs the Intrabeam system (Zeiss Surgical, Oberkochen, Germany), which was developed at University College, London, and is a completely portable unit that can be used in a standard operating theater (Fig. 43.2).

Intrabeam has a miniature X-ray-source at the tip of a 10-cm long probe which measures 3.2 mm in diameter. Accelerated electrons strike a gold target resulting in an almost isotropic X-ray distribution around the tip. Energy levels can be set at 30, 40, or 50 kV with currents of 5, 10, 20, and 40A (50KeV is normally used). A notable feature is that the X-ray unit is small and lightweight (weight = 1.8 kg; dimensions: X-ray generator body 7 × 11 × 14 cm). It is combined with a floor stand with a balanced support that provides 6 degrees of freedom to gain access to target sites throughout the body. This flexibility enables radiation therapy to be administered in any operating theater from any direction. The X-rays are of low energy and therefore no special wall, floor, or ceiling shielding is required and treatment can be carried out in a conventional operating theater which normally has adequate shielding for intraoperative diagnostic radiology.

Mobile Accelerator with Electrons at a Maximum Energy of 9–12 MeV
This is a limited energy device that permits the use of an accelerating "in-axis" structure directly inserted into the warhead. It characteristically emits low levels of environmental irradiation over a wide dosage range although some stray radiation comes from both patient and bed-generated *bremsstrahlung* (10). These stray rays, which constitute no more than 0.5% of the total electron dose, are absorbed by additional lead barriers placed around the operating table and a lead shield (15-cm thick) beneath the surgical bed corresponding to the axis of the electron field (a beam stopper). A principal feature of this apparatus is the high dose per impulse, with values of

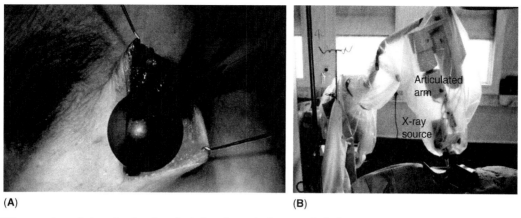

(A)   **(B)**

Figure 43.2 TARGIT—operative technique showing the spherical applicator in the tumor bed after wide local excision (A) and the articulated arm holding the XRS in a transparent sterile enclosure with the patient covered with blue drapes and a (black) shield to protect the theater staff from radiation (B). *Abbreviations*: TARGIT, TARGeted Intraoperative radioTherapy; XRS, x-ray source.

2.5–12 cGy per impulse (compared with 0.06 cGy per impulse for traditional accelerators). Ionization cameras for low-dose dosimetry cannot therefore be used and chemical dosimeters containing an iron sulfate solution (Fricke's method) are preferred. Radiochromic film can also be used to calibrate monitor cameras. Electron-beam collimation is achieved through lightweight cylindrical applicators with a diameter varying between 4 cm and 12 cm and terminal angles of between 0° and 45°. The diameter of the applicator determines its length, since uniformity of distribution in the treatment field is due to scattering from the applicator walls (no scatter filters). This scattering effect also impacts upon dose rate: smaller applicator diameters are associated with a higher dose output because more electrons are scattered from the walls to reach the beam field. Dosimetric procedures must be performed in a water puppet at a maximal dose depth for flat applicators and a depth corresponding to the beam axis for angular applicators. As these are high-energy beams, the chest wall needs to be protected with a thick lead shield that is placed between the breast tissue and the chest wall, after dissecting the breast tissue off the chest wall.

RATIONALE FOR USE OF IORT IN BREAST CONSERVATION TREATMENT

Modern understanding of breast cancer pathology suggests that occult/latent lesions in the areas of the breast remote from the index quadrant are not the reason for local relapse, which almost always occurs at the site of the original excision. Indeed, a cancer is just as likely to develop in the contralateral breast as a recurrence outside the index quadrant in the ipsilateral breast, yet prophylactic radiotherapy will never routinely be considered to the other side. If that is indeed the case, then carefully targeted high-dose radiotherapy at the time of surgery may obviate the need for external beam WBRT, thus saving both machine and patient time. These findings support the employment of more limited radiotherapy aimed at the elimination of residual cancer cells in the vicinity of the primary tumor. In addition, it opens up the possibility of conservation surgery for breast cancer among women in most developing countries and indeed in many parts of the developed world, journey times are so long and/or tiring as to render breast conserving surgery a nonfeasible option. Furthermore, by coapting the walls of the excision cavity to the applicator after lumpectomy, the conformal geometry is much better than the simulations required for external beam treatment, which should in theory lead to better local control of disease.

Translational research has shown that postoperative wound fluid normally stimulates cancer cell growth, motility, and invasiveness (properties which are commensurate with the need to heal a wound). TARGIT has been found to abrogate this effect of surgical wounding. Thus, in addition to reaching the appropriate tissue, TARGIT is also applied at an opportune time. This biological rationale is to some extent borne out in the clinic. The first pilot series that used TARGIT was started in 1998 and accrued 300 patients. These patients received TARGIT, as well as external beam radiotherapy. The actuarial local recurrence rate in this unselected group of patients has been very low: 1.73% at five years. From the case mix, the estimated local recurrence in this group of patients should be double this rate. The ongoing TARGIT-B trial will determine whether TARGIT boost is superior to a conventional externally delivered boost dose to the tumor bed.

The Electron IntraOperative Treatment (ELIOT, a full-dose intraoperative radiotherapy with electrons) which was developed at the European Institute of Oncology in Milan and the Mobitron system differ from TARGIT (Intrabeam); first in terms of significantly higher capital costs and second, the need for a special shielded operation room. Xoft is a hybrid method which incorporates elements of both Intrabeam and MammoSite (Hologic), but its physical dose, dosimetry and dose rate are different and clinical experience in its use is very limited.

In 1995, the author's group presented data from whole-organ analysis of mastectomy specimens in which an analysis of tumor location at different sites in the breast was performed in three dimensions (11,12). This analysis indicated that when a mastectomy specimen harboring a presumed unifocal cancer is examined meticulously, additional cancers distributed throughout the breast are found in approximately two-thirds of the cases. If it is believed that these other cancers could give rise to clinical tumors, then the Halsted mastectomy should never have been abandoned (Fig. 43.3). In reality, the premise behind Halsted's operation has prevailed even after introduction of breast conservation surgery, as the whole breast was

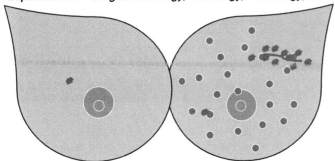

Br J Cancer 1996;74:820-824
British journal of cancer (1996) 74, 820–824
© 1996 Stockton press all rights reserved 0007–0920/96 $12.00

Multicentricity of breast cancer: whole-organ analysis and clinical implications

JS Vaidya', JJ Vyas', RF Chinoy[2], N Merchant[3], OP Sharma[3] and I Mittra'

Departments of 'Surgical Oncology,' Pathology, [3]Radiology, Tata Memorial Hospital, Bombay, 400 012, India.

Breast cancer is frequently multicentric...

But most recurrences occur near the primary tumour

So, it makes sense to target radiotherapy to the tumour bed

Figure 43.3 The original study that suggested that while a breast may harbor many other tumors (green dots), local recurrences (red stars) usually appear at the site of the primary tumor; recurrences in other quadrants are not dissimilar to new tumors in the contralateral breast.

essentially treated with radical radiotherapy instead of radical surgery.

Evidence from randomized trials of breast conserving surgery showed that even when radiotherapy is omitted, the location of early recurrence in the conserved breast is mainly around the site of primary excision, suggesting that these other more distant cancers generally remain dormant.

We published our findings and hypothesized that these foci of tumor in other parts of the breast may not need treatment with radiotherapy (which generated much discussion in the *Lancet*) (12–14). The authors conceived a randomized trial to test whether omission of radiation treatment for these cancers results in equivalent local control. For this purpose, a new technique called TARGIT was developed and evaluated (9,15) and a large multicenter randomized clinical trial namely TARGIT-A was subsequently undertaken (16,17). Contemporaneously, groups in Milan (18), the United States (19), and other parts of Europe (20) were also evaluating this concept of partial breast irradiation (PBI).

This is particularly relevant with increasing trends for use of screening mammography in which breast cancers are more frequently found in very early stages. It is well documented that there is a significant degree of overdiagnosis in screening programs which is estimated between 10% and 50% (21,22). Thus, consideration of overtreatment is an ethical imperative and follows the principle of *primum non nocere*. When the whole breast is treated, either by surgery (mastectomy) or radiotherapy, there are some unintended consequences. The psychological impact of mastectomy is evident even before surgery is performed (23) and can persist despite immediate breast reconstruction (24). It can be argued that not all patients require WBRT. Since local recurrence after breast-conserving surgery occurs mainly in the area around the original primary tumor (12,14), radiotherapy directed to peritumoral tissue by TARGIT might be an appropriate method to prevent local relapse in selected patients with early-stage breast cancer.

Very Little "Elsewhere" Recurrence Without WBRT

A recent paper suggested that mastectomy rates in patients undergoing PBI (not TARGIT) were higher than for those receiving external beam WBRT (3.95% *vs.* 2.4%, respectively) (25). However, the reported differences were very small in absolute terms (1.55%); more importantly, this study has provided corroboration of our proposal that other malignant foci in the breast do not progress. In this study, almost 7000 patients were treated exclusively with brachytherapy after breast-conserving surgery. Sixty-three percent (12,26), that is, approximately 5000 of these patients would be expected to have cancers other than the main tumor; these cancers were therefore left untreated when only the peri-tumoral tissues were treated with partial breast irradiation. Our hypothesis would be falsified if 90% of these cancers grew within five years resulting in 4500 patients requiring mastectomy. In the event, fewer than 400 of these patients needed a mastectomy. Even if it is assumed that these mastectomies were all performed for local recurrence outside the index quadrant, it must be concluded that other 4100 untreated cancers in the breast did not progress and remained dormant in these patients.

The multicenter randomized TARGIT-A trial involved 2232 patients and results were published in 2010. At four years, almost 99% of patients randomized to TARGIT did not have a recurrence, suggesting that something in the internal milieu and/or microenvironment of these patients maintained tumor dormancy. Thus, there are now available several thousand women with mature follow-up in whom it appears that most malignant foci outside the index quadrant of the presenting tumor do not progress in the absence of WBRT.

It is evident that if radiotherapy is omitted following a lumpectomy, recurrence rates can reach up to 9% even for those patients aged above 70 years (27) and this rate may be higher for younger patients. If localized radiotherapy is to be employed, it is important to use the most effective technique that has been properly assessed in randomized trials.

Over the past decade, several methods for delivering PBI have been developed and evaluated. The TARGIT technique aims to avoid a geographic or temporal miss by irradiating the tumor bed while the tissues are exposed during surgery thus delivering radiation at the right time and in the right place.

The relative biological effect of a single IORT dose is estimated to be 1.5–2.5 times higher than that of the dose delivered with external beam radiotherapy. More specifically, the equivalence of IORT to standard 2-Gy fractionation can be estimated using the linear-quadratic model and computing the survival fraction of clonogenic units with different (α/β) ratios. For example, a total dose of 60 Gy given with 2 Gy fractionation is equivalent biologically to a single dose of intraoperative radiotherapy of 22.3 Gy (28). Formulae for radio-biological equivalence (linear-quadratic model, biological equivalent dose, etc.) cannot accurately predict the therapeutic or toxic effects of a single dose of high-intensity IORT.

The hypothesis that irradiation of the tumor bed using low-energy X-rays is equivalent to a conventional six-week course of external beam radiation of the whole breast in terms of local relapse rates is tested in the TARGIT-A trial launched in March 2000 (17). The original recruitment target was achieved in early 2010 (2232 patients). TARGIT-A trial was pragmatic and compared two treatment policies in patients with early breast cancer who have undergone local excision of a good prognosis tumor. The conventional policy is for each patient to receive a radical course of external beam radiotherapy (with or without a boost) according to local treatment guidelines. The experimental arm involved TARGIT given as a single dose. It was recognized that some patients randomized to this treatment and found subsequently to have unfavorable features on pathological examination of the excised lesion, would need to have additional external beam therapy (i.e., without the boost provided by the targeted dose). This was estimated to occur in 15–20% of cases and was taken into account in the power calculations. Thus, it should be remembered that the TARGIT-A trial was designed from the outset to compare two policies: risk-adjusted radiotherapy versus one-size-fits-all radiotherapy rather than a dogmatic comparison of intraoperative radiotherapy versus EBRT.

Due to this pragmatic nature the TARGIT-A trial had similar results in each of the ASTRO groups, including those that were thought to be unsuitable for PBI (28). In Fig. 43.4 it is clearly seen that in patients that fall in the "suitable," "cautionary," or "unsuitable" by the ASTRO criteria, the differences in local recurrence were very low and the 95% CI crossed zero.

SURGICAL ASPECTS AND WORKFLOW
TARGIT Procedure
Details of the original technique are published elsewhere and an operative video is available at the following http://youtube/GVlHGpvRf8A. The procedure has been widely used in over 150 centers throughout the world over the last 12 years and more than 2000 patients have been treated. A single prophylactic dose of intravenous antibiotics (Augmentin (GSK GlaxoSmithKline) 1.5 g) is given at the induction of anesthetic. Sentinel lymph node biopsy is performed in the usual way and WLE can be carried out with meticulous hemostasis while waiting for intraoperative assessment. Hemostasis is very important because even a tiny ooze from the capillaries can lead to accumulation of blood during radiotherapy which could potentially cause a distortion of the cavity around the applicator and change the dose that the target tissues receive. In addition, a slight increase in the temperature of 1–2°C during irradiation can induce bleeding so it is essential that a thorough hemostasis be achieved.

The diameter of the cavity is now measured with a disposable tape measure cut to 4 or 5 cm. This together with a judgment of how the breast tissue wraps around the applicator will determine the size of the latter; inserting the applicators in the wound and visualizing apposition is very useful. The usual size of the applicator is 3.5, 4.0, 4.5, or 5.0 cm.

A purse string is now taken with a strong Prolene (Ethicon) (no.1) mounted on a large needle. This step is very important and needs to be undertaken carefully as the dosage to target tissues depends on this. This suture needs to be skillfully placed: it must pass through the breast parenchyma and appose it to the applicator, but at the same time must not draw the dermis too close to the applicator surface (at least 1 cm away). When the skin edge falls inward on to the applicator surface, a fine Prolene suture (4/0) through the dermis can gently retract the skin to ensure that it is out of the path. However, the subcutaneous breast tissue that formed the anterior tumor bed should remain in contact with the applicator, to ensure adequate irradiation. Under no circumstance should anything be placed between the applicator and the target tissue in an attempt to increase the distance to the skin. Sometimes in the lower inner quadrant, the ribs are in close proximity. Here it may be possible to insert a piece of wet gauze between the muscle and the rib, so that the distance between them is at least 1 cm. Again, the final position should ensure that the target tumor bed is in contact with the applicator surface. It is important for the surgeon to understand the radiobiological principles and undergo proper training before undertaking this operation.

The Intrabeam X-ray source is not sterile and must be wrapped in a sterile polyethylene bag. A commercial drape is available with predesigned holes and tapes to cover the equipment. Once the applicator is in place, the purse string is tightened carefully. Care is taken to ensure that all breast tissue in the cavity is in apposition and no part of the skin is less than a distance of 1 cm from the applicator. Prolene stitches that slightly retract the skin away from the applicator are useful for

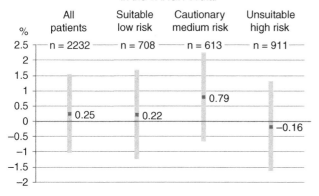

Absolute difference in Local Recurrence (LR) rate
LR of TARGIT group *minus* LR of EBRT group
in the TARGIT-A trial

Figure 43.4 The absolute difference in local recurrence between the two randomised groups (TARGIT minus EBRT in the TARGIT-A trial) for all patients, patients considered 'suitable' 'cautionary' and 'unsuitable' as per the ASTRO categories for partial breast irradiation. The red box represents the absolute difference in local recurrence and the vertical lines are the 95% confidence intervals at 4 years. The data as of Lancet 2010 publication.

the edges of the wound but placement of wound retractors is *not* recommended because they can inadvertently draw breast tissue away from the applicator. Before starting treatment, a lead sheet covers the wound around the applicator. This blocks most of the extraneous radiation and greatly reduces levels in the operating theater with near-zero levels in outside corridors. The heart and the lungs are indirectly protected by the distance through which the radiation needs to travel (the chest wall) and no additional measures are required unless the chest wall is very thin. If the rib or the lungs are expected to be within 1 cm of the applicator surface (as can happen in very medial tumors in thin women) then a similar barrier can be placed between the pectoralis muscle and the rib/chest wall. The anesthesiologist and the physicist, both wearing lead gowns, sit or stand behind the patient or just outside the theater close to the patient and the monitoring equipment. The surgeon and nurses unscrub and leave the theater using the time for other work. Once the radiotherapy is complete, the sheet is removed, the purse string cut, and the applicator removed. Hemostasis is reconfirmed and the wound closed.

Delivering TARGIT with Intrabeam increases the operating time by 45 minutes on average (range 34–60 minutes).

When TARGIT is performed, it usually involves orchestration of several teams and individuals: the patient, her companion and friend, the breast care nurse, the surgeon, the radiation oncologist, the radiologist and radiographers, nuclear medicine staff, theater staff with nurses and circulating staff trained in all the processes, the anesthetist, the medical/ radiation physicists, the pathologist for immediate assessment of the sentinel node, the courier/porters to take the sample to the pathologist and to the radiologist for specimen X-ray, secretarial staff, hospital administrators, and clinical governance staff. During the period, frequently the patient will have an injection of radiocolloid for localization of the sentinel node in the nuclear medicine department, insertion of a guide wire for localization of the tumor in the radiology department, followed by general anesthesia, sentinel node biopsy which undergoes intraoperative assessment, wire-guided WLE which is examined by a specimen mammogram to assess adequate excision, TARGIT with Intrabeam described earlier, followed by a closure of the wound. With such meticulous orchestration, the local treatment for breast cancer is complete within a day and the patient is able to go home the same day, or the following morning and in over 80% of cases, will not need any further surgery or radiotherapy and when performed in properly selected cases, enjoy excellent local control and freedom from the side effects of conventional radiotherapy.

An update of the TARGIT-A trial will be presented which will include an analysis of local recurrence with a more mature follow up, analysis of overall survival, and whether predictive markers such as hormone receptors help in the selection of patients for TARGIT.

ELIOT Technique

With the ELIOT technique, in order to minimize radiation exposure of the chest wall and ensure that maximal doses of radiation are delivered to the breast parenchyma, protective plates are positioned between the breast and the pectoral muscle. A dedicated lead disk (5 mm thickness) and an aluminum disk (4 mm thickness) are commonly used for this purpose to collectively shield and protect the chest wall. The electron beam energy is selected on the basis of the thickness of the target volume, and the optimum dose distribution within the gland is attained if the thickness of the irradiated target remains as uniform as possible. It is important to reconstruct the breast parenchyma in order to expose the appropriate portion of the gland to the radiation beam as well as avoid excessive inhomogeneity in the target volume. For this purpose, the breast tissue is dissected away from the skin and from the chest wall. Following mobilization and undermining of the breast parenchyma, the gland is sutured in accordance with the defect resulting from the surgical extirpation of the tumor (Fig. 43.3). The anatomy and thickness of the breast are partially restored, protecting the underlying thoracic wall. However, the tissue at the edge of the dissected gland—the target of radiation- may well have poor vascularity and low oxygen saturation, at least for a short duration—that coincides with the timing of radiation and may well reduce its effectiveness. The precise thickness of the breast tissue is measured with a special device and biologically effective electron energy is selected. The skin must be held away from the collimator to avoid inadvertent irradiation of the skin in the vicinity of the surgical breach (Fig. 43.4). If the skin lies in contiguity with the Perspex collimator, its margin will receive approximately 5% of the total dose. A special piece of equipment has been developed that completely spares the skin from radiation exposure during the delivery of ELIOT. This consists of a metallic ring with a variable diameter that is adjusted according to an individual patient's anatomy (Fig. 43.5). This ring is connected to fine nontraumatic metallic hooks, which anchor the skin margins and gently retract the skin away from the radiation field. A wet sterile gauze can also be placed between the skin and the collimator to create a further tissue-equivalent barrier that can absorb low-energy electrons scattered around the edge of the collimator. Once the breast tissue has been sutured and the skin edges securely fixed, the sterile collimator can be positioned to ensure that the entire target volume is included within the radiation field. The portion of breast tissue that is to be irradiated (the clinical target volume) corresponds to a zone of 4–5 cm around the surgical resection site. However, depending on the breast size tumor location and glandular transposition, up to 10 cm of breast parenchyma may be irradiated. The collimator diameter is selected on the basis of the area to be treated and should cover both the tumor bed and a safe margin. The thickness of the target tissue will determine the energy of the electron beam.

The applicator is placed in direct contact with the breast tissue, and the linear accelerator can be manipulated under remote control to allow positioning of the collimator within the operating field. Care should be taken to avoid any herniation of breast tissue into the collimator, which will expose the superficial part of the gland to excessive radiation. The remote control of the linear accelerator facilitates accurate positioning of the collimator by the radiation technologist, and the connection to the distal part of the applicator is made in exactly the desired position.

Once the applicator is in position, a series of mobile shields are placed around the operating table to protect against scattering of X-rays. All personnel leave the operating room and

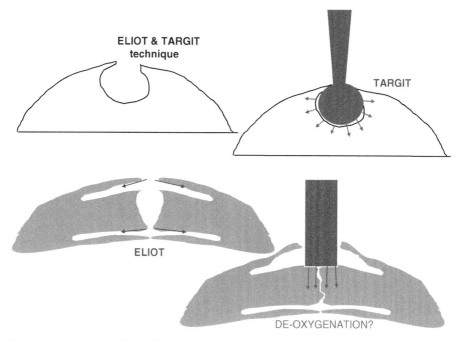

Figure 43.5 The difference between the operative technique of TARGIT and ELIOT. For TARGIT, there is no additional dissection of breast tissue and the radiation is delivered from within the breast and the lumpectomy cavity. For ELIOT, the breast tissue needs to be dissected off the skin and off the chest wall; a lead shield is placed between the breast and the chest wall and the breast tissue is brought together and radiation is delivered from the front. The immediate, albeit temporary, reduction in vascularity of the dissected breast tissue at the tumor bed-edge of the recently dissected tissue may, in theory, reduce the effectiveness of radiotherapy.

the radiation equipment is switched on via the control panel. Radiation is delivered in two consecutive phases, each of which represents half of the prescribed dose. Using this method, the dose delivered in the first phase can be controlled and the dose in the second phase adjusted if necessary. In practice, any difference between planned and delivered dosage is rarely more than ±1.5%. The radiation is completed in 2–4 minutes, but the whole procedure including the dissection and set up can be expected to take about 30–40 minutes.

After radiation treatment has been completed, the applicator is removed immediately from the surgical wound and the linear accelerator withdrawn from the area of the operating table. The sutures within the breast parenchyma are cut in order to allow removal of the lead and aluminum disks. The breast tissue is then reconstructed once more and the skin and subcutaneous tissues closed using an absorbable monofilament material. The postoperative course is usually uneventful.

The authors (JV, JT) have shown that the relatively small volume of tissue that is irradiated in TARGIT leads to a significant change in the properties of the wound fluid. Normal wound fluid is stimulatory to cancer cells, but the wound fluid that collects after TARGIT is not (4). One can also speculate as to how TARGIT might modify the systemic response to the trauma of surgery. The low-dose rate and smaller volume of tissue irradiated in the TARGIT technique may be critically important and the technique of IORT is generally less traumatic to the normal breast tissues. As originally described in the TARGIT technique, we do not mobilize tissues and the tumor bed is wrapped around the spherical applicator of an appropriate size, using a carefully placed purse-string suture. By contrast, the ELIOT technique requires extensive mobilization of tissues before radiotherapy is delivered, which may have unintended consequences such as devascularization and

deoxygenation making the tissues less sensitive to radiotherapy. By the time WBRT is delivered, wound healing will have improved vascularity and oxygenation; consequently, the effectiveness of external beam radiation therapy would not be affected. However, this remains a speculation.

The devil may well be in the detail; several factors may have played a part in achieving the low recurrence rates that we have seen with the TARGIT technique. These include immediate delivery of radiation to well-vascularized tissues at the right time and delivery of an optimum dose to the minimum required volume of tissue at a dose rate that will allow normal tissue to heal.

Before considering the results of the randomized trials TARGIT-A, and ELIOT in terms of managing our patients in the future, we must re-emphasize three points: First, these results apply only to the population that participated in the trials. Second, the design and technique of the ELIOT trial did not allow addition of WBRT in patients found to be at higher risk postoperatively. The design of the TARGIT trial was pragmatic and risk adjusted, so that the experimental approach using TARGIT is a policy and not a single treatment. WBRT was added to the TARGIT treatment on the basis of predefined indications by each center, namely when postoperative pathology implied risk of local recurrence was greater than anticipated before surgery. Finally, these results only apply to the specific technology that delivers a specified dose of radiation (with a specific spectrum) over a given time period and may not be transferable to situations employing other technologies.

The TARGIT-B trial (to be launched in late 2012) will determine whether a tumor bed boost with TARGIT achieves superior local control than conventional external beam boost in women below 45 years and those with higher risk tumors. Further substudies will also assess the economic and social costs alongside clinical efficacy. Standardized international models are perhaps the most suitable system for the development and evaluation of these technically complex treatment methods, where personnel training and specificity of equipment and apparatus are critical determinants of the outcome.

It can be said that the recent development of IORT demonstrates how innovation and scientific progress are driven by thinking "outside the box" and design and conduct of appropriate randomized controlled trials not only can improve our treatments, but also give us insights into the natural history of the disease.

ACKNOWLEDGMENTS

The authors thank Prof. Michael Baum for participating in the discussion and sharing his views about several issues described in this chapter and Prof. Max Bulsara for the statistical analysis. The author (JSV) retains copyright for the figures.

REFERENCES

1. Darby S, McGale P, Correa C, et al. Effect of radiotherapy after breast-conserving surgery on 10-year recurrence and 15-year breast cancer death: meta-analysis of individual patient data for 10,801 women in 17 randomised trials. Lancet 2011; 378: 1707–16.
2. Bentzen SM, Agrawal RK, Aird EG, et al. The UK Standardisation of Breast Radiotherapy (START) trial A of radiotherapy hypofractionation for treatment of early breast cancer: a randomised trial. Lancet Oncol 2008; 9: 331–41.
3. Calvo FA, Micaily B, Brady LW. Intraoperative radiotherapy. A positive view. Am J Clin Oncol 1993; 16: 418–23.
4. Belletti B, Vaidya JS, D'Andrea S, et al. Targeted intraoperative radiotherapy impairs the stimulation of breast cancer cell proliferation and invasion caused by surgical wounding. Clin Cancer Res 2008; 14: 1325–32.
5. Vaidya JS, Tobias JS, Baum M, et al. Intraoperative radiotherapy for breast cancer. Lancet Oncol 2004; 5: 165–73.
6. Abe M. History of intraoperative radiation therapy. In: Dobelbower RRJ, Abe M, eds. Intraoperative Radiation Therapy. Boca Raton: CRC Press, 1989: 2–9.
7. Willet CG, Gunderson LL, Busse PM, et al. IOERT treatment factors. Technique, equipment. In: Gunderson LL, et al. eds. Current Clinical Oncology: Intraoperative Irradiation: Techniques and Results. Totowa, NJ: Humana Press, 1999: 65–85.
8. Biggs DS, Thomson ES. Radiation properties of a miniature X-ray device for radiosurgery. Br J Radiol 1996; 69: 544–7.
9. Vaidya JS, Baum M, Tobias JS, Morgan S, D'Souza D. The novel technique of delivering targeted intraoperative radiotherapy (Targit) for early breast cancer. Eur J Surg Oncol 2002; 28: 447–54.
10. Piermattei A, DelleCanne S, Azario L, et al. Linac Novac7 electron beam calibration using GAF-Chromic film. PhysicaMedica 1999; 15: 277–83.
11. Vaidya JS, Vyas JJ, Mittra I, Chinoy RF. Multicentricity and its influence on conservative breast cancer treatment strategy. Hong kong International Cancer Congress 1995; Abstract 44.4.
12. Vaidya JS, Vyas JJ, Chinoy RF, et al. Multicentricity of breast cancer: whole-organ analysis and clinical implications. Br J Cancer 1996; 74: 820–4.
13. Sacchini V. Multicentricity and recurrence of breast cancer. Lancet 1996; 348: 1256–7.
14. Baum M, Vaidya JS, Mittra I. Multicentricity and recurrence of breast cancer. Lancet 1997; 349: 208.
15. Vaidya JS, Baum M, Tobias JS, et al. Targeted intra-operative radiotherapy (Targit): an innovative method of treatment for early breast cancer. Ann Oncol 2001; 12: 1075–80.
16. Vaidya JS, Joseph DJ, Tobias JS, et al. Targeted intraoperative radiotherapy versus whole breast radiotherapy for breast cancer (TARGIT-A trial): an international, prospective, randomised, non-inferiority phase 3 trial. Lancet 2010; 376: 91–102.
17. Vaidya JS, Baum M, Tobias JS, Houghton J. Targeted Intraoperative Radiothearpy (TARGIT)- trial protocol. Lancet 1999.[Available from: http://www.thelancet.com/protocol-reviews/99PRT-47].
18. Veronesi U, Orecchia R, Luini A, et al. A preliminary report of intraoperative radiotherapy (IORT) in limited-stage breast cancers that are conservatively treated. Eur J Cancer 2001; 37: 2178–83.
19. Baglan KL, Martinez AA, Frazier RC, et al. The use of high-dose-rate brachytherapy alone after lumpectomy in patients with early-stage breast cancer treated with breast-conserving therapy. Int J Radiat Oncol Biol Phys 2001; 50: 1003–11.
20. Polgar C, Sulyok Z, Fodor J, et al. Sole brachytherapy of the tumor bed after conservative surgery for T1 breast cancer: five-year results of a phase I-II study and initial findings of a randomized phase III trial. J Surg Oncol 2002; 80: 121–8.
21. Jorgensen KJ, Gotzsche PC. Overdiagnosis in publicly organised mammography screening programmes: systematic review of incidence trends. BMJ 2009; 339: b2587.
22. Vaidya JS. Women undergoing screening mammography experience a higher incidence of invasive breast cancer, without a corresponding reduction in symptomatic breast cancer. Br Med J (Clin Res Ed) 2009. [Available from: http://www.bmj.com/rapid-response/2011/11/02/women-undergoing-screening-mammography-experience-higher-incidence-invasiv].
23. Jones L, Law P, Vaidya JS. "Cancer" is described as the diagnosis by three times as many patients scheduled for mastectomy compared with breast conserving surgery. Eur J Cancer Suppl 2008; 6: 2.
24. Metcalfe KA, Semple J, Quan ML, et al. Changes in psychosocial functioning 1 year after mastectomy alone, delayed breast reconstruction, or immediate breast reconstruction. Ann Surg Oncol 2012; 19: 233–41.
25. Smith GL, Xu Y, Buchholz TA, et al. Association between treatment with brachytherapy vs whole-breast irradiation and subsequent mastectomy, complications, and survival among older women with invasive breast cancer. JAMA 2012; 307: 1827–37.
26. Holland R, Veling SH, Mravunac M, Hendriks JH. Histologic multifocality of Tis, T1-2 breast carcinomas. Implications for clinical trials of breast-conserving surgery. Cancer 1985; 56: 979–90.
27. Hughes KS, Schnapper LA, Cirrincione C, et al. CALGB, ECOG, RTOG. Lumpectomy plus tamoxifen with or without irradiation in women age 70 or older with early breast cancer. J Clin Oncol 2010; 28: Abstr 507.
28. Smith BD, Arthur DW, Buchholz TA, et al. Accelerated partial breast irradiation consensus statement from the American Society for Radiation Oncology (ASTRO). J Am Coll Surg 2009; 209: 269–77.

44 Systemic hormonal therapies for early-stage breast cancer

Stephen R.D. Johnston

INTRODUCTION

Endocrine manipulation has been recognized as a treatment modality for breast cancer for over 100 years. Estrogen is an important promoter in the pathogenesis of breast cancer, and response to hormonal therapy is largely dependent on the presence of estrogen receptor (ER), a protein which can be detected in about 70% of primary breast cancers. Historically, treatments over 50 years ago for advanced breast cancer involved surgical removal of endocrine glands such as the ovaries, adrenal glands, or the pituitary hypophysis. However, a better understanding of the pharmacological mechanisms that result in estrogenic deprivation and which yield an antiproliferative effect on breast cancer cells has enabled the development of effective medical therapeutics (Table 44.1). These therapies quickly replaced surgical ablative procedures in the management of advanced breast cancer. Over the last 30 years, systemic hormonal therapies are now routinely given for early-stage ER-positive breast cancer in the adjuvant setting, and have transformed management of the disease.

This chapter reviews the advances that have been made with a variety of systemic hormonal therapies, all of which have enhanced the survival of women with ER-positive breast cancer. In addition, this chapter discusses the current guidance that is available for the optimal use of systemic hormonal therapies, and looks to the future as we start to classify ER-positive breast cancer into different intrinsic subtypes for which novel hormonal strategies involving combination with targeted biological agents may soon be evaluated in the adjuvant setting.

THE PHARMACOLOGY OF SYSTEMIC HORMONAL THERAPIES

In order to understand how systemic hormonal therapies work in breast cancer, it is important to appreciate how estrogen interacts with the ER protein to influence gene transcription and cell growth, while also being aware of where estrogen is synthesized in the body in both pre- and postmenopausal women. Estrogen exerts its effect on gene expression and cellular growth by diffusing into the cell and binding nuclear ER, which in turn activates receptor dimerization, association with co-activator and co-repressor proteins (to a greater or lesser extent, respectively), and subsequent DNA binding of liganded ER within promoter regions of DNA upstream of estrogen-regulated target genes (Fig. 44.1). Gene transcription is activated through two separate transactivation domains within ER, termed AF-1 in the aminoterminal A/B region and AF-2 in the carboxy-terminal E region (1). Some of the key estrogen-regulated genes include those involved in cell proliferation and growth, thus explaining the growth promoting and mitogenic effects that estrogen has in ER-positive breast cancer cells. At a cellular level, therefore, pharmacological approaches to hormonal manipulation include either antiestrogens that compete for ER in the breast tumor or estrogen deprivation approaches which lower systemic estrogen levels.

Antiestrogens

Hormonal manipulation with antiestrogens is achieved at a cellular level by competing with estrogen for ER within the breast tumor. Thus at its simplest level, tamoxifen functions as a competitive antiestrogen to inhibit estrogen action. Tamoxifen-bound ER still dimerizes and binds DNA, but the downstream effects are different as a result of the altered conformational shape of the tamoxifen–ER complex compared with estradiol (Fig. 44.1). This results in a change in the receptor bound balance of co-activators and co-repressors such that tamoxifen-liganded ER may block gene transcription through the AF-2 domain, while AF-1 mediated gene transcription may still occur (2). This may explain the partial agonist activity of tamoxifen in some tissues (i.e., bone, endometrium), while at the same time tamoxifen's ability to antagonize estrogen-regulated gene transcription in other tissues (i.e., breast). Furthermore, it provides a mechanistic understanding for the drug's toxicity profile which is discussed in the following text.

Alternative anti-estrogenic agents known as "selective estrogen receptor modulators" (SERMs), and "pure" antiestrogens or "selective estrogen receptor downregulators" such as fulvestrant, have been developed (3). These drugs have little or no estrogenic agonist effects, and have been utilized in the advanced breast cancer setting when breast cancer returns after prior antiestrogen or aromatase inhibitor (AI) therapy. These drugs were developed with the aim of retaining both the antagonist activity of tamoxifen within the breast and the agonist profile in bone and the cardiovascular system, yet at the same time eliminating unwanted agonist effects on the gynecological tract, in particular the uterus. While this profile could be more attractive than tamoxifen for early breast cancer, they have not been fully evaluated in this setting. On the other hand, their profile has made some of the SERMs attractive drugs to develop as chemopreventive agents, although this will not be discussed in this chapter.

Nonsteroidal SERMs fall into two broad categories, namely those that are structurally similar to the triphenylethylene structure of tamoxifen (first-generation SERMs such as tore-mifene) and those that are structurally different and more related to the benzothiophene structure of raloxifene (Fig. 44.2). A third class of antiestrogenic agents includes the steroidal anti-estrogen fulvestrant which is a structural derivative of estradiol

Table 44.1 Medical Endocrine Treatments for Breast Cancer

Antiestrogens:
  Tamoxifen, toremifene
  Other selective estrogen receptor modulators; raloxifene,
  lasofoxifene
  Steroidal "pure" anti-estrogens: fulvestrant
Estrogen deprivation therapies:
  Luteinizing hormone releasing hormone analogs; goserelin
  Aromatase inhibitors; letrozole, anastrozole, exemestane
Other agents:
  Progestogens; medroxyprogesterone acetate,
  megestrol acetate
  Androgens
  Corticosteroids
  Estrogens; diethylbestrol

with a long hydrophobic side-chain at the 7-alfa position (Fig. 44.2) (4). Pharmacologically these latter compounds are pure antiestrogens which not only impair ER dimerization but also induce ER degradation and as such have been termed selective estrogen receptor downregulators (SERDs) (Fig. 44.1) (5,6). They would appear to behave as potent antiestrogens in all tissues including the breast, uterus, and probably bone. The best known selective estrogen receptor downregulator is fulvestrant, which to date has only been utilized in advanced postmenopausal ER-positive breast cancer (7), and will not be discussed further in this chapter.

Estrogen Deprivation
An alternative approach to the anti-estrogen strategy is to lower systemic estrogen levels (estrogen deprivation). The net

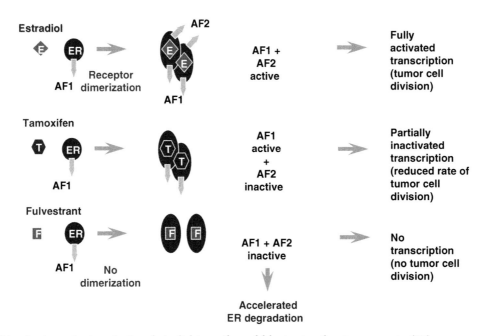

Figure 44.1 Differential molecular mechanism of action of estradiol, tamoxifen, and fulvestrant on the estrogen receptor (ER).

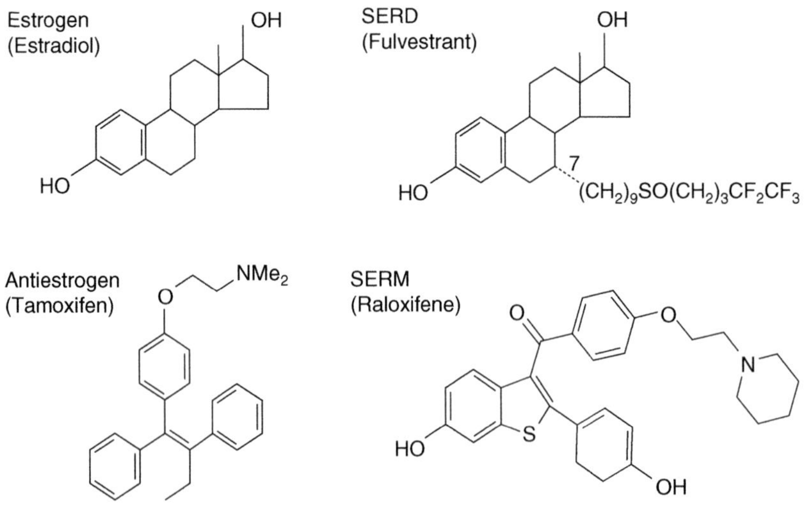

Figure 44.2 Examples of chemical structure of estrogens, antiestrogens, selective estrogen receptor modulator (SERM), and selective estrogen receptor downregulators (SERDS).

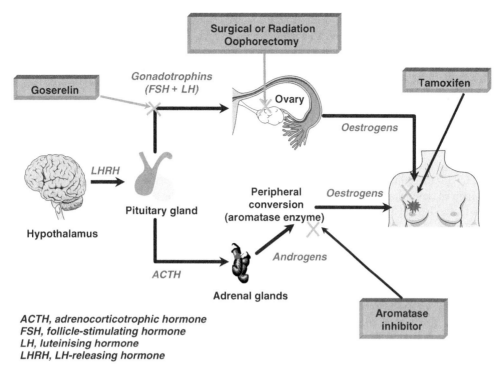

ACTH, adrenocorticotrophic hormone
FSH, follicle-stimulating hormone
LH, luteinising hormone
LHRH, LH-releasing hormone

Figure 44.3 Source of estrogen biosynthesis, and strategies to induce estrogen deprivation in pre-and postmenopausal women.

effect upon the ER-positive cell is similar to an antiestrogen, namely to deprive the cell of its mitogenic signal by removing the liganded estrogen. How estrogen deprivation is achieved depends on where systemic estrogens are being synthesized in the body. In premenopausal women with functional intact ovaries, the source of circulating estrogens is dependent on an intact pituitary axis which releases luteinizing hormone and follicle-stimulating hormone in a cyclical fashion. In postmenopausal women, estrogen biosynthesis switches to the peripheral aromatization of androgens into estrogens once ovarian function has finally ceased (Fig. 44.3). Thus, in premenopausal women estrogen deprivation occurs by the use of luteinizing hormone releasing hormone (LHRH) agonists, whereas in postmenopausal women it is achieved by the use of AIs which block estrogen synthesis in non-ovarian tissues such as fat, muscle, and indeed the breast itself.

Role of Adjuvant Hormonal Therapies in Early Breast Cancer

As discussed within this chapter, both of these pharmacological approaches to hormonal therapy in early breast cancer (i.e., anti-estrogens or estrogen deprivation) have been extensively investigated within the context of large scale international trials of adjuvant endocrine therapy over the last two decades. The details for each approach in both pre- and postmenopausal women are outlined later, and these strategies have undoubtedly yielded substantial gains in overall survival for women with ER-positive breast cancer. However, several key issues and unanswered questions remain, namely the best choice of endocrine agents and the optimal strategies in the postmenopausal setting, the appropriate duration of endocrine therapy, and the true role of ovarian suppression in premenopausal women. In addition, the molecular classification of breast cancer has now allowed us to better estimate endocrine responsiveness in ER-positive breast cancer, introducing another tool in addition to

established guidelines for decision making in the adjuvant setting; in particular, this has allowed us to address the issue of whether endocrine therapy alone is enough for many patients. This will be discussed later in the chapter.

ANTIESTROGENS IN EARLY BREAST CANCER: TAMOXIFEN

The triphenylethylene non-steroidal antiestrogen tamoxifen (Fig. 44.2) was first synthesized in the 1960s and found to have clinical activity in postmenopausal women with advanced breast cancer (8). As outlined earlier, tamoxifen antagonizes the effects of estrogen in breast cancer cells by binding ER, inducing G1 cell cycle arrest, and inhibiting tumor growth (Fig. 44.1). Preclinical studies showed that tamoxifen prevented the growth of ER-positive breast tumor xenografts *in vivo* (9); at the same time, it stimulated uterine growth (10) and supported the growth of endometrial xenografts *in vivo* (11). During early clinical trials in the adjuvant setting with tamoxifen a similar spectrum of estrogenic and antiestrogenic effects emerged in patients, with vaginal dryness and hot flushes the most frequently reported antiestrogenic toxicities (12). Due to the estrogenic activity of tamoxifen in the liver, total serum cholesterol levels were reduced by 10–15% (13). Likewise, bone mineral density was preserved in tamoxifen-treated postmenopausal women, although in premenopausal women this effect was less apparent (14,15). In postmenopausal patients, tamoxifen functioned as an estrogen on the endometrium, with endometrial thickening and hyperplasia together with an increased risk of endometrial cancer (16). This toxicity profile appeared to be acceptable and manageable, and through the 1980s, several large placebo-controlled studies were undertaken to assess the benefit of tamoxifen in the early breast cancer setting.

The initial 1998 meta-analysis of all clinical trials found that five years of tamoxifen in women with an early-stage ER-positive breast cancer significantly reduced the risk of recurrence (47%

reduction in annual odds) and death (26% reduction in annual odds) (17). This benefit was greatest in women with ER-rich tumors and occurred across all age groups, irrespective of nodal involvement. In addition, tamoxifen's antiestrogenic effects on normal breast epithelial cells resulted in a 50% reduction in new contralateral breast cancers, evidence which provided much of the impetus to develop tamoxifen in chemoprevention. At the same time, the estrogenic effects of tamoxifen therapy on bone and cholesterol were seen to be of clinical benefit for these women in terms of reducing risk from osteoporosis and cardiovascular disease (13,14). In the adjuvant setting tamoxifen's increased risk of endometrial cancer has been perceived as small in relation to the substantial benefit from reduction in breast cancer–related events (18). However, both in adjuvant and metastatic therapy with tamoxifen, breast epithelial cells and established tumors adapt to chronic antiestrogen exposure and develop resistance to tamoxifen, which may relate to the partial agonist effect of tamoxifen in stimulating tumor growth (19,20).

In the next 2005 overview of the effects of chemotherapy and hormonal therapy for early-stage breast cancer by the Early Breast Cancer Trialists' Collaborative Group (EBCTCG), a 50% reduction in the risk of relapse and a 31% reduction in the annual breast cancer death rate were reported for five years of adjuvant tamoxifen at 15 years of follow-up (21). Although the risk of distant recurrence is greatest during the first decade, it can still continue through the second decade (22), raising the question about the magnitude of carry-over effect from initial therapy, or indeed the need for extended adjuvant therapy beyond five years in those women at a greater risk (Fig. 44.4). In the 2011 meta-analysis the EBCTCG updated their analysis of long-term outcomes in 21,457 women with early-stage breast cancer from 20 randomized trials of five years of tamoxifen versus observation or placebo (23). They showed that five years of tamoxifen reduced the recurrence rate substantially in years 0–4 during therapy [rate ratio (RR)

0.53], and also in years 5–9 (RR 0.68) and throughout the first 15 years (RR 0.70, p < 0.00001). Most importantly, the relapse curves do not converge after year 10, with a continued annual absolute gain from the annual reduction in breast cancer mortality through to year 15. Furthermore, the benefit only occurs in those with ER-positive tumors, being maximal in those with rich expression of the receptor. As such, five years of tamoxifen probably cures many patients rather than simply delays an inevitable recurrence.

These mature data from the meta-analysis regarding a well established treatment such as tamoxifen give confidence to both clinicians and patients in the beneficial effects of endocrine therapy on improving overall survival from breast cancer; so how long do patients need to take tamoxifen? Studies of duration such as NSABP-14 have compared 5 to 10 years of tamoxifen and shown no advantage beyond five years, indeed perhaps a slight disadvantage in terms of disease-free survival (DFS) (24). However, this study only examined node-negative patients. In two further trials (adjuvant tamoxifen- to offer more?; aTTOm and Adjuvant Tamoxifen, Longer Against Shorter; ATLAS) preliminary results have suggested a small reduction in breast cancer recurrence for those patients randomized to continue tamoxifen, although no significant difference was observed for breast cancer–specific or overall mortality (25,26). Further follow-up of these studies is required to reliably assess the longer term effects on recurrence and overall effects, if any, on mortality.

While tamoxifen remains the most appropriate sole treatment option for many premenopausal and perimenopausal women, postmenopausal women may have other options. Some women will still relapse despite therapy and tamoxifen has either unacceptable short-term vasomotor toxicities or increased long-term risks such as venous thrombosis and endometrial cancer. The incorporation of AIs into the treatment of postmenopausal early-stage ER-positive breast cancer

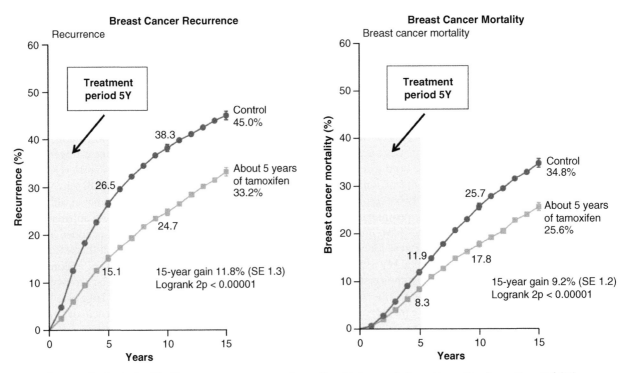

Figure 44.4 Prolonged reduction in the risk of breast cancer recurrence and mortality with 5 years of adjuvant tamoxifen. *Source:* From Ref. (21).

has now led to further improvements in outcomes over tamoxifen as discussed in the next section. The key issue is how AIs should be incorporated as adjuvant therapy in early breast cancer, and whether indeed a role for tamoxifen still remains in postmenopausal breast cancer.

ESTROGEN DEPRIVATION IN POSTMENOPAUSAL WOMEN: AROMATASE INHIBITORS

The oral AIs that are used in clinical practice include anastrozole (Arimidex), letrozole (Femara), and exemestane (Aromasin). All three drugs reduce serum estrogen levels in post-menopausal women by preventing the conversion of adrenal androgens (androstenedione and testosterone) into estradiol (E1) and estrone (E2) by the cytochrome P450 enzyme aromatase (27). While aromatase is highly expressed in the placenta and in the granulosa cells of ovarian follicles, it is also present in lower levels in several non-glandular tissues including fat, liver, and muscle. At the menopause mean plasma E2 levels fall from about 400–600 pmol/L to around 25–50 pmol/L. While estrogens are synthesized in the ovary in premenopausal women, following the menopause estrogens come solely from peripheral aromatase conversion, particularly in subcutaneous fat; indeed plasma E2 levels correlate with body mass index in postmenopausal women (28). AIs are indicated only for postmenopausal women to prevent the peripheral conversion of androgens into estrogens, and on their own are not effective in reducing the much higher levels of circulating E1/E2 seen in premenopausal women. Unlike tamoxifen, they have no partial agonist activity. Anastrozole and letrozole are both non-steroidal AIs (Fig. 44.5) and have similar pharmacokinetics with half-lives approximating 48 hours (29,30) allowing a once daily schedule. The half-life of exemestane which is a steroidal aromatase inactivator is 27 hours (Fig. 44.5) (31).

Between 1995 and 2000, the three third-generation AIs established themselves clinically when a series of randomised controlled trials (RCTs) involving more than 2000 women demonstrated clinical superiority over megestrol acetate as a second-line therapy after tamoxifen (32–34). Although the benefit was often small, these initial trials confirmed a very low

incidence of serious side effects with AIs, in particular less weight gain and thromboembolic events than with progestins. As such AIs became the standard therapy for postmenopausal women with advanced breast cancer which relapsed or progressed after tamoxifen (35). While pharmacodynamic studies in advanced breast cancer had suggested greater estrogen suppression for patients treated with letrozole compared with anastrozole (36), an open randomized trial in over 600 patients suggested no overall significant differences in efficacy (37).

The establishment of the efficacy and tolerability of AIs in advanced breast cancer encouraged the development of a number of trials examining their use in the adjuvant setting (27). In general, these therapeutic studies have either evaluated primary "up-front" AI therapy for five years compared with five years of tamoxifen, or a so-called "switch" strategy of initial tamoxifen for two to three years followed either by an AI for two to three years or continued tamoxifen through to year 5. The absolute benefits of these approaches have been assessed in a meta-analysis of all the adjuvant trials of AIs versus the previous standard of care, namely five years of tamoxifen (38). The key message is that AIs produce significantly lower recurrence rates compared with tamoxifen, either as initial monotherapy or following two to three years of tamoxifen; however, the true impact on long-term survival is less clear at this stage. The 2010 American Society of Clinical Oncology (ASCO) guidelines on adjuvant endocrine therapy for women with ER-positive breast cancer recommend incorporating AI therapy at some point during adjuvant treatment (39), while recognizing that the optimal timing and duration of therapy remain unresolved questions. So what are the benefits, and what has been learned from all the trials of adjuvant AIs to date?

Aromatase Inhibitors Used "Up-front"

Two large studies have assessed the efficacy of AIs compared with tamoxifen as "up-front" adjuvant endocrine therapy in postmenopausal women with early breast cancer (Table 44.2) (40–44). The Arimidex, Tamoxifen, Alone or in Combination (ATAC) trial was the first large study to investigate the role of AIs as adjuvant therapy for early-stage breast cancer. Over four years, 9366 postmenopausal women from 21 countries were

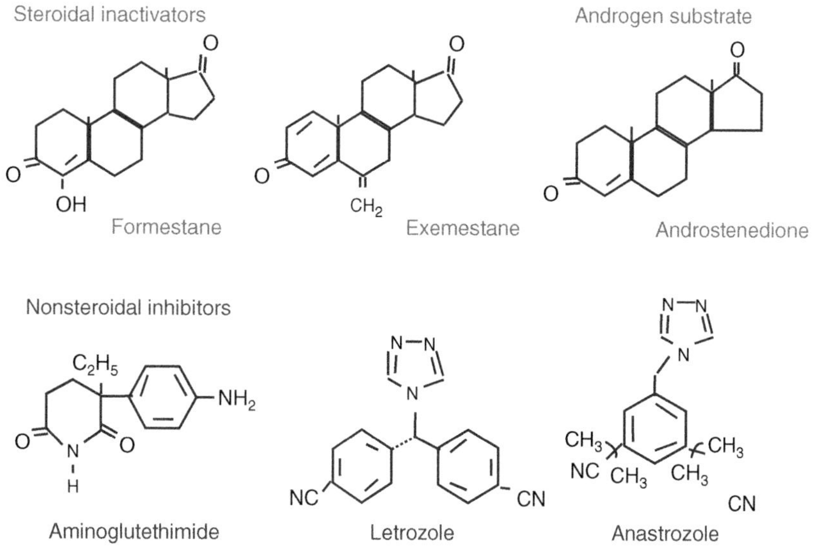

Figure 44.5 Structures of steroidal and nonsteroidal aromatase inhibitors.

enrolled. The hypotheses tested were that anastrozole was non-inferior or superior to tamoxifen, or that the combination of anastrozole and tamoxifen was superior to tamoxifen alone. The combination treatment was discontinued following the initial analysis because it showed no efficacy or tolerability benefits over tamoxifen alone (40). Following a median follow-up of 100 months (41), anastrozole compared with tamoxifen was associated with a significantly improved DFS in hormone receptor–positive patients [hazard ratio (HR) 0.85, p = 0.003]. In the most recent 10-year analysis, the absolute differences in time to recurrence in hormone receptor–positive patients increased over time, being 2.7% at five years and 4.3% at 10 years (Fig. 44.6) (42). In addition, recurrence rates remained significantly lower on anastrozole compared with tamoxifen after treatment completion (HR 0.81, p = 0.03), although the carry-over effect was smaller after eight years. However, these differences in preventing or delaying disease recurrence did not result in a difference in overall survival between the two treatments (HR 0.95, 95% CI 0.84–1.06) (42).

Differences in toxicity profile demonstrated a higher incidence of thromboembolic and cardiovascular events with tamoxifen, and more musculoskeletal events and fractures with anastrozole (43). A bone substudy of the main trial confirmed that AI therapy was associated with an accelerated bone loss over the five-year treatment period, although no patients with normal bone mineral density at baseline became osteoporotic at five years (44). Indeed once therapy is completed, the risk of fractures diminishes quickly while the benefit of treatment in reducing recurrence is maintained (Fig. 44.6).

The BIG 1-98 trial assessed the efficacy of "up-front" AI therapy with letrozole for five years versus tamoxifen, as well as switching strategies (see the next section). It recruited 8028 women who were randomized to one of four treatment arms. In 2005, the first analysis at a median follow-up of 25.8 months reported that five years of letrozole demonstrated a significant improvement both in DFS (HR 0.81, p = 0.003) and distant disease-free survival (DDFS) (HR 0.73 p = 0.001) over tamoxifen (45). These results led to the unblinding of the tamoxifen-alone arm, and 25.2% of patients selectively crossed over to letrozole which has complicated subsequent intention to treat (ITT) analyses of the monotherapy arms. The updated report at a median follow-up of 76 months (46) included both an ITT analysis and a censored analysis at the time of cross-over, and still demonstrated a statistically significant improvement in DFS and DDFS in favor of letrozole over tamoxifen, within addition a non-significant improvement in overall survival (HR 0.87, 95% CI 0.75–1.02, p = 0.08). In terms of toxicity, endometrial cancer, vaginal bleeding and thromboembolism were more common with tamoxifen, while musculoskeletal events and hypercholesterolemia were higher with letrozole.

The meta-analysis of both of these studies showed an absolute five-year reduction in the recurrence of 2.9% (9.6% for AI *vs.* 12.6% for tamoxifen, 2p < 0.00001), with an absolute 3.9% reduction at 8 years (38). This was associated with only a 1.1% reduction in breast cancer mortality at five years which was non-significant.

Table 44.2 Comparative Efficacy of Up-Front 5 Years' AIs *Vs.* 5 Years' Tamoxifen in Early Breast Cancer

Study (Reference)	ATAC (41)	BIG-198 (46)
Number of patients	6241	4922
Median follow-up (months)	100	76
DFS	HR 0.90 p = 0.025	HR 0.88 p = 0.03
Five year DFS difference (%)	2.8	2.9
Time to distant recurrence	HR 0.86 p = 0.022	HR 0.85 p = 0.05
Overall survival	HR 1.00 p = 0.99	HR 0.87 p = 0.08

p ≤ 0.05 = significant.
Abbreviations: AI, aromatase inhibitor; ATAC, Arimidex, tamoxifen, alone, or in combination; DFS, disease-free survival; HR, hazard ratio.

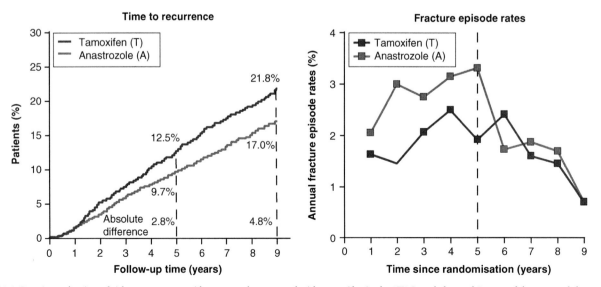

Figure 44.6 Ongoing reduction of risk or recurrence with anastrozole compared with tamoxifen in the ATAC study beyond 5 years of therapy, and the associated reducing risk of fractures once therapy was completed. *Source*: From Ref. (42).

Table 44.3 Comparative Efficacy of 2–3 Years Tamoxifen Followed by a Switch to 2–3 Years Aromatase Inhibitor *Vs.* 5 Years Tamoxifen Alone

Study (reference)	IES (48)	ARNO 95 (49)	ITA (50)	ABCSG 8 (49)
Number of patients	4724	979	448	3714
Median follow-up(months)	55.7	30.1	64	72
DFS	HR 0.76	HR 0.66	HR 0.56	HR 0.79
	p = 0.0001	p = 0.49	p = 0.01	p = 0.038
Overall survival	HR 0.83[a]	HR 0.53	HR 0.56	HR 0.77
	p = 0.05	p = 0.045	p = 0.1	p = 0.025

$p \leq 0.05$ = significant.
[a]In a subset of estrogen receptor-positive patients only.
Abbreviations: DFS, disease-free survival; HR, hazard ratio.

Switching from Tamoxifen to AIs Compared with Tamoxifen Alone

In terms of a switching strategy, several trials have evaluated a switch to an AI after two to three years of tamoxifen compared to five years tamoxifen alone (in an attempt to pre-empt the development of resistance to tamoxifen, and to minimize long term side effects of either therapy if given alone for five years) (Table 44.3) (47–51). The largest of these studies was the Intergroup Exemestane Study (IES) which compared switching to exemestane after two to three years of tamoxifen with tamoxifen for five years. This study demonstrated not only a statistically significant improvement in DFS (HR 0.68, p < 0.001) (47), but also in overall survival in an updated analysis of those with ER-positive disease (HR 0.86, p < 0.04) (48). These findings were also confirmed in a meta-analysis of three separate trials with the tamoxifen-anastrozole switch compared with tamoxifen alone [the Austrian Breast and Colorectal Cancer Study Group (ABCSG 8), Arimidex-Nolvadex (ARNO 95) and Italian Tamoxifen Anastrozole (ITA) studies (49,50). This meta-analysis included over 4000 patients with a mean follow-up of 30 months, which is shorter than for the IES study. Despite this limited follow-up, the combined analysis still showed a significant improvement in DFS (HR 0.59, p < 0.0001) from switching to anastrozole and was also associated with a statistically significant reduction in breast cancer mortality and death from any cause (HR 0.71, p < 0.037) (51).

These individual studies seem to suggest significantly better outcomes in terms of disease-free and overall survival by a switching strategy when compared with tamoxifen alone. In addition to lesser long-term toxicity with tamoxifen, there appears to be a substantial gain in efficacy, presumably by preventing relapses that were destined to occur during continued tamoxifen usage by utilizing a non-cross-resistant therapy. Moreover, it has been questioned by some whether early relapses on tamoxifen could be prevented by an up-front AI strategy, and it remains unclear which approach (tamoxifen with early switch to an AI, or AI upfront) will yield better oncological outcomes and overall tolerability. However, two large trials (BIG 1–98 and TEAM) have now provided direct data on these comparisons (see the next section).

Switching Tamoxifen to AIs Compared with AI Upfront

The Breast International Group (BIG) 1–98 study was the first clinical trial to report a direct comparison between the use of an upfront AI and a switching strategy (46). At a median follow-up of 76 months, there was no significant difference in disease-free recurrence, overall survival, or time to distant recurrence between the switching (tamoxifen to letrozole) and the letrozole monotherapy arms. However, there were fewer early relapses among women who were assigned to letrozole alone compared with the switch of tamoxifen followed by letrozole. This trend was greatest in node-positive patients with a 1.4% difference in breast cancer recurrence in node-negative patients (3.5% *vs.* 4.9%), and a 2.3% absolute difference in node-positive patients (12.4% *vs.* 14.7%) at five years. Interestingly, there was no significant difference in breast cancer recurrence between the letrozole followed by a reverse-switch to tamoxifen and the letrozole monotherapy arm. The clinical significance of these findings is that patients who commence an AI but experience side effects or toxicity may be safely switched over to tamoxifen to complete adjuvant endocrine therapy, without compromising on the anti-tumor efficacy of an AI.

The second study to provide a direct comparison was the Tamoxifen Exemestane Adjuvant Multicentre (TEAM) trial which randomized 9779 postmenopausal women with ER-positive early breast cancer to either exemestane for five years or tamoxifen for 2.5–3 years followed by exemestane (52). At a median follow-up of 5.1 years, there was no difference in either disease-free or overall survival, a result very similar to that observed in the BIG 1–98 study.

Which is the Best Strategy for AIs: Up-Front or Switch?

So what are we to conclude from these large well-conducted studies as to which strategy is the best? From the meta-analysis of all these studies the addition of an AI in either strategy (up-front or switch) clearly improves DFS compared with five years of tamoxifen. Moreover, delaying relapse does not appear to translate into a substantial survival advantage, although a modest benefit that was evident from a meta-analysis of all switching studies (yielding an absolute gain in overall survival of 1.7% at eight years) (38). Biomarker studies in many of these trials have attempted to determine whether conventional indicators of hormone responsiveness such as absolute ER and PR levels (53–55), co-expression of human epidermal growth factor receptor 2 (HER2) (53), proliferation as assessed by Ki-67 labelling index (56), or indeed the 21-gene recurrence score (57) can identify those patients who benefit more from an AI than tamoxifen. While confirming the prognostic role of different biomarkers, none of these individual studies has

Table 44.4 Comparative Efficacy of Extended Adjuvant Therapy of 5 Years Tamoxifen Followed by 3–5 Years Aromatase Inhibitor *Vs.* 5 Years Tamoxifen Alone

Study (reference)	MA-17 (62)	NSABP B-33 (66)	ABCSG-6a (65)
Number of patients	5170	1562	852
Median follow-up (months)	64	30	62
Disease-free survival	HR 0.68	HR 0.68	HR 0.62
	p = 0.0001	p = 0.07	p = 0.031
Overall survival	HR 0.98	NR	HR 0.89
	p = 0.853		p = 0.57

Abbreviations: HR, hazard ratio; NR, not recorded.

identified patients with a differential response between tamoxifen and AI therapy. At the present time, the two direct comparisons between up-front AI or switch strategy (BIG 1–98 and TEAM) have shown no significant differences between these approaches, although in the letrozole study fewer recurrences were seen with AI up front compared with switching for higher risk node-positive patients (46). Therefore, tumor burden in conjunction with other inherent risk factors related to disease biology (higher grade or proliferation score, lower levels of ER or PR, co-expression of HER2) might be used in clinical decision making to favor up-front AIs as opposed to a switch strategy.

Patient-related factors and toxicity concerns should also be considered when making a decision between these: up-front AI use or a switch strategy. In general, the third-generation AIs are well tolerated, and in the clinical trial setting different side effect profiles of tamoxifen and AIs do not appear to impact on a patient's quality of life (58). Assessing an individual's risk or history of venous thrombosis may influence whether tamoxifen is appropriate, while assessment of joint arthropathies or risk of osteoporosis may determine the optimal timing for starting an AI. Current ASCO guidelines recommend that postmenopausal women who receive an AI should have their bone mineral density evaluated with calcium and vitamin D supplementation or bisphosphonate use depending on the result (59). Thus, clinicians and patients have a choice on when and how to use an AI which is dependent on the level of risk from the cancer and general health issues for each individual woman—with only marginal differences in efficacy outcomes (particularly in relation to survival).

In terms of which is the best AI to use, the only reported comparison to date is the MA.27 study where five years of adjuvant exemestane yielded similar results to five years of adjuvant anastrozole (60). A trial comparing the two nonsteroidal AIs letrozole and anastrozole (FACE) has completed recruitment, and results are awaited. Tolerability profiles between the different AIs are very similar, and to date there is no evidence to suggest that one agent is substantially better overall than another.

Duration of Adjuvant Endocrine Therapy with AIs

ER-positive breast cancer has a chronic relapsing nature, with the risk of recurrence continuing indefinitely; indeed in the tamoxifen overview, approximately half of all recurrences occurred between 5 and 15 years after surgery despite five years of adjuvant tamoxifen treatment (21,23). Therefore, there is a clear rationale for considering extended adjuvant

endocrine therapy beyond five years in an attempt to reduce long-term risk of recurrence further. The MA-17 study (61) was a double blind, placebo controlled trial of over 5000 patients designed to test whether five years of letrozole therapy in postmenopausal women who had completed five years of adjuvant tamoxifen could further improve DFS between years 5 and 10 from the time of diagnosis. The trial demonstrated a significant improvement for DFS in patients who continued treatment with letrozole after completion of five years of tamoxifen. The four-year DFS rates (i.e., year 9 since initial diagnosis) were 93% *vs.* 87% respectively (61). Furthermore, after a median follow-up of 30 months among higher risk lymph node–positive patients, overall survival was statistically significantly improved with letrozole (HR 0.61, 95% CI 0.38–0.98; p = 0.04) (62). Subsequent analyses of this trial have suggested that this benefit was greatest in those with ER-positive, PR-positive tumors (63), and that benefits may also accrue if the switch to extended adjuvant letrozole occurred a few years after completion of tamoxifen (64). Two separate, smaller studies with either anastrozole (65) or exemestane (66) as extended adjuvant therapy after completion of five years of tamoxifen have shown similar quantitative results in terms of reduction in risk of recurrence, with hazard ratios of 0.62 and 0.68, respectively (Table 44.4).

These data confirm that risk of recurrence in ER-positive breast cancer does indeed persist well beyond completion of five years of adjuvant tamoxifen. Careful consideration should be given to offering longer duration of adjuvant therapy with AIs for those deemed to be at greatest risk. While all of these studies examined treatment following five years of tamoxifen, increasingly clinical practice is to either use AI therapy up front in higher risk node-positive patients, or a switch approach of AIs following an initial two to three years of tamoxifen. How can we translate data from extended adjuvant therapy studies into current guidelines for AI usage today? Can we safely use AIs beyond a total duration of five years without, for example, compromising bone health? The answer at present is unknown, although safety data relating to the optimal duration of AIs indicate that therapy should be given for a maximum of five years. Indeed, the ASCO guidelines recommend that AI therapy should not exceed five years outside the setting of clinical trials, and that in the sequential setting patients should receive an AI after two to three years of tamoxifen for a total of five years of adjuvant endocrine therapy. The guidelines recognize that this may yield "an unfamiliar pattern of different durations of adjuvant treatment based on the treatment strategy used"; Furthermore, neither five years' up-front AI nor sequential switch strategies (*two to three* years tamoxifen followed by two to three years of an AI) have been compared against the longer overall duration of the extended adjuvant therapy regimens where treatment duration was up to 8–10 years. Two trials (MA.17R and NSABP B-42) are addressing whether longer durations of AI therapy improve outcomes without compromising safety and will report at a future date.

ESTROGEN DEPRIVATION IN PREMENOPAUSAL WOMEN: OVARIAN SUPPRESSION

LHRH agonists, which initially stimulate and then exhaust the LHRH receptors in the pituitary, cause reversible suppression of ovarian function and are currently used as an alternative to ovarian ablation for treatment of advanced breast cancer in premenopausal women. The EBCTCG (21) reviewed trials involving almost 8000 women with ER-positive or ER unknown early breast cancer who were randomized to ovarian ablation (surgery/irradiation) or ovarian suppression with an LHRH agonist. Overall, there were definite benefits of ovarian ablation/suppression both in terms of recurrence and breast cancer mortality. However, effects of ovarian treatment appear smaller in those trials where both groups received chemotherapy, (than in trials where neither did) and chemotherapy-induced amenorrhea probably attenuated any additional effect of ovarian suppression. For example, in the Intergroup 0101 trial, the addition of the LHRH agonist goserelin to CAF chemotherapy for premenopausal women with ER-positive node-positive breast cancer appeared to have a greater effect on improved DFS in women below 40 compared to those above 40 years (67).

Likewise, the International Breast Cancer Study Group (IBCSG) trial VIII randomized premenopausal women with node-negative ER-positive early breast cancer to either adjuvant CMF chemotherapy and goserelin for two years, or CMF followed by goserelin for 18 months (68). The addition of goserelin had only minimal impact on five-year DFS, and once again the benefit was maximal in women aged below 40 years with a hazard ratio of 0.34.

A meta-analysis evaluated only those trials where ER status was known and that used LHRH agonists as a method for ovarian suppression (69). The primary endpoints were any recurrence or death after recurrence, with a median follow-up time of 6.8 years. In particular, a benefit was observed when LHRH agonists were used after chemotherapy (either alone or with tamoxifen) in women aged below 40 years in whom chemotherapy is less likely to induce permanent amenorrhea. Optimum duration of use of reversible ovarian suppression is unknown, although studies in general have utilized two to three years of LHRH agonist with five years of tamoxifen.

While the standard of care for ER-positive premenopausal breast cancer remains tamoxifen alone for five years, prospective trials to address the added role (if any) of ovarian suppression compared with tamoxifen alone have been undertaken (Fig. 44.7). The SOFT (Suppression of Ovarian Function Trial) randomized trial will assess the role of ovarian suppression/ablation in combination with the AI exemestane, compared with ovarian suppression plus tamoxifen or tamoxifen alone. Over 3000 women were randomized into this study which completed accrual in January 2011. The TEXT trial (Tamoxifen and Exemestane Trial) assesses an LHRH agonist with the

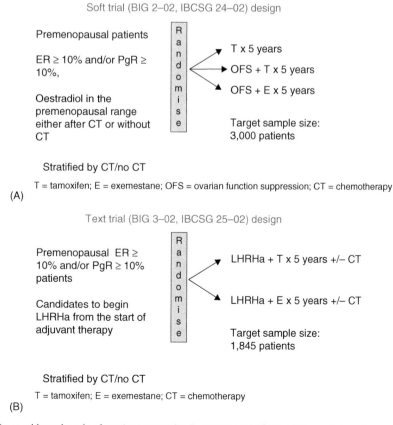

Figure 44.7 Design of two studies to address the role of ovarian suppression in premenopausal ER-positive early breast cancer; (**A**) the Suppression of Ovarian Function Trial (SOFT) study and (**B**) the Tamoxifen and Exemestane Trial (TEXT) study. *Abbreviations*: ER, estrogen receptor; OFS, ovarian function suppression; PR, progesterone.

addition of either tamoxifen or exemestane for five years, and accrual of over 2600 women was completed in March 2011 (chemotherapy is optional with this trial). It is hoped that both these trials will provide important additional information about the optimal endocrine therapy for premenopausal women with ER-positive early breast cancer.

ADJUVANT ENDOCRINE THERAPY: ROLE OF DECISION-MAKING TOOLS

One of the most important issues in the current management of ER-positive early breast cancer is not the choice of strategy for systemic hormonal therapy, but rather the threshold for using adjuvant chemotherapy in addition to adjuvant endocrine therapy to gain further clinical benefit. With increased understanding of the various intrinsic subtypes of breast cancer and their differential prognoses (70), there is ongoing debate among oncologists about the relative benefit of adjuvant chemotherapy versus endocrine therapy and whether for many patients with endocrine responsive breast cancer a hormonal approach alone would be sufficient to maximize a patient's chance of cure.

Clinicopathological Factors Used in Deciding Adjuvant Therapy

Historically, clinicians have used various established risk factors related to disease burden and tumor grade to make decisions about adjuvant therapy, namely the size and histological grade of a tumor, lymph node involvement, and the receptor status for both hormone (ER and PR) and growth factor receptors (HER2). Until recently, it was deemed that most women with early-stage ER-positive breast cancer would gain further proportional benefit in terms of reducing risk of recurrence and improving overall survival, by the addition of chemotherapy to hormonal systemic therapies. As such, only those women with small (T1), well, or moderately differentiated (grades 1 and 2) breast cancer that was node-negative and ER-positive were spared administration of cytotoxic chemotherapy in addition to endocrine therapy. There was an urgent need to estimate risk more accurately and determine the magnitude of benefit for different systemic treatment approaches.

Decision making tools such as Adjuvant! Online (71) have been used to estimate the risk of 10-year recurrence-free and overall survival for individual patients based on several key clinical (age and morbidity) and pathological (tumor size, grade, nodal burden, and ER status) features. The tool demonstrates an absolute benefit from the addition of chemotherapy or hormonal therapy, or a combination thereof in terms of gain in recurrence-free or overall survival. The web site, Adjuvant! Online, can therefore be helpful in informing patients of their level of risk, together with the relative magnitude of benefit that can be gained from each systemic therapy. However, the tool has some limitations and does not take account of the aspects of nodal burden (other than 0, 1–3, >4 nodes), or more importantly tumor biology (i.e., there is no assessment of quantitative level of ER, presence of PR, and of HER2 status). Over the years, it has become obvious that the focus in decision making needs to shift to an assessment of tumor biology rather than tumor size and nodal burden alone; this has been reflected by gradual changes in the international guidelines that are available to

clinicians, such as the St Gallen International Expert Consensus on the Primary Therapy of Early Breast Cancer.

Molecular Tools to Assess Endocrine Responsiveness in Early Breast Cancer

The previous St Gallen Consensus guidelines in 2007 and 2009 had started to characterize what might be considered truly endocrine responsive breast cancer based on levels of receptor expression for both ER and PR, with a relative absence of proliferation markers (72). It was noted, however, that endocrine responsiveness occurs as a continuum, although it was easy to recognize very endocrine-sensitive disease based on high levels of both ER and PR, with absence of HER2 and low proliferation. The indications for recommending chemotherapy were inversely related to the level of endocrine responsiveness, although this still left a zone of uncertainty, albeit that proliferation seemed to be a key biological feature in determining the level of endocrine responsiveness. In the 2009 Guidelines, the addition of adjuvant chemotherapy to endocrine therapy was only recommended if other risk features related to tumor burden were present in so-called endocrine responsive tumors (i.e., tumor size above 5 cm, greater than four nodes, and extensive vascular invasion) (73). At that time, gene arrays were only just evolving, but it was recognized that a multigene prognostic signature could be used if doubt remained about the use of adjuvant chemotherapy accepting that these were only providing information about prognosis and not predicting endocrine resistance or chemo-sensitivity (73).

In the latest set of St Gallen Consensus Guidelines published in 2011 (74), a new approach has been adopted for the classification of patients with early breast cancer based on the recognition of the intrinsic biological subtypes (Table 44.5) (70). Within these guidelines, the ability to subclassify ER-positive breast cancer into luminal A or luminal B subtypes is based on an approximation using clinicopathological determination (i.e., ER, PR, HER2, and proliferation assessed for example by Ki-67). Luminal subtypes are not always that easily identified using standard pathological criteria of proliferation and tumor grade. While many luminal A cancers have low proliferation scores and probably minimal benefit from adjuvant chemotherapy, not all luminal B cancers will have a high proliferation index. Likewise, controversy exists about the correct cut-off and reproducibility for the Ki-67 assay, although attempts have been made to standardize this in recent years (75). Various new gene expression assays such as the PAM-50 might ultimately identify those ER-positive cancers with different prognoses and altered levels of endocrine responsiveness (76). In addition, the genomic grade index (GGI) is a multigene signature that serves as a surrogate for histological grade and represents a strong prognostic tool (77). Studies to date have shown that GGI can separate very clearly luminal B tumors with a high GGI, and luminal A cancers with a low GGI (78). In practice, this tool might help identify those ER-positive grade 1 or 2 node-negative tumors that carry a higher intrinsic risk, and for whom adjuvant endocrine therapy alone will be insufficient.

At present the most widely used genomic assay in clinical practice is the 21-gene signature (Oncotype DX) which can be used to predict prognosis and recurrence risk in patients with ER-positive breast cancer using data generated from the

Table 44.5 Definitions of Intrinsic Subtypes of Breast Cancer Based on Clinicopathological Features, as Described within the 2011 St Gallen Consensus Guidelines

Intrinsic Subtype (1)	Clinicopathological Definition	Notes
Luminal A	"Luminal A" ER and/or PR positive (76) HER2 negative (77) Ki-67 low (<14%)	This cut-off point for Ki-67 labeling index was established by comparison with PAM50 intrinsic subtyping (7). Local quality control of Ki-67 staining is important
Luminal B	"Luminal B (HER2 negative)" ER and/or PR-positive HER2 negative Ki-67 high	Genes indicative of higher proliferation are markers of poor prognosis in multiple genetic assays (78). If reliable Ki-67 measurement is not available, some alternative assessment of tumor proliferation such as grade may be used to distinguish between "luminal A" and "luminal B (HER2 negative)"
	"Luminal B (HER2 positive)" ER and/or PR positive Any Ki-67 HER2 over-expressed or amplified	Both endocrine and anti-HER2 therapy may be indicated.
Erb-B2 overexpression	"HER2 positive (non luminal)" HER2 over-expressed or amplified ER and PR absent	
"Basal-like"	"Triple negative (ductal)" ER and PR absent HER2 negative	Approximately 80% overlap between "triple negative" and intrinsic "basal-like" subtypes but "triple negative" also includes some special histological types such as (typical) medullary and adenoid cystic carcinoma with low risks of distant recurrence. Staining for basal keratins (79) although shown to aid selection of true basal-like tumors, is considered insufficiently reproducible for general use

Source: From Ref. (74).

NSABP-B14 trial (79). The assay measures expression of 16 genes related to endocrine responsiveness, proliferation, and invasion in addition to five reference control genes. More recently, the assay was used to predict risk of recurrence in the ATAC study which confirmed its utility for predicting the risk of distant recurrence regardless of whether treatment was with tamoxifen or anastrozole (57). However, the assay is increasingly being used in clinical practice to determine whether adjuvant chemotherapy is of added benefit in ER-positive early breast cancer. The assay is based on data generated from the randomized SWOG trial which investigated the addition of anthracycline-based chemotherapy regimen (CAF) to endocrine therapy in women with ER-positive node-positive disease (80). The assay is increasingly being used to identify good prognosis ER-positive breast cancer with a low recurrence score where the addition of chemotherapy to endocrine treatment may yield no additional benefit (81). This could allow women with endocrine responsive disease and a good prognosis to avoid chemotherapy. This concept has been tested prospectively in two important clinical trials to assess whether this can further refine and guide adjuvant treatment decisions: the Trial Assigning IndividuaLized Options for Treatment (Rx) (TAILORx) where the Oncotype DX assay is being used in over 10,000 patients and the Microarray in Node-negative Disease May Avoid ChemoTherapy (MINDACT) trial using the MammaPrint assay in 6000 patients.

As we come to understand breast cancer subtypes better, it is hoped that these molecular profiling tools will allow us to stratify women with ER-positive early-stage breast cancer much more effectively into those where endocrine therapy alone is sufficient therapy versus those where the addition of chemotherapy has a real role to play, and those with truly

endocrine-sensitive disease where the optimal strategy for endocrine therapy alone discussed earlier is all that is required to cure the disease.

Current guidelines are therefore starting to make recommendations for systemic therapy based on these profiling classifications (74).

UNDERSTANDING ENDOCRINE RESPONSE: FUTURE OPPORTUNITIES IN EARLY ER-POSITIVE BREAST CANCER

Decision making is becoming much more individualized in early ER-positive breast cancer, yielding better outcomes and rationalizing the use of systemic chemotherapy to those with more endocrine non-responsive disease that might really benefit. In addition to the role of multigene signatures, other innovative approaches are being utilized to better predict response to endocrine therapy in ER-positive breast cancer patients.

Predicting Endocrine Response Preoperatively

In a short-term preoperative study of the biological effects of two weeks of endocrine therapy with an AI in ER-positive postmenopausal breast cancer, an anti-proliferative signal (as determined by a decrease in Ki-67) was shown to be strongly correlated with relapse-free survival (82). This approach is now being tested prospectively in the United Kingdom (UK) Pre-operative Endocrine Therapy Individualising Care (POETIC) study in which Ki-67 values after two weeks of AI therapy will be used to determine whether changes in this proliferation index can predict for benefit from adjuvant endocrine therapy (Fig. 44.8). Likewise, this trial is also an opportunity to assess whether gene expression signatures can

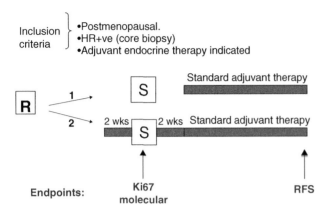

Figure 44.8 Design of the UK Pre-operative Endocrine Therapy Individualising Care (POETIC) study. *Abbreviations*: RFS, relapse-free survival.

identify a patient with a responding ER-positive breast cancer more effectively than the Ki-67 index.

Preventing Endocrine Resistance: Novel Combinations

While predicting response or resistance to adjuvant endocrine therapy may be helpful, it still leaves unanswered questions about what molecular pathways cause endocrine resistance, and how in future this may be overcome or prevented. In recent years a clear rationale has developed for combining signal transduction inhibitors (STIs) with endocrine therapies, not only to enhance endocrine responsiveness, but also to delay the emergence of acquired resistance to hormonal therapy. Continuous exposure to endocrine therapy over time with either tamoxifen or estrogen deprivation, permits ER signaling in breast cancer to become more dependent on alternate growth factor signaling pathways, allowing cells to escape the antiproliferative effects of endocrine therapy alone. This mechanism undoubtedly may be the cause of relapse during adjuvant endocrine therapy in a number of cases.

Preclinical studies to investigate mechanisms of resistance to estrogen deprivation have demonstrated persistence of an active ER pathway (83). A number of intracellular signaling pathways may "cross-talk" and activate ER including the HER family pathway (84), and the phosphatidylinositol 3-kinase (PI3K)/ Akt/ mammalian target of rapamycin (mTOR) pathway (85). These findings have led to much interest in the concept of combining various growth factor receptor antagonists or signaling inhibitors with AIs to enhance endocrine responsiveness and delay, or even reverse resistance. To date, attempts to combine AIs with the EGFR tyrosine kinase inhibitor (TKI) gefitinib or the HER2 targeted TKI lapatinib in ER-positive HER2-negative breast cancer have been disappointing in unselected patients (86–89). This approach only appears to be successful when there is known dual target expression (i.e., ER-positive; HER2 positive) (89,90).

The most notable success in this area has been the BOLERO-2 study, which represents the single most significant development in this field (91). In this phase III randomized trial, 724 patients with ER-positive advanced breast cancer were enrolled, all of whom had evidence of recurrence or progression while receiving prior nonsteroidal AI therapy. BOLERO-2 addressed the treatment of ER-positive breast cancer that had developed acquired endocrine resistance to a nonsteroidal AI. The response to exemestane alone as the control arm was very similar to the

data seen in the previous EFECT study of fulvestrant versus exemestane (92), namely a median PFS (centrally assessed) of only 4.1 months. In contrast, those treated with the combination of everolimus and exemestane had a median PFS of 10.6 months. The objective response rate was significantly better for the combination (7% *vs.* 0.4%, p < 0.001), although grade 3/4 adverse events, particularly stomatitis (8% *vs.* 1%), were more common in the combination group.

The magnitude of the clinical benefit seen for the addition of everolimus to endocrine therapy with exemestane was substantial, probably because this trial correctly identified the best group of patients to target with the combination (those with acquired endocrine resistance following prior hormonal responsiveness). The challenge is to ascertain how these findings can be translated into the early breast cancer setting, and how those patients with ER-positive breast cancer at risk of developing resistance to estrogen deprivation can be identified from the outset. Preclinical experiments have already shown that PI3K/Akt/mTOR intracellular signaling can become activated during long-term estrogen deprivation (85). However, there will probably be a few untreated ER-positive tumors that may already have an activated pathway which could cause "de-novo" endocrine resistance and an early relapse during adjuvant endocrine therapy. Therefore, in theory these cases could represent those who may benefit very well from the combination. In a phase II neoadjuvant study of letrozole plus everolimus, some patients had ER-positive tumors with activated PIK3CA mutations at exon 9; in these tumors the combination of letrozole plus everolimus had a significantly greater antiproliferative effect than letrozole alone (93).

More research on biomarker selection is urgently needed to confirm these findings in untreated ER-positive breast cancer. Adjuvant studies involving appropriate combinations of signaling agents with endocrine therapy are being planned, but will only succeed if those ER-positive tumors that are destined to relapse early can be identified at the time of primary diagnosis. It is likely that either multigene signatures or assays used to identify key oncogenic abnormalities in relevant pathways will be used to select these patients for such trials. Affirmative results will represent a significant further step in advances that have been made with adjuvant endocrine therapy over the last 20–30 years. These novel hormonal systemic strategies may in turn improve cure rates in ER-positive early breast cancer.

CONCLUSION

Hormonal systemic therapies for early-stage breast cancer have had the biggest single impact on enhancing survival from the disease, with tamoxifen alone being responsible for saving many thousands of lives. In postmenopausal women, enormous progress has been made by incorporation of estrogen deprivation with AIs into the treatment of early-stage ER-positive breast cancer. Large well-conducted trials have established "upfront" or "switch" strategies that are now widely used in clinical practice. Increasingly, extended adjuvant therapy is being considered, as "longer may be better" for some women who have an ongoing risk of recurrence beyond year five. For others "less may be more" and molecular profiling may inform us of those women who do not need chemotherapy. As such, we are refining how to use our therapies beyond the "one strategy fits all" approach of yesteryear. Endocrine therapy will continue to evolve, and current research is now exploring novel approaches to enhance endocrine responsiveness even further through combination approaches with novel targeted therapies.

REFERENCES

1. Kumar V, Green S, Stack G, et al. Functional domains of the human estrogen receptor. Cell 1987; 51: 941–51.
2. Tzukerman MT, Esty A, Santisomere D, et al. Human estrogen receptor transcriptional capacity is determined by both cellular and promoter context and mediated by two functionally distinct intramolecular regions. Mol Endocrinol 1994; 8: 21–30.
3. Johnston SRD. Endocrine Manipulation in advanced breast cancer - recent advances with SERMs therapies. Clin Cancer Res 2001; 4376–87.
4. Wakeling AE. Similarities and distinctions in the mode of action of different classes of antioestrogens. Endocr Relat Cancer 2000; 7: 17–28.
5. Dauvois S, Daniellan PS, White R, et al. Antiestrogen ICI 164,384 reduces cellular estrogen content by increasing its turnover. Proc Natl Acad Sci USA 1992; 89: 4037–41.
6. Parker MG. Action of pure antiestrogens in inhibiting estrogen receptor function. Breast Cancer Res Treat 1993; 26: 131–7.
7. Johnston SRD. Fulvestrant and the sequential endocrine cascade for advanced breast cancer. Br J Cancer 2004; s15–18.
8. Cole MP, Jones CTA, Todd IDH, et al. A new antiestrogenic agent for breast cancer; an early appraisal of ICI 46,474. Br J Cancer 1971; 270–5.
9. Osborne CL, Hobbs K, Clark GM, et al. Effects of estrogens and antiestrogens on growth of human breast cancer cells in athymic nude mice. Cancer Res 1985; 584–90.
10. Jordan VC, Robinson SP. Species specific pharmacology of antiestrogens; role of metabolism. Fed Proc 1987; 46: 1870–4.
11. Gottardis MM, Ricchio MD, Satyaswaroop PG, et al. Effect of steroidal and nonsteroidal antiestrogens on the growth of a tamoxifen-stimulated human endometrial carcinoma (EnCa101) in athymic mice. Cancer Res 1990; 50: 3189–92.
12. Love RR, Cameron L, Connell BL, et al. Symptoms associated with tamoxifen-treatment in postmenopausal women. Arch Intern Med 1991; 151: 1842–7.
13. Rutquivst LE, Mattsson A. Cardiac and thrombembolic morbidity among postmenopausal women with early-stage breast cancer in randomised trials of adjuvant tamoxifen. J Natl Cancer Inst 1993; 85: 1398–406.
14. Love RR, Mazess RB, Barden HS, et al. Effects of tamoxifen on bone mineral density in postmenopausal women with breast cancer. N Engl J Med 1992; 326: 852–6.
15. Powles TJ, Hickish T, Kanis JA, et al. Effect of tamoxifen on bone mineral density measured by dual-energy x-ray absorptiometry in healthy premenopausal and postmenopausal women. J Clin Oncol 1996; 14: 78–84.
16. Fisher B, Costantini JP, Redmond CK, et al. Endometrial cancer in tamoxifen-treated breast cancer patients; findings from the National Surgical Adjuvant Breast and Bowel Project (NSABP) B-14. J Natl Cancer Inst 1994; 86: 527–37.
17. Early Breast Cancer Trilaists Group. Tamoxifen for Early Breast Cancer; an overview of the randomised trials. Lancet 1998; 351: 1451–67.
18. Fisher B, Costantini JP, Redmond CK, et al. Endometrial cancer in tamoxifen-treated breast cancer patients; findings from the National Surgical Adjuvant Breast and Bowel Project (NSABP) B-14. J Natl Cancer Inst 1994; 86: 527–37.
19. Osborne CK, Fuqua SAW. Mechanisms of tamoxifen resistance. Breast Cancer Res Treat 1994; 32: 49–55.
20. Johnston SRD. Acquired tamoxifen resistance in human breast cancer; potential mechanisms and clinical implications. Anticancer Drugs 1997; 8: 911–30.
21. Early Breast Cancer Trialists' Collaborative Group (EBCTCG). Effects of chemotherapy and hormonal therapy for early breast cancer on recurrence and 15-year survival: an overview of the randomised trials. Lancet 2005; 365: 1687–717.
22. Dignam JJ, Dukic V, Anderson SJ, et al. Hazard of recurrence and adjuvant treatment effects over time in lymph node negative breast cancer. Breast Cancer Res Treat 2009; 116: 595–602.
23. Early Breast Cancer Trialists' Collaborative Group (EBCTCG). Relevance of breast cancer hormone receptors and other factors to the efficacy of adjuvant tamoxifen: patient-level meta-analysis of randomised trials. Lancet 2011; 378: 771–84.
24. Fisher B, Dignam J, Bryant J, Wolmark N. Five versus more than five years of tamoxifen for lymph node-negative breast cancer: updated findings from the National Surgical Adjuvant Breast and Bowel Project B-14 randomized trial. J Natl Cancer Inst 2001; 93: 684–90.
25. Peto R. ATLAS (Adjuvant Tamoxifen, Longer Against Shorter); international rndomised trial of 10 versus 5 years of adjuvant tamoxifen among 11 500 women - preliminary results. San Antonio Breast Cancer Symposium; 2007; Late breaking abstract 48.
26. Gray RG, Rea DW, Handley A, et al. aTTom (adjuvant tamoxifen- to offer more?): Randomised trial of 10 versus 5 years of adjuvant tamoxifen among 6,934 women with etrogen receptor positive (ER+) or ER untested breast cancer- preliminary results. J Clin Oncol 2008; 26: abstract 513.
27. Smith IE, Dowsett M. Aromatase inhibitors in breast cancer. N Engl J Med 2003; 2431–42.
28. Longcope C, Baker R, Johnston CC Jr. Androgen and estrogen metabolism: relationship to obesity. Metabolism 1986; 35: 235–7.
29. Lamb HM, Adkins JC. Letrozole. A review of its use in postmenopausal women with advanced breast cancer. Drugs 1998; 56: 1125–40.
30. Wiseman LR, Adkins JC. Anastrozole. A review of its use in the management of postmenopausal women with advanced breast cancer. Drugs Aging 1998; 13: 321–32.
31. Lonning PE. Pharmacological profiles of exemestane and formestane, steroidal aromatase inhibitors used for treatment of postmenopausal breast cancer. Breast Cancer Res Treat 1998; 49: S45–52.
32. Buzdar A, Jonat W, Howell A, et al. Anastrozole, a potent and selective aromatase inhibitor, versus megestrol acetate in postmenopausal women with advanced breast cancer: results of overview analysis of two phase III trials. Arimidex Study Group. J Clin Oncol 1996; 14: 2000–11.
33. Dombernowsky P, Smith I, Falkson G, et al. Letrozole, a new oral aromatase inhibitor for advanced breast cancer: double-blind randomized trial showing a dose effect and improved efficacy and tolerability compared with megestrol acetate. J Clin Oncol 1998; 16: 453–61.
34. Kaufmann M, Bajetta E, Dirix LY, et al. Exemestane is superior to megestrol acetate after tamoxifen failure in postmenopausal women with advanced breast cancer: results of a phase III randomized double-blind trial. The Exemestane Study Group. J Clin Oncol 2000; 18: 1399–411.
35. Hamilton A, Piccart M. The third-generation non-steroidal aromatase inhibitors: a review of their clinical benefits in the second-line hormonal treatment of advanced breast cancer. Ann Oncol 1999; 10: 377–84.
36. Geisler J, Haynes B, Anker G, Dowsett M, Lonning PE. Influence of letrozole and anastrozole on total body aromatization and plasma estrogen levels in postmenopausal breast cancer patients evaluated in a randomized, Cross-Over Study. J Clin Oncol 2002; 20: 751–7.
37. Rose C, Vtoraya O, Pluzanska A, et al. Letrozole (Femara) vs anastrozole (Arimidex): second-line treatment in postmenopausal women with advanced breast cancer. Proc Am Soc Clin Oncol 2002; 21: abstract 131.
38. Dowsett M, Cuzick J, Ingle J, et al. Meta-analysis of breast cancer outcomes in adjuvant trials or aromatase inhibitors vs tamoxifen. J Clin Oncol 2010; 509–18.
39. Burstein HJ, Prestrud AA, Seidenfeld J, et al. American Society of Clinical Oncology Clinical Practice Guideline: update on adjuvant endocrine therapy for women with hormone-receptor-positive breast cancer. J Clin Oncol 2010; 28: 3784–96.
40. The ATAC Trialists Group. Anastrozole alone or in combination with tamoxifen versus tamoxifen alone for adjuvant treatmnet of postmenopausal women with early breast cancer: first results of the ATAC randomised trial. Lancet 2002; 359: 2131–9.
41. The Arimidex, Tamoxifen, Alone or in combination (ATAC) Trialists' Group. Effect of anastrozole and tamoxifen as adjuvant treatment for early-stage breast cancer: 100-month analysis of the ATAC trial. Lancet Oncol 2008; 9: 45–53.
42. Cuzick J, Sestak I, Baum M, et al. Effect of anastrozole and tamoxifen as adjuvant treatment for early stage breast cancer: 10-year analysis of the ATAC trial. Lancet Oncol 2010; 11: 1135–41.
43. The ATAC (Arimidex, Tamoxifen, Alone or in Combination) Trialists' Group. Anastrozole alone or in combination with Tamoxifen versus Tamoxifen alone for adjuvanat treatment of postmenopausal women with early stage breast cancer. Cancer 2003; 98: 1802–10.
44. Eastell R, Adams JE, Coleman RE, et al. Effect of anastrozole on bone mineral density; 5-year resulst from the anastrozole, tamoxifen, alone or in combination trial 18233230. J Clin Oncol 2008; 26: 1051–8.

45. The Breast International Group (BIG) 1-98 Collaborative Group. A comparison of letrozole and tamoxifen in postmenopausal women with early breast cancer. N Engl J Med 2005; 353: 2747–57.

46. The BIG 1-98 Collaborative Group. Letrozole therapy alone or in sequence with tamoxifen in women with breast cancer. N Engl J Med 2009; 766–76.

47. Coombes RC, Hall E, Gibson LJ, et al. A randomised trial of exemestane after two to three years of tamoxifen therapy in postmenopausal women with primary breast cancer. N Engl J Med 2004; 1081–92.

48. Coombes RC, Kilburn LS, Snowdon CF, et al. Survival and safety of exemestane versus tamoxifen after 2-3 years' tamoxifen treatment (Intergroup Exemestane Study): a randomised controlled trial. Lancet 2007; 369: 559–70.

49. Jackesz R, Jonat W, Gnant M, et al. Switching of postmenopausal women with endocrine-responsive early breast cancer to anastrozole after 2 years adjuvant tamoxifen; combined resulst of ABCSG trial 8 and ARNO 95 trial. Lancet 2005; 366: 455–62.

50. Boccardo F, Rubagotti A, Puntoni M, et al. Switching to anastrozole versus continued tamoxifen treatment of early breast cancer. preliminary results of the Italian Tamoxifen Anastrozole (ITA) trial. J Clin Oncol 2005; 23: 5138–47.

51. Jonat W, Gnant M, Boccardo F, et al. Effectiveness of switching form adjuvant tamoxifen to anastrozole in postmenopausal women with hormone-sensitive early-stage breast cancer: a meta-analysis. Lancet Oncol 2006; 7: 991–6.

52. Van de Velde CJH, Rea D, Seynaeve C, et al. Adjuvant tamoxifen and exemestane in early breast cancer (TEAM): a randomised phase 3 trial. Lancet 2011; 377: 321–31.

53. Dowsett M, Allred C, Knox J, et al. Relationship between quantitative estrogen and progesterone receptor expression and human epidermal growth factor 2 (HER-2) status with recurrence in the Arimidex, Tamoxifen, Alone or in Combination Trial. J Clin Oncol 2008; 26: 1059–65.

54. Viale G, Regan MM, Maiorano E, et al. Prognostic and predictive value of centrally reviewed expression of estrogen and progesterone receptors in a randomised trial comparing letrozole and tamoxifen adjuvant therapy for postmenopausal early breast cancer: BIG 1-98. J Clin Oncol 2007; 25: 3846–52.

55. Bartlett JMS, Brookes CL, Billingham LJ, et al. A prospectively planned pathology study within the TEAM trial confirms that progesterone receptor expression is prognostic, but is not predictive for differentail response to exemestane vs tamoxifen. SABCS. 2008.

56. Viale G, Giobbie-Harder A, Regan MM, et al. Prognostic and predictive value of centrally reviewed Ki-67 labelling index in postmenopausal women with endocrine-responsive breast cancer: results form Breast International Group trial 1-98 comparing adjuvant tamoxifen with letrozole. J Clin Oncol 2008; 26: 5569–75.

57. Dowsett M, Cuzick J, Wale C, et al. Prediction of risk of distant recurrence using the 21-gene recurrence score in node-negative and node-positive postmenopausal patients with breast cancer treated with anastrozole or tamoxifen: a TransATAC study. J Clin Oncol 2010; 28: 1829–34.

58. Buzdar A, Howell A, Cuzick J, et al. Comprehensive side-effect profile of anastrozole and tamoxifen as adjuvant treatment for early-stage breast cancer: long-term safety analysis of the ATAC trial. Lancet Oncol 2006; 7: 633–43.

59. Hillner BE, Ingle JN, Chlebowski RT, et al. American Society of Clinical Oncology 2003 update on the role of bisphosphonates and bone health issues in women with breast cancer. J Clin Oncol 2003; 21: 4042–57.

60. Goss PE, Ingle JN, Chapman J-AW, et al. Final analysis of NCIC MA.27; a randomised phase III trial of exemestane versus anastrozole in postmenopausal women with hormone receptor positive primary breast cancer. Presented at San Antonio Breast Cancer Symposium 2010; abstract S1-1.

61. Goss PE, Ingle JN, Martino S, et al. A randomized trial of letrozole in postmenopausal women after five years of tamoxifen therapy for early-stage breast cancer. N Engl J Med 2003; 349: 1793–802.

62. Goss PE, Ingle JN, Martino S, et al. Randomised trial of letrozole following tamoxifen as extended adjuvant therapy in receptor-positive breast cancer: updated findings from NCIC CTG MA.17. J Natl Cancer Inst 2005; 97: 1262–71.

63. Goss PE, Ingle JN, Martino S, et al. Efficacy of letrozole extended adjuavnt therapy according to estrogen receptor and progesterone receptor status of the primary tumour: National Cancer Institute of Canada Trials Group MA.17. J Clin Oncol 2006; 25: 2006–11.

64. Goss PE, Ingle JN, Pater JL, et al. Late extended adjuvant treatment with letrozole improved outcome in women with early stage breast cancer who completes 5 years of tamoxifen. J Clin Oncol 2008; 26: 1948–55.

65. Jakesz R, Greil R, Gnant M, et al. Extended adjuvant therapy with anastrozole among postmenopausal breast cancer patients; results from the randomised Austrian Breast and Colorectal Cancer Study Group Trial 6a. J Natl Cancer Inst 2007; 99: 1845–53.

66. Mamounas EP, Jeong J-H, Wickerham L, et al. Benefit from exemestane as extended adjuvant therapy after 5 years of adjuvant tamoxifen; intention-to-treat analysis of the National Surgical Adjuvant Breast and Bowel Project B-33 Trial. J Clin Oncol 2008; 26: 1965–71.

67. Davidson NE, O'Neill AM, Vukov AM, et al. Chemoendocrine therapy for pre-menopausal women with axillary lymph-node positive, steroid hormone receptor positive breast cancer: resulst from INT 0101 (E5188). J Clin Oncol 2005; 23: 2973–82.

68. International Breast Cancer Study Group. Adjuvant chemotherapy followed by goserelin versus either modality alone for pre-menopausal lymph node negative breast cancer - a randomised trial. J Natl Cancer Inst 2003; 95: 1833–46.

69. Cuzick J, Ambroisine L, Davidson N, et al. Use of luteinising-hormone-releasing hormone agonists as adjuvant treatment in premenopausal patients with hormone-receptor-positive breast cancer: a meta-analysis of individual patient data from randomised adjuvant trials. Lancet 2007; 369: 1711–23.

70. Sotiriou C, Pusztai L. Gene expression signatures in breast cancer. N Engl J Med 2009; 360: 790–800.

71. Ravdin PM, Siminoff LA, Davis GJ, et al. Computer program to assist in making decisions about adjuvant therapy for women with early breast cancer. J Clin Oncol 2001; 19: 980–91.

72. Goldhirsch A, Wood WC, Gelber RD, et al. 10th St Gallen conference. Progress and promise; highlights of the international expert consensus on the primary therapy of early breast cancer 2007. Ann Oncol 2007; 18: 1133–44.

73. Goldhirsch A, Ingle JN, Gelber RD, et al. Panel members. Thresholds for therapies; highlights of the international expert consensus on the primary therapy of early breast cancer 2009. Ann Oncol 2009; 20: 1319–29.

74. Goldhirsch A, Wood WC, Coates RD, et al. Strategies for subtypes - dealing with the diversity of breast cancer; highlights of the St Galen International Expert Consensus on the Primary Therapy of Early Breast Cancer 2011. Ann Oncol 2011; 22: 1736–47.

75. Dowsett M, Nielsen TO, A'Hern R, et al. Ki-67 in breast cancer: recommendations from the International Ki-67 Breast Cancer Working Group. J Natl Cancer Inst 2011; 103: 1656–64.

76. Cheang MCU, Chia SK, Voduc D, et al. Ki-67 index, HER2 status, and prognosis of patients with luminal B breast cancer. J Natl Cancer Inst 2009; 101: 736–50.

77. Sotoriou C, Wirapati P, Loi S, et al. Gene expression profiling in breast cancer: understanding teh molecular basis of histiligical grade to improve prognosis. J Natl Cancer Inst 2006; 98: 262–72.

78. Loi S, Haibe-Kains B, Desmedt C, et al. Definition of clinically distinct molecular subtypes in estrogen receptor-positive breast carcinomas through genomic grade. J Clin Oncol 2007; 25: 1239–46.

79. Paik S, Shak S, Tang G, et al. A multigene assay to predict recurrence of tamoxifen-treated, node-negative breast cancer. N Engl J Med 2004; 351: 2817–26.

80. Albain K, Barlow WE, Shak S, et al. Prognostic and predictive value of the 21-gene recurrence score assay in postmenopausal women with node-positive, oestrogen-receptor positive breast cancer on chemotherapy; a retrospective analsysi of a randomised trial. Lancet Oncol 2010; 11: 55–65.

81. Lo SS, Mumby PB, Norton J, et al. Prospective multicenter study of the impact of the 21-gene recurrence score assay on medical oncologist and patient adjuvant breast cancer treatment selection. J Clin Oncol 2010; 28: 1671–6.

82. Dowsett M, Smith IE, Ebbs SR, et al. Prognostic value of Ki-67 expression after short-term pre-surgical endocrine therapy for primary breast cancer. J Natl Cancer Inst 2007; 99: 167–70.

83. Martin LA, Farmer I, Johnston SR, et al. Enhanced estrogen receptor (ER) alpha, ERBB2, and MAPK signal transduction pathways operate during the adaptation of MCF-7 cells to long term estrogen deprivation. J Biol Chem 2003; 278: 30458–68.

84. Nicholson RI, McClelland RA, Robertson JF, Gee JM. Involvement of steroid hormone and growth factor cross-talk in endocrine response in breast cancer. Endocr Relat Cancer 1999; 6: 373–87.

85. Campbell RA, Bhat-Nakshatri P, Patel NM, et al. Phosphatidylinositol 3-kinase/AKT-mediated activation of estrogen receptor alpha: a new model for anti-estrogen resistance. J Biol Chem 2001; 276: 9817–24.

86. Smith IE, Walsh G, Skene A, et al. A phase II placebo-controlled trial of neo-adjuvant anastrozole alone or with gefitinib in early breast cancer. J Clin Oncol 2007; 25: 3816–22.

87. Osborne CK, Neven P, Dirix LY, et al. Gefitinib or placebo in combination with tamoxifen in patients with hormone receptor-positive metastatic breast cancer: a randomized phase II study. Clin Cancer Res 2011; 17: 1147–59.

88. Cristofanilli M, Valero V, Mangalik A, et al. Phase II, randomized trial to compare anastrozole combined with gefitinib or placebo in postmenopausal women with hormone receptor-positive metastatic breast cancer. Clin Cancer Res 2010; 16: 1904–14.

89. Johnston SRD, Pippen J, Pivot X, et al. Lapatinib combined with letrozole versus letrozole and placebo as first-line therapy for postmenopausal hormone-receptor-positive metastatic breast cancer. J Clin Oncol 2009; 27: 5538–846.

90. Kaufman B, Mackey JR, Clemens MR, et al. Trastuzumab plus anastrozole versus anastrozole alone for the treatment of postmenopausal women with human epidermal growth factor receptor 2-positive, hormone receptor-positive metastatic breast cancer: results form the randomized TAnDEM study. J Clin Oncol 2009; 27: 5529–37.

91. Baselga J, Campone M, Piccart M, et al. Everolimus in postmenopausal hormone-receptor-positive advanced breast cancer. N Engl J Med 2012; 366: 520–9.

92. Chia S, Gradishar W, Mauriac L, et al. Double-blind, randomised placebo controlled trial of fulvestrant compared with exemestane after prior non-steroidal aromatase inhibitor therapy in postmenopausal women with hormone receptor positive advanced breast cancer: results form EFECT. J Clin Oncol 2008; 26: 1664–70.

93. Baselga J, Semiglazov V, Van Dam P, et al. Phase II randomised study of neo-adjuvant everolimus plus letrozole compared with placebo plus letrozole in patients with estrogen receptor-positive breast cancer. J Clin Oncol 2009; 27: 2630–7.

45 Adjuvant chemotherapy and biological therapies for early-stage breast cancer

Sausan Abouharb and Francisco J. Esteva

Breast cancer cells can metastasize early in tumor development, resulting in disease recurrence at distant sites even if the primary tumor and regional lymph nodes are eradicated completely by surgery and radiotherapy. Understanding breast cancer as a systemic disease dates back to laboratory and clinical studies conducted in the 1960s and 1970s (1,2). Bonadonna et al. (3) completed a landmark clinical trial in which 12 months of combination chemotherapy consisting of cyclophosphamide, methotrexate, and fluorouracil was evaluated as adjuvant treatment for patients who had undergone radical mastectomy for primary breast cancer with positive axillary lymph nodes. Follow-up showed a significant drop in rates of recurrence and increases in both disease-free survival (DFS) and overall survival (OS) rates (4).

Since then many studies have evaluated the role of adjuvant cytotoxic chemotherapy in the treatment of early breast cancer. Evidence supporting the role of adjuvant chemotherapy was presented in the Oxford overview completed by the Early Breast Cancer Trialists' Collaborative Group (EBCTCG) (5). This report was the result of a meta-analysis of data from more than 100,000 women with early breast cancer in 123 randomized trials comparing polychemotherapy versus no chemotherapy as well as different polychemotherapy regimens. The Oxford overview has concluded that women with early-stage breast cancer, who are enrolled in a clinical trial, benefit from adjuvant chemotherapy. It has also determined that anthracycline- and taxane-based regimens provide higher efficacy than alkylator-based chemotherapy. Furthermore, the addition of taxane increases the effectiveness of anthracycline-based chemotherapy (Fig. 45.1).

European and North American guidelines recommend adjuvant chemotherapy for patients with positive axillary lymph node disease (who are otherwise healthy) and for patients with negative lymph nodes whose tumors are larger than 1 cm or are associated with other adverse prognostic factors (6). Ravdin et al. (7) used actuarial analysis to project outcomes of patients who receive or do not receive adjuvant therapy. This analysis was based on the estimates of prognosis derived from the Surveillance, Epidemiology, and End Results (SEER) database for patients living in the United States together with estimates of the efficacy of adjuvant therapy based on 1998 overviews of randomized trials of adjuvant therapy (8,9). Radvin and colleagues developed a publicly available software known as Adjuvant! Online (www.adjuvantonline.com) for assessing the risks and benefits of adjuvant therapy. The program has four major components: (*i*) patient information [e.g., age, menopausal status, estrogen receptor (ER) status, tumor size, number of positive axillary lymph nodes, and comorbidities], which is used to estimate a patient's prognosis; (*ii*) estimated efficacy of endocrine therapy and chemotherapeutic regimens (i.e., cyclophosphamide, methotrexate, and fluorouracil (CMF)-like; anthracycline based, or anthracycline and taxane); (*iii*) projected outcomes of the patient's DFS and OS rates in a numerical and graphical form, based on the efficacy estimates; (*iv*) a tool bar to save patient information and print results (Fig. 45.2). Patients included in the initial program analysis had a history of invasive, unilateral, and noninflammatory disease; had undergone definitive surgery; and had undergone axillary staging with at least six nodes sampled. For inclusion in the analysis, patients must have had known information on tumor size, number of nodes, sampled, and number of nodes positive for tumor. Adjuvant! Online is a helpful tool because there are many clinical situations in which decisions can be made regarding the options of chemotherapy, endocrine therapy, both, or no additional therapy. Regardless, the anticipated degree of benefit cannot be completely known for each patient, preventing her from being able to make a truly informed decision.

The fundamental purpose of Adjuvant! Online is to estimate the individualized net benefit that could be gained from an adjuvant systemic therapy by estimating a patient's reduced risk of negative outcomes (i.e., death or disease relapse). Estimates of prognosis are generated from SEER data, whereas estimates of therapy efficacy are based on the proportional risk reductions from the 1998 overview summary (8,9). For example, if a woman has a 60% risk of dying of breast cancer at 10-year follow-up and can be given adjuvant therapy to achieve a proportional risk reduction of 25%, her breast cancer mortality rate will be reduced by 15% (60% × 25%). The 15% mortality rate would thus reduce her annual risk of breast cancer-related death from 8.8% to 6.6%.

A limitation of Adjuvant! Online is that it does not take into account the human epidermal growth factor receptor 2 (HER2) status of the patient's primary tumor. Now that trastuzumab monoclonal antibody therapy for HER2-overexpressing breast cancer is available, the choice of adjuvant chemotherapy is currently based on the HER2 status of the primary tumor. Therefore, the predictive utility of Adjuvant! Online is more relevant for patients with HER2-negative tumors. Another limitation of Adjuvant! Online is its reliance on the SEER database, which does not collect information about which adjuvant therapy was used, relapse status, or reliable cause of death. In addition, estimates of breast cancer-related mortality are derived indirectly from total survival after adjustment for expected age-adjusted natural mortality.

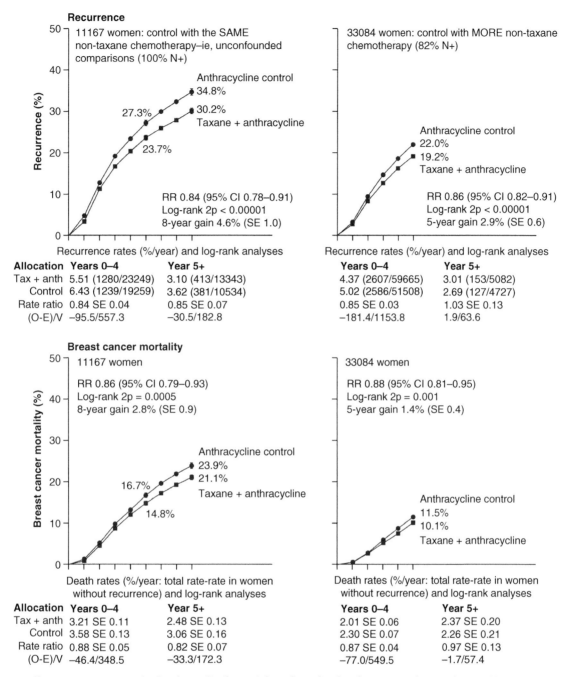

Figure 45.1 Rates of breast cancer recurrence (top) and mortality (bottom) for anthracycline-based regimens with taxane (Tax+anth) or without taxane (control). Control treatment usually consisted of four cycles of anthracycline and cyclophosphamide (left); some women received additional cycles of non-taxane chemotherapy (right). *Source*: From Ref. (5).

In this chapter we summarize the clinical trials that have been conducted to address the drug types, doses, and schedules; number of drugs; and treatment duration used for adjuvant chemotherapy candidates regardless of ER, progesterone (PR), or HER2 status. We then discuss a more targeted approach to the treatment of patients with breast cancer that is ER positive, PR positive, or both; HER2 positive; or triple negative. Finally, we discuss novel therapies in development.

CMF THERAPY

The first randomized trial of adjuvant chemotherapy was launched in Milan by Dr Gianni Bonadonna and collaborators in the early 1970s. Results from three successive trials of CMF versus observation for patients with node-positive breast cancer at the time of mastectomy revealed reduced relative risks (RRs) of

relapse [hazard ratio (HR) 0.71, 95% CI 0.56–0.91, P = 0.005] and death (HR 0.79, 95% CI 0.63–0.98, P = 0.04) among patients who had been treated with 6 or 12 cycles of CMF (4). Because the 12-cycle CMF treatment was just as efficacious as the six-cycle one, the latter became routinely used worldwide for patients with early-stage breast cancer (4).

By the early 1980s, the "classical" CMF regimen had become the standard adjuvant chemotherapy for treatment of early-stage breast cancer. Designed to resemble the mustargen, oncovin, procarbazine, prednisone (MOPP) combination therapy used to treat Hodgkin's disease (10), the CMF regimen (oral 100 mg/m² cyclophosphamide on days 1–14, intravenous 40 mg/m² methotrexate on days 1 and 8, and intravenous 600 mg/m² 5-fluorouracil on days 1 and 8) was given every four weeks. The rationale for using this combination emerged

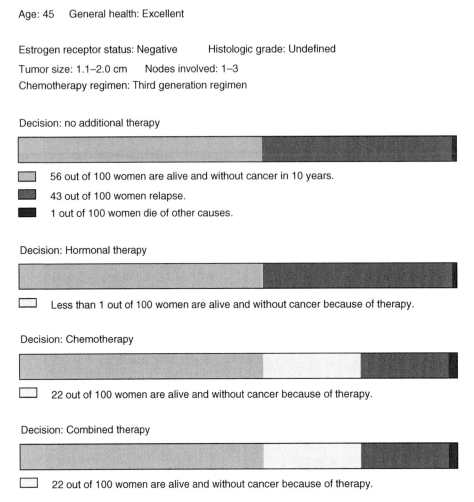

Age: 45   General health: Excellent

Estrogen receptor status: Negative   Histologic grade: Undefined

Tumor size: 1.1–2.0 cm   Nodes involved: 1–3

Chemotherapy regimen: Third generation regimen

Decision: no additional therapy

- 56 out of 100 women are alive and without cancer in 10 years.
- 43 out of 100 women relapse.
- 1 out of 100 women die of other causes.

Decision: Hormonal therapy

- Less than 1 out of 100 women are alive and without cancer because of therapy.

Decision: Chemotherapy

- 22 out of 100 women are alive and without cancer because of therapy.

Decision: Combined therapy

- 22 out of 100 women are alive and without cancer because of therapy.

Figure 45.2 Example of Adjuvant! Online report.

from the fact that these drugs were non–cross-resistant and that each was moderately effective as a single agent in treating advanced breast cancer. The EORTC Breast Cancer Cooperative Group discussed several aspects of this schedule (11). Fourteen days of cyclophosphamide tablets could cause nausea and vomiting, especially when higher doses (150–200 mg/m^2) were used, and some patients would not comply with the cyclophosphamide regimen. The variability in patients' ability to absorb oral medication and uncertainties about bioavailability were additional concerns. The bone marrow suppression that can occur with the use of methotrexate and fluorouracil was a concern as well.

In a trial conducted by Engelsman et al. (11), 254 patients with advanced breast cancer were randomly allocated to receive the classical CMF schedule or a modified schedule (600 mg/m^2 cyclophosphamide, 40 mg/m^2 methotrexate, and 600 mg/m^2 5-fluorouracil all given intravenously on day 1 every three weeks). The objective response rates for the classical and modified CMF regimens were 48% and 29%, respectively (P = 0.003); median duration of response was 11 months for both regimens. Time to progression and median survival time were longer in the classical CMF arm. Mucositis and alopecia were encountered more frequently when the cyclophosphamide was taken orally, but nausea and vomiting were more troublesome when it was given intravenously. The overall improved results seen with the classical CMF schedule were likely due to the higher dose intensity achieved per unit of time as well as to better tolerability.

Over the years, various CMF-like regimens have been developed with different dosages, routes, and schedules (Table 45.1). That being said, there have been no randomized trials directly comparing exclusively intravenous CMF on days 1 and 8, to the classic regimen that includes oral cyclophosphamide days 1–14 in addition to IV 5-FU and methotrexate on days 1 and 8. Currently there is no evidence that cyclophosphamide has different toxicities or effectiveness when administered orally and intravenously (12). A review (13) of the history of CMF (dating back almost 30 years) has pointed to the great success of this combination therapy, which remained unchallenged until the mid-1980s when anthracyclines appeared, and then again in the 1990s when taxanes entered the field.

The Early Breast Cancer Trialists' Collaborative Group conducted a meta-analysis of CMF-based (first generation) and anthracycline-based (second generation) regimens. That overview showed that compared with CMF schedules, anthracycline-based regimens produced a 12% proportional reduction in risk recurrence (P = 0.006; absolute benefit 3.2%) and an 11% proportional reduction in risk of mortality (P = 0.02; absolute benefit 2.7%) (8). However, the patient population in this meta-analysis included both pre- and postmenopausal women (about 70% of the women in this analysis were younger than 50 years) with hormone receptor–positive or –negative disease. As a specific example, among the women younger than 50 years, there was a 13% reduction in risk of recurrence (P = 0.01) and a nonsignificant (P = 0.09) reduction in risk of

Table 45.1 Adjuvant Chemotherapy Regimens Recommended for HER2-Negative Breast Cancer

Regimen	Comments
Third Generation	
AC-T	Dose-dense AC followed by paclitaxel, every 2 wks; doxorubicin as the anthracycline
AC-T	Four cycles of AC followed by 12 cycles of weekly paclitaxel
TC	Four cycles; docetaxel as the taxane
First and Second Generation	
AC	Doxorubicin as the anthracycline
FAC, CAF	Doxorubicin as the anthracycline
FEC, CEF	
CMF	
AC-T	AC followed by docetaxel, every 3 wks
EC	
A-T-C	Doxorubicin followed by paclitaxel followed by cyclophosphamide, every 2 wks, with filgrastim support
FEC-T	FEC followed by docetaxel or by weekly paclitaxel

Abbreviations: A, anthracycline; C, cyclophosphamide or carboplatin; E, epirubicin; F, fluorouracil; H, trastuzumab; M, methotrexate; T, taxane.

mortality with anthracycline-based regimens compared with CMF schedules (9).

Comparisons of CMF regimens with taxane-based (third generation) regimens in the adjuvant setting have not been conclusive which is mainly attributable to no direct comparison having been performed to date.

The National Surgical Adjuvant Breast and Bowel Program (NSABP) is a large cooperative group in the United States led by Dr Bernard Fisher (14). NSABP randomized trials, B-13 and B-19, evaluated CMF regimens and regimens with only methotrexate and fluorouracil for their effectiveness in treating women with ER-negative, node-negative tumors. Among patients younger than 49 years, CMF clearly resulted in better DFS and OS. For patients older than 50 years differences in effectiveness were less clear, although both types of regimens were beneficial.

Follow-up of Trial MA5 of the National Cancer Institute of Canada's Clinical Trials Group (15) demonstrated that patients with HER2-enriched tumors derived a greater benefit from cyclophosphamide, epirubicin, and fluorouracil (CEF) than CMF. On the other hand, patients with chemotherapy-sensitive, basal-like tumors received no added benefit from CEF over CMF, suggesting that a non-anthracycline regimen may be adequate for treating this tumor subtype (HR 1.1 for relapse-free survival and 1.3 for OS).

The International Breast Cancer Study Group Trials VIII and IX enrolled 2257 patients with node-negative, operable breast cancer (16). These trials compared three or six courses of a CMF regimen, endocrine therapy, and both together. Results showed that compared with patients with ER-positive disease, women with triple negative tumors (303 patients, 13% of the cohort) who had undergone chemotherapy received a statistically significantly greater benefit than those who did not (HR 0.58, 95% CI 0.29–1.17, interaction P = 0.24). In addition, the magnitude of the benefit obtained from CMF chemotherapy was the largest for patients with triple negative, node negative breast cancer (16).

Much has been discovered about CMF regimens over the past 35 years or so, including their side effects, toxicity and safety profiles, potential roles in triple negative breast cancer, and economic value. Nonetheless, more studies are needed to further evaluate their role in treating certain tumor types and to explore their use in combination with taxanes (e.g., PARP).

ANTHRACYCLINES

The anthracycline class of medication works by inhibiting DNA and RNA synthesis through intercalation between DNA base pairs and by inhibition of toposiomerase II, thereby preventing the relaxation of supercoiled DNA. The first anthracycline discovered was daunorubicin, which was shortly followed by doxorubicin. Other agents in this class include epirubicin, idarubicin, valrubicin, and mitoxantrone (17).

The first adjuvant anthracycline-based regimens incorporated fluorouracil, doxorubicin (or epirubicin), and cyclophosphamide (FAC or FEC). In one of the first clinical trials initiated at The University of Texas MD Anderson Cancer Center, 220 patients with stage II–III breast cancer were treated with FAC. At a median follow-up of 133 months, the estimated 10-year DFS rate for women with stage II or stage III disease was 58% and 36%, respectively. The corresponding 10-year OS rates were 62% and 40%, suggesting a higher OS rate compared with historical control subjects (18). Doses higher than the conventional FAC doses (500/50/500 mg/m^2 every three weeks for six cycles) did not improve outcomes (19,20).

In a comparison of FAC and CMF regimens as adjuvant chemotherapy for operable breast cancer, the former was found to be superior (21). In that study, patients had been randomly allocated to receive either FAC (500/50/500 mg/m^2) or CMF (600/60/600 mg/m^2) every three weeks for six cycles. In the prospectively formed subset of node negative patients, the rates of DFS and OS were statistically superior in the FAC arm (p = 0.041 and 0.034, respectively for DFS and OS), but this advantage was not seen with the subset of node-positive patients. The relative risks for disease recurrence and death were significantly lower with FAC than CMF treatment (recurrence: RR 1.2, P = 0.03; death: RR 1.3, P = 0.05) (21). This result was due mainly to the difference observed in the node negative population. Although the clinical toxicity of FAC was greater than that of CMF, the levels were manageable and clinically acceptable.

In the Trial MA5 of the National Cancer Institute of Canada Clinical Trials Group, 710 women with axillary node-positive breast cancer were randomly assigned to receive CEF or CMF (22). After a median follow-up of 10 years, the relapse-free survival rates were 52% and 45%, respectively (P = 0.007) and the 10-year OS rates were 62% and 58% (P = 0.085) (22), which demonstrated the benefit of using anthracyclines over first-generation chemotherapy. In the French Adjuvant Study Group 05 trial, FEC with different doses of epirubicin (50 vs. 100 mg/m²) given every three weeks to 565 women with lymph node–positive breast cancer resulted in five-year DFS rates of 55% vs. 66% (P = 0.03) and OS rates of 65% vs. 77% (P = 0.007), favoring the higher epirubicin dose (23).

The NSABP evaluated the safety and efficacy of four cycles of anthracycline (doxorubicin; 60 mg/m²) and cyclophosphamide (600 mg/m²) (AC) in the adjuvant setting. The NSABP trials B-15 and B-23 randomly allocated patients with early-stage breast cancer to four cycles of AC (three months) or six cycles of CMF (6 months). Both trials showed equivalent DFS and OS rates (24,25) and a similar quality of life (26).

Anthracyclines are the backbone of most breast cancer regimens (Table 45.1) (8,27). The overview analysis by the EBCTCG demonstrated that, compared with standard treatment with CMF, regimens incorporating doxorubicin or epirubicin reduced the annual risk of recurrence of breast cancer by 12% and the annual risk of death by 11%. In another study, six months of anthracycline-based polychemotherapy (i.e., FAC) reduced the annual breast cancer death rate by about 38% for women younger than 50 years and about 20% for those aged 50–69, irrespective of nodal status, hormonal status, and tumor characteristics (28).

Be it acute or chronic, cardiovascular toxicity is seen among patients treated with anthracyclines. More attention and focus should be given to this toxicity because some patients are now also being exposed to trastuzumab at different times during their treatment course for early breast cancer; cardiovascular toxicity is also a known side effect of trastuzumab treatment (29). Baseline and follow-up echocardiograms should be performed to monitor these patients' cardiac function; however, delayed cardiac toxicity can also occur years later. In addition, secondary acute myeloid leukemias can develop in a small percentage of women treated with anthracyclines and can be challenging to treat (30).

TAXANES

Relatively new therapeutic agents, the taxanes (i.e., paclitaxel and docetaxel) stabilize and prevent disaggregation of microtubules and disrupt the mitotic spindle, resulting in cell death (31). Taxanes have non–cross-resistance with anthracyclines and other conventional agents (32).

Taxanes have been incorporated into clinical trials. A randomized trial conducted by the Cancer and Leukemia Group B (CALGB 9344) showed that the addition of four cycles of paclitaxel after four cycles of AC (with doxorubicin) increased survival among patients with node-positive breast cancer (33). The results were similar to those of the NSABP B-28 trial, which randomly assigned 3060 patients with positive axillary nodes to receive four cycles of AC, with or without four cycles of subsequent paclitaxel (33). At a median follow-up of 64 months, the addition of paclitaxel significantly improved the five-year DFS rate (76% vs. 72%) but not the OS rate (85% for both arms) and reduced the hazard for a DFS event by 17% (P = 0.006). Moreover, levels of toxicity were considered acceptable (33).

The CALGB 9741 trial (34) evaluated dose-dense treatment versus conventional schedules as well as sequential versus concurrent combination chemotherapy, as adjuvant treatment of node-positive primary breast cancer. In the trial, 2005

female patients were randomly assigned to one of four treatment arms, with four cycles of each chemotherapeutic agent: (*i*) anthracycline followed by taxane and then cyclophosphamide, every two weeks with granulocyte-colony stimulating factor (G-CSF); (*ii*) AC followed by taxane, every two weeks with filgrastim; (*iii*) anthracycline followed by taxane and then cyclophosphamide, every three weeks; (*iv*) AC followed by taxane, every three weeks. No differences were noted between the concurrent and sequential arms. The dose-dense regimen raised the DFS rate (RR 0.74, P = 0.010) and OS rate (RR 0.69, P = 0.013), with the four-year DFS rate being 82% for the dose-dense regimens and 75% for the other three.

Trials have investigated the efficacy of more intensive anthracycline regimens, with or without docetaxel, for node-positive patients and have shown statistically significant improvements in OS for those regimens that included a taxane (35,36). In the PACS 01 trial (35), 1999 patients were randomly allocated to receive either six cycles of FEC or three cycles of FEC followed by three cycles of docetaxel. Compared with treatment schedules using FEC alone, FEC followed by docetaxel significantly improved the five-year DFS and OS rates: DFS rates were 73.2% and 78.4%, respectively (P = 0.012), and the corresponding OS rates were 86.7% and 90.7% (P = 0.017), thereby resulting in a 27% reduction in the RR of death.

ECOG E1199 was a large, four-arm trial led by the North American Intergroup that randomly assigned 4950 women to receive AC followed by a taxane (paclitaxel or docetaxel) given every one or three weeks (37). At a median follow-up of 63.8 months, no statistically significant difference in DFS or OS was observed between the taxanes or between the frequencies of administration. However, paclitaxel given weekly was superior to paclitaxel given every three weeks in terms of DFS (P = 0.006) and OS (P = 0.01). Docetaxel given every three weeks was superior to paclitaxel every three weeks for DFS (P = 0.02) but not in OS (P = 0.25) (37). On the basis of these findings, as well as those of the CALBG trial 9741 described earlier, the weekly paclitaxel regimen was recommended (6).

Large randomized trials involving treatments for metastatic breast cancer have discovered that the combination of docetaxel, the anthracycline doxorubicin, and cyclophosphamide (TAC) has antitumor activity that is superior to that of FAC, although survival is not significantly different between treatment groups (38,39). In 2005, a phase III multicenter prospective randomized trial was published that compared TAC with FAC (with doxorubicin as the anthracycline) (36). Patients with early-stage breast cancer, axillary lymph node–positive disease were randomly assigned to receive either TAC (75/50/500 mg/m²) or FAC (500/50/500 mg/m²) every three weeks for six cycles. The superiority of TAC was apparent in all planned subgroup analyses. The estimated rates of DFS at five years were 75% for the TAC group and 68% for the FAC group (P = 0.001). This difference was mainly due to the greater number of patients in the FAC group who had experienced relapse of breast cancer at distant sites. Compared with adjuvant FAC, adjuvant TAC was associated with a 28% reduction in risk of relapse after adjustment for nodal status (HR 0.72, 95% CI 0.59–0.88). The estimated OS rates at five years were 87% and 81% in the TAC and FAC groups, respectively (36). On the other hand, the incidence of grade 3 or 4 neutropenia and febrile neutropenia was significantly higher in the TAC group than in the FAC group (grade 3 or 4: 65.5% *vs.* 49.3%, P < 0.001; febrile: 24.7% *vs.* 2.5%, P < 0.001). Overall, adjuvant chemotherapy with TAC rather than FAC significantly improved the rates of DFS and OS among women with operable node-positive breast cancer, albeit at the expense of increased toxicity.

As described, TAC was found to be a superior adjuvant therapy compared with FAC among women with node-positive breast cancer. In a similar comparison, 1060 women with axillary node negative breast cancer and at least one high-risk feature for recurrence were randomly assigned to treatment with TAC (75/50/500 mg/m^2) or FAC (500/50/500 mg/m^2) every three weeks for six cycles after surgery (40). At a median follow-up of 77 months, the DFS rates were 87.8% in the TAC arm and 81.8% in the FAC arm, representing a 32% reduction in the risk of disease recurrence with TAC (HR 0.68, 95% CI 0.49–0.93, P = 0.01 by log-rank test). Subgroup analyses by receptor status, menopausal status, and the number of high-risk factors (e.g., age, tumor size, and grade) suggested that the DFS benefits of TAC over FAC were consistent with the overall study. The difference in OS rates was not significant (TAC 95.2%, FAC 93.5%, (HR 0.76; 95% CI 0.45–1.26). Rates of grade 3 and grade 4 adverse events were 28.2% for patients who received TAC and 17% for those who received FAC (p < 0.001). Neutropenic fever was observed in 9.6% and 2.3% of patients who were receiving TAC and FAC, respectively (p < 0.001). Most of the TAC-induced toxic effects were ameliorated with the use of G-CSF as the primary prophylaxis.

The NSABP-30 trial assessed the use of TAC, anthracycline with docetaxel, or AC followed by docetaxel in patients with node-positive breast cancer. AC followed by docetaxel showed a significant advantage in DFS (P = 0.006), but not in OS (HR 0.91, 95% CI 0.75–1.11) when compared with the TAC regimen, and significant increases in both DFS (p = 0.001) and OS (p = 0.034) when compared with the regimen of anthracycline with docetaxel. The combination of anthracycline with docetaxel was not inferior to TAC. Based on this study, it seems that the sequential use of four cycles of AC followed by four cycles of docetaxel is superior to AT or TAC. However, the benefit of the sequential approach could also be attributed to the number of cycles (six for AC→T *vs.* four for AT and four for TAC) (41).

The US Oncology Research 9735 A phase III trial compared AC against the combination of taxane and cyclophosphamide (TC) (42). In this trial, 1016 patients with stage I–III operable invasive breast cancer were randomly assigned to receive four cycles of standard AC every three weeks or four cycles of TC every three weeks as adjuvant chemotherapy. At five years, patients who had received TC had a DFS superior to that of patients who had received AC (86% *vs.* 80%, P = 0.015) and a different toxicity profile (42). At seven years, TC remained superior (DFS: 81% *vs.* 75%, P = 0.033; OS: 87% *vs.* 82%, P = 0.032) (43).

Yet another trial determined that FEC followed by weekly paclitaxel was superior to FEC alone among 1246 randomly assigned women with lymph node-positive disease (44). The estimated five-year DFS rate was 78.5% in the FEC plus paclitaxel arm and 72.1% in the FEC only arm (p = 0.006). A 23% reduction in risk of relapse (P = 0.022) was noted in the arm containing paclitaxel, but at a median follow-up of 66 months no significant difference in OS was noted between the two treatment arms (44).

Results of the TACT multicenter, open-label, phase III randomized controlled trial were published in 2009 (45). This study investigated whether sequential docetaxel after anthracycline chemotherapy would improve patient outcome compared with standard of care. A total of 4162 women with node-positive or high risk node negative, operable early breast cancer were randomly assigned to receive a control regimen, or FEC (600/60/600 mg/m^2) every three weeks for four cycles followed by docetaxel (100 mg/m^2) every three weeks for four cycles. The control regimen was either FEC (600/60/600 mg/m^2) every three weeks for eight cycles, or epirubicin (60 mg/m^2) every three weeks for four cycles followed by CMF (600/40/600 mg/m^2) for four cycles. However, the trial results did not show any overall gain from the addition of docetaxel to standard-of-care anthracycline-based chemotherapy.

TACT II is an ongoing phase III trial that has recruited approximately 4400 patients with early-stage breast cancer who have undergone surgery. Four treatment arms are being assessed in this study: epirubicin (every two weeks or every three weeks) followed by CMF or capecitabine. Results of this study are yet to be reported and published.

It remains unclear whether all patients need dose-dense regimens or taxanes, or how many cycles indeed are sufficient (Table 45.1). Efforts are ongoing to identify gene expression profiles that would help select patients for specific chemotherapies using taxanes (46). A popular combination is FEC plus docetaxel for women with involvement of four or more nodes. Provisional results from the TACT I trial suggested that the benefit from adding four cycles of docetaxel to one of two standard anthracycline-containing regimens is minimal for unselected patients (45).

Finally, retrospective studies indicate that aberrant HER2 expression may correlate with the benefit gained from the use of paclitaxel in the adjuvant setting (47) and that modulation of topoisomerase II gene expression due to deletion or amplification may predict response to anthracycline-based chemotherapy (48). Coamplification of HER2 and the topoisomerase II amplicon is associated with higher response rates to anthracyclines (48). However, reports from various trials have been inconsistent, and the topoisomerase II assay has not been validated for clinical use (49).

ADJUVANT CHEMOTHERAPY FOR ER-/PR-POSITIVE BREAST CANCER

According to the results of the EBCTCG meta-analysis (5), adjuvant chemotherapy is effective regardless of the hormone receptor status of the primary tumor. However, the benefit of adjuvant chemotherapy is extremely low in some patients with node negative breast cancer that is ER positive, PR positive, or both. Several molecular assays have been developed to identify women with ER-positive/PR-positive breast cancer who may not need adjuvant chemotherapy.

For example, the Oncotype DX test measures the expression of 21 genes using RT-PCR (16 cancer genes and five control genes) (Fig. 45.3) (50). The assay was validated using archival breast cancer tissue from the NSABP B-14 trial. In that study, patients with node-negative, ER-positive/PR-positive breast cancer had been randomly assigned to treatment with tamoxifen or placebo. Oncotype DX could categorize the patients who had received tamoxifen into three groups based

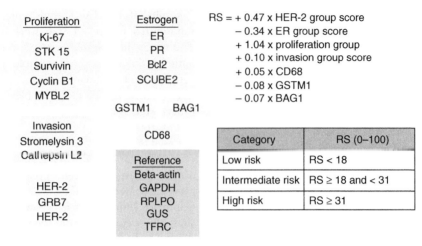

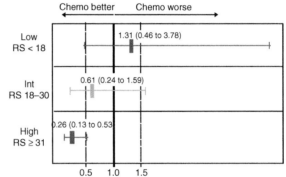

Figure 45.3 Genes included in Oncotype DX score. *Source*: From Ref. (53).

on their recurrence scores (low (< 18), intermediate (18–30), or high (≥31)) (51). Another study evaluated the predictive role of the assay for patients with node-negative, ER-positive/PR-positive breast cancer who had been randomly allocated to receive tamoxifen or CMF on the NSABP B-20 trial (52). Both NSABP trials demonstrated that tamoxifen was more effective among patients with a low Oncotype DX recurrence score, whereas CMF was more effective for patients with a high score (Fig. 45.4).

Several other molecular assays have been developed to identify women who may not need adjuvant chemotherapy. The TAILORx trial randomly allocated patients with node-negative, ER-positive/PR-positive breast cancer who had an intermediate recurrence score to chemotherapy or no chemotherapy (all patients received endocrine therapy) (53). Outcome data from TAILORx are expected to be available within the next few years. The MammaPrint® (Agendia, Amsterdam, The Netherlands) assay (54), which is based on a 70-gene profile using cDNA microarrays, can predict prognosis based on retrospective clinical trials. The MINDACT trial randomly assigned patients with early stage, ER-positive/PR-positive breast cancer to chemotherapy or no chemotherapy on the basis of clinico-pathological features and MammaPrint data; the results from this trial should also be available within the next few years. Assessment of HOXB13/IL17BR expression by RT-PCR (55) is another approved molecular test for assessing prognosis among breast cancer patients. These microarrays require fresh-frozen tissue, whereas the Oncotype DX assay can measure gene expression in formalin-fixed, paraffin-embedded tumor tissue (50,56).

The 21-gene Oncotype DX assay is also predictive of benefit from adjuvant chemotherapy for patients with node-positive breast cancer. A North American trial randomly assigned premenopausal women with node-positive, ER-positive breast cancer to a tamoxifen-only arm or a cyclophosphamide, doxorubicin, and fluorouracil (CAF) arm before or concurrently with tamoxifen. The use of CAF followed by tamoxifen maximized DFS rates. However, application of the Oncotype DX assay to archival primary tissue showed that only patients with a high recurrence score derived benefit from CAF chemotherapy (57). The RxPONDER prospective clinical trial was launched in 2011 in the United States to determine the role of chemotherapy for patients with node-positive breast

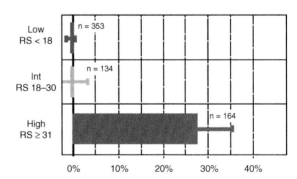

Figure 45.4 (A) Relative and (B) absolute risk of chemotherapy (chemo) benefit as a function of recurrence score (RS) risk category in low, intermediate (int), and high recurrence score groups. *Source*: From Ref. (52).

cancer (up to three positive lymph nodes) and a low Oncotype DX recurrence score. In the near future, patients with low-risk breast cancer may be able to avoid chemotherapy regardless of the size of the primary tumor and the degree of nodal involvement.

TRASTUZUMAB

The discovery of the *her2* oncogene (58,59) and the correlation of *her2* gene amplification or HER2 protein overexpression with poor prognosis (60) led to the development of HER2 targeted therapies for breast cancer (61). The HER2 status of the primary tumor or metastatic deposit should be assessed for all patients with breast cancer using immunohistochemistry, fluorescence *in situ* hybridization, or chromogenic *in situ* hybridization techniques (62–64). If the tumor is HER2 positive, the patient should be considered for trastuzumab as adjuvant therapy and for participation in clinical trials of novel HER2-directed treatments (65,66).

Trastuzumab (Herceptin) is a monoclonal antibody directed against the extracellular domain of HER2 (67–69). For patients with HER2-positive, early-stage breast cancer, trastuzumab improves DFS and OS rates independent of age, axillary node metastases, and ER/PR status (68,70–72). Two American trials (NSABP B-31 and Intergroup N9831) reported a reduction in risk of recurrence of about 50% (HR 0.48, p < 0.0001) and have shown an early survival benefit favoring trastuzumab over chemotherapy alone at two years (HR 0.67, p = 0.015) (70). The European HERA trial showed similar reductions in risk of recurrence (HR 0.54, p < 0.0001) (71) and death (HR 0.66, p = 0.0115) (71). In the American trials, trastuzumab was given concurrently with an anthracycline-based chemotherapy (AC followed by paclitaxel, with or without trastuzumab) and was thereafter continued as a single-agent therapy for a total of 52 weeks, whereas in the HERA trial, trastuzumab was prescribed only after completion of a chemotherapy (with any anthracycline)-based regimen of four or more cycles.

The international study BCIRG 006 demonstrated a significant improvement in DFS and OS for patients undergoing a non–anthracycline-based regimen (docetaxel, carboplatin, and trastuzumab) compared with those receiving an anthracycline-based regimen (AC plus trastuzumab) and five-fold lower cardiotoxicity compared with chemotherapy consisting of AC followed by both paclitaxel and trastuzumab (72). In the Finnish trial FinHer (73), 1010 women were randomly allocated to either nine weeks of vinorelbine or three cycles of docetaxel (both followed by three cycles of FEC). The 232 patients with HER2-positive cancer were further randomly assigned to receive trastuzumab or not for nine weeks during the initial portion (i.e., vinorelbine or docetaxel) of the chemotherapy. At a median follow-up of three years, the addition of trastuzumab was associated with a reduction in risk of recurrence (89% *vs.* 78%, HR 0.42, P = 0.01).

The risk of cardiac toxicity in the adjuvant setting ranges from 0.5% to 4% (70,74–76). Patients should undergo a baseline echocardiogram or cardiac scan to assess left ventricular ejection fraction (LVEF) before trastuzumab-based therapy is initiated. Serial LVEF evaluations are recommended every three months while the patients are receiving trastuzumab, with a close follow-up in the first two years after completion of therapy. In the event of cardiac toxicity, trastuzumab should be discontinued and LVEF reassessed in four weeks, although this

decision should be individualized and take into account the risk of recurrence and pre-existing cardiac morbidity.

Table 45.2 lists the three most commonly used trastuzumab-based regimens in the adjuvant setting. Trastuzumab should be administered for a total of 52 weeks. However, the optimal duration of this therapy remains unknown and is the subject of ongoing trials.

TRIPLE-NEGATIVE BREAST CANCER

The term "triple-negative breast cancer" has been used to describe tumors that are ER/PR negative and HER2 normal (i.e., not amplified). Some of these tumors resemble the basal subtype defined by gene expression profiling (77,78). It is well known that this category of tumors carries a relatively worse prognosis and continues to be a challenge to treat. Patients with involvement of axillary lymph nodes are treated with adjuvant chemotherapy, which is usually recommended for tumors greater than 1 cm in size (regardless of nodal status). The treatment of patients with T1a/b tumors (0.1–1 cm in diameter) should be personalized. The choice of adjuvant chemotherapy regimen for this aggressive group of tumors is unresolved. Although anthracycline- and taxane-based chemotherapy regimens are generally favored, CMF may also be a good option for these patients (79,80). Predictive markers of response have been proposed but none is validated for routine clinical use (81). Novel chemotherapies and biologics are under clinical development for patients with anthracycline- and taxane-refractory breast cancer (82).

Poly(adenosine) diphosphate (ADP)-ribose polymerase (PARP) inhibitors are being investigated for treatment of patients with BRCA 1/2 mutations and patients with triple-negative breast cancer (83,84). PARP plays a key role in the repair of base damage via the base-excision repair pathway. An elaborate set of signaling pathways detects single- and double-stranded DNA breaks and mediates DNA repair, or apoptosis if the damage is too great. Pharmacological inhibition of PARP induces cell death in tumors with mutations in certain DNA repair pathways, such as the BRCA pathways, and when combined with chemotherapies that cause DNA damage.

NOVEL TARGETED THERAPIES

Drug resistance is one of the most important challenges in oncology, and occurs even in the setting of a well-selected group of patients (e.g., HER2 positive) treated with a highly targeted therapy (e.g., trastuzumab). Approximately 15–20% of patients develop metastatic disease despite adjuvant trastuzumab-based chemotherapy. Proposed mechanisms of resistance include but are not limited to activation of the PI3K/Akt/mTOR pathway (85,86), insulin-like growth factor type I receptor (IGF-IR) activation through dimerization with HER proteins (87,88), Src signaling (89), and upregulation of erythropoietin receptors (90).

Lapatinib (Tykerb) is a reversible, small-molecule tyrosine kinase inhibitor directed against HER2 and epidermal growth factor receptor (91–95). The combination of lapatinib and capecitabine was shown to improve DFS rates compared with capecitabine alone for heavily pretreated patients with metastatic breast cancer (96). Clinical trials are now evaluating the role of lapatinib in the adjuvant setting.

Pertuzumab is a monoclonal antibody directed against HER2 that prevents formation of heterodimers between HER2 and other members of the HER family (87,97,98). The binding

Table 45.2 Adjuvant Chemotherapy Regimens with Trastuzumab for HER2-Positive Breast Cancer

Regimen	Comments
AC-TH	AC followed by paclitaxel or docetaxel and concurrent H
TCH	Docetaxel, carboplatin, and H
A-H	Anthracycline-based chemotherapy followed by H sequentially

Abbreviations: A, anthracycline; C, cyclophosphamide or carboplatin; H, trastuzumab; T, taxane.

sites of trastuzumab and pertuzumab localize to different domains of the HER2 protein. Preclinical studies from our group and others have demonstrated a synergistic interaction between pertuzumab and trastuzumab (98,99), and this combination is being explored in clinical trials (97).

Overexpression of IGF-IR is associated with poor prognosis and resistance to a variety of drugs, such as trastuzumab, and to endocrine therapy (87,88). Approaches to inhibiting IGF-IR have included the use of monoclonal antibodies, small-molecule tyrosine kinase inhibitors, and IGF-binding proteins. Intracellular transduction pathways activated by growth factor receptors such as HER2 and IGF-IR are potential therapeutic targets; both the mitogen-activated protein kinase and the PI3K/Akt/mTOR pathways have been well characterized in breast cancer cells (100). Clinical trials are testing a variety of inhibitors directed against different aspects of these signaling pathways (101). Post-receptor signaling pathways are not linear, but rather form complex networks with much cross-talk. Multiple compensatory mechanisms exist with some functional redundancy, and blocking a single protein (e.g., mTOR) often leads to activation of more proximal steps (e.g., Akt) and potentially increased cell proliferation (100,102). One approach to overcoming the compensatory loops is to use multiple inhibitors and to target central signaling nodes critical for sustained growth-inhibitory effects.

Novel approaches target not only cancer cells but also the tumor microenvironment and new vessel formation. Preclinical and clinical studies have shown that blocking angiogenesis improves the efficacy of cytotoxic chemotherapy. Bevacizumab is a recombinant, humanized monoclonal antibody against vascular endothelial growth factor. A phase II trial of trastuzumab and bevacizumab showed this combination to be highly effective for patients with HER2 overexpressing metastatic breast cancer that failed prior therapies (103). Randomized clinical trials are ongoing in the adjuvant setting to determine the safety and efficacy of bevacizumab in combination with chemotherapy, endocrine therapy, and trastuzumab for all types of breast cancer.

REFERENCES

1. Schiebel HM. Combined adjuvant chemotherapy with radical mastectomy for carcinoma of the breast. N C Med J 1966; 27: 57–62.
2. Schabel FM. Concepts for systemic treatment of micrometastases. Cancer 1975; 35: 15–24.
3. Bonadonna G, Brusamolino E, Valagussa P, et al. Combination chemotherapy as an adjuvant treatment in operable breast cancer. N Engl J Med 1976; 294: 405–10.
4. Bonadonna G, Moliterni A, Zambetti M, et al. 30 years' follow up of randomised studies of adjuvant CMF in operable breast cancer: cohort study. BMJ 2005; 330: 217.
5. Peto R, Davies C, Godwin J, et al. Comparisons between different polychemotherapy regimens for early breast cancer: meta-analyses of long-term outcome among 100,000 women in 123 randomised trials. Lancet 2012; 379: 432–44.
6. Carlson RW, Brown E, Burstein HJ, et al. NCCN Task Force Report: Adjuvant Therapy for Breast Cancer. J Natl Compr Canc Netw 2006; 4: S1–26.
7. Ravdin PM, Siminoff LA, Davis GJ, et al. Computer program to assist in making decisions about adjuvant therapy for women with early breast cancer. J Clin Oncol 2001; 19: 980–91.
8. Early Breast Cancer Trialists' Collaborative Group. Polychemotherapy for early breast cancer: an overview of the randomised trials. Lancet 1998; 352: 930–42.
9. Early Breast Cancer Trialists' Collaborative Group. Tamoxifen for early breast cancer: an overview of the randomised trials. Lancet 1998; 351: 1451–67.
10. Moore MR, Jones SE, Bull JM, et al. MOPP chemotherapy for advanced Hodgkin's disease. Prognostic factors in 81 patients. Cancer 1973; 32: 52–60.
11. Engelsman E, Klijn JC, Rubens RD, et al. "Classical" CMF versus a 3-weekly intravenous CMF schedule in postmenopausal patients with advanced breast cancer. An EORTC Breast Cancer Co-operative Group Phase III Trial (10808). Eur J Cancer 1991; 27: 966–70.
12. O'Shaughnessy JA. Oral alkylating agents for breast cancer therapy. Drugs 1999; 58: 1–9.
13. Munzone E, Curigliano G, Burstein HJ, et al. CMF revisited in the 21st century. Ann Oncol 2012; 23: 305–11.
14. Fisher B, Dignam J, Mamounas EP, et al. Sequential methotrexate and fluorouracil for the treatment of node-negative breast cancer patients with estrogen receptor-negative tumors: eight-year results from National Surgical Adjuvant Breast and Bowel Project (NSABP) B-13 and first report of findings from NSABP B-19 comparing methotrexate and fluorouracil with conventional cyclophosphamide, methotrexate, and fluorouracil. J Clin Oncol 1996; 14: 1982–92.
15. Cheang MC, Voduc KD, Tu D, et al. Responsiveness of intrinsic subtypes to adjuvant anthracycline substitution in the NCIC.CTG MA.5 randomized trial. Clin Cancer Res 2012; 18: 2402–12.
16. Colleoni M, Cole BF, Viale G, et al. Classical cyclophosphamide, methotrexate, and fluorouracil chemotherapy is more effective in triple-negative, node-negative breast cancer: results from two randomized trials of adjuvant chemoendocrine therapy for node-negative breast cancer. J Clin Oncol 2010; 28: 2966–73.
17. Hortobagyi GN. Anthracyclines in the treatment of cancer. An overview. Drugs 1997; 54: 1–7.
18. Buzdar AU, Kau SW, Smith TL, et al. Ten-year results of FAC adjuvant chemotherapy trial in breast cancer. Am J Clin Oncol 1989; 12: 123–8.
19. Hortobagyi GN, Bodey GP, Buzdar AU, et al. Evaluation of high-dose versus standard FAC chemotherapy for advanced breast cancer in protected environment units: a prospective randomized study. J Clin Oncol 1987; 5: 354–64.
20. Esteva FJ, Hortobagyi GN. Locally advanced breast cancer. Hematol Oncol Clin North Am 1999; 13: 457–72.
21. Martin M, Villar A, Sole-Calvo A, et al. Doxorubicin in combination with fluorouracil and cyclophosphamide (i.v. FAC regimen, day 1, 21) versus methotrexate in combination with fluorouracil and cyclophosphamide (i.v. CMF regimen, day 1, 21) as adjuvant chemotherapy for operable breast cancer: a study by the GEICAM group. Ann Oncol 2003; 14: 833–42.
22. Levine MN, Pritchard KI, Bramwell VH, et al. Randomized trial comparing cyclophosphamide, epirubicin, and fluorouracil with cyclophosphamide, methotrexate, and fluorouracil in premenopausal women with node-positive breast cancer: update of National Cancer Institute of Canada Clinical Trials Group Trial MA5. J Clin Oncol 2005; 23: 5166–70.
23. French Adjuvant Study Group. Benefit of a high-dose epirubicin regimen in adjuvant chemotherapy for node-positive breast cancer patients with poor prognostic factors: 5-year follow-up results of French Adjuvant Study Group 05 randomized trial. J Clin Oncol 2001; 19: 602–11.
24. Fisher B, Brown AM, Dimitrov NV, et al. Two months of doxorubicin-cyclophosphamide with and without interval reinduction therapy compared with 6 months of cyclophosphamide, methotrexate, and fluorouracil in positive-node breast cancer patients with tamoxifen-nonresponsive tumors: results from the National Surgical Adjuvant Breast and Bowel Project B-15. J Clin Oncol 1990; 8: 1483–96.
25. Fisher B, Dignam J, Wolmark N, et al. Tamoxifen and chemotherapy for lymph node-negative, estrogen receptor-positive breast cancer. J Natl Cancer Inst 1997; 89: 1673–82.
26. Land SR, Kopec JA, Yothers G, et al. Health-related quality of life in axillary node-negative, estrogen receptor-negative breast cancer patients undergoing AC versus CMF chemotherapy: findings from the National Surgical Adjuvant Breast and Bowel Project B-23. Breast Cancer Res Treat 2004; 86: 153–64.
27. Gianni L, Norton L, Wolmark N, et al. Role of anthracyclines in the treatment of early breast cancer. J Clin Oncol 2009; 27: 4798–808.
28. Early Breast Cancer Trialists' Collaborative Group (EBCTCG). Effects of chemotherapy and hormonal therapy for early breast cancer on recurrence and 15-year survival: an overview of the randomised trials. Lancet 2005; 365: 1687–717.

29. Guarneri V, Lenihan DJ, Valero V, et al. Long-term cardiac tolerability of trastuzumab in metastatic breast cancer: the M.D. Anderson Cancer Center experience. J Clin Oncol 2006; 24: 4107–15.

30. Patt DA, Duan Z, Fang S, et al. Acute myeloid leukemia after adjuvant breast cancer therapy in older women: understanding risk. J Clin Oncol 2007; 25: 3871–6.

31. Schiff PB, Fant J, Horwitz SB. Promotion of microtubule assembly in vitro by taxol. Nature 1979; 277: 665–7.

32. Esteva FJ, Valero V, Pusztai L, et al. Chemotherapy of metastatic breast cancer: what to expect in 2001 and beyond. Oncologist 2001; 6: 133–46.

33. Mamounas EP, Bryant J, Lembersky B, et al. Paclitaxel after doxorubicin plus cyclophosphamide as adjuvant chemotherapy for node-positive breast cancer: results from NSABP B-28. J Clin Oncol 2005; 23: 3686–96.

34. Citron ML, Berry DA, Cirrincione C, et al. Randomized trial of dose-dense versus conventionally scheduled and sequential versus concurrent combination chemotherapy as postoperative adjuvant treatment of node-positive primary breast cancer: first report of Intergroup Trial C9741/Cancer and Leukemia Group B Trial 9741. J Clin Oncol 2003; 21: 1431–9.

35. Roche H, Fumoleau P, Spielmann M, et al. Sequential adjuvant epirubicin-based and docetaxel chemotherapy for node-positive breast cancer patients: the FNCLCC PACS 01 Trial. J Clin Oncol 2006; 24: 5664–71.

36. Martin M, Pienkowski T, Mackey J, et al. Adjuvant docetaxel for node-positive breast cancer. N Engl J Med 2005; 352: 2302–13.

37. Sparano JA, Wang M, Martino S, et al. Weekly paclitaxel in the adjuvant treatment of breast cancer. N Engl J Med 2008; 358: 1663–71.

38. Nabholtz JM, Falkson C, Campos D, et al. Docetaxel and doxorubicin compared with doxorubicin and cyclophosphamide as first-line chemotherapy for metastatic breast cancer: results of a randomized, multicenter, phase III trial. J Clin Oncol 2003; 21: 968–75.

39. Nabholtz JM, Mackey JR, Smylie M, et al. Phase II study of docetaxel, doxorubicin, and cyclophosphamide as first-line chemotherapy for metastatic breast cancer. J Clin Oncol 2001; 19: 314–21.

40. Martin M, Segui MA, Anton A, et al. Adjuvant docetaxel for high-risk, node-negative breast cancer. N Engl J Med 2010; 363: 2200–10.

41. Swain SM, Jeong J-H, Geyer CE, et al. NSABP-B30: Definitive analysis of patient outcome from a randomized trial evaluating different schedules and combinations of adjuvant therapy containing doxorubicin, docetaxel, and cyclophosphamide in women with operable, node positive breast cancer. Breast Cancer Res Treat 2008; 102: A75.

42. Jones SE, Savin MA, Holmes FA, et al. Phase III trial comparing doxorubicin plus cyclophosphamide with docetaxel plus cyclophosphamide as adjuvant therapy for operable breast cancer. J Clin Oncol 2006; 24: 5381–7.

43. Jones S, Holmes FA, O'Shaughnessy J, et al. Docetaxel With Cyclophosphamide Is Associated With an Overall Survival Benefit Compared With Doxorubicin and Cyclophosphamide: 7-Year Follow-Up of US Oncology Research Trial 9735. J Clin Oncol 2009; 27: 1177–83.

44. Martin M, Rodriguez-Lescure A, Ruiz A, et al. Randomized phase 3 trial of fluorouracil, epirubicin, and cyclophosphamide alone or followed by Paclitaxel for early breast cancer. J Natl Cancer Inst 2008; 100: 805–14.

45. Ellis P, Barrett-Lee P, Johnson L, et al. Sequential docetaxel as adjuvant chemotherapy for early breast cancer (TACT): an open-label, phase III, randomised controlled trial. Lancet 2009; 373: 1681–92.

46. Hess KR, Anderson K, Symmans WF, et al. Pharmacogenomic predictor of sensitivity to preoperative chemotherapy with paclitaxel and fluorouracil, doxorubicin, and cyclophosphamide in breast cancer. J Clin Oncol 2006; 24: 4236–44.

47. Hayes DF, Thor AD, Dressler LG, et al. HER2 and response to paclitaxel in node-positive breast cancer. N Engl J Med 2007; 357: 1496–506.

48. Pritchard KI, Messersmith H, Elavathil L, et al. HER-2 and topoisomerase II as predictors of response to chemotherapy. J Clin Oncol 2008; 26: 736–44.

49. Esteva FJ, Hortobagyi GN. Topoisomerase II{alpha} amplification and anthracycline-based chemotherapy: the jury is still out. J Clin Oncol 2009; 27: 3416–17.

50. Esteva FJ, Sahin AA, Coombes K, et al. Multi-gene RT-PCR assay for redicting recurrence in node negative breast cancer patients - M. D. Anderson Clinical Validation Study. Breast Cancer Res Treat 2003; 82: A17.

51. Paik S, Shak S, Tang G, et al. A multigene assay to predict recurrence of tamoxifen-treated, node-negative breast cancer. N Engl J Med 2004; 351: 2817–26.

52. Paik S, Tang G, Shak S, et al. Gene expression and benefit of chemotherapy in women with node-negative, estrogen receptor-positive breast cancer. J Clin Oncol 2006; 24: 3726–34.

53. Sparano JA, Paik S. Development of the 21-gene assay and its application in clinical practice and clinical trials. J Clin Oncol 2008; 26: 721–8.

54. Ross JS, Hatzis C, Symmans WF, et al. Commercialized multigene predictors of clinical outcome for breast cancer. Oncologist 2008; 13: 477–93.

55. Jansen MP, Sieuwerts AM, Look MP, et al. HOXB13-to-IL17BR expression ratio is related with tumor aggressiveness and response to tamoxifen of recurrent breast cancer: a retrospective study. J Clin Oncol 2007; 25: 662–8.

56. Sotiriou C, Pusztai L. Gene-expression signatures in breast cancer. N Engl J Med 2009; 360: 790–800.

57. Albain KS, Barlow WE, Shak S, et al. Prognostic and predictive value of the 21-gene recurrence score assay in postmenopausal women with node-positive, oestrogen-receptor-positive breast cancer on chemotherapy: a retrospective analysis of a randomised trial. Lancet Oncol 2010; 11: 55–65.

58. King CR, Kraus MH, Aaronson SA. Amplification of a novel v-erbB-related gene in a human mammary carcinoma. Science 1985; 229: 974–6.

59. Schechter AL, Hung MC, Vaidyanathan L, et al. The neu gene: An erbB-homologous gene distinct from and unlinked to the gene encoding the EGF receptor. Science 1985; 229: 976–8.

60. Slamon DJ, Clark GM, Wong SG, et al. Human breast cancer: correlation of relapse and survival with amplification of the HER-2/neu oncogene. Science 1987; 235: 177–82.

61. Nahta R, Esteva FJ. HER-2-targeted therapy: lessons learned and future directions. Clin Cancer Res 2003; 9: 5078–84.

62. Wolff AC, Hammond ME, Schwartz JN, et al. American Society of Clinical Oncology/College of American Pathologists guideline recommendations for human epidermal growth factor receptor 2 testing in breast cancer. J Clin Oncol 2007; 25: 118–45.

63. Esteva FJ, Sahin AA, Cristofanilli M, et al. Molecular prognostic factors for breast cancer metastasis and survival. Semin Radiat Oncol 2002; 12: 319–28.

64. Esteva FJ, Hortobagyi GN, Sahin AA, et al. Expression of erbB/HER receptors, heregulin and P38 in primary breast cancer using quantitative immunohistochemistry. Pathol Oncol Res 2001; 7: 171–7.

65. Esteva FJ. Monoclonal antibodies, small molecules, and vaccines in the treatment of breast cancer. Oncologist 2004; 9: 4–9.

66. Morrow PK, Wulf GM, Ensor J, et al. Phase I/II study of trastuzumab in combination with everolimus (RAD001) in patients with HER2-overexpressing metastatic breast cancer who progressed on trastuzumab-based therapy. J Clin Oncol 2011; 29: 3126–32.

67. Nahta R, Esteva FJ. Herceptin: mechanisms of action and resistance. Cancer Lett 2006; 232: 123–38.

68. Johnson PH, Esteva FJ. The use of HER2 modulation in the adjuvant setting. Curr Oncol Rep 2007; 9: 9–16.

69. Nahta R, Esteva FJ. Trastuzumab: triumphs and tribulations. Oncogene 2007; 26: 3637–43.

70. Romond EH, Perez EA, Bryant J, et al. Trastuzumab plus adjuvant chemotherapy for operable HER2-positive breast cancer. N Engl J Med 2005; 353: 1673–84.

71. Smith I, Procter M, Gelber RD, et al. 2-year follow-up of trastuzumab after adjuvant chemotherapy in HER2-positive breast cancer: a randomised controlled trial. Lancet 2007; 369: 29–36.

72. Perez EA, Suman VJ, Davidson NE, et al. Cardiac safety analysis of doxorubicin and cyclophosphamide followed by paclitaxel with or without trastuzumab in the North Central Cancer Treatment Group N9831 adjuvant breast cancer trial. J Clin Oncol 2008; 26: 1231–8.

73. Joensuu H, Kellokumpu-Lehtinen PL, Bono P, et al. Adjuvant docetaxel or vinorelbine with or without trastuzumab for breast cancer. N Engl J Med 2006; 354: 809–20.

74. Tan-Chiu E, Yothers G, Romond E, et al. Assessment of cardiac dysfunction in a randomized trial comparing doxorubicin and cyclophosphamide followed by paclitaxel, with or without trastuzumab as adjuvant therapy in node-positive, human epidermal growth factor receptor 2-overexpressing breast cancer: NSABP B-31. J Clin Oncol 2005; 23: 7811–19.

75. Gianni L, Dafni U, Gelber RD, et al. Treatment with trastuzumab for 1 year after adjuvant chemotherapy in patients with HER2-positive

early breast cancer: a 4-year follow-up of a randomised controlled trial. Lancet Oncol 2011; 12: 236–44.

76. Slamon D, Eiermann W, Robert N, et al. Adjuvant trastuzumab in HER2-positive breast cancer. N Engl J Med 2011; 365: 1273–83.

77. Perou CM, Sorlie T, Eisen MB, et al. Molecular portraits of human breast tumours. Nature 2000; 406: 747–52.

78. Carey LA, Dees EC, Sawyer L, et al. The triple negative paradox: primary tumor chemosensitivity of breast cancer subtypes. Clin Cancer Res 2007; 13: 2329–34.

79. Colleoni M, Cole BF, Viale G, et al. Classical cyclophosphamide, methotrexate, and fluorouracil chemotherapy is more effective in triple-negative, node-negative breast cancer: results from two randomized trials of adjuvant chemoendocrine therapy for node-negative breast cancer. J Clin Oncol 2010; 28: 2966–73.

80. Munzone E, Curigliano G, Burstein HJ, et al. CMF revisited in the 21st century. Ann Oncol 2011; 23: 305–11.

81. Juul N, Szallasi Z, Eklund AC, et al. Assessment of an RNA interference screen-derived mitotic and ceramide pathway metagene as a predictor of response to neoadjuvant paclitaxel for primary triple-negative breast cancer: a retrospective analysis of five clinical trials. Lancet Oncol 2010; 11: 358–65.

82. Dean-Colomb W, Esteva FJ. Emerging agents in the treatment of anthracycline- and taxane-refractory metastatic breast cancer. Semin Oncol 2008; 35: S31–8; quiz S40.

83. Comen EA, Robson M. Poly(ADP-ribose) polymerase inhibitors in triple-negative breast cancer. Cancer J 2010; 16: 48–52.

84. O'Shaughnessy J, Osborne C, Pippen JE, et al. Iniparib plus chemotherapy in metastatic triple-negative breast cancer. N Engl J Med 2011; 364: 205–14.

85. Esteva FJ, Guo H, Zhang S, et al. PTEN, PIK3CA, p-AKT, and p-p70S6K status: association with trastuzumab response and survival in patients with HER2-positive metastatic breast cancer. Am J Pathol 2010; 177: 1647–56.

86. Nagata Y, Lan KH, Zhou X, et al. PTEN activation contributes to tumor inhibition by trastuzumab, and loss of PTEN predicts trastuzumab resistance in patients. Cancer Cell 2004; 6: 117–27.

87. Nahta R, Yuan LX, Zhang B, et al. Insulin-like growth factor-I receptor/human epidermal growth factor receptor 2 heterodimerization contributes to trastuzumab resistance of breast cancer cells. Cancer Res 2005; 65: 11118–28.

88. Huang X, Gao L, Wang S, et al. Heterotrimerization of the growth factor receptors erbB2, erbB3, and insulin-like growth factor-i receptor in breast cancer cells resistant to herceptin. Cancer Res 2010; 70: 1204–14.

89. Zhang S, Huang WC, Li P, et al. Combating trastuzumab resistance by targeting SRC, a common node downstream of multiple resistance pathways. Nat Med 2011; 17: 461–9.

90. Liang K, Esteva FJ, Albarracin C, et al. Recombinant human erythropoietin antagonizes trastuzumab treatment of breast cancer cells via Jak2-mediated Src activation and PTEN inactivation. Cancer Cell 2010; 18: 423–35.

91. Wood ER, Truesdale AT, McDonald OB, et al. A unique structure for epidermal growth factor receptor bound to GW572016 (Lapatinib): relationships among protein conformation, inhibitor off-rate, and receptor activity in tumor cells. Cancer Res 2004; 64: 6652–9.

92. Esteva FJ, Yu D, Hung MC, et al. Molecular predictors of response to trastuzumab and lapatinib in breast cancer. Nat Rev Clin Oncol 2010; 7: 98–107.

93. Zhang D, Pal A, Bornmann WG, et al. Activity of lapatinib is independent of EGFR expression level in HER2-overexpressing breast cancer cells. Mol Cancer Ther 2008; 7: 1846–50.

94. Nahta R, Yuan LX, Du Y, et al. Lapatinib induces apoptosis in trastuzumab-resistant breast cancer cells: effects on insulin-like growth factor I signaling. Mol Cancer Ther 2007; 6: 667–74.

95. Esteva FJ, Pusztai L. Optimizing outcomes in HER2-positive breast cancer: the molecular rationale. Oncology 2005; 19: 5–16.

96. Geyer CE, Forster J, Lindquist D, et al. Lapatinib plus capecitabine for HER2-positive advanced breast cancer. N Engl J Med 2006; 355: 2733–43.

97. Nahta R, Hung MC, Esteva FJ. The HER-2-targeting antibodies trastuzumab and pertuzumab synergistically inhibit the survival of breast cancer cells. Cancer Res 2004; 64: 2343–6.

98. Nahta R, Hung MC, Esteva FJ. The HER-2-targeting antibodies trastuzumab and pertuzumab synergistically inhibit the survival of breast cancer cells. Cancer Res 2004; 64: 2343–6.

99. Scheuer W, Friess T, Burtscher H, et al. Strongly enhanced antitumor activity of trastuzumab and pertuzumab combination treatment on HER2-positive human xenograft tumor models. Cancer Res 2009; 69: 9330–6.

100. O'Reilly KE, Rojo F, She QB, et al. mTOR inhibition induces upstream receptor tyrosine kinase signaling and activates Akt. Cancer Res 2006; 66: 1500–8.

101. Nahta R, Hortobagyi GN, Esteva FJ. Signal transduction inhibitors in the treatment of breast cancer. Curr Med Chem 2003; 3: 201–16.

102. Meric-Bernstam F, Esteva FJ. Potential role of mammalian target of rapamycin inhibitors in breast cancer therapy. Clin Breast Cancer 2005; 6: 357–60.

103. Pegram M, Chan D, Cichmann RA, et al. Phase II combined biological therapy targeting the HER2 proto-oncogene and the vascular endothelial growth factor (VEGF) using trastuzumab and bevacizumab as first-line treatment of HER2-amplified breast cancer. Breast Cancer Res Treat 2006; 100: A201.

46 Primary systemic therapy in breast cancer

Lisardo Ugidos, Andreas Makris, and Jenny C. Chang

INTRODUCTION

Preoperative, primary, or neoadjuvant systemic therapy refers to the use of pharmacological treatments before surgical locoregional treatment of breast cancer. Although initially used in locally advanced disease, neoadjuvant approaches have been increasingly championed for treatment of operable tumors, with the goal of increasing the breast-conserving surgery (BCS) rates. Additionally, primary therapy constitutes a powerful *in vivo* model, providing information about not only clinical, but pathological and molecular predictors of response. Since the primary tumor remains *in situ*, neoadjuvant therapy allows for monitoring of treatment effects through serial biopsies or imaging. Initial experience was focused on chemotherapy and endocrine therapies but other targeted therapies, including trastuzumab, have broadened the spectrum of preoperative therapies.

CHEMOTHERAPY

Introduction

Neoadjuvant chemotherapy was initially used for non-operable disease, particularly cases of locally advanced breast cancer (LABC) and inflammatory breast cancer. Initial experience with non-randomized trials in LABC showed high overall response rates (1–5), allowing many of these tumors to become operable and established this modality as the treatment of choice in this setting.

Subsequently, primary chemotherapy was used for treatment of women with large but operable breast cancers who would otherwise have needed mastectomy as surgical treatment. One of the most important studies to demonstrate the feasibility of this approach was conducted in Milan by Bonnadonna et al. (4) and they reported that 81% of responders were eligible to be treated with BCS.

Further support in favor of the preoperative approach included the theoretical benefit of "earlier" treatment of micrometastases and maintenance of an intact blood supply in unoperated tumors. This support came from a series of elegant preclinical experiments by Fisher et al. showing that surgical resection in mice led to an increase in the growth rate of micrometastases that could be prevented by pretreatment with chemotherapy or endocrine therapy (6–8).

Adjuvant Vs. Neoadjuvant Chemotherapy

While adjuvant chemotherapy was becoming established for routine treatment of high-risk early breast cancer (9), several trials were being conducted in the 1980s and early 1990s comparing chemotherapy given prior to or after surgery (10–16) (summarized in Table 46.1). The largest of these trials was the National Surgical Adjuvant Breast and Bowel Project (NSABP) trial B-18, which enrolled 1523 patients with stage I–III operable breast cancer (13% with tumors larger than 5 cm and 26% with node-positive disease) (15). Patients were randomized to receive four cycles of AC (doxorubicin 60 mg/m^2 and cyclophosphamide 600 mg/m^2 every three weeks) either preoperatively or postoperatively. Tamoxifen was administered to women 50 years of age or older, after completion of chemotherapy. In the preoperative arm, the clinical overall response rate (ORR) (including complete and partial clinical responses) was 80%, with a complete clinical response (cCR) rate of 36%. The pathological complete response (pCR) rate in the breast was 9% (13% if residual non-invasive carcinoma was included). Significant downstaging was also demonstrated in the axilla with node-negative disease at surgery documented in 58% of neoadjuvant patients compared with 42% of postoperative adjuvant patients (p < 0.0001). Importantly, BCS rates were also improved with preoperative chemotherapy: 68% versus 60% (p = 0.001). This reduction in the need for mastectomy established preoperative therapy as a clinically useful approach for the treatment of large but operable breast cancers. Rather disappointingly, disease-free survival (DFS) and overall survival (OS) rates were not significantly different for the two groups of patients.

In the latest update of this trial, with a median of follow-up of 16 years, DFS and OS were similar in both arms (17). The 8-year and 16-year survival estimates were 72% and 55%, respectively, in the postoperative group compared with 72% and 55%, respectively, in the preoperative group (HR 0.94, p = 0.56). The 8-year and 16-year DFS estimates were 55% and 39% in the postoperative group compared with 58% and 42% in the preoperative group, respectively (HR 0.93, p = 0.27). Nevertheless, DFS conditional on being event-free for 5 years showed a trend for benefit in favor of the preoperative group (HR 0.81, p = 0.053). There was a higher but not statistically significant rate of ipsilateral breast tumor recurrence with preoperative versus postoperative chemotherapy (13 vs.10%, p = 0.21). In subset analysis, there was a trend in favor of preoperative AC for OS and DFS in patients younger than 50 years of age (HR 0.81; p = 0.06 and HR 0.85; p = 0.09 respectively). Of note, women achieving a pCR had superior DFS and OS compared with patients who did not achieve this (DFS HR 0.47; p < 0.0001; OS HR 0.32; p < 0.0001).

The observation that pCR was associated with improved survival rates led to trials to determine whether treatment with more effective chemotherapy which increased pCR rates could result in improved survival. In the European Organisation for Research and Treatment of Cancer (EORTC) 10902 clinical

Table 46.1 Clinical trials comparing neoadjuvant versus adjuvant chemotherapy.

Study	N pts	Stage	Treatment	ORR	cCR	pCR	BCS rate	DFS	OS
S6 trial[10]	390	T2-3 N0-1	CAF x4 (pre vs postsurgery)	65%	–	–	82 vs 77%	–	64.6% vs 60.2% at 10 yr
Powles et al.[11]	212	Operable	MMM x4 – surgery – MMM x4 vs surgery – MMM x8[a]	85%	18%	10%	88% vs 71%[b] (p<0.005)	–	–
Mauriac et al.[12]	272	T2-3 N0-1	EVM x3 MTv x3 (pre vs postsurgery)	–	33%	–	63% vs 0%[c]	No difference at 10 yr	No difference at 10 yr
Deo et al.[13]	101	T4b N0-2	CEF x3 –surgery – CEF x3 vs surgery – CEF x6	66%	14%	4%	–	61% vs 76% at 25 mo	76% vs 82% at 25 mo
ABCSG-07[14]	423	T1-3 N0-1	CMF x3 – surgery – CMF x3 vs surgery – CMF x6[d]	62%	12.3%	6%	65.5% vs 59.5%	69.5% vs 77.4% at 9 yr[e,b]	No difference at 9 yr
NSABP B-18[15,17]	1523	T1-3 N0-1	AC x4 (pre vs postsurgery)	80%	36%	9%	68 vs 60%[b]	58 vs 55% at 8 yr	72 vs 72% at 8 yr
EORTC 10902[16,18]	698	T1c-4b N0-1	FEC x4 (pre vs postsurgery)	49%	6.6%	4.4%	23 vs 18%	48 vs 50% at 10 yr	64 vs 66% at 10 yr

[a]All patients received tamoxifen for 5 years starting concurrently with chemotherapy.
[b]Statistically significant.
[c]All patients were treated with mastectomy in the adjuvant group.
[d]Node-positive patients received 3 cycles of EC (epirubicin and cyclophosphamide) instead of the last 3 cycles of CMF.
[e]Only distant metastases-free survival.

Abbreviations: N pts, Number of randomized patients; ORR, clinical overall response rate; cCR, clinical complete response; pCR pathologic complete response; BCS, breast-conserving surgery; DFS, disease-free survival; OS, overall survival; CAF, cyclophosphamide, doxorubicin and 5-fluorouracil; MMM, mitomycin, mitoxantrone and methotrexate; EVM x3 MTv x3, epirubicin-vincristine-methotrexate followed by mitomycin-thiotepa-vindesine; CEF, cyclophosphamide, epirubicin and 5-fluorouracil; CMF, cyclophosphamide, methotrexate and 5-fluorouracil; AC, doxorubicin and cyclophosphamide; FEC, 5-fluorouracil, epirubicine and cyclophosphamide.

trial, 698 women with T1c-4b N0-1 breast cancer were randomized to receive four cycles of FEC (fluorouracil 600 mg/m², epirubicin 60 mg/m², and cyclophosphamide 600 mg/m² every 21 days) pre- or postoperatively (16). In the preoperative group, 23% of patients were treated with BCS instead of pre-planned mastectomy (18% in the postoperative arm). The cCR and pCR rates were 6.6% and 4.4%, respectively. In a later update (18), with a median follow-up of 10 years, there were no significant differences in DFS (50% in the postoperative and 48% in the preoperative group, HR 1.12, p = 0.30) or in OS (66% in the postoperative and 64% in the preoperative group, HR 1.09, p 0.54). As seen in the B18 protocol, patients who achieved a pCR had a significantly higher OS over those who had residual disease (HR 0.86, p = 0.008).

Two published meta-analyses have corroborated the similar efficacy in the long-term outcome of neoadjuvant and adjuvant chemotherapy. In the first one, nine randomized studies, including a total of 3946 patients, were evaluated (19). No statistically significant differences were observed between neoadjuvant and adjuvant therapy arms associated with death (RR 1.00, 95% CI 0.90–1.12), disease progression (RR 0.99, 95% CI 0.91–1.07), or distant disease recurrence (RR 0.94, 95% CI 0.83–1.06). However, neoadjuvant therapy was significantly associated with an increased risk of locoregional disease recurrence (RR 1.22, 95% CI 1.04–1.43); this observation might be attributed to more patients in the neoadjuvant arm being treated with radiotherapy without local surgery in a number of trials. In the second meta-analysis, data from 5500 women in 14 randomized studies with operable breast cancer were evaluated (20). There were no statistically significant differences in OS (HR 0.98, 95% CI 0.87–1.09). Once again, a significant difference in locoregional recurrence in favor of adjuvant chemotherapy was found. However, in three studies, more than one-third of patients received just radiotherapy and no surgery after complete tumor regression. After excluding these studies from the analysis, the remaining eight studies demonstrated no difference in locoregional recurrence rate (HR 1.12, 95% CI 0.92–1.37). Furthermore, the mastectomy rate was significantly lower among patients treated with neoadjuvant chemotherapy (RR 0.71, 95% CI 0.67–0.75), and patients with a pCR had improved OS (HR 0.48, 95% CI 0.33–0.69).

Taxanes

After proving their clinical benefit in metastatic disease, taxanes (mainly paclitaxel and docetaxel) were introduced in adjuvant and neoadjuvant trials. Several phase II studies demonstrated promising clinical and pathological response rates using docetaxel as primary therapy (alone or in combination with anthracyclines) in locally advanced disease, with overall clinical response, cCR, and pCR rates of 85–95%, 3–25% and 1–24% respectively (21–27). In addition, small phase II trials with paclitaxel showed activity in the preoperative setting, with cCR rates of 17–40% (28–30). In particular, one study of 20 patients demonstrated a pCR of 25% when paclitaxel was administered alone.

These results led to large comparative trials to determine whether the addition of taxanes in preoperative treatment would improve outcomes and to establish the optimal sequence with anthracyclines (sequentially or concurrent). These trials are summarized in Table 46.2.

Combination schedules with anthracyclines were tested since they were more active in the adjuvant setting. In a phase II trial, 407 patients with unresectable stage III disease were randomized to four cycles of FAC (fluorouracil, doxorubicin, and cyclophosphamide) versus the same number of cycles of the concurrent combination AT: docetaxel (75 mg/m²) plus doxorubicin (50 mg/m²) (31). The ORRs were 62% for AT and 55% for FAC (p = 0.0056) and the respective cCR rates were 16% and 6%. Nonetheless, the trial failed to demonstrate an improvement in the pCR rate (16 and 11%, no statistically significant difference) from a combined regimen.

In a randomized single-center phase III trial (the Aberdeen trial) 162 patients with operable or locally advanced (IIB and III stages) breast cancer were treated with four cycles of an anthracycline-containing regimen (CVAP: cyclophosphamide 1000 mg/m², doxorubicin 50 mg/m², vincristine 1.5 mg/m², and prednisolone 40 mg for 5 days) every 21 days (32). Non-responders were treated with four cycles of docetaxel 100 mg/m² every 21 days. Responders were randomized to further cycles of CVAP versus four cycles of docetaxel. In the non-responders' group, addition of docetaxel yielded ORR, cCR, and pCR rates of 47%, 11%, and 1.8%, respectively. A clinical response rate of 47% for docetaxel in patients unresponsive to CVAP was encouraging and suggested that patients not responding to an anthracycline schedule should be switched to docetaxel. Among the patients responding to four cycles of CVAP, those who received four cycles more had ORR, cCR, and pCR rates of 64%, 33%, and 15.4%, respectively. By contrast, ORR, cCR, and pCR rates for those who switched to docetaxel were significantly better (85%, 56%, and 30.8%, respectively). Patients receiving docetaxel had an increased BCS rate (67% vs. 48%, p < 0.01) and an increased OS at a median follow-up of 3 years (78% of CVAP alone group were alive compared with 93% of patients who received docetaxel, p = 0.04) (33). Though the "standard" regimen used in this trial is not popular, this was an important result suggesting that despite patients responding (at least clinically) to an anthracycline schedule, they had a better outcome if they switched to a non–cross-resistant regimen. However, given the small size of this trial, it is important for this observation to be confirmed in other trials of similar design.

The largest trial comparing addition of sequential docetaxel in the neoadjuvant setting was the NSABP B-27. A total of 2411 patients with operable stage II breast cancer (44% with tumors >4 cm and 30% with positive clinical nodes) were randomized into three arms: group I, four cycles of AC (doxorubicin 60 mg/m² with cyclophosphamide 600 mg/m²) followed by surgery; group II, four cycles of AC followed by 4 cycles of docetaxel (100 mg/m²) every 21 days and then surgery; group III, four cycles of AC followed by surgery, and then 4 cycles of docetaxel (100 mg/m²) as postoperative adjuvant therapy (34). Of note, all patients started treatment with tamoxifen for 5 years at the start of neoadjuvant chemotherapy.

The cCR rate for the groups treated with only four cycles of AC preoperatively was 40%, but reached 63.6% when docetaxel was added (p < 0.01). Among the patients in group II who did not achieve a cCR after treatment with AC, 42.9% were characterized as complete responders after treatment with docetaxel. The pCR rate was 12.9% and 14.4% respectively for groups I and III, and 26.1% for group II (p < 0.01).

Table 46.2 Clinical trials comparing taxanes versus anthracyclin-containing schedules in the neoadjuvant chemotherapy.

Study	N pts	Stage	Treatment	ORR	cCR	pCR	BCS rate	DFS	OS
Vinholes et al.[31]	406	Stage III unresectable	FAC x4 – S vs AT x4 – S	55% vs 62%[a]	6% vs 16%[a]	11% vs 16%	–	–	–
Aberdeen trial[32,33]	162	Stage IIB-III operable	CVAP x8 – S (R) vs CVAP x4 – D x4 – S (R) vs CVAP x4 – D x4 – S (NR)[b]	64% vs 85% vs 47%	33% vs 56% vs 11%	15.4% vs 30.8% vs 1.8%	48% vs 67%[a,c]	–	–
NSABP B-27[17,34]	2411	T1-3 N0-1 operable	AC x4 – S vs AC x4 – D x4 – S vs AC x4 – S – D x4[d]	85.5% vs 90.7%[a,c]	40% vs 63.6%[a,c]	12.9% vs 26.1%a vs 14.4%	61.6% vs 63.7%[c]	59% vs 62% vs 62% at 8 yr	74% vs 75 % vs 75% at 8 yr
Buzdar et al.[35,36]	174	T1-3 N0-1	FAC x4 – S – FAC x4 vs 3wP x4 – S – FAC x4	79% vs 80%	24% vs 27%	14% vs 8%	–	83% vs 86% at 4-yr	–
Green et al.[37]	258	T1-3 N0-1	WkP x12 – FAC x4 – S vs 3wP x4 – FAC x4 – S	77% vs 71%	34% vs 24%	28.2% vs 15.7%[a]	47% vs 38%[a]	–	–

[a]Statistically significant.

[b](R) = Responders to initial 4 cycles of CVAP; (NR) = Non-responders to initial 4 cycles of CVAP.

[c]Comparing non-docetaxel schedules versus docetaxel-containing schedules.

[d]All patients received tamoxifen for 5 years starting concurrently with chemotherapy.

Abbreviations: N pts, Number of patients; ORR, clinical overall response rate; cCR, clinical complete response; pCR, pathologic complete response; BCS, breast-conserving surgery; DFS, disease-free survival; OS, overall survival; FAC, 5-fluorouracil, doxorubicin and cyclophosphamide; AT, doxorubicin and docetaxel; AC, doxorubicin and cyclophosphamide; S, surgery; D, docetaxel; WkP, weekly paclitaxel; 3wP, 3-weekly paclitaxel.

Moreover, the addition of preoperative docetaxel increased the proportion of patients with negative axillary lymph nodes from 50.8% in groups I and III combined to 58.2% in group II (p < 0.001). The BCS rates were similar among those who received preoperative AC only and those who received both preoperative AC and preoperative docetaxel (61.6% vs. 63.7%, p = 0.33) indicating that despite the increased response rates a similar proportion of patients could avoid mastectomy. At the latest update on follow-up at a median of 8.5 years, OS, DFS, and relapse-free survival rates were similar for the three groups (17). The 5-year and 8-year OS estimates were 82% and 74% for group I, 83% and 75% for group II, and 82% and 75% for group III, respectively. The five- and eight-year DFS estimates were 68% and 59% for group I, 71% and 62% for group II, and 70% and 62% for group III, respectively. The pCR rate was a highly significant predictor of improved DFS (HR 0.49, p < 0.0001) and OS (HR 0.36, p = 0001), as was pathological nodal status (p < 0.001). This study confirms that the addition of docetaxel to AC improves clinical and pathological responses and improves the chance of pCR. However, long-term outcomes were not significantly different.

With respect to paclitaxel, a phase III trial from MD Anderson compared four cycles of 3-weekly paclitaxel (250 mg/m^2 as a 24-hour infusion) versus four cycles of FAC (fluorouracil, doxorubicin and cyclophosphamide). A total of 174 patients with T1-3 N0-1 breast cancer were included (35). No statistically significant differences were found in ORR (80% for paclitaxel and 79% for FAC), cCR (27% and 24%), or pCR (8% and 14%) and the BCS rate was similar in both arms. After surgery, all patients received four further cycles of FAC. At a median follow-up of 60 months, the four-year DFS was not significantly different (83% with preoperative FAC and 86% with preoperative paclitaxel) (36).

Weekly paclitaxel has been shown to be more effective than 3-weekly paclitaxel in the metastatic setting. Thus, a phase III neoadjuvant trial was undertaken to compare two schedules of paclitaxel: weekly paclitaxel for 12 weeks (80 mg/m^2 dose) for clinically node-negative disease, and 150 mg/m^2 for 3 weeks and 1 week off for clinically node-positive disease versus paclitaxel as a 24-h infusion at 225 mg/m^2 every 3 weeks for 4 cycles (Table 46.2) (37). A total of 258 patients were enrolled. Clinical response rates were similar for both arms (with a trend to better cCR rate with weekly paclitaxel, 34 vs. 24%) but BCS rate improved in the weekly group (47 vs. 38%, p = 0.05). Also, the pCR rate in the breast and axilla was significantly higher when paclitaxel was administered in a weekly regimen (28.2 vs. 15.7%, p = 0.02). These data are consistent with the results of studies from metastatic (38) and adjuvant (39) settings.

In conclusion, the addition of docetaxel or paclitaxel to anthracycline-containing chemotherapy improves clinical and pathological response rates. However, long-term outcomes in terms of DFS and OS are not improved (apart from the small Aberdeen trial).

Concurrent Vs. Sequential Anthracycline and Taxane-Containing Schedules

The trials discussed in the previous section suggest that the addition of taxanes to anthracyclines improves response rates. Taxanes can be given either concurrently or sequentially with anthracyclines. In this section we discuss trials that help to determine whether either of these approaches is superior to the other.

In the Anglo-Celtic phase III trial, 363 patients with locally advanced and inflammatory breast cancer were randomized to six cycles of AC versus AD (doxorubicin 60 mg/m^2 and docetaxel 75 mg/m^2) every three weeks (40). No differences were found between pCR rates for the anthracycline alone (AC) compared with the concurrent anthracycline/taxane regimen (17% and 20%, respectively, p = 0.42). In an updated analysis, with a median follow-up of 99 months, there was no significant difference between the two groups for either DFS (p = 0.20) and OS (p = 0.24) (41).

In a similar study with paclitaxel, 200 patients with T2-3 N0-1 breast cancer were randomized to receive preoperative treatment with either AP (concurrent doxorubicin 60 mg/m^2 plus paclitaxel 200 mg/m^2 as a 3-hour infusion) or AC every three weeks, for four cycles (42). The pCR rates provided by independent pathologists were similar between the two groups (8% and 6%). BCS was performed in 58% and 45% of patients in the AP and AC arms, respectively. Once again, no survival advantage was found for the taxane-containing regimen.

A meta-analysis involving 2455 patients from seven trials comparing neoadjuvant schedules with or without taxanes found no significant differences in pCR rates (p = 0.11) (43). However, when only studies with sequential regimens were included, there was a favorable advantage from addition of taxanes (RR 1.73, 95% CI 1.12–2.68, p = 0.013), but no improvement was found for concurrent schedules.

Dose-Dense Treatments

In the adjuvant setting, dose-dense chemotherapy regimens containing anthracyclines and taxanes are clearly superior to standard schedules, improving DFS and in some cases OS (44). However, results for preoperative trials evaluating these schedules are not so clear.

In a EORTC-NCIC-SAKK multicenter trial, 448 patients with locally advanced breast cancer were randomly treated with a conventional CEF regimen (cyclophosphamide 75 mg/m^2 orally on days 1–14, epirubicin 60 mg/m^2 intravenously days on 1, 8, and fluorouracil 500 mg/m^2 days 1, 8 each 28 days) for six cycles versus EC (epirubicin 120 mg/m^2 IV day 1 and cyclophosphamide 830 mg/m^2 IV day 1), with granulocyte colony-stimulating factor, every 14 days for six cycles (45). Clinical complete response rates were similar in both arms (31.3 and 26.5% respectively). After chemotherapy, 382 patients received local therapy (surgery, radiotherapy, or both). Nineteen patients (14%) in CEF and 15 patients (10%) in EC had a pCR. After a median follow-up of 5.5 years, the median progression-free survival rates were 34 and 33.7 months (p = 0.68), and the 5-year OS rates were 53%, and 51% for CEF and EC, respectively (p = 0.94).

In the GeparDuo phase III trial, four cycles of concurrent dose-dense doxorubicin and docetaxel (50 mg/m^2 and 75 mg/m^2, respectively) every 14 days, were compared with four cycles of AC every 21 days followed by four cycles of docetaxel 100 mg/m^2 every 21 days (46). A total of 913 patients with operable or locally advanced disease were included. The primary objective, the pCR rate, was notably higher for the sequential regimen (14.3%) compared with the concurrent dose-dense scheme (7%, OR 2.22, p < 0.001). Clinical response (85% vs. 75%) and

BCS rates (75% vs. 65%) were also significantly improved for the sequential compared with the concurrent groups.

Therefore, in conclusion, dose-dense chemotherapy does not appear to be superior to conventional dose treatments in the preoperative setting.

Duration of Primary Chemotherapy

Neoadjuvant studies with anthracyclines (with or without taxanes) have often employed schedules from the adjuvant setting, sometimes with different durations of treatment. Most currently used schedules are between 12 and 24 weeks, and may be divided before or after surgery.

In an Austrian Breast Cancer Study Group (ABCSG) trial of 292 patients with stage I–III disease, three cycles versus six cycles of concurrent preoperative epirubicin (75 mg/m^2) and docetaxel (75 mg/m^2) every 3 weeks were compared (47). The six-cycle arm achieved a significantly higher pCR rate (18.6% vs. 7.7%, respectively; p = 0.0045), a higher percentage of patients with negative axillary status (56.6% vs. 42.8%, respectively; p = 0.02), and a trend toward a greater chance of BCS (75.9% vs. 66.9%, respectively; p = 0. 10).

Another smaller study enrolling 176 patients, compared four (ED4) or six (ED6) cycles of concurrent epirubicin and docetaxel, using the same doses as the previous trial (48). The pCR rate was 11% with ED4 and 24% with ED6 (p = 0.047). The BCS rate was 47% for the ED4 group compared with 58% for the ED6 group.

In the GeparTrio trial, patients who responded to two cycles of TAC regimen (docetaxel 75 mg/m^2, doxorubicin 50 mg/m^2, and cyclophosphamide 500 mg/^{2}, every 21 days), were randomized to receive four versus six further cycles (49). A total number of 1390 patients were assessed in these arms. Rates of pCR were not statistically significantly different between the two groups (21% with six TAC cycles and 23.5% with eight TAC cycles, p = 0.27). The rates of BCS were similar in both arms (67.5% vs. 68.5%, respectively, p = 0.68).

A meta-analysis of the German Breast Group, including data from seven neoadjuvant trials (50), demonstrated in a multivariable analysis that pCR became more likely with an increase in the number of cycles (p = 0.009), with higher cumulative anthracycline doses (p = 0.002), higher cumulative taxane doses (p = 0.009), and capecitabine-containing regimens (p = 0.022). Interestingly, the association of pCR with the number of cycles was more pronounced in patients with hormone receptor (HR)-positive tumors, as compared with HR-negative tumors (p = 0.039).

In conclusion, the optimal duration of preoperative chemotherapy is unknown and perhaps should be tailored for different schedules in different subsets of patients. However, for concurrent anthracyclines and taxanes six cycles may be optimal.

Tailoring Therapy Based on Response

Another important question regarding neoadjuvant treatment is whether chemotherapy should be changed for patients whose tumors do not respond to the initial chemotherapy. As previously discussed, the Aberdeen trial (32) showed that non-responders to an anthracycline-containing regimen had a clinical response rate of 47% when docetaxel was sequentially added, and some of them avoided mastectomy.

In the GeparTrio study, patients who did not respond to two cycles of TAC (docetaxel 75 mg/m^2, doxorubicin 50 mg/m^2, and cyclophosphamide 500 mg/^{2}, every 21 days), were randomized to four further cycles of TAC or four cycles of NX (vinorelbine 25 mg/m^2 days 1 and 8, capecitabine 2000 mg/m^2 days 1–14, every 21 days) (49,51). The cCR rate was similar in the two arms (22.5% for TAC and 21.9% for NX). A pCR was reached in 7.3% and 3.1% with TAC and NX, respectively. Of note, responders to the two initial cycles of TAC presented a pCR rate of 22.6%.

In conclusion, after the failure of an anthracycline-containing schedule, taxane-based preoperative chemotherapy might improve the clinical response. There is no evidence of benefit from adding other chemotherapy agents if no response is reached for an anthracycline plus taxane regimen.

Predictors of Response to Primary Chemotherapy

One of the most relevant conclusions of the large clinical trials and meta-analyses in the neoadjuvant setting is that patients achieving cCR and especially pCR in the breast, have better long-term outcomes (17–20). Different definitions of pCR have been used, but the most accepted is the absence of invasive carcinoma in the breast and axillary nodes (some authors include absence of in situ carcinoma too). The response in the axillary nodes seems to be important since a pathologically positive node status after neoadjuvant chemotherapy is associated with inferior DFS and OS (52,53). One retrospective study which included 122 patients showed that the number of residual positive axillary nodes and the size of nodal metastases were correlated with distant DFS and OS. Compared with patients with negative nodes, even the presence of lymph node micrometastasis (≤2 mm) was associated with worsened DFS and OS (54).

Thus, the goal of preoperative chemotherapy should be to achieve a pCR in both the breast and axilla which can then become a surrogate marker to perform smaller and faster clinical trials. In some of the neoadjuvant chemotherapy trials, clinical features such as size of the primary tumor were correlated with clinical response (55). Furthermore, pCR rates were 50% in patients with tumors less than 2 cm compared with only 18% for tumors more than 5 cm in size. In addition, the presence of clinical axillary node disease before treatment was found to influence the response to chemotherapy. A clinico-pathological analysis was performed in 1234 patients included in the NSABP B-18 trial (56). Patients with negative lymph nodes in the preoperative group more frequently exhibited a pCR in terms of the primary tumor compared with those who had positive lymph nodes (29% vs. 11%; p < 0.0001). In both treatment groups, the OS and DFS were significantly better for lymph node–negative patients (p < 0.001).

In the aforementioned study, it was also found that poor nuclear grade was significantly associated with a pCR compared with a more favorable nuclear grade (26% vs. 14%) (56). Other differentiation features, such as the number of mitosis or histological grade appear to be correlated with responsiveness to chemotherapy (57,58). Undifferentiated tumors are more sensitive to chemotherapy which translates in higher pCR rates in some cases.

Hormone receptor expression is an important prognostic and predictive factor in breast cancer. In the European Cooperative Trial in Operable breast cancer (ECTO) trial, two adjuvant arms and one neoadjuvant chemotherapy arm with CMF, doxorubicin, and paclitaxel were evaluated. Interestingly, it was found on multivariate analysis that only estrogen receptor (ER) status was significantly associated with pCR (OR for ER negative, 5.77, p < 0.0001) (59).

In a pooled analysis of 1731 patients treated with preoperative chemotherapy (91% with anthracyclines, 66% with taxanes), a significantly higher pCR rate was found in women with ER-negative compared with ER-positive tumors (24 vs. 8%, p < 0.001) (60). These findings have been corroborated by other clinical trials and meta-analyses, and show that patients with ER-negative tumors have a higher chance of achieving a pCR (34,36,43).

Histological type might also play a role in selecting patients with a greater chance of a pCR after neoadjuvant chemotherapy. In a study involving more than 900 patients, those with invasive lobular carcinoma (ILC) (n = 122) were less likely to have a pCR compared with those with invasive ductal carcinoma (IDC) (3% vs. 15%, respectively, p < 0.001) in a retrospective analysis of six clinical trials (61). Patients with a lobular phenotype tended to be older and have more ER-positive tumors. In another study, pathological features of 457 patients (8% with ILC) were analyzed (62). ILC was an independent predictor for a poor clinical response (p = 0.02) and ineligibility for BCS after neoadjuvant chemotherapy (p = 0.03). Other factors predicting a poor response to chemotherapy (favorable histological grade, ER positivity, low Ki67 expression) were more frequent in lobular than in ductal carconimas.

The expression of C-erb2 (HER2) has been recognized as a marker of chemosensitivity in some small neoadjuvant studies, especially for anthracycline-containing regimens (63). One study enrolled 79 patients treated with six cycles of two different schedules of FEC chemotherapy (one with epirubicin 50 mg/m^2 and the other with 100 mg/m^2) and initially reported that HER2-positive tumors seemed to have better clinical ORR to FEC100 than HER2-negative tumors (100% vs. 69%, p = 0.07) (64). In a further report, with 119 treated in the FEC100 arm, only ER status and Ki67 were predictive markers for response, but not HER2 (65). In a subanalysis of the German Breast Cancer Group (GEPARTRIO) trial, *ERBB2* gene expression was strongly predictive of pCR (p = 0.017), cCR (p = 0.05), and also OS (p = 0.037) (66). In contrast, another possible marker of sensitivity to anthracyclines, *TOP2A* (topoisomerase II), did not correlate with clinical or pathological response.

The role of Ki67 expression, a marker of cell proliferation, has been particularly controversial. Although its role as a prognostic factor is well recognized (67), early studies suggesting that it might be a predictor of clinical or pathological response in the neoadjuvant setting were conflicting (68,69). Nevertheless, the largest retrospective analysis, involving 552 patients treated with neoadjuvant chemotherapy (60% anthracyclines and taxanes), showed that 70.7% of tumors had a high proliferative rate in the initial core biopsy (with an immunohistochemical cut-off value of 13%). Ki67 was found to be an independent predictor for pCR (OR 3.5; 95% CI, 1.4–10.1), OS (HR 8.1; 95% CI, 3.3–20.4) and distant DFS (HR 3.2; 95% CI, 1.8–5.9) (70).

As mentioned previously, the German Breast Group published a detailed analysis of 3332 women included in the seven neoadjuvant trials in order to determine which patients, tumors, and treatments characteristics were associated with a pCR (50). Higher pCR rates were observed in younger patients, lower stage disease, ductal subtype carcinomas, higher grade tumors, and hormone receptor–negative and HER2-positive tumors (p for trend or interaction < 0.001 for each of these factors).

In conclusion, patients with small ER-negative, poorly differentiated, axillary node–negative and highly proliferative breast tumors may be more likely to achieve a pCR with neoadjuvant chemotherapy.

New Drugs in Primary Chemotherapy

Although anthracyclines and taxanes remain the standard of care for both adjuvant and neoadjuvant chemotherapy schedules, other drugs used in the metastatic setting have been evaluated in clinical trials.

Vinorelbine, a semisynthetic vinca alkaloid, has been studied in a phase III trial. A total of 451 patients were randomized to six cycles of AC or VE (vinorelbine 25 mg/m^2 on days 1 and 8 and epirubicin 60 mg/m^2 on day 1, 3 weekly) (71). Clinical and pathological responses were similar for both arms of the study (cCR 20 and 24%, pCR 12% for both), though toxicity profiles were very different.

Capecitabine, an oral fluoropyrimidine, has been tested in two preoperative trials. In the first one, 209 patients with axillary node–positive breast cancer were treated with AC chemotherapy or TX (docetaxel 75 mg/m^2 on day 1 plus capecitabine 1000 mg/m^2 orally twice daily on days 1–14 every three weeks), for four cycles (72). Compared with AC, TX significantly increased the pCR rate (21% vs. 10%, respectively, p = 0.024) and the ORR (84% vs. 65%, p = 0.003). At a median follow-up of 37 months, there was no significant difference in DFS (p = 0.932). In the second trial, 1421 patients received four cycles of EC chemotherapy and were then randomized to three separate arms: (A) four cycles of docetaxel 100 mg/m^2, (B) four cycles of docetaxel plus capecitabine (TX; docetaxel 75 mg/m^2 plus capecitabine 1800 mg/m^2), or (C) four cycles of docetaxel 75 mg/m^2 followed by four cycles of capecitabine 1800 mg/m^2 (73). Following definitive surgery, pCR rates were 22.3% for arm A, 19.5% for arm B, and 22.3% for arm C (p = 0.298). BCS rates were 70.1%, 68.4%, and 65.3%, respectively (p = 0.781). Although addition of capecitabine was negative in this study, a further meta-analysis found that inclusion of capecitabine had a favorable impact on pCR rates (50).

Platinum compounds are DNA-damaging agents that have been evaluated in the metastatic and adjuvant settings, especially for triple negative (TN) breast cancers in which DNA-repair systems seem to be disrupted. The combination of carboplatin with docetaxel was studied in 74 patients with stage II/III breast cancer (74). The pCR rate was 26.8%, but notably higher in the TN subset (54.6%). On multivariate analysis, tumor subtype was an independent predictor of pCR. In a phase III trial, 200 patients received epirubicin plus paclitaxel, with or without cisplatin (i.e., ET vs. PET) in a weekly schedule (75). More patients in the PET arm achieved a pCR or near pCR compared to the ET arm (p = 0.02). At a median follow-up of 74 months, the 5-year distant DFS and OS were 73% and 55% (p = 0.04), versus 82% and 69% (p = 0.07) for PET and ET groups respectively. In a subset analysis, PET was significantly better than ET only for high-grade or highly proliferating tumors.

In conclusion, drugs other than anthracyclines and taxanes have demonstrated efficacy in the neoadjuvant setting, and might be alternatives in selected cases, although their use is not the standard of care.

ENDOCRINE THERAPY
Introduction
Primary systemic therapy has focused mainly on chemotherapy schedules but experience with primary endocrine therapy has been steadily accumulating particularly in older postmenopausal women. Initial experience was with tamoxifen but subsequently AIs have replaced this as the agent of first choice. The development of primary endocrine therapy has taken a different course to that of chemotherapy in that the latter was initially used for treatment of locally more aggressive disease in younger women while the former tended to be employed initially as treatment for elderly frail patients.

Experience with Tamoxifen
Tamoxifen has been the most widely used endocrine therapy for treatment of breast cancer and for many years was the treatment of choice in the adjuvant setting (76). Initial reports in the early 1980s on the use of tamoxifen as primary therapy in elderly patients (often medically unfit) with locally advanced disease indicated rates of response ranging from 33% to 68% (77). Tamoxifen was being used as an alternative to surgery in these patients who were often not selected on the basis of ER status.

Following these reports a number of randomized trials were conducted which compared either tamoxifen alone versus surgery (78,79) or tamoxifen alone versus surgery plus tamoxifen (80,81). In the former it had been hoped that tamoxifen would replace surgery for elderly women while in the latter it was seen as an addition to surgery. In the two trials comparing tamoxifen with surgery (78,79) women with operable tumors above the age of 70 years were recruited. Though the sample sizes of 116 and 135 are small and need to be treated with some caution, no differences in OS were observed. However, Robertson and colleagues did find a high local failure rate with tamoxifen alone (43% vs. 24%) and suggested that surgery should be incorporated into any optimal treatment plan (79). With these two trials it should be emphasized that patients having surgery did not receive tamoxifen.

Two subsequent trials compared tamoxifen alone with surgery and adjuvant tamoxifen as would have been standard of care. In one of these, a randomized study of 381 patients conducted by Bates et al., no differences were observed in OS rates, but local failure was higher for patients receiving tamoxifen alone (35% vs. 20.5%) (80). A similar result was found in the other trial which enrolled 473 women, and reported a local failure rate of 25% in the tamoxifen alone arm compared with 5% for combined treatment (81).

These trials are consistent in the association between tamoxifen treatment alone and a high local failure rate. However, it should be noted that patients were often not selected on the basis of ER status and some patients would have been ER negative/poor and therefore unlikely to respond to endocrine therapy.

Tamoxifen Vs. Aromatase Inhibitors
In the adjuvant setting AIs have demonstrated superior efficacy to tamoxifen in postmenopausal women either as upfront therapy or as part of a switch/sequencing strategy (82). It therefore seemed logical that a series of trials would be undertaken to compare AIs with tamoxifen in the neoadjuvant setting. Most experience has been with the nonsteroidal AIs, letrozole and anastrozole, with less experience using the steroidal AI exemestane. These trials are summarized in Table 46.3.

Eirmann et al. reported the PO24 trial, which was a double-blind multinational trial comparing letrozole with tamoxifen for four months prior to surgery in women with ER-positive and/or PR-positive primary breast tumors (83). A total of 337 postmenopausal women were recruited, and the ORR was significantly higher for letrozole than tamoxifen (55% vs. 36%, p < 0.001). BCS rates were also improved with letrozole (45% vs. 35%, p = 0.02). As a result of these data, letrozole has largely replaced tamoxifen as the agent of choice for primary endocrine therapy in postmenopausal women. In a further analysis of tumor samples from this study, Ellis et al. reported on response to letrozole in relation to ER as well as erbB1 and/or erbB2 status (84). Clinical responses to letrozole were markedly superior compared with tamoxifen for those tumors overexpressing erbB1 and/or erbB2 [88% vs. 21% (p = 0.0004)].

Two large randomized trials have compared anastrozole with tamoxifen in the neoadjuvant setting. In the IMPACT trial, 330 postmenopausal women with ER-positive primary breast tumors were randomized to receive anastrozole, tamoxifen, or the combination for 12 weeks (85). This was the neoadjuvant equivalent to the much larger adjuvant trial Arimidex and Tamoxifen Alone or in Combination (ATAC) which compared the same options in the adjuvant setting for a total treatment period of five years (86). Objective clinical response rates were 37% for anastrozole, 36% for tamoxifen, and 39% for the combination with ultrasound measurements also showing no significant differences. Of the 124 patients judged to have required mastectomy at baseline, 44% received BCS in the anastrozole group, and 31% after preoperative tamoxifen (p = 0.23).

In the Pre-Operative "Arimidex" Compared to Tamoxifen (PROACT) trial, 451 postmenopausal women with ER-positive primary breast cancer were randomized to either anastrozole or tamoxifen for a period of 12 weeks prior to surgery (87). The protocol allowed women in this study to receive concomitant chemotherapy which was 29% and 32% for the anastrozole and tamoxifen groups respectively. For the

Table 46.3 Phase III clinical trials of neoadjuvant hormone therapy.

Study	N pts	Treatment	ORR	BCS rate
P024[83]	337	L vs T (16 wk)	55% vs 36%[a]	45% vs 35%[a]
IMPACT[85]	330	A vs T vs T+A (12 wk)	37% vs 36% vs 39%	46% vs 22% vs 26%
PROACT[87]	451	A vs T (12 wk)	39.5% vs 35.4%	43% vs 30.8%[a]
Semiglazov et al[88]	451	E vs T (12 wk)	76% vs 40%[a]	37% vs 20%[a]

[a]Statistically significant.
Abbreviations: N pts, Number of patients; cCR, clinical complete response; BCS, breast-conserving surgery; T, tamoxifen; L, letrozole; A, anastrozole; E, exemestan.

primary endpoint of ultrasound response rate, no significant differences were found between anastrozole (39.5%) and tamoxifen (35.4%) but BCS rates were higher for patients in the anastrozole group (43% vs. 31%, p = 0.04).

Semiglazov and colleagues have reported the only randomized trial of exemestane versus tamoxifen (88) with 151 women with ER-positive tumors treated for three months prior to surgery. Both clinical response rates (76% vs. 40%, p = 0.05) and BCS rates (36.8% vs. 20%, p = 0.05) were significantly in favor of exemestane.

Duration of Endocrine Therapy

The optimal duration of primary endocrine therapy is unknown but may well be longer than for chemotherapy. For the latter, duration of treatment is limited to some extent by tolerability which is not an issue with endocrine therapy. The pCR rates to primary endocrine therapy have generally been very low (3%) and more prolonged therapy could potentially increase both rates of pCR as well as BCS (83,89).

No randomized trial of different durations of primary endocrine therapy has been undertaken to date. However, Carpenter et al. reported an interesting non-randomized study at the annual meeting of the American Society of Clinical Oncology in 2010 (90). In this multicenter United Kingdom (UK) trial, women with primary ER-positive and/or PR-positive breast tumors >2 cm that were not conservable, were treated with letrozole for up to 12 months. The primary endpoint was the time at which a patient became eligible for BCS.

Primary Chemotherapy Vs. Aromatase Inhibitors

There is a paucity of studies comparing these two approaches of primary chemotherapy with AIs. The most important study addressing this issue was reported by Semiglazov et al. who performed a randomized phase II trial of exemestane for three months or four 3-weekly cycles of doxorubicin with paclitaxel (89). A total of 121 patients were randomized and eligible women were postmenopausal with ER-positive and/or PR-positive tumors. Clinical objective response rates were 64% for both arms and though the pCR rates were higher for chemotherapy (6% vs. 3%), these results were not significantly different. Furthermore, BCS rates were higher for exemestane (33% vs. 24%, p = 0.058) and not unexpectedly, endocrine therapy was better tolerated.

The pilot phase of the UK randomized trial NEOCENT has been completed. This trial also compared primary chemotherapy with endocrine therapy and incorporated a translational component to identify predictors of response and resistance to treatment.

Predictors of Response to Preoperative
Aromatase Inhibitors

As discussed earlier for the IMPACT trial, no differences were found in response rates among anastrozole, tamoxifen, or the combination (85). However, Dowsett and colleagues have reported on changes in the proliferation marker Ki67 at baseline, after two weeks of primary endocrine treatment and at the time of surgery (91). Significant reductions in Ki67 expression were seen both at two weeks (76%, 59.5%, and 64% for anastrozole, tamoxifen, and the combination respectively) and at the time of surgery (81%, 62%, and 61%, respectively). The reduction in Ki67 at two weeks for anastrozole compared

with tamoxifen accurately predicted results of the adjuvant ATAC trial, showing a small but significant benefit in favor of anastrozole (92).

The POETIC trial is nearing completion in the UK and aims to recruit 4000 patients in a multicenter phase III trial with the aim of determining whether Ki67 at two weeks after starting preoperative endocrine therapy can be used to predict which patients will do well with adjuvant endocrine therapy alone and who will require additional treatments (93).

Conclusion

Primary endocrine therapy with AIs is an appropriate option for frail elderly patients with inoperable hormone receptor–positive disease. It may be used to downstage tumors to allow for BCS as with neoadjuvant chemotherapy. However, for those patients who are medically fit, surgery should be included in the treatment plan. Future studies are needed to identify and address patients who are best managed with either neoadjuvant endocrine therapy or chemotherapy.

ANTI HER2 THERAPY
Introduction

The human epidermal growth factor receptor 2 (HER2, codified by *ERBB2* gene) is a transmembrane protein-kinase receptor member of the family of HER receptors and plays an important role in breast cancer (94,95). Although it was known as a poor prognostic factor for many years, molecular classifications from the 2000s' decade have emphasized the importance of *ERBB2*- enriched breast cancers (96). Drugs designed specifically against HER2 have been developed. Trastuzumab, the first monoclonal antibody evaluated, demonstrated an important clinical benefit in metastatic and early stage disease as adjuvant treatment (97,98). Lately, other anti-HER2 drugs have been assessed in preclinical and clinical trials.

Trastuzumab

Several one-armed phase II trials of operable and locally advanced disease with patient numbers ranging from 31 to 94 have evaluated the efficacy of trastuzumab combined with different chemotherapy schedules (99–104). Clinical response rates have ranged from 70% to 100%, with cCR and pCR rates of 46–62% and 12–47%, respectively. All of these studies showed a greater benefit in patients with ER-negative tumors. In the GEPARQUATTRO phase III trial (where patients were randomized to receive capecitabine added or not to an anthracycline and docetaxel-containing schedule), 445 HER2-positive patients were treated with concurrent trastuzumab every three weeks (105). The pCR rate, as defined by the absence of residual invasive or *in situ* disease in the breast, was 31.7%.

Some phase III trials have corroborated evidence for the benefit of adding trastuzumab to conventional chemotherapy versus chemotherapy alone. Summarized data from these trials are included in Table 46.4. In a study by Buzdar et al., patients with stage II/IIIA HER2-positive breast tumors were randomized to receive weekly paclitaxel followed by FEC (fluorouracil, epirubicin, and cyclophosphamide), or the same regimen with weekly trastuzumab during 24 weeks of treatment (106). Initially 33 patients were enrolled (10 in the only-chemotherapy arm and 23 in the trastuzumab arm), but later 22 more were treated with the combination. Clinical response was near 100%

Table 46.4   Comparative clinical trials including anti-HER2 therapy in the neoadjuvant setting.

Study	N pts	Treatment	ORR	cCR	pCR
Buzdar et al.[106]	64	WkP – FEC vs WkP – FEC + T	94% vs 100%	47% vs 91%	26.3% vs 65.2%[a]
NOAH[107]	235	AP – P – CMF vs AP – P – CMF + T	–	–	22% vs 43%
NeoALTTO[112]	455	WkP + L vs WkP + T vs WkP + T + L	52.6% vs 29.5% vs 67.1%[b]	–	24.7% vs 29.5% vs 51.3%[a]
NeoSphere[115]	417	T+D vs T+Pe+D vs Pe+D vs T+Pe	80% vs 88% vs 71% vs 68%	–	29% vs 45.8%[a] vs 17.8% vs 24%

[a]Statistically significant
[b]ORR at 6 weeks of only targeted therapy (without chemotherapy).
Abbreviations: N pts, Number of patients; ORR, overall clinical response rate; cCR, clinical complete response; pCR, pathologic complete response; BCS, breast-conserving surgery; DFS, disease-free survival; OS, overall survival; WkP, weekly paclitaxel; FEC, fluoruracil, epirubicine and cyclophosphamide; AP, doxorubicin and paclitaxel; P, paclitaxel; CMF, cyclophosphamide, metothrexate, and fluoruracil; D, docetaxel; CT, chemotherapy; T, trastuzumab; L, lapatinib; Pe, pertuzumab.

in both arms, with cCR in 21 of the 23 patients initially treated with trastuzumab. The pCR rate in breast and nodes was 26.3% in the chemotherapy-alone arm and 65.2% in the trastuzumab plus chemotherapy arm. After 34 patients had completed therapy, the Data Monitoring Committee stopped the trial because of the superiority of the combination. With a median follow-up of 36.1 months, DFS was significantly better among patients randomized to chemotherapy plus trastuzumab, with a DFS at three years of 100% (but the small number of patients included should be taken into account).

In the NOAH phase III trial, 235 patients with HER2-positive locally advanced breast cancer were randomized to a more prolonged regimen of chemotherapy (three cycles of doxorubicin with paclitaxel every 21 days, followed by four cycles of paclitaxel every 21 days, and then three cycles of cyclophosphamide, methotrexate, and fluorouracil every 28 days) with or without trastuzumab (followed by adjuvant trastuzumab to complete one year) (107). A cohort of women with HER2-negative tumors was used as the comparator group. Comparing the chemotherapy-alone arm and the combination, pCR rates in the breast were 22% and 43%, respectively and 19% and 38%, in the axilla respectively. Results in the HER2-negative cohort with chemotherapy were similar to those for HER2-positive patients receiving chemotherapy only. After a median follow-up of 3.2 years, DFS was 71% in the trastuzumab arm and 56% in the non-trastuzumab group (HR 0.59, 95% CI 038–0.90; p = 0.013) but no significant differences were found in OS.

Although administering trastuzumab concurrently with adjusted doses of anthracyclines does not appear to have significant cardiac toxicity, some trials have explored the use of non-anthracycline combinations (102,108). Clinical and pathological responses are similar to those previously reported for anthracycline regimens, so these might be an alternative option for patients at high cardiovascular risk.

In conclusion, trastuzumab-based therapy is regarded as the standard of care in the neoadjuvant setting for patients with HER2-positive breast cancer.

Other HER2-Directed Therapies

The dual HER1 (EGFR) and HER2 inhibitor lapatinib has been shown to be active and safe in advanced breast cancer when administered alone or in combination with other agents (109,110). Results of adjuvant trials are promising, and some randomized trials in the neoadjuvant setting are ongoing.

In a phase II trial, patients with HER2-positive inflammatory breast cancer received lapatinib at 1500 mg/day for 14 days, and then the same dose in combination with weekly paclitaxel (80 mg/m²) for 12 weeks (111). The clinical response rate was 78.1% (with cCR 9%) and the pCR was 9.4%.

Some phase III trials have been performed with new anti-HER2 therapies (summarized in Table 46.4). The NeoALTTO study compared three arms of neoadjuvant treatment: either lapatinib 1500 mg/d, or trastuzumab 4 mg/kg loading dose followed by 2 mg/kg IV weekly, or lapatinib 1000 mg/d with trastuzumab for a total of six weeks. Patients subsequently continued on the same targeted therapy plus weekly paclitaxel 80 mg/m² for a further 12 weeks (112). After surgery, all patients received adjuvant anthracycline-containing chemotherapy and trastuzumab. A total of 455 patients were recruited into this NeoALTTO study. The pCR rate was significantly higher for the combination arm (lapatinib plus trastuzumab) compared with either trastuzumab or lapatinib alone (51.3% vs. 29.5% vs. 24.7%, respectively; p < 0.01 for both). The corresponding ORRs at 6 weeks (biological window) were 67.1% (combination), 30.2% (trastuzumab), and 52.6% (lapatinib).

Interestingly, a phase II trial using the combination of lapatinib and weekly trastuzumab for 12 weeks as exclusive neoadjuvant treatment in women with HER2-positive breast cancers showed a pathological response rate (pRR, defined as pCR and residual disease less than 1 cm in breast) of 53% and pCR of 28% (113). This study suggests that some patients might benefit from targeted therapy alone, avoiding undesirable effects of chemotherapy.

Pertuzumab is an antiHER2 antibody that binds a different epitope from trastuzumab and thus avoids heterodimerization of HER2 with other receptors. Promising results have been obtained in the metastatic setting (114). The NeoSphere phase III trial included 417 patients in four possible treatment arms: four cycles of docetaxel with trastuzumab every 21 days (TH), the same schedule with the addition of pertuzumab (840 mg loading dose and then 420 meg every 21 days) (THP), docetaxel with pertuzumab (TP), or both anti-HER2 therapies without chemotherapy (HP) (115). After surgery, all patients received FEC chemotherapy and trastuzumab. The ORR was 80%, 88%, 68%, and 71% for TH, THP, HP, and TP arms, respectively. The pCR rates in the breast were 29%, 46%, 18%, and 24% respectively and were significantly superior for the three-drug combination.

In conclusion, the combination of trastuzumab with other anti-HER2 drugs aimed at more complete blockage of the receptor appears promising in the context of neoadjuvant treatment of HER2-positive breast cancer. A proportion of patients may be satisfactorily treated with only anti-HER2 targeted therapies, but more extensive understanding of the intrinsic biology of these tumors is needed.

Predictors of Response to Anti-HER2 Therapy

HER2 measurement is performed using immunohistochemistry and/or fluorescent *in situ* hybridization (FISH) methods in accordance with consensus guidelines (116). Nevertheless, only a proportion of patients with HER2-positive breast cancer respond to anti-HER2 therapy. The cause of this resistance may lie in the underlying molecular mechanisms of HER2, whose pathway activation occurs via receptor heterodimerization with other HER family members (HER1 or EGFR, HER3, HER4) (117).

To illustrate this point, activation of HER2 upregulates the PI3K/AKT/mTOR pathway that is related to cell proliferation and survival in breast cancer (118). Other reasons for such upregulation are mutations in genes encoding the PI3K catalytic domain (*PIK3CA*) and loss of the phosphatase and tensin homolog (*PTEN*) tumor suppressor gene. Loss of PTEN is associated with trastuzumab resistance *in vitro* (119). These observations are corroborated by data from two preoperative trials (120). Patients with locally advanced HER2-overexpressing tumors were treated with trastuzumab for three weeks, or lapatinib for six weeks, followed by docetaxel and trastuzumab for 12 weeks. Low PTEN levels or activating mutations in *PIK3CA* conferred resistance to the trastuzumab regimen (p = 0.015), whereas low PTEN expressing tumors were associated with a high pathological response to lapatinib (p = 0.007). A combination of lapatinib and trastuzumab is supported by results of translational data.

More studies *in vivo*, examining resistance to anti-HER2 therapies in the preoperative setting, are necessary and this represents an optimal model to implement translational research. A combination of different anti-HER2 drugs is supported by preclinical and clinical studies, and addition of other targeted therapies might improve results further.

ASSESMENT OF RESPONSE TO PRIMARY TREATMENT
Introduction

Clinical examination of any residual tumor mass at completion of neoadjuvant therapy is traditionally used for evaluation of response to treatment. However, even when a cCR has occurred, viable tumor cells may be seen on pathological examination, thus emphasizing the importance of surgical resection of the original tumor site (121,122). Nevertheless, assessment of final clinical response remains important as a guide to surgical management. In addition to clinical examination, the assessment of response radiologically has also proven to be a useful adjunct and is now routinely performed.

Mammography and Ultrasound

Initial attempts to use mammography to predict pathological response after primary treatment showed limited accuracy (123). One retrospective study reviewed data on 189 patients treated with a neoadjuvant doxorubicin-containing schedule (124). Size estimates by clinical examination, mammography, and ultrasound revealed only moderate correlation with residual pathological tumor size (Spearman correlation coefficient, rho (p) 0.41 and 0.42 respectively). An accuracy to within one centimeter was obtained with ultrasound in 75% of patients, 66% with physical examination, and 70% with mammography. The rate of false-positive and false-negative reports after chemotherapy was respectively 20% and 57% for physical examination, 65% and 10% for ultrasound, and 46% and 20% for mammography.

A prospective study compared the three methods of assessment in 141 consecutive breast cancer patients treated with primary chemotherapy (125). According to World Health organization (WHO) criteria, the grade of response based on mammography and ultrasound was less marked than that seen on clinical examination. Residual tumor size assessed clinically had a stronger correlation with pathological findings (p = 0.68) than residual disease assessed by ultrasonography (p = 0.29) and mammography (p = 0.33). The pCR rate in this study was 2.1% (three cases); two of these achieved a cCR on clinical palpation, a single case was recognized by mammography, and none by ultrasonography.

In conclusion, the accuracy of evaluation with mammography and ultrasound can be variable and should be interpreted carefully in conjunction with physical examination. All modalities tend to overestimate the extent of residual disease, with particular difficulty in distinguishing between active disease and post-treatment fibrosis. Magnetic resonance imaging (MRI) may be a more sensitive technique in this context, allowing for more accurate and confident delineation of residual tumor.

Magnetic Resonance

Conventional MRI is an important tool in screening high-risk patients. In the neoadjuvant setting, MRI can provide useful information to aid surgical management of patients. Different patterns of tumor growth and response to chemotherapy have been identified on MRI. In a small study involving 33 patients treated with neoadjuvant doxorubicin and cyclophosphamide, four patterns of growth were described (126).

1. Circumscribed mass (ORR 77%)
2. Diffuse tissue infiltration (37.5%)
3. Patchy enhancement (20%)
4. Septal spread (25%)

In another study, 25 patients were evaluated with MRI after neoadjuvant chemotherapy. A concentric shrinkage pattern was found in 48% who were subsequently good candidates for BCS, in contrast to 52% in whom a dendritic shrinkage pattern was observed (127). In this latter group, positive margins were frequently seen after BCS, necessitating subsequent mastectomy. On pathological examination, tumors that were ER positive and HER2 negative with a low nuclear grade and displaying a papillary-tubular pattern tended to show a dendritic pattern of shrinkage.

The correlation of MRI to pathological response has also been evaluated in several studies. In a prospective study of 33 patients, residual tumor size on MRI was closely correlated with microscopic pathological disease, with a Spearman coefficient of 0.982 (128). A similar prospective study (n = 52 patients) showed a coefficient "r" of 0.89 for MRI measurements compared with 0.60 for clinical measurements (129). Of note, the accuracy of MRI appears to be less when there is improved response in terms of change in tumor size and this was also found in a third study involving 29 patients (130). Thus the correlation between tumor size measured by MRI and histopathology was 0.83 (p < 0.0007) in 12 tumors without regressive changes and 0.48 (p < 0.051) in 17 tumors with a significant change in tumor size in response to chemotherapy.

A meta-analysis of 25 studies has demonstrated a pooled sensitivity and specificity for MRI in predicting pathological response of 63% and 91% respectively (131). The I^2 index was highly significant, confirming strong evidence for between-study heterogeneity. Different variables were assessed, with statistically significant differences in sensitivity or specificity among studies that used different magnetic field strengths (less vs. more than 1 tesla). Nonetheless, specificity in studies with a pCR rate higher than 20% was lower than for studies with a pCR rate less than 20% (p = 0.003) with no significant differences observed for sensitivity.

An important concern is the differential pattern of response between the various biological subtypes of breast cancer (132). In one study addressing this issue, 188 patients were evaluated with MRI before and after neoadjuvant chemotherapy. Residual disease on final pathology was present in 66% of TN tumors, 61% of HER2-positive tumors, and 93% of ER-positive/HER2-negative tumors. The breast response index (representing the relative change in tumor stage) showed significant correlation with breast cancer subtype, MRI, and age (Pearson's coefficient 0.465; p < 0.001). On subset analysis, this index was only significant for TN tumors (p < 0.001) and HER2-positive tumors (p < 0.05).

Additionally, there is emerging evidence that functional MRI techniques which provide information about tumor vascularity may help identify early responders to neoadjuvant chemotherapy (133). In a study of 28 patients with primary breast cancer who underwent anthracycline based chemotherapy, reductions in MRI-derived vascular parameters (Ktrans, kep, rBV, and rBF) after just two cycles were significantly correlated with final pathological response (p < 0.01) (134).

In conclusion, MRI may be more accurate than physical examination or other imaging modalities in determining tumor response to primary treatment and suitability for BCS. However, response based primarily on MRI images should be interpreted with caution and in conjunction with clinical examination particularly in view of early evidence suggesting that responses may be influenced by different biological subtypes. Newer functional MRI techniques which provide information about tumor vascularity and cellularity may prove to be more useful in identifying responders to not only conventional chemotherapy schedules but also targeted biological therapies.

SENTINEL NODE BIOPSY

Sentinel lymph node biopsy (SLNB) is a well-established procedure in patients with clinically negative axillary nodes for whom trials have demonstrated no significant differences in long-term outcome compared with axillary lymph node dissection (ALND) (135). The main concern in the neoadjuvant setting is whether it should be performed before or after preoperative systemic treatment.

In the NSABP B-27 trial, 428 patients underwent SLNB and ALND after neoadjuvant chemotherapy (136). The success rate for identification and removal of sentinel nodes was 84.8% and the reported false-negative rate was 10.7%. Similar results were found in a French multicenter study in which 195 patients were assessed (137). The sentinel node identification rate was 90% and the false-negative rate was 11.5%. Of note, those patients without palpable axillary nodes before preoperative chemotherapy had a higher sentinel node detection rate compared with patients with suspicious axillary nodes prior to commencing chemotherapy (94.6% vs. 81.5%, p = 0.008).

Three separate meta-analyses have evaluated the role of SLNB after neoadjuvant chemotherapy. Sample sizes for each meta-analysis ranged from 1273 to 2148 patients and the number of studies included ranged from 21 to 27. The summary identification rate ranged from 89.6% to 91%, and the false-negative rate from 8.4 to 12% (138–140).

Three studies enrolling a small number of patients with operable breast cancer demonstrated that all the patients who were node negative in the SLNB before chemotherapy, remained node negative in ALND after treatment (141–143).

SLNB undertaken prior to chemotherapy will minimize the risk of a false-negative result and may allow more accurate initial staging (144–146). Nonetheless, there are concerns about possible delays in commencement of definitive treatment when SLNB precedes primary chemotherapy. These delays could be a consequence of either scheduling issues or wound complications. Seroma formation occurs not infrequently in SLNB cases and aspiration of clinically significant seromas increases the chance of introducing infection at the surgical site.

No direct comparisons of the efficacy of SLNB before or after neoadjuvant chemotherapy have been performed. So far, data suggest that both approaches are feasible in clinical practice.

Current trials are evaluating the role of repeat SLNB in patients with a positive sentinel node prior to chemotherapy but no clinical or sonographic evidence of nodal disease after a course of primary chemotherapy.

REFERENCES

1. Swain SM, Sorace RA, Bagley CS, et al. Neoadjuvant chemotherapy in the combined modality approach of locally advanced nonmetastatic breast cancer. Cancer Res 1987; 47: 3889–9.
2. Perloff M, Lesnick GJ, Korzun A, et al. Combination chemotherapy with mastectomy or radiotherapy for stage III breast carcinoma: a Cancer and Leukemia Group B study. J Clin Oncol 1988; 6: 261–9.
3. Hortobagyi GN, Ames FC, Buzdar AU, et al. Management of stage III primary breast cancer with primary chemotherapy, surgery, and radiation therapy. Cancer 1988; 62: 2507–16.
4. Bonadonna G, Veronesi U, Brambilla C, et al. Primary chemotherapy to avoid mastectomy in tumors with diameters of three centimeters or more. J Natl Cancer Inst 1990; 82: 1539–45.
5. Schwartz GF, Birchansky CA, Komarnicky LT, et al. Induction chemotherapy followed by breast conservation for locally advanced carcinoma of the breast. Cancer 1994; 73: 362–9.
6. Fisher B, Gunduz N, Saffer EA. Influence of the interval between primary tumor removal and chemotherapy on kinetics and growth of metastases. Cancer Res 1983; 43: 1488–92.
7. Fisher B, Gunduz N, Coyle J, et al. Presence of a growth-stimulating factor in serum following primary tumor removal in mice. Cancer Res 1989; 49: 1996–2001.

8. Fisher B, Saffer B, Rudock C, et al. Effect of local or systemic treatment prior to primary tumor removal on the production and response to a serum growth-stimulating factor in mice. Cancer Res 1989; 49: 2002–4.

9. Early Breast Cancer Trialists' Collaborative Group. Polychemotherapy for early breast cancer: an overview of the randomized trials. Lancet 1996; 352: 930–42.

10. Broët P, Scholl SM, de la Rochefordière A, et al. Short and long-term effects on survival in breast cancer patients treated by primary chemotherapy: an updated analysis of a randomized trial. Breast Cancer Res Treat 1999; 58: 151–6.

11. Powles TJ, Hickish TF, Makris A, et al. Randomized trial of chemoendocrine therapy started before or after surgery for treatment of primary breast cancer. J Clin Oncol 1995; 13: 547–52.

12. Mauriac L, MacGrogan G, Avril A, et al. Neoadjuvant chemotherapy for operable breast carcinoma larger than 3 cm: a unicentre randomized trial with a 124-month median follow-up. Ann Oncol 1999; 10: 47–52.

13. Deo SV, Bhutani M, Shukla NK, et al. Randomized trial comparing neoadjuvant versus adjuvant chemotherapy in operable locally advanced breast cancer (T4b N0-2 M0). J Surg Oncol 2003; 84: 192–7.

14. Taucher S, Steger GG, Jakesz R, et al. The potential risk of neoadjuvant chemotherapy in breast cancer patients–results from a prospective randomized trial of the Austrian Breast and Colorectal Cancer Study Group (ABCSG-07). Breast Cancer Res Treat 2008; 112: 309–16.

15. Fisher B, Brown A, Mamounas E, et al. Effect of preoperative chemotherapy on local-regional disease in women with operable breast cancer: findings from National Surgical Adjuvant Breast and Bowel Project B-18. J Clin Oncol 1997; 15: 2483–93.

16. van der Hage JA, van de Velde CJ, Julien JP, et al. Preoperative chemotherapy in primary operable breast cancer: results from the European Organization for Research and Treatment of Cancer trial 10902. J Clin Oncol 2001; 19: 4224–37.

17. Rastogi P, Anderson SJ, Bear HD, et al. Preoperative chemotherapy: updates of National Surgical Adjuvant Breast and Bowel Project Protocols B-18 and B-27. J Clin Oncol 2008; 26: 778–85.

18. van Nes JG, Putter H, Julien JP, et al. Preoperative chemotherapy is safe in early breast cancer, even after 10 years of follow-up; clinical and translational results from the EORTC trial 10902. Breast Cancer Res Treat 2009; 115: 101–13.

19. Mauri D, Pavlidis N, Ioannidis JP. Neoadjuvant versus adjuvant systemic treatment in breast cancer: a meta-analysis. J Natl Cancer Inst 2005; 97: 188–94.

20. Mieog JS, van der Hage JA, van de Velde CJ. Neoadjuvant chemotherapy for operable breast cancer. Br J Surg 2007; 94: 1189–200.

21. von Minckwitz G, Costa SD, Eiermann W, et al. Maximized reduction of primary breast tumor size using preoperative chemotherapy with doxorubicin and docetaxel. J Clin Oncol 1999; 17: 1999–2005.

22. Valero V, Esteva FJ, Sahin AA, et al. Phase II trial of neoadjuvant chemotherapy with docetaxel and doxorubicin, surgery, adjuvant CMF, and radiotherapy +/− tamoxifen in locally advanced breast cáncer (abstract 253). Breast Cancer Res Treat 2000; 64: 69.

23. Ardavanis A, Pateras C, Pissakas G, et al. Sequential epirubicin and docetaxel followed by surgery and postoperative chemo-radiotherapy for locally advanced breast cáncer (abstract 1779). Proc Am Soc Clin Oncol 2001; 20: 8b.

24. Bines J, Vinholes J, del Giglio A, et al. Induction chemotherapy with weekly docetaxel (Taxotere) in unfavorable locally advanced breast cáncer (abstract 1881). Proc Am Soc Clin Oncol 2001; 20: 33b.

25. Baltali E, Altundağ MK, Onat DA, et al. Neoadjuvant chemotherapy with taxotere-epirubicin-5-fluorouracil (TEF) in local-regionally advanced breast cancer: a preliminary report. Tumori 2002; 88: 474–7.

26. Estévez LG, Cuevas JM, Antón A, et al. Weekly docetaxel as neoadjuvant chemotherapy for stage II and III breast cancer: efficacy and correlation with biological markers in a phase II, multicenter study. Clin Cancer Res 2003; 9: 686–92.

27. Gradishar WJ, Wedam SB, Jahanzeb M, et al. Neoadjuvant docetaxel followed by adjuvant doxorubicin and cyclophosphamide in patients with stage III breast cancer. Ann Oncol 2005; 16:1297–304.

28. Ezzat AA, Ibrahim EM, Ajarim DS, et al. Phase II study of neoadjuvant paclitaxel and cisplatin for operable and locally advanced breast cancer: analysis of 126 patients. Br J Cancer 2004; 90: 968–74.

29. Taillibert S, Antoine E, Mousseau M, et al. Preliminary results of a multicenter clinicobiological phase II study combining epirubicin, cyclophosphamide and paclitaxel as induction chemotherapy for women with stage II and III breast cancer (abstract 1809). Proc Am Soc Clin Oncol 2001; 20: 15b.

30. Cristofanilli M, Gonzalez-Angulo AM, Buzdar AU, et al. Paclitaxel improves the prognosis in estrogen receptor negative inflammatory breast cancer: the M. D. Anderson Cancer Center experience. Clin Breast Cancer 2004; 4: 415–19.

31. Vinholes J, Bouzid K, Salas F, et al. Preliminary Results of a Multicentre Phase III Trial of Taxotere and Doxorubicin (AT) Versus 5-Fluorouracil, Doxorubicin and Cyclophosphamide (FAC) in Patients (Pts) with Unresectable Locally Advanced Breast Cancer (ULABC). Proc Am Soc Clin Oncol 2001; 20: abstract 101.

32. Smith IC, Heys SD, Hutcheon AW, et al. Neoadjuvant chemotherapy in breast cancer: significantly enhanced response with docetaxel. J Clin Oncol 2002; 20: 1456–66.

33. Heys SD, Hutcheon AW, Sarkar TK, et al. Neoadjuvant docetaxel in breast cancer: 3-year survival results from the Aberdeen trial. Clin Cancer Res 2002; 3: S69–74.

34. Bear HD, Anderson S, Brown A, et al. The effect on tumor response of adding sequential preoperative docetaxel to preoperative doxorubicin and cyclophosphamide: preliminary results from National Surgical Adjuvant Breast and Bowel Project Protocol B-27. J Clin Oncol 2003; 21: 4165–74.

35. Buzdar AU, Singletary SE, Theriault RL, et al. Prospective evaluation of paclitaxel versus combination chemotherapy with fluorouracil, doxorubicin, and cyclophosphamide as neoadjuvant therapy in patients with operable breast cancer. J Clin Oncol 1999; 17: 3412–17.

36. Buzdar AU, Singletary SE, Valero V, et al. Evaluation of paclitaxel in adjuvant chemotherapy for patients with operable breast cancer: preliminary data of a prospective randomized trial. Clin Cancer Res 2002; 8: 1073–9.

37. Green MC, Buzdar AU, Smith T, et al. Weekly paclitaxel improves pathologic complete remission in operable breast cancer when compared with paclitaxel once every 3 weeks. J Clin Oncol 2005; 23: 5983–92.

38. Seidman AD, Berry D, Cirrincione C, et al. Randomized phase III trial of weekly compared to every-3-weeks paclitaxel for metastatic breast cancer, with trastuzumab for all HER-2 overexpressors and random assignment to trastuzumab or not in HER-2 non-overexpressors: final results of Cancer and Leukemia Group B protocol 9840. J Clin Oncol 2006; 26: 1642–9.

39. Sparano JA, Wang M, Martino S, et al. Weekly paclitaxel in the adjuvant treatment of breast cancer. N Engl J Med 2008; 358: 1663–71.

40. Evans TR, Yellowlees A, Foster E, et al. Phase III randomized trial of doxorubicin and docetaxel versus doxorubicin and cyclophosphamide as primary medical therapy in women with breast cancer: an anglo-celtic cooperative oncology group study. J Clin Oncol 2005; 23: 2988–95.

41. Mansi JL, Yellowlees A, Lipscombe J, et al. Five-year outcome for women randomized in a phase III trial comparing doxorubicin and cyclophosphamide with doxorubicin and docetaxel as primary medical therapy in early breast cancer: an Anglo-Celtic Cooperative Oncology Group study. Breast Cancer Res Treat 2010; 122: 787–94.

42. Diéras V, Fumoleau P, Romieu G, et al. Randomized parallel study of doxorubicin plus paclitaxel and doxorubicin plus cyclophosphamide as neoadjuvant treatment of patients with breast cancer. J Clin Oncol 2004; 22: 4958–65.

43. Cuppone F, Bria E, Carlini P, et al. Taxanes as primary chemotherapy for early breast cancer: meta-analysis of randomized trials. Cancer 2008; 113: 238–46.

44. Citron ML, Berry DA, Cirrincione C, et al. Randomized trial of dose-dense versus conventionally scheduled and sequential versus concurrent combination chemotherapy as postoperative adjuvant treatment of node-positive primary breast cancer: first report of Intergroup Trial C9741/Cancer and Leukemia Group B Trial 9741. J Clin Oncol 2003; 21: 1431–9.

45. Therasse P, Mauriac L, Welnicka-Jaskiewicz M, et al. Final results of a randomized phase III trial comparing cyclophosphamide, epirubicin, and fluorouracil with a dose-intensified epirubicin and cyclophosphamide + filgrastim as neoadjuvant treatment in locally advanced breast cancer: an EORTC-NCIC-SAKK multicenter study. J Clin Oncol 2003; 21: 843.

46. von Minckwitz G, Raab G, Caputo A, et al. Doxorubicin with cyclophosphamide followed by docetaxel every 21 days compared with doxorubicin and docetaxel every 14 days as preoperative treatment in

operable breast cancer: the GEPARDUO study of the German Breast Group. J Clin Oncol 2005; 23: 2676–85.

47. Steger GG, Galid A, Gnant M, et al. Pathologic complete response with six compared with three cycles of neoadjuvant epirubicin plus docetaxel and granulocyte colony-stimulating factor in operable breast cancer: results of ABCSG-14. J Clin Oncol 2007; 25: 2012–18.

48. Han S, Kim J, Lee J, et al. Comparison of 6 cycles versus 4 cycles of neoadjuvant epirubicin plus docetaxel chemotherapy in stages II and III breast cancer. Eur J Surg Oncol 2009; 35: 583–7.

49. von Minckwitz G, Kümmel S, Vogel P, et al. Intensified neoadjuvant chemotherapy in early-responding breast cancer: phase III randomized GeparTrio study. J Natl Cancer Inst 2008; 100: 552–62.

50. von Minckwitz G, Untch M, Nüesch E, et al. Impact of treatment characteristics on response of different breast cancer phenotypes: pooled analysis of the German neo-adjuvant chemotherapy trials. Breast Cancer Res Treat 2011; 125: 145–56.

51. von Minckwitz G, Blohmer JU, Raab G, et al. In vivo chemosensitivity-adapted preoperative chemotherapy in patients with early-stage breast cancer: the GEPARTRIO pilot study. Ann Oncol 2005; 16: 56–63.

52. Pierga JY, Mouret E, Laurence V, et al. Prognostic factors for survival after neoadjuvant chemotherapy in operable breast cancer: the role of clinical response. Eur J Cancer 2003; 39: 1089–96.

53. Hennessy BT, Hortobagyi GN, Rouzier R, et al. Outcome after pathologic complete eradication of cytologically proven breast cancer axillary node metastases following primary chemotherapy. J Clin Oncol 2005; 23: 9304–11.

54. Klauber-DeMore N, Ollila DW, Moore DT, et al. Size of residual lymph node metastasis after neoadjuvant chemotherapy in locally advanced breast cancer patients is prognostic. Ann Surg Oncol 2006; 13: 685.

55. Bonadonna G, Valagussa P, Brambilla C, et al. Primary chemotherapy in operable breast cancer: eight-year experience at the Milan Cancer Institute. J Clin Oncol 1998; 16: 93–100.

56. Fisher ER, Wang J, Bryant J, et al. Pathobiology of preoperative chemotherapy: findings from the National Surgical Adjuvant Breast and Bowel (NSABP) protocol B-18. Cancer 2002; 95:681–95.

57. Fernandez-Sanchez M, Gamboa-Dominguez A, Uribe N, et al. Clinical and pathological predictors of response to neoadjuvant anthracycline chemotherapy in locally advanced breast cancer. Med Oncol 2006; 23: 171–83.

58. Prisack HB, Karreman C, Modlich O, et al. Predictive biological markers for response of invasive breast cancer to anthracycline/cyclophosphamide-based primary (radio-)chemotherapy. Anticancer Res 2005; 25: 4615–21.

59. Gianni L, Baselga J, Eiermann W, et al. Feasibility and tolerability of sequential doxorubicin/paclitaxel followed by cyclophosphamide, methotrexate, and fluorouracil and its effects on tumor response as preoperative therapy. Clin Cancer Res 2005; 11: 8715–21.

60. Guarneri V, Broglio K, Kau SW, et al. Prognostic value of pathologic complete response after primary chemotherapy in relation to hormone receptor status and other factors. J Clin Oncol 2006; 24: 1037–44.

61. Cristofanilli M, Gonzalez-Angulo A, Sneige N, et al. Invasive lobular carcinoma classic type: response to primary chemotherapy and survival outcomes. J Clin Oncol 2005; 23: 41–8.

62. Mathieu MC, Rouzier R, Llombart-Cussac A, et al. The poor responsiveness of infiltrating lobular breast carcinomas to neoadjuvant chemotherapy can be explained by their biological profile. Eur J Cancer 2004; 40: 342–51.

63. Paik S, Bryant J, Park C, et al. erbB-2 and response to doxorubicin in patients with axillary lymph node-positive, hormone receptor-negative breast cancer. J Natl Cancer Inst 1998; 90: 1361–70.

64. Petit T, Borel C, Ghnassia J-P, et al. Chemotherapy response of breast cancer depends on HER-2 status and anthracycline dose intensity in the neoadjuvant setting. Clin Cancer Res 2001; 7: 1577–81.

65. Petit T, Wilt M, Velten M, et al. Comparative value of tumour grade, hormonal receptors, Ki-67, HER-2 and topoisomerase II alpha status as predictive markers in breast cancer patients treated with neoadjuvant anthracycline-based chemotherapy. Eur J Cancer 2004; 40: 205–11.

66. Rody A, Karn T, Gätje R, et al. Gene expression profiling of breast cancer patients treated with docetaxel, doxorubicin, and cyclophosphamide within the GEPARTRIO trial: HER-2, but not topoisomerase II alpha and microtubule-associated protein tau, is highly predictive of tumor response. Breast 2007; 16: 86–93.

67. Jones RL, Salter J, A'Hern R, et al. The prognostic significance of Ki67 before and after neoadjuvant chemotherapy in breast cancer. Breast Cancer Res Treat 2009; 116: 53.

68. Burcombe RJ, Makris A, Richman PI, et al. Evaluation of ER, PgR, HER-2 and Ki-67 as predictors of response to neoadjuvant anthracycline chemotherapy for operable breast cancer. Br J Cancer 2005; 92: 147–55.

69. Faneyte IF, Schrama JG, Peterse JL, et al. Breast cancer response to neoadjuvant chemotherapy: predictive markers and relation with outcome. Br J Cancer 2003; 88: 406–12.

70. Fasching PA, Heusinger K, Haberle L, et al. Ki67, chemotherapy response, and prognosis in breast cancer patients receiving neoadjuvant treatment. BMC Cancer 2011; 11: 486.

71. Chua S, Smith IE, A'Hern RP, et al. Neoadjuvant vinorelbine/epirubicin (VE) versus standard adriamycin/cyclophosphamide (AC) in operable breast cancer: analysis of response and tolerability in a randomised phase III trial (TOPIC 2). Ann Oncol 2005; 16: 1435–41.

72. Lee KS, Ro J, Nam BH, et al. A randomized phase-III trial of docetaxel/capecitabine versus doxorubicin/cyclophosphamide as primary chemotherapy for patients with stage II/III breast cancer. Breast Cancer Res Treat 2008; 109: 481–9.

73. von Minckwitz G, Rezai M, Loibl S, et al. Capecitabine in addition to anthracycline- and taxane-based neoadjuvant treatment in patients with primary breast cancer: phase III GeparQuattro study. J Clin Oncol 2010; 28: 2015–23.

74. Chang HR, Glaspy J, Allison MA, et al. Differential response of triple-negative breast cancer to a docetaxel and carboplatin-based neoadjuvant treatment. Cancer 2010; 116: 4227–37.

75. Frasci G, D'Aiuto G, Comella P, et al. Preoperative weekly cisplatin, epirubicin, and paclitaxel (PET) improves prognosis in locally advanced breast cancer patients: an update of the Southern Italy Cooperative Oncology Group (SICOG) randomised trial 9908. Ann Oncol 2010; 21: 707–16.

76. Early Breast Cancer Trialists' Collaborative Group. Tamoxifen for early breast cancer: an overview of the randomised trials. Lancet 1998; 351: 1451–67.

77. Beresford MJ, Ravichandran D, Makris A, et al. Neoadjuvant endocrine therapy in breast cancer. Cancer Treat Rev 2007; 33: 48–57.

78. Gazet JC, Markopoulos C, Ford HT, et al. Prospective randomised trial of tamoxifen versus surgery in elderly patients with breast cancer. Lancet 1988; 1: 679–81.

79. Robertson JF, Todd JH, Ellis IO, et al. Comparison of mastectomy with tamoxifen for treating elderly patients with operable breast cancer. BMJ 1988; 297: 511–14.

80. Bates T, Riley DL, Houghton J, et al. Breast cancer in elderly women: a Cancer Research Campaign trial comparing treatment with tamoxifen and optimal surgery with tamoxifen alone. The Elderly Breast Cancer Working Party. Br J Surg 1991; 78: 591–4.

81. Mustacchi G, Milani S, Pluchinotta A, et al. Tamoxifen or surgery plus tamoxifen as primary treatment for elderly patients with operable breast cancer: The G.R.E.T.A. Trial. Group for Research on Endocrine Therapy in the Elderly. Anticancer Res 1994; 14: 2197–200.

82. Jakesz R, Kaufmann M, Boccardo F, et al. Meta-analysis of breast cancer outcomes in adjuvant trials of aromatase inhibitors versus tamoxifen. J Clin Oncol 2010; 28: 509–18.

83. Eiermann W, Paepke S, Appfelstaedt J, et al. Preoperative treatment of postmenopausal breast cancer patients with letrozole: a randomized double-blind multicenter study. Ann Oncol 2001; 12: 1527–32.

84. Ellis MJ, Coop A, Singh B, et al. Letrozole is more effective neoadjuvant endocrine therapy than tamoxifen for ErbB-1- and/or ErbB-2-positive, estrogen receptor-positive primary breast cancer: evidence from a phase III randomized trial. J Clin Oncol 2001; 19: 3808–16.

85. Smith IE, Dowsett M, Ebbs SR, et al. Neoadjuvant treatment of postmenopausal breast cancer with anastrozole, tamoxifen, or both in combination: the Immediate Preoperative Anastrozole, Tamoxifen, or Combined with Tamoxifen (IMPACT) multicenter double-blind randomized trial. J Clin Oncol 2005; 23: 5108–16.

86. Baum M, Budzar AU, Cuzick J, et al. Anastrozole alone or in combination with tamoxifen versus tamoxifen alone for adjuvant treatment of postmenopausal women with early breast cancer: first results of the ATAC randomised trial. Lancet 2002; 359: 2131–9.

87. Cataliotti L, Buzdar AU, Noguchi S, et al. Comparison of anastrozole versus tamoxifen as preoperative therapy in postmenopausal women with hormone receptor-positive breast cancer: the Pre-Operative "Arimidex" Compared to Tamoxifen (PROACT) trial. Cancer 2006; 106: 2095–103.

88. Semiglazov V, Kletsel A. Exemestane (E) vs tamoxifen (T) as neoadjuvant endocrine therapy for postmenopausal women with ER+ breast cancer (T2N1-2, T3N0-1, T4N0M0). J Clin Oncol 2005; 23: 16S.

89. Semiglazov VF, Semiglazov VV, Dashyan GA, et al. Phase 2 randomized trial of primary endocrine therapy versus chemotherapy in postmenopausal patients with estrogen receptor-positive breast cancer. Cancer 2007; 110: 244–54.

90. Carpenter R, Doughty JC, Cordiner C, et al. A multicenter study to determine the optimum duration of neoadjuvant letrozole on tumor regression to permit breast-conserving surgery: final analyses. J Clin Oncol 2010; 28:abstract 670.

91. Dowsett M, Smith IE, Ebbs SR, et al. Short-term changes in Ki-67 during neoadjuvant treatment of primary breast cancer with anastrozole or tamoxifen alone or combined correlate with recurrence-free survival. Clin Cancer Res 2005; 11: 951s–8s.

92. Dowsett M, Smith IE, Ebbs SR, et al. Prognostic value of Ki67 expression after short-term presurgical endocrine therapy for primary breast cancer. J Natl Cancer Inst 2007; 99: 167–70.

93. Smith I. Neoadjuvant therapy: what, when, and why. Eur J Cancer 2012; 48: S41.

94. Slamon DJ, Godolphin W, Jones LA, et al. Studies of the HER-2/neu proto-oncogene in human breast and ovarian cancer. Science 1989; 244: 707–12.

95. Tommasi S, Paradiso A, Mangia A, et al. Biological correlation between HER-2/neu and proliferative activity in human breast cancer. Anticancer Res 1991; 11: 1395–400.

96. Perou CM, Sørlie T, Eisen MB, et al. Molecular portraits of human breast tumours. Nature 2000; 406: 747–52.

97. Liao C, Yin F, Huang P, et al. A meta-analysis of randomized controlled trials comparing chemotherapy plus trastuzumab with chemotherapy alone in HER-2-positive advanced breast cancer. Breast J 2011; 17: 109–11.

98. Viani GA, Afonso SL, Stefano EJ, et al. Adjuvant trastuzumab in the treatment of her-2-positive early breast cancer: a meta-analysis of published randomized trials. BMC Cancer 2007; 7: 153.

99. Bines J, Murad A, Lago S, et al. Multicenter Brazilian study of weekly docetaxel and trastuzumab as primary therapy in stage III, HER-2 overexpressing breast cancer. Proc Am Soc Clin Oncol 2003; 22: abstract 268.

100. Hurley J, Doliny P, Reis I, et al. Docetaxel, cisplatin, and trastuzumab as primary systemic therapy for human epidermal growth factor receptor 2-positive locally advanced breast cancer. J Clin Oncol 2006; 24: 1831–8.

101. Harris LN, You F, Schnitt SJ, et al. Predictors of resistance to preoperative trastuzumab and vinorelbine for HER2-positive early breast cancer. Clin Cancer Res 2007; 13: 1198–207.

102. Sikov WM, Dizon DS, Strenger R, et al. Frequent pathologic complete responses in aggressive stages II to III breast cancers with every-4-week carboplatin and weekly paclitaxel with or without trastuzumab: a Brown University Oncology Group Study. J Clin Oncol 2009; 27: 4693–700.

103. Anton A, Ruiz A, Plazaola A, et al. Phase II clinical trial of liposomal-encapsulated doxorubicin citrate and docetaxel, associated with trastuzumab, as neoadjuvant treatment in stages II and IIIA HER2-overexpressing breast cancer patients. GEICAM 2003-03 study. Ann Oncol 2011; 22: 74–9.

104. Untch M, Fasching PA, Konecny GE, et al. Pathologic complete response after neoadjuvant chemotherapy plus trastuzumab predicts favorable survival in human epidermal growth factor receptor 2-overexpressing breast cancer: results from the TECHNO trial of the AGO and GBG study groups. J Clin Oncol 2011; 29: 3351–7.

105. Untch M, Rezai M, Loibl S, et al. Neoadjuvant treatment with trastuzumab in HER2-positive breast cancer: results from the GeparQuattro study. J Clin Oncol 2010; 28: 2024–31.

106. Buzdar AU, Valero V, Ibrahim NK, et al. Neoadjuvant therapy with paclitaxel followed by 5-fluorouracil, epirubicin, and cyclophosphamide chemotherapy and concurrent trastuzumab in human epidermal growth factor receptor 2-positive operable breast cancer: an update of the initial randomized study population and data of additional patients treated with the same regimen. Clin Cancer Res 2007; 13: 228–33.

107. Gianni L, Eiermann W, Semiglazov V, et al. Neoadjuvant chemotherapy with trastuzumab followed by adjuvant trastuzumab versus neoadjuvant chemotherapy alone, in patients with HER2-positive locally advanced breast cancer (the NOAH trial): a randomised controlled superiority trial with a parallel HER2-negative cohort. Lancet 2010; 375: 377–84.

108. Guiu S, Liegard M, Favier L, et al. Long-term follow-up of HER2-overexpressing stage II or III breast cancer treated by anthracycline-free neoadjuvant chemotherapy. Ann Oncol 2011; 22: 321–8.

109. Geyer CE, Forster J, Lindquist D, et al. Lapatinib plus capecitabine for HER2-positive advanced breast cancer. N Engl J Med 2006; 355: 2733–43.

110. Johnston S, Pippen J Jr, Pivot X, et al. Lapatinib combined with letrozole versus letrozole and placebo as first-line therapy for postmenopausal hormone receptor-positive metastatic breast cancer. J Clin Oncol 2009; 27: 5538–46.

111. Boussen H, Cristofanilli M, Zaks T, et al. Phase II study to evaluate the efficacy and safety of neoadjuvant lapatinib plus paclitaxel in patients with inflammatory breast cancer. J Clin Oncol 2010; 28: 3248–55.

112. Baselga J, Bradbury I, Eidtmann H, et al. Lapatinib with trastuzumab for HER2-positive early breast cancer (NeoALTTO): a randomised, open-label, multicentre, phase 3 trial. Lancet 2012; 379: 633–40.

113. Chang JC, Mayer IA, Forero-Torres A, et al. TBCRC 006: A multicenter phase II study of neoadjuvant lapatinib and trastuzumab in patients with HER2-overexpressing breast cancer. J Clin Oncol 2011; 29(Suppl): abstract 505.

114. Baselga J, Cortés J, Kim SB, et al. Pertuzumab plus trastuzumab plus docetaxel for metastatic breast cancer. N Engl J Med 2012; 366: 109–19.

115. Gianni L, Pienkowski T, Im Y-H, et al. Efficacy and safety of neoadjuvant pertuzumab and trastuzumab in women with locally advanced, inflammatory, or early HER2-positive breast cancer (NeoSphere): a randomised multicentre, open-label, phase 2 trial. Lancet Oncol 2012; 13: 25–32.

116. Wolff AC, Hammond ME, Schwartz JN, et al. American Society of Clinical Oncology/College of American Pathologists guideline recommendations for human epidermal growth factor receptor 2 testing in breast cancer. J Clin Oncol 2007; 25: 118–45.

117. Waterman H, Yarden Y. Untangling the ErbB signalling network. Nat Rev Mol Cell Biol 2001; 2: 127–37.

118. Sabatini DM. mTOR and cancer: insights into a complex relationship. Nat Rev Cancer 2006; 6: 729–34.

119. Nagata Y, Lan KH, Zhou X, et al. PTEN activation contributes to tumor inhibition by trastuzumab, and loss of PTEN predicts trastuzumab resistance in patients. Cancer Cell 2004; 6: 117–27.

120. Dave B, Migliaccio I, Gutierrez MC, et al. Loss of phosphatase and tensin homolog or phosphoinositol-3 kinase activation and response to trastuzumab and lapatinib in human epidermal growth factor receptor 2-overexpressiong locally advanced breast cancer. J Clin Oncol 2001; 29: 166–73.

121. Veronesi U, Bonadonna G, Zurrida S, et al. Conservation surgery after primary chemotherapy in large carcinomas of the breast. Ann Surg 1995; 222: 612–18.

122. Gralow JR, Burstein HJ, Wood W, et al. Preoperative therapy in invasive breast cancer: pathologic assessment and systemic therapy issues in operable disease. J Clin Oncol 2008; 26: 814–19.

123. Vinnicombe SJ, MacVicar AD, Guy RL, et al. Primary breast cancer: mammographic changes after neoadjuvant chemotherapy, with pathologic correlation. Radiology 1996; 198: 333–40.

124. Chagpar AB, Middleton LP, Sahin AA, et al. Accuracy of physical examination, ultrasonography, and mammography in predicting residual pathologic tumor size in patients treated with neoadjuvant chemotherapy. Ann Surg 2006; 243: 257–64.

125. Fiorentino C, Berruti A, Bottini A, et al. Accuracy of mammography and echography versus clinical palpation in the assessment of response to primary chemotherapy in breast cancer patients with operable disease. Breast Cancer Res Treat 2001; 69: 143–51.

126. Esserman L, Kaplan E, Partridge S, et al. MRI phenotype is associated with response to doxorubicin and cyclophosphamide neoadjuvant chemotherapy in stage III breast cancer. Ann Surg Oncol 2001; 8: 549–59.

127. Nakamura S, Kenjo H, Nishio T, et al. Efficacy of 3D-MR mammography for breast conserving surgery after neoadjuvant chemotherapy. Breast Cancer 2002; 9: 15–19.

128. Cheung YC, Chen SC, Su MY, et al. Monitoring the size and response of locally advanced breast cancers to neoadjuvant chemotherapy (weekly paclitaxel and epirubicin) with serial enhanced MRI. Breast Cancer Res Treat 2003; 78: 51–8.

129. Partridge SC, Gibbs JE, Lu Y, et al. Accuracy of MR imaging for revealing residual breast cancer in patients who have undergone neoadjuvant chemotherapy. AJR Am J Roentgenol 2002; 179: 1193–9.

130. Wasser K, Sinn HP, Fink C, et al. Accuracy of tumor size measurement in breast cancer using MRI is influenced by histological regression induced by neoadjuvant chemotherapy. Eur Radiol 2003; 13: 1213–23.

131. Yuan Y, Chen XS, Liu SY, et al. Accuracy of MRI in prediction of patho-logic complete remission in breast cancer after preoperative therapy: a meta-analysis. AJR Am J Roentgenol 2010; 195: 260–8.

132. Loo CE, Straver ME, Rodenhuis S, et al. Magnetic resonance imaging response monitoring of breast cancer during neoadjuvant chemother-apy: relevance of breast cancer subtype. J Clin Oncol 2011; 29: 660–6.

133. Martincich L, Montemurro F, De Rosa G, et al. Monitoring response to primary chemotherapy in breast cancer using dynamic contrast-enhanced magnetic resonance imaging. Breast Cancer Res Treat 2004; 83: 67–76.

134. Ah-See ML, Makris A, Taylor NJ, et al. Early changes in functional dynamic magnetic resonance imaging predict for pathologic response to neoadjuvant chemotherapy in primary breast cancer. Clin Cancer Res 2008; 14: 6580–9.

135. Fraile M, Rull M, Julián FJ, et al. Sentinel node biopsy as a practical alter-native to axillary lymph node dissection in breast cancer patients: an approach to its validity. Ann Oncol 2000; 11: 701–5.

136. Mamounas EP, Brown A, Anderson S, et al. Sentinel node biopsy after neoadjuvant chemotherapy in breast cancer: results from National Sur-gical Adjuvant Breast and Bowel Project Protocol B-27. J Clin Oncol 2005; 23: 2694–702.

137. Classe JM, Bordes V, Campion L, et al. Sentinel lymph node biopsy after neoadjuvant chemotherapy for advanced breast cancer: results of Gan-glion Sentinelle et Chimiotherapie Neoadjuvante, a French prospective multicentric study. J Clin Oncol 2009; 27: 726–32.

138. Xing Y, Foy M, Cox DD, et al. Meta-analysis of sentinel lymph node biopsy after preoperative chemotherapy in patients with breast cancer. Br J Surg 2006; 93: 539–46.

139. Kelly AM, Dwamena B, Cronin P, et al. Breast cancer sentinel node iden-tification and classification after neoadjuvant chemotherapy-systematic review and meta analysis. Acad Radiol 2009; 16: 551–63.

140. van Deurzen CH, Vriens BE, Tjan-Heijnen VC, et al. Accuracy of sentinel node biopsy after neoadjuvant chemotherapy in breast cancer patients: a systematic review. Eur J Cancer 2009; 45: 3124–30.

141. Sabel MS, Schott AF, Kleer CG, et al. Sentinel node biopsy prior to neo-adjuvant chemotherapy. Am J Surg 2003; 186: 102–5.

142. Schrenk P, Hochreiner G, Fridrik M, et al. Sentinel node biopsy per-formed before preoperative chemotherapy for axillary lymph node stag-ing in breast cancer. Breast J 2003; 9: 282–7.

143. Ollila DW, Neuman HB, Sartor C, et al. Lymphatic mapping and sentinel lymphadenectomy prior to neoadjuvant chemotherapy in patients with large breast cancers. Am J Surg 2005; 190: 371–5.

144. Sabel MS, Schott AF, Kleer CG, et al. Sentinel node biopsy prior to neo-adjuvant chemotherapy. Am J Surg 2003; 186: 102–5.

145. Menard J-P, Extra J-M, Jacquemier J, et al. Sentinel lymphadenectomy for the staging of clinical axillary node negative breast cancer before neoadjuvant chemotherapy. Eur J Surg Oncol 2009; 35: 916–20.

146. Cox CE, Cox JM, White LB, et al. Sentinel node biopsy before neoadju-vant chemotherapy for determining axillary status and treatment prog-nosis in locally advanced breast cancer. Ann Surg Oncol 2006; 13: 483–90.

47 Breast cancer in the elderly

R.C.F. Leonard and G.A. Thomas

INTRODUCTION

Breast cancer is, like most cancers, a disease associated with advancing age. In general, the biology of the disease is influenced by age in that proportionately more young patients present with aggressive, often oestrogen receptor (ER)-negative disease, whereas older postmenopausal women present with proportionately less aggressive, ER-positive disease. However, as discussed later in the chapter, these differences are not always as clearly defined and minimal intervention should be approached cautiously. There is also the associated paradox that older women's (greater than 70 years of age at diagnosis) mortality from the disease remains higher than younger women, i.e. that age, *per se*, is an adverse prognostic factor for breast cancer-specific survival (1).

This paradox may be explained by factors such as access to appropriate surgical care, inadequate staging, and underutilization of complex, often toxic, adjuvant treatments such asdrug and radiation therapies, which improve the outcomes of the treatment of early-stage disease.

There are two interrelated issues which have conspired to consistently to impair management of breast cancer in older women:

- The inherent complexity of assessing risk of any intervention in women whose age and pre-existing comorbid disease may lead to serious complications associated with treatments.
- The attitudes of the various health professionals whose caution may inappropriately deprive the patient of effective and safe treatment, in the context of uncertainties relating to age and co-morbidity.

However, there may be age-related differences in the molecular phenotype of breast cancer that could be used to tailor treatment more effectively for the elderly patient. In addition to the treatment offered to the patient, several other factors have been found to relate to prognosis, which are associated with the clinical presentation and biology of disease. Among these are tumor size, node status and ER status (2). Durbecq et al. (3) reviewed 2723 consecutive patients operated at the Institut Jules Bordet in Brussels. Their findings suggested that elderly women with breast cancer (aged over 70 years) presented withlarger tumors (>5 cm), suggesting that elderly women are less likely to seek medical advice promptly after identifying a lump in their breast.

The ER represents a critical growth and survival pathway in most breast tumors; agents that block the ER signalling pathway (endocrine therapies) have been shown to be highly effective in the treatment of breast cancer and have been the most widely used adjuvant therapies for 'early-stage' disease. The benefit of endocrine therapy for patients with ER-negative disease is negligible, but women with ER-positive disease have more than 40% proportional reduction in the odds of recurrence and a corresponding 22% reduction in the odds of death when given endocrine therapy after 'curative' surgery (4).

The probability of a patient presenting with an ER-positive tumor is also affected by age. Eppenberger-Castori et al. (5) studied an American collection of 800 samples and a European collection of 3000 samples of breast cancers to 'explore the hypothesis that ageing not only increases breast cancer incidence but also alters breast cancer biology'. The study concluded that breast cancer is indeed significantly affected by patient age at clinical presentation. Breast tumors arising in older patients had slower growth rates and were more likely to be ER-positive. Nonetheless, there may be no directassociation between ER status and proliferation index, and other effects ofage at clinical presentation on tumor biology may exist.

In younger women, especially those who are premenopausal, a significant contributor to increased survival rates for breast cancer has also been the use of cytotoxic chemotherapy either following, or prior to, surgery. The odds reduction in death from combination chemotherapy given for several months, either pre or post surgery, is significant in both ER-positive and ER-negative disease and is similar in magnitude to the endocrine effect (*albeit* for ER-positive disease only). Unlike endocrine therapy, side-effects can be life-threatening as well as debilitating and it cannot be employed without judicious considerationof co-morbid factors. Importantly, chemotherapy-associated survival benefits tend to be proportionately greater in young, premenopausal women and decrease progressively in the older age cohorts of postmenopausal women.

This chapter focuses on the treatment options for the older breast cancer patients and presents evidence suggesting that age is a major factor in treatment decisions, and that age may also determinethe basic biology of the disease. A clearer understanding of the way in which age interacts with biology and physiology should lead to a better management decisions and improved quality of life for the increasing population of elderly breast cancer patients, who will constitute the predominant clinical group.

BREAST CANCER MORBIDITY AND MORTALITY

Government policy in the United Kingdom (UK), as in other countries, is strongly influenced by recognition of rapidly growing numbers of people living for many years beyond retirement age. Age and cancer risk are co-associates for most of the common epithelial malignancies, particularly those of breast , lung, bowel and prostate. Statistics that specifically address care and survival of older women with breast cancer have been lacking

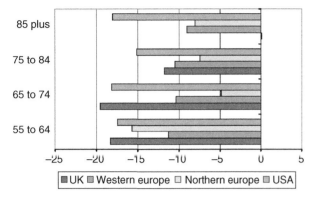

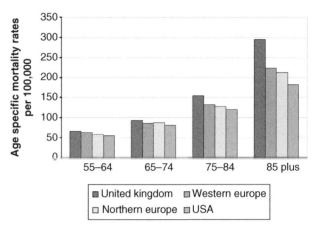

Figure 47.1 Change in mortality from 1995–1997 to 2003–2005. Note no change in UK for 85 yrs and over age group. *Source*: From Ref. (6).

Figure 47.2 Comparative outcome data for UK versus Northern, Western Europe, and USA age-specific mortality. *Source*: From Ref. (6).

hitherto but are now the subject of intensive study in Western countries. The North West Cancer Intelligence Unit has, in the past few years, produced data that give cause for concern in terms of overall outcome measures and in particular with comparative statistics for other European countries and North America (6).

These data demonstrate not only a poorer age-related breast cancer specific survival but worsening of relative survival with advancing age compared with neighbors in Western Europe. In cohort studies conducted later, there is evidence for some improvement in outcomes has been some improvement in outcomes,with satisfactory metrics for younger age cohorts within the UK, but once again, the UK fares badly against comparators when considering elderly groups alone (Figs 47.1 and 47.2).

PATHOLOGY AND AGE

The incidence of breast cancer shows a bimodal distribution and an exponential rise with age until the menopause at around 50 years of age, after which there is a slower rate of increase in those aged over 50. About 80% of all breast cancers arise in women aged over 50 years at diagnosis, and the 10-year probability of developing invasive breast cancer increases from less than 1.5% at age 40 years, to 3% at age 50 years and over 4% by age 70 years, yielding a cumulative lifetime risk of 13.2% or 1.8 (7). The consensus hypothesis for the age-associated increase in cancer incidence involves the accumulation of errors in somatic cells as a result of intrinsic damage attributable to extrinsic factors such as reactive oxygen species or ionizing radiation (8,9). Although this may explain the rise in cancer incidence with attained age, these factors donot necessarily have any bearing on the prognosis of cancer at different ages. It has been stated that, stage for stage, older patients with breast cancer do as well or slightly better than their younger counterparts. Certainly for ER-positive, node-negative tumors, long-term disease-free survival seems to be significantly different between cohorts of women aged below46 years at diagnosis and aged over 69 years at diagnosis. Ten-year disease-free survival reaches a plateau at less than 30% for the early-onset group and more than 70% for the late-onset group. Even when the data are adjusted for the age-associated differences in proliferation in young-onset versus older-onset breast cancers, significant differences in outcome persist, suggesting that intrinsic, as yet unknown, biological factors affect the disease-free and overall survival (7).

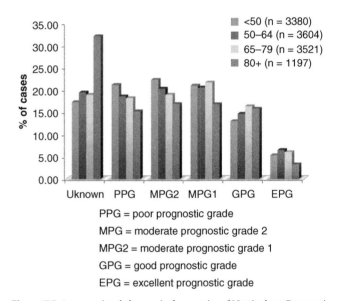

Figure 47.3 Age-associated changes in frequencies of Nottingham Prognostic Index. Redrawn from Figure 9, in the 3rd year report of the Breast Cancer clinical outcome measures report (http://www.wmciu.nhs.uk/documents/Bccomyear3report.pdf).

This contention is further supported by the finding of significant age-related differences in the distribution of the Nottingham Prognostic Index (NPI); younger women showing a higher proportion of tumors with poor and moderate prognostic NPI grade, whereas patients aged 80+ show a high frequency of tumors with excellent prognosis (Fig. 47.3).

These findings suggest that there should be differences in the biology of breast cancer in younger patients as opposed to older patients, and that an improved understanding of pathobiological mechanisms may enable treatments to be tailored more appropriately to the patient's age-associated tumor characteristics. Nonetheless, the Nottingham Prognostic Index data are based both on stage and grade with the former being influenced by delays in presentation and diagnosis rather than being a reflection of inherent biological difference *per se*.

Medullary and inflammatory breast cancers were more commonly observed in younger age groups, whereas papillary, lobular and mucinous cancers were more commonly observed in the older age groups. Cheung et al. (10) reviewed a total of 2078 tumors from 2061 consecutive patients aged over 70 years at diagnosis and operated at the Nottingham Breast Cancer Centre between 1987 and 2006. In total, 1976 patients had invasive breast cancer, with most (1738; 88%) having invasive ductal carcinoma. The proportion of patients with grade 3 carcinoma was substantially less in this older-population when compared with young patients (17.1% in the elderly group compared with 45.3% in the young group), and the proportion of grade 1 was substantially higher in the older group (62.7% compared with 37.5%). ER-positive disease is more common in the elderly population, with a higher proportion being strongly ER-positive, which is consistent with the coorelation between ER status correlates and grade. Her2 positivity rates were markedly reduced in patients aged over 70 years when compared with those under 50 years (7% vs 15%). Proliferation rates of tumors in the elderly (measured by ki67 immunocy to chemistry) were significantly lower, although this finding is entirely consistent with the higher proportion of grade 3 cases in younger cohorts and the mitotic index isone of the criteria used in forgrading tumors. Immunophenotyping, supported by molecular biological studies, now permits us to dissect out different subgroups among the breast cancer population. The Sorlie classification using a molecular classifier from RNA analyses (11) separates breast cancer subtypes as follows: luminal A and B (both ER-positive), and basal-like, Her2 positive and normal breast-like (all ER-negative). Within the luminal type, B type tumors display a clinically more aggressive phenotype than luminal A. Cheang et al. (12) studied a cohort of 4046 patients with primary invasive breast cancer referred to the British Columbia Cancer Agency between 1986 and 1992. They used classical immunophenotyping to distinguish five types of breast cancer: ER/PgR positive, Her2 negative, equivalent to luminal A in the Sorlie classification, luminal B (either positive for ER or PgR and Her2 positive), and core basal (ER/PgR/Her2 positive, but cytokeratin 5/6 and/or EGFR positive). The final subtype is negative for all five markers (5NP: ER, PgR, Her2, cytokeratin 5/6 and EGFR). The luminal B classification used by Cheang et al. (11) differsfrom that used by Sorlie et al. (10), in that only 30-50% of the luminal B tumors in the Sorlie classification are positive for Her2. Figure 47.3 shows the frequency of the different subtypes of breast cancer identified by Cheang et al. (11) in relation to the age of the patient at diagnosis. There is a clear increase in luminal A tumors with age, whereas the frequency of both core basal and 5NP subtypes decrease with age. This may be related partly to the finding that 87% of core basal and 64.4% of 5NP are classified as grade 3, and grade 3 is more common in the younger age groups. Interestingly, the core basal group showed a hazard ratio of 1.62 for risk of death from breast cancer (95% confidence interval 1.31–2.00), whereas the 5NP showed no prognostic significance. Dubecq et al. (3) subdivided 61% (1661) of their 2723 consecutive breast cancers into four subtypes: luminal A (ER-positive/Her2 negative, grade 1 and 2), luminal B (ER-positive/Her2 negative/grade 3), Her2 positive and ER/Her2 negative. Their results are broadly concordantwith those of Cheang et al. (12), indicating that lower-grade ER-positive tumors increase in frequency with age, whereas ER/Her2-negative and Her2-positive subtypes, associated with higher-grade tumors, are less common in the older age groups.

Nonetheless, not all breast cancer in the elderly is indolent and a significant proportion of breast cancer in the over 70's is associated with a more aggressive phenotype and a poorer prognosis: 19% of the series reported by Durbecq et al. (3) were ER positive but grade 3, and 17% were ER/Her2 negative.

AGE AND BIOLOGICAL FEATURES OF BREAST CANCER

It has long been known that the ER contentof breast cancers is higher in postmenopausal women compared with premenopausal women, reflecting biological differences between these groups of cancers taken as a whole (11–13). A study by Diab et al. (14) evaluated 50,828 patients from the San Antonio Breast Cancer Database and 256,287 patients from a large American database registry project, the Surveillance, Epidemiology and End Results (SEER). These workers confirmed the association between increasing age at diagnosis and the presence of more favorable biological tumor characteristics, including hormone receptor positivity, low proliferation rate, normal p53, absence of expression of c-erbB2 and epidermal growth factor receptor (EGFR), and low ploidy. Similar patterns of tumor marker expression were found in the study by Daidone et al. (15) evaluating 14,007 breast cancer patients. By contrast, in a much more detailed study of genes associated with ER signaling, Quong et al. (16), confirmed an age-dependent increase in ER positivity, but no age dependency in the expression of ER responsive genes such as progesterone receptor (PR), cathepsin D, pS2 and Bcl2 was found. Therefore, these findings provide evidence that perhaps the ER signaling pathway was not as intact in the older patient as mightbe predicted by the level of ER immunohistochemical staining. ER-positive, PR-negative breast cancers are less responsive to hormonal therapies than ER- and PgR-positive breast cancers. Therefore, these findings provide evidence for justifying different treatment modalities in the older patient. Expression of ER-inducible genes is dependent upon the interaction of ERα and the Sp1 promoter which can be disrupted by mutational changes or inactivation of the Sp1 protein's binding domain. Loss of Sp1 function is also a consequence of oxidative stress, and loss of DNA binding with a decrease in Sp1 protein concentration is associated with aging in many organ systems (17,18), including the breast (Quong et al. (16)). This appears to be linked to loss of binding of Sp1 to DNA rather than a loss of intracellular Sp1 expression *per se*. Loss of Sp1 DNA binding also correlated with an age-associated increase in phospho-Erk5, which is involved in a redox-activated signalling pathway (19). In contrast, these investigators did not find a similar age-associated alteration in AP1 DNA binding, which has been associated with tamoxifen resistance (20), suggesting a different mechanism for tamoxifen resistance in older patients.

Collectively, these studies clearly show that, in general, late-onset has different biological features from young-onset breast cancer, particularly in respect to estrogen signaling pathways in breast epithelial cells.

The pathological behaviorof a tumor is driven largely by its innate biology. Many molecular studies do not take account of basic pathological criteria like the histological grade of a tumor when seeking to identify age related differences. Comparing a grade 1 breast cancer with a grade 3 cancer is like comparing an apples with oranges. A critical review of the papers purporting to show age-related differences realeed that many of these were more likely related to the histological characteristics of prevalent tumors invarious age groups rather than age *per se* (1).

CLINICAL TREATMENT OF BREAST CANCER IN THE ELDERLY: ASSESSMENT

It should be borne in mind that interventions might include surgery under general anaesthesia followed by months of debilitating cytotoxic chemotherapy. Accurate assessment of risk and benefit is critical in deciding treatment in elderly patients. A study by the Breast International Group was designed to identify how oncologists assessed their elderly patients. The age of 70 years was the average cut-off commonly used to define a patient as elderly and only 2% of the oncologists collaborated on a regular basis with a consultant geriatrician. Oncologists rarely carried out any geriatric assessment before proposing adjuvant chemotherapy to an elderly patient. The most frequently used instruments were the activities of daily living scale (61%), a co-morbidity scale (49%) and the mini-mental state evaluation (38%) (21). These findings were confirmed by a French cohort study (22). Evaluation of patients' fitness for treatment was based primarily on the Eastern Cooperative Oncology Group (ECOG) performance status and medicine for the elderly clinicians were only very rarely involved (23). This is despite evidence to show that traditional oncological measures of function, such as the Karnofsky and ECOG performance status scales, are poor predictors in the elderly (22,23). The best evidence that we have is that 'comprehensive geriatric assessment' scales provide the best estimation of an individual's functional reserve and life expectancy. Although time-consuming, they has been used very effectively in general care of the elderly (24,25). However, to date in oncology there are no prognostic validation studies based on such measures (26). Alternatively, Gosney (27) suggested that a stepwise approach that first identifies frail individuals should be used to target resources. Those identified as fit should be treated as individuals 20 years younger within the current evidence, and those identified as frail elderly should undergo a more thorough multidisciplinary assessment.

It is the authors' belief that attitudes of clinicians, not always based on solid evidence, is a dominant factor in determining the management of the elderly breast cancer patient. This is discussed in some detail in the following section.

ATTITUDES OF CLINICIANS

A retrospective cohort study involving case note review was undertaken, based on the North Western Cancer Registry database of women aged over 65 years, resident in Greater Manchester with invasive breast cancer registered over a 1-year period (n = 480). Adjusting for tumor characteristics associated with age by logistic regression analyses, older women were less likely to receive standard management than younger women for all indicators investigated. Compared to women aged 65–69 years, women aged over 80 years with operable (stage I–IIIa) breast cancer had increased odds of not receiving triple assessment, not receiving primary surgery, not undergoing axillary node surgery and not undergoing tests for steroid receptors. Women aged 75–79 years had increased odds of not receiving radiotherapy following breast-conserving surgery compared to women aged

65–69 years. These results demonstrated that older women in the UK are less likely to receive standard management for breast cancer, compared to younger women and this disparity cannot be explained by differences in tumor characteristics (28).

One of the authors led a study to investigate the attitudes, perceptions, and practices of breast cancer specialists with reference to the effect of patient age on management decisions in breast cancer, and attempted to identify national consensus on this issue (29). One hundred thirty-three relevant specialists, including 75 surgeons and 43 oncologists, participated in a virtual consultation using e-mailed questionnaires and open-ended discussion documents, culminating in the development of proposed consensus statements sent to participants for validation.

A strong consensus was seen in favor of incorporating minimum standards of diagnostic services, treatment, and care for older patients with breast cancer into relevant national guidance, endorsed by professional bodies. Similarly, an overwhelming majority of participants agreed that simple, evidence-based protocols or guidelines on standardizing assessment of biological and chronological age should be produced by the National Institute for Health and Clinical Excellence and the Scottish Medicines Consortium, developed in collaboration with specialist geriatricians, and endorsed by professional bodies. A further recommendation that all breast cancer patient treatment and diagnostic procedures be undertaken in light of up-to-date, relevant scientific data met with majority support. This study was successful in gauging national specialist opinion regarding the effect of patient age on management decisions in breast cancer in the UK.

Respondents to the invitation process received a semi-quantitative baseline questionnaire—partly factual, partly attitudinal—developed in collaboration with the steering group and validated in a previous national consultation on prospective HER-2 testing (30), to provide an initial gauge of situation, opinions, and issues. Feedback from the questionnaire was used to inform the selection of topics for the key national discussion stage of the consultation. An open-ended discussion document was prepared providing a narrative of findings from the baseline survey and seeking national participants' views.

About 80% of respondents were confident or very confident that they could evaluate social and emotional dimensions of patients when making management decisions. Of the remainder, about half said a lack of relevant training meant that they were not fully confident about effectively evaluating social and emotional dimensionsof patients, whereas the others believed that there was a lack of time for them to adequately manage the complexity of these dimensions in addition to the usual clinical assessments.

Three-quarters of respondents worked in a multidisciplinary team evaluating whether patients were suitable for treatment. Most teams included a breast surgeon (96%), clinical oncologist (91%), and specialist nurse (90%). Themajority of teams (62%) included a medical oncologist, whereas 42% included an anaesthetist. A geriatrician was included in only a small minority (8%) of teams.

ATTITUDES CONCERNING CHEMOTHERAPY IN OLDER PATIENTS

Factors restricting a recommendation of treatment with chemotherapy for patients with early-stage disease were poor general health or fitness for treatment (cited by 100% of respondents), and comorbidity. Lack of relevant data in the elderly and reluctance of carers to suggest chemotherapy to patients, were also cited by the overwhelming majority of respondents. Other factors cited by a very large majority were a perception of inaccuracy of "Adjuvant! Online" data for breast cancer in patients aged over 70 years , negative perceptions among older people regarding chemotherapy, poor general medical and geriatric medicine skills among surgeons, the absence of a trained nurse to advise on the assessment of older cancer patients and tumor characteristics associated with age (81%).

Other than poor general health, the key factor in assessing fitness for chemotherapy in patients was comorbidity. Comorbid conditions considered by respondents when making decisions regarding treatment in patients were heart disease and chronic obstructive pulmonary disease, each cited by all respondents. Nearly all respondents also mentioned diabetes (98%), hypertension (98%), arthritis (98%), renal failure (98%), stroke (98%), and previous malignancy (96%) as being very common and contraindicating morbidities. Comorbidity was thus a very frequently used reason to not provide older women with toxic or risky treatments. Older women being perceived as more likely than younger women to not want therapy was also cited as an important issue. Regardless of comorbidity, respondents' main areas of toxicity concern were (in order of perceived importance):heart (cited by 89% of respondents), bone marrow (67%), and kidney (47%). Around a quarter (23%) of respondents cited neurological toxicity concerns. Most respondents took the biological and chronological age and some used formal scoring of patients including tools such as mini-mental score, Karnofsky fitness score, and the geriatric assessment scale called the Instrument Assessing Daily Living (IADL).

Over half of the respondents pointed to a difference in standards between private and NHS care. Some respondents pointed out that more treatments may be offered in the private sector because patients might feel they can demand therapies when they are paying and may be more persuasive if they are highly educated, wealthy, or from a higher social class.

A strong consensus for trials issues restricting the recommendation for chemotherapy could be easily addressed to achieve the most benefit to patients. Three-quarters of the respondents cited a lack of relevant data in the elderly population. However, as we shall see later, despite such enthusiasm to study chemotherapy in the elderly, the application of this kind of research has proved to be rather problematical. A consensus was also evident in favor of a simple protocol or guidelines to standardise the approach to the assessment of biological and chronological age. Many respondents advocated the help of geriatricians in the development of such guidelines. Asked what the ideal objective tool for assessing patients' health status or fitness for treatment should be, more than a third of respondents cited specific approaches including comprehensive geriatric assessment and cognitive function and physical condition assessment tools. A significant minority said more research was needed to make a judgment. Many respondents suggested that this development should be with in the context of clinical trials.

There was no clear consensus on what should be considered best practice when assessing patients' health status or fitness for treatment.

SUMMARY OF ATTITUDES AND ASSESSMENT

The elderly are more vulnerable tonutritional complications of cancer and cancer treatment. Higher rates of locally advanced and metastatic disease at presentation may be explained by a combination of decreased breast awareness and reduced screening in older women.

Among those women who receive chemotherapy, older women tend to receive a lower dose intensity (31), despite a number of studies showing good tolerance and efficacy of chemotherapy in the elderly with breast cancer.In addition, they are less likely to be offered the opportunity to participate in research. A study of patients enrolled in 164 Southwest Oncology Group trials in the USA found that patients aged 65 years and over were under-represented in trials. This was especially apparent in breast cancer trials, where only 9% of patients enrolled were 65 years or older, despite 49% of breast cancer patients being in that age group (32). Elderly patients themselves, however, are keen for treatment. Research by Extermann and Hurria (33) has recently shown that the elderly are very willing to have chemotherapy, despite 17% considering that alopecia isirreversible and 30% that vomiting is unavoidable.

TREATMENT
The Challenges of Obtaining Evidence for Differing Treatments in the Elderly Patient

It is well recognized that there are difficulties in setting up successful trialsof therapy in older women with breast cancer. To an important degree, this is due to a 'protective' attitude towards older patients by clinicians. Contrariwise, patients do not necessarily agree with this. Thus the reason for the failure of older women to benefit from treatment regimes other than tamoxifen may, as we have seen above, result from the attitude of those treating the patient, rather than the patient.

Thus there is a lack of firm evidence in the elderly population for many of the interventions that have been demonstrated in younger patients in recent decades. In turn, this lack of a firm evidence base has discouraged funders from supporting these, sometimes, expensive therapies. The Early Breast Cancer Trialist's Collaborative Group (EBCTCG: 34) data assessing the benefits of tamoxifen and/or chemotherapy concluded that the trials of chemotherapy included 'too few women aged over 70 to be reliably informative' despite evidence that the magnitude of benefit was possibly similar to the 60–69 years of age group. Furthermore, none of these studies was primarily aimed at addressing the treatment of older women. Recently published audits from different national settings continue to show the wide variations in practice in all aspects of the treatment of older women with breast cancer, particularly in the use of systemic therapy as an adjuvant to or an alternative to primary surgery (35–37).

Surgery

The surgical aspects of breast cancer are dealt with in other chapters. In this section we will cover aspects that are relevant to the older patient.

Surgery remains the mainstay of treatment for early breast cancer even in the elderly patient. Surgical and anaesthetic risks carry a low morbidity for most patients. (38) Although mastectomy is relevantly more frequent, most patients choose conservation/radiotherapy if given the choice(39). Axillary staging by sentinel node biopsy has reduced the extent of axillary surgery for many women. Although the complication rate from axillary clearance is not higher than in younger women, one randomized trial suggested there was no survival advantage in women allocated axillary surgery versus simple mastectomy alone (all had adjuvant tamoxifen: 40).

The question of whether surgery can be omitted in favor of primary endocrine therapy alone has been reported in a Cochrane review (41). Whereas there is no evidence of a survival gain for surgery there is inferior local control over the following 1–2 years if surgery is omitted. This is therefore relevant to the particularly frail patient whose medium term survival is poor.

It has also been debated as to whether the aromatase inhibitors might be an alternative to surgery, being probably more potent than tamoxifen (42). Unfortunately a well-designed randomized trial to address this (ESTEeM) failed adequately to recruit, seemingly a common theme in recent randomised trials in the elderly (43). Details of this trial are described later in this chapter. Even with in the setting of clinical research, to a 'protective' attitude towards older patients by clinicians. Contrariwise, patients do not necessarily agree with this. Thus the reason for the failure of older women to benefit from treatment regimes other than endocrine therapy may result from the attitude of those treating the patient, rather than attitude of the patient herself.

For the present it seems reasonable to take the approach that for most patients whose life expectancy is more than just one or two years, surgery supported by sentinel node biopsy is optimal. For a much smaller minority with a much shorter life expectancy, primary endocrine therapy with an aromatase inhibitor may be preferred.

Adjuvant Endocrine Therapy

After the publication of several small studies showing the efficacy of tamoxifen as an alternative to surgery in the early 1980s this strategy gained widespread acceptance, particularly in the UK. A small number of randomized controlled trials were carried out and these have recently been the subject of a Cochrane Review (44). This analysis showed no significant survival benefit when primary endocrine therapy with tamoxifen was compared with surgery and adjuvant tamoxifen. However, there was a significant advantage in favor of surgery in terms of local disease control. In the middle of the 1980's the first of the EBCTCG meta-analyses was published. This in many ways was a watershed discovery that once and for all unequivocally showed the benefit for adjuvant endocrine therapy for early stage breast cancer. Although most of the data again emanated from randomized trials in younger women, a subgroup analysis showed that in the age group 70–75 years, surgery seemed to have a significant benefit in terms of survival and local control, whereas in the over 75 years age group surgery had no effect on survival.

This seemed to be due to competing mortality from co-morbid conditions. At that time, the ER assay was a biochemical technique and required unfixed tissue. Therefore as in other countries, very few UK centres produced ER data and few older women were assessed in the trials.

When the immuno-histochemical assay on routinely available formalin fixed paraffin embedded material emerged in the 1990's it became clear that there was an increasing trend for the older patients to have ER-rich types of breast cancer and hence potentially could benefit from adjuvant endocrine therapy. Subsequent quinquennial meta-analyses by the EBCTCG have sustained the recognition that for ER rich breast cancer at any age, endocrine therapy provides important protection against distant and local relapse and against new contralateral disease.

Thus for premenopausal women, ovarian suppression was confirmed to be effective whilst for all women tamoxifen provided a convenient, well-tolerated, relatively safe therapy, and was most effective when given over a minimum of 5 years. In the latter part of the 1990's the arrival of 3 well-tolerated and quite specific aromatase inhibitors became available for trial and quickly established a place as an alternative and possibly more potent inhibitor of breast cancers in the metastatic setting when compared against standard anti-hormones, particularly high dose progestational agents. The mode of action of these new agents necessitated that they could be tested in only postmenopausal women. Several very large international trials in the adjuvant setting, involving in total tens of thousands of patients, then confirmed a relative benefit over tamoxifen in terms of disease-free survival in middle-aged and older women.

They have therefore effectively replaced tamoxifen as first choice of therapy in advanced disease and are replacing it or being used in sequence with tamoxifen in early stage disease.

For many years, in cases where older women were perceived to be too frail to undergo general anaesthesia and surgery as the main treatment for their breast cancers, primary endocrine therapy was seen to be an attractive and preferable option. However, as discussed earlier, although the short-term results are impressive, longer term evaluation revealed a high rate of local failure.

We lack firm evidence for the best selection of patients for such an approach as compared against conventional surgical treatment supported by endocrine therapy. In 2008 the ESTEeM (Endocrine or Surgical Therapy for Elderly women with Mammary cancer) trial was set up to address this question by comparing surgery/anastrozole against anastrozole alone as primary treatment for ER-positive breast cancer in women aged 75 years and older. As is so often the case (see later under chemotherapy) when the treatment arms of a randomized trial are radically different, it proved to be impossible adequately to recruit patients into the trial. Despite the remaining lack of data, however, there does seem to be a trend to accept that local failure is an unacceptable risk and more elderly women are being offered surgery than was the practice 10 years ago.

Neoadjuvant Endocrine Therapy

Based on such clinical observations as noted above, neoadjuvant hormone manipulation has been evaluated in the older breast cancer patient, potentially allowing less extensive surgery. Many non-randomised studies and several international randomized trials have shown that primary endocrine therapy is effective as a prelude to surgery in reducing tumor size and reducing the need for mastectomy, particularly desirable in reducing the trauma in an older patient. Furthermore such studies have sustained the belief that again, aromatase inhibitors are the most effective agents when compared against tamoxifen.

When compared against chemotherapy, again the effectiveness of aromatase inhibitors has been shown to be impressive. In a study of 121 postmenopausal women with hormone-sensitive breast cancer, patients were randomised to receive either neoadjuvant doxorubicin and paclitaxel for four cycles or neoadjuvantan astrozole or exemestane for 3 months before surgery. Thirty-two per cent of the endocrine group and 20% of the chemotherapy group were over 70 years of age (45). There was a trend forincreasing rates of breast conservation in favor of endocrine treatment with no differences in local recurrence rates at 34 months. Endocrine treatment was. of course, better tolerated. The optimum duration of neoadjuvanthormone treatment is yet to be defined, but patients not responding by 3 months are unlikely to benefit from further treatment.

Data from a series of phase 2 studies at the Edinburgh Breast Unit suggests that neoadjuvant aromatase inhibitors produce ongoing shrinkage in the primary cancer over 12 months in those showing response at 3 months (45). In the neoadjuvant setting, an astrozole has been compared with tamoxifen in the IMPACT trial (46), whereas in the 'PO24' trial the efficacy of letrozole and tamoxifen was evaluated preoperatively (47). In the latter trial, none of the patients was considered to be a candidate for breast-conserving surgery and 14% were inoperable. The effect on proliferation was evaluated by the Ki67 labelling index. In the IMPACT trial, the mean age was 73 years and in PO24 the mean age was 67 years. In both there was a significantly higher rate of breast-conserving surgery in the aromatase inhibitor group, whereas data suggested that Ki67 levels after 2 weeks' treatment may predict for longterm outcome (48). This is being tested in the POETIC (Perioperative Endocrine Therapy) trial. Fulvestrant, an estrogen receptor antagonist with no agonist effects, in effect, a 'cleaner' agent than tamoxifen, has been studied in the neoadjuvant setting in the NEWEST trial. The biological and clinical activity of two doses of the drug, namely the approved dose of 250 mg/month vs a high dose of 500 mg/month, were evaluated in a phase II randomised multicentre trial. In total, 211 patients with a mean age of 67 years participated. The high dose regimen reduced the mean Ki67 labelling index and levels of ER expression significantly more than the approved dose over a 16 weekperiod (49).

Adjuvant Radiotherapy

Adjuvant radiotherapy is the current standard of care for patients with early breast cancer following breast-conserving surgery, and in patients with a high risk of local recurrence following mastectomy. The EBCTCG studies have demonstrated considerable benefit both in terms of local control and overall survival. Radiotherapy following breast-conserving surgery was associated with proportional reductions in local recurrence across all age groups. However, the absolute benefits of treatment were lower in older patients as their overall risk of local recurrence was less (absolute reductions in 5-year local recurrence risk for post-BCS radiotherapy: 22, and 11% for those aged <50, and >70 years, respectively: data from reference 50).

As with chemotherapy the observations on UK practice show that radiotherapy use after surgery falls quite dramatically with advancing age, especially in women aged 70 years and older. According to the Oxford overview analysis, 5-year local recurrence risks were 7 vs 26% (p<0.00001) and a 15-year breast cancer mortality risks 30.5 vs 35.9% (p<0.0002), in those who underwent radiotherapy following surgery compared with those undergoing breast-conserving surgery alone (51). There is reasonable concern about the risk of coronary heart disease that has been observed with older radiation techniques in recent decades where there was unequivocal evidence of a higher rate of excess mortality from heart disease and even lung cancer. However with modern equipment, that risk is almost certainly much reduced.

One important large randomised trial has directly addressed the role of adjuvant radiotherapy following breast-conserving surgery in older women (52) In this study women aged 70 years or more with T1 N0 hormone receptor-positive breast cancers who had undergone breast-conserving surgery and were being treated with tamoxifen, were randomized to receive radiotherapy or not. At the most recent update (at a median follow up of 10.5 years), the rate of local or regional recurrence was 9% in those treated with tamoxifen alone, and 2% in those who also received radiotherapy (p<0.001). There were no significant differences between the two groups in overall survival.

It is also the case however, that aromatase inhibitors have a favorable impact on local recurrence when compared with tamoxifen. Taken together with recent trends for falling local recurrence rates, these factors are likely to further reduce the already low local recurrence rates seen in older patients, and may mean that the absolute benefits of radiotherapy in this population in the future will be smaller still.

More recently, the PRIME II (post-operative radiotherapy in minimum-risk elderly phase II) trial has recruited women aged 65 or over with low-risk breast cancer (less than 3 cm, grade I or II, node negative and hormone receptor positive), treated by breast-conserving surgery and adjuvant endocrine therapy (53). Patients were randomised to receive post-operative breast radiotherapy or no radiotherapy, and the trial was designed to detect a difference in local recurrence rates of at least 5%.

Despite concerns about side-effects, post-operative radiotherapy remains the standard of care in older patients undergoing breast-conserving surgery, except in those very frail patients with a limited life expectancy. However, it is frequently reported that older patients are much more likely to be treated with breast-conserving surgery alone (54,55). The reasons are likely to be multi-factorial, including issues relating to the attitudes of the doctors treating the elderly patient, service practicalities and patients' wishes. However, older patients with tumors at higher risk for local recurrence and reasonable life-spans should be offered irradiation as part of their treatment plan.

In an attempt to make radiotherapy less of an ordeal for patients, and cheaper to deliver, two studies have compared a previous standard schedule of 50 Gy in 25 fractions with shorter schedules of 15–16 fractions over 21 and 22 days, respectively (56,57). There were no significant differences in efficacy between the treatment strategies, with the shorter fractionation schedule providing convenience to patients and reduced healthcare expenditure. In the future, hypo-fractionation, partial breast irradiation, brachytherapy and intra-operative radiotherapy, may all mean that radiotherapy can be more efficiently delivered. This may be particularly relevant to older women where reduction in treatment time and reduced frequency of hospital visits is to be encouraged. However, less than 20% of patients were aged 70 or over in these studies.

Adjuvant Chemotherapy

The current life expectancy of a 70-year-old woman in the UK is 16 years. Therefore many older women with breast cancer are at risk of recurrence and death from breast cancer in their projected lifetime, and may potentially benefit from chemotherapy (58). As discussed above, older women are more likely to have low-grade, ER-positive tumors. As a consequence, endocrine therapy hasbeen the mainstay of adjuvant systemic therapy for the older age group. However, a significant proportion of older women do still present with tumors with adverse prognostic features, suggesting a significant risk of disease recurrence, and therefore the need to consider other treatment options.

In the Oxford overview of the Early Breast Cancer Trialists' Collaborative Group, published in 2005, the benefits of polychemotherapy were seen to decrease progressively with increasing age. The reductions in risk of death for polychemotherapy compared with no chemotherapy were respectively 30% and 13% for the age groups 40–49, and 70 and over. (59). In this analysis, the benefit for patients aged 70 or over was of the same order as for younger postmenopausal women, but the result was not significant as the number of older women in the analysis was too small (only 1200 women included in the trials analysed were aged 70 years or over) (59). Further evidence for the value of this treatment modality is required, as without this, the value of programmes such as Adjuvant! Online may be limited in this patient population, as the predictive estimates are based on clinical trials where older patients are under-represented.

In an attempt to redress this, two contemporary trials, Adjuvant cytotoxic ChemoTherapy In Older women (ACTION: 60) and Chemotherapy Adjuvant Study for women at Advanced age (CASA), planned to examine the benefits of adjuvant chemotherapy in women aged over 70 years and 65 years, respectively, with ER-negative or high-risk ER-positive tumors. Both trials included chemotherapy and no chemotherapy arms, in an attempt to quantify the absolute gains from chemotherapy. Unfortunately both trials closed due to poor recruitment. Therefore, the available data suggest that there may be a benefit to adjuvant systemic chemotherapy in some older women with breast cancer, but which patients benefit and the magnitude of the benefit are unknown. The Cancer and Leukemia Group B (CALGB) 49907 study tookas a premise that adjuvant chemotherapy is of benefit in older women, and has compared two treatment regimens (61). Women aged 65 or older with invasive T1–T4 breast cancer (ER-positive or negative) and node positive or negative, were randomised to receive standard chemotherapy (six cycles of CMF or four cycles of AC, according to physician choice), or six cycles of oral capecitabine. Accrual stopped at 633 patients, at which point 61% of patients were aged 70 years or over. After a median follow-up of 2 years, patients randomised to capecitabine were 2.4 times more likely to experience relapse (adjusted $p < 0.0003$) and 2.1 times more likely to die ($p < 0.02$) than those receiving standard chemotherapy. This trial shows

that there is a benefit to giving patients over 65 with a good performance status standard polychemotherapy compared with single agent capecitabine chemotherapy. An unplanned subset analysis in this trial showed that the major benefit for standard chemotherapy was in patients with hormone receptor-negative tumors.

Toxicity is likely to be a key factor when considering adjuvant chemotherapy in older patients. In a large retrospective review of four CALGB trials of adjuvant chemotherapy, treatment-related mortality was found to be related to age: 0.2% (<50 years), 0.7% (51–64 years) and 1.5% (over 65 years) ($p < 0.001$) (62). Age is also a significant risk factor for congestive cardiac failure in women receiving adjuvant chemotherapy for breast cancer (HR, 1.79 per 10 years) (63). The US Oncology group has compared an anthracycline (doxorubicin/cyclophosphamide) with a non-anthracycline (docetaxel/cyclophosphamide) regimen in the adjuvant treatment of operable breast cancer (64). The non-anthracycline arm was found to be superior to the anthracycline treatment, including in the 16% of patients who were aged 65 or over at study entry. Owing to the low risks of cardio toxicity and acceptable neutropaenic sepsis rate, this regimen has become popular with many oncologists treating older women.

ASSESSING RISK OF CHEMOTHERAPY TOXICITY

In a study of patients aged 65 years or older with cancer investigators from seven institutions completed a pre-chemotherapy assessment that captured socio-demographics, tumor and treatment variables, laboratory test results, and geriatric assessment variables (function, co-morbidity, cognition, psychological state, social activity and support, and nutritional status). Patients were followed through the chemotherapy course to capture grade 3 (severe), grade 4 (life-threatening or disabling), and Grade 5 (death) as defined by the National Cancer Institute Common Terminology Criteria for Adverse Events. In total, 500 patients with a mean age of 73 years (range, 65 to 91 years) with stage I to IV lung (29%), gastrointestinal (27%), gynecological (17%), breast (11%), genitourinary (10%), or other (6%) cancer joined this prospective study. Grade 3 to 5 toxicity occurred in 53% of the patients. A predictive model for grade 3 to 5 toxicity was developed that consisted of geriatric assessment variables, laboratory test values, and patient, tumor, and treatment characteristics. A scoring system identified older adults at low (30%), intermediate (52%), or high risk (83%) of chemotherapy toxicity. They concluded that a risk stratification schema can establish the risk of chemotherapy toxicity in older adults (65). For further discussion of the treatment options, and their evidence base, for the elderly patient, the reader is referred to a recently published review by Ring et al, (66).

CONCLUSION

It is clear that there are many reasons why the treatment offered to elderly patients may be different from that offered to a younger patient. Not all of these are associated with evidence that this treatment dichotomy, where the diversion happens around the age of 70 years, should occur. Treating physicians clearly have their own biases in what the older patient will tolerate, so we need to have more objective tools identified by evidence-based studies to aid in treatment decision-making for the older patient. The evidence isthat we are probably significantly under-treating many patients, and in others we are causing a reduced quality of life with no clinical benefit. It is also likely that the biology of the tumor in the elderly patient is different from what appears to be a similar tumor in the younger patient . Given the significant co-morbities that come with age, better targeted agents, that do not have the inherent problems of current cytotoxic chemotherapy, may prove to be useful in the future in this increasing population.

It is important also to recognise the potential for better selection of individual patient's risk based on a deeper understanding of the biology of their particular tumor. Promising studies of molecular profiling (e.g., Oncotype-Dx or Mammaprint: reviewed in reference 67) are emerging, again in younger populations but it is likely that genetic profiles identified in tumors from a younger population may be equally relevant in an older women. Thus trials such as the 'TAILOR-x' trial in the USA and the MINDACT in Europe could be the first of several initiatives that will sustain the importance of such individual fine tuning to help treatment selection, especially when it concerns the use of toxic chemotherapies or molecularly targeted agents.

Finally, although this is a chapter concerning breast cancer treatment, many of the issues raised here are found in patients with other cancers. Breast cancer is not the only tumor type to show different age-associated molecular pathological patterns. Similar findings have also been made in thyroid cancer (68), colorectal cancer (69), rhabdomyosarcoma (70) and acute myeloid leukaemia (71). In cancer research we tend to concentrate solely on the cancer tissue itself, forgetting that the tissue in which it grows is subject to influences from a large number of circulating factors, as well as locallyproduced factors, all of which may show large fluctuations asthe body's physiology changes with the ageing process. Perhaps therefore it is time to consider how age can affect not just the doctor's attitude, and the patients ability to cope with the appropriate treatment regimes, but also the biology of the tumor itself.

REFERENCES

1. Thomas GA, Leonard RCF. Breast cancer in the elderly. Clin Oncol 2009; 21: 79–80.
2. Thomas GA, Leonard RCF. How age affects the biology of breast cancer. Clin Oncol 2009; 21: 81–85.
3. Durbecq V, Ameye L, Veys I, et al. A significant proportion of elderly patients develop hormone-dependant "luminal-B" tumors associated with aggressive characteristics. Crit Rev Oncol Hematol 2008; 67: 80–92.
4. Hawkins RA, White G, Bundred NJ, et al. Prognostic significance of oestrogen and progesterone receptor activities in breast cancer. Br J Surg 1987; 74: 1009–13.
5. Eppenberger-Castori S, Moore DH Jr, Thor AD, et al. Age associated biomarker profiles of human breast cancer. Int J Biochem Cell Biol 2002; 34: 1318–30.
6. Moller H, Flatt G and Moran A. High cancer mortality rates in the elderly in the UK. Cancer Epidemiol 2011; 35: 407–12.
7. Benz CC. Impact of aging on the biology of breast cancer. Crit Rev Oncol Hematol 2008; 66: 65–74.
8. Chung YM, Lee SB, Kim HJ, et al. Replicative senescence induced by romo1-derived reactive oxygen species. J BiolChem 2008; 283: 33763–71.
9. Burhans WC, Weinberger M. DNA replication stress, genome instability and aging. Nucleic Acids Res 2007; 35: 7545–56.
10. Cheung KL, Wong AWS, Parker H, et al. Pathological features of breast cancer in the elderly based on needle core biopsiesda large series from a single centre. Crit Rev Oncol Hematol 2008; 67: 263–7.
11. Sorlie T, Perou CM, Tibshirani R, et al. Gene expression patterns of breast carcinomas distinguish tumor subclasses with clinical implications. Proc Natl Acad Sci USA 2001; 98: 10869–74.
12. Cheang MC, Voduc D, Bajdik C, et al. Basal-like breast cancer defined by five biomarkers has superior prognostic value than triple-negative phenotype. Clin Cancer Res 2008; 14: 1368–76.
13. Clark GM, Osbourne CK, McGuire WL. Correlations between estrogen receptor, progesterone receptor and patient characteristics in human breast cancer. J ClinOncol 1984; 2: 1102–109.
14. Diab SG, Elledge RM, Clark GM. Tumor characteristics and clinical outcome of elderly women with breast cancer. J Natl Cancer Inst 2000; 92: 550–6
15. Daidone MG, Coradini D, Martelli G, Veneroni S. Primary breast cancer in elderly women: biological profile and relation with clinical outcome. Crit Rev Oncol Hematol 2003; 45: 313–25.
16. Quong J, Eppenberger-Castori S, Moore D, et al. Age-dependent changes in breast cancer hormone receptors and oxidant stress markers. Breast Cancer Res Treat 2002; 76: 221–36.
17. Ammedola R, Mesuraca M, Russo T, Cimino F. Sp1 DNA binding efficiency is highly reduced in nuclear extracts from aged rat tissues. J Biol Chem 1992; 267: 17944–8.
18. Ammedola R, Mesuraca M, Russo T, Cimino F. The DNA binding efficiency of Sp1 is affected by redox changes. Eur J Biochem 1994; 225: 483–9.
19. Abe J, Knushara M, Ulevitch RJ, Berk BC, Lee J-D. Big mitogen activated protein kinase 1 (BMK-1) is a redox-sensitive kinase. J Biol Chem 1996; 271: 16586–90.
20. Johnston SRD, Lu B, Scott GK, et al. Increased activated protein-1 DNA binding and c-Jun NH2-terminal kinase activity in human breast tumors with acquired tamoxifen resistance. Clin Cancer Res 1999; 5: 251–6.
21. Biganzoli L, Goldhirsch A, Straehle C, et al. Adjuvant chemotherapy in elderly patients with breast cancer: a survey of the Breast International Group. Ann Oncol 2004; 15: 207–10.
22. Freyer G, Braud A-C, Chaibi P, et al. Dealing with metastatic breast cancer in elderly women: results from a French study on a large cohort carried out by the 'Observatory on Elderly Patients'. Ann Oncol 2006; 17: 211–16.
23. Extermann M, Overcash J, Lyman GH, et al. Comorbidity and functional status are independent in older cancer patients. J ClinOncol 1998; 16: 1582–7.
24. Repetto L, Fratino L, Audisio RA, et al. Comprehensive geriatric assessment adds information to Eastern Cooperative Oncology Group performance status in elderly cancer patients: an Italian Group for Geriatric Oncology study. J Clin Oncol 2002; 20: 494–502.
25. Muss HB, Biganzoli L, Sargent DJ, et al. Adjuvant therapy in the elderly. Making the right decision. J Clin Oncol 2007; 25: 1870–5.
26. Maas HAAM, Janssen-Heijnen MLG, OldeRikkert MGM, et al. Comprehensive geriatric assessment and its clinical impact on oncology. Eur J Cancer 2007; 43: 2161–9.
27. Gosney M. Contribution of the geriatrician to the management of cancer in older patients. Eur J Cancer 2007; 43: 2153–60.
28. Lavelle K, Moran A, Howell A et al. Older women with operable breast cancer are less likely to have surgery. Br J Surg 2007; 94: 1209–15.
29. Leonard RC, Barrett-Lee P, Gosney MA, Willett AM, Reed MW, Hammond PJ. Effect of patient age on management decisions in breast cancer: consensus from a national consultation. Oncologist 2010; 15: 657–64.
30. Dowsett M, Hanby AM, Laing R, Walker R, National HER2 Consultation Steering Group. Her2 testing in the UK: consensus from a national consortium. J Clin Pathol 2007; 60: 685–9.
31. Lyman GH, Dale DC, Crawford J. Incidence and predictors of low dose-intensity in adjuvant breast cancer chemotherapy: a nationwide study of community practices. J Clin Oncol 2003; 21: 4524–34.
32. Hutchins LF, Unger JM, Crowley JJ, et al. Underrepresentation of patients 65 years of age or older in cancer treatment trials. N Engl J Med 1999; 341: 2061–7.
33. Extermann M, Hurria A. Comprehensive geriatric assessment for older patients with cancer. J Clin Oncol 2001; 83: 378–82.
34. Early Breast Cancer Trialist's Collaborative Group (EBCTCG). Chemotherapy and hormonal therapy for early breast cancer: effects on recurrence and 15-year survival in an overview of the randomised trials. 2002. [Available from: http://www.ctsu.ox.ac.uk/ inebctcg].
35. Wyld L, Garg DK, Kumar ID, Brown H, Reed MW. Stage and treatment variation with age in postmenopausal women with breast cancer: compliance with guidelines. Br J Cancer 2004; 90: 1486–91.

36. Lavelle K, Todd C, Moran A, et al. Non-standard management of breast cancer increases with age in the UK: a population based cohort of women 1⁄4 65 years. Br J Cancer 2007; 96: 1197–203.

37. Mustacchi G, Cazzaniga ME, Pronzato P, et al. Breast cancer in elderly women: a different reality? Results from the NORA study. Ann Oncol 2007; 18: 991–6.

38. Wyld L, Reed M. The role of surgery in the management of olderwomen with breast cancer. Eur J Cancer 2007; 43: 2253–63.

39. Sandison AJP, Gold DM, Wright P, Jones PA. Breast conservation or mastectomy: treatment choice of women age 70 years or older. Br J Surg 1996; 83: 994–6.

40. International Breast Cancer Study Group. Randomized trial comparing axillary clearance versus no axillary clearance in older patients with breast cancer: first results of international breast cancer study group trial 10–93. J Clin Oncol 1996; 24: 337–44.

41. Hind D, Wyld L, Reed MWR. Surgery, with or without tamoxifen, vstamoxifen alone for older women with operable breast cancer: cochrane review. Br J Cancer 2007; 96: 1025–9.

42. Crivellari D, Sun Z, Coates AS, et al. Letrozole compared with tamoxifenfor elderly patients with endocrine-responsive early breast cancer: the BIG 1–98 trial. J ClinOncol 2008; 26: 1972–9.

43. Reed MW, Wyld L, Ellis P, et al. Breast cancer in older women: trials and tribulations. Clin Oncol 2009; 21: 99–102.

44. Semiglazov VF, Semiglazov V, Ivanov V, et al. The relative efficacy of neoadjuvant endocrine therapy vs. chemotherapy in postmenopausal women with ER positive breast cancer. Proc Am Soc Clin Oncol 2004; 22: 519.

45. Renshaw L, Murray J, Young O, et al. Is there an optimal duration of neoadjuvant therapy? Breast Cancer Res Treat 2004; 88(Suppl 1): S36.

46. Smith I, Dowsett M, on behalf of IMPACT Trialists. Comparison of anastrozolevstamoxifen alone and in combination as neoadjuvant treatment of estrogen receptor-positive (ER.) operable breast cancer in post-menopausal women: the IMPACT trial. Breast Cancer Res Treat 2003; 82(Suppl 1): S6.

47. Eiermann W, Paepke S, Appfelstaedt J, et al. Preoperative treatment of postmenopausal breast cancer patients with letrozole: a randomized double-blind multicenter study. Ann Oncol 2001; 12: 1527–32.

48. Ellis MJ, Coop A, Singh B, et al. Letrozole inhibits tumor proliferation more effectively than tamoxifen, independent of HER1/2 expression status. Cancer Res 2003; 63: 6523–31.

49. Kuter I, Hegg R, Singer CF, et al.; On behalf of the NEWEST investigators. Fulvestrant 500 mg vs 250 mg: first results from NEWEST, a randomized, phase II neoadjuvant trial in postmenopausal women with locally advanced, estrogen receptor positive breast cancer (abstract 23). 30th Annual San Antonio Breast Cancer Symposium. 2007.

50. Early Breast Cancer Trialists' Collaborative Group (EBCTCG). Effects of radiotherapy and of differences in the extent of surgery for early breast cancer on local recurrence and 15-year survival: an overview of the randomised trials. Lancet 2005a; 366: 2087–106.

51. Hughes KS, Schnaper LA, Cirrincione C, et al. Lumpectomy plus tamoxifen with or without irradiation in women age 70 or older with early breast cancer. N Engl J Med 2004; 351: 971–7.

52. Arimidex, Tamoxifen, Alone or in Combination (ATAC) Trialists' Group. Effect of anastrozole and tamoxifen as adjuvant treatment for early-stage breast cancer: 100-month analysis of the ATAC trial. Lancet Oncol 2008; 9: 45–53.

53. Kunkler I. PRIME II breast cancer trial. Clin Oncol 2004; 16: 447–8.

54. Lavelle K, Todd C, Moran A, Howell A, Bundred N, Campbell M. Non-standard management of breast cancer increases with age in the UK: a population based cohort of women X65 years. Br J Cancer 2007; 96: 1197–203.

55. Schonberg MA, Marcantonio ER, Li D, Silliman RA, Ngo L, McArthy EP. Breast cancer among the oldest old: tumor characteristics, treatment choices and survival. J Clin Oncol 2010; 28: 2038–45.

56. Whelan TJ, Pignol JP, Levine MN, et al. Long-term results of hypofractionated radiation therapy for breast cancer. N Engl J Med 2010; 362: 513–20.

57. START Trialist's Group. The UK Standardisation of Breast Radio-therapy (START) Trial B of radiotherapy hypofractionation for treatment of early breast cancer: a randomised trial. Lancet 2008; 371: 1098–107.

58. Office for National Statistics. Current interim life tables: United Kingdom (2006–2008). 2010. [Available from: http://www.statistics.gov.uk/statbase] (Accessed 30 June 2010).

59. Early Breast Cancer Trialists' Collaborative Group (EBCTCG). Effects of chemotherapy and hormonal therapy for early breast cancer on recurrence and 15-year survival: an overview of the randomised trials. Lancet 2005b; 365: 1687–717.

60. Leonard R, Ballinger R, Cameron D, et al. Adjuvant Chemotherapy in Older Women (ACTION) Study – What did we learn from the Pilot Phase? B J Cancer 2011; 105: 1260–6.

61. Muss HB, Berry DA, Cirrincione CT, et al. Adjuvant chemotherapy in older women with early-stage breast cancer. N Engl J Med 2009; 360: 2055–65.

62. Muss HB, Woolf S, Berry D, et al. Adjuvant chemotherapy in older and younger women with lymph-node positive breast cancer. JAMA 2005; 293: 1073–81.

63. Mustacchi G, Cazzaniga ME, Pronzato P, et al. Breast cancer in elderly women: a different reality? Results from the NORA study. Ann Oncol 2007; 18: 991–6.

64. Jones SE, Holmes F, O'Shaughnessy J, et al. Extended follow-up and analysis by age of the US Oncology Adjuvant trial 9735: docetaxel/cyclophosphamide is associated with an overall survival benefit compared to doxorubicin/cyclophosphamide and is well-tolerated in women 65 or older (abstract 12). Breast Cancer Res Treat 2007; 106: S5.

65. Hurria A, Togawa K, Mohile SG, et al. Predicting chemotherapy toxicity in older adults with cancer: a prospective multicenter study. J Clin Oncol 2011; 29: 3457–65.

66. Ring A, Reed M, Leonard R et al. The treatment of early breast cancer in women over the age of 70. Br J Cancer 2011; 105: 189–93.

67. O'Toole SA, Selinger CI, Millar EK et al. Molecular assays in breast cancer pathology. Pathology 2011; 43: 116–27.

68. Powell NG, Jeremiah J, Morishita M, et al. Frequency of BRAF T1794A mutation in thyroid papillary carcinoma relates to age of patient at diagnosis and not to radiation exposure. J Pathol 2005; 205: 558–64.

69. Arai T, Sugai T, Kasahara I, et al. Age-related alteration in the association of microsatellite instability with absent hMLH1 expression and histological types of colorectal carcinoma. Pathol Int 2006; 56: 597–603.

70. Parham DM, Ellison DA. Rhabdomyosarcomas in adults and children. Arch Pathol Lab Med 2006; 130: 1454–65.

71. Chou W-C, Tang J-L, Lin L-I. Nucleophosmin mutations in de novo acute myeloid leukemia: the age-dependent incidences and the stability during disease evolution. Cancer Res 2006; 66: 3310–16.

48 Breast cancer and pregnancy

Christobel Saunders and Angela Ives

INTRODUCTION

Breast cancers associated with pregnancy are uncommon. However, as women increasingly choose to delay pregnancy until their 30s and 40s, when the incidence of breast cancer rises, this is likely to lead to an increased risk of pregnancy-associated breast cancer (PABC). It will also lead to an increase in women diagnosed with breast cancer before they have a chance to start a family.

A diagnosis of breast cancer is a life-changing event for any woman. For young women and their families it can be devastating. Women aged under 45 years constitute fewer than 15% of new cases of breast cancer diagnosed annually in Australia and the United Kingdom (1,2). Nonetheless, both in the developed world and internationally, the incidence of breast cancer in premenopausal women is increasing (3). In 2008, the age-specific incidence rates per 100,000 were very similar for women aged 20–44 years in Australia, the United Kingdom, and the United States (3–5). The age-specific incidence rates for breast cancer in less developed countries are lower than in the developed world for all age groups but incidence rises in similar increments for both groups as age increases and it appears that a relatively high proportion of breast cancers occurs in younger women (Fig. 48.1) (6).

It is recognized that breast cancer in young women has distinct physical and psychological outcomes compared with breast cancer in older women (7). Moreover, a diagnosis of breast cancer in a younger woman is associated with variable physical and psychological profiles depending on whether the diagnosis is made during or shortly after pregnancy or when pregnancy occurs subsequent to the breast cancer diagnosis.

This chapter describes what we know to date about breast cancer and pregnancy in these two important groups of younger women and what additional research is needed to not only assist clinicians in advising their patients but also to allow women to make informed choices about their cancer treatment and reproductive life.

PREGNANCY AS A RISK FACTOR FOR BREAST CANCER

Pregnancy can have both positive and negative influences on the risk and histological type of breast cancer. Early age at first pregnancy and multiparity generally reduce the long-term risk of developing breast cancer. Late age at first pregnancy and/or late age at last pregnancy also modify the risk of developing breast cancer. For premenopausal women, the risk of developing breast cancer is also influenced by the time since last pregnancy. There is a transient increased risk of developing breast cancer in the five years after completing a pregnancy after which the chance of developing breast cancer declines (8,9).

Women with a family history of breast cancer also have a short-term increased risk of developing breast cancer after a pregnancy (10).

PREGNANCY ASSOCIATED WITH BREAST CANCER

PABC or gestational breast cancer has been defined traditionally as, "breast cancer diagnosed when a woman is pregnant or in the first twelve months postpartum" (11). This definition of PABC is contentious as some clinicians and researchers argue that only women diagnosed with breast cancer during pregnancy should be defined as having PABC. Others argue, however, that breast cancer diagnosed up to one year postpartum, or when lactation occurs, should be included in the definition of PABC as the natural history of breast cancer suggests that the cancer would have been present before delivery and thus during the pregnancy. While it is unlikely that the associated pregnancy causes the breast cancer, little is known about what effect pregnancy or lactation has on the developing cancer (12–14).

There are significant and distinct challenges in the management of PABC. It appears to have a worse prognosis than breast cancer diagnosed in other young women; the epidemiological data are sparse and often conflicting. As PABC is an uncommon event, an individual clinician's experience of PABC may be limited. It is mandatory, therefore, that a multidisciplinary approach be taken to the oncology and obstetric care of women diagnosed with PABC.

Epidemiology

PABC is reported to affect between 0.76% and 3.8% of all women diagnosed with breast cancer (15–19). A large but historical study of 45,000 women presenting with breast cancer between 1850 and 1950 reported PABC in 2.9% of cases (15). More pertinently, 7–14% of premenopausal women diagnosed with breast cancer are diagnosed around the time of a pregnancy (20–22).

In a review of PABC, Wallack reported that about 10–39 per 100,000 pregnancies were complicated by a diagnosis of breast cancer (15,16). These women were older mothers falling in the age range of 32–37 years (16). Although this review was published in 1983, the median age of women diagnosed with PABC has not changed. Reports from the German Breast Group and a case series from the MD Anderson Cancer Center, United States, report a median age of 33 years (23,24).

Outcomes and Survival

Women diagnosed with PABC are generally reported to have worse outcomes than other premenopausal women diagnosed with breast cancer. PABC is thought to be more aggressive and

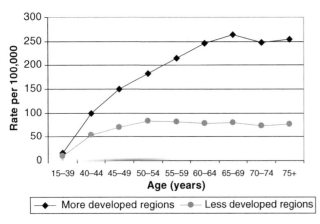

Figure 48.1 Age-specific breast cancer incidence rates as of 2008 for the more and less developed regions in the world. *Source*: From Ref. (6).

advanced at diagnosis (larger tumors and more positive lymph nodes) than non-PABC (25–28). Until the time when age and disease stage were taken into account, there appeared to be no difference in survival between PABC and non-PABC (11,21,29). Both survival comparison studies (PABC vs. non-PABC) based at major/tertiary institutions and those undertaken in smaller units demonstrate poorer outcomes for women diagnosed during pregnancy (25–28). In 2008, Rodriguez et al. reported that women diagnosed with breast cancer while pregnant or within nine months postpartum were more likely to die than similar aged women diagnosed with breast cancer when surgery type, stage, hormone receptor status, and race were controlled for (hazard ratio 1.14, 95% CI 1.00–1.29, p = 0.046) (30). It was suggested that there is an increased incidence of inflammatory breast cancer during pregnancy, but no specific pathological differences have so far been found (27).

Johansson et al. (31) have recently published a paper demonstrating that women who were four to six months postpartum at breast cancer diagnosis were four times more likely to die than those with no recently associated pregnancy and that women who were diagnosed with breast cancer when pregnant or within three months postpartum were twice as likely to die than non-PABC cases. This and other data (12–14,28,32–34), support the findings of a cohort study of women diagnosed with breast cancer under the age of 45 years in Western Australia. This as-yet unpublished work found that women diagnosed with PABC, when up to 12 months postpartum, were 48% more likely to die than other young women diagnosed with breast cancer, whereas those diagnosed when pregnant were only 3% more likely to die than other young women diagnosed with breast cancer (35). This finding suggests that the deleterious effect of pregnancy on cancer survival may be cumulative; that is, the further a woman is into the pregnancy or postpartum when she is diagnosed with breast cancer, the worse her survival may be (36).

Management

Women diagnosed with breast cancer during pregnancy are generally managed on an ad hoc basis. We are aware of four sets of guidelines or protocols that have been published with regard to the management of breast cancer and pregnancy. The Royal College of Obstetricians and Gynaecologists (London) and Canadian Society of Obstetricians and Gynaecologists have published evidence-based guidelines on how

physicians can counsel women diagnosed with breast cancer regarding concurrent and subsequent pregnancy (37,38). The MD Anderson Cancer Center in the United States has developed a protocol for the management of breast cancer during pregnancy that includes patient counseling, surgical and adjuvant therapy guidelines, and obstetric advice (24). International consensus guidelines have also been published by an expert panel (Fig. 48.2) (39,40).

Investigation and Diagnosis of Pregnancy-Associated Breast Cancer

Family History

A family history of breast cancer is a risk factor for almost half of all women diagnosed with breast cancer when less than 40 years of age. Up to 9% of these women will have a BRCA1 or BRCA2 mutation, predisposing them to the disease (41–43). It is important, therefore, that genetic counseling be considered for all very young women diagnosed with breast cancer, whether associated with pregnancy or not.

Diagnostic Delays

While the symptoms of PABC are the same as for non-PABC, the "milk rejection" sign has been identified as a unique presentation of breast cancer during lactation (44–46). It is often stated that women with PABC present at a late stage, thus leading to worse outcomes. However, reports from literature have shown that the time from identification of an initial symptom by the woman to breast cancer diagnosis can range from a few days to months though generally, breast cancer is diagnosed in women who are pregnant or lactating within two months of first noticing symptoms (35,47). This time of breast cancer diagnosis in pregnant and lactating women is comparable with that of all women. Delay of breast cancer diagnosis in any woman by a month, however, may increase the risk of nodal involvement, although the magnitude of this increased risk is likely to be extremely small (less than 1%) (48).

Breast cancer can be masked by engorgement of the pregnant or lactating breast and sometimes cancer symptoms can be attributed to pregnancy or lactation. Therefore, a cancer can be asymptomatic for a longer period, potentially leading to more advanced disease stage at presentation (19). This advanced presentation is likely due to delays in diagnosis as the pathology of PABC and non-PABC appears similar. However, tumor cells may behave differently during pregnancy due to physiological changes in the maternal system. Therefore, physiological mechanisms resulting in delayed manifestation of the symptoms cannot be absolutely excluded as a reason for advanced presentation.

Any new breast symptoms persisting for longer than two to four weeks should be taken seriously. Primary care physicians and obstetricians play an important role in the early detection of PABC by promoting breast awareness in their premenopausal patients. As recommended for non-pregnant women with breast symptoms, clinicians should offer prompt and appropriate referral of pregnant and lactating women with breast abnormalities to a multidisciplinary team for assessment (38,49).

The breast abnormality of a pregnant or lactating woman referred for further investigation should be reviewed in the same way as a non-pregnant woman presenting with a breast

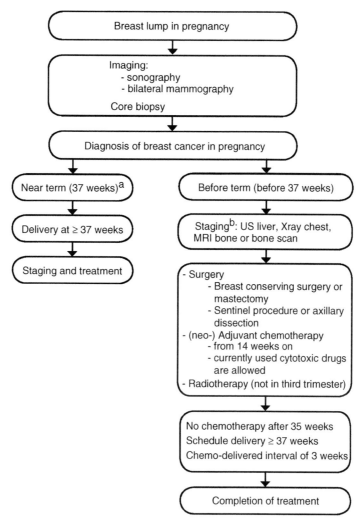

Figure 48.2 Algorithm for treatment of breast cancer diagnosed during pregnancy. [a]A wait policy of 2–4 weeks is allowed to attain fetal maturity; [b]as far as this will change clinical practice. *Source*: Adapted from Ref. (40).

abnormality. It should be assessed by clinical history, a clinical examination, and imaging and pathology; that is, with "triple assessment" (40,49). The physiological changes in the pregnant or lactating breast may mask the appearance of a lump, but it is inappropriate to delay investigation on the basis that the abnormality may be related to pregnancy or lactation (50–52).

There are, however, difficulties with assessing the pregnant/lactating breast. As pregnancy progresses, the intense hormonal milieu causes greater volume and firmness that can make clinical and imaging findings of the breast more difficult to interpret (53).

Imaging
Imaging of the breast during pregnancy and lactation is not always straightforward. Historically, two reasons are cited for this: first, the fear of inducing a fetal abnormality and secondly, interpretation of a mammogram or breast ultrasound during pregnancy or lactation may be difficult due to the breast's increased density and vascularity.

A number of studies on breast imaging during pregnancy or lactation have been reported in the literature but most are small in size (54–59). Samuels suggested that ultrasound is the most useful imaging modality during pregnancy, but clinicians should not be reluctant to use mammography when a breast mass is suspicious of cancer (54–58,60). It is generally assumed that all mammograms undertaken on young women demonstrate increased opacity of the breast parenchymal tissue (density). Samuels, however, makes the point that mammograms from one-third of women under 35 years of age do not demonstrate increased density (57). Digital mammography has been shown to be more sensitive in younger women with dense breast tissue than film screen mammography (61). When used appropriately, digital mammography may be associated with an up to 75% reduction in radiation dose compared to film mammography and is recommended for younger women when available (61).

When a woman is pregnant, it is important to consider whether mammography will alter breast cancer management. In a series reported by Liberman, no concomitant clinically undetected carcinoma was detected with mammography of the ipsilateral or contralateral breast, but two groups have each reported unsuspected contralateral disease in one case (55,58).

The safety of magnetic resonance imaging (MRI) during pregnancy is unknown. The *American Journal of Roentgenology* White Paper on Magnetic Resonance Safety states that MRI scans may be performed at any stage in pregnancy if warranted by the risk–benefit ratio for the mother (62). The usefulness, accuracy, and safety of contrast-enhanced breast MRI during pregnancy and lactation are uncertain as there is no

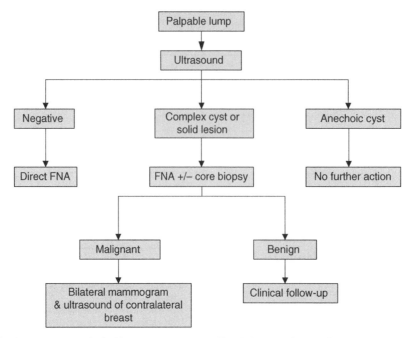

Figure 48.3 Algorithm for the investigation of palpable mass in pregnancy. *Abbreviation*: FNA, fine needle aspiration. *Source*: Adapted from Ref. (58).

published literature on this issue. There is concern that there may be high levels of background parenchymal enhancement which may obscure parenchymal abnormalities during pregnancy and lactation (63,64). Talele et al. reported on the use of contrast-enhanced MRI in a lactating woman with a palpable mass, which demonstrated generalized increase in Gadolinium uptake bilaterally which hampered tumor detection (64). Other published work has demonstrated that this may not be the case and that lesion detection did not appear to be a problem and multifocal disease could be identified (58,65). Taylor and colleagues, however, have warned of the potential for overestimation of lesion size (58).

Even if MRI can be safely performed during pregnancy, there are practical difficulties in positioning the woman prone in a standard breast coil during the later stages of pregnancy. A special "frame" may be needed to support the woman as she lies prone during scanning. While there are no known recorded adverse effects following MRI or the administration of gadolinium during pregnancy, there are ongoing theoretical concerns regarding the effects of exposure of the fetus to high magnetic fields during pregnancy and of exposure to free gadolinium ions (62). Currently, it is recommended that MRI should not be used as a routine examination during pregnancy, particularly in the first trimester (66,67), and that contrast-enhanced MRI should only be used in exceptional circumstances during pregnancy but is safe to use during lactation (67).

A proposed algorithm for the investigation of pregnant women with a palpable breast abnormality is given (Fig. 48.3).

Pathology

It is important that clinicians clearly specify on pathology request forms when a breast sample is taken from a woman who is pregnant or lactating to allow the most accurate appraisal of the pathology specimen by the pathologist. Fine needle aspiration cytology can be ambiguous because of cellular changes within the pregnant or lactating breast (68).

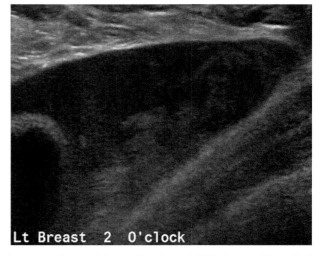

Figure 48.4 Ultrasound image of a galactocele following core biopsy during breast feeding. *Source*: Courtesy of Kulawansa S, Taylor D, McCallum D, Galloway J, Saunders C, Breast Clinic, Royal Perth Hospital, Australia.

A number of cytological differences, however, have been reported in breast cancers diagnosed during pregnancy and lactation compared with those diagnosed in the non-pregnant/non-lactational breast. This includes crowding and overlapping of nuclei, dyscohesion, and pleomorphic nuclei with irregular nuclear membranes, coarse nuclear chromatins, and mitoses (69). Core biopsy is considered to give more accurate information, and although 14G core biopsy is considered safe, a vacuum-assisted biopsy may potentially cause problems with milk fistula or galactocele (Fig. 48.4) (70–72).

Several studies have been published which report the pathology of PABC (17,73–77). Many of these are limited to a basic description of tumor type, size, and histological grade. Only one study has reviewed in more detail the morphological and immunochemical features of just 14 PABC cases (75). Shousha's small study reported some differences in the pathology of PABC when compared with 13 non-PABC controls. These differences included a higher incidence of totally or partly mucinous tumors in the lactational breast which were also MUC2 positive. However, larger studies are needed to investigate this further (75).

Pathologically, there are no discernable differences in tumor type between PABC and breast cancer diagnosed in non-pregnant young women. In previously published studies, invasive ductal carcinoma was the most common histological type found in women diagnosed with PABC (17,47,75,78–80). Where histological grade was reported, over 95% of women had grade 2 or 3 disease (75,76,80). Middleton also reported that high-grade ductal carcinoma *in situ* was associated with 72% of PABC cases (79). Except for one published report of a high incidence of inflammatory breast cancer in pregnant women (27), most case series report a similar incidence of inflammatory breast cancer in women diagnosed with PABC and non-PABC, with rates between 1.5% and 4% (26,81,82).

Women diagnosed with PABC are generally reported to have larger tumors, with lesions less than 20 mm in diameter found in only 20–35% of PABC cases (74,76–78). In Shousha's study, only one of 14 cases had a tumor less than 20 mm (75). Higher mitotic rates, less tubule formation, and increasing levels of lymphocytosis have been identified in PABC (13,35). In an age- and stage-matched case–control study of PABC versus non-PABC, the most unexpected and highly significant finding was that a negative lymph node status at diagnosis conveyed a survival advantage for non-PABC cases but not for PABC cases (35). Ishida reported similar findings but assumed that pregnancy itself was the poor prognostic factor (17). This suggests that prognosis in PABC depends not only on conventional histopathological factors such as tumor size and lymph node status, but also on other molecular markers, and this warrants further research.

The number of women with lymph node involvement reported in the literature is similar for young women diagnosed with PABC and non-PABC (75,77). The proportion of women diagnosed with PABC who had positive lymph nodes ranged from 58% to 80%; the number of cases in these studies varied from 13 to 192 (17,74–77). A high percentage of PABC cases with the adverse prognostic marker lymphovascular invasion was reported in some studies (17,79,83). PABC is commonly reported as being estrogen receptor (ER) and/or progesterone receptor (PR) negative (27,76,77,79,80). A potential bias may occur because the older ligand binding assay used to identify ER and PR status yields more false-negative results when high circulating levels of estrogen and progesterone downregulate receptors (84). When immunohistochemistry techniques are used, there appears to be no difference in the numbers of hormone receptor–positive tumors diagnosed in women with PABC and in similar aged women with non-PABC (84). Shousha also reports that most pregnant women had ER- and PR-negative tumors but women with lactational breast cancers were more likely to be ER and PR positive (75–77,79).

Overexpression of c-erbB-2 has been variably reported to differ in PABC (76,77,79). One study suggests overexpression of c-erb-2 and p53 mutations are more common in lactational carcinomas but not in breast cancers diagnosed during pregnancy (75–77). As might be expected in a cohort of very young women, PABC has been associated with a higher rate of BRCA allelic mutations than sporadic breast cancer (85,86).

Results from studies that have reviewed the pathological characteristics of PABC are inconclusive. This is attributable to either small sample sizes, failure to compare tumors of women diagnosed with PABC to those of similar aged women diagnosed with breast cancer, or review of only major characteristics such as tumor type and lymph node status (17,75,79,87). A larger case–control study is required.

Treatment

Multidisciplinary Approach

The initial management of PABC is best carried out in a specialist referral center where a multidisciplinary approach can be utilized. The team should include those involved in the management of both breast cancer and obstetric care so that mother and child receive the most appropriate care to optimize morbidity, mortality, psychosocial, and supportive outcomes. The management of PABC will depend on the stage of pregnancy or whether the woman is postpartum when diagnosed with breast cancer.

Local Treatment: Surgery and Radiotherapy

Mastectomy is often the preferred surgical treatment of breast cancer diagnosed during pregnancy, whatever the tumor size may be (72,88). While breast conserving surgery and adjuvant radiotherapy are routine treatment for non-PABC, this is largely contraindicated during pregnancy because radiotherapy to the breast, chest wall, or axillary lymph nodes may be harmful to the fetus (39,51). One group, however, has reported that in selected women and with excellent shielding, the breast can be irradiated during pregnancy without damage to the fetus (89).

When early-stage PABC is diagnosed in late pregnancy, radiotherapy can be performed after the delivery of the child. PABC diagnosed in postpartum lactating and non-lactating women can be managed with local treatment in the same way as other women but lactation should be ceased prior to treatment (72). Sentinel node biopsy is now the standard alternative to axillary dissection in early breast cancer for women without clinically obvious axillary nodal involvement. This remains controversial in pregnant women, but may be an option in a selected few (90,91).

Adjuvant Systemic Therapy

In theory, chemotherapy agents are all potentially teratogenic and mutagenic. The damage they cause to the fetus depends on the type of drug used, the dose given, and the stage of pregnancy when administered. The teratogenic properties of these agents are species specific and no trials of chemotherapy have been undertaken in pregnant humans because it would be unethical to do so (92).

Adjuvant chemotherapy administered during the first trimester of pregnancy results in unacceptably high levels of spontaneous abortion, fetal death, and fetal abnormality (51,93). A number of chemotherapy agents can be safely administered in the second and third trimester with no significant differences in reported rates of malformation (4% vs. 3%). Adjuvant chemotherapy during pregnancy may be associated with low birth weight and early delivery although the precise pathogenesis of this is unclear (24,94).

There are specific chemotherapeutic agents that should be avoided throughout pregnancy, including antimetabolites such as methotrexate (95). For optimal antineoplastic effect, a number of chemotherapy drugs are administered in combination. The most commonly recommended cytotoxic drugs for use in the treatment of breast cancer during pregnancy are adriamycin and cyclophosphamide or fluorouracil (5-FU), adriamycin, and cyclophosphamide (39,92). Other cytotoxic drug regimens are also employed which increasingly include a taxane (96). When chemotherapy is administered in the second or third trimester, fetal growth and development can be seriously affected. The drug combinations used can cause intrauterine growth retardation, pancytopenia, sepsis, neutropenia, preeclampsia, and reversible heart failure (92,97).

Case reports of other chemotherapy drugs administered inadvertently in the treatment of breast cancer during pregnancy have been published and report no negative effects to the fetus (98–103). Trastuzumab has been used during pregnancy for women who had c-erb-B2-positive advanced disease; the only side effect documented was reversible anhydramnios (101,103–111). However, this agent is not recommended for routine use during pregnancy. Interestingly, a case study from Italy reported the use of taxanes in a pregnant woman with metastatic breast cancer without detriment to fetal health (100).

When chemotherapy is administered during pregnancy, it should be discontinued at least two to three weeks prior to delivery or at the very latest by 35 weeks gestation. This reduces the chance of myelosuppression for both the mother and fetus at delivery. It also gives the placenta the chance to remove drug residues from the fetal organ systems as the neonatal liver and kidneys cannot initially metabolize and excrete cytotoxic drugs (92).

More than 25 cases of severe congenital abnormalities have been reported following use of tamoxifen during pregnancy but no congenital anomaly has been specifically associated with tamoxifen use (99,112,113). Although there have been at least 35 healthy babies born after therapeutic use and 85 after prophylactic use in breast cancer prevention trials during pregnancy, tamoxifen remains contraindicated in pregnancy (92,99,113).

Breast feeding is contraindicated once adjuvant systemic therapy has commenced, as drugs can pass freely from mother to child via breast milk and their effects on the infant are unknown (92).

To date, no long-term effects have been reported in the offspring of women diagnosed with breast cancer and treated with adjuvant systemic therapy during pregnancy (92,114). Long term follow up has demonstrated normal growth and development of children exposed to antineoplastic agents in utero. There is no clear evidence to corroborate the concerns of delayed malignancy or infertility affecting such children, but increasing recognition of the role of epigenetics in embryo development warrants continued vigilance over this matter.

Termination of Pregnancy

Historically, most women diagnosed with breast cancer during pregnancy were advised to terminate the pregnancy. There is no evidence suggesting that termination of pregnancy conveys any survival benefit to a woman. On the contrary, termination of pregnancy has been shown in one study to adversely affect breast cancer outcome (25). However, results of this study may be biased as it is possible that women with more advanced disease or poorer prognostic features were more likely recommended for a termination and this group would have a reduced chance of survival with or without termination (71,72). Termination can be medically indicated in those women who present with advanced or inflammatory breast cancer early on in pregnancy when urgent systemic treatment is required (16,72,115,116).

In the contemporary era, when breast cancer can be managed safely during pregnancy, a woman choosing to continue a concurrent pregnancy can do so in the knowledge there will be minimal impact on her child's wellbeing. Nonetheless, there are complex psychosocial issues surrounding PABC such as bearing and raising a child when the mother has an uncertain prognosis and a potentially life-threatening disease.

Ultimately, when women find themselves in this difficult dilemma and are given adequate information and support, they should be able to make an informed choice about their breast cancer management and the outcome of pregnancy. As Byrd succinctly said in 1968, "*In the face of general enthusiasm for terminating the pregnancy, we believe the evidence is that the cancer should be terminated*" (117).

Psychosocial Issues

Women diagnosed with breast cancer during or just after completion of pregnancy are forced to deal with two conflicting events simultaneously. Thus, a pregnant woman who is diagnosed with breast cancer must make decisions that can affect both her and her unborn child's morbidity and mortality. A decision to protect the health of her unborn child at the expense of her own after a diagnosis of breast cancer (or vice versa) is not taken lightly (118,119). The decisions she makes at this time will be unique to her and will be based not only on information provided to her about treatment options but on her life experiences, beliefs, values, and needs.

Breast cancer treatment chosen by the mother can have a psychological impact on the relationship with her child. This is not only the case for a woman diagnosed with breast cancer when she is pregnant but also for women who have young babies at the time of diagnosis. These psychological issues have not been well researched (120). Parental concerns regarding transmission of inheritable mutations to offspring are an important issue which may need to be addressed through formal referral for genetic counseling.

Practical difficulties can be a source of stress and concern for younger women diagnosed with breast cancer. Looking after a household, particularly with young children, is challenging for a woman who is also coping with breast cancer treatment (120,121). The resultant stress can be compounded when the woman is socially isolated. Financial difficulties are common when a woman is unable to work and her partner may be forced to take time off work to look after other children while she undergoes treatment (120–123).

PREGNANCY AFTER BREAST CANCER
Epidemiology
It is estimated that 7% of premenopausal women remain fertile and only 3–4% become pregnant following a diagnosis of breast cancer (51,124–126), despite the minimal effect of pregnancy on the outcome of the disease (124,126–129). The

proportion of women who become pregnant after a diagnosis of breast cancer is likely to be lower than expected for two reasons. First, underreporting of pregnancy terminations and missed abortions may occur. Secondly, no formal population-based study has been undertaken to determine how many women remain fertile following a diagnosis of breast cancer.

Outcomes and Survival

The literature to date indicates that breast cancer survivors who subsequently conceive have equivalent survival, and in some studies better survival, compared with those women who do not become pregnant after a diagnosis of breast cancer (21,73,128,130–134). These findings suggest that a subsequent pregnancy may provide some survival benefit. Sankila reported that women diagnosed with breast cancer under the age of 40 years had improved 10-year survival if they had a full-term pregnancy subsequently compared with those who did not (92%, 95% CI 85–99 vs. 60%, 95% CI 54–66) (126). These results are susceptible to bias, as generally only a select group of women with favorable prognosis tumors are likely to become pregnant after a diagnosis of breast cancer. This bias is often referred to as the "healthy mother" effect (126).

Management

The diagnosis and management options for women who become pregnant after a diagnosis of breast cancer are the same as for other young women diagnosed with breast cancer.

Contraception and Pregnancy After Breast Cancer Diagnosis

Contraceptive advice should be offered to pre- and perimenopausal women following a diagnosis of breast cancer. Mechanical contraception is preferred, as the oral contraceptive pill may cause a small increased risk of recurrence (135,136).

With increasing numbers of women delaying pregnancy until their late 30s and early 40s, it is important that those who are pre- or perimenopausal and recently diagnosed with breast cancer be asked about the possibility of pregnancy before commencing treatment. Some women will accidentally become pregnant while receiving adjuvant systemic treatment. If this occurs, the woman and her partner should discuss the implications and options with the relevant clinicians; experiences of

other women gleaned from case reports will be useful in the decision-making process for these women. When tamoxifen is prescribed as long-term adjuvant treatment, it is very important that premenopausal women use contraception as tamoxifen is known to induce ovulation in premenopausal women and cause fetal malformation (99).

Pregnancy is often discouraged in the first two years following the completion of breast cancer treatment (82,137). This is to ensure the woman does not become pregnant while on systemic treatment as well as to minimize the chance of an early recurrence being complicated by pregnancy. However, research has shown that many women choose not to wait for this length of the period before conceiving, without detriment to survival (128). Thus, it is appropriate to recommend after discussion with their oncologist, that women with a good prognosis tumor and who have completed treatment can attempt conception within the first two years (128).

Fertility After Breast Cancer Diagnosis

It is widely recognized that both cytotoxic and hormonal treatments will affect fertility (51,138,139). Of the adult women who undergo chemotherapy, 64% will experience some symptoms of ovarian failure (93,134,140,141). Many women who receive chemotherapy for breast cancer will become permanently amenorrheic, particularly those aged over 40 years (Fig. 48.5) (142,143). In women with ER-positive tumors, temporary or permanent ovarian suppression may be an aim of treatment, although survival gains must be weighed against morbidity and patient concerns (93,144,145).

Infertility can be devastating for a woman who wishes to conceive a child. Various strategies have been proposed to protect the fertility of a woman undergoing chemotherapy. One is reversible chemical sterilization with GnRH analogues such as goserelin, which potentially protects the ovarian follicles during chemotherapy. Cryopreservation of ovarian tissue is unlikely to prove to be of any clinical utility and remains highly experimental and is not currently a viable option in routine clinical practice (146,147). Undergoing a cycle of in vitro fertilization with embryo (or less successfully egg) capture prior to chemotherapy may be an option.

It is important that the issue of fertility be discussed with the premenopausal woman at, or shortly after a diagnosis of breast

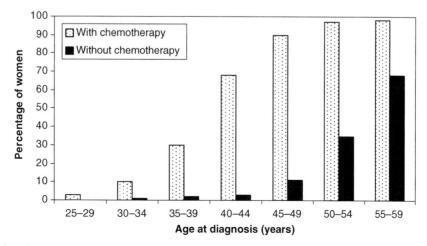

Figure 48.5 Estimated number of women who become menopausal after chemotherapy depending on their age at diagnosis. *Source:* Adapted from Ref. (142).

cancer. If a woman wishes to become pregnant then it is important that she be referred to a fertility specialist to discuss her options and to undergo any necessary procedures before adjuvant systemic therapy commences (148). A decision aid has been developed in Australia to assist women in deciding what choices they want to make about their fertility following treatment for breast cancer (149).

Psychosocial Issues

Any woman diagnosed with breast cancer can experience psychological distress. Younger women diagnosed with breast cancer are reported to be at an increased risk of psychological issues. It is therefore recommended that specific concerns of young women be assessed regularly, including at the long-term follow-up of their disease (150). It is also recommended that young women who are identified as having persistent or severe symptoms of psychological distress which disrupts their daily life and relationships should be referred to an appropriate psychosocial service (151).

KEY POINTS
Pregnancy-associated breast cancer

- More advanced disease at diagnosis
- More difficult to detect abnormalities through imaging in the pregnant and lactating breast
- Survival worse for women diagnosed with PABC when compared with similar aged women diagnosed with breast cancer
- Psychosocial issues related to dealing with two conflicting events simultaneously
- Treatment issues, in particular, timing of adjuvant therapies diagnosed for women while pregnant
- The pregnancy should be managed by an obstetrician based at a tertiary center
- Good communication between the multidisciplinary team which should include both obstetrics and oncology health professionals

Pregnancy and contraception following a diagnosis of breast cancer

- Women who conceive after a diagnosis of breast cancer are likely to have better prognosis tumors (e.g., "Healthy mother" effect)
- Timing of a potential future pregnancy: currently a two-year delay following the completion of cancer treatment but this may not be necessary for women who have completed treatment and have good prognosis tumors
- Fertility advice should be provided at the time of breast cancer diagnosis for all younger women, and before adjuvant therapy is commenced
- Women should be referred to a fertility specialist before adjuvant therapy commences to discuss their future fertility options if they feel their family is not complete

CONCLUSION
Published research suggests that young women diagnosed with breast cancer when pregnant can receive treatments similar to that of other non-pregnant women of similar age without detriment to either their own health or that of their unborn child. A multidisciplinary approach which includes both oncological and obstetric heath professionals is important to provide the best care for mother and child. There are two key areas, where further research is needed to understand how pregnancy may influence breast cancer. First, why survival appears poorer for those women who are diagnosed with breast cancer when they have recently completed a full-term pregnancy when compared with other young women, diagnosed with breast cancer, who have no associated pregnancy. Second, why the survival for women who are pregnant at the time of breast cancer diagnosis is similar to that of other young women diagnosed with breast cancer who have no associated pregnancy.

Premenopausal women who are diagnosed with breast cancer and who may want to consider pregnancy after completing their cancer treatment should be referred for fertility advice and treatment if they opt for that. It should not be assumed that women who already have children think their family is complete. Until recently, it was recommended that women wait at least two years after completing their cancer treatment before considering pregnancy because of the risk of early recurrence. For some women this additional delay may further reduce their already depleted ovarian reserve. A study published in 2007 has suggested that women who have good prognosis tumors may consider conception when they have completed adjuvant treatments, after consulting with their oncologist (128).

Survival has improved significantly in the last 20 years for all women diagnosed with breast cancer. Psychosocial issues are therefore likely to be important measures of quality of life as survivorship increases. It is important that the long-term effects of breast cancer, including fertility, contraception, and early menopause, are discussed soon after diagnosis so that women can make informed choices about their potential future needs.

Further collaborative research involving clinical, psychosocial, and biomedical aspects is needed (i) to better understand the effect of pregnancy on breast cancer and vice versa; (ii) to ensure that these women, their families, and treating clinicians are well informed; (iii) to reduce the psychological and social morbidities for young women diagnosed with breast cancer.

REFERENCES
1. Australian Institute of Health and Welfare. ACIM (Australian Cancer Incidence and Mortality) Books. Canberra: AIHW, 2010.
2. Cancer Research UK. Breast Cancer - UK Incidence Statistics. 2011.
3. Australian Institute of Health and Welfare, National Breast and Ovarian Cancer Centre. Breast Cancer in Australia: An Overview, 2009. Cat. no. CAN 46, 2009.
4. Horner MJ, Ries LAG, Krapcho M, et al. SEER Cancer Statistics Review, 1975–2006. Bethesda: National Cancer Institute, 2009.
5. Jemal A, Bray F, Center MM, et al. Global cancer statistics. CA Cancer J Clin 2011; 61: 69–90.
6. Ferlay J, Shin HR, Bray F, et al. Cancer Incidence and Mortality Worldwide. GLOBOCAN 2008. Lyon, France: International Agency for Research on Cancer, 2010.
7. Shannon C, Smith IE. Breast cancer in adolescents and young women. Eur J Cancer 2003; 39: 2632–42.
8. Albrektsen G, Heuch I, Hansen S, Kvale G. Breast cancer risk by age at birth, time since birth and time intervals between births: exploring interaction effects. Br J Cancer 2005; 92: 167–75.
9. Lambe M, Hsieh C, Trichopoulos D, et al. Transient increase in the risk of breast cancer after giving birth. N Engl J Med 1994; 331: 5–9.

10. Albrektsen G, Heuch I, Thoresen S, Kvale G. Family history of breast cancer and short-term effects of childbirths on breast cancer risk. Int J Cancer 2006; 119: 1468–74.

11. Petrek JA, Dukoff R, Rogatko A. Prognosis of pregnancy-associated breast cancer. Cancer 1991; 67: 869–72.

12. Phillips KA, Milne RL, Friedlander ML, et al. Prognosis of premenopausal breast cancer and childbirth prior to diagnosis. J Clin Oncol 2004; 22: 699–705.

13. Daling JR, Malone KE, Doody DR, Anderson BO, Porter PL. The relation of reproductive factors to mortality from breast cancer. Cancer Epidemiol Biomarkers Prev 2002; 11: 235–41.

14. Kroman N, Wohlfahrt J, Andersen KW, et al. Time since childbirth and prognosis in primary breast cancer: population based study. BMJ 1997; 315: 851–5.

15. White TT. Carcinoma of the breast in the pregnant and nursing patient. Am J Obstet Gynecol 1955; 69: 1277–86.

16. Wallack MK, Wolf JA, Bedwinek J, et al. Gestational carcinoma of the female breast. Curr Probl Cancer 1983; 7: 1–58.

17. Ishida T, Yokoe T, Kasumi F, et al. Clinicopathologic characteristics and prognosis of breast cancer patients associated with pregnancy and lactation: analysis of case-control study in Japan. Jpn J Cancer Res 1992; 83: 1143–9.

18. Gallenberg MM, Loprinzi CL. Breast cancer and pregnancy. Semin Oncol 1989; 16: 369–76.

19. Bunker M, Peters M. Breast cancer associated with pregnancy or lactation. Am J Obstet Gynecol 1963; 85: 312–21.

20. Applewhite RR, Smith LR, De Vincenti F. Carcinoma of the breast associated with pregnancy and lactation. Am Surg 1973; 39: 101–4.

21. Nugent P, O'Connell TX. Breast cancer and pregnancy. Arch Surg 1985; 120: 1221–4.

22. Treves N, Holleb AI. A report of 549 cases of breast cancer in women 35 years of age or younger. Surg Gynecol Obstet 1958; 107: 271.

23. Loibl S, Bontenbal M, Ring A, et al. Breast cancer during pregnancy: a prospective and retrospective European registry (GBG-20/BIG02-03). Eur J Cancer 2010; 8: 499.

24. Berry DL, Theriault RL, Holmes FA, et al. Management of breast cancer during pregnancy using a standardized protocol. J Clin Oncol 1999; 17: 855–61.

25. Clark R, Chua T. Breast cancer and pregnancy: the ultimate challenge. Clin Oncol 1989; 1: 11–18.

26. Clark RM, Reid J. Carcinoma of the breast in pregnancy and lactation. Int J Radiat Oncol Biol Phys 1978; 4: 693–8.

27. Bonnier P, Romain S, Dilhuydy JM, et al. Influence of pregnancy on the outcome of breast cancer: a case-control study. Societe Francaise de Senologie et de Pathologie Mammaire Study Group. Int J Cancer 1997; 72: 720–7.

28. Guinee VF, Olsson H, Moller T, et al. Effect of pregnancy on prognosis for young women with breast cancer. Lancet 1994; 343: 1587–9.

29. Ezzat A, Raja MA, Berry J, et al. Impact of pregnancy on non-metastatic breast cancer: a case control study. Clin Oncol 1996; 8: 367–70.

30. Rodriguez AO, Chew H, Cress R, et al. Evidence of poorer survival in pregnancy-associated breast cancer. Obstet Gynecol 2008; 112: 71–8.

31. Johansson AL, Andersson TM, Hsieh CC, et al. Increased mortality in women with breast cancer detected during pregnancy and different periods postpartum. Cancer Epidemiol Biomarkers Prev 2011; 20: 1865–72.

32. Kroman N, Mouridsen HT. Prognostic influence of pregnancy before, around, and after diagnosis of breast cancer. Breast 2003; 12: 516–21.

33. Lethaby AE, O'Neill MA, Mason BH, et al. Overall survival from breast cancer in women pregnant or lactating at or after diagnosis. Auckland Breast Cancer Study Group. Int J Cancer 1996; 67: 751–5.

34. Stensheim H, Moller B, van Dijk T, Fossa SD. Cause-specific survival for women diagnosed with cancer during pregnancy or lactation: a registry-based cohort study. J Clin Oncol 2009; 27: 45–51.

35. Ives A. Breast Cancer and Pregnancy: How does a Concurrent or Subsequent Pregnancy Affect Breast Cancer Diagnosis, Management and Outcomes? The University of Western Australia, 2009.

36. Albrektsen G, Heuch I, Thoresen S, Kvale G. Clinical stage of breast cancer by parity, age at birth, and time since birth: a progressive effect of pregnancy hormones? Cancer Epidemiol Biomarkers Prev 2006; 15: 65–9.

37. Helewa M, Levesque P, Provencher D, et al. Breast cancer, pregnancy, and breastfeeding. J Obstet Gynaecol Can 2002; 24: 164–80; quiz 181-4.

38. Davies MC, Jones AL. Pregnancy and Breast Cancer. Green-top Guideline No 12, 2nd edn. London: Royal College of Obstetricians and Gynaecologists, 2011.

39. Loibl S, von Minckwitz G, Gwyn K, et al. Breast carcinoma during pregnancy. International recommendations from an expert meeting. Cancer 2006; 106: 237–46.

40. Amant F, Deckers S, Van Calsteren K, et al. Breast cancer in pregnancy: recommendations of an international consensus meeting. Eur J Cancer 2010; 46: 3158–68.

41. Loman N, Johannsson O, Kristoffersson U, et al. Family history of breast and ovarian cancers and BRCA1 and BRCA2 mutations in a population-based series of early-onset breast cancer. J Natl Cancer Inst 2001; 93: 1215–23.

42. Samphao S, Wheeler AJ, Rafferty E, et al. Diagnosis of breast cancer in women age 40 and younger: delays in diagnosis result from underuse of genetic testing and breast imaging. Am J Surg 2009; 198: 538–43.

43. Chang ET, Milne RL, Phillips KA, et al. Family history of breast cancer and all-cause mortality after breast cancer diagnosis in the Breast Cancer Family Registry. Breast Cancer Res Treat 2009; 117: 167–76.

44. Goldsmith HS. Milk-rejection sign. A clinical observation. Cancer 1966; 19: 1185–6.

45. Goldsmith HS. Milk-rejection sign of breast cancer. Am J Surg 1974; 127: 280–1.

46. Saber A, Dardik H, Ibrahim IM, Wolodiger F. The milk rejection sign: a natural tumor marker. Am Surg 1996; 62: 998–9.

47. Woo JC, Yu T, Hurd TC. Breast cancer in pregnancy: a literature review. Arch Surg 2003; 138: 91–8; discussion 99.

48. Nettleton J, Long J, Kuban D, et al. Breast cancer during pregnancy: quantifying the risk of treatment delay. Obstet Gynecol 1996; 87: 414–18.

49. National Breast and Ovarian Cancer Centre. The Investigation of a New Breast Symptom. A Guide for General Practitioners, 2nd edn. Sydney: 2005.

50. Bernik S, Bernik T, Whooley B, Wallack M. Carcinoma of the breast during pregnancy: a review and update on treatment options. Surg Oncol 1998; 7: 45–9.

51. Saunders CM, Baum M. Breast cancer and pregnancy. J R Soc Med 1993; 86: 162–5.

52. Damrich D, Glasser G, Dolan M. The characteristics and evaluation of women presenting with a breast mass during pregnancy. Prim Care Update OBS/GYNS 1998; 5: 21–3.

53. Gemignani M, Petrek J. Pregnancy associated breast cancer: diagnosis and treatment. Breast J 2000; 6: 68–73.

54. Ahn BY, Kim HH, Moon WK, et al. Pregnancy and lactation-associated breast cancer: mammographic and sonographic findings. J Ultrasound Med 2003; 22: 491–7; quiz 498-9.

55. Liberman L, Giess CS, Dershaw DD, et al. Imaging of pregnancy-associated breast cancer. Radiology 1994; 191: 245–8.

56. Max MH, Klamer TW. Pregnancy and breast cancer. South Med J 1983; 76: 1088–90.

57. Samuels TH, Liu FF, Yaffe M, Haider M. Gestational breast cancer. Can Assoc Radiol J 1998; 49: 172–80.

58. Taylor D, Lazberger J, Ives A, et al. Reducing delay in the diagnosis of pregnancy-associated breast cancer: how imaging can help us. J Med Imaging Radiat Oncol 2011; 55: 33–42.

59. Robbins J, Jeffries D, Roubidoux M, Helvie M. Accuracy of diagnostic mammography and breast ultrasound during pregnancy and lactation. AJR Am J Roentgenol 2011; 196: 716–22.

60. Bock K, Hadji P, Ramaswamy A, et al. Rationale for a diagnostic chain in gestational breast tumor diagnosis. Arch Gynecol Obstet 2006; 273: 337–45.

61. Pisano ED, Gatsonis C, Hendrick E, et al. Diagnostic performance of digital versus film mammography for breast-cancer screening. N Engl J Med 2005; 353: 1773–83.

62. Kanal E, Borgstede J, Barkovich A, et al. American College of Radiology white paper on MR safety: 2004 update and revisions. Am J Roentgenol 2004; 182: 1111–14.

63. Heywang-Kobrunner S, Schereer I, Dershaw D. Differential diagnosis and diagnostic work up and the young patient. In: Heywang-Kobrunner S, Schereer I, Dershaw D, eds. Diagnostic Breast Imaging: Mammography, Sonography, Magnetic Resonance Imaging and Interventional Procedures. New York: Thieme, 1997.

64. Talele AC, Slanetz PJ, Edmister WB, et al. The lactating breast: MRI findings and literature review. Breast J 2003; 9: 237–40.

65. Espinosa LA, Daniel BL, Vidarsson L, et al. The lactating breast: contrast-enhanced MR imaging of normal tissue and cancer. Radiology 2005; 237: 429–36.

66. Kuhl CK. Current status of breast MR imaging. Part 2. Clinical applications. Radiology 2007; 244: 672–91.

67. Chen MM, Coakley FV, Kaimal A, Laros RK Jr. Guidelines for computed tomography and magnetic resonance imaging use during pregnancy and lactation. Obstet Gynecol 2008; 112: 333–40.

68. Novotny DB, Maygarden SJ, Shermer RW, Frable WJ. Fine needle aspiration of benign and malignant breast masses associated with pregnancy. Acta Cytol 1991; 35: 676–86.

69. Mitre BK, Kanbour AI, Mauser N. Fine needle aspiration biopsy of breast carcinoma in pregnancy and lactation. Acta Cytol 1997; 41: 1121–30.

70. Petrek JA. Pregnancy safety after breast cancer. Cancer 1994; 74: 528–31.

71. Gemignani M, Petrek J, Brogen P. Breast cancer and pregnancy. Surg Clin North Am 1999; 79: 1157–69.

72. Gwyn K, Theriault R. Breast cancer during pregnancy. Oncology (Huntingt) 2001; 15: 39–46; discussion 46, 49–51.

73. Holleb AI, Farrow JH. The relation of carcinoma of the breast and pregnancy in 283 patients. Surg Gynecol Obstet 1962; 115: 65–71.

74. King RM, Welch JS, Martin JK Jr, Coulam CB. Carcinoma of the breast associated with pregnancy. Surg Gynecol Obstet 1985; 160: 228–32.

75. Shousha S. Breast carcinoma presenting during or shortly after pregnancy and lactation. Arch Pathol Lab Med 2000; 124: 1053–60.

76. Reed W, Sandstad B, Holm R, Nesland JM. The prognostic impact of hormone receptors and c-erbB-2 in pregnancy-associated breast cancer and their correlation with BRCA1 and cell cycle modulators. Int J Surg Pathol 2003; 11: 65–74.

77. Aziz S, Pervez S, Khan S, et al. Case control study of novel prognostic markers and disease outcome in pregnancy/lactation-associated breast carcinoma. Pathol Res Pract 2003; 199: 15–21.

78. Gentilini O, Masullo M, Rotmensz N, et al. Breast cancer diagnosed during pregnancy and lactation: biological features and treatment options. Eur J Surg Oncol 2005; 31: 232–6.

79. Middleton LP, Amin M, Gwyn K, et al. Breast carcinoma in pregnant women: assessment of clinicopathologic and immunohistochemical features. Cancer 2003; 98: 1055–60.

80. Ring AE, Smith IE, Jones A, et al. Chemotherapy for breast cancer during pregnancy: an 18-year experience from five London teaching hospitals. J Clin Oncol 2005; 23: 4192–7.

81. Anderson JM. Inflammatory carcinomas of the breast. Ann R Coll Surg Engl 1980; 62: 195–9.

82. Petrek JA. Breast cancer and pregnancy. J Natl Cancer Inst Monogr 1994: 113–21.

83. Ring AE, Smith IE, Ellis PA. Breast cancer and pregnancy. Ann Oncol 2005; 16: 1855–60.

84. Elledge RM, Ciocca DR, Langone G, McGuire WL. Estrogen receptor, progesterone receptor, and HER-2/neu protein in breast cancers from pregnant patients. Cancer 1993; 71: 2499–506.

85. Shen T, Vortmeyer AO, Zhuang Z, Tavassoli FA. High frequency of allelic loss of BRCA2 gene in pregnancy-associated breast carcinoma. J Natl Cancer Inst 1999; 91: 1686–7.

86. Johannsson O, Loman N, Borg A, Olsson H. Pregnancy-associated breast cancer in BRCA1 and BRCA2 germline mutation carriers. Lancet 1998; 352: 1359–60.

87. Reed W, Hannisdal E, Skovlund E, et al. Pregnancy and breast cancer: a population-based study. Virchows Arch 2003; 443: 44–50.

88. Rosner D, Yeh J. Breast cancer and related pregnancy: suggested management according to stages of the disease and gestational stages. J Med 2002; 33: 23–62.

89. Kal HB, Struikmans H. Breast cancer and pregnancy. Breast 2008; 17: 7.

90. Gentilini O, Cremonesi M, Trifiro G, et al. Safety of sentinel node biopsy in pregnant patients with breast cancer. Ann Oncol 2004; 15: 1348–51.

91. Dubernard G, Garbay JR, Rouzier R, Delaloge S. Safety of sentinel node biopsy in pregnant patients. Ann Oncol 2005; 16: 987; author reply 987–8.

92. Cardonick E, Iacobucci A. Use of chemotherapy during human pregnancy. Lancet Oncol 2004; 5: 283–91.

93. Reichman BS, Green KB. Breast cancer in young women: effect of chemotherapy on ovarian function, fertility, and birth defects. J Natl Cancer Inst Monogr 1994; 16: 125–9.

94. Zemlickis D, Lishner M, Degendorfer P, et al. Fetal outcome after in utero exposure to cancer chemotherapy. Arch Intern Med 1992; 152: 573–6.

95. Williams SF, Schilsky RL. Antineoplastic drugs administered during pregnancy. Semin Oncol 2000; 27: 618–22.

96. Halaska MJ, Pentheroudakis G, Strnad P, et al. Presentation, management and outcome of 32 patients with pregnancy-associated breast cancer: a matched controlled study. Breast J 2009; 15: 461–7.

97. Pan PH, Moore CH. Doxorubicin-induced cardiomyopathy during pregnancy: three case reports of anesthetic management for cesarean and vaginal delivery in two kyphoscoliotic patients. Anesthesiology 2002; 97: 513–15.

98. Andreadis C, Charalampidou M, Diamantopoulos N, et al. Combined chemotherapy and radiotherapy during conception and first two trimesters of gestation in a woman with metastatic breast cancer. Gynecol Oncol 2004; 95: 252–5.

99. Barthelmes L, Gateley CA. Tamoxifen and pregnancy. Breast 2004; 13: 446–51.

100. De Santis M, Lucchese A, De Carolis S, et al. Metastatic breast cancer in pregnancy: first case of chemotherapy with docetaxel. Eur J Cancer Care (Engl) 2000; 9: 235–7.

101. Fanale MA, Uyei AR, Theriault RL, et al. Treatment of metastatic breast cancer with trastuzumab and vinorelbine during pregnancy. Clin Breast Cancer 2005; 6: 354–6.

102. Gonzalez-Angulo AM, Walters RS, Carpenter RJ Jr, et al. Paclitaxel chemotherapy in a pregnant patient with bilateral breast cancer. Clin Breast Cancer 2004; 5: 317–19.

103. Watson WJ. Herceptin (trastuzumab) therapy during pregnancy: association with reversible anhydramnios. Obstet Gynecol 2005; 105: 642–3.

104. Bader AA, Schlembach D, Tamussino KF, et al. Anhydramnios associated with administration of trastuzumab and paclitaxel for metastatic breast cancer during pregnancy. Lancet Oncol 2007; 8: 79–81.

105. Berveiller P, Mir O, Sauvanet E, et al. Ectopic pregnancy in a breast cancer patient receiving trastuzumab. Reprod Toxicol 2008; 25: 286–8.

106. Pant S, Landon MB, Blumenfeld M, et al. Treatment of breast cancer with trastuzumab during pregnancy. J Clin Oncol 2008; 26: 1567–9.

107. Sekar R, Stone PR. Trastuzumab use for metastatic breast cancer in pregnancy. Obstet Gynecol 2007; 110: 507–10.

108. Shrim A, Garcia-Bournissen F, Maxwell C, et al. Favorable pregnancy outcome following Trastuzumab (Herceptin) use during pregnancy–Case report and updated literature review. Reprod Toxicol 2007; 23: 611–13.

109. Shrim A, Garcia-Bournissen F, Maxwell C, et al. Trastuzumab treatment for breast cancer during pregnancy. Can Fam Physician 2008; 54: 31–2.

110. Waterston AM, Graham J. Effect of adjuvant trastuzumab on pregnancy. J Clin Oncol 2006; 24: 321–2.

111. Witzel ID, Muller V, Harps E, et al. Trastuzumab in pregnancy associated with poor fetal outcome. Ann Oncol 2008; 19: 191–2.

112. Cullins SL, Pridjian G, Sutherland CM. Goldenhar's syndrome associated with tamoxifen given to the mother during gestation. JAMA 1994; 271: 1905–6.

113. Braems G, Denys H, De Wever O, et al. Use of tamoxifen before and during pregnancy. Oncologist 2011; 16: 1547–51.

114. Aviles A, Niz J. Long-term follow-up of children born to mothers with acute leukemia during pregnancy. Med Pediatr Oncol 1988; 16: 3–6.

115. DiFronzo LA, O'Connell TX. Breast cancer in pregnancy and lactation. Surg Clin North Am 1996; 76: 267–78.

116. Cardonick E, Dougherty R, Grana G, et al. Breast cancer during pregnancy: maternal and fetal outcomes. Cancer J 2010; 16: 76–82.

117. Byrd BF, Bayer DS, Robertson JC, et al. Treatment of breast tumors associated with pregnancy and lactation. Ann Surg 1962; 155: 940–7.

118. Eisinger F, Noizet A. Breast cancer and pregnancy: decision making and the point of view of the mother. Bull Cancer 2002; 89: 755–7.

119. Zanetti-DAllenbach R, Tschudin S, Lapaire O, et al. Psychological management of pregancy-related breast cancer. Breast 2006; 15: S53–9.

120. Coyne E, Borbasi S. Holding it all together: breast cancer and its impact on life for younger women. Contemp Nurse 2006; 23: 157–69.

121. Dunn J, Steginga S. Young women's experience of breast cancer: defining young and identifying concerns. Psychooncology 2000; 9: 137–46.

122. Arndt V, Merx H, Sturmer T, et al. Age-specific detriments to quality of life among breast cancer patients one year after diagnosis. Eur J Cancer 2004; 40: 673–80.

123. Mor V, Allen S, Malin M. The psychosocial impact of cancer on older versus younger patients and their families. Cancer 1994; 74: 2118–27.

124. Kroman N, Jensen M, Wolfahrt J, Mouridsen H. Should women be advised against pregnancy after breast-cancer treatment? Lancet 1997; 350: 319–22.

125. Surbone A, Petrek J. Pregnancy after breast cancer. The relationship of pregnancy to breast cancer development and progression. Crit Rev Oncol Hematol 1998; 27: 169–78.

126. Sankila R, Heinavaara S, Hakulinen T. Survival of breast cancer patients after subsequent term pregnancy: "healthy mother effect". Am J Obstet Gynecol 1994; 170: 818–23.

127. Azim HA Jr, Santoro L, Pavlidis N, et al. Safety of pregnancy following breast cancer diagnosis: a meta-analysis of 14 studies. Eur J Cancer 2011; 47: 74–83.

128. Ives A, Saunders C, Bulsara M, Semmens J. Pregnancy after breast cancer: population based study. BMJ 2007; 334: 194.

129. Kroman N, Jensen MB, Wohlfahrt J, Ejlertsen B. Pregnancy after treatment of breast cancer–a population-based study on behalf of Danish Breast Cancer Cooperative Group. Acta Oncol 2008; 47: 545–9.

130. Ribeiro G, Jones DA, Jones M. Carcinoma of the breast associated with pregnancy. Br J Surg 1986; 73: 607–9.

131. Ribeiro GG, Palmer MK. Breast carcinoma associated with pregnancy: a clinician's dilemma. BMJ 1977; 2: 1524–7.

132. Harvey JC, Rosen PP, Ashikari R, et al. The effect of pregnancy on the prognosis of carcinoma of the breastfollowing radical mastectomy. Surg Gynecol Obstet 1981; 153: 723–5.

133. Peters MV. The effect of pregnancy in breast cancer. In: Forrest APM, Kunkler PB, eds. Prognostic Factors in Breast Cancer. Baltimore: Williams and Wilkins, 1968: 65–80.

134. Sutton R, Buzdar AU, Hortobagyi GN. Pregnancy and offspring after adjuvant chemotherapy in breast cancer patients. Cancer 1990; 65: 847–50.

135. Moore HCF, Foster RS Jr. Breast cancer and pregnancy. Semin Oncol 2000; 27: 646–53.

136. Two cases of breast cancer in young women. Eur J Surg Oncol 1996; 22: 108–13.

137. Isaacs JH. Cancer of the breast in pregnancy. Surg Clin North Am 1995; 75: 47–51.

138. Surbone A, Petrek JA. Childbearing issues in breast carcinoma survivors. Cancer 1997; 79: 1271–8.

139. Donegan WL. Breast cancer and pregnancy. Obstet Gynecol 1977; 50: 244–52.

140. Gadducci A, Cosio S, Genazzani AR. Ovarian function and childbearing issues in breast cancer survivors. Gynecol Endocrinol 2007; 23: 625–31.

141. Petrek JA, Naughton MJ, Case LD, et al. Incidence, time course, and determinants of menstrual bleeding after breast cancer treatment: a prospective study. J Clin Oncol 2006; 24: 1045–51.

142. Goodwin PJ, Ennis M, Pritchard KI, et al. Risk of menopause during the first year after breast cancer diagnosis. J Clin Oncol 1999; 17: 2365–70.

143. Richards MA, O'Reilly SM, Howell A, et al. Adjuvant cyclophosphamide, methotrexate, and fluorouracil in patients with axillary node-positive breast cancer: an update of the Guy's/Manchester trial. J Clin Oncol 1990; 8: 2032–9.

144. Bao T, Davidson NE. Adjuvant endocrine therapy for premenopausal women with early breast cancer. Breast Cancer Res 2007; 9: 115.

145. Early Breast Cancer Trialists' Collaborative Group (EBCTCG). Effects of chemotherapy and hormonal therapy for early breast cancer on recurrence and 15-year survival: an overview of the randomised trials. Lancet 2005; 365: 1687–717.

146. Meadors B, Robinson D. Fertility options after cancer treatment: a case report and literature review. Prim Care Update OB/GYNS 2002; 9: 51–4.

147. Oktay K, Buyuk E, Davis O, et al. Fertility preservation in breast cancer patients: IVF and embryo cryopreservation after ovarian stimulation with tamoxifen. Hum Reprod 2003; 18: 90–5.

148. Lee SJ, Schover LR, Partridge AH, et al. American Society of Clinical Oncology recommendations on fertility preservation in cancer patients. J Clin Oncol 2006; 24: 2917–31.

149. Peate M. Fertility Decision Aid to Assist Women Diagnosed with Breast Cancer [email 2 April 2009]. Sydney: 2009.

150. Clinical Practice Guidelines for the Management and Support of Younger Women with Breast Cancer. Camperdown, NSW: National Breast Cancer Centre, 2004.

151. National Breast Cancer Centre, National Cancer Control Initiative. Clinical Practice Guidelines for the Psychosocial Care of Adults with Cancer. Camperdown, NSW: National Breast Cancer Centre, 2003.

49 Male breast cancer

Maisam Z. Fazel and Vassilis Pitsinis

INTRODUCTION

Breast cancer in men is rare representing only 0.6–1% of all breast cancers and less than 0.1% of all male cancers (1,2). As a result, there is a paucity of clinical and epidemiological studies relating to its management. However, it is known that male breast cancer (MBC) has important variations as compared with the female counterpart: MBC has a different hormonal receptor status with higher estrogen receptor (ER) and progesterone receptor (PR) expression and histological variations showing a predominance of invasive ductal carcinoma. Differences also exist in the age at diagnosis, frequency of lymph node involvement, and survival (3,4).

EPIDEMIOLOGY AND RISK FACTORS
Age of Diagnosis
Various studies estimate the age at diagnosis of MBC to be later in life compared with that of female breast cancer (FBC). Comparing a million cases of FBC with 6000 MBC cases in the United States (US) from 1973 to 2005, the median age of diagnosis was found to be 67 versus 61 years for FBC (5). Furthermore, while examining the trends in incidence and age at diagnosis, it has been found that the incidence of MBC increases in a linear fashion with age, peaking at the age of 71 years. In contrast, the age-specific rates for FBC increase rapidly till the age of 50 and then continue to increase at a much slower rate (5). Thus, MBC has a unimodal age-frequency distribution, whereas FBC demonstrates a bimodal age-frequency distribution with peak incidences at 52 and 71 years, respectively (1,3). The bimodal nature of the latter is believed to relate to estrogen exposure (3).

Race
African-Caribbean men have been shown to have a higher incidence of MBC (3). In contrast to Caucasian men, African-Caribbean men with breast cancer tend to have an early onset and present with higher tumor grade, negative hormone receptor expression, and a more advanced stage at diagnosis. Part of this is thought to be due to reduced access to healthcare and sociocultural factors (3,6) but tumor biology may also be responsible for this variation.

Genetics
A family history of breast cancer confers an overall relative risk of 2.5 with 20% of cases having a first-degree relative with the disease (7). The association of MBC mirrors FBC in terms of risk and is around 5–10% (8,9). Furthermore, the BRCA2 mutation appears to have a much more enhanced role compared with FBC in terms of the risk of cancer development (10,11).

Endocrine Risk Factors
Exogenous Exposure
There is no doubt that exogenous estrogens increase the risk of breast cancer in men, with several cases of breast cancer having been reported in men treated for prostate cancer (12). In addition, transsexuals taking estrogens have been shown to have an increased risk of developing mammary tumors (13).

Endogenous Exposure
The incidence of MBC also increases in conditions that elevate endogenous exposure to estrogen or decrease androgen exposure. Men with Klinefelter's syndrome (an additional X chromosome to the normal XY karyotype) have testicular dysgenesis, gynecomastia, low testosterone concentrations, and increased gonadotrophin levels. The risk of breast cancer in these individuals is 20–50 times higher than XY men. Similarly, among individuals with Kleinefelter's syndrome, breast cancer mortality rates are similar to those in women (14,15).

Obesity leads to increased levels of circulating estrogens and has been shown to double the risk of developing MBC. (16,17).

Other testicular abnormalities resulting in decreased androgen production implicated in MBC include mumps, undescended testes (which cause a 12-fold increase in risk) as well as a congenital inguinal hernia resulting in unilateral or bilateral orchidectomy (18). Studies have also associated liver cirrhosis with MBC due to the effect on circulating androgens (19).

Lifestyle and Environmental Risk Factors
Lifestyle
In terms of lifestyle factors, body mass index is statistically significantly associated with MBC (17). As with FBC, a relationship also exists between the risk of developing breast cancer and the degree of physical inactivity. This relationship persists even after adjustment for body mass index and is especially linked to physical inactivity during adolescence (20). Several studies have also suggested that excessive alcohol consumption may increase MBC risk with a 16% increase noted per 10 g daily alcohol intake (21,22).

Interestingly, studies examining gynecomastia in MBC have not shown a higher incidence of MBC compared with the general male population (16).

Environmental Risk Factors
Radiation exposure is known to increase the risk of MBC. Male atomic bomb survivors demonstrated an eight times increase in the risk per sievert (23). Harmful effects have also

been associated with lengthy exposure to diagnostic radiographs and radiotherapy.

In addition, a heightened frequency of breast cancer has been reported in men who work in hot environments, such as blast furnaces, steel works, and rolling mills. Some evidence implicates occupational exposure to petrol and exhaust fumes as a risk factor. In a pension fund study of 12,880 controls and 230 patients with MBC there was a 2.5-fold increase in risk in men with more than three months' employment in such work environment (24).

CLINICAL PRESENTATION
Symptoms

The most common symptom is a lump, which is the presenting feature in 75% of the cases. Pain is associated with a lump in only 50% of patients. In contrast to FBC, nipple involvement usually occurs early in the course of the disease presenting with ulceration, retraction, or discharge. Paget's disease of the male breast is very rare presenting in about 1% of cases. Even more rare is occult disease presenting with axillary lymphadenopathy alone (16).

Histopathology

Since male breast tissue is rudimentary, it does not usually differentiate and undergo lobule formation unless exposed to increased concentrations of endogenous or exogenous estrogen. Thus, the predominant histological type of disease is invasive ductal carcinoma, which forms more than 90% of cases. The relative percentage in women is 80%. Much rarer tumor types include invasive papillomas and medullary lesions.

In terms of tumor grade, 15% are grade 1, 55% grade 2, and 30% grade 3. Lobular carcinoma is very rare and accounts proportionally for only 1% of the cases. These occur predominantly in men with Kleinefelter's syndrome, but also in genotypically normal men with no previous history of estrogen exposure. On the other hand, around 12% of FBCs are lobular (1).

MBC is much more likely to be ER positive with 90% of tumors being ER positive and 92–96% being PR positive. With regards to the human epidermal growth factor receptor 2 (HER2), the data are less clear. In one study comparing HER2 overexpression between MBC and FBC, 58 male cases were compared with 202 female cases. Only one case of MBC showed overexpression on immunostaining but no amplification was seen, compared with 26% of FBC tumors showing overexpression and 27% manifesting amplification (25).

MANAGEMENT OF MALE BREAST CANCER
Assessment

The rarity of MBC together with the low index of suspicion often results in a significant delay in presentation and subsequent diagnosis. Retrospective reviews show a delay in the range of 6–10 months (26,27). This delay coupled with a scarcity of breast tissue in men results in more than 40% of cases presenting with stage III/IV disease (4). Furthermore, at the point of diagnosis, 7% of men have evidence of distant metastatic disease versus 5.6% of women. The size of the presenting tumor is also different with only 10% of the men presenting with a tumor size of less than 1 cm compared with 20% women (1).

Triple assessment forms the cornerstone for detecting MBC. During clinical examination, it is important to note that gynecomastia can obscure an underlying malignant mass (28). The axilla must be carefully examined as cases of occult MBC presenting solely with axillary node metastases have been reported (29).

Mammography, with a sensitivity of 92% and a specificity of 90% in MBC (30), is valuable in the diagnostic workup as it helps triage the cases which need further cytological evaluation. Typical features of a malignant lesion include a mass which is often but not always spiculate. The mass tends to be eccentric to the nipple, in contrast to gynecomastia which tends to be concentric to the nipple (31). Calcifications are less common than in women, but when present calcifications that will be accepted as benign in women can indicate malignant disease in men (32).

Ultrasound scanning typically reveals a hypoechoic mass with irregular or indistinct margins. Color flow Doppler may reveal vascular flow within the peripheries of the lesion with scanty vessels. Cysts are rare in male breast tissue; thus, all cysts should be thoroughly evaluated for complexity as neoplastic papillary lesions frequently manifest as complex cystic lesions (33). As in FBC, ultrasonography also plays a role in staging the axilla, accompanied by cytological assessment where indicated.

As the vast majority of lesions in MBC are palpable, the role of magnetic resonance imagining (MRI) is not established. Other imaging modalities such as thallium scanning (TI-201) and galactograms remain confined to the research arena (34).

Cytology remains the primary pathological sampling technique due to its versatility and reliability. Several studies comparing fine-needle aspiration (FNA) findings from breast lesions to subsequent core or excision biopsy results have revealed a sensitivity and specificity approaching 100% respectively (35,36). A core biopsy is indicated where FNA is inadequate or equivocal (37).

Surgery
Breast

The vast majority of cases continue to be treated with complete resection of the breast tissue. As with FBC, the extent of surgery has become less aggressive over the years, from radical mastectomy to modified radical mastectomy and now simple mastectomy with no effect on survival or local recurrence rates (26,38). However, given the later presentation and thus increased stage, radical or modified radical mastectomy is more likely to be required compared with the female counterparts.

The role of breast conservation surgery in MBC is less clear. The relatively larger tumor size, retroareolar location, paucity of breast tissue, and a higher rate of chest wall infiltration are factors which may render breast conservation technically less appropriate. In a Canadian study of 229 patients, those who underwent breast conservation surgery had a higher local recurrence rate compared with the patients who underwent a mastectomy (39). Similarly, in a French study of 31 cases of ductal carcinoma *in situ*, the local recurrence rate was significantly higher post lumpectomy compared with mastectomy (40).

By contrast, a study from the Brigham and Women's Hospital in Boston found no evidence of local recurrence at 67 months in any of the seven men with breast cancer treated with a lumpectomy. The authors suggest that men without overt nipple–areolar involvement can safely undergo wide excision to clear margins with reasonable local recurrence rates and acceptable cosmesis. Thus, breast conservation surgery may be a feasible and oncologically sound approach in carefully selected patients. Unfortunately, validation of such data is unlikely to be possible because of the small number of MBCs.

Axilla

The surgical management of the axilla in MBC has also evolved over the years. Axillary dissection was the standard of care for many years but was associated with well-documented morbidity such as lymphedema, paresthesia, persistent pain, and reduced shoulder mobility.

The first case of sentinel lymph node biopsy in men was published in 1999 (41). Since then there has been a growing interest in this technique in MBC. Several small studies have shown that the dual localization technique using blue dye and a radioisotope yields identification rates between 96% and 100% (42,43).

As men tend to present with breast cancers at a more advanced stage, there has been some concern that this may adversely impact the false-negative rate when using the sentinel lymph node biopsy technique (44). However, subsequent studies in women have shown that though the false-negative rate increases with the primary tumor size, this increase is not statistically significant (45). Thus, sentinel lymph node biopsy should be considered as the initial axillary staging procedure in clinically node-negative cases.

Reconstruction

Unlike in female breast reconstruction where volume replacement is the primary goal to achieve a good esthetic outcome, the rationale for breast reconstruction in men post breast cancer surgery is often to provide adequate skin coverage. This is particularly needed as 40% of cases present with stage III or IV disease making primary skin closure challenging (4).

To address this, various fasciocutaneous and myocutaneous flaps have been proposed (46). In the simplest cases, Di Benedetto recommends the use of thoracic flaps, based on the superficial thoracic artery, or thoracoepigastric fasciocutaneous flaps, based on the intercostal perforators. The latter are easy to harvest and offer a good and stable covering of the lost tissue area with very quick postoperative recovery.

However, when very large and deep excisions are required, myocutaneous flaps such as latissimus dorsi flaps or transverse rectus abdominis muscle flaps are preferred as these provide an appropriate thickness for the newly reconstructed thoracic wall. Other less well-known flaps have also been described, including the use of a deltopectoral flap (47) as well as a transverse thoracoepigastric flap (48).

Spear et al. (49) recommend the use the transverse rectus abdominis myocutaneous flap, as not only does this afford adequate cover of the post mastectomy defect, but it also has the added advantage of providing hair-bearing skin similar to that in a male chest.

Radiotherapy

In FBC, postmastectomy radiation to the chest wall and axillary lymph nodes is used to decrease locoregional recurrence and to improve survival (50).

However, the data surrounding the rate of local recurrence post surgery in MBC is limited and very variable (51,52). This, together with the fact that the lack of breast tissue prevents a large surgical margin, has been the rationale for the frequent use of post mastectomy radiation in all stages of MBC.

Cobalt-60 or 4 MV photons are usually the energy source of choice for patients receiving radiotherapy. The dose delivered to the chest wall is usually 45–65 Gy while 45–54 Gy is administered to supraclavicular, axillary, and internal mammary lymph nodes as appropriate. Some patients receive a boost with to the scar. The regimen duration tends to involve daily sessions lasting between three and six weeks.

Where data relating to the use of adjuvant radiotherapy is available, it tends to be derived from small retrospective studies. The scenario is further complicated by a variety for radiation doses, regimens, and sources being used. For example, one study (7) demonstrated that the addition of radiation decreased the incidence of local recurrence in MBC. Of the 89 patients retrospectively evaluated, 57 had postoperative radiotherapy. The local recurrence-free survival rate was significantly superior (75%) in patients receiving radiation and surgery compared with those receiving surgery alone (68%). There was no difference in overall survival. Similarly, a study examining data from 20 French units over 30 years showed an overall locoregional recurrence rate of 7.3% in the irradiated group versus 13% in the non-irradiated group (52).

On the other hand, Stierer's retrospective analysis of 169 MBC patients produced contrasting results (51). Sixty-four patients were treated with adjuvant chest wall radiation after surgery. There was no difference in the rates of local recurrence in patients treated with or without postmastectomy radiation. Unfortunately, the findings from both these studies are limited as the patients were not matched for tumor size, nodal status, stage, or median follow-up, factors which would affect the risk of recurrence and the interpretation of the results.

An interesting study from Johns Hopkins suggested that postmastectomy radiation should be reserved for high-risk disease alone, as is the case in FBC (53). In this retrospective study, the case notes of 44 men treated for breast cancer were reviewed. Of the 34 patients with stage I/II disease, 28 underwent surgery alone. At five-year follow-up, only one had suffered an isolated locoregional recurrence (3.5%). Of the remaining 10 patients with stage III disease, three underwent surgery alone and none suffered a local failure. Thus, the isolated local recurrence rate (before distant failure) was seen in only 6%, and only 3% among those with stages I/II disease treated with surgery alone. The authors concluded that risk stratification should be employed to determine the benefit of adjuvant chest wall radiation in men. This is especially relevant as breast cancer tends to occur at an older age in men, who are thus potentially at a greater risk from cardiovascular and pulmonary comorbidities.

Although breast conservation surgery is relatively infrequent in MBC, where employed, it has followed adjuvant radiotherapy in an attempt to reduce the local recurrence rate. Typically, the radiation technique used is whole-breast irradiation for a dose of 45 Gy, while the tumor bed receives a total dose of 60 Gy, similar to the technique used in women with breast carcinoma. This practice has shown promise as demonstrated in a study from the Brigham and Women's Hospital (54). In this study, of the six men who underwent breast conserving surgery for invasive disease followed by adjuvant radiotherapy, there were no local recurrences at a median follow-up of 67 months.

Chemotherapy

As with radiation therapy, the role of chemotherapy in treating MBC suffers from a paucity of robust data. As a result, there may a risk of undertreating MBC. In a study from the US National Cancer Database, only 27% of men were treated with adjuvant chemotherapy as compared with 41% of age- and stage-matched women with breast cancer (55).

Several small retrospective studies in MBC have suggested that the use of adjuvant chemotherapy is associated with a reduced risk of relapse (56,57). However, any benefit derived must be balanced against the potential for associated toxicities.

The chemotherapy regimens frequently used include cyclophosphamide, methotrexate, 5-fluorouracil (CMF), or anthracycline-based regimens, often 5-fluorouracil, adriamycin, cyclophosphamide (FAC). Taxanes have been used with anthracyclines but the data on this are too limited to allow any conclusion to be drawn regarding greater efficacy (58).

In one of the few prospective studies conducted in this area, 24 men with breast cancer at the US National Cancer Institute were given adjuvant CMF for node-positive stage II breast cancer (59). The five-year actuarial survival rate of this group was 80%, notably better than that of historical controls of similar stage.

Giordano published the MD Anderson Cancer Center experience in 2005 and reported the results of chemotherapy given to 32 men with breast cancer. A median of six cycles were given: 84% in an adjuvant setting, 6% in a neoadjuvant setting, and 9% received chemotherapy on either side of their primary surgery (sandwich technique). Furthermore, 81% received had anthracycline-based regimens, 9% had additional taxanes, and 16% had CMF. For men with node-positive disease, adjuvant chemotherapy was associated with a lower risk of death (hazard ratio 0·78), although this difference was not significant. Furthermore, the 11 node-positive patients who were treated with adjuvant chemotherapy were estimated to have a greater than 85% of five-year survival rate, substantially better than the survival rates of historical controls. Although this study did not show a statistically significant survival advantage in using chemotherapy, it estimated a 22% risk reduction, similar to that seen in women (60).

It is very unlikely that adequately powered randomized studies will ever be performed to evaluate the role of chemotherapy in treating MBC. Thus, drawing on the experience of using chemotherapy in women, supported by some of the small studies outlined above, it seems reasonable to recommend use of chemotherapy for men with intermediate or high-grade disease, particularly those with ER-negative tumors.

Trastuzamab

The HER2 receptor appears to be less frequently overexpressed in MBC compared with women (61). Although no male specific data exist, given the benefit that trastuzumab therapy provides to women with HER2-positive breast cancer, it will be prudent to consider its use in men with high-risk HER2-positive disease. Indeed, a case of a man with metastatic breast cancer was published demonstrating a successful response to treatment with trastuzumab (62).

Endocrine Therapy

As MBC is ER positive in approximately 90% of cases, adjuvant hormonal therapy in men has become an integral part of treatment. Tamoxifen is generally accepted as the standard of care for adjuvant hormonal therapy in MBC. This antiestrogen is known to reduce the recurrence rate and to improve survival in women with ER-positive breast cancer.

While no clinical trials have assessed the use of adjuvant tamoxifen in men, many retrospective studies have compared the outcomes of men treated with adjuvant tamoxifen and those who received no hormonal therapy. In one notable study from Toronto, Goss et al. reported improved disease-free and overall survival rates in men treated with adjuvant tamoxifen, even though this was often prescribed for less than two years (39). In another study, the five-year survival rate of 39 male patients with stage II and III breast cancer treated with adjuvant tamoxifen was 61% versus 44% in the control group, suggesting significant benefit from tamoxifen (26). Again, these male patients received tamoxifen for only one to two years. This is in contrast to the standard treatment duration for women, where clinical trials have shown that the optimum length of tamoxifen therapy is five years. Thus, both studies may be underestimating the true benefit of tamoxifen in men, which might be improved with more prolonged therapy.

However, there appears to be a high rate of tamoxifen-related side effects among male patients, leading to poor compliance and a higher than expected rate of discontinuation. In the largest retrospective study of its kind, researchers from MD Anderson Cancer Center discovered that the most common significant side effects included sexual dysfunction, weight gain, hot flushes, thromboembolic events and neurocognitive deficits. As a result, 20% of men discontinued tamoxifen during the treatment period (63).

Over the past 10–15 years, the new-generation aromatase inhibitors (anastrozole, letrozole, and exemestane) have shown superior efficacy compared with tamoxifen in the treatment of postmenopausal women with breast cancer both in the adjuvant and metastatic setting. These agents act by inhibiting aromatase, the enzyme that produces estrogen via peripheral aromatization of circulating androgens. In men, 80% of estrogen arises from peripheral aromatization while the remaining 20% is derived from the testicular production of estrogen, which is independent of aromatase (64). This potentially limits the efficacy of aromatase inhibitors.

Interestingly, although the first-generation aromatase inhibitor aminoglutethimide was seen to be ineffective in men with advanced breast cancer (65), it was found to be effective in men who had undergone previous orchidectomy (66). A possible explanation is that aminoglutethimide does not lower the continued secretion of estrogens by the testes even when aromatization is blocked. However, in orchidectomized patients, all of their estrogen is produced by the peripheral aromatase system.

In MBC, there is only one published series reporting the use of the third-generation aromatase inhibitor anastrozole. Five patients who had received tamoxifen previously were prescribed anastrozole. None of the patients had undergone orchidectomy (67). Although there were no responses to treatment, three patients had disease stabilization: two of which showed stable disease for longer than 24 weeks.

There is minimal data on the use of the pure antiestrogen fulvestrant in men. Unlike tamoxifen, fulvestrant has no agonist estrogenic activity. One case report from Nottingham showed clinical benefit in two ER-positive cases of advanced metastatic MBC (16).

Therefore in the absence of large scale studies, tamoxifen remains the first-line hormone therapy at the present time.

Metastatic Disease

Previously, the management of metastatic MBC consisted of surgery to produce hormonal status modifications, such as orchidectomy, adrenalectomy, or hypophysectomy. Although traumatic, these interventions did produce a positive response in 55–80% of cases, depending on the procedure performed (68). Indeed gonadal ablation remains an effective therapeutic intervention in metastatic MBC. Naturally, these procedures were only effective in those patients with hormone responsive breast carcinomas. Nowadays, medical forms of hormonal manipulation have replaced surgical ablation with equal success. There have even been reports of complete response to luteinising hormone releasing hormone analogues, with or without antiandrogens (69). Other possibilities include androgens, progestins, corticosteroids, and high doses of estrogens. These have shown response rates of up to 75% (57). Third-generation aromatase inhibitors have also been used with case reports suggesting a beneficial role for letrozole in metastatic MBC (64).

As most men will respond to hormonal manipulation, systemic chemotherapy is often reserved as a second-line treatment strategy in metastatic MBC. There has been only one study comparing the efficacy of chemotherapy with hormonal therapy in MBC; this found superior response rates in patients treated with hormonal therapy (65).

Chemotherapy can provide a palliative role in cases of hormone-refractory MBC. Response rates reported range from as low as 13% for the single agent fluorouracil to as high as 67% for a combination regimen including FAC (68). As with the treatment of women with advanced breast cancer, sequential use of endocrine therapy and chemotherapy is preferred to simultaneous use of these two modalities of treatment (58).

As HER2 gene amplification is rare in MBC, the activity of trastuzumab in HER2 overexpressing MBC without gene amplification is unknown. There is only one reported case of the successful use of trastuzumab in metastatic MBC (62). No data exist about the activity or tolerance of bevacizumab or other angiogenesis inhibitors.

PROGNOSIS

The age-adjusted incidence of MBC is increasing. The reason remains unclear. However, the rate of increase in incidence does not appear to decrease after the age of 50 years as is observed in women. This difference most likely is due to the lack of, or a more gradual change in, the hormonal milieu than occurs in women at menopause (1,70).

Mortality from breast cancer has improved over the last three decades. In general, men are frequently diagnosed with more advanced-stage cancer than women, particularly in regions where women are routinely screened with mammography (5). Intercurrent illness plays a major role in the overall survival of men with breast cancer, reflecting the fact that men are diagnosed at an older age. A study shows that approximately 40% of men with breast cancer die from causes unrelated to their breast cancer (1).

Survival

Studies put the overall 5- and 10-year survival rates for MBC at 63% and 41%, respectively. This ranges from a 78% five-year survival for stage I disease to a 19% rate for stage IV disease. The overall five-year survival rates were found to be lower stage-by-stage for men compared to women with breast carcinoma. However, these differences disappear when relative survival rates (which adjust for the expected survival rate in terms of race, gender and age) are taken into account.

When comparing men with women the relative five-year survival is nearly the same at 96% respectively for stage I disease, 84% for both in stage II disease, 52% versus 55% respectively for stage III, and 24% versus 18% respectively for stage IV disease (1).

Factors Affecting Prognosis

Patient age greater than 65 years, a larger tumor size, lymph node involvement, and a high tumor grade were all found to be independently associated with a higher risk of death (1). Conversely, ER and PR positivity is associated with a significantly reduced risk of death. Data on HER2 positivity in MBC is sparse and it is therefore difficult to draw any conclusion about the effect of HER2 status on prognosis (5). Studies have failed to show any significant correlation between Ki-67 expression and MBC prognosis suggesting Ki-67 does not play a dominant role in the survival of MBC patients (2).

Ethnicity

Despite the fact that Afro-Caribbean men have a higher incidence of breast cancer than white Caucasians, their survival rates are similar. However compared with men of other ethnicity (Asian, Pacific, Hispanic) both these ethnic groups have substantially decreased survival rates: the overall five-year survival rates are 66% for Caucasians, 57% for Afro-Caribbeans, and 75% for men of other ethnicity. For breast cancer-specific survival, the five -year survival rates are higher: 83%, 72%, and 89% respectively. Although these data suggest differences in survival rates, these differences may be due to factors reflected in the race or ethnicity, rather than genetics per se. They may reflect a "healthy immigrant" effect. For example, men who emigrate to the US may be in better overall health and are better able to survive a breast cancer diagnosis. Future studies exploring socioeconomic status, comorbidities, and detailed treatment data (including access to treatment) may explain the racial differences in breast cancer survival rates (71).

SUMMARY

Much of the rationale for the management of MBC has been extrapolated from studies involving FBC, with reasonable justification. More studies focussing specifically on male breast cancer are needed but are likely to be challenging to undertake in view of the relatively scarcity of this disease.

REFERENCES

1. Giordano SH, Cohen DS, Buzdar AU, Perkins G, Hortobagyi GN. Breast carcinoma in men: a population-based study. Cancer 2004; 101: 51–7.
2. Xia Q, Shi YX, Liu DG, Jiang WQ. Clinicopathological characteristics of male breast cancer: analysis of 25 cases at a single institution. Nan Fang Yi Ke Da Xue Xue Bao 2011; 31: 1469–73.
3. Anderson WF, Althuis MD, Brinton LA, Devesa SS. Is male breast cancer similar or different than female breast cancer? Breast Cancer Res Treat 2004; 83: 77–86.
4. Donegan WL, Redlich PN. Breast cancer in men. Surg Clin North Am 1996; 76: 343–63.
5. Korde LA, Zujewski JA, Kamin L, et al. Multidisciplinary meeting on male breast cancer: summary and research recommendations. J Clin Oncol 2010; 28: 2114–22.
6. Chen VW, Correa P, Kurman RJ, et al. Histological characteristics of breast carcinoma in blacks and whites. Cancer Epidemiol Biomarkers Prev 1994; 3: 127–35.
7. Erlichman C, Murphy KC, Elhakim T. Male breast cancer: a 13-year review of 89 patients. J Clin Oncol 1984; 2: 903–9.
8. Brinton LA, Richesson DA, Gierach GL, et al. Prospective evaluation of risk factors for male breast cancer. J Natl Cancer Inst 2008; 100: 1477–81.
9. Martin AM, Weber BL. Genetic and hormonal risk factors in breast cancer. J Natl Cancer Inst 2000; 92: 1126–35.
10. Palli D, Falchetti M, Masala G, et al. Association between the BRCA2 N372H variant and male breast cancer risk: a population-based case-control study in Tuscany, Central Italy. BMC Cancer 2007; 7: 170.
11. Thorlacius S, Tryggvadottir L, Olafsdottir GH, et al. Linkage to BRCA2 region in hereditary male breast cancer. Lancet 1995; 346: 544–5.
12. McClure JA, Higgins CC. Bilateral carcinoma of male breast after estrogen therapy. J Am Med Assoc 1951; 146: 7–9.
13. Symmers WS. Carcinoma of breast in trans-sexual individuals after surgical and hormonal interference with the primary and secondary sex characteristics. Br Med J 1968; 2: 83–5.
14. Hultborn R, Hanson C, Köpf I, et al. Prevalence of Klinefelter's syndrome in male breast cancer patients. Anticancer Res 1997; 17: 4293–7.
15. Swerdlow AJ, Schoemaker MJ, Higgins CD, Wright AF, Jacobs PA. Cancer incidence and mortality in men with Klinefelter syndrome: a cohort study. J Natl Cancer Inst 2005; 97: 1204–10.
16. Agrawal A, Ayantunde AA, Rampaul R, Robertson JFR. Male cancer: a review of clinical management. Breast Cancer Res Treat 2007; 103: 11–21.
17. Krause W. Male breast cancer–an andrological disease: risk factors and diagnosis. Andrologia 2004; 36: 346–54.
18. Thomas DB, Jimenez LM, McTiernan A, et al. Breast cancer in men: risk factors with hormonal implications. Am J Epidemiol 1992; 135: 734–48.
19. Sørensen HT, Friis S, Olsen JH, et al. Risk of breast cancer in men with liver cirrhosis. Am J Gastroenterol 1998; 93: 231–3.
20. Lahmann PH, Friedenreich C, Schuit AJ, et al. Physical activity and breast cancer risk: the European Prospective Investigation into Cancer and Nutrition. Cancer Epidemiol Biomarkers Prev 2007; 16: 36–42.
21. Guénel P, Cyr D, Sabroe S, et al. Alcohol drinking may increase risk of breast cancer in men: a European population-based case-control study. Cancer Causes Control 2004; 15: 571–80.
22. Keller AZ. Demographic, clinical and survivorship characteristics of males with primary cancer of the breast. Am J Epidemiol 1967; 85: 183–99.
23. Ron E, Ikeda T, Preston DL, Tokuoka S. Male breast cancer incidence among atomic bomb survivors. J Natl Cancer Inst 2005; 97: 603–5.
24. Hansen J. Elevated risk for male breast cancer after occupational exposure to gasoline and vehicular combustion products. Am J Ind Med 2000; 37: 349–52.
25. Bloom KJ, Govil H, Gattuso P, Reddy V, Francescatti D. Status of HER-2 in male and female breast carcinoma. Am J Surg 2001; 182: 389–92.
26. Ribeiro GG, Swindell R, Harris M, Banerjee SS, Cramer A. A review of the management of the male breast carcinoma based on an analysis of 420 treated cases. Breast 1996; 5: 141–6.
27. Joshi MG, Lee AK, Loda M, et al. Male breast carcinoma: an evaluation of prognostic factors contributing to a poorer outcome. Cancer 1996; 77: 490–8.
28. Günhan-Bilgen I, Bozkaya H, Ustün EE, Memiş A. Male breast disease: clinical, mammographic, and ultrasonographic features. Eur J Radiol 2002; 43: 246–55.
29. Gu G-L, Wang S-L, Wei X-M, Ren L, Zou F-X. Axillary metastasis as the first manifestation of male breast cancer: a case report. Cases J 2008; 1: 285.
30. Stewart RA, Howlett DC, Hearn FJ. Pictorial review: the imaging features of male breast disease. Clin Radiol 1997; 52: 739–44.
31. Doyle S, Steel J, Porter G. Imaging male breast cancer. Clin Radiol 2011; 66: 1079–85.
32. Dershaw DD, Fleischman RC, Liberman L, et al. Use of digital mammography in needle localization procedures. AJR Am J Roentgenol 1993; 161: 559–62.
33. Yang WT, Whitman GJ, Yuen EH, Tse GM, Stelling CB. Sonographic features of primary breast cancer in men. AJR Am J Roentgenol 2001; 176: 413–16.
34. Ozdemir A, Oznur II, Vural G, et al. TL-201 scintigraphy, mammography and ultrasonography in the evaluation of palpable and nonpalpable breast lesions: a correlative study. Eur J Radiol 1997; 24: 145–54.
35. Rosen DG, Laucirica R, Verstovsek G. Fine needle aspiration of male breast lesions. Acta Cytol 2009; 53: 369–74.
36. Wauters CAP, Kooistra BW, de Kievit-van der Heijden IM, Strobbe LJA. Is cytology useful in the diagnostic workup of male breast lesions? A retrospective study over a 16-year period and review of the recent literature. Acta Cytol 2010; 54: 259–64.
37. Westenend PJ. Core needle biopsy in male breast lesions. J Clin Pathol 2003; 56: 863–5.
38. Borgen PI, Wong GY, Vlamis V, et al. Current management of male breast cancer. A review of 104 cases. Ann Surg 1992; 215: 451–7; discussion 457–9.
39. Goss PE, Reid C, Pintilie M, Lim R, Miller N. Male breast carcinoma: a review of 229 patients who presented to the Princess Margaret Hospital during 40 years: 1955–1996. Cancer 1999; 85: 629–39.
40. Cutuli B, Dilhuydy JM, De Lafontan B, et al. Ductal carcinoma in situ of the male breast. Analysis of 31 cases. Eur J Cancer 1997; 33: 35–8.
41. Hill AD, Borgen PI, Cody HS. Sentinel node biopsy in male breast cancer. Eur J Surg Oncol 1999; 25: 442–3.
42. Rusby JE, Smith BL, Dominguez FJ, Golshan M. Sentinel lymph node biopsy in men with breast cancer: a report of 31 consecutive procedures and review of the literature. Clin Breast Cancer 2006; 7: 406–10.
43. Boughey JC, Bedrosian I, Meric-Bernstam F, et al. Comparative analysis of sentinel lymph node operation in male and female breast cancer patients. J Am Coll Surg 2006; 203: 475–80.
44. Schlag PM, Bembenek A. Specification of potential indications and contraindications of sentinel lymph node biopsy in breast cancer. Recent Results Cancer Res 2000; 157: 228–36.
45. Wong SL, Chao C, Edwards MJ, et al. Accuracy of sentinel lymph node biopsy for patients with T2 and T3 breast cancers. Am Surg 2001; 67: 522–6; discussion 527–8.
46. Di Benedetto G, Pierangeli M, Bertani A. Carcinoma of the male breast: an underestimated killer. Plast Reconstr Surg 1998; 102: 696–700.
47. Nakao A, Saito S, Naomoto Y, Matsuoka J, Tanaka N. Deltopectoral flap for reconstruction of male breast after radical mastectomy for cancer in a patient on hemodialysis. Anticancer Res 2002; 22: 2477–9.
48. Cagliá P, Veroux PF, Cardillo P, et al. Carcinoma of the male breast: reconstructive technique. G Chir 1998; 19: 358–62.
49. Spear SL, Bowen DG. Breast reconstruction in a male with a transverse rectus abdominis flap. Plast Reconstr Surg 1998; 102: 1615–17.
50. Clarke M, Collins R, Darby S, et al. Effects of radiotherapy and of differences in the extent of surgery for early breast cancer on local recurrence and 15-year survival: an overview of the randomised trials. Lancet 2005; 366: 2087–106.
51. Stierer M, Rosen H, Weitensfelder W, et al. Male breast cancer: Austrian experience. World J Surg 1995; 19: 687–92; discussion 692-3.
52. Cutuli B, Cohen-Solal-le Nir C, de Lafontan B, et al. Breast-conserving therapy for ductal carcinoma in situ of the breast: the French Cancer Centers' experience. Int J Radiat Oncol Biol Phys 2002; 53: 868–79.
53. Chakravarthy A, Kim CR. Post-mastectomy radiation in male breast cancer. Radiother Oncol 2002; 65: 99–103.
54. Golshan M, Rusby J, Dominguez F, Smith BL. Breast conservation for male breast carcinoma. Breast 2007; 16: 653–6.
55. Scott-Conner CE, Jochimsen PR, Menck HR, Winchester DJ. An analysis of male and female breast cancer treatment and survival among demographically identical pairs of patients. Surgery 1999; 126: 775–80; discussion 780–1.

56. Izquierdo MA, Alonso C, De Andres L, Ojeda B. Male breast cancer. Report of a series of 50 cases. Acta Oncol 1994; 33: 767–71.

57. Patel HZ, Buzdar AU, Hortobagyi GN. Role of adjuvant chemotherapy in male breast cancer. Cancer 1989; 64: 1583–5.

58. Fentiman IS, Fourquet A, Hortobagyi GN. Male breast cancer. Lancet 2006; 367: 595–604.

59. Bagley CS, Wesley MN, Young RC, Lippman ME. Adjuvant chemotherapy in males with cancer of the breast. Am J Clin Oncol 1987; 10: 55–60.

60. Early Breast Cancer Trialists' Collaborative Group. Polychemotherapy for early breast cancer: an overview of the randomised trials. Lancet 1998; 352: 930–42.

61. Rudlowski C. Male breast cancer. Breast Care (Basel) 2008; 3: 183–9.

62. Hayashi H, Kimura M, Yoshimoto N, et al. A case of HER2-positive male breast cancer with lung metastases showing a good response to trastuzumab and paclitaxel treatment. Breast Cancer 2009; 16: 136–40.

63. Pemmaraju N, Munsell MF, Hortobagyi GN, Giordano SH. Retrospective review of male breast cancer patients: analysis of tamoxifen-related side-effects. Ann Oncol 2012; 23: 1471–4.

64. Nahleh ZA. Hormonal therapy for male breast cancer: a different approach for a different disease. Cancer Treat Rev 2006; 32: 101–5.

65. Lopez M, Di Lauro L, Lazzaro B, Papaldo P. Hormonal treatment of disseminated male breast cancer. Oncology 1985; 42: 345–9.

66. Harris AL, Dowsett M, Stuart-Harris R, Smith IE. Role of aminoglutethimide in male breast cancer. Br J Cancer 1986; 54: 657–60.

67. Giordano SH, Valero V, Buzdar AU, Hortobagyi GN. Efficacy of anastrozole in male breast cancer. Am J Clin Oncol 2002; 25: 235–7.

68. Jaiyesimi IA, Buzdar AU, Sahin AA, Ross MA. Carcinoma of the male breast. Ann Intern Med 1992; 117: 771–7.

69. Doberauer C, Niederle N, Schmidt CG. Advanced male breast cancer treatment with the LH-RH analogue buserelin alone or in combination with the antiandrogen flutamide. Cancer 1988; 62: 474–8.

70. La Vecchia C, Levi F, Lucchini F. Descriptive epidemiology of male breast cancer in Europe. Int J Cancer 1992; 51: 62–6.

71. O'Malley CD, Prehn AW, Shema SJ, Glaser SL. Racial/ethnic differences in survival rates in a population-based series of men with breast carcinoma. Cancer 2002; 94: 2836–43.

50 Trends in the use of contralateral prophylactic mastectomy

Todd M. Tuttle

INTRODUCTION

Patients with unilateral breast cancer are at increased risk for developing cancer in the contralateral breast. As a result, some patients choose contralateral prophylactic mastectomy (CPM) to prevent cancer in the contralateral breast. Several studies have reported that the CPM rates have markedly increased in recent years in the United States. Similar trends have not yet been observed in Europe. Young age, white race, and lobular histology are associated with higher CPM rates. The risk of contralateral breast cancer is reduced by about 95% after CPM. Since the risk of systemic metastases usually exceeds the risk of contralateral breast cancer, most patients will not experience any survival benefit from CPM. Moreover, CPM is irreversible and not risk free. Alternatives to CPM include surveillance with clinical breast examination, mammography, and possibly breast magnetic resonance imaging (MRI). Endocrine therapy with tamoxifen or aromatase inhibitors significantly reduces the risk of contralateral breast cancer and may be more acceptable than CPM for some patients.

CPM TRENDS

CPM is the removal of the normal intact breast among women with unilateral breast cancer. The Surveillance Epidemiology and End Results (SEER) registry began coding CPM in 1998. At that time, the proportion of patients who underwent CPM in the United States was very low (1). However, the CPM rate among all surgically treated patients with invasive breast cancer increased 150% from 1998 to 2003 in the United States. These trends were observed for all cancer stages and continued to increase at the end of the study period with no plateau. Among the SEER registries, Atlanta had the highest CPM rates, while Connecticut had the lowest rates. Although significant geographic variations were observed between different SEER registries, no general geographic trends were identified. Similar findings were observed in the SEER database among patients with ductal carcinoma in situ (DCIS) (2).

Other studies using different databases have confirmed these findings. Using the American College of Surgeons' National Cancer Data Base (NCDB), Yao et al. reported similar increases in CPM rates from 1998 to 2007; in 2007, the rates were still increasing with no plateau effect (3). In a study using the New York State Cancer Registry, McLaughlin et al. reported that CPM use more than doubled from 1995 to 2005 (4). Single-institutional studies have also demonstrated marked increases in CPM rates (5–7).

In contrast, similar trends have not been observed in Europe. In a single-center study from Switzerland, Güth et al. reported that the CPM rates at an academic surgery center did not

increase from 1995 to 2009 (8). The authors concluded that CPM rates were a "trend made in the USA." Another study supports this viewpoint. In an international registry of women with unilateral breast cancer and BRCA mutation, Metcalfe et al. reported that 49% of women in the United States underwent CPM (9). In contrast, the CPM rates from Europe and Israel were only about 10% or less.

Various patients, tumors, and treatment factors are significantly associated with CPM rates (Table 50.1). Younger women are much more likely to receive CPM (1,3). White race, higher education level, private health insurance, and family history of breast cancer have also been associated with higher CPM rates (1,3,5,7). In the SEER study, the presence of infiltrating lobular histology was one of the strongest predictors of CPM (1). Yet, recent studies indicate that the risk of contralateral breast cancer is not significantly increased for infiltrating lobular histology as compared with infiltrating ductal histology (10). Multicentric breast cancer has also been associated with higher CPM rates (11). BRCA testing is significantly associated with CPM, even among patients who do not have BRCA mutations. In one single-center study, the CPM rate was 40% among those patients who tested negative (12). Several studies have reported that preoperative MRI is associated with CPM (5,7,11). Patients treated at comprehensive cancer programs or teaching facilities are more likely to receive CPM (3).

REASONS FOR INCREASED CPM RATES

This trend toward more aggressive breast cancer surgery is curious and counterintuitive in the modern era of minimally invasive surgery. The following section of this chapter is largely speculative because the exact reasons for increased CPM rates in the United States are unknown. However, many factors probably contribute to increased CPM use. Public awareness of genetic breast cancer and increased BRCA testing may partially explain these observations. Improvements in mastectomy (including skin-sparing and nipple-sparing mastectomy) and reconstruction techniques and access to breast reconstruction probably contribute to increased CPM rates. Moreover, symmetric reconstruction is often easier to achieve after bilateral mastectomy as compared to unilateral mastectomy. Additionally, the native and reconstructed breast age differently, so symmetric outcomes may diminish over time.

Several studies have reported that preoperative breast MRI is associated with higher CPM rates (5,7). The proposed explanation is that MRI findings introduce concern about the opposite breast. For example, a patient is diagnosed with a unilateral breast cancer, and clinical breast examination and

Table 50.1 Factors Associated with CPM

Patient
    Young age
    White race
    Private insurance
    Family history of breast cancer
Tumor
    Infiltrating lobular histology
    Multicentric disease
    Size
Treatment
    BRCA testing
    MRI
    Breast reconstruction
    Facility type

mammography of the contralateral breast are normal. The patient is an ideal candidate for breast-conserving treatment. However, an MRI is obtained, which demonstrates an occult indeterminate lesion in the contralateral breast. Next, the patient gets called back to obtain a second-look (targeted) ultrasound to characterize this MRI finding. The ultrasound imaging is normal, so the patient gets called back again for an MRI-guided biopsy, which is negative for cancer. However, the patient decides to have bilateral mastectomy to avoid this stressful scenario again. Preoperative breast MRI probably contributes to increased CPM rates, but the observed CPM trends in the United States preceded the widespread use of breast MRI (1,3).

Obesity rates in the United States have markedly increased over the past two decades (13). An obese woman with large breasts may encounter many lifestyle problems after unilateral mastectomy without reconstruction. Also, a plastic surgeon may have technical challenges in achieving a symmetric reconstruction after unilateral mastectomy for an obese woman with large breasts. For some women, bilateral mastectomy with or without reconstruction may provide effective local breast cancer treatment, avoid future radiographic surveillance, and relieve symptoms from macromastia. Nevertheless, it is not known whether increasing obesity rates are contributing to current CPM trends.

Another possible explanation for the increased CPM rates is that some patients may considerably overestimate their risk of contralateral breast cancer. Previous studies have reported that healthy women substantially overestimate their risk of developing breast cancer and that women with early breast cancer markedly overestimate their risk of recurrence (14,15). In a recent survey of 350 mastectomy patients, Han et al. reported that the most common reason for CPM was worry about contralateral breast cancer (16).

However, the rates of metachronous contralateral breast cancer have declined in the United States in recent decades (17). The increased use of adjuvant therapies likely explains these findings. The Early Breast Cancer Trialists' Collaborative Group recently updated their meta-analyses and reported that the annual rate of contralateral breast cancer was about 0.4% for patients with estrogen receptor-positive breast cancer treated with tamoxifen (18). The annual rate of contralateral breast cancer was about 0.5% for patients with estrogen receptor-negative

breast cancer. Thus, the 10-year cumulative risk of contralateral breast cancer is about 4% to 5%. Abbott et al. recently published the results of a prospective single-center study designed to determine patients' perceived risk of contralateral breast cancer (19). Patients completed a standardized survey prior to surgical consultation and were asked to estimate their risk of contralateral breast cancer. Patients substantially overestimated their 10-year cumulative risk of contralateral breast cancer, with a perceived risk of 31.4%. Also, an increased perceived risk of contralateral breast cancer was significantly associated with measurements of psychological distress.

Moreover, some patients may overestimate the oncologic benefits of CPM. In a review of open-ended comments from women who underwent CPM, Altschuler et al. recorded comments such as "I do not worry about recurrence," and I am "free of worries about breast cancer" (20). Such comments suggest a lack of understanding of the benefits of CPM, since removal of the normal contralateral breast does not treat systemic metastases from the known ipsilateral breast cancer.

OUTCOMES AFTER CPM

Several studies have demonstrated that CPM is effective in reducing the risk of contralateral breast cancer (21–25). In a study of 745 breast cancer patients with a family history of breast cancer, McDonnell et al. reported that CPM reduced the incidence of contralateral breast cancer by more than 90% (22). In a retrospective study of 239 patients, Goldflam et al. reported that only one contralateral breast cancer (0.4%) developed after CPM (25). Depending upon the statistical methods used, CPM reduces the risk of contralateral breast cancer by about 90%.

However, the effectiveness of CPM in reducing breast cancer mortality is not as clear. The only plausible way that CPM improves breast cancer survival is by reducing the risk of a potentially fatal contralateral breast cancer. Using the SEER database, Bedrosian et al. identified patients with unilateral breast cancer diagnosed between 1998 and 2003 (26). The authors concluded that CPM is associated with a small improvement (4.8%) in 5-year breast cancer-specific survival rates for young women with early-stage estrogen receptor-negative breast cancer. However, the cumulative incidence of contralateral breast cancer was less than 1% in this study, so the apparent survival benefit is most likely due to selection bias. In a retrospective single-center study, Boughey et al. reported that CPM was associated with improved overall survival and disease-free survival rates (27). However, a Cochrane review of published CPM studies concluded "there is insufficient evidence that CPM improves survival" (28).

Despite the results of retrospective or cancer registry studies, CPM is not likely to improve breast cancer survival rates for patients who do not have BRCA mutations. For these patients, the 10-year cumulative risk of contralateral breast cancer is about 4% to 5%; most metachronous contralateral breast cancers are stage I or IIA with a 10-year mortality rate of about 10% to 20% (29). Thus, the 20-year mortality rate from a contralateral breast cancer is about 1% or less. In addition, many patients die from systemic metastases from their known ipsilateral breast cancer or from other causes during 20-year follow-up. Finally, CPM does not prevent all contralateral breast cancers. Thus, CPM will not decrease breast cancer mortality rates for most breast cancer patients without BRCA mutations.

On the other hand, for patients with BRCA-associated unilateral breast cancer, the annual risk of contralateral breast cancer is about 4% per year with a cumulative 10-year risk of contralateral breast cancer of about 40% (30). Thus, the possibility of developing a potentially fatal contralateral breast cancer is substantially higher among breast cancer patients with a BRCA mutation. The relative risk reduction of CPM is similar for patients with and without BRCA mutations. In a cohort of patients with unilateral breast cancer and BRCA1 or BRCA2 mutations, van Sprundel et al. reported that CPM reduced the risk of contralateral breast cancer by 91% (24). Using Markov modeling, Schrag et al. estimated that CPM would increase life expectancy by 0.6 to 2.1 years for a 30-year-old patient with a BRCA mutation (31). Clearly, randomized trials comparing CPM with no CPM for either selected (BRCA mutations) or heterogeneous patients are not feasible.

CPM is an irreversible procedure and is not risk free. Severe complications after CPM may potentially delay recommended adjuvant therapy and may require additional surgical procedures and subsequent loss of reconstruction. The overall complication rate after bilateral mastectomy and reconstruction is about 15% to 20% (25,32). About half of the complications are secondary to the prophylactic mastectomy. Even without complications, these operations are long (often 5–6 hours) and require 2 to 3 days of inpatient hospital care, drainage catheters, and 3- to 4-week overall recovery.

Despite potential risks and complications, most patients are satisfied with their decision to undergo CPM (33–35). The greatest reported benefit contributing to patient satisfaction is a reduction in breast cancer-related concerns. Frost et al. reported that 83% of patients were either satisfied or very satisfied with their decision to undergo CPM at a mean of 10 years after surgery (33). A minority of women have negative psychosocial outcomes following CPM, most often related to high levels of psychological distress, sexual function, and body image or poor cosmetic outcome (20). Montgomery et al. reported that the most common reasons for regret after CPM were a poor cosmetic outcome and diminished sense of sexuality (34).

ALTERNATIVES TO CPM

Patients with unilateral breast cancer have options that are less drastic than CPM. Surveillance with clinical breast examination, mammography, and potentially breast MRI may detect cancers at earlier stages (36,37). Several prospective randomized trials have demonstrated that tamoxifen, given as adjuvant therapy for estrogen receptor-positive breast cancer, significantly reduces the rate of contralateral breast cancer (38–40). In the National Surgical Adjuvant Breast and Bowel Project (NSABP) B-14 study, 2,892 women with node-negative, estrogen receptor-positive breast tumors were randomly assigned to either tamoxifen (20 mg/day) or placebo for at least 5 years (38). After an average follow-up of 53 months, 55 second contralateral breast cancers developed in placebo-treated women and 28 developed in the tamoxifen-treated women ($p = .001$). Aromatase inhibitors may reduce the risk of contralateral breast cancer as much as, or even more than, tamoxifen (41). The ATAC (Arimidex, Tamoxifen Alone, or in Combination) trial demonstrated that anastrozole was superior to tamoxifen in preventing contralateral breast cancer in postmenopausal

women. Ovarian ablation and cytotoxic chemotherapy also reduce the risk of contralateral breast cancer (30,42,43).

CONCLUSIONS

Increasingly more patients in the United States with invasive breast cancer and DCIS undergo CPM to prevent contralateral breast cancer. Patient, tumor, and treatment factors are associated with increased use. Indeed, CPM does reduce the risk of contralateral breast cancer, but does not impact breast cancer survival rates. Controversy exists about whether the physician or patient should initiate the discussion of CPM. If a patient appropriately chooses breast-conserving surgery, CPM is not a relevant treatment. For patients who undergo mastectomy, CPM may be a reasonable option, particularly if a patient has a BRCA mutation, has a strong family history, and is obese or if imaging of the contralateral breast is difficult. Several studies have demonstrated that many patients are not well informed about the risk of contralateral breast cancer or the benefits of CPM. Physicians need to provide breast cancer patients with accurate information on the risk of contralateral breast cancer and on the risks and benefits of CPM. In addition, physicians should encourage appropriate patients to consider less drastic options (e.g., endocrine therapy) to reduce the risk of contralateral breast cancer.

Presently, no study has prospectively evaluated the complex decision-making processes that lead to CPM. Future research should include development of models and instruments to elucidate these processes. Also, the surgeon's role and influence in the choice of breast cancer surgery should be evaluated. Finally, decision aids should be developed for breast cancer patients and physicians.

REFERENCES

1. Tuttle TM, Habermann EB, Grund EH, et al. Increasing use of contralateral prophylactic mastectomy for breast cancer patients: a trend toward more aggressive surgical treatment. J Clin Oncol 2007; 25: 5203–9.
2. Tuttle TM, Jarosek S, Habermann E, et al. Increasing rates of contralateral prophylactic mastectomy among patients with ductal carcinoma in situ. J Clin Oncol 2009; 27: 1362–7.
3. Yao K, Stewart AK, Winchester DJ, Winchester DP. Trends in contralateral prophylactic mastectomy for unilateral cancer: a report from the National Cancer Data Base, 1998-2007. Ann Surg Oncol 2010; 17: 2554–62.
4. McLaughlin CC, Lillquist PP, Edge SB. Surveillance of prophylactic mastectomy: trends in use from 1995 through 2005. Cancer 2009; 115: 5404–12.
5. Sorbero ME, Dick AW, Burke Beckjord E, et al. Diagnostic breast magnetic resonance imaging and contralateral prophylactic mastectomy. Ann Surg Oncol 2009; 16: 1597–605.
6. Jones NB, Wilson J, Kotur L, et al. Contralateral prophylactic mastectomy for unilateral breast cancer: an increasing trend at a single institution. Ann Surg Oncol 2009; 16: 2691–6.
7. King TA, Sakr R, Patil S, et al. Clinical management factors contribute to the decision for contralateral prophylactic mastectomy. J Clin Oncol 2011; 29: 2158–64.
8. Güth U, Myrick ME, Viehl CT, et al. Increasing rates of contralateral prophylactic mastectomy-a trend made in USA? Eur J Surg Oncol 2012; 38: 296–301.
9. Metcalfe KA, Lubinski J, Ghadirian P, et al. Hereditary Breast Cancer Clinical Study Group. Predictors of contralateral prophylactic mastectomy in women with a BRCA1 or BRCA2 mutation: the Hereditary Breast Cancer Clinical Study Group. J Clin Oncol 2008; 26: 1093–7.
10. Gao X, Fisher SG, Emami B. Risk of second primary cancer in the contralateral breast in women treated for early-stage breast cancer: a population-based study. Int J Radiat Oncol Biol Phys 2003; 56: 1038–45.

11. Stucky CC, Gray RJ, Wasif N, et al. Increase in contralateral prophylactic mastectomy: echoes of a bygone era? Surgical trends for unilateral breast cancer. Ann Surg Oncol 2010; 17: 330–7.
12. Yi M, Hunt KK, Arun BK, et al. Factors affecting the decision of breast cancer patients to undergo contralateral prophylactic mastectomy. Cancer Prev Res 2010; 3: 1026–34.
13. Mitchell NS, Catenacci VA, Wyatt HR, Hill JO. Obesity: overview of an epidemic. Psychiatry Clin North Am 2011; 34: 717–32.
14. Black WC, Nease RF Jr, Tosteson AN. Perceptions of breast cancer risk and screening effectiveness in women younger than 50 years of age. J Natl Cancer Inst 1995; 87: 720–31.
15. Rakovitch E, Franssen E, Kim J, et al. A comparison of risk perception and psychological morbidity in women with ductal carcinoma in situ and early invasive breast cancer. Breast Cancer Res Treat 2003; 77: 285–93.
16. Han E, Johnson N, Glissmeyer M, et al. Increasing incidence of bilateral mastectomies: the patient perspective. Am J Surg 2011; 201: 615–18.
17. Nichols HB, Berrington de González A, et al. Declining incidence of contralateral breast cancer in the United States from 1975 to 2006. J Clin Oncol 2011; 29: 1564–9.
18. Early Breast Cancer Trialists' Collaborative Group (EBCTCG). Davies C, Godwin J, Gray R, et al. Relevance of breast cancer hormone receptors and other factors to the efficacy of adjuvant tamoxifen: patient-level meta-analysis of randomised trials. Lancet 2011; 378: 771–84.
19. Abbott E, Rueth N, Pappas-Varco S, et al. Perceptions of contralateral breast cancer: an overestimation of risk. Ann Surg Oncol 2011; 18: 3129–36.
20. Altschuler A, Nekhlyudov L, Rolnick S, et al. Positive, negative, and disparate women's differing long-term psychosocial experiences of bilateral or contralateral prophylactic mastectomy. Breast J 2008; 14: 25–3.
21. Peralta EA, Ellenhorn JD, Wagman LD, et al. Contralateral prophylactic mastectomy improves the outcome of selected patients undergoing mastectomy for breast cancer. Am J Surg 2000; 180: 439–45.
22. McDonnell SK, Schaid DJ, Myers JL, et al. Efficacy of contralateral prophylactic mastectomy in women with a personal and family history of breast cancer. J Clin Oncol 2001; 19: 3938–43.
23. Herrinton LJ, Barlow WE, Yu O, et al. Efficacy of prophylactic mastectomy in women with unilateral breast cancer: a cancer research network project. J Clin Oncol 2005; 23: 4275–86.
24. van Sprundel TC, Schmidt MK, Rookus MA, et al. Risk reduction of contralateral breast cancer and survival after contralateral prophylactic mastectomy in BRCA1 or BRCA2 mutation carriers. Br J Cancer 2005; 93: 287–92.
25. Goldflam K, Hunt KK, Gershenwald JE, et al. Contralateral prophylactic mastectomy. Predictors of significant histologic findings. Cancer 2004; 101: 1977–86.
26. Bedrosian I, Hu CY, Chang GJ. Population-based study of contralateral prophylactic mastectomy and survival outcomes of breast cancer patients. J Natl Cancer Inst 2010; 102: 401–9.
27. Boughey JC, Hoskin TL, Degnim AC, et al. Contralateral prophylactic mastectomy is associated with a survival advantage in high-risk women with a personal history of breast cancer. Ann Surg Oncol 2010; 17: 2702–9.
28. Lostumbo L, Carbine NE, Wallace J. Prophylactic mastectomy for the prevention of breast cancer. Cochrane Database Syst Rev 2010: CD002748.
29. Houssami N, Ciatto S, Martinelli F, et al. Early detection of second breast cancers improves prognosis in breast cancer survivors. Ann Oncol 2009; 20: 1505–20.
30. Metcalfe K, Lynch HT, Ghadirian P, et al. Contralateral breast cancer in BRCA1 and BRCA2 mutation carriers. J Clin Oncol 2004; 22: 2328–35.
31. Schrag D, Kuntz KM, Garber JE, et al. Life expectancy gains from cancer prevention strategies for women with breast cancer and BRCA1 or BRCA2 mutations. JAMA 2000; 283: 617–24.
32. Woerdeman LA, Hage JJ, Smeulders MJ, et al. Skin-sparing mastectomy and immediate breast reconstruction by use of implants: an assessment of risk factors for complications and cancer control in 120 patients. Plast Reconstr Surg 2006; 118: 321–30.
33. Frost MH, Slezak JM, Tran NV, et al. Satisfaction after contralateral prophylactic mastectomy: the significance of mastectomy type, reconstructive complications, and body appearance. J Clin Oncol 2005; 23: 7849–56.
34. Montgomery LL, Tran KN, Heelan MC, et al. Issues of regret in women with contralateral prophylactic mastectomies. Ann Surg Oncol 1999; 6: 546–52.
35. Geiger AM, West CN, Nekhlyudov L, et al. Contentment with quality of life among breast cancer survivors with and without contralateral prophylactic mastectomy. J Clin Oncol 2006; 24: 1350–6.
36. Ciatto S, Ambrogetti D, Bonardi R, et al. Prognostic impact of early detection of contralateral primary breast cancer. Tumori 1990; 76: 370–3.
37. Mellink WA, Holland R, Hendriks JH, et al. The contribution of routine follow-up mammography to an early detection of asynchronous contralateral breast cancer. Cancer 1991; 67: 1844–8.
38. Fisher B, Redmond C. New perspective on cancer of the contralateral breast: a marker for assessing tamoxifen as a preventive agent. J Natl Cancer Inst 1991; 83: 1278–80.
39. Stewart HJ. The Scottish trial of adjuvant tamoxifen in node-negative breast cancer. Scottish Cancer Trials Breast Group. J Natl Cancer Inst Monogr 1992; 117–20.
40. Rutqvist LE, Cedermark B, Glas U, et al. Contralateral primary tumors in breast cancer patients in a randomized trial of adjuvant tamoxifen therapy. J Natl Cancer Inst 1991; 83: 1299–306.
41. Baum M, Budzar AU, Cuzick J, et al. Anastrozole alone or in combination with tamoxifen versus tamoxifen alone for adjuvant treatment of postmenopausal women with early breast cancer: first results of the ATAC randomised trial. Lancet 2002; 359: 2131–9.
42. Meakin JW, Hayward JL, Panzarella T, et al. Ovarian irradiation and prednisone following surgery and radiotherapy for carcinoma of the breast. Breast Cancer Res Treat 1996; 37: 11–19.
43. Early Breast Cancer Trialists' Collaborative Group. Tamoxifen for early breast cancer: an overview of the randomised trials. Lancet 1998; 351: 1451–67.

51 The principles of breast reconstructive surgery

Animesh J.K. Patel, Rosanna C. Ching, John R. Benson,
and Charles M. Malata

INTRODUCTION

Increasing numbers of women are diagnosed with breast cancer each year, with estimates of the lifetime risk in western society being 1 in 8 (1). As screening regimes have the potential to pick up cancers earlier, there has been an inevitable increase in the number of patients undergoing surgery for early-stage breast cancers.

Surgical management of invasive and in situ disease can range from wide local excision to total mastectomy. With the emergence of oncoplastic techniques, more patients now have the choice of cancer excision while preserving the breast shape and thus avoiding mastectomy. However, many patients with early breast cancer undergo mastectomy either because of an unfavorable location of the tumor (proximity to the nipple) and its aggressiveness or because the patient prefers this option to breast conservation (perhaps because of a perceived minimization of risk of future disease in the same breast).

Similarly, patients at high risk of breast cancer (e.g., those with a genetic predisposition such as BRCA tumor suppressor gene mutation carriers, those with affected first-degree relatives, and those who have had previous contralateral breast cancer) may choose to have mastectomy as a risk-reducing procedure. These issues relating to future risk have resulted in a rise in the number of patients undergoing mastectomy. Although not all mastectomy patients wish to have a breast reconstruction, a significant number will request this as an option (2) and a variety of techniques are available in the reconstructive surgeon's armamentarium to achieve that aim. For those patients considering risk-reducing mastectomy, the decision to have a mastectomy is perhaps influenced by the availability of reliable and realistic techniques for immediate reconstruction at the same time as mastectomy. Breast reconstruction can free a woman from having to wear an external breast prosthesis, and can go some way to re-establishing self-confidence in her own body image.

The goal of the reconstructive surgeon following breast cancer extirpative surgery can vary from simple wound coverage to the complexities of creating a breast mound that has an esthetically pleasing surface, shape, and volume. In the case of unilateral surgery, the ultimate aim is to achieve symmetry with the contralateral breast. The female breast has unique physical and psychological functions, which collectively contribute to femininity. Reconstructive techniques available today cannot reconstitute the physiological function of the mammary gland. However, the restoration of body image that is lost after mastectomy is surgically achievable and goes a long way in helping restore a woman's self-esteem after having to face the consequences of losing a breast and what it symbolizes.

Although in the planning and execution of breast reconstruction, the reconstructive surgeon must work closely with the breast oncological surgeon, the patient's wishes and expectations are paramount. At the same time, it is important that women understand the limitations of current techniques and the appropriateness of particular procedures in their individual case.

Reconstructive techniques used in breast surgery following mastectomy can be broadly divided into those that use alloplastic materials (i.e., breast implants) and those that use autologous techniques (i.e., the patient's own tissues). There are also techniques that combine these two basic approaches.

Breast implants or prostheses are either saline-filled or silicone-filled medical devices that are available in a variety of shapes and sizes to suit an individual patient but are all designed to augment breast size. The prosthesis requires adequate soft tissue coverage and therefore a pocket for the implant to be placed in must be developed. Often the pocket is expanded to size using a temporary expander or inflatable implant, which is then subsequently exchanged for a fixed-volume implant. In addition to temporary expanders and simple/fixed-volume implants, a further type of prosthesis is also available, which combines the features of a fixed-volume implant and those of an expander. This is called an "expandable implant" or a "permanent expander" (3) and is a popular choice in contemporary breast reconstruction.

Autologous techniques include the use of pedicled and free flaps. A flap is defined as a block of tissue that is "moved" or transferred from one part of the body (donor site) to another (recipient site). A pedicled flap survives by keeping its blood supply intact during flap movement. In free flaps (also known as free tissue transfers), the flap's vascular pedicle, containing its blood supply, is surgically divided at the donor site and then reanastomosed to blood vessels at the recipient site using microsurgical techniques. The main advantage of autologous flaps is that they more closely resemble native breast tissue in their feel and consistency. They also reduce or eliminate the need for prostheses, which being foreign materials carry their own risks. A pertinent consideration in breast reconstruction is that they withstand the effects of radiotherapy better than implant-based or implant-only techniques. Commonly used pedicled flaps in breast reconstruction include the latissimus dorsi (LD) myocutaneous flap and the pedicled transverse rectus abdominis myocutaneous (TRAM) flap. As will be discussed below, often the LD flap alone has insufficient volume to create the breast mound, and an implant or expander is often necessary to provide supplementary volume. Although still used by some surgeons, the pedicled TRAM has largely fallen out of favor and been superseded by free tissue transfer techniques, most commonly using cognate abdominal tissue (i.e., the free TRAM flap) and its modifications. Other free flaps that have been used successfully for breast reconstruction include buttock flaps using the superior and inferior gluteal arteries and flaps using tissue harvested from the thigh. Each potential donor site has its merits and the choice of which to use must be made on an individual patient basis taking account of tissue availability and the requirements for reconstruction, in terms of size and volume.

HISTORY OF BREAST RECONSTRUCTION

The Austrian-German surgeon Vincenz Czerny is credited with describing the first breast reconstruction (4). In 1893, he used a lipoma excised from the flank to restore the breast in a patient who had undergone resection of a fibroadenoma in the setting of chronic interstitial mastitis. The fat autograft was deemed successful, and Czerny noted persistence of the transplanted lipoma with a satisfactory cosmetic appearance of the breast 1 year after surgery. Since that time, however, other surgeons have found retention rates for fat grafts to be poor, especially when a large volume of tissue is transferred. Therefore, autologous fat grafting is not a viable option at the present time for total breast reconstruction.

In 1896, an Italian surgeon, called Iginio Tansini, reported using a flap of tissue from the back, which was pedicled at the axilla, to reconstruct a radical mastectomy defect (5). The publication described a skin flap that had a narrow superior base in the axilla. As might be expected, such a tissue flap was susceptible to vascular embarrassment in its most distal part, which led Tansini to more thoroughly investigate the vascular supply of these tissues. He realized the importance of including the LD muscle to make a musculocutaneous unit and published the results of this principle in 1906 (6). Although he appreciated how muscle provided soft tissue bulk to complement the skin paddle, which provided basic cover at the mastectomy site, the technique served mainly to resurface the (radical) mastectomy defect and was effectively a chest wall reconstruction, rather than a breast reconstruction per se. It was not until the 1970s that the concept of using an LD myocutaneous flap to recreate a breast mound (being complemented by a prosthesis to provide additional volume) was realized (7–9).

The silicone breast prosthesis was introduced in the early 1960s by Cronin and Gerow (10) and began to be used for postmastectomy reconstruction shortly thereafter. However, outcomes were often suboptimal owing in part to the radicalism of the extirpative surgery, which was prevalent at the time for breast cancer patients. Wide excision of skin, soft tissues, and pectoral muscle, as in Halsted's radical mastectomy, prevented adequate soft tissue coverage of the prostheses and consequently these reconstructions suffered from an esthetic point of view. The next landmark step in the evolution of breast reconstructive techniques came in 1982 with Chemodir Radovan's description of using tissue expansion prior to placement of the definitive prosthesis (11). This resulted in a larger, expanded pocket in which to place the prosthesis and also attempted to reconstruct the deficiency in the breast skin envelope following mastectomy.

Throughout the early 20th century, a number of plastic surgical techniques were used, which included flaps that were waltzed in multiple stages from a distant donor site to the defect over a period of months (12). These fell out of favor with the emergence and better understanding of other locoregional pedicled flaps and free tissue transfer techniques that offered singe-stage reconstruction.

By the 1970s, the LD flap combined with a silicone prosthesis had become a popular option in breast reconstruction. Nonetheless, this was not a completely autologous reconstruction and suffered from risks of using a foreign body such as implant infection, extrusion, and the development of peri-implant capsular contracture.

The recognition that a breast mound with overlying skin could be created with autologous tissue alone was a significant step forward and became a reality in 1982 when Carl Hartrampf (of Atlanta, Georgia, US) used abdominal tissue to reconstruct a breast mound at the mastectomy defect (13). This pedicled TRAM flap subsequently gained popularity and utilized a transverse ellipse of skin and adipose tissue along with the underlying rectus abdominis muscle, which once raised is passed through a subcutaneous tunnel to the anterior chest wall region.

Of interest, prior to this pedicled TRAM flap described by Hartrampf, Holmstrom had described the "free abdominoplasty flap" in 1979, which transferred abdominal tissue as a free tissue transfer with reestablishment of blood supply by microsurgical reanastomosis at the recipient mastectomy site (14). As microsurgery was only just emerging at the time and few surgeons possessed the necessary skills, the potential of this free flap was temporarily overlooked in favor of Hartrampf's pedicled TRAM flap.

Although a totally autologous reconstruction, the pedicled TRAM was initially plagued with complications not only at the recipient site with wound healing problems, partial flap failures, and fat necrosis but also, more importantly, at the donor site where significant rates of abdominal wall bulges and herniae occurred (15,16).

Microsurgical expertise improved with time and it was appreciated that although the rectus abdominis muscle had a dual blood supply, it was the deep inferior epigastric (DIE) vessels that were dominant in supplying the overlying abdominal skin and adipose tissue (17,18).

Consequently, the free TRAM flap based on the DIE vessels became increasingly popular for breast reconstruction. Although requiring microsurgical expertise, it resulted in lower rates of fat necrosis in the reconstructed breast but donor site problems remained similar to those for patients undergoing pedicled TRAM flap reconstructions.

The anatomy of perforating vessels from the main trunk of the DIE vessel was further delineated, and it became evident that the adipocutaneous portion of the flap could be raised on the same vessels while preserving much of the rectus abdominis muscle and rectus sheath. This description of the deep inferior epigastric perforator (DIEP) flap was arguably the most significant advance in refining abdominal flap breast reconstruction and culminated in the realization that the skin and fat of the abdomen could be harvested as a flap based solely on the perforating vessels from the DIE system. This permitted total muscle and fascia preservation, thus combining the advantages of using autologous tissue from the abdomen based on the dominant DIE system while minimizing morbidity relating to disruption of the anterior abdominal wall (19). This DIEP flap was first described in 1989 by Koshima (20), but its specific use in breast reconstruction was first described simultaneously by Allen and Blondeel in 1994 (21,22), spawning the concept of perforator-based flap reconstructions. In a similar way, myocutaneous buttock flaps, based on the superior and inferior gluteal vascular systems, have been modified to preserve the gluteal muscles and harvest exclusively the adipocutaneous components of these flaps (23). Although there is a steep learning curve with these perforator flaps, and more prolonged initial operating times, there are clear advantages in terms of reduced donor site morbidity.

The DIEP flap, however, is technically challenging for surgeons with a definite learning period. Consequently, some surgeons prefer the "muscle-sparing TRAM (MS TRAM)" as an attempt to avoid the tedious dissection of perforators. This method includes harvesting part of the muscle around the DIEP perforators, which facilitates and shortens time for dissection, while still minimizing donor site morbidity (24,25).

TIMING OF BREAST RECONSTRUCTION

Breast reconstruction performed at the same time as the mastectomy is known as "immediate" breast reconstruction (IBR), and is offered routinely in many centers around the world. Indeed, the British National Mastectomy and Breast Reconstruction Audit (2) recommends that immediate reconstruction should be offered to the majority of patients undergoing mastectomy. IBR has numerous advantages (26); breast cancer resection and reconstruction are carried out under a single general anesthetic; the patient does not have to live without a breast for any time, minimizing problems with loss of femininity, body image, and self-esteem; skin-sparing mastectomy with preservation of the breast skin envelope and inframammary fold can be performed with a more esthetically pleasing reconstruction (27–29). Despite initial concerns, IBR does not compromise the adequacy of mastectomy and is oncologically safe (except in some cases of inflammatory breast cancer or where there is extensive skin involvement) (30). Although uncommon, it can potentially be associated with delay in receiving adjuvant treatments if there is prolonged healing or other problems (31). An added advantage of immediate autologous flap reconstruction is that they can better tolerate adjuvant therapies, namely external beam radiotherapy.

Delayed breast reconstruction is performed months or years after mastectomy. It has a number of potential advantages (Table 51.1), not least being the fact that cancer treatments have been completed. It also staggers surgery and entails two relatively smaller and separate procedures.

Table 51.1 Delayed Breast Reconstruction—Advantages and Disadvantages

Advantages
    Staggers the surgeries: shorter recovery times
    No risk of masking recurrence
    All the adjuvant treatment has been completed
Disadvantages
    Difficult to achieve excellent cosmesis
    Adverse effects of prior radiotherapy
    Multiple operations, hospitalization, time off work
    Possibly more expensive overall

Meticulous planning is important for the successful execution of both immediate and delayed breast reconstruction, but factors to be taken into consideration are somewhat different for these two scenarios.

Successful immediate reconstruction also requires close consultation with the oncological surgeon. For example, in the case of an implant-based reconstruction, it is important to ensure that the mastectomy skin flaps are left adequately perfused at the end of the mastectomy prior to reconstruction. They should therefore not be too thin so as to provide viable, healthy tissue with minimal risk of poor wound healing. Necrosis of thinner mastectomy flaps may lead to wound breakdown and implant exposure. By contrast, mastectomy flaps that are too thick may contain residual breast tissue, thus rendering the mastectomy oncologically "incomplete." Furthermore, as the prosthesis will be placed in a submuscular pocket, it is important to not violate the pectoralis major muscle during mastectomy (especially medially) as this structure is required to provide soft tissue coverage of the prosthesis. Hence, a patient who is known to have locally advanced disease with infiltration of the muscle is not a candidate for an immediate implant-only reconstruction. Another important consideration is that the breast surgeon should not disrupt the inframammary fold or indeed cross the midline during mastectomy. It is important that the breast boundaries are clearly marked on the patient preoperatively in order to guide the breast surgeon but more importantly to aid reconstruction.

Undertaking a delayed breast reconstruction can be more challenging as there may be few clues to guide the surgeon in correctly positioning the inframammary fold (if this was not preserved during mastectomy) together with the medial and lateral breast borders. Hence accurate preoperative planning is essential for a good esthetic outcome. The boundaries of the opposite breast are important in this regard. If the reconstruction is unilateral, the opposite breast will serve as a guide for preoperative marking of these critical borders. As the breast skin envelope is deficient in a delayed reconstruction (by definition), it will need to be augmented, and for implant-based reconstructions, this can be attained through a period of tissue expansion. If autologous flaps are used, the extent of skin deficiency must be calculated and incorporated into the flap planning such that the flap that is raised has an adequate skin component to compensate. It is best to overestimate the amount of skin needed.

IMPLANT-BASED (ALLOPLASTIC) BREAST RECONSTRUCTION

Alloplastic breast reconstruction remains the most common form of postmastectomy reconstruction (32), which is perhaps not surprising considering its relative lack of surgical complexity. Breast prostheses are available in a wide variety of shapes and sizes, with many used in breast reconstruction being biodimensional nowadays. (Fig. 51.1). Anatomically, the breast prosthesis is placed in a surgically created pocket underneath the pectoralis major muscle. Careful planning is required to ensure an appropriately sized pocket is created and that it is sited in the correct anatomical position on the chest wall. As well as having a layer of partial muscle coverage for the prosthesis, it is important that the overlying skin and soft tissues are sufficiently pliable to accommodate the prosthesis. A good quality, well-vascularized soft tissue envelope will maximize the chances of primary wound

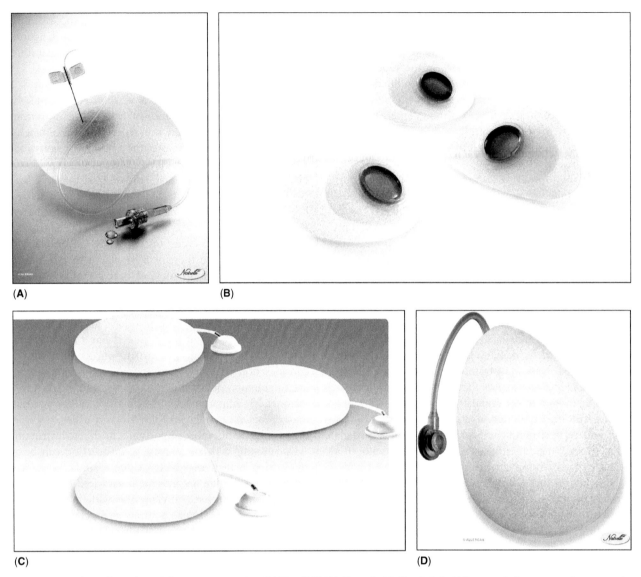

Figure 51.1 Commonly used prostheses in breast reconstruction: (**A**) Natrelle™ 133 (formally McGhan® Style 133) anatomical temporary tissue expander with integrated port; (**B**) Mentor Siltex™ Contour Profile® temporary breast tissue expanders with integrated port—low (Style 6100), medium (Style 6200), and tall (Style 6300) height prostheses; (**C**) Mentor Siltex® Contour Profile® Becker expandable implants—round (Becker 25 and Becker 50) and anatomical (Becker 35) shapes; and (**D**) Natrelle™ 150 (formally McGhan® Style 150) short height expandable implant.

healing at the postsurgical scar and will help maintain longevity of the prosthetic reconstruction. Table 51.2 lists the advantages and disadvantages of prosthetic breast reconstruction.

For the small-breasted patient, an implant-based reconstruction may be undertaken as a single-stage procedure (3,33), but patients with moderate-to-large breasts will usually require a period of tissue expansion to create a pocket of sufficient size to accommodate the definitive prosthesis and to expand the overlying breast skin envelope. Most commonly, this is achieved by placing a tissue expander in a "submuscular pocket" (deep to the pectoralis major muscle), which is inflated to the desired size over time. In a second procedure, the tissue expander is exchanged for a fixed-volume implant. Alternatively, an "expandable implant" (34), such as the Siltex® Contour Profile® Becker 35 (35,36) or the Natrelle™ 150 (formally McGhan® Style 150 (37)), can be employed. These are "hybrid" devices that, in addition to an outer silicone gel component, also have an inner inflatable pocket that can be expanded with saline to the desired size. Such

Table 51.2 Prosthetic Breast Reconstruction—Advantages and Disadvantages

Advantages
  Simple
  Quick
  No extra scars/no donor sites
  Faster recovery
  Cheaper initially: short term
Disadvantages
  Small-to-moderate size breasts only
  Cannot withstand radiotherapy
  Complications: infection, exposure, extrusion, capsular contracture
  Multistage, frequent revisions
  Patient acceptance variable
  Ptosis difficult to achieve
  Poor projection in nipple-areola area
  More expensive if combined with an acellular dermal matrix

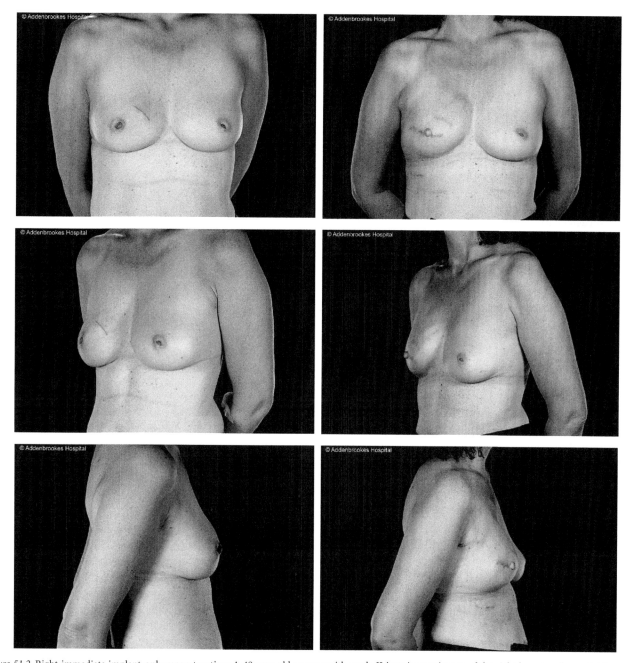

Figure 51.2 Right immediate implant-only reconstruction: A 49-year-old woman with grade II invasive carcinoma of the right breast underwent skin-sparing mastectomy and immediate prosthetic reconstruction with a permanent expander. No adjuvant radiotherapy was required. Postoperative images show her following nipple reconstruction, before areolar tattooing. Note the excellent reconstructive breast contour on the oblique and lateral views and the superomedial rippling. The lack of projection in the nipple areolar area is a typical feature of implant-only reconstruction. This is ideal for small-to-moderate-sized breasts with no glandular or nipple ptosis as shown here.

an expandable implant does not necessarily need to be exchanged, hence their alternative name of "permanent expanders" (3).

Any patient undergoing mastectomy is suitable for an alloplastic reconstruction (Fig. 51.2), but the technique is ideally suited to the patient with small-to-moderate–sized breasts with minimal ptosis and sufficient chest wall soft tissue to ensure adequate coverage of the prosthesis. Many patients choose to undergo this form of reconstruction as it is associated with a shorter operating time and faster postoperative recovery and does not violate another body site. This contrasts with autologous flap reconstruction where there is potential donor site morbidity. Moreover, for those patients who have a paucity of tissue or previous surgical intervention in potential donor areas,

an implant-only reconstruction may be optimal. In addition, when undergoing bilateral postmastectomy reconstruction, an implant-only reconstruction can produce a symmetrical reconstruction and is often the procedure of choice for patients undergoing bilateral reconstruction following risk-reducing mastectomies. For patients with larger breasts, prosthetic reconstruction can be feasible when a reduction of the opposite ("target" breast) is simultaneously performed.

Immediate Alloplastic Breast Reconstruction
Successful immediate implant-only reconstruction relies on close collaboration between the oncological and reconstructive surgeons (see Table 51.3 for indications). In this setting, the

Table 51.3 Indications for Immediate Prosthetic Breast Reconstruction

Simple (fixed-volume) implants
  Patient choice
  Patient acceptance of foreign material
  Small volume breasts (A/B cup size)
  No ptosis
  No radiotherapy planned or likely
  Adequate soft tissue cover
  Lack of donor tissues primarily or secondary to previous surgery
  Nonsmoker, ideally young with good muscle
  Unwilling to tolerate extra scars
  Bilateral reconstructions
Expanders (temporary or permanent)
  Patient choice
  Patient acceptance of foreign material
  Small-to-moderate volume breasts (A–C cup size)
  No or minimal ptosis
  Lack of donor tissues: primarily or secondary to previous surgery
  No radiotherapy planned or likely
  Well-vascularized, healthy soft tissue and skin envelope
  Unwilling to tolerate extra scars
  Unfit for major surgery
  Flexibility
  Preferably nonsmokers
  Bilateral reconstructions

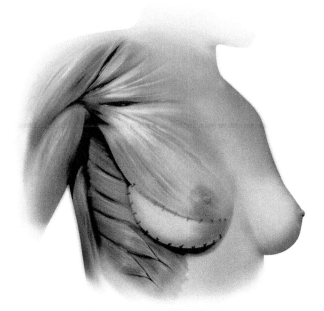

Figure 51.3 Illustration of Strattice™ Reconstructive Tissue Matrix *in situ* for coverage of the lower pole of the breast prothesis (courtesy LifeCell Corporation, Branchburg, New Jersey, US).

mastectomy can be carried out using a skin-sparing approach with excision of the nipple-areola complex (NAC) and underlying glandular tissue and preservation of the remaining overlying skin envelope. There are many incision patterns for skin-sparing mastectomy (26–28). The incision can be drawn as a transverse ellipse to give greater access for the mastectomy and allow for a neater skin closure by eliminating "dog ears." Once the mastectomy has been completed, the skin flaps must be assessed for their viability and the mastectomy cavity or pocket inspected for hemostasis. A submuscular pocket is then created.

• The senior author's approach is to find the lateral edge of the pectoralis major muscle and elevate the muscle using a combination of electrocautery and blunt dissection to create the pocket. If total submuscular coverage is desired, especially in the case of thin skin flaps, an inferolateral space (deep to the serratus anterior fascia or muscle) will also need to be elevated, as the pectoralis major does not cover this area. Alternatively, if the fascia inferior to the pectoralis major muscle has been damaged or is tenuous (as in thin patients), a strip of an acellular dermal matrix (ADM), for example, Alloderm® Regenerative Tissue Matrix (RTM) or Strattice™ Reconstructive Tissue Matrix (LifeCell Corporation, Branchburg, New Jersey, USA), can be used to cover the implant in this region (Fig. 51.3).

• An alternative approach is to split the pectoralis muscle away from its lateral edge and develop a pocket from there. The advantage of this approach is that once in the submuscular plane, deep to the pectoralis major, careful dissection laterally can elevate the serratus anterior fascia and muscle in the same plane and ensure an even pocket, thus allowing total musculo-fascial coverage of the implant. This, however, can lead to poor pro-

jection but is useful in separating the implant from the axillary clearance where this has been performed. Dissection may also be more difficult.

Once hemostasis is ensured, suction drains are placed in both the submuscular and subcutaneous pockets. Care must be taken to limit the pocket to the boundaries/dimensions of the original breast, and these dimensions (the breast "foot-print") will then govern the choice of size for the tissue expander to be used. The most important dimension is the breast width.

Patients with large breasts must be counseled that an alloplastic reconstruction is limited by the maximum size of implants available, and the reconstruction may not be able to recreate a breast of the same original size. Furthermore, implant-based reconstructions ultimately lack the ptosis associated with native tissues, and larger-breasted patients may require contralateral balancing surgery to achieve a symmetrical result (38) or possible reduction of the breast skin envelope (27,29,39).

If a small breast (A or B cup size) is being reconstructed, there may be a sufficient skin envelope to perform a single-stage reconstruction with a fixed-volume prosthesis, but similar principles in terms of choosing the most appropriate implant apply. This situation rarely occurs in routine practice. It is more applicable if the patient is undergoing bilateral breast reconstruction for very small breasts or unilateral reconstruction of the relatively larger of two small breasts.

Delayed Alloplastic Breast Reconstruction

Many patients do not undergo immediate reconstruction, either as a result of their own choice or from not being offered it at the time of mastectomy. Sometimes IBR is not available and rarely it is deemed oncologically inappropriate to undertake an immediate procedure. In such cases of delayed reconstruction, many patients choose to have an implant-only–based technique. Selection criteria are similar to immediate implant-only reconstruction, but the main difference is the deficiency of any skin envelope and this has to be recreated. The other difference is loss of the inframammary fold and other breast borders, which is not infrequent. The site of the new inframammary fold and medial and lateral breast borders must be determined preoperatively (foot-print), and for unilateral reconstruction, the contralateral breast should serve as a template for this. To create a pocket sufficient to accommodate the definitive prosthesis, the skin and soft tissues must be surgically stretched by use of a breast tissue expander.

Tissue Expansion

In those cases where a single-stage implant-based reconstruction with a fixed-volume prosthesis cannot be achieved, the submuscular pocket and the overlying soft tissue and skin envelope must undergo a period of tissue expansion, and this always pertains whenever a delayed implant-based reconstruction is being carried out. Tissue expansion is a technique that reconstructive surgeons have employed for many years, and this relies on the viscoelastic properties of skin and soft tissues and is dependent upon cellular proliferation within the stretched tissues (40,41). In 1982, Radovan successfully applied the concept to postmastectomy breast reconstruction with the use of a silicone shell implant with an expandable saline component connected via a tube to a remote port. This port was placed in a subcutaneous pocket and allowed for percutaneous injection of saline at regular intervals to inflate the prosthesis thus expanding the overlying soft tissue. Since that time, although the concept has remained the same, the devices themselves have undergone numerous modifications. Current expanders for breast reconstruction are available with either remote or integrated ports and manufactured in both round and anatomical shapes. Those with integrated ports, such as the Natrelle™ 133 (usually a butterfly needle, size 19 or 21 French gauge) (formally McGhan® Style 133) and Mentor Siltex® Contour Profile® Breast Expanders Style 6100, 6200, 6300, have a metallic backing at the port site. Hence when the patient attends the clinic, the port can be readily located by means of a magnet and a small cannula (usually a size 19 or 21G butterfly needle) accurately placed prior to expansion.

Nowadays, tissue expanders and fixed-volume implants are available in different shapes and sizes and, specific to breast surgery, these are round or 'tear-drop' shaped (bio-dimensional/anatomical/contour profile) prostheses. These latter anatomical prostheses have more volume in the inferior portion, which leads to better projection in the lower pole of the breast. The upper portion of the prosthesis is much thinner and hence the patient has a more natural looking upper pole (excessive fullness of the upper pole is often associated with the use of round expanders or implants) (3, 32).

Despite being the simplest method for breast reconstruction, implants by virtue of being prosthetic carry inherent risks (Table 51.2), which include infection and extrusion. The importance of a well-vascularized, healthy soft tissue and skin envelope is crucial to promote primary wound healing and minimize the risk of extrusion. Periprosthetic infection is disastrous for implant-based reconstruction and usually necessitates removal of the prosthesis. After some months of healing, reimplantation can be undertaken (>6 months later) once

the tissues have settled. Careful planning and a meticulous operative technique, which limits the dissection of the implant pocket to the predetermined breast borders, will minimize the risk of incorrect implant placement. Moreover, a pocket that is just large enough to accommodate the implant will reduce the chance of in-situ implant rotation or displacement.

Capsular Contracture and the Effect of Radiotherapy on Implant-Based Reconstruction

After placement of a breast prosthesis, the body will mount a tissue reaction to it, as it is a foreign object. This results in a thin layer of scar-like tissue forming around the prosthesis, known as a capsule. In most patients, this remains as a thin layer that is neither palpable nor visible. However, in others the capsule thickens and contracts for reasons that are not entirely clear. This results in worsening degrees of capsular contracture, which Baker originally divided into four grades depending on clinical firmness of the breast following cosmetic augmentation. The Baker classification has been modified by Spear to include breast reconstruction (42), and a commonly used version is based on clinical assessment of the breast capsule, as follows:

(I) impalpable, not visible;
(II) palpable, not visible;
(III) palpable and visible; and
(IV) causing symptoms, such as pain, often associated with visible distortion of the breast.

Severe capsular contracture (grade III/IV) typically requires revisional surgery in the form of capsulectomy and implant exchange.

The reasons for development of severe capsular contracture in patients with breast implants have not been fully elucidated. However, the incidence appears to be influenced by pocket location (submuscular placement is associated with lower rates) and implant surface (textured implants have lower rates compared with smooth implants) (43,44). Furthermore, subclinical infection and hematoma formation have also been implicated as causative factors, and most notably in breast reconstruction significantly increased rates are seen in patients receiving external beam radiotherapy as part of cancer treatment. In the authors' unit, a review of patients having immediate prosthesis-based breast reconstructions suggested a 30% incidence of severe (grade III/IV) capsular contracture at 5 years in patients undergoing postoperative radiotherapy compared with those without radiotherapy for whom the incidence of severe capsular contracture was zero (45). These risks need to be discussed with patients who are likely to require postoperative radiotherapy (e.g., those with locally advanced or aggressive tumors or those at a risk of local or regional recurrence following mastectomy), and close liaison with the oncologist and breast surgeon is essential. In such patients, it is often more appropriate to avoid an implant-based reconstruction and instead carry out an immediate reconstruction using autologous flaps. If none of these are suitable or acceptable to patients, a delayed reconstruction is preferable.

Similarly, preoperative radiotherapy can have deleterious effects on the native tissues of the breast with induction of perivascular inflammation leading to endarteritis obliterans in the skin and soft tissues. This results in reduced tissue vascularity and is associated with high rates of complications such

Table 51.4 Indications/Advantages of Autologous Tissue Reconstruction

Patient choice
Large or ptotic breasts
Adjuvant radiotherapy is planned: can tolerate postoperative radiotherapy
Previous radiotherapy
Best possible cosmetic result is demanded by the patient
Most durable and natural
Best cosmesis
No artificial materials

Table 51.5 Main Types of Autologous Tissue Reconstruction

Latissimus dorsi myocutaneous flap
Abdominal flaps
   Pedicled transverse rectus abdominis myocutaneous (TRAM) flap
   Free TRAM flap
   Deep inferior epigastric artery perforator (DIEP) flap
   Superficial inferior epigastric artery (SIEA) flap
Gluteal flaps
   Superior gluteal myocutaneous flap
   Inferior gluteal myocutaneous flap
   Superior gluteal artery perforator (SGAP) flap
   Inferior gluteal artery perforator (IGAP) flap
Taylor-Ruben's peri-iliac flap
Thigh flaps
   Transverse upper/myocutaneous gracilis flap (TUG/TMG)
   Lateral transverse thigh flap
   Anterolateral thigh (ALT) flap

as poor wound healing, skin necrosis, infection, and implant extrusion (46,47). For these reasons, the use of implants in patients who have had previous radiotherapy may not be appropriate, unless supplemented by autologous flaps, such as the LD myocutaneous flap, which will bring in healthy, well-vascularized tissue to aid primary healing, and these discussions must be had with patients before choosing the mode of reconstruction. In previously irradiated patients undergoing implant-based reconstruction, it is important that the expander is minimally filled at surgery and the inflation protocol is more protracted (start later, i.e., at 3 weeks, and inflate with small volumes and less frequently).

AUTOLOGOUS TISSUE BREAST RECONSTRUCTION

The main indications for autologous tissue breast reconstruction are listed in Table 51.4, most of which are relative. Autologous tissue is generally more durable than prosthetic material and results in a more natural looking breast. The use of autologous tissue provides opportunity to avoid artificial materials. Furthermore, they provide versatility in creating ptosis, the anterior axillary fold, lateral fullness, and filling out the infraclavicular hollow. These aspects of breast reconstruction are much less likely to be achieved with a prosthesis-based reconstruction.

The critical issues in selecting one technique (Table 51.5) over another are beyond the scope of this chapter but briefly include (*i*) patient's choice, (*ii*) availability of donor tissues (patient body habitus), (*iii*) recovery period, (*iv*) likely requirement for adjuvant radiotherapy, (*v*) the presence of previous scars, and finally, (*vi*) the surgeon's experience and preference. Implant-based reconstructions should generally be avoided in patients for whom radiotherapy is planned (45).

THE LD MYOCUTANEOUS FLAP

The LD is a large flat muscle that has a proximal attachment (insertion) to the floor of the bicipital groove of the humerus and has distal attachments (origins) to the angle of the scapula, spinous processes of lower thoracic vertebrae and integrates with the lumbar fascia at the level of the posterior iliac crest. The vascular pedicle is the thoracodorsal vessels from the subscapular axis, and this enters the muscle 8 cm (roughly a hand's breadth) below the axilla. During flap harvest, it is essential to be conversant with the vascular anatomy of this area to ensure flap viability. This is also of particular importance when the patient is undergoing, or has undergone, axillary dissection, as the thoracodorsal vessels are encountered in this surgery. This is also of relevance to immediate reconstruction in the lateral position when the flap is being harvested with the patient on their side. Under these circumstances, some reconstructive surgeons themselves identify it for the ablative surgeon.

When designing an LD flap, a skin paddle needs to be harvested with the muscle. For immediate reconstruction following skin-sparing mastectomy with a periareolar incision, this will reconstruct the area where the NAC has been removed. In the case of a delayed reconstruction (Figure 51.4B), a larger skin paddle is required. Various designs of skin paddle have been described, but the authors prefer to draw a transverse skin paddle at such a location where there is sufficient skin excess so that tension-free primary closure can be achieved. It is preferable to place the resultant scar in the brassiere line (as shown in Figs. 51.4A and 51.4B), with the aim that it will be concealed when the patient is wearing a brassiere or swimwear. In delayed reconstruction where a large skin paddle is needed, or in a totally autologous LD reconstruction, the skin paddle is orientated obliquely in the crease line in order to allow a wider skin paddle to be harvested (maximum width of about 10 cm).

For immediate reconstruction (Figure 51.4A), it is possible to perform mastectomy and/or axillary clearance at the same time as the flap is being raised, with the patient placed in the lateral decubitus position. If a skin-sparing mastectomy is being undertaken, a small skin paddle on the LD muscle will be required to reconstruct the skin defect in the breast envelope. Careful planning is required to ensure the skin paddle of the flap is sited such that it will inset appropriately at the recipient site. Nonetheless, the exact position may be less critical when division of the LD tendon is carried out, which allows greater flexibility in terms of flap positioning and inset. In the case of a delayed reconstruction (Fig. 51.4B), a larger skin paddle is required, the length of which should approximate to the width of the breast to be reconstructed. The vertical width of the skin paddle should not be excessive and allow primary closure of the back wound. Although a larger skin paddle will be required in a delayed reconstruction, skin from the back alone may be insufficient to fully reconstruct the breast skin envelope. In these circumstances, the skin can be further increased in extent by the use of a tissue expander. In contrast, in immediate reconstruction, a fixed volume (standard) implant may sometimes be used.

In the case of delayed reconstruction, the mastectomy scar on the anterior chest will need to be excised with elevation

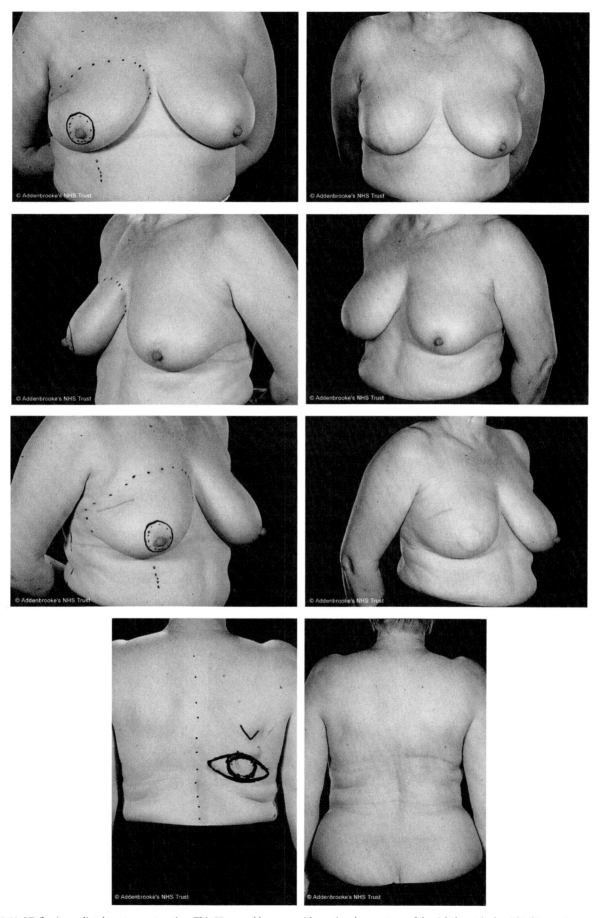

Figure 51.4A LD flap immediate breast reconstruction: This 57-year-old woman with previous lumpectomy of the right breast had a right skin-sparing mastectomy for DCIS with immediate reconstruction with an LD flap and expandable implant. She later declined nipple reconstruction. The LD skin paddle is orientated horizontally so as to leave a scar that can be hidden in the brassiere line. Note the moderately large-sized and ptotic breasts that were successfully reconstructed with this technique. *Abbreviations*: DCIS, Ductal carcinoma *in situ*; LD, Latissimus dorsi.

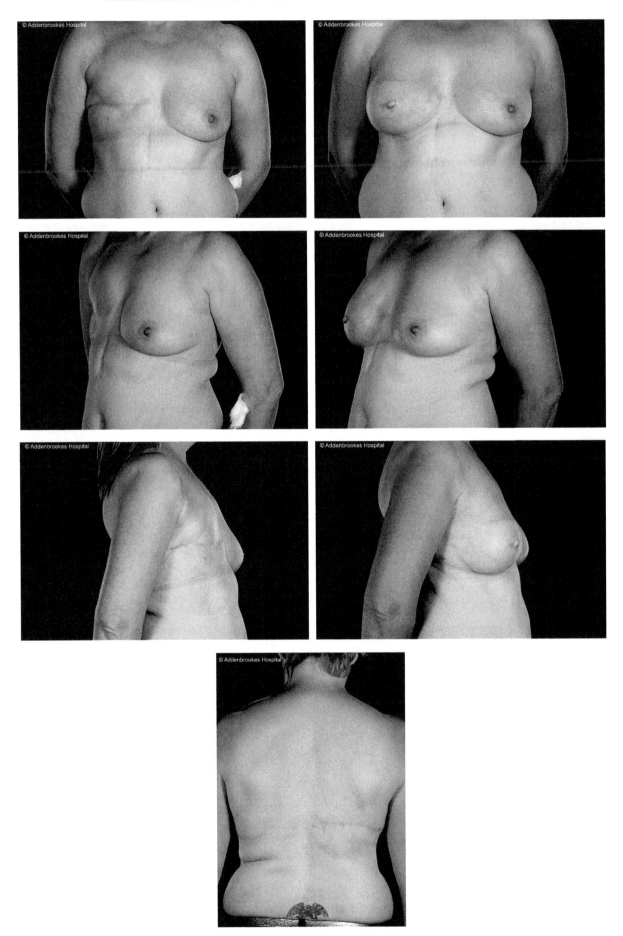

Figure 51.4B LD flap delayed breast reconstruction: A 48-year-old woman who underwent a delayed reconstruction of the right breast with an LD myocutaneous flap and tissue expander, 12 months after her mastectomy. The delayed option requires a larger skin paddle to be harvested, as shown in this patient. The downside of delayed breast reconstruction with autologous flaps is the obvious patch effect. *Abbreviation*: LD, Latissimus dorsi.

of mastectomy flaps such that a pocket is surgically created to allow inset of the flap. The LD flap is transferred to the site of the mastectomy defect through a subcutaneous tunnel high in the axilla, and care must be taken to ensure the vascular pedicle is not placed under any tension, kinked, twisted or avulsed during this maneuver (48). Adequate perfusion of the flap should be checked at this stage. Transposition of the flap can be aided by dividing the proximal tendinous attachment, and this allows for greater flexibility in movement and inset of the flap (49) and possibly improved cosmetic results (50).

A standard LD myocutaneous flap alone will generally not provide sufficient tissue to completely reconstruct the volume deficit following the mastectomy. There are two ways in which satisfactory volume replacement can be achieved. First, a "total autologous" or "extended" LD flap can be used (51,52). Six areas of fat are potentially available to safely harvest with the LD flap, but this extended technique is only suitable for selected patients. These fatty zones are as follows:

1. Fat deep to the skin paddle
2. A layer of fat below the superficial (Scarpa's) fascia covering the entire surface of the muscle
3. Suprascapular fat
4. Fat adjacent to the anterior edge of the flap
5. Suprailiac fat (so-called love handles)
6. Fat on the deep surface of the muscle.

This technique is suitable for patients who have an excess of adipose tissue in the region of the back but is very much dependent on individual body habitus.

The method for additional volume replacement that is most commonly used, however, is to supplement the LD flap with a prosthesis—an implant-assisted LD flap. Once the flap is transposed and the LD muscle has been inset to the periphery of the predetermined breast borders, the prosthesis (expander or implant) is placed deep to it. In the case of an immediate reconstruction of a small breast, this can be achieved using a fixed-volume implant. In the case of delayed reconstruction or immediate reconstruction of a larger breast, tissue expansion may be required and similar principles to implant-only reconstruction with tissue expanders or expandable implants apply. The volume of an LD flap based reconstruction can also be increased by the use of fat injections (performed either at the same time or later) (53).

Vascular compromise or total failure of an LD flap is very unusual. If it does occur, it may be due to unrecognized injury to the vascular pedicle, excessive tension on the pedicle, or inadvertent twisting/kinking. Hence careful transposition of the flap from the back to the anterior chest wall, ensuring the pedicle is lying tension free without any twists or kinks, is essential to minimize these potential problems. The tunnel must be adequate and must not have a "sharp" edge over which the pedicle may be stretched or kinked. Sometimes if an expander filled with saline has been used, the pressure of the filled prosthesis may be sufficient to produce external pressure on the flap's pedicle. This can be relieved by removing fluid from the injection port in the immediate or early postoperative period.

One of the more common sequelae of LD flap harvest is the potential space that is left behind at the donor site; it is not uncommon for patients to develop seromas that require serial needle aspiration postoperatively. The use of suction drains may reduce the incidence of seroma formation to some degree, and other measures such as quilting of the donor site at the time of wound closure may also help (54).

Limitations of shoulder function following LD flap breast reconstructions are reported, but early postoperative physiotherapy can help minimize these functional problems (55). Although certain groups of patients rely on the function of the LD muscle (such as wheelchair-bound patients or those who undertake activities such as rock climbing (56)), for the majority of patients, the remaining stabilizing muscles are sufficient to avoid any compromise in shoulder function. However, these factors must be borne in mind when counseling the young, physically active female patient who is being considered for breast reconstruction. These effects may be compounded when undergoing a bilateral LD-based reconstruction, leading to a synergistic deficit in function (57).

Overall, the LD muscle is an extremely reliable flap for breast reconstruction with an anatomically consistent, robust blood supply and a low incidence of significant long-term donor site morbidities. It is useful in the setting of both immediate and delayed breast reconstruction. As often used in conjunction with a prosthesis, the LD flap provides total muscular coverage of the implant, which is effectively sandwiched between two well-vascularized muscles, namely the pectoralis major below and the LD muscle above. This anatomical arrangement maximizes the opportunity for primary wound healing. and possibly reduces capsular contracture rates.

ABDOMINAL FLAPS
Abdominal pedicled and free flaps are based on blood vessels that supply the rectus abdominis muscles and the overlying adipocutaneous tissue. In addition to this, the lower abdominal skin and fat also receive blood supply from the superficial inferior epigastric (SIE) system, which derives from the femoral vessels.

The rectus abdominis muscles are a paired set of muscles that are vertically oriented either side of the midline, from the xiphisternum to pubis. The rectus abdominis muscle has a dual blood supply. Superiorly this is from the superior epigastric artery (a continuation of the internal thoracic artery) and inferiorly from the deep inferior epigastric (DIE) artery, a branch of the external iliac artery. These vessels enter the deep surface of the muscle, and their terminal branches anastomose with each other. From these deeper vessels, small perforating blood vessels traverse the rectus abdominis muscle and enter the overlying skin and adipose tissue, creating a network of vessels that connect across the anterior abdominal wall. An understanding of this intricate vascular network is essential in the planning and execution of the TRAM, SIEA and DIEP flaps.

The Pedicled TRAM Flap
The pedicled TRAM flap (13) is based on the superior epigastric vessels and uses a transverse adipocutaneous paddle (as would be removed during an abdominoplasty) attached to the rectus muscle to recreate the breast. Once raised, the flap is passed through a subcutaneous tunnel in the hypogastrium to the breast and inset into the mastectomy defect (Fig. 51.5A). It is important to position the muscle pedicle carefully without kinking it. Since its original description, the pedicled TRAM flap has been associated with significant complications, both at donor

and at recipient sites. At the donor site, removal of one of the rectus abdominis muscles and its attached rectus sheath leaves a defect that typically requires a synthetic mesh to reestablish the integrity of the anterior abdominal wall. This carries the inherent risk of hernia formation, but with meticulous technique during inset of the mesh and closure of the abdominal donor site, the development of bulges and herniae can be reduced and any functional compromise minimized (58). At the site of the flap inset, partial flap necrosis in the early postoperative period has been described, while late fat necrosis tends to occur at the periphery of flaps in those areas farthest away from the vascular pedicle (59). These areas of fat necrosis lead to suboptimal final results (60).

The Free TRAM and DIEP Flaps

Improvements in abdominal flap breast reconstruction came about with realization that the adipocutaneous component of the TRAM flap was better perfused by the perforating vessels that arise from branches of the deep inferior epigastric (DIE) vessels. A flap based on these vessels, however, necessitates the use of microsurgery to vessels at the recipient site. This refinement of the TRAM flap had a steep learning curve but successful free flap transfer resulted in improved outcomes at the recipient site (Fig. 51.5A). Nonetheless, a free TRAM flap still harvests a portion of the rectus abdominis and rectus sheath with continued risk of donor site problems. Further refinements came with improved understanding of the anatomy of DIE perforators, and how the flap could be raised as an adipocutaneous unit with only a small amount of muscle (the so-called MS TRAM flap) (24) or even without the need to sacrifice any of the rectus muscle or rectus sheath at all (DIEP flap) (Figs. 51.5B–C) (21,22). It should be noted that even if the muscle bellies are left intact, the nerve supply to the rectus abdominis muscle must be protected to minimize functional loss.

When dissecting the perforators through the rectus abdominis muscle, often a split in the muscle along the line of its fibers is all that is necessary to visualize and further dissect the perforators. However, anatomy of these perforating vessels is variable. The DIE vessels can have one of three arrangements (61). Most commonly, the vessel divides into medial and lateral trunks and perforators arise from these. Lateral row perforators tend to have a shorter, more vertical route through the muscle, whereas medial row perforators (although often of a larger caliber) tend to have a more oblique and longer intramuscular course, necessitating more dissection. The other two anatomic variations are the presence of only one trunk or existence of three trunks. Regardless of type, these trunks gradually decrease in size as they travel superiorly and will eventually anastomose with branches of the superior epigastric system.

Once the perforators are identified, dissection will proceed in an inferior direction, and the main trunks will be followed back to the DIE vessels. After the recipient site vessels have been prepared, the DIE artery and vein can be ligated and divided prior to reanastomosis at the recipient site mastectomy defect.

From the surgical viewpoint, the transverse ellipse of skin and fat that makes up the flap is divided into four zones as originally described by Hartrampf, although this classification has been subsequently modified following emergence of the DIEP flap (62). The area overlying the pedicle is termed zone 1,

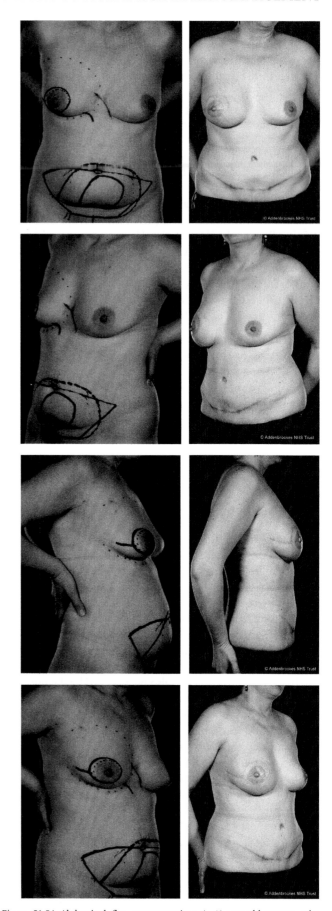

Figure 51.5A Abdominal flap reconstruction: A 41-year-old woman who underwent a right-sided skin-sparing mastectomy with immediate left pedicled TRAM flap reconstruction of the right breast. The position of the subcutaneous epigastric tunnel is shown between her breasts in the preoperative images. The tumor dictated a large skin resection and replacement, hence the target-like appearance of the right breast following nipple-areolar reconstruction. *Abbreviation*: TRAM, transverse rectus abdominis myocutaneous.

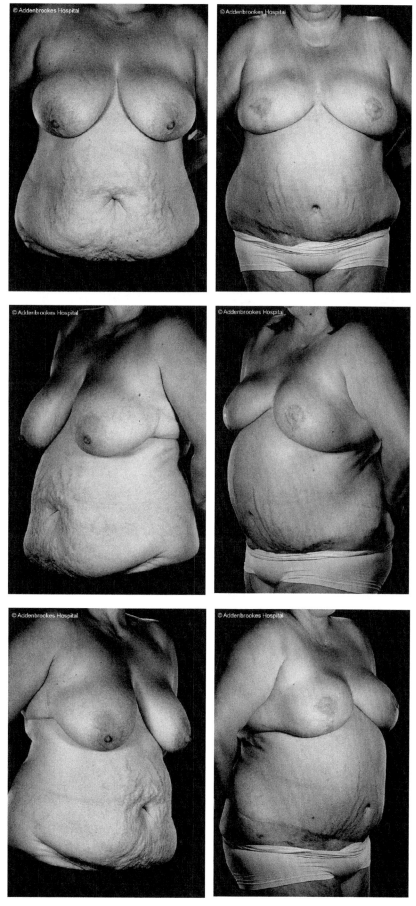

Figure 51.5B Abdominal flap immediate breast reconstruction: A 49-year-old woman with Cowden's syndrome and large ptotic breasts elected to proceed with bilateral risk-reducing mastectomies, which were performed using the Lejour skin reduction pattern and reconstructed using a DIEP flap for the right breast and an SIEA flap for the left breast. The postoperative breast mounds show an improvement in appearance, mimicking an esthetic breast procedure, without sacrificing breast volume or symmetry. *Abbreviations*: DIEP, deep inferior epigastric perforator; SIEA, superficial inferior epigastric artery.

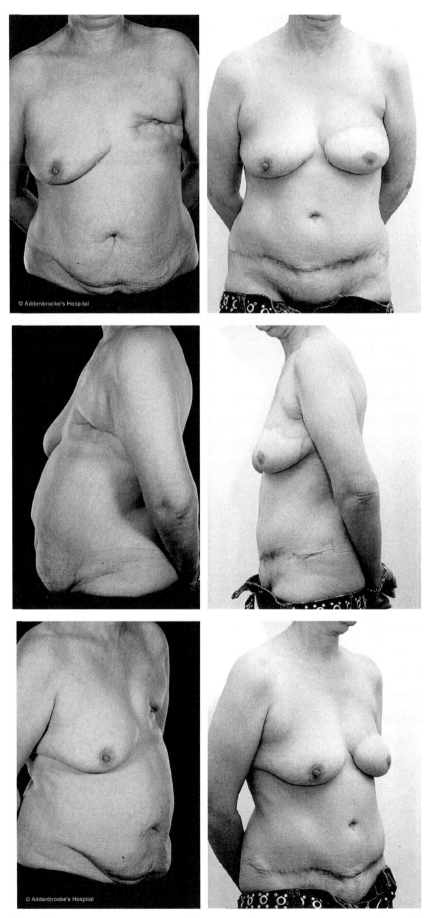

Figure 51.5C Abdominal flap delayed breast reconstruction: A 58-year-old woman with a severe postmastectomy and postradiation deformity presented for delayed breast reconstruction. Despite the small breast volume, she declined implant-based reconstructions. She therefore underwent a free DIEP flap to the left breast with excellent cosmesis. The abdominal flap was able to restore the chest contour and addressed the large skin deficit. Postoperative results after NAC tattoo. *Abbreviations*: DIEP, deep inferior epigastric perforator; NAC, nipple-areola complex.

whereas the zone farthest away from the pedicle is zone 4. The areas of the flap nearest to the pedicle are often best vascularized, usually some or all of zone 4 has to be discarded as it will be relatively poorly vascularized in comparison. Depending on which specific perforators are chosen to base the flap on, be it lateral or medial rows, zones 2 and 3 are either ipsilateral or across the midline, respectively. Therefore the nomenclature is interchangeable depending on the precise vascular anatomy of the flap.

The free TRAM and DIEP flaps utilize the same abdominal tissue as used in Hartrampf's original pedicled TRAM flap, which corresponds to the tissue that is removed during an abdominoplasty or apronectomy operation. Hence if a patient has undergone either of these procedures in the past, this precludes a free TRAM/DIEP flap. Furthermore, if there has been any previously documented injury to the DIE vessels, then likewise this flap should not be attempted. If such an injury is suspected (e.g., from previous trauma or surgery), it may be pertinent to undertake radiological imaging of these vessels even though successful flap harvest is possible in patients with pre-existing abdominal scars (63,64). In fact, because of the variability of the specific DIE perforators, many surgeons choose to routinely carry out radiological imaging of the DIE and its perforators prior to surgery. Not only does this confirm the presence of the main trunks but also provides a roadmap of the perforators, which allows judgment on which are the best perforators to be utilized in the flap. This can be done using one of the several imaging modalities—duplex sonography, CT, or MR angiography (65).

The Superficial Inferior Epigastric Artery Flap

In some cases, especially those in which only half of the abdominal tissue is required, a flap based on the superficial inferior epigastric (SIE) vessels can be raised (66,67). The SIE vessels typically supply the ipsilateral skin and fat only and therefore flaps based solely on these vessels cannot reliably cross the midline (68). However, the caliber of these vessels, in particular the superficial inferior epigastric artery (SIEA), is highly variable and often of insufficient size to be reliably dissected. Indeed, anatomic and clinical reviews suggest that the artery is useable in fewer than 50% of dissections (17,69). In those patients where a sizable or prominent SIEA and vein are identified during flap harvest surgery, the flap can be raised without disruption of the rectus sheath (Fig. 51.5B), but it must be remembered that vascularity across the midline is not guaranteed, and consequently only half of the lower abdominal skin and fat can be safely harvested. The limiting factor from a technical viewpoint is the size of the artery; if it is pulsatile and clearly visible without (surgical) loupe magnification, it is possible to harvest the flap. It is the senior author's practice to look for the SIE vessels in every patient undergoing lower abdominal flap breast reconstruction in case the artery is large enough to support a flap. However, an SIE artery flap is not formally planned at the outset, except in patients who have lost significant amounts of weight (70).

The SIE vein can also prove useful if present and can be dissected to provide additional venous drainage for a TRAM or DIEP flap. Therefore, routine preservation of the SIE vein is recommended (71).

ALTERNATIVE FREE FLAP RECONSTRUCTIONS

If a patient declines a prosthesis-based reconstruction, and it is decided to proceed with a flap-based reconstruction, there will be instances where the first choice of an abdominal free flap is not available or tissue volume is insufficient for the size of reconstruction required. In these circumstances, alternative donor sites can be considered.

Flaps raised from the buttock area are based on blood supply from the superior and inferior gluteal vessels. Before development of the perforator concept, these flaps were raised as musculocutaneous units, taking portions of the gluteus maximus muscle with it (72,73). This can potentially result in morbidity at the donor site, which might be manifest as problems with gait, for example. However, the main problem with the gluteal myocutaneous flaps was the reach of the pedicle. It was shortened by the presence of muscle and often vein grafts were needed (72,73). The shorter vascular pedicles also hindered flap inset as the recipient site routinely used at that time was the thoracodorsal vessels. When raised as perforator flaps, there is no muscle to sacrifice with consequent advantages of fewer donor problems and longer pedicles. The superior gluteal artery perforator (SGAP) flap harvests tissue from the upper part of the buttock (74), whereas the inferior gluteal artery perforator (IGAP) flap uses tissue from the lower buttock (75). The IGAP flap is often preferred because of better scarring and lower donor site deficit. With particular regard to the reconstruction, buttock tissue tends to be firmer than abdominal tissue, and although providing more projection than a DIEP/TRAM flap, the tissue is more difficult to shape. At the donor site, the SGAP flap leaves a conspicuous scar across the upper buttock and can leave a flattened or depressed contour. In contrast, the IGAP flap can be harvested in such a way so that the donor scar is placed in the lower gluteal crease (75). Criticisms of gluteal flaps include difficulty in simultaneously harvesting the flap and performing mastectomy for immediate reconstruction due to patient positioning, difficult perforator dissection, constrained flap inset and potential buttock asymmetry.

If a patient's body habitus is such that they have minimal abdominal or buttock tissue, an alternative flap option is the transverse upper/myocutaneous gracilis flap (76,77), which utilizes adipocutaneous tissue from the upper medial thigh and the gracilis muscle. The gracilis is a thin, long muscle in the adductor compartment of the thigh whose arterial supply arises from the adductor artery, a branch of the profunda femoris. Harvest of the muscle leaves minimal donor site morbidity. This flap is particularly useful when carrying out reconstruction of a small breast, although problems with donor site healing are reported (78).

MISCELLANEOUS ASPECTS OF BREAST RECONSTRUCTION

Free Flap Microsurgery

Recipient Vessels

The authors' preferred choice for recipient vessels in free tissue breast reconstruction is the internal thoracic (internal mammary) vessels. The traditional technique for preparing these recipient vessels is to remove the third costal cartilage and prepare the vessels between the second and fourth costal cartilages (79,80). However, a cartilage-sparing approach is preferred (81), and the vessels can be prepared without excising any costal cartilage (82).

If the internal thoracic vessels are not available, options include the thoracodorsal or circumflex scapular vessels in the axilla and indeed these are the vessels of choice for many reconstructive surgeons (83,84). The disadvantage is that microsurgery has to be performed in the axillary region and hence an adequate length of pedicle is required. If the pedicle is short, as in a SIE artery flap, the thoracodorsal vessels may not be appropriate; however, with DIEP flaps, pedicle length is not an issue and microsurgery can be carried out at either recipient location.

Perioperative Management

Successful free flap breast reconstruction is not only reliant on factors associated with surgery per se, but careful preparation of patients and postoperative management are essential. Surgery involves prolonged general anaesthesia, and hence a patient's comorbidities and their suitability for a free flap procedure must be assessed. Flap planning involves selecting the most appropriate flap for individual patients, and adjuncts such as the handheld Doppler, duplex sonography, or angiography (CT/MRI) can be used to evaluate perforating vessels in the flap being planned.

Intraoperatively, careful dissection and meticulous tissue handling are necessary to avoid mechanical and thermal damage to the delicate blood vessels that will perfuse the flap. Once raised, microsurgery to reanastomose the flap's pedicle to recipient vessels must be undertaken with a precise technique to ensure successful flap perfusion. A suboptimal microsurgical technique will encourage thrombus formation at the site of the anastomosis, which can lead to flap failure.

Postoperatively, these patients must be nursed in heated rooms (>70°F) and be kept well hydrated (to ensure maximal perfusion of the flap) and also pain free to minimize sympathetically driven vasoconstriction. Regular assessment with accurate recording of respiratory and hemodynamic parameters is essential for optimal recovery; oxygen saturation, respiratory rate, pulse rate, systemic blood pressure, temperature, and hourly urine output measurements must all be recorded. Any deviation from normal values or changes in trends should be identified and acted upon promptly. An accurate, noninvasive measure of fluid balance in patients undergoing free flap surgery is urine output, which should be a minimum level of 0.5–1 ml/kg/hr to maintain hyperdynamic circulation within the flap.

Free Flap Monitoring

Monitoring perfusion of the free flap is absolutely vital for early detection of any signs that indicate a failing flap. Clinical assessment is one of the most accurate and reliable methods but must be carried out by trained nursing staff. Clinical signs that are readily assessable on inspection include the color and capillary refill times. Palpation of the flap will allow assessment of temperature and turgor as well as the presence of swelling or hematoma, either of which could cause external compression of the flap's pedicle, especially the vein. As these flaps contain perforating vessels that reach the skin, clinical assessment can be supplemented by the use of a handheld Doppler probe to auscultate arterial and venous signals from the perforators.

The skin paddle of a healthy flap will be of normal color (relative to donor site skin), be soft and warm to the touch, and have a capillary refill time of approximately 2 seconds. By contrast, a pale, flaccid skin paddle with a delayed capillary refill time and which fails to bleed if scratched with a needle suggests impaired arterial inflow. A problem with the venous outflow may be evident from a mottled appearance, swelling, and increased turgor in the presence of a brisk capillary refill time. When scratched, a flap with a venous congestion will rapidly ooze dark blood. A common cause for flap congestion is external compression of the pedicle vein by hematoma. Tight dressings may also contribute to external compression of the pedicle, and the initial maneuver is to release dressings and sutures, which may provide relief. Any suspicion of a failing flap should prompt immediate surgical exploration to maximize the chance of salvage. The patient must return to the operating theater without delay for examination of the micro-anastomoses and flap pedicle. If necessary, the microsurgical anastomoses will need to be redone, and the earlier this intervention is carried out, the higher is the chance of the flap surviving.

Free flap failure is generally uncommon with the latest figures from the United Kingdom (UK) National Mastectomy and Breast Reconstruction Audit (2), suggesting that the national rate for complete flap failure is 2%. To maximize success rates with this surgery, it should only be undertaken in units well rehearsed in the care of these patients, where microsurgery is carried out on a regular basis and where systems are in place to identify and manage postoperative problems quickly and efficiently.

Acellular Dermal Matrices (ADMs)

In patients with moderately large breasts or those with poor soft tissue coverage, an alternative to using a LD flap with a prosthesis is to use an Acellular Dermal Matrix (ADM), such as Alloderm® Regenerative Tissue Matrix (RTM) or Strattice™ Reconstructive Tissue Matrix, human- and porcine-derived biosynthetic materials respectively." (Fig. 51.5) (85–87).

These materials can be used to provide coverage and support to the lower pole of the breast prosthesis. By creating a pocket underneath the pectoralis major (starting from its lateral edge rather than splitting the muscle as mentioned above), the superomedial part of the prosthesis will be covered. Instead of elevating some of the serratus anterior fascia or muscle to provide inferolateral coverage of the prosthesis, the ADM can be sutured to the periphery of the defect in this lower pole and acts as a sling to cover and provide support and coverage for the prosthesis. The other edge of the ADM sheet is sutured to the free lateral edge of the pectoralis major muscle, thereby totally covering the prosthesis. The material acts as a scaffold into which there is vascular ingrowth, shown experimentally (88) and clinically (89), and with time the material is said to incorporate with the native tissue. The advantage over trying to achieve total submuscular coverage under serratus inferolaterally is that the breast can have a more natural, ptotic appearance and the projection will not be constrained by a submuscular pocket, which would otherwise lack ptosis and projection. However, the material is thinner than muscle and is initially avascular, requiring time for the vascular in growth. The significant cost associated with these products also needs to be factored into decision making.

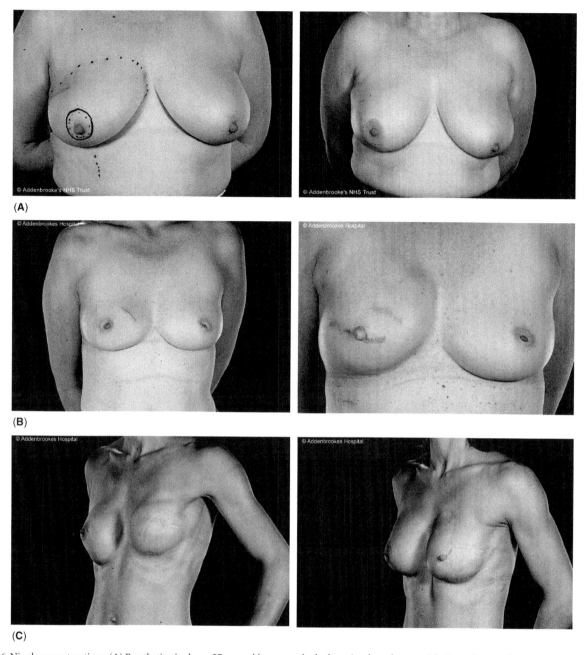

Figure 51.6 Nipple reconstructions: (A) Prosthetic nipple—a 57-year-old woman who had previously undergone right immediate LD flap and expandable implant reconstruction. (B) C-V flap nipple reconstruction—Pre- and postoperative images of a 49-year-old woman following C-V flap nipple reconstruction undertaken 6 months after her initial implant-only breast mound reconstruction. No adjuvant radiotherapy was needed. (C) Double-opposing tabs method of nipple reconstruction—a 39-year-old patient was referred to the Cambridge Breast Unit for a second opinion regarding management of local tumor recurrence. She required LD flap chest wall reconstruction and insisted on implant replacement and simultaneous contralateral revision breast augmentation. Nipple reconstruction was achieved with double-opposing tabs, an ideal solution for patients with high oblique scars. *Abbreviation*: LD, Latissimus dorsi.

The use of AlloDerm RTM (predominantly in United States) has raised the suggestion that it may have a protective effect on adverse capsular contracture (90) although a recent meta-analysis suggests that ADMs may be associated with higher complication rates overall compared with implant-only reconstruction (91). Further long-term outcome reports are awaited.

This option may prove useful in those patients who do not want a complex free flap procedure and want to avoid harvest of the LD muscle. It combines the relative simplicity of an implant-only reconstruction but allows for total coverage of the prosthesis and encourages a more natural-looking implant-based reconstruction. Its place in breast reconstruction has yet to be established.

NAC Reconstruction

Often the final stage in breast reconstruction is NAC. As an alternative to a prosthetic nipple (Fig. 51.6A), reconstruction of the NAC can be carried out surgically with autologous grafts or local flaps.

Some surgeons will prefer to undertake this as part of the breast reconstruction procedure; the main advantage of this approach being that it reduces the overall number of surgical

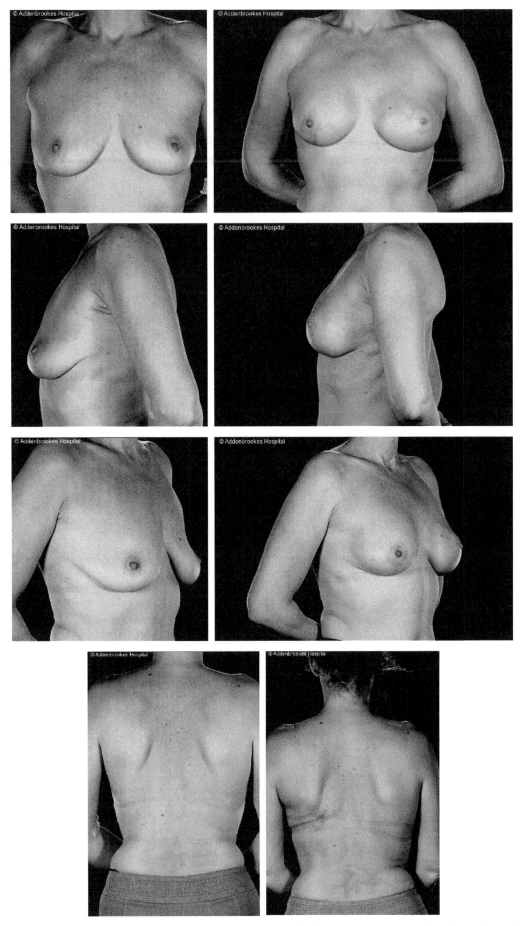

Figure 51.7 Contralateral balancing surgery: This 50-year-old woman underwent a left Lejour pattern mastectomy for DCIS and immediate reconstruction with an LD flap and expandable implant and a simultaneous contralateral balancing Lejour augmentation-mastopexy. Note that the postlactational atrophy has been corrected by implant augmentation of the contralateral breast to improve symmetry. The donor site scar is totally hidden when the patient is wearing a bra. *Abbreviations*: DCIS, Ductal carcinoma *in situ*; LD, Latissimus dorsi.

procedures that the patient must undergo. However, NAC reconstruction at the same time as the breast reconstruction should only be carried out if the reconstructive surgeon is confident on the location of the ideal position for the NAC. This may be possible in the case of immediate reconstruction following skin-sparing mastectomy (92).

In the authors' practice, NAC reconstruction is carried out once the primary reconstruction has settled into its final position and the patient has completed any adjuvant treatment. Autologous breast reconstructions tend to sit proud on the chest wall initially and over the subsequent months develop a degree of ptosis (encouraged by massaging) until they rest in what will ultimately be their natural position. It is at this time that NAC reconstruction can be positioned with confidence. This is usually 3 months postoperatively or more than 6 months if the patient has received adjuvant radiotherapy.

Nipple reconstruction can be carried out either by the use of local tissue flaps, such as the CV flap or double-opposing tabs (Figs. 51.6B, C), or by using free grafts (93). The CV flap technique is one of the commonly-used local flap procedures, and involves using a single C-shaped flap, and two V-shaped flaps (or modifications thereof) that are sutured to each other to create the nipple. Grafts can be harvested from the opposite nipple (if it is large enough) or other sites such as the earlobe and labia. Grafts rely on receiving blood supply and nutrition from the recipient bed and hence there is a risk of graft failure with this technique. Local flap techniques, on the other hand, are more reliable in terms of vascularity but are prone to shrinkage with time. Hence these should be made at least twice the predicted size of the eventual nipple to allow for this change.

Often the reconstructed breast skin is insensate and nipple reconstruction can be undertaken without anesthetic. However, if required, a solution containing lidocaine and adrenaline is the local anesthetic of choice.

Areolar reconstruction is often carried out with intradermal tattooing although some surgeons do use full-thickness skin grafts (e.g., from the inner thigh where the skin is often darker to mimic the darker pigmentation of the areola). If an autologous nipple reconstruction has been undertaken, it is sensible to wait for these surgical scars to heal before commencing tattooing (for a period of at least 3 months). Decisions regarding which pigment to use are made in conjunction with the patient, and for unilateral reconstruction, it is based on the color of the contralateral NAC. Intradermal tattooing is generally a safe procedure with a low risk of complications, but patients must be warned of the need for multiple sessions to achieve the final outcome; pigment retention and hence fading of color are highly variable and unpredictable (91). Any history of adverse reactions to tattoo pigment should be ascertained before starting this treatment.

The Contralateral Breast

Excellent results can be achieved for unilateral breast reconstruction, but as previously mentioned, the ultimate goal is to achieve symmetry with the contralateral breast. In some cases, depending on the size and volume of the contralateral breast, this may not be possible without carrying out a balancing procedure. If a patient is displeased with their breast size and/or shape prior to reconstructive surgery, balancing surgery can be planned either at the same time as the primary reconstruction or at a later date. Options for symmetrizing surgery include breast augmentation, breast reduction, or uplift (mastopexy) surgery to the contralateral breast.

Careful planning of contralateral surgery may facilitate ipsilateral reconstruction. For example, a patient with large breasts, who might otherwise benefit from reductional surgery, may be able to undergo contralateral reduction and hence require a smaller flap size overall. This would be particularly useful in the case of a patient having autologous flap reconstruction but with a relative paucity of tissue at the desired donor site. A patient with significant breast ptosis may desire an uplift, and skin-reducing mastectomy incisions could be used on the reconstructed side and a mastopexy (with matching skin incisions) carried out contralaterally.

Similarly, in patients with small breasts, the reconstruction can be planned to incorporate contralateral augmentation should the patient desire a larger breast size (Fig. 51.7). There are several advantages of simultaneous contralateral surgery at the time of the primary reconstructive procedure; patients have symmetrization carried out under a single general anesthetic; it avoids waiting for a second procedure and allows for supervised training in such procedures.

SUMMARY

The techniques available for postmastectomy breast reconstruction vary from comparatively simple implant-only–based reconstruction to complex microsurgical procedures utilizing the patient's own tissues. The decision on choice of procedure is dependent on many factors including the wishes and expectation of patients.

Early reconstructive procedures were limited in esthetic outcomes and often resulted in suboptimal appearance. An important factor that has led to improvement in cosmetic outcome is the evolution of techniques for extirpative surgery. The radical mastectomy of Halsted is rarely performed nowadays due to smaller tumor size at presentation and neoadjuvant therapies. Preservation of local musculature and much of the breast skin envelope has left the reconstructive surgeon with more native tissue at their disposal, and improvements in reconstructive techniques have permitted more esthetic and natural forms of breast reconstruction.

In the absence of radiotherapy, implant-based reconstruction can yield excellent results for smaller-breasted women and is acceptable to many. For the more challenging breast reconstruction involving larger, more ptotic breasts and when radiotherapy is anticipated, autologous flap-based techniques are more appropriate. Moreover, reconstruction using the patient's own tissues remains the current gold standard for breast reconstruction and is associated with superior cosmetic results that are maintained in the longer term.

ACKNOWLEDGMENTS

Siltex® Contour Profile® Becker 35 and Siltex® Contour Profile® Breast Expanders Style 6100, 6200, 6300—Mentor Corporation, a part of Johnson & Johnson. Natrelle™ 150 and Natrelle™ 133—Allergan, UK. Alloderm® Regenerative Tissue Matrix and Strattice™ Reconstructive Tissue Matrix—LifeCell Corporation, Branchburg, New Jersey, US.

REFERENCES

1. Cancer Research UK. http://info.cancerresearchuk.org/cancerstats/types/breast/incidence. [accessed on 22 October 2012.]
2. National Mastectomy and Breast Reconstruction Audit 2011, Fourth Annual Report. [Available from: http://www.ic.nhs.uk/services/national-clinical-audit-support-programme-ncasp/audit-reports/mastectomy-and-breast-reconstruction] [accessed on 22 October 2012.]
3. Hodgson EL, Malata CM. Implant-based breast reconstruction following mastectomy. Breast Dis 2002; 16: 47–63.
4. Goldwyn RM. Vincenz Czerny and the beginnings of breast reconstruction. Plast Reconstr Surg 1978; 61: 673–81.
5. Tansini I. Nuovo processo per l'amputazione della mammella per cancre. La Riforma Medica 1896; 12: 3. Reprinted in Langenbeck's Archiv fur Klinische Chirurgie 1896.
6. Maxwell GP. Iginio Tansini and the origin of the latissimus dorsi musculocutaneous flap. Plast Reconstr Surg 1980; 65: 686–92.
7. Olivari N. The latissimus flap. Br J Plast Surg 1976; 29: 126–8.
8. Schneider WJ, Hill HL, Brown RG. Latissimus dorsi myocutaneous flap for breast reconstruction. Br J Plast Surg 1977; 30: 277–81.
9. Bostwick J 3rd, Vasconez LO, Jurkiewicz MJ. Breast reconstruction after a radical mastectomy. Plast Reconstr Surg 1978; 61: 682–93.
10. Cronin TD, Gerow FJ. Augmentation mammoplasty: a new 'natural feel' prosthesis. In: Proceedings of the 3rd International Congress of Plastic Surgery. Washington DC. Excerpta Medica Int. Congr. Ser. Number 66. Amsterdam, Excerpta Medica Foundation, 1963. 41–9.
11. Radovan C. Breast reconstruction after mastectomy using the temporary expander. Plast Reconstr Surg 1982; 69: 195–208.
12. Orticochea M. Use of the buttock to reconstruct the breast. Br J Plast Surg 1973; 26: 304–9.
13. Hartrampf CR, Scheflan M, Black PW. Breast reconstruction with a transverse abdominal island flap. Plast Reconstr Surg 1982; 69: 216–25.
14. Holmström H. The free abdominoplasty flap and its use in breast reconstruction. An experimental study and clinical case report. Scand J Plast Surg 1979; 13: 423–7.
15. Paige KT, Bostwick J 3rd, Bried JT, Jones G. A comparison of morbidity from bilateral, unipedicled and unilateral, unipedicled TRAM flap breast reconstructions. Plast Reconstr Surg 1998; 101: 1819–27.
16. Zienowicz RJ, May JW Jr. Hernia prevention and aesthetic contouring of the abdomen following TRAM flap breast reconstruction by the use of polypropylene mesh. Plast Reconstr Surg 1995; 96: 1346–50.
17. Boyd JB, Taylor GI, Corlett R. The vascular territories of the superior epigastric and the deep inferior epigastric systems. Plast Reconstr Surg 1984; 73: 1–16.
18. El-Mrakby HH, Milner RH. The vascular anatomy of the lower anterior abdominal wall: a microdissection study on the deep inferior epigastric vessels and the perforator branches. Plast Reconstr Surg 2002; 109: 539–43.
19. Blondeel N, Vanderstraeten GG, Monstrey SJ, et al. The donor site morbidity of free DIEP flaps and free TRAM flaps for breast reconstruction. Br J Plast Surg 1997; 50: 322–30.
20. Koshima I, Soeda S. Inferior epigastric artery skin flaps without rectus abdominis muscle. Br J Plast Surg 1989; 42: 645–8.
21. Allen RJ, Treece P. Deep inferior epigastric perforator flap for breast reconstruction. Ann Plast Surg 1994; 32: 32–8.
22. Blondeel PN, Boeckx WD. Refinements in free flap breast reconstruction: the free bilateral deep inferior epigastric perforator flap anastomosed to the internal mammary artery. Br J Plast Surg 1994; 47: 495–501.
23. Weiler-Mithoff E, Hodgson EL, Malata CM. Perforator flap breast reconstruction. Breast Dis 2002; 16: 93–106.
24. Nahabedian MY, Tsangaris T, Momen B. Breast reconstruction with the DIEP flap or the muscle-sparing (MS-2) free TRAM flap: is there a difference? Plast Reconstr Surg 2005; 115: 436–44.
25. Elliott LF, Seify H, Bergey P. The 3-hour muscle-sparing free TRAM flap: safe and effective treatment review of 111 consecutive free TRAM flaps in a private practice setting. Plast Reconstr Surg 2007; 120: 27–34.
26. Malata CM, McIntosh SA, Purushotam AD. Immediate breast reconstruction after mastectomy for cancer: review. Br J Surg 2000; 87: 1455–72.
27. Toth BA, Lappert P. Modified skin incisions for mastectomy: the need for plastic surgical input in preoperative planning. Plast Reconstr Surg 1991; 87: 1048–53.
28. Cunnick GH, Mokbel K. Skin-sparing mastectomy. Am J Surg 2004; 188: 78–84.
29. Malata CM, Hodgson EL, Chikwe J, Canal AC, Purushotham AD. An application of the LeJour vertical mammaplasty pattern for skin-sparing mastectomy: a preliminary report. Ann Plast Surg 2003; 51: 345–50.
30. Cunnick GH, Mokbel K. Oncological considerations of skin-sparing mastectomy. Int Semin Surg Oncol 2006; 3: 14.
31. Azzawi K, Ismail A, Forouhi P, Earl H, Malata CM. Influence of neoadjuvant chemotherapy on outcomes of immediate breast reconstruction. Plastic & Reconstructive Surgery 2010; 126: 1–11. [accessed on 22 october 2012.]
32. American Society of Plastic Surgeons, Report of the 2010 Plastic Surgery Statistics. [Available from: http://www.plasticsurgery.org/Documents/news-resources/statistics/2010-statisticss/Patient-Ages/2010-reconstructive-demographics-breast-surgery-statistics.pdf] was accessed on 22 October 2012.
33. Spear SL, Spittler CJ. Breast reconstruction with implants and expanders. Plast Reconstr Surg 2001; 107: 177–87.
34. Mahdi S, Jones T, Nicklin S, McGeorge DD. Expandable anatomical implants in breast reconstructions: a prospective study. Br J Plast Surg 1998; 51: 425–30.
35. Hsieh F, Shah A, Malata CM. Experience with the Mentor Contour Profile Becker-35 expandable implants in reconstructive breast surgery. J Plast Reconstr Aesthet Surg 2010; 63: 1124–30.
36. Scuderi N, Alfano C, Campus GV, et al. Multicenter study on breast reconstruction outcome using Becker implants. Aesthetic Plast Surg 2011; 35: 66–72.
37. Gui GP, Tan SM, Faliakou EC, et al. Immediate breast reconstruction using biodimensional anatomical permanent expander implants: a prospective analysis of outcome and patient satisfaction. Plast Reconstr Surg 2003; 111: 125–38.
38. Losken A, Carlson GW, Bostwick J 3rd, et al. Trends in unilateral breast reconstruction and management of the contralateral breast: the Emory experience. Plast Reconstr Surg 2002; 110: 89–97.
39. Di Candia M, Lie KH, Forouhi P, Malata CM. Experience with the Wise mammaplasty skin resection pattern in skin-sparing mastectomy and immediate breast reconstruction for large breast volumes. Int J Surg 2011; 9: 41–5.
40. Mustoe TA, Bartell TH, Garner WL. Physical, biomechanical, histologic, and biochemical effects of rapid versus conventional tissue expansion. Plast Reconstr Surg 1989; 83: 687–91.
41. Malata CM, Williams NW, Sharpe DT. Tissue expansion: an overview. J Wound Care 1995; 4: 37–44.
42. Spear SL, Baker JL Jr. Classification of capsular contracture after prosthetic breast reconstruction. Plast Reconstr Surg 1995; 96: 1119–23.
43. Malata CM, Feldberg L, Coleman DJ, Foo IT, Sharpe DT. Textured or smooth implants for breast augmentation? Three year follow-up of a prospective randomised controlled trial. Br J Plast Surg 1997; 50: 99–105.
44. Hakelius L, Ohlsén L. Tendency to capsular contracture around smooth and textured gel-filled silicone mammary implants: a five-year follow-up. Plast Reconstr Surg 1997; 100: 1566–9.
45. Whitfield GA, Horan G, Irwin MS, et al. Incidence of severe capsular contracture following implant-based immediate breast reconstruction with or without postoperative chest wall radiotherapy using 40 Gray in 15 fractions. Radiother Oncol 2009; 90: 141–7.
46. Dickson MG, Sharpe DT. The complications of tissue expansion in breast reconstruction. A review of 75 cases. Br J Plast Surg 1987; 40: 629–35.
47. Nahabedian MY, Tsangaris T, Momen B, Manson PN. Infectious complications following breast reconstruction with expanders and implants. Plast Reconstr Surg 2003; 112: 467–76.
48. Martano A, Malata CM. Accidental latissimus dorsi flap pedicle avulsion during immediate breast reconstruction: salvage by conversion to free flap. J Plast Reconstr Aesthet Surg 2012; 65: 1107–10.
49. Hammond DC. Latissimus dorsi flap breast reconstruction. Plast Reconstr Surg 2009; 124: 1055–63.
50. Gerber B, Krause A, Reimer T, Müller H, Friese K. Breast reconstruction with latissimus dorsi flap: improved aesthetic results after transection of its humeral insertion. Plast Reconstr Surg 1999; 103: 1876–81.
51. Germann G, Steinau HU. Breast reconstruction with the extended latissimus dorsi flap. Plast Reconstr Surg 1996; 97: 519–26.
52. Delay E, Gounot N, Bouillot A, Zlatoff P, Rivoire M. Autologous latissimus breast reconstruction: a 3-year clinical experience with 100 patients. Plast Reconstr Surg 1998; 102: 1461–78.
53. Sinna R, Delay E, Garson S, Delaporte T, Toussoun G. Breast fat grafting (lipomodelling) after extended latissimus dorsi flap breast reconstruction:

A preliminary report of 200 consecutive cases. J Plast Reconstr Aesthet Surg 2010; 63: 1769–77.

54. Titley OG, Spyrou GE, Fatah MF. Preventing seroma in the latissimus dorsi flap donor site. Br J Plast Surg 1997; 50: 106–8.

55. Forthomme B, Heymans O, Jacquemin D, et al. Shoulder function after latissimus dorsi transfer in breast reconstruction. Clin Physiol Funct Imaging 2010; 30: 406–12.

56. Spear SL, Hess CL. A review of the biomechanical and functional changes in the shoulder following transfer of the latissimus dorsi muscles. Plast Reconstr Surg 2005; 115: 2070–3.

57. Losken A, Nicholas CS, Pinell XA, Carlson GW. Outcomes evaluation following bilateral breast reconstruction using latissimus dorsi myocutaneous flaps. Ann Plast Surg 2010; 65: 17–22.

58. Atisha D, Alderman AK. A systematic review of abdominal wall function following abdominal flaps for postmastectomy breast reconstruction. Ann Plast Surg 2009; 63: 222–30.

59. Kroll SS, Gherardini G, Martin JE, et al. Fat necrosis in free and pedicled TRAM flaps. Plast Reconstr Surg 1998; 102: 1502–7.

60. Garvey PB, Buchel EW, Pockaj BA, et al. DIEP and pedicled TRAM flaps: a comparison of outcomes. Plast Reconstr Surg 2006; 117: 1711–19.

61. Moon HK, Taylor GI. The vascular anatomy of rectus abdominis musculocutaneous flaps based on the deep superior epigastric system. Plast Reconstr Surg 1988; 82: 815–32.

62. Holm C, Mayr M, Höfter E, Ninkovic M. Perfusion zones of the DIEP flap revisited: a clinical study. Plast Reconstr Surg 2006; 117: 37–43.

63. Hsieh F, Kumiponjera D, Malata CM. An algorithmic approach to abdominal flap breast reconstruction in patients with pre-existing scars: results from a single surgeon's experience. J Plast Reconstr Aesth Surg 2009; 62: 1650–60.

64. Di Candia M, Al-Asfoor A, Mickute Z, Kumiponjera D, Hsieh F, Malata CM. Previous multiple abdominal surgery: A valid contraindication to abdominal free flap breast reconstruction? E-Plasty 2012; 12: e31: 286-303. Epub July 23. PMID: 22848775.

65. Mathes DW, Neligan PC. Preoperative imaging techniques for perforator selection in abdomen-based microsurgical breast reconstruction. Clin Plast Surg 2010; 37: 581–91.

66. Grotting JC. The free abdominoplasty flap for immediate breast reconstruction. Ann Plast Surg 1991; 27: 351.

67. Arnez ZM, Khan U, Pogorelec D, Planinsek F. Breast reconstruction using the free superficial inferior epigastric artery (SIEA) flap. Br J Plast Surg 1999; 52: 276–9.

68. Holm C, Mayr M, Höfter E, Ninkovic M. The versatility of the SIEA flap: a clinical assessment of the vascular territory of the superficial epigastric inferior artery. J Plast Reconstr Aesthet Surg 2007; 60: 946–51.

69. Allen RJ, Heitland AS. Superficial inferior epigastric artery flap for breast reconstruction. Semin Plast Surg 2002; 16: 35.

70. Gusenoff JA, Coon D, De La Cruz C, Rubin JP. Superficial inferior epigastric vessels in the massive weight loss population: implications for breast reconstruction. Plast Reconstr Surg 2008; 122: 1621–6.

71. Blondeel PN, Arnstein M, Verstraete K, et al. Venous congestion and blood flow in free transverse rectus abdominis myocutaneous and deep inferior epigastric perforator flaps. Plast Reconstr Surg 2000; 106: 1295–9.

72. Shaw WW. Breast reconstruction by superior gluteal microvascular free flaps without silicone implants. Plast Reconstr Surg 1983; 72: 490–501.

73. Codner MA, Nahai F. The gluteal free flap breast reconstruction. Making it work. Clin Plast Surg 1994; 21: 289–96.

74. Allen RJ, Tucker T Jr. Superior gluteal artery perforator free flap for breast reconstruction. Plast Reconstr Surg 1995; 95: 1207–12.

75. Allen RJ, Levine JL, Granzow JW. The in-the-crease inferior gluteal artery perforator flap for breast reconstruction. Plast Reconstr Surg 2006; 118: 333–9.

76. Arnez ZM, Pogorelec D, Planinsek F, et al. Breast reconstruction by the free transverse gracilis (TMG) flap. Br J Plast Surg 2004; 57: 20–6.

77. Schoeller T, Wechselberger G. Breast reconstruction by the free transverse gracilis (TMG) flap. Br J Plast Surg 2004; 57: 481–2.

78. Fattah A, Figus A, Mathur B, Ramakrishnan VV. The transverse myocutaneous gracilis flap: technical refinements. J Plast Reconstr Aesthet Surg 2010; 63: 305–13.

79. Ninković M, Anderl H, Hefel L, Schwabegger A, Wechselberger G. Internal mammary vessels: a reliable recipient system for free flaps in breast reconstruction. Br J Plast Surg 1995; 48: 533–9.

80. Majumder S, Batchelor AG. Internal mammary vessels as recipients for free TRAM breast reconstruction: aesthetic and functional considerations. Br J Plast Surg 1999; 52: 286–9.

81. Parrett BM, Caterson SA, Tobias AM, Lee BT. The rib-sparing technique for internal mammary vessel exposure in microsurgical breast reconstruction. Ann Plast Surg 2008; 60: 241–3.

82. Malata CM, Moses M, Mickute Z, Di Candia M. Tips for successful microvascular abdominal flap breast reconstruction utilizing the "total rib preservation" technique for internal mammary vessel exposure. Ann Plast Surg 2011; 66: 36–42.

83. Moran SL, Nava G, Behnam AB, Serletti JM. An outcome analysis comparing the thoracodorsal and internal mammary vessels as recipient sites for microvascular breast reconstruction: a prospective study of 100 patients. Plast Reconstr Surg 2003; 111: 1876–82.

84. Banwell M, Trotter D, Ramakrishnan V. The thoracodorsal artery and vein as recipient vessels for microsurgical breast reconstruction. Ann Plast Surg 2012; 68: 542–3.

85. Sbitany H, Sandeen SN, Amalfi AN, Davenport MS, Langstein HN. Acellular dermis-assisted prosthetic breast reconstruction versus complete submuscular coverage: a head-to-head comparison of outcomes. Plast Reconstr Surg 2009; 124: 1735–40.

86. Spear SL, Parikh PM, Reisin E, Menon NG. Acellular dermis-assisted breast reconstruction. Aesthetic Plast Surg 2008; 32: 418–25.

87. Bain C, Lancaster K, Mohanna P, Farhadi J, Ho-Asjoe M. Can Acellular Dermal Matrix (ADM) replace the latissimus dorsi flap in breast reconstruction? Presented at BAPRAS Winter Scientific Meeting. Royal College of Surgeons of England, London, UK, 01 December 2010.

88. Connor J, McQuillan D, Sandor M, et al. Retention of structural and biochemical integrity in a biological mesh supports tissue remodeling in a primate abdominal wall model. Regen Med 2009; 4: 185–95.

89. Katerinaki E, Zanetto U, Sterne GD. Histological appearance of Strattice tissue matrix used in breast reconstruction. J Plast Reconstr Aesthet Surg 2010; 63: e840–1.

90. Salzberg CA, Ashikari AY, Koch RM, Chabner-Thompson E. An 8-year experience of direct-to-implant immediate breast reconstruction using human acellular dermal matrix (AlloDerm). Plast Reconstr Surg 2011; 127: 514–12.

91. Kim JY, Davila AA, Persing S, et al. A meta-analysis of human acellular dermis and submuscular tissue expander breast reconstruction. Plast Reconstr Surg 2012; 129: 28–41.

92. Delay E, Mojallal A, Vasseur C, Delaporte T. Immediate nipple reconstruction during immediate autologous latissimus breast reconstruction. Plast Reconstr Surg 2006; 118: 1303–12.

93. Tyrone JW, Losken A, Hester TR. Nipple areola reconstruction. Breast Dis 2002; 16: 117–22.

Index

Printed and bound by CPI Group (UK) Ltd, Croydon, CR0 4YY

23/10/2024

01778247-0010